Neonatal respiratory disorders

Neonatal respiratory disorders

Second edition

Edited by

Anne Greenough MD, FRCP, DCH
Professor of Clinical Respiratory Physiology and
Honorary Consultant Paediatrician
King's College School of Medicine and Dentistry
London, UK

Anthony D Milner MD, FRCP, DCH
Professor of Neonatology
Department of Child Health
United Medical and Dental School of Guy's and
St Thomas' Hospitals
London, UK

ARNOLD

A member of the Hodder Headline Group

LONDON

First published in Great Britain in 2003 by
Arnold, a member of the Hodder Headline Group,
338 Euston Road, London NW1 3BH

http://www.arnoldpublishers.com

Distributed in the United States of America by
Oxford University Press Inc.,
198 Madison Avenue, New York, NY10016
Oxford is a registered trademark of Oxford University Press

British Library Cataloguing in Publication Data
A catalogue record for this book is available from the
British Library

Library of Congress Cataloging-in-Publication Data
A catalog record for this book is available from the
Library of Congress

ISBN 0 340 80813 6

1 2 3 4 5 6 7 8 9 10

Commissioning Editor: Joanna Koster
Development Editor: Sarah Burrows
Project Editor: Anke Ueberberg
Production Controller: Deborah Smith
Cover Design: Stewart Larking

Typeset in 10/12 Minion by Charon Tec Pvt Ltd., Chennai, India
Printed and bound in Italy

What do you think about this book? Or any other Arnold title?
Please send your comments to feedback.arnold@hodder.co.uk

To our very much loved daughter Antonia, for her unfailing good humor and patience while Mummy and Daddy 'wrote the book'.

Contents

List of contributors

Steven H Abman MD
Professor of Pulmonary and Critical Care, Director,
Pediatric Heart Lung Center, Department of Pediatrics,
University of Colorado School of Medicine and
The Children's Hospital, Denver, CO, USA

Jalal M Abu-Shaweesh MD
Assistant Professor of Pediatrics, Case Western Reserve
University, Cleveland, OH, USA

David Albert
Consultant Paediatric Otolaryngologist, Portland Hospital
Consulting Suite, London, UK

Terry M Baird MD
Assistant Professor of Pediatrics, Case Western Reserve
University, Cleveland, OH, USA

Edward Baker
Senior Lecturer and Honorary Consultant, Paediatric
Cardiology, Department of Congenital Heart Disease,
Guy's Hospital, London, UK

Eduardo Bancalari MD
Professor of Pediatrics, Director, Division of Neonatology,
University of Miami School of Medicine, Miami, FL, USA

Jacques de Blic MD
Service de Pneumologie et d'Allergologie Pédiatriques,
Necker Enfants Malades Hospital, Paris, France

Mark Davenport
Consultant Paediatric Surgeon, Paediatric Surgery, King's
College Hospital, London, UK

Peter RF Dear MD FRCP FRCPCH DCH
Consultant in Neonatal Medicine, Regional Neonatal
Intensive Care Unit, St James's University Hospital,
Leeds, UK

Sean P Devane
Consultant Neonatologist, Children Nationwide Regional
Neonatal Intensive Care Centre, King's College Hospital,
London, UK

Steven M Donn MD
Professor of Pediatrics, Director, Neonatal-Perinatal
Medicine, University of Michigan Health System, Mott
Children's Hospital, Ann Arbor, MI, USA

Amanda Fife
Consultant Microbiologist, South London Public Health
Laboratory and Department of Infection, Guy's, King's

and St Thomas' School of Medicine, Department of
Microbiology, King's College Hospital, London, UK

Grenville F Fox MBChB MRCP FRCPCH
Consultant Neonatologist, Guy's and St Thomas' Hospital
Trust, Guy's Hospital, London, UK

Anne Greenough
Professor of Clinical Respiratory Physiology,
Department of Child Health, King's College Hospital,
London, UK

Henry L Halliday MD FRCPE FRCP FRCPCH
Professor, The Nuffield Department of Child Health,
Queen's University of Belfast, Institute of Clinical Science,
Belfast, Northern Ireland

Simon Hannam
Consultant and Honorary Senior Lecturer in Neonatal
Medicine, Department of Child Health, King's College
Hospital, London, UK

Alison A Hislop PhD
Reader in Developmental Vascular Biology, Vascular
Biology and Pharmacology Unit, Institute of Child Health,
Great Ormond Street Hospital, London, UK

Jan Johansson MD PhD
Professor, Department of Veterinary Medical Chemistry,
Swedish University of Agricultural Sciences, Uppsala,
Sweden, Karolinska Institutet, Stockholm, Sweden

John Karani
Consultant Radiologist, Department of Diagnostic
Radiology, King's College Hospital, London, UK

John P Kinsella MD
Professor of Neonatology, Department of Pediatrics,
University of Colorado School of Medicine and
The Children's Hospital, Denver, CO, USA

Hugo Lagercrantz
Professor, Karolinska Institutet, Astrid Lindgren Children's
Hospital, Department of Woman and Child Health,
Neonatal Unit, Karolinska Hospital, Stockholm, Sweden

Susan Leech
Consultant Paediatrician, Department of Child Health,
King's College Hospital, London, UK

Andrew Lyon MA MB FRCP FRCPCH
Consultant Neonatologist, Neonatal Unit, Simpson Centre
for Reproductive Health, Edinburgh, UK

Richard J Martin MD
Professor of Pediatrics, Case Western Reserve University;
and Director, Division of Neonatology, Rainbow Babies
and Children's Hospital, Cleveland, OH, USA

Anthony D Milner
Professor of Neonatology, Department of Child Health,
United Medical and Dental School of Guy's and St Thomas'
Hospitals, London, UK

Neena Modi MBChB MD FRCP FRCPCH
Reader and Consultant in Neonatal Medicine, Division of
Paediatrics, Obstetrics & Gynaecology, Faculty of
Medicine, Imperial College, Hammersmith Hospital and
Chelsea and Westminster Hospital, London, UK

Kypros H Nicolaides
Director, Harris Birthright Research Centre for Fetal
Medicine, King's College Hospital, London, UK

Annette Parker MCSP
Superintendent Physiotherapist, Physiotherapy
Department, Taunton and Somerset Hospital,
Taunton, Somerset, UK

Gerrard F Rafferty
Lecturer in non-Clinical Respiratory Physiology,
Department of Child Health, Guy's, King's & St Thomas'
School of Medicine, London, UK

Janet M Rennie MA MD FRCP FRCPCH DCH
Consultant and Honorary Senior Lecturer in
Neonatal Medicine, King's College Hospital,
London, UK

N R Clifford Roberton MA MB FRCP
Emeritus Consultant Paediatrician, Addenbrooke's
Hospital, Cambridge, UK

Bengt Robertson MD PhD
Professor, Laboratory for Surfactant Research,
Department of Surgical Sciences, Karolinska Institute,
Stockholm, Sweden

David I Rushton MB ChB FRCPCH FRCPath
Consultant Perinatal and Paediatric Pathologist,
Birmingham Women's Hospital, UK

Andreas Schulze MD
Professor of Pediatrics, Head, Division of Neonatology,
Department of Obstetrics and Gynecology, Division of
Neonatology, Klinikum Grosshadern, München, Germany

Thomas H Shaffer
Director, Nemours Lung Center, Department of Research,
Alfred I. duPoint Hospital for Children, Wilmington,
DE, USA; and Professor of Physiology and Pediatrics
and Director, Respiratory Physiology Section, Temple
University School of Medicine, Departments of Physiology
and Pediatrics, Temple University Children's Hospital,
Philadelphia, PA, USA

Ilene RS Sosenko MD
Professor of Pediatrics, Associate Director for Clinical
Development and Outreach, Division of Neonatology,
University of Miami School of Medicine, Miami, FL, USA

Pinchi Srinivasan MD
Fellow in Neonatology, Department of Pediatrics,
State University of New York, Stony Brook, NY, USA

Ben Stenson MB MD FRCP FRCPCH
Consultant Neonatologist, Simpson Centre for
Reproductive Health Pavilion, Edinburgh, UK

Dafydd V Walters
Professor of Child Health, St George's Hospital Medical
School, University of London, London, UK

Ronny Wickstrom
Karolinska Institutet, Astrid Lindgren Children's Hospital,
Department of Woman and Child Health, Neonatal Unit,
Karolinska Hospital, Stockholm, Sweden

Marla R Wolfson
Associate Professor of Physiology and Pediatrics,
Temple University School of Medicine, Department of
Physiology and Pediatrics, Temple University Children's
Hospital, Philadelphia, PA, USA

Thomas E Wiswell MD
Attending Neonatologist and Professor of Pediatrics,
Health Sciences Center, State University of New York,
Stony Brook, NY, USA

Preface

Respiratory disorders remain a major problem in neonatal intensive care. As a consequence, this is an area of intensive research. In writing the second edition we, therefore, felt it important to involve leading researchers from all over the world to contribute in their specialist areas. Our aim is for this book to provide a comprehensive and up-to-date statement on the physiology, pathology, management and outcome of respiratory problems facing neonatal clinicians on a daily basis.

Anne Greenough MD, FRCP, DCH
Anthony D Milner MD, FRCP, DCH

Acknowledgments

We would like to acknowledge the enormous debt we owe to all who contributed chapters to this book and to their secretaries. We are particularly grateful to Sue Williams in the Department of Child Health at Guy's, King's and St Thomas' School of Medicine whose excellent secretarial, administrative and interpersonal relationship skills, patience and goodwill enabled this second edition to be completed. We are enormously grateful to Dr Paul Cheeseman who spent many hours meticulously scanning in all the figures, to Dr John Karani who additionally provided the legends to all the chest radiographs and Dr Johan Smith who provided key imaging pictures. We also acknowledge the help received from all Edward Arnold staff, particularly Sarah Burrows and Dr Joanna Koster.

Anne Greenough MD, FRCP, DCH
Anthony D Milner MD, FRCP, DCH

Abbreviations

μ	heavy chain of IgM molecule
ΨL	surrogate light chain of the immunoglobulin molecule, formed during B-cell development
a/AO$_2$	arterial/alveolar oxygen
A/C	assist control
AaDO$_2$	alveolar-arterial oxygen difference
AC	alternating current
AchR	acetylcholine receptor
ACT	activated clotting time
ADH	antidiuretic hormone
AFI	amniotic fluid index
AHA/AAP	American Heart Association/American Academy of Pediatrics
ALE	acquired lobar emphysema
ALTE	acute life-threatening event
AMPA	alpha-amino-3-hydroxyl-5-methyl-4-isoxazole-propionate
AP	anteroposterior
ARDS	acute respiratory distress syndrome; adult respiratory distress syndrome
AREC	assistence respiratoire extracorporelle
ARF	acute renal failure
ATD	asphyxiating thoracic dystrophy
ATP	adenosine triphosphate
ATS	American Thoracic Society
AVP	arginine vasopressin
AWD	abdominal wall defects
B-1 cells	atypical, self-renewing B cells with a less diverse receptor repertoire than conventional B cells, secreting mainly IgM
BAL	bronchoalveolar lavage
BCG	bacille Calmette–Guérin
bFGF	basic fibroblast growth factor
BLES	bovine liquid extract surfactant
BPD	bronchopulmonary dysplasia
bpm	beats per minute; breaths per minute
BUN	blood urea nitrogen
Cμ	gene segment coding for the constant region of the IgM heavy chain
C1 esterase	inhibitor of the classical pathway of complement activation
C3, C4, C8, C9	complement component
CAM	cystic adenomatoid malformation of the lung
cAMP	cyclic adenosine monophosphate
CBFV	cerebral blood flow velocity
CBS	captive bubble system
CC10	Clara cell 10 kDa protein
CCAM	congenital cystic adenomatoid malformation of the lung
CD	clusters of differentiation representing cell surface molecules
CDH	congenital diaphragmatic hernia
CDR3	complementarity determining region 3 – hypervariable loop at the end of variable domain of antibodies or T-cell receptors
CFTR	cystic fibrosis transmembrane regulator
cGMP	cyclic guanosine monophosphate
CHAOS	congenital high airway obstruction
CHARGE	coloboma of the iris and retina, heart disease, atresia choanae, retarded growth, genital hypoplasia, ear defects
CI	confidence interval
CK	creatine kinase
CLD	chronic lung disease
CMV	conventional mechanical ventilation;
CMV	cytomegalovirus
CNEP	continuous negative extrathoracic pressure
CNS	central nervous system
CO$_2$	carbon dioxide
CoNS	coagulase-negative staphylococci
CPAP	continuous positive airways pressure
CPL	congenital pulmonary lymphangiectasis
CR3	complement receptor 3
CRD	carbohydrate recognition domain
CRP	C-reactive protein
CRT	capillary refill time
CSF	cerebrospinal fluid
CT	computerized tomography
CVP	central venous pressure
CVS	chorion villus sampling
CXR	chest X-ray
DC	direct current
DIC	disseminated intravascular coagulation
DNA	deoxyribonucleic acid
DPPC	dipalmitoylphosphatidylcholine

DTPA	diethylene triamine pentaacetic acid	HFFI	high-frequency flow interrupter
EA	early amniocentesis	HFJV	high-frequency jet ventilation
EBV	Epstein–Barr virus	HFO	high-frequency oscillation
ECG	electrocardiograph	HFOV	high-frequency oscillatory ventilation
ECHO	echocardiograph	HFPPV	high-frequency positive pressure
ECMO	extracorporeal membrane oxygenation		ventilation
EDHF	endothelium-derived hyperpolarizing	HIV	human immunodeficiency virus
	factor	HLA	human leukocyte antigen – genetic
EEG	electroencephalograph		designation for MHC
EFA	essential fatty acid	HMD	hyaline membrane disease
EGF	epidermal growth factor	HNF-3β	hepatocyte nuclear factor-3β
ELBW	extremely low birthweight	HRCT	high-resolution computed tomography
ELSO	Extracorporeal Life Support	HSV	herpes simplex virus
	Organization	I:E	inspiratory:expiratory
EMG	electromyograph	ICH	intracranial hemorrhage
ENaC	epithelial sodium channel	ID	internal diameter
ENG	electroneurogram	IFD	infant flow driver
ENT	ear, nose and throat	IFN	interferon
EOG	electro-oculograph	Ig	immunoglobulin
EPI	echoplanar imaging	IL	interleukin
EPIMRI	echoplanar magnetic resonance imaging	ILCOR	International Liaison Committee on
EPO	erythropoietin		Resuscitation
ERS	European Respiratory Society	IMV	intermittent mandatory ventilation
ET	endotracheal tube	iNO	inhaled nitric oxide
ET-1	endothelin-1	IPPV	intermittent positive pressure ventilation
EXIT	*ex utero* intrapartum treatment	IQ	intelligence quotient
Factor B	component of the alternative pathway of	IRDS	idiopathic RDS
	complement activation	ITPV	intratracheal pulmonary ventilation
FB	fiberoptic bronchoscope	IVC	inferior vena cava
FBM	fetal breathing movements	IVH	intraventricular hemorrhage
Fc	fragment crystallizable – contains the	IVIG	intravenous immunoglobulin
	majority of the constant regions of the	JCT	J chest tube
	IgG molecule	KGF	keratinocyte growth factor
Fcγreceptor	receptor for the constant arm of the IgG	L:S	lecithin:sphingomyelin (ratio)
	molecule	LFT	lung function test
FDLE	fetal distal lung epithelial	LPC	lysophosphatidylcholine
$FEV_{0.5}$	forced expiratory volume in half a second	LPEP/LVET	left ventricular pre-ejection period to
$FEV_{0.75}$	forced expiratory volume in three-		ejection time
	quarters of a second	L/T	lung–thorax
FG	French gauge	LV	liquid ventilation
FiO_2	inspired oxygen concentration	M3G	morphine-3-glucuronide
FPEFVL	forced partial expiratory flow–volume	M6G	morphine-6-glucuronide
	loop	MAP	mean airway pressure
FRC	functional residual capacity	MAS	meconium aspiration syndrome
FSP	familial spontaneous pneumothorax	MCT	medium chain triglyceride
FVC	forced vital capacity	MDI	metered drug inhaler
GA	gestational age	MHC	major histocompatibility complex
GABA	gamma-aminobutyric acid	MRA	magnetic resonance angiography
GBS	group B streptococcus	MRI	magnetic resonance imaging
G-CSF	granulocyte-colony stimulating factor	mRNA	messenger ribonucleic acid
GER	gastroesophageal reflux	MRSA	methicillin-resistant *Staphylococcus*
GI	gastrointestinal		*aureus*
GM-CSF	granulocyte-macrophage colony-	MUPG	3-methoxy-4-hydroxyphenylethylene
	stimulating factor		glycol
GMP	guanosine 3,5-monophosphate	MV	mechanical ventilation
HB_IR	Hering–Breuer inflation reflex	Na^+	sodium ion

NADH	nicotinamide adenine dinucleotide	PKA	protein kinase A
NANCi	inhibitory non-adrenergic, non-cholinergic	PLV	partial liquid ventilation
nCPAP	nasal continuous positive airways pressure	PMA	postmenstrual age
NEC	necrotizing enterocolitis	PO_2	partial pressure of oxygen
nHFOV	nasal high-frequency oscillatory ventilation	PPHN	persistent pulmonary hypertension of the newborn
NICHD	National Institute of Child Health and Human Development	ppm	parts per million
NICU	neonatal intensive care unit	PPROM	preterm premature rupture of the membranes; prolonged preterm rupture of the membranes
NIDCAP	Neonatal Individualized Developmental Care and Assessment Program		
NIH	National Institutes of Health	PPT	partial prothrombin time
nIPPV	nasal intermittent positive pressure ventilation	PROM	premature rupture of the membranes
		PSV	pressure support ventilation
NK cell	natural killer cell	PT	prothrombin time
NMDA	N-methyl-D-aspartate	PTV	patient-triggered ventilation
NO	nitric oxide	PVL	periventricular leukomalacia
NO_2	nitrogen dioxide	PVR	pulmonary vascular resistance
NOS	nitric oxide synthase	RDS	respiratory distress syndrome
nSIMV	nasal synchronized intermittent mandatory ventilation	REM	rapid eye movement
		RIP	respiratory inductive plethysmography
nSIPPV	nasal synchronized intermittent positive pressure ventilation	RIS	respiratory insufficiency syndrome
		RMU	respiratory mechanical unloading
NTB	necrotizing tracheobronchitis	ROP	retinopathy of prematurity
OD	outside diameter	RPR	rapid plasma reagent
OH	oligohydramnios	RQ	respiratory quotient
OR	odds ratio	RR	relative risk; respiratory rate
$PaCO_2$	arterial carbon dioxide tension	RSV	respiratory syncytial virus
PAF	platelet activating factor	SaO_2	oxygen saturation
P_{ao}	pressure at the airway opening	SAVI	synchronized assisted ventilation for infants
PaO_2	arterial oxygen tension		
PAP	pulmonary alveolar proteinosis	SCID	severe combined immunodeficiency
PAV	proportional assist ventilation	SD	standard deviation
PBS	pulsating bubble surfactometer	sGC	smooth muscle guanylate cyclase
PC	phosphatidylcholine	SIADH	syndrome of inappropriate antidiuretic hormone secretion
PCA	postconceptional age		
PCO_2	partial pressure of CO_2	SIDS	sudden infant death syndrome
PCR	polymerase chain reaction	sIg	secretory immunoglobulin
PCV	packed cell volume; patient-controlled ventilation	SIMV	synchronized intermittent mandatory ventilation
PDA	patent ductus arteriosus	SIPPV	synchronized intermittent positive pressure ventilation
PDE	phosphodiesterase		
PDGF-AA	platelet-derived growth factor	SLN	superior laryngeal nerve
P_{di}	diaphragmatic pressure	SMA	spinal muscular atrophy
P_E	expiratory pressure	SOD	superoxide dismutase
PEEP	positive end expiratory pressure	SP	substance P
P_{EMAX}	maximal static expiratory pressure	SP-A, B, C	surfactant proteins A, B, C
$P_{ET}CO_2$	endotracheal carbon dioxide pressure	STOP-ROP	supplemental therapeutic oxygen for prethreshold retinopathy of prematurity
PFC	perfluorochemical		
PG	phosphatidylglycerol; prostaglandin	SVC	superior vena cava
PHA	phytohemagglutinin	SVD	spontaneous vaginal delivery
P_I	inspiratory pressure	T_4	thyroxine
PIA	L-N-phenylisopropyladenosine	$TcCO_2$	transcutaneous CO_2
PIE	pulmonary interstitial emphysema	TcO_2	transcutaneous oxygen
P_{IMAX}	maximal static inspiratory pressure	T_E	expiratory time
PIP	peak inflating pressure; peak inspiratory pressure	TGF-β	transforming growth factor-beta
		TGV	thoracic gas volume

THAM	tris(hydroxymethyl)aminomethane
T_I	inspiratory time
TLC	total lung capacity
TLV	total liquid ventilation
TNF	tumour necrosis factor
TOF	tracheoesophageal fistula
t_{PTEF}/t_E	relationship between the time to reach peak expiratory flow and total expiratory flow time
TRH	thyrotropin-releasing hormone
tTdT	Terminal deoxynucleotidyl transferase – enzyme inserting nucleotides into the gene segments in T-cell receptor and immunoglobulin variable regions
TTF	thyroid transcription factor
TTN	transient tachypnea of the newborn
TwP_{di}	twitch transdiaphragmatic pressure
UAC	umbilical artery catheter
UKOS	United Kingdom Oscillation Study
URTI	unspecific respiratory tract infection
US	ultrasound
UVC	umbilical venous catheter(ization)

V	volume
VA	venoarterial
VCV	volume-controlled ventilation
V-D-J	Variable-diversity-joining gene segments which recombine during development of the T-cell receptor and immunoglobulin molecule
VDRL	Venereal Disease Research Laboratories
VEGF	vascular epidermal growth factor; vascular endothelial growth factor
VG	volume guarantee
V_I	inspiratory volume
V_{max}	maximum flow
VILI	ventilator-induced lung injury
VLBW	very low birthweight
VLM	ventrolateral medulla
V/Q	ventilation–perfusion
V-region	variable region gene segments of the immunoglobulin molecule
V_T	tidal volume
VV	venovenous

PART 1

Development and physiology of the respiratory system

Fetal and postnatal anatomical lung development

ALISON A HISLOP

There are major changes in the function of the lung at the moment of birth. The lung has to be ready to function efficiently at this time, although it has grown while not fulfilling its postnatal function. The lung at birth is not a miniature version of the adult lung, but has grown sufficiently to support the respiratory needs of the infant. The primary function of the lung is gas exchange and the airways and blood vessels are arranged to produce a distribution system for the air and blood to a large surface area within a relatively small chest volume.

During infancy and childhood, as the body surface increases the lung grows in size, increasing the size of airways and the surface area for gas exchange in the alveolar region with a concomitant increase in the size of blood vessels and number of capillaries. The structure of the components also mature.

FETAL STAGES OF LUNG DEVELOPMENT

The classic descriptions of lung growth have divided fetal development into four major stages based on the appearance of the lung tissue. These are embryonic, pseudoglandular, canalicular and alveolar; the last is sometimes divided into an earlier saccular or terminal sac phase and a later alveolar stage (Table 1.1, Figure 1.1). The alveolar stage continues after birth and in some species is entirely postnatal. There is also considerable individual variation and one stage gradually merges into the next. Within each phase, development of specific structures is of major importance. During the embryonic period the main hilar connections of the airways and the pulmonary circulation are made. During the pseudoglandular phase the pre-acinar airways with their accompanying arteries and veins develop. During the canalicular phase the blood–gas barrier thins and the maturation of the surfactant system begins. In the alveolar phase alveoli multiply and by birth up to half the adult number are present.

Development of the airways

The lung appears as a ventral diverticulum from the endodermal foregut in the fourth week after ovulation. The complete lining epithelium of the lung is derived from the endoderm. This bud is formed within the splanchnic mesoderm surrounding the gut and the dorsal aorta; it is from this mesenchyme that the airway walls and blood vessels are derived. A division produces the left and right bronchi by 26–28 days of gestational age and segmental airways are present by 6 weeks. Further division of airways into the surrounding mesenchyme continues until the end of the pseudoglandular stage (17 weeks of gestation) by which time all pre-acinar airways to the level of the terminal bronchiolus are present. The majority of divisions occur during the tenth to fourteenth weeks of gestation[5] (Figures 1.1 and 1.2).

During the canalicular period (16–27 weeks of gestation) the pre-acinar airways increase in diameter and length. The peripheral airways continue to divide to form the prospective respiratory bronchioli (two to three generations in humans) and beyond these the prospective alveolar ducts. The mesenchymal region between the

Table 1.1 *Phases of lung development in man*

Embryonic	0–7 weeks of gestation	Lung buds form. Blood vessels connect to the heart
Pseudoglandular	6–17 weeks of gestation	Pre-acinar airways and blood vessels develop
Canalicular	16–27 weeks of gestation	Respiratory (intra-acinar) region develops. Thinning of peripheral epithelium and mesenchyme. Type I and II pneumonocytes
Alveolar	27 weeks to term	Development of saccules and then alveoli
Postnatal	Up to 18 months	Alveoli and small blood vessels multiply. All structures increase in size

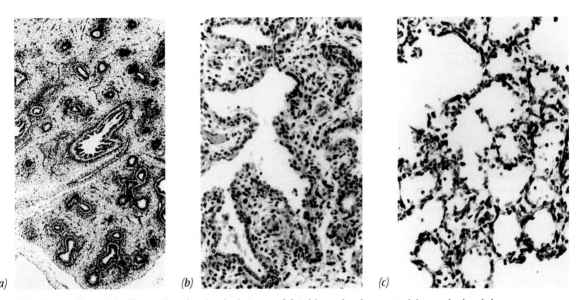

(a) (b) (c)

Figure 1.1 *Photomicrographs illustrating the classical stages of fetal lung development: (a) pseudoglandular, 6–17 weeks of gestation; (b) canalicular, 16–27 weeks of gestation; (c) alveolar, 27 weeks to term.*

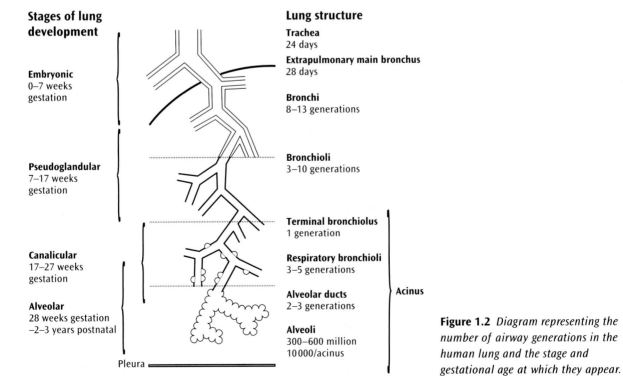

Stages of lung development

Embryonic
0–7 weeks
gestation

Pseudoglandular
7–17 weeks
gestation

Canalicular
17–27 weeks
gestation

Alveolar
28 weeks gestation
–2–3 years postnatal

Pleura

Lung structure

Trachea
24 days

Extrapulmonary main bronchus
28 days

Bronchi
8–13 generations

Bronchioli
3–10 generations

Terminal bronchiolus
1 generation

Respiratory bronchioli
3–5 generations

Alveolar ducts
2–3 generations

Alveoli
300–600 million
10 000/acinus

Acinus

Figure 1.2 *Diagram representing the number of airway generations in the human lung and the stage and gestational age at which they appear.*

airways thins and capillaries come to lie beneath the epithelium of the peripheral airways, apparently causing the epithelium to become thinner. The larger airways (prospective bronchi) are lined by columnar epithelium, but the distal bronchioli are lined by cuboidal cells. At the level of the prospective respiratory bronchioli, part of the wall is lined by flattened cells, as are the prospective alveolar ducts which at this stage are sac shaped (saccules). By 20–22 weeks of gestation, type I and II alveolar epithelial cells can be identified lining all saccular air spaces. The type I cells are flat and elongated and cover the majority of the surface. The type II cells maintain a cuboidal shape and develop lamellar bodies around 24 weeks of gestation, which is 4–5 weeks before surfactant can be detected in the amniotic fluid. By the end of the canalicular stage, the air to blood barrier is thin enough to support gas exchange (about 0.6 μm) but the gas exchange units are the large thin-walled saccules. True alveoli develop later (p. 7).

Increase in airway size in the prenatal period is linear and continuous with antenatal growth. After the first year of life, there is a slowing in growth, there being an approximately twofold increase between 22 weeks of gestation and 8 months postnatal age and a two- to threefold increase between birth and adulthood.[20] A previous study, measuring airway length and diameter in children from birth to adulthood, had reported symmetrical growth throughout the lung.[17] Tracheal size does not differ between sexes during early life,[12] but adult males have a larger trachea than females. Girls have wider and/or shorter airways than boys during early childhood and this may explain their lesser tendency to wheeze, but by adulthood males have relatively large airways. This may be a factor in the relative decline in reversible obstructive airways disease in teenage boys.

Airway wall structure

As successive airways form, their walls first develop airway wall smooth muscle closely followed by cartilage, submucosal glands and connective tissue. These structural elements of the airway wall appear from the hilum towards the periphery and by 24 weeks of gestation the airways have the same structure as they do in the adult.[5,6] Smooth muscle cells are present in human trachea and lobar bronchi by 6 weeks of gestation and extend along the airway pathway as the peripheral airways divide (Figure 1.3). Only the ultimate lung buds do not have any airway smooth muscle.[13,35] As in adult lungs, fetal airway smooth muscle expresses contractile smooth muscle specific myofilaments such as smooth muscle α-actin and smooth muscle myosin. *In vitro* studies of peripheral explants of first trimester human lung have shown that fetal airway smooth muscle cells have spontaneous tone and peristalsis-like contractions which cause active

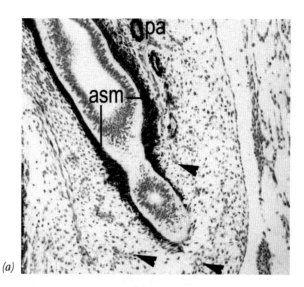

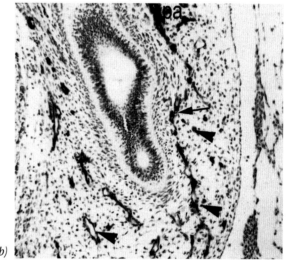

Figure 1.3 *Photomicrograph of peripheral airway bud in a 44-day-old fetus immunostained for (a) α smooth muscle actin and (b) CD31 (endothelial marker). Airway smooth muscle (asm) α smooth muscle positive, is seen to the penultimate branch. Capillaries (arrowheads), positive for CD31 are seen as far as the peripheral bud and coalesce alongside the airway (arrowed). A muscle wall, one cell thick and α smooth muscle positive which is derived from adjacent bronchial smooth muscle cells surrounds the pulmonary artery (pa).*

movement of intraluminal fluid.[35] The movements are sensitive to acetylcholine and isoproterenol, suggesting that neurohumoral factors modulate smooth muscle activity.[35] Postnatally there is reactivity to methacholine and subsequent bronchodilation after addition of metaproterenol in healthy infants less than 15 months of age.[47] During fetal life and in the newborn, the amount of muscle within a given sized airway is generally less than in the adult (Figure 1.4).[20] During the first year of life, particularly in the first few weeks after birth, there is a rapid increase in bronchial smooth muscle mass relative to airway size. This rapid increase is probably related to the change to air breathing since it occurs at a similar postnatal age and therefore an earlier gestational age in babies that are born prematurely (Figure 1.4). Airway smooth muscle mass increases above normal in artificially ventilated babies.[20]

Cartilage first appears in the sixth gestational week in the trachea, the tenth week in the main bronchi and the twelfth week in segmental bronchi and by 24 weeks of gestation extends as far as in the adult. There is a progressive increase in the total cartilage mass through infancy and childhood as airways increase in size. The submucosal glands are responsible for producing most of the mucus found in the airways. They appear in the trachea of the human at 10 weeks of gestation and gradually extend towards the periphery of the lung, reaching their adult position by the canalicular stage, but it is only at 13 years of age that the glands have the adult appearance. During childhood there is relatively more submucosal gland mass within the airway wall than in the adult.[34]

Airway epithelium

The epithelial cells develop by differentiation and maturation of the primitive endodermal cells. As well as producing the fluid and mucus for the ciliary escalator to remove particles from inside the lung, the epithelium is a source of smooth muscle inhibitory factor(s), and can also generate endothelin, which is a contractile agonist as well as a smooth muscle cell mitogen.[46]

Ciliated cells are found from the trachea to the respiratory bronchioli and at all levels are the most numerous cells. They first appear at 11 weeks of gestation.[25] They do not divide, but originate from basal or secretory cells. Mucus-secreting or goblet cells are found from the trachea to the end of the bronchioli. The presence of intracellular mucus has been demonstrated in the human fetal lung at 13 weeks of gestation but at this age the cells are sparse. At birth, there is still a relatively low number of goblet cells, less than 10 percent of the total number of epithelial cells. After birth, there is a rapid increase in the number of goblet cells, reaching up to 40 percent of the total in the bronchi by 3 months of age.[20] Basal cells are found in the larger airways and can be identified from 12 to 14 weeks of gestation and have been considered to be a stem cell. In the terminal bronchioli a further cell type, the Clara cell, is found. They are progenitors for the ciliated cells in peripheral airways.[16] They produce Clara cell 10 kDa protein (CC10) which has immunomodulatory and anti-inflammatory activity and may play a role in controlling airway inflammation. Clara cells also produce surfactant apoprotein, under β-adrenergic control.

Bronchial blood vessels

The airways are supplied with oxygenated blood via the bronchial arteries, which appear from 8 weeks of gestation. They arise from the descending aorta as small branches, probably by angiogenesis, and supply the extrapulmonary bronchi and extend down the intrapulmonary airway wall alongside the cartilage plates. They divide to form a subepithelial plexus and an adventitial plexus on either side of the bronchial smooth muscle and cartilage. By birth they extend to the end of the bronchioli. True

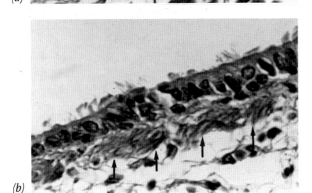

(a)

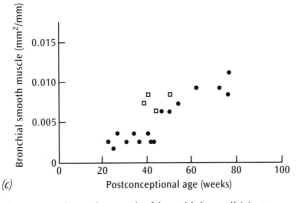

(b)

(c)

Figure 1.4 *Photomicrograph of bronchiolar wall (a) at term and (b) at 8 months of age (×800). The bronchial smooth muscle at arrows increases with age. (c) The area of bronchial smooth muscle/mm of airway perimeter in small bronchi related to postconceptional age. ●, Normal fetus and infant; □, premature infant.*

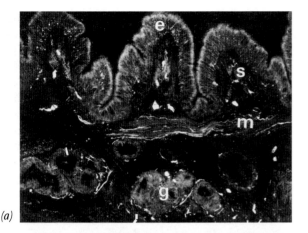

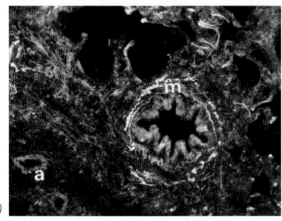

Figure 1.5 *Nerve fibers in (a) bronchus (×125) and (b) bronchiolus (×200) supplying epithelium (e), submucosal region (s), bronchial smooth muscle (m), submucosal gland (g) and pulmonary artery (a). Taken from, Hislop et al. (1990)[22]. With permission from Official Journal of the American Thoracic Society. American Lung Association.*

bronchial veins drain the trachea and upper bronchi and return blood to the right atrium while the veins in the more peripheral airways drain via the pulmonary veins to the left atrium.[3]

Innervation

The nerves of the lung develop from neural crest cells which migrate via the vagus to the future trachea and lung before it separates from the gut. There is progressive extension and increase in complexity of the nerve supply.[45] By 4 months of gestation the trachea has a nerve supply to smooth muscle, submucosal glands and epithelium and there are nerves present in all but the smallest airways, arteries and veins. By term and in the neonate, the distribution and density of nerves are similar to that seen in the adult, with parasympathetic (cholinergic) excitatory nerves and inhibitory non-adrenergic, non-cholinergic

(NANCi) nerve fibres forming a meshwork within the airway wall (Figure 1.5).[22] Sensory nerves are also found in the epithelium. There are few nerves within the air spaces of the alveolar region of the lung.

DEVELOPMENT OF ALVEOLI

At the beginning of the alveolar stage of fetal lung development, the peripheral airspaces or saccules have discrete bundles of elastin at intervals around their luminal edge forming small crests or subdivisions (Figure 1.6).[18] Between 28 and 32 weeks of gestation, these crests elongate sufficiently to form primitive alveoli.[18,28] The walls of these alveoli are still thicker than in the adult, having a double capillary supply and mesenchymal tissue between the epithelial layers. With age, the crests increase in length, become thinner by loss of interstitial matrix and have only a single capillary network.[7] By 34 weeks of gestation, mature cup-shaped alveoli line the elongated saccules, now called alveolar ducts, and they are also found lining part of the walls of the respiratory bronchioli.

Counts of the alveoli (Figure 1.6) show an increase with gestational age and by term between one-third and one-half of the adult number is present, around 150 million[18] (adult number 300–600 million[2]). The increase in lung volume seen in late fetal life is due mainly to the increase in number of the alveoli. The alveolar surface area increases and shows a linear relationship to age and body weight. After birth the alveolar region of the lung grows rapidly and it is likely that the adult number is almost complete by 18 months of age.[28,51] Males generally have a greater number of alveoli[48] than females at all ages over 1 year, independent of weight as well as age. Lung volume (as measured by the vital capacity) continues to increase until the early 20s in normal adults by increase in size of alveoli.

DEVELOPMENT OF THE PULMONARY VASCULATURE

The pulmonary arteries are connected to the heart at the aortic sac and the pulmonary veins to the left atrium by 5 weeks of gestation. There is a circulation between the two via a capillary plexus in the lung bud mesenchyme. In the adult lung the arteries run alongside the airways and branch with them, suggesting that their growth might be regulated by the airways. In addition to these conventional arteries there are extra, smaller, supernumerary arteries, which are alongside the airway branches. They supply the alveolar region more directly and are two to three times greater in number than the conventional arteries. The veins have a similar number of branches, both conventional and supernumerary, but they run independently of the airways

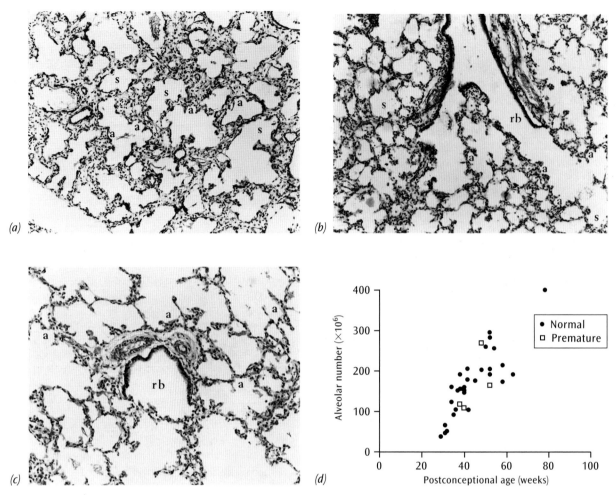

Figure 1.6 *Alveolar development. (a) Photomicrograph of lung at 28 weeks of gestation. Saccules (s) with shallow alveoli (a) are separated by relatively thick interstitium (×187). (b) The lung at 34 weeks of gestation. A respiratory bronchiolus (rb) leads into an alveolar duct lined by alveoli (a). Some saccules are still present (s) (×187). (c) Lung at term. Alveoli are mature in shape and thin walled (×187).[18] (With permission from Elsevier Science.) (d) Number of alveoli related to postconceptional age in normal and premature infants and fetuses.*

between acini and segments. Early studies on the development of the arteries and veins showed that they grow at the same time as the airways so that all pre-acinar vessels are present by the seventeenth week of gestation, the end of the pseudoglandular stage. The supernumerary arteries and veins, which will be associated with the alveoli (not developed by this time), also grow during this period. This suggests a genetic influence on blood vessel development.[21] Recent studies of human fetal lungs, using specific immunostaining, have shown that the pulmonary blood vessels initially form *de novo* as endothelial tubes in the mesenchyme around the peripheral airways (Figure 1.3), the process of vasculogenesis, rather than by inward growth of existing arteries, angiogenesis.[13] As the airways divide towards the periphery from 6 to 17 weeks of gestation, the intrapulmonary arteries form by continuous coalescence of the endothelial tubes alongside the airway. The veins derive independently from the same mesenchyme but coalesce to run between the airways. The capillaries in the mesenchyme are continuous between the arteries and veins.

Arteries and veins develop alongside the respiratory airways in the canalicular stage. At this time the capillaries in the mesenchyme come to lie under the epithelium, producing the blood–gas barrier (see above). Later, as alveoli form in late fetal life (after 30 weeks of gestation) and after birth, there is a rapid increase in the number of small pre- and post-capillary vessels. At birth, the pattern of branching of the arteries and veins is the same as in the adult. They increase in size with age as the lung increases in volume and the number of vessels at the periphery increases. Between birth and adulthood, the surface area of the lung increases about 20-fold and the capillary volume 35-fold to maintain efficient gas exchange. This increase may be by sprouting angiogenesis or alternatively by intussusception of tissue within an existing sheet so increasing its surface area and complexity.[7]

Vessel wall structure

Smooth muscle cells are found around the newly formed arteries soon after they line up alongside the airways (Figure 1.3). Muscle cells initially appear to derive from the bronchial smooth muscle cells of the adjacent airway. As the arteries increase in size, further putative muscle cells are recruited from the mesenchyme and increase the thickness of the muscle wall.[13] Elastic laminae and collagen are laid down between the layers of muscle cells. By half-way through fetal life the structure of the pulmonary arteries is the same as it is in the adult.[21] The veins are relatively thin walled, with only two to three layers of muscle even at the hilum. Both arteries and veins are surrounded by a thick adventitia made up of collagen.

During fetal life, blood flow is directed away from the lung due to high pulmonary artery resistance. Immediately after birth, pulmonary vascular resistance falls, and there is a decrease in the wall thickness of the small muscular arteries in the first few days. In the larger vessels the low adult level is reached by 3 months of age.[15] Studies on neonatal pigs have shown that the rapid thinning at the periphery is due to reorganization of the shape and orientation of both pulmonary vascular smooth muscle and endothelial cells.[14] The rapid dilation of the pulmonary vasculature is stimulated by the rise in arterial oxygen partial pressure and the alveolar stretching. Endothelial-derived relaxation factor or nitric oxide[27] plays an important role in vascular dilatation. The enzyme nitric oxide synthase is present in the endothelial cells at birth, increases in amount at 2–3 days of age, suggesting a role in the adaptation process.[23] Nitric oxide is used successfully in treatment of infants with persistent pulmonary hypertension of the newborn.

THE LUNG AT BIRTH

At birth, the lung has a small volume, but this is related to body weight. It has the adult number of airways with an airway wall consisting of the components found in the adult lung. Within the respiratory portion of the lung the majority of respiratory airways are present and there are up to half the adult number of alveoli present. The alveoli, though smaller than in the adult, have a blood–gas barrier of mature thickness. The blood supply to the lung is complete save for the blood vessels that will supply the enlarging alveolar region. Before birth the lung is filled with liquid and only 8–10 percent of the total cardiac output flows through the pulmonary circulation. At birth, fluid is replaced by air and a drop in pulmonary arterial resistance allows total blood flow to pass through the capillary bed.

During infancy, lung volume increases as alveoli continue to multiply. The airways continue to grow at the same rate as before birth but the relative amount of bronchial smooth muscle increases and goblet cell number increases. Premature delivery in the last trimester does not seem to affect normal alveolar multiplication (Figure 1.6)[19] or growth in airway size. The airways are small for postnatal age and will thus have a relative increase in smooth muscle mass and mucus secreting cells (Figure 1.4).[20] These structural changes are accentuated by ventilator therapy.[19] Infants who go on to develop bronchopulmonary dysplasia (BPD) have a reduced number of alveoli beyond the age when normal alveolar development is complete.[29]

FACTORS AFFECTING LUNG GROWTH

The earliest event in lung morphogenesis, the commitment of foregut endoderm cells to form the lung bud, appears to be critically dependent on the transcription factor, hepatocyte nuclear factor-3β (HNF-3β).[1] Other transcription factors are also involved in early differentiation. Gli proteins are implicated in the mesenchymal–epithelial cell interactions that characterize much of lung branching morphogenesis.[40] Inhibition of thyroid transcription factor (TTF-1) in fetal mouse lung explants results in restricted branching morphogenesis.[39]

Subsequent airway branching events and pulmonary vasculogenesis involve reciprocal epithelial–mesenchymal interactions mediated by growth factors and their receptors as well as extracellular matrix proteins and their cognate receptors on cells. Airway branching requires the presence of both the endodermal tube lined by epithelial cells and the surrounding mesenchyme. An airway tube will continue to grow in length but will not branch if its mesenchyme is stripped away,[38] whereas mesenchyme transplanted from an area of active branching will stimulate an otherwise dormant epithelial tube to divide. In general, receptor tyrosine kinases and their ligands, basic fibroblast growth factor (bFGF), platelet derived growth factor (PDGF-AA) and epidermal growth factor (EGF), positively modulate lung growth and branching morphogenesis while transforming growth factor-beta (TGF-β) family members have an inhibitory effect on branching morphogenesis. The initialization of capillary vasculogenesis is possibly dependent upon the vascular epidermal growth factor (VEGF) produced by the epithelial cells.[44] Interplay may also occur between growth factors and physical stimuli such as spontaneous airway contractions and fetal breathing movements. However, much of the integration of positive and negative signaling pathways is still unknown.[50]

Recent epidemiological evidence showing a relationship between adult airway function and birth weight suggests that intrauterine nutrition in humans may be more important than recognized previously.[4] Malnutrition will affect lung growth both pre- and postnatally and will have the greatest effect at the time of rapid alveolar development.[11,42] This suggests that in humans the most relevant time will be during late fetal life and up to 2 years of age. In addition to calorie intake, vitamin A (retinoic acid) has been shown to be essential for normal alveolar development;[31] vitamin A deficiency decreases alveolar septal development. More importantly, vitamin A supplementation leads to redevelopment of alveoli in rats with elastase-induced emphysema[32] and retinoic acid treatment given to young rats with dexamethasone-induced failure of alveolar development induced new septal formation.[33]

Maternal smoking during pregnancy leads to an increased risk of low birthweight, preterm delivery, and sudden death in infancy.[9] Functional studies in human infants shortly after birth show diminished airflows[10] and reduced specific conductance[37] in those whose mothers smoked during pregnancy. Recent measurements in preterm infants have shown that these changes are evident at least 7 weeks before term.[24] Animal studies have shown maternal exposure to cigarette smoke results in offspring with small lungs and decreased airspaces,[31] reduces elastin production[30] and leads to an increase in collagen around airways.[43]

Glucocorticoids may be administered before birth to accelerate maturation and prevent surfactant deficiency syndrome (p. 256). They are also used to reduce inflammation postnatally (p. 412). The use of glucocorticoids may affect lung growth, especially since lung morphogenesis is regulated by glucocorticoid-affecting growth factors.[36] Structural studies in sheep and rats[26,41] treated with prenatal and postnatal dexamethasone have shown accelerated alveolar wall thinning and maturation, at the expense of subsequent normal alveolar development.[49] Too few alveolar septae will eventually lead to alveoli that are too large and more smoothly contoured, an apparent emphysematous appearance.[8] Glucocorticoids have been shown to reduce elastin, decrease procollagen mRNA and reduce cross-linking, all of which may alter the stability of the alveoli and the caliber of the peripheral airways, possibly leading to enhanced 'small airways disease' in the long term. The clinical effects of such events may not become apparent until the aging process is well established. The largely experimental data in relation to glucocorticoids shows that therapeutic intervention at critical stages of development may have unwanted or unexpected sequelae at a later stage in development. Lung growth *in utero* is also influenced by a number of biophysical factors (p. 452). These biophysical factors include the space available in the chest cavity, fluid in the lungs and the amniotic sac, pressures within the chest cavity and fetal breathing movements, all of which interact to contribute to overall lung growth (p. 456).

ACKNOWLEDGMENT

The author wishes to thank the British Heart Foundation for their continued support.

REFERENCES

1 Ang, S.-L., Rossan, J. (1994) HNF-3β is essential for node and notochord development in mouse development. *Cell* **78**, 561–574.

2 Angus, G.E., Thurlbeck, W.M. (1972) Number of alveoli in the human lung. *Journal of Applied Physiology* **32**, 483–485.

3 Baile, E.M. (1996) The anatomy and physiology of the bronchial circulation. *Journal of Aerosol Medicine* **9**, 1–6.

4 Barker, D.J.P. (1991) The intrauterine environment and adult cardiovascular disease. In Bock, G., Whelan, J. (eds), *The Childhood Environment and Adult Disease*. Chichester: John Wiley & Sons, pp. 3–15.

5 Bucher, U., Reid, L. (1961) Development of the intrasegmental bronchial tree: the pattern of branching and development of cartilage at various stages of intra-uterine life. *Thorax* **16**, 207–218.

6 Bucher, U., Reid, L. (1961) Development of the mucus-secreting elements in human lung. *Thorax* **16**, 219–225.

7 Burri, P.H. (1997) Structural aspects of prenatal and postnatal development and growth of the lung. In McDonald, J.A. (ed.), *Lung Growth and Development*. New York: Marcel Dekker, pp. 1–35.

8 Burri, P.H., Hislop, A.A. (1998) Structural considerations. *European Respiratory Journal* **12**, Suppl 27, 59s–65s.

9 Cook, D.G., Strachan, D.P. (1999) Summary of effects of parental smoking on the respiratory health of children and implications for research. *Thorax* **54**, 357–366.

10 Dezateux, C., Stocks, J., Dundas, I., Fletcher, M.E. (1999) Impaired airway function and wheezing in infancy. *American Journal of Respiratory and Critical Care Medicine* **159**, 403–410.

11 Gaultier, C. (1991) Malnutrition and lung growth. *Pediatric Pulmonology* **10**, 278–286.

12 Griscom, N.T., Wohl, M.E.B., Fenton, T. (1989) Dimensions of the trachea to age 6 years related to height. *Pediatric Pulmonology* **6**, 186–190.

13 Hall, S.M., Hislop, A.A., Pierce, C., Haworth, S.G. (2000) Prenatal origins of human intrapulmonary arteries: formation and maturation. *American Journal of Respiratory Cell and Molecular Biology* **23**, 194–203.

14 Haworth, S.G. (1988) Pulmonary vascular remodelling in neonatal pulmonary hypertension. State of the art. *Chest* **93**, 133S–138S.

15 Haworth, S.G., Hislop, A.A. (1981) Normal structural and functional adaptation to extra-uterine life. *Journal of Pediatrics* **98**, 915–918.

16 Hermans, C., Bernard, A. (1999) Lung epithelium-specific proteins – characteristics and potential applications as markers. *American Journal of Respiratory and Critical Care Medicine* **159**, 646–678.

17 Hislop, A., Muir, D.C.F., Jacobsen, M., Simon, G., Reid, L. (1972) Postnatal growth and function of the pre-acinar airways. *Thorax* **27**, 265–274.

18 Hislop, A., Wigglesworth, J.S., Desai, R. (1986) Alveolar development in the human fetus and infant. *Early Human Development* **13**, 1–11.

19 Hislop, A., Wigglesworth, J.S., Desai, R., Aber, V. (1987) The effects of preterm delivery and mechanical ventilation on human lung growth. *Early Human Development* **15**, 147–164.

20 Hislop, A.A., Haworth, S.G. (1989) Airway size and structure in the normal fetal and infant lung and the effect of premature delivery and artificial ventilation. *American Review of Respiratory Disease* **140**, 1717–1726.

21 Hislop, A.A., Reid, L.M. (1977) Formation of the pulmonary vasculature. In Hodson, W.A. (ed.), *Development of the Lung*. New York: Marcel Dekker, pp. 37–86.

22 Hislop, A.A., Wharton, J., Allen, K.M., Polak, J., Haworth, S.G. (1990) Immunohistochemical localization of peptide-containing nerves in the airways of normal young children. *American Journal of Respiratory Cell and Molecular Biology* **3**, 191–198.

23 Hislop, A.A., Springall, D.R., Buttery, L.D.K., Pollock, J.S., Haworth, S.G. (1995) Abundance of endothelial nitric oxide synthase in newborn intrapulmonary arteries. *Archives of Disease in Childhood* **12**, F17–F21.

24 Hoo, A.F., Henschen, M., Dezateux, C., Costeloe, K., Stocks, J. (1998) Respiratory function among preterm infants whose mothers smoked during pregnancy. *American Journal of Respiratory and Critical Care Medicine* **158**, 700–705.

25 Jeffery, P.K., Reid, L. (1977) The ultrastructure of the airway lining and its development. In Hodson, W.A. (ed.), *Development of the Lung*. New York: Marcel Dekker, pp. 87–134.

26 Johnson, J.W.C., Mitzner, W., Beck, J.C. *et al.* (1981) Long-term effects of betamethasone on fetal development. *American Journal of Obstetrics and Gynecology* **141**, 1053–1061.

27 Kinsella, J.P., Ivy, D.D., Abman, S.H. (1994) Ontogeny of NO activity and response to inhaled NO in the developing ovine pulmonary circulation. *American Journal of Physiology* **267**, H1955–H1961.

28 Langston, C., Kida, C., Reed, M., Thurlbeck, W.M. (1984) Human lung growth in late gestation and in the neonate. *American Review of Respiratory Disease* **129**, 607–613.

29 Margraf, L.R., Tomashefski, J.F.J., Bruce, M.C., Dahms, B.B. (1991) Morphometric analysis of the lung in bronchopulmonary dysplasia. *American Review of Respiratory Disease* **143**, 391–400.

30 Maritz, G.S., Woolward, K. (1992) Effect of maternal nicotine exposure on neonatal lung elastic tissue and possible consequences. *South African Medical Journal* **81**, 517–519.

31 Massaro, G.D., Massaro, D. (1996) Formation of pulmonary alveoli and gas exchange surface area: quantitation and regulation. *Annual Reviews in Physiology* **58**, 73–92.

32 Massaro, G.D., Massaro, D. (1997) Retinoic acid treatment abrogates elastase-induced pulmonary emphysema in rats. *Nature Medicine* **3**, 675–677.

33 Massaro, G.D., Massaro, D. (2000) Retinoic acid treatment partially rescues failed septation in rats and in mice. *American Journal of Physiology* **278**, L955–L960.

34 Matsuba, K., Thurlbeck, W.M. (1972) A morphometric study of bronchial and bronchiolar walls in children. *American Review of Respiratory Disease* **105**, 908–913.

35 McCray, P.B. (1993) Spontaneous contractility of human fetal airway smooth muscle. *American Journal of Respiratory Cell and Molecular Biology* **8**, 573–580.

36 Melnick, M., Choy, H.A., Jaskoll, T. (1996) Glucocorticoids, tumor necrosis factor-alpha, and epidermal growth factor regulation of pulmonary morphogenesis: a multivariate in vitro analysis of their related actions. *Developmental Dynamics* **205**, 365–378.

37 Milner, A.D., Marsh, M.J., Ingram, D.M. *et al.* (1999) Effects of smoking in pregnancy on neonatal lung function. *Archives of Disease in Childhood Fetal and Neonatal Edition* **80**, F8–F14.

38 Minoo, P., Ring, R.J. (1994) Epithelial-mesenchymal interactions in lung development. *Annual Reviews in Physiology* **56**, 13–45.

39 Minoo, P., Hamdan, H., Bu, D., Warburton, D., Stepanik, P., deLemos, R. (1995) TTF-1 regulates lung epithelial morphogenesis. *Developmental Biology* **172**, 694–698.

40 Motoyoma, J., Liu, J., Mo, R., Ding, Q., Post, M., Hui, C.C. (1998) Essential function of Gli2 and Gli3 in the formation of the lung, trachea and esophagus. *Nature Genetics* **20**, 54–57.

41 Pinkerton, K.E., Willet, K.E., Peake, J.L., Sly, P.D., Jobe, A.H., Ikegami, M. (1997) Prenatal glucocorticoid and T4 effects on lung morphology in preterm lambs. *American Journal of Respiratory and Critical Care Medicine* **156**, 624–630.

42 Sekhon, H.S., Thurlbeck, W.M. (1995) Lung cytokinetics after exposure to hypobaria and/or hypoxia and undernutrition in growing rats. *Journal of Applied Physiology* **79**, 1299–1309.

43 Sekhon, H.S., Jia, Y., Raab, R., Kuryatov, A., Pankow, J.F., Whitsett, J.A. (1999) Prenatal nicotine increases pulmonary a7 nicotine receptor expression and alters fetal lung development in monkeys. *Journal of Clinical Investigation* **103**, 637–647.

44 Shannon, J.M., Deterding, R.R. (1997) Epithelial-mesenchymal interactions in lung development. In McDonald, J.A. (ed.), *Lung Growth and Development*. New York: Marcel Dekker, pp. 81–118.

45 Sparrow, M.P., Weichselbaum, M., McCray, P.B. (1999) Development of the innervation and airway smooth muscle in human fetal lung. *American Journal of Respiratory Cell and Molecular Biology* **20**, 550–560.

46 Spina, D. (1998) Epithelium smooth muscle regulation and interactions. *American Journal of Respiratory and Critical Care Medicine* **158**, S141–S145.

47 Tepper, R.S. (1987) Airway reactivity in infants: a positive response to metacholine and metaproterenol. *Journal of Applied Physiology* **62**, 1155–1159.

48 Thurlbeck, W.M. (1975) Postnatal growth and development of the lung. *American Review of Respiratory Disease* **3**, 803–844.

49 Tschanz, S.A., Damke, B.M., Burri, P.H. (1995) Influence of postnatally administered glucocorticoids on rat lung growth. *Biology of the Neonate* **68**, 229–245.

50 Warburton, D., Zhao, J., Berberich, M.A., Bernfield, M. (1999) Molecular embryology of the lung: then, now, and in the future. *American Journal of Physiology* **276**, L697–L704.

51 Zeltner, T.B., Burri, P.H. (1986) The postnatal development and growth of the human lung. II Morphology. *Respiration Physiology* **67**, 269–282.

2

Surfactant

BENGT ROBERTSON AND JAN JOHANSSON

The first breaths result in an enormous expansion of the air–liquid interface of the respiratory system, from about $2\,cm^2$ (estimated surface area of the larynx) to some 2–$3\,m^2$ in a full-term newborn baby when all alveoli have become recruited.[4] The work required to expand the inner respiratory surface is directly related to surface tension.[123] Gruenwald,[31] on the basis of port-mortem pulmonary pressure–volume recordings and histological observations of lung expansion patterns, postulated that 'the addition of surface active substances to the air or oxygen which is being spontaneously breathed in or introduced by a respirator might aid in relieving the initial atelectasis of newborn infants'. These observations anticipated the physicochemical demonstration of surface-active material in lung tissue by Pattle[86] and Clements.[13]

SURFACTANT FUNCTION

There are three fundamentally different basic concepts concerning the organization of the surface-active material in the airspaces, linked to divergent physiological concepts. According to most workers in the field, alveoli communicate with ambient air throughout the ventilatory cycle and their surface is coated with a continuous wet lining layer, which may undergo phase transition (with solidification) during surface compression.[14] An alternative concept was introduced by Brian Hills,[44] who claimed that the alveolar surface is essentially dry, and that the surface-active material adsorbs directly to the alveolar epithelium, except for small bulging water pools at the alveolar corners. The third concept implies that the

alveoli are stabilized by complete bubbles, in the neonatal period as well as later in life.[102] In this theoretical model, the alveolar opening to alveolar ducts and respiratory bronchioles are closed by a thin film of surfactant (at least a bilayer), which may disrupt and reform during ventilation to facilitate gas exchange. Each of these ideas can be supported by morphological observations. Our bias goes with the first alternative, especially as recent low temperature electron microscopy images of the peripheral airspaces of rat lungs have documented a continuous lining layer, concave in the corners.[5] In our opinion, the terminal airspaces do not need closed bubble films for stability. Once the alveoli have become expanded with air, their total surface area is much larger than that of the exit route (the conductive airways), allowing only limited centripetal surface flux during expiration. The gradual loss of respiratory surface area that may nevertheless occur during regular breathing or mechanical ventilation can probably be compensated for by alveolar recruitment maneuvers in the form of intermittent sighing.

LIFE CYCLE OF PULMONARY SURFACTANT

Lung surfactant comprises several different intracellular and extracellular structural entities, including lamellar bodies, tubular myelin, large and small vesicles and surface associated layers (Figure 2.1). There is continuity between these forms and they are mainly composed of lipids and a few specific proteins. The biochemical composition of lung surfactant is often illustrated as the

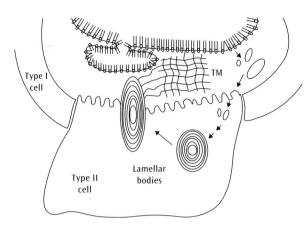

Figure 2.1 *Schematic presentation of the life cycle of surfactant showing an alveolar type II cell containing lamellar bodies, a secreted lamellar body swelling to tubular myelin, an air–water interfacial monolayer of phospholipids with an associated bilayer and subphase vesicles. Some desorbed surfactant is degraded by alveolar macrophages (not shown) but the major part is recycled by type II cells and degradation by alveolar macrophages are indicated by arrows. TM, tubular myelin.*

percentages of various compounds, where dipalmitoyl-phosphatidylcholine (DPPC) constitutes about 35 percent of the total mass, other lipid components including unsaturated phosphatidylcholine (PC) and phosphatidylglycerol (PG) and neutral lipids about 55 percent and proteins about 10 percent of the surface-active material. Such a static model, however, does not do justice to the versatility of the surfactant system during various phases of its life cycle. Lamellar bodies isolated from lung tissue by density gradient centrifugation contain the surfactant lipids and the surfactant proteins A, B and C (SP-A, SP-B and SP-C, see below). Whereas SP-B and SP-C are highly enriched in lamellar bodies, constituting about 50 percent of total protein, the SP-A content is very low, about 1 percent. Transition to tubular myelin implies a change in the chemical composition, in that SP-A becomes more abundant and apparently added from other sources (direct secretion from type II cells and/or Clara cells[82]). SP-A constitutes about 50 percent of the protein in extracellular surfactant purified from lung lavage fluid.[80] This is consistent with the postulated role of SP-A as an important 'organizer' of the tubular myelin. It has been documented by immunoelectron microscopy that SP-A is located in the corners of the tubular myelin structures, apparently splinting the lattice.[124]

Direct transition from tubular myelin to the surface film can be demonstrated by electron microscopy.[73] The surface film likely adsorbs as a mixture of saturated and unsaturated PC and PG and the insertion of the lipids into the surface 'monolayer' is apparently promoted by the hydrophobic surfactant proteins.[78,79] Selective adsorption of DPPC to the air–water interface, also mediated by the hydrophobic surfactant proteins, may

occur.[107,108] The surface film probably is refined by selective squeeze-out of unsaturated lipids,[85] and at expiration to functional residual capacity it probably consists of nearly pure DPPC, which is solid at normal body temperature and therefore avoids the destabilizing effect of surface tension in a system of alveoli of different size.[103] The desorbed material, ultrastructurally characterized as 'small vesicles', contains less DPPC and less surfactant proteins, and is less surface active than the material organized as lamellar bodies, tubular myelin or 'large vesicles'.[95] Desorbed surfactant is taken up by alveolar type II cells (Figure. 2.1) or, to a minor extent, degraded by alveolar macrophages.

The life cycle of surfactant is tightly regulated to ensure maximal economy, especially in the neonatal period. The type II cells recycle desorbed surfactant material. It has been estimated that in the neonatal rabbit lung about 95 percent of alveolar PC molecules is recycled before being catabolized or removed from the alveolar spaces by other routes; in adult rabbits the corresponding figure is about 20 percent.[47,48] There is negative feedback regulation of surfactant production mediated by SP-A binding to type II cells.[117] Surfactant secretion is at least to some extent triggered by stretch receptors and by β-adrenergic receptors on alveolar type II cells which increase in number towards the end of gestation. Several other secretagogs stimulating the release of surfactant into the alveolar spaces have been identified.[71,101]

PHYSICAL PROPERTIES OF SURFACTANT FILMS

The molecular mechanisms involved in the sorting of surfactant material at the air–liquid interface of the lung are not well understood. SP-A enhances surface adsorption of lipid extract surfactant at low surfactant concentrations ($\leqslant 0.2$ mg/ml), and seems to promote selective removal of non-saturated phospholipids during cyclic film compression. These effects of SP-A are amplified in the presence of calcium.[107] SP-B and SP-C individually accelerate the adsorption of phospholipids from the hypophase.[19,78,79] SP-B, which is composed of two subunits, has the ability to crosslink phospholipid membranes and may be important for generation of a 'surface-associated surfactant reservoir'.[109] The presence of multilayers in the wall of a captive bubble can be demonstrated in wash-out experiments (Figure 2.2). For a review of various methods to evaluate surface tension see reference 100.

Methods to assess surface tension

The classical *in vitro* experiments documenting the capacity of surfactant films to reduce the contractile force of an air–liquid interface (usually referred to as surface tension)

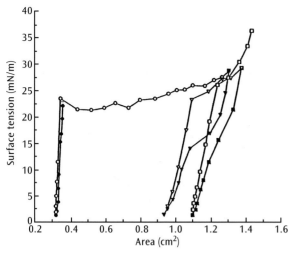

Figure 2.2 *Surface-tension-area isotherms obtained with a film of bovine lipid extract surfactant (BLES), after washout of surfactant material from the hypophase. Recordings were made with a captive bubble surfactometer at 37°C. During the first film compression (filled circles) only a small area change is required to produce near zero minimum surface tension, indicating a film highly enriched in DPPC. During first bubble area expansion (open circles) surface tension remains around 25 mN/m because of adsorption of material from the surface-associated reservoir. The bubble surface can be expanded to three to four times the original area, without losing its capacity to generate near zero surface tension on compression. This indicates that the bubble initially was coated with a multilayer of surfactant lipids. From Schürch and Bachofen,[104] with permission.*

to very low levels during surface compression were performed with a Langmuir-Wilhelmy balance.[13] The same type of instrument was used by Avery and Mead[3] to demonstrate the absence of surfactant material in the lungs of babies with RDS (hyaline membrane disease). Later on, Enhorning[23] developed a device, usually referred to as the pulsating bubble surfactometer (PBS), for evaluation of dynamic surface tension of a bubble formed in a liquid sample (for example, amniotic fluid, fetal lung liquid or lung lavage fluid) and communicating with ambient air. The Langmuir-Wilhelmy balance and the PBS both have the potential problem of film leakage, which may lead to underestimation of film stability during surface compression.[96]

Film leakage is avoided with the captive bubble system (CBS) invented by Schürch et al.[106] In the CBS, the bubble is closed, floating against a ceiling of agarose, and there is no exit for the surface film during surface compression. Surface tension is determined from the shape of the bubble profile, which becomes flatter when surface tension is reduced below the equilibrium level. Using this machine, Schürch et al.[107,108] demonstrated that preparations of surfactant isolated from mammalian

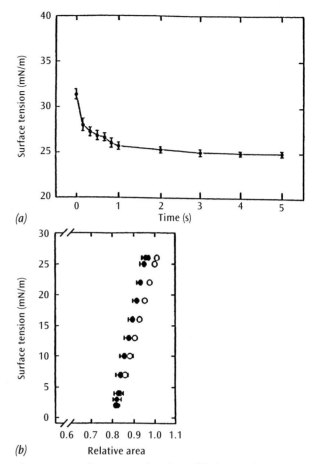

(a)

(b)

Figure 2.3 *Surface properties of modified natural surfactant (Curosurf, diluted to 1 mg/ml) containing only lipids and the hydrophobic proteins SP-B and SP-C, recorded with a captive bubble surfactometer at 37°C. Data are given as mean and sem. (a) Time course for adsorption as reflected by surface tension measurements immediately after bubble formation in the sample chamber (n = 4). An equilibrium surface tension of about 25 mN/m is established within approximately 1 second. (b) Surface tension plotted against relative surface area during the first compression cycle (n = 5). Only 20 percent surface compression is required to reduce surface tension to about 2 mN/m, indicating selective adsorption of DPPC. Adapted from Schürch et al.[108]*

lungs by extraction with organic solvents (containing only lipids and the two hydrophobic proteins SP-B and SP-C) adsorb extremely rapidly to the bubble surface, and that a minimum surface tension of nearly 0 mN/m, indicating phase transition with solidification of the surface film, is recorded after only about 20 percent surface compression (Figure 2.3). These are precisely the surface properties required for adequate lung adaptation at birth. The fast adsorption rate matches the rapid enlargement of the surface area in the lungs during the first breaths, and the low compressibility of the surface film (due to selective adsorption of DPPC and/or selective squeeze-out of non-DPPC components) effectively stabilizes the alveoli during expiration. Schürch *et al.*[105] measured alveolar surface tension *in situ* by observing the shape of droplets of liquid applied onto the alveolar surface. They found that alveolar surface tension dropped to very low levels (nearly 0 mN/m) at the end of expiration. Under these experimental conditions alveolar surface tension is unrelated to alveolar size but depends on the degree of surface compression.[103]

SURFACTANT PROTEINS

There are four proteins associated with lung surfactant, which are thought to be important regulators of surfactant activity. These proteins are called SP-A, SP-B, SP-C and SP-D from their order of discovery.[92] SP-C is the only one of the surfactant proteins that is expressed exclusively in alveolar type II cells. The other three surfactant proteins are expressed also in Clara cells, and SP-A and SP-D in the gastrointestinal tract and the Eustachian tube.[42]

SP-A and SP-D

STRUCTURE

SP-A is a large (about 650 kDa) glycoprotein that, like SP-D, from a structural point of view belongs to the calcium-dependent collectin (collagenous lectin) family of proteins. Other collectins include the serum proteins mannan-binding protein, CL-43 and conglutinin. The collectins share a common architecture composed of N-terminal triple helical collagen-like helices to which C-terminal lectin-like globular heads, or carbohydrate recognition domains (CRDs) are linked. There is one globular head for each polypeptide chain in the triple helix, thus making three lectin domains that each can bind one carbohydrate moiety per collagen stem.[45] SP-A contains six triple-helical collagen stems and thus contains in total 18 polypeptide chains. The six collagen-like stems of SP-A are arranged in a flower bouquet-like manner, with the lectin domains located in the periphery and parts of the collagen-like helices being held together laterally (Figure 2.4). The overall structures of SP-A and the complement factor C1q are very similar, although C1q does not belong to the collectin family.

SP-D shares the presence of collagen-like stems and lectin CRDs with SP-A, but the quaternary structure of SP-D is different from that of SP-A and more closely related to that of the bovine serum protein conglutinin. SP-D is an X-shaped molecule composed of four triple-helical stems that are held together in the N-terminal parts and radiate towards the periphery and end with the CRDs[45] (Figure 2.4). Native SP-D is thus composed of 12 polypeptide chains and has a total molecular mass of

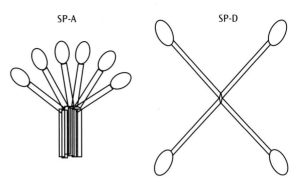

Figure 2.4 *Structural properties of SP-A and SP-D. Each elongated stem represents a collagen-like helix of three polypeptide chains and each oval 'head' represents three carbohydrate recognition domains.*

about 500 kDa. SP-D is a glycoprotein, like SP-A, but the N-linked carbohydrate chains are bound to different sites.

FUNCTION

The collectins can via their CRDs target carbohydrate structures on invading pathogens, mainly bacteria but also fungi, viruses, and potential allergens, resulting in the agglutination and enhanced clearance of the foreign material.[37] The distances between the three CRDs of each trimeric unit of SP-D are well suited to bind carbohydrates located on the surfaces of microorganisms, but too long to bind to the more closely spaced carbohydrates on eukaryotic cells.[38] This probably also applies to SP-A, although no experimental high-resolution structural data is available. These features strongly suggest that a main function of the surfactant proteins SP-A and SP-D is to bind microorganisms invading the airways. They, thus, belong to the non-clonal and innate host defense, which is functional in the absence of, and prior to, the development of the adaptive antibody-based immune system. The trimeric structure imposed by the collagen-like stem is a prerequisite for the proper function of collectins; the carbohydrate affinity of a single CRD is weak but the trimeric organization permits a trivalent and hence stronger interaction between collectin and carbohydrate-containing surface. The further assembly into larger entities enables the collectins to cross-link several target particles and perhaps also to interact simultaneously with target and with host cells.[37]

In addition to their binding of carbohydrates, both SP-A and SP-D, in contrast to what is known for most other collectins, also bind phospholipids. SP-A binds to several phospholipid classes but with a preference for DPPC,[9,64,88] while SP-D specifically binds phosphatidylinositol (PI),[77,89] a relatively minor compound of the surfactant lipids in most species. SP-A was discovered as a component of surfactant isolated from animal lungs, and was thus anticipated to be involved in the organization of surfactant lipids and reduction of alveolar surface tension. The essential role of SP-A for formation of tubular myelin structures *in vitro*[113,129] and *in vivo*[58] is in keeping with this notion. However, SP-A knockout mice show no evidence of respiratory disorders (p. 18). The presence of SP-A in surfactant preparations enhances resistance to inactivation by exogenous components,[16,112] possibly by formation of large lipid aggregates that are less susceptible to disruption by inhibitory agents. SP-A may thus be important for reduction of surface tension under stress conditions, for example when plasma proteins leak into the airways. It remains to be established whether the tight association of SP-A with surfactant lipids is of importance for the surface tension reduction by surfactant under certain conditions that are not encountered in the SP-A knockout mice. Alternatively, the association of SP-A with surfactant may be important for its innate host defense activities. Although SP-D binds PI, very little SP-D segregates with surfactant during purification, that is, most SP-D is recovered in the soluble supernatant after centrifugal precipitation of surfactant.[65] It is possible that SP-D binds PI because of the structural similarity between the inositol moiety of the PI head group and carbohydrates normally recognized by SP-D.

SP-B

STRUCTURE

SP-B is a comparatively small protein with a molecular mass of 17 kDa, composed of two identical polypeptide chains that are held together by a disulphide bond.[50] SP-B belongs to the family of saposin-like proteins, which include also the lysosomal sphingolipid activating proteins (saposins) and the membranolytic NK-lysin from white blood cells and amebapores from *Entamoeba histolytica*.[68] The pairwise sequence similarities between different saposin-like proteins is low but they all share the presence of unpolar residues at positions which are buried in the interior of the folded proteins and the location of half-cystines that form three intrachain disulphide bridges. The three-dimensional structures of the different saposin-like proteins are therefore similar, whilst their surfaces differ substantially.[55] This is reflected in that the saposin-like proteins perform widely different specific functions, but they all interact with lipids. SP-B is the only one of the saposin-like proteins that is a covalent dimer. This specific feature is, however, not necessary for the function of SP-B, as replacement of the Cys residue that forms the interchain disulphide bridge with Ser does not lead to detectable respiratory problems in transgenic mice.[6] The mutant (Cys48Ser) SP-B, however, is less surface active than the wild-type protein *in vitro*, which can be compensated for by increasing the concentration of the mutant protein.[6,132]

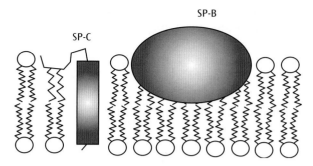

Figure 2.5 *Structural properties and lipid interactions of SP-B and SP-C. The SP-B structure is built up from two identical subunits held together by a disulphide bond and is depicted as an elongated molecule in which the poles are positively charged and the central region is mainly polar. SP-B is here located in the superficial parts of a phospholipid bilayer, but other localizations are also possible, see text for details. SP-C consists mainly of a transmembranous α-helix and an N-terminal region, which harbors two palmitoyl groups bound to Cys residues via thioester bonds.*

SP-B contains about 45 percent α-helical secondary structure. This is in good agreement with the suggested presence of four to five amphipathic helices, that is, α-helices in which one part of the circumference is unpolar and the other part is polar.[2] Most experimental data suggest that SP-B is a peripheral membrane protein, that is, that it interacts with the superficial parts of phospholipid bilayers and lacks transmembranous segments[119] (Figure 2.5). The tertiary structure of SP-B has not been experimentally determined, and different models of its structure and lipid interactions have been proposed.[15,43,54,63] The SP-B polypeptide sequence has been modeled on the NK-lysin structure. The ensuing molecular model is elongated and each end is strongly positively charged, while the central region mainly contains unpolar residues.[131] It is likely that association of SP-B to a phospholipid bilayer is mediated, on the one hand, via interactions between the central unpolar region of the protein and the lipid acyl chains and, on the other hand, between the positively charged poles of SP-B and the phospholipid head groups, preferentially the head groups of negatively charged phospholipids. The model structure of SP-B can be located differently in a phospholipid bilayer, either superficially (Figure 2.5), or at the edges of bilayer disks, or even in a transmembranous manner. It is possible that SP-B/phospholipid interactions are dynamic and that SP-B can adopt different locations under different circumstances.

FUNCTION

SP-B is unique among the saposin-like proteins in being soluble only in organic solvents or detergents. SP-B is tightly associated with surfactant lipids and removal of SP-B from lipids requires chromatographic separation in organic solvents. In line with this, SP-B has profound effects on lipid organization.[87] SP-B is required for tubular myelin formation *in vitro* and *in vivo*[113,129] and induces bilayer disk formation when added to lipid vesicles.[94] SP-B is also able to cross-link and fuse lipid vesicles and accelerates the spreading of lipids to an air–water interface.[10,18,19,78] SP-B in a surface-associated lipid layer is more effective than SP-C in promoting insertion of additional lipids from the subphase.[79] SP-B carries a strong net positive charge and interacts preferentially with negatively charged phospholipids,[88,130] of which PG is the most abundant in surfactant. In pure palmitic acid monolayers at high surface pressure, SP-B induces a fluid network around condensed domains.[70] Oviedo and coworkers[83] recently showed that the immunoreactivity of SP-B is more pronounced in anionic than in zwitterionic phospholipid bilayers, and the authors suggested that the conformation of SP-B may be modulated by the surrounding lipids.

SP-C

STRUCTURE

SP-C is the smallest of the surfactant proteins with a molecular mass of 4 kDa. Strictly speaking, SP-C is not a protein but a 35-residue peptide composed of only one secondary structure element. SP-C is extremely hydrophobic, more so than SP-B, and behaves chromatographically like a long chain fatty acid.[32] The very hydrophobic nature is caused by a long stretch of aliphatic residues with branched side chains, primarily valine, which is branched at the β-carbon, and two palmitoylated Cys residues. The polyvaline region covers the middle and C-terminal parts of SP-C and the palmitoylcysteines are present in the N-terminal part of the peptide. The three-dimensional structure of SP-C encompasses an α-helix covering positions 9–34, that is, the entire polyvaline part. This helix perfectly matches the size of a fluid bilayer composed of DPPC, which makes it very likely that SP-C is a transmembranous peptide[52] (Figure 2.5). This conclusion was drawn already from infrared spectroscopy studies, which showed that the SP-C helix is oriented in parallel with the lipid acyl chains in a phospholipid bilayer.[84,118] It is likely, but not experimentally proven, that the two palmitoyl groups and the helix interact with the same bilayer. This would leave essentially only the N-terminal three to four residues located outside the phospholipid bilayer plane. Alternatively, it is possible that the SP-C helix and the palmitoyl groups interact with two different lipid layers; this would enable SP-C to bind two lipid entities together.[93] The short distance (at the most 10–15 Å) from the start of the helix to the palmitoyl groups, however, is expected to give

strong repulsive forces between two phospholipid layers. The functional roles of the palmitoyl groups of SP-C are not known. Removal of the palmitoyl groups by chemical methods yields a less surface-active peptide.[97,127] The presence of the acyl groups has been suggested to influence the orientation of SP-C relative to the phospholipid plane.[17] Comparison of a palmitoylated and non-palmitoylated synthetic analog of SP-C in the PBS showed that the presence of the palmitoyl groups increased the mechanical stability of the peptide/lipid mixtures, facilitated the respreading of lipids to the interface and increased the amount of surface-associated lipid material.[34]

SP-C is a particularly clear example of a protein that can take on different conformations.[53] The soluble α-helical structure of SP-C converts in about 2 weeks into an insoluble aggregate in which SP-C shows β-strand conformation.[114] The SP-C polyvaline α-helix is kinetically very stable from tight interactions between the valine side chains,[60] but once it opens up into a non-helical structure, it does not refold again but forms β-sheet aggregates. This is in agreement with the early observation that synthetic peptides with the SP-C amino acid sequence do not fold properly into a helical conformation, but form insoluble aggregates,[51] although α-helical conformation has been observed for SP-C expressed in a baculovirus system.[121] The α-helix → β-sheet conversion of SP-C is associated with formation of amyloid fibrils. This is not an uncommon feature of polypeptide chains, in fact a number of different proteins have recently been found to forms fibrils under partly denaturing *in vitro* conditions, although they are not known to form amyloid under physiological conditions. Formation of SP-C aggregates and fibrils is, however, not limited to *in vitro* situations, but occurs in association with pulmonary alveolar proteinosis (PAP).[33] In bronchoalveolar lavage fluid from PAP patients, but not from healthy controls, abundant insoluble aggregates can be isolated which exhibit the characteristic properties of amyloid by light and electron microscopy, and are composed of SP-C. The PAP-associated fibrils appear to contain a significant amount of non-palmitoylated SP-C, while SP-C isolated from healthy individuals is almost entirely composed of the dipalmitoylated peptide. This suggests that removal of the palmitoyl chains can occur in PAP and that depamitoylated SP-C is more prone to form fibrils. Removal of one or both of the palmitoyl groups *in vitro* destabilizes the SP-C peptide and results in faster unfolding of the α-helical conformation and formation of insoluble aggregates.[35] It is not known what factor(s) may cause removal of the palmitoyl groups in PAP.

SP-C is the only known transmembrane helix composed of almost exclusively a polyvaline stretch. It is possible that the high short-term stability given by the polyvaline design is required for SP-C function and cannot be mimicked by amino acid sequences usually found in transmembrane helices. SP-C contains positively charged residues only at the N-terminal end of the helix and, as pointed out by Amrein and coworkers,[1] the SP-C helix constitutes a strong dipole. Maybe the stable polyvaline segment is required for stabilization of this inherently unstable helix. Further studies are needed in order to fully understand the biological significance of the very unusual structural features of SP-C.

FUNCTION

SP-C is found in lamellar bodies and in alveolar surfactant, but the preferred location of SP-C in alveolar surfactant is not known. From the size of SP-C, it appears that the peptide would preferentially be located in a phospholipid bilayer, and when SP-C is placed in a phospholipid monolayer the helix axis makes a 70 degrees tilt relative to a normal to the monolayer plane so that the unpolar polyvaline part can interact with the fatty acyl chains.[26] Although SP-C has a number of documented *in vitro* effects on the organization and behavior of lipid vesicles and monolayers,[120] the function of SP-C at a molecular level is not understood. *In vitro*, SP-C dramatically accelerates the spreading and adsorption of phospholipids to an air–water interface, decreases the surface tension achieved by lipid mixtures under dynamic conditions, and organizes the collapse phase obtained by area compression.[17,19,61,116,122] From their different structures, it would seem likely that SP-B and SP-C perform different functions in the surfactant system, but many of the *in vitro* effects on lipid behavior are similar for SP-B and SP-C. Notable exceptions are that only SP-B is able to fuse lipid vesicles[81] and that SP-C appears to be more effective than SP-B in promoting reinsertion of collapse-phase lipids into the surface film.[97]

'Knockout' models

SP-A

Ablation of the genes coding for the surfactant proteins in mice has generated important, and partly unexpected, information about their specific functions. Knockout of the SP-A gene makes the mice unable to form tubular myelin, however, without respiratory dysfunction.[58] In line with this, blockage of SP-A in newborn rabbits by monoclonal antibodies does not lead to respiratory distress.[57] As expected from the SP-A collectin properties, however, SP-A knockout results in increased susceptibility to infection with group B streptococci[67] and Pseudomonas aeruginosa (for a review see reference 58).

SP-D

As SP-A and SP-D both are collectins and similar in structure, it is rather surprising that knockout of SP-D does not produce any detectable increased susceptibility to infections. SP-D knockout does, however, produce alveolar accumulation of lipids and proteins, which

increases with age but does not lead to respiratory failure.[7,59] The histological picture seen as a result of SP-D deficiency is similar to that seen in association with alveolar lipoproteinosis, and suggests that SP-D modulates surfactant clearance by alveolar macrophages. Knockout of the gene coding for granulocyte macrophage colony-stimulating factor (GM-CSF) also yields alveolar lipoproteinosis,[21] but the underlying mechanisms seem to differ between SP-D and GM-CSF deficiency.

SP-B

Knockout, or blockage by antibodies, of SP-B leads to lethal neonatal respiratory distress with decreased lung compliance, leakage of plasma proteins into the airspaces, and hyaline membranes.[12,30,99] In SP-B knockout mice, lamellar bodies are abnormal and tubular myelin structures are absent, implying disturbed intracellular as well as alveolar surfactant metabolism. This strongly suggests that SP-B and/or proSP-B is central to surfactant function. In the SP-B knockout mice (as well as in children with genetic deficiency of SP-B, see below) the normal proteolytic processing of proSP-C into the mature SP-C is disturbed, causing accumulation of a processing intermediate and to abnormally low levels of mature SP-C in the alveolar spaces.[12,125] A likely explanation to these disturbances is that proteolysis of proSP-C normally partly takes place in lamellar bodies, and that the malformation of these organelles in SP-B knockout mice leads to a block in the processing of proSP-C. It is unclear to what extent the disturbances in the generation of SP-C contribute to the phenotype of the SP-B knockout mice.

SP-C

The structural properties of SP-C suggest that it is functionally important. However, studies on SP-C knockout mice have given contradictory results, depending on the strain of mice used. In a first series of experiments, SP-C gene targeted outbred Swiss black mice had normal lung function and development. The only detectable abnormality was reduced captive bubble stability at low surfactant concentrations compared to surfactant from wild-type mice.[27] Apparently lack of SP-C in the fetal and neonatal lung can be compensated for. Considering that SP-C and SP-B have similar *in-vitro* activity (see above), it is likely that SP-B, which is present in normal amounts in SP-C knockout mice, can at least to some extent replace SP-C. In more recent studies, SP-C knockout congenic 129/Sv mice developed chronic interstitial lung disease[27a] similar to the pathological findings reported in human patients with familial SP-C deficiency,[75] as further discussed below.

ONTOGENY OF THE SURFACTANT SYSTEM

There has been a continuous interest in developmental aspects of the surfactant system since it was first discovered that levels of surfactant components in amniotic fluid could serve as markers of fetal lung maturation, predicting the risk of RDS in cases of threatened premature birth.[28] The clinical significance of this concept was amplified with Liggins and Howie's pioneering observation[69] that fetal lung maturation can be accelerated by maternal treatment with corticosteroids (p. 256). Gluck and coworkers[28] showed that the lecithin:sphingomyelin (L:S) ratio was a useful parameter for this purpose ('lecithin' is the trivial name for PC). The L:S ratio normally reaches mature levels at a gestational age of about 36 weeks, but there is a large individual scatter, especially as accelerated fetal lung maturation may occur in a variety of fetoplacental disease conditions. More accurate information on fetal lung maturity can be obtained by analyzing the entire phospholipid profile in amniotic fluid, where particularly the appearance of PG signals that the fetal lung is ready for the first breath, at least as far as the surfactant system is concerned. A number of other tests are now available for antenatal evaluation of lung maturity, including biophysical measurements of surfactant activity as reflected by, for example, stable microbubbles, lamellar body counts and assessment of SP-A and SP-B in amniotic fluid. In principle, these tests can also be applied to gastric aspirates obtained at birth.[11,40]

Surfactant proteins

All surfactant proteins are expressed in fetal lung epithelium, but at different stages of development. SP-C expression starts during the second trimester, while the SP-B, SP-A and SP-D expression starts during the second half of the third trimester. The temporal pattern of SP-C expression during development hence does not correlate with that of pulmonary surfactant maturation. It is not known whether this reflects a function of SP-C not related to surfactant, or that SP-C expression is driven by transcription factors different than those involved in the expression of the other surfactant proteins in the fetal lung.

Alveolar pool

The normal alveolar pool size of surfactant phospholipids in a full-term neonatal lung has been estimated to about 100 mg/kg,[49] which is about 10 times larger than the corresponding figure for the normal adult lung, or for the lungs of a newborn baby with RDS.[41] Large amounts of surfactants apparently have to be secreted into the fetal airspaces towards the end of gestation to prepare the baby for the first breath. This is because the fetal lungs are filled with fluid at a volume approximately corresponding to functional residual capacity (about 30 ml/kg). Kobayashi et al.[56] assessed, in experiments on preterm newborn rabbits, the amount of surfactant that

had to be instilled into the liquid-filled airspaces at birth to ensure adequate air expansion of the lungs and concluded that the 'critical concentration' of surfactant is about 3.5 mg/ml. This is strikingly similar to the estimated normal pool size of alveolar phospholipids in the full term neonatal lung[49] divided by the volume of fetal lung liquid in the alveolar compartment. The normal pool size of surfactant lipids in the neonatal lung also matches the recommended clinical dose of surfactant in a baby with RDS (100 mg/kg).[39] The infant may need so much surfactant at birth because there is so much water in the lungs. This water must be removed from the airspaces to leave room for air expansion and gas exchange. Postnatal resorption of lung liquid is not instantaneous and during transition from liquid-filled to completely air-expanded airspaces there is probably a stage of mild hyperexpansion and foaming, both in conducting airways and alveoli. This phenomenon has been studied by Scarpelli,[102] who claimed that alveoli are stabilized by bubbles not only in the immediate neonatal period but also later in life. This intriguing concept has not been generally accepted.

Lung fluid resorption and surfactant

The fetal lung is a secretory organ, producing lung liquid at a rate of about 70 ml/kg/h near term (Chapter 3). The surge of catecholamines at birth triggers a switch from lung liquid production to resorption through sodium-channels, reversing the flow of water across the lung epithelium. The sodium channels can be blocked by amiloride.[76] Resorbed lung water accumulates in the interstitial compartment, visible in histological sections as perivascular 'cuffs' during the first few hours after birth, and is further drained by lymphatics. The drainage of liquid from the neonatal rabbit lung is reflected in a fall in wet weight from approximately 25 mg/kg at birth to 21 mg/kg at 1 hour and 12 mg/kg at 24 hours[29] (for review see references 8 and 126).

It has been claimed that the transepithelial movement of lung liquid at birth is directly influenced by surfactant, and that the wet lung syndrome, also known as transient tachypnea of the newborn, is caused by mild surfactant deficiency[22] (p. 272). Although the idea seems attractive, it underestimates the role of active transepithelial water transport and has not been supported by animal experimental data. Of course, stabilization of the alveoli after fetal lung liquid has been transported to the interstitial compartment is a vital function of surfactant, but this does not mean that surfactant provides a driving force for transepithelial flux of water. Knockout of the αENaC subunit of the sodium channels referred to above results in failure to drain the fetal lung liquid and the mice die in the neonatal period from respiratory failure.[46]

Song et al.[110] carried out a series of experiments on newborn rabbits to clarify the functional significance of surfactant and sodium channels for clearance of fetal lung liquid at birth. Animals were delivered at a gestational age of 27.5 days (immature lungs, surfactant deficient) or 29.5 days (nearly mature, surfactant sufficient) and tracheotomized. Experimental animals were treated with 1 mM amiloride or saline, and immature animals were in addition treated with modified porcine surfactant (Curosurf, Chiesi Pharmaceutici, Parma, Italy; dose 150 mg/kg). As expected, the drainage of water from the lungs, reflected by decreased wet weight and extravascular lung water content, was more effective in the 29.5 day than in the 27.5 day animals, and was not influenced in the immature animals by treatment with surfactant. Another anticipated finding was that amiloride caused a significant delay in clearance of lung water from the lungs of the nearly mature animals; no such effect was seen in the immature animals (in which the sodium channels probably were poorly developed). Surfactant increased the compliance of the immature lungs (again an expected finding), but had no influence on lung water content. These data together argue against a role of surfactant in the transepithelial clearance of lung liquid at birth.

NEONATAL DISEASES RELATED TO SURFACTANT DYSFUNCTION

RDS (Chapter 19)

Pool sizes of alveolar surfactant lipids in a preterm baby with RDS are only about 10 mg/kg,[41] and the situation is further complicated by structural immaturity, delayed postnatal resorption of fetal lung liquid,[91] epithelial disruption with a leakage of plasma proteins into the airspaces and inactivation of surfactant leading to a vicious cycle. The clinical condition may require artificial ventilation unless the defective supply of surfactant is compensated for by continuous positive airways pressure and/or administration of exogenous surfactant. Babies with RDS show different allelic profiles in the locus for SP-A on chromosome 10 compared to healthy subjects but the significance of this finding remains to be defined.[25]

Surfactant protein deficiency

Pathophysiological aspects of SP-B deficiency have been discussed above. In human babies, this condition is usually caused by a frameshift mutation on chromosome 2, leading to premature stop in the translation of proSP-B and complete absence of mature SP-B in the airspaces.[74] As in SP-B knockout mice, there is a defective proteolytic processing of proSP-C, leading to reduced levels of SP-C

and accumulation of a processing intermediate in the airspaces.[125] A genetic defect in proSP-C that leads to significantly reduced amounts of mature SP-C and possibly aggregation of variant forms of proSP-C has recently been detected in association with familial interstitial lung disease.[75] Moreover, reduced levels of SP-C are associated with acute lung injury in Belgian White and Blue calves.[20] No clinical association between alveolar lipoproteinosis and SP-D deficiency has been reported, but the histopathological appearance of the lungs of SP-D−/− mice[7,59] suggests that similar pathogenic mechanisms might be involved in the knockout model and the human disease.

Meconium aspiration syndrome (Chapter 23)

Inactivation of surfactant is an important element in the pathophysiology of inflammatory lung disease such as meconium aspiration syndrome (MAS),[72,111] bacterial and viral pneumonia, and the 'adult' form of acute respiratory distress syndrome – a disease that may occur also in newborn babies.[90] In MAS the aspirated material is in itself a potent inactivator of surfactant and the disease is further complicated by physical airway obstruction. Large doses of exogenous surfactant may be required to counterbalance surfactant inactivation,[24] and removal of aspirated material by airway lavage with diluted surfactant may potentiate the therapeutic effect of exogenous surfactant in MAS.[66] It also seems possible to increase the resistance to inactivation by adding non-ionic polymers (e.g. dextran, polyethylene glycol) to the exogenous surfactant (for review see reference 115). 'Spiking' surfactant with SP-A has also been considered for the same purpose,[16,112] but may be problematic since addition of SP-A to recombinant SP-C surfactant attracts granulocytes and stimulates the release of pro-inflammatory cytokines when instilled into the airways of ventilated preterm lambs.[62]

Future applications

Current efforts in surfactant research will widen the indications for surfactant therapy and lead to the development of a new generation of surfactant substitutes. These new preparations mimic the organic solvent extract surfactants from animals in that they contain only analogs of the native hydrophobic proteins mixed with DPPC, PG and other well-defined lipids.[100] It should be possible to tailor specific surfactants to fit the requirements of babies with different forms of lung disease. For example, resistance to inactivation by meconium varies between different surfactants and should be maximized in surfactants designed for use in MAS, and bacteriostatic effects may be important in babies with bacterial pneumonia, initially masquerading as RDS. Interaction with bacteria differ between surfactants[98] and may be related to the presence of antibacterial peptides such as prophenin which has been isolated from modified porcine surfactant.[128] Curosurf, which contains about 0.1 mg/ml of prophenin, is bacteriostatic to group B streptococci, an important pathogen causing severe lung disease in the neonatal period. No such bacteriostatic effect was demonstrated for the modified bovine surfactant Survanta (Abbott, North Chicago, IL), which instead stimulated the proliferation of *Escherichia coli* under the same *in vitro* conditions (culturing in nutrient-free media).[98]

In general, understanding of the basic physiology of pulmonary surfactant at birth and later in life is a prerequisite for rational design of surfactant substitutes for clinical use. The hydrophobic protein components of artificial surfactants do not have to be structurally similar to the native SP-B and/or SP-C, although proper α-helical folding of the SP-C analog seems to be essential. Two synthetic surfactants based on the 21-residue artificial polypeptide KL4,[15] or modified recombinant SP-C,[36] have recently been evaluated in clinical trials for treatment of neonatal and adult (acute) RDS respectively, but final results are not yet available.

ACKNOWLEDGMENTS

This work was supported by the Swedish Research Council (project nos 3351 and 10371) and the King Oscar II Jubilee Foundation.

REFERENCES

1 Amrein, M., Knebel, D., Kroll, S., Galla, H.-J., Sieber, M. (2000) Scanning probe microscopy in pulmonary surfactant research. *Applied Cardiopulmonary Pathophysiology* **9**, 188–192.

2 Andersson, M., Curstedt, T., Jörnvall, H., Johansson, J. (1995) An amphipathic helical motif common to tumourolytic polypeptide NK-lysin and pulmonary surfactant polypeptide SP-B. *Federation of European Biochemical Societies Letters* **362**, 328–332.

3 Avery, M.E., Mead, J. (1959) Surface properties in relation to atelectasis and hyaline membrane disease. *American Medical Association Journal of Diseases of Children* **97**, 517–523.

4 Bangham, A.D. (1987) Lung surfactant: how it does and does not work. *Lung* **165**, 17–25.

5 Bastacky, J., See, C.Y., Goerke, J. *et al.* (1995) Alveolar lining layer is thin and continuous: low-temperature scanning electron microscopy of rat lung. *Journal of Applied Physiology* **79**, 1615–1628.

6 Beck, D.C., Ikegami, M., Na, C.L. *et al.* (2000) The role of homodimers in surfactant protein B function in vivo. *Journal of Biological Chemistry* **275**, 3365–3370.

7 Botas, C., Poulain, F., Akiyama, J. *et al.* (1998) Altered surfactant homeostasis and alveolar type II cell morphology in mice lacking surfactant protein D. *Proceedings of the National Academy of Sciences of the United States of America* **95**, 11869–11874.

8 Carlton, D.P., Bland, R.D. (1995) Surfactant and lung fluid balance. In Robertson, B., Taeusch, H.W. (eds), *Surfactant Therapy for Lung Disease*. New York: Marcel Dekker, 33–46.

9 Casals, C., Miguel, E., Pérez-Gil, J. (1993) Tryptophan fluorescence study on the interaction of pulmonary surfactant protein A with phospholipid vesicles. *Biochemical Journal* **296**, 585–593.

10 Chang, R., Nir, S., Poulain, F.R. (1998) Analysis of binding and membrane destabilization of phospholipid membranes by surfactant apoprotein B. *Biochimica et Biophysica Acta* **1371**, 254–264.

11 Chida, S. (1995) A stable microbubble test for antenatal and early neonatal diagnosis of surfactant deficiency. In Robertson, B., Taeusch, H.W. (eds), *Surfactant Therapy for Lung Disease*. New York: Marcel Dekker, 107–120.

12 Clark, J.C., Wert, S.E., Bachurski, C.J. *et al.* (1995) Targeted disruption of the surfactant protein B gene disrupts surfactant homeostasis, causing respiratory failure in newborn mice. *Proceedings of the National Academy of Sciences of the United States of America* **92**, 7794–7798.

13 Clements, J.A. (1957) Surface tension of lung extracts. *Proceedings of the Society for Experimental Biology and Medicine* **95**, 170–175.

14 Clements, J.A. (1977) Functions of the alveolar lining. *American Review of Respiratory Disease* **115**, 67–71.

15 Cochrane, C.G., Revak, S.D. (1991) Pulmonary surfactant protein B (SP-B): structure–function relationships. *Science* **254**, 566–568.

16 Cockshutt, A., Weitz, J., Possmayer, F. (1990) Pulmonary surfactant-associated protein A enhances the surface activity of lipid extract surfactant and reverses inhibition by blood proteins in vitro. *Biochemistry* **29**, 8424–8429.

17 Creuwels, L.A.J.M., Demel, R.A., van Golde, L.M.G., Benson, B.J., Haagsman, H.P. (1993) Effect of acylation on structure and function of surfactant protein C at the air–liquid interface. *Journal of Biological Chemistry* **268**, 26752–26758.

18 Creuwels, L.A., van Golde, L.M.G., Haagsman, H.P. (1996) Surfactant protein B: effects on lipid domain formation and intermembrane lipid flow. *Biochimica et Biophysica Acta* **1285**, 1–8.

19 Curstedt, T., Jörnvall, H., Robertson, B., Bergman, T., Berggren, P. (1987) Two hydrophobic low-molecular-mass protein fractions of pulmonary surfactant. Characterization and biophysical activity. *European Journal of Biochemistry* **168**, 255–262.

20 Danlois, F., Zaltash, S., Johansson, J. *et al.* (2000) Very low surfactant protein C contents in newborn Belgian White and Blue calves with respiratory distress syndrome. *Biochemical Journal* **351**, 779–787.

21 Dranoff, G., Crawford, A.D., Sadelain, M. *et al.* (1994) Involvement of granulocyte-macrophage colony-stimulating factor in pulmonary homeostasis. *Science* **264**, 713–716.

22 Egan, E.A. (1989) Surfactant and fetal lung liquid absorption at birth. In Shapiro, D.L., Notter, R.H. (eds), *Surfactant Replacement Therapy*. New York: Alan R Liss, 91–98.

23 Enhorning, G. (1977) Pulsating bubble technique for evaluating pulmonary surfactant. *Journal of Applied Physiology* **43**, 198–203.

24 Findlay, R.D., Taeusch, H.W. Walther, F.J. (1996) Surfactant replacement therapy for meconium aspiration syndrome. *Pediatrics* **97**, 48–52.

25 Floros, J., Hoover, R.R. (1998) Genetics of the hydrophilic surfactant proteins A and D. *Biochimica et Biophysica Acta* **1408**, 312–322.

26 Gericke, A., Flach, C.R., Mendelsohn, R. (1997) Structure and orientation of lung surfactant SP-C and

L-α-dipalmitoylphosphatidylcholine in aqueous monolayers. *Biophysical Journal* **73**, 492–499.

27 Glasser, S.W., Burhans, M.S., Korfhagen, T.R. *et al.* (2001) Altered stability of pulmonary surfactant in SP-C-deficient mice. *Proceedings of the National Academy of Sciences of the United States of America* **98**, 6366–6371.

27a Glasser, S.W., Detmer, E.A., Ikegami, M., Na, C-L., Stahlman, M.T., Whitsett, J.A. (2003) Pneumanitis and emphysema in SP-C gene targeted mice. *Journal of Biological Chemistry.*(in press)

28 Gluck, L., Kulovich, M.V., Borer, R.C. Brenner, P.H., Anderson, G.G., Spellacy, W.N. (1971) Diagnosis of the respiratory distress syndrome by amniocentesis. *American Journal of Obstetrics and Gynecology* **109**, 440–445.

29 Grossmann, G., Robertson, B. (1975) Lung expansion and the formation of the alveolar lining layer in the fullterm newborn rabbit. *Acta Paediatrica Scandinavia* **64**, 7–16.

30 Grossmann, G., Suzuki, Y., Robertson, B. *et al.* (1997) Pathophysiology of neonatal lung injury induced by monoclonal antibody to surfactant protein B. *Journal of Applied Physiology* **82**, 2003–2010.

31 Gruenwald, P. (1947) Surface tension as a factor in the resistance of neonatal lungs to aeration. *American Journal of Obstetrics and Gynecology* **53**, 996–1007.

32 Gustafsson, M., Curstedt, T., Jörnvall, H., Johansson, J. (1997) Reverse-phase HPLC of the hydrophobic pulmonary surfactant proteins: detection of a surfactant protein C isoform containing Nε-palmitoyl-lysine. *Biochemical Journal* **326**, 799–806.

33 Gustafsson, M., Thyberg, J., Näslund, J., Eliasson, E., Johansson, J. (1999) Amyloid fibril formation by pulmonary surfactant protein C. *Federation of European Biochemical Societies Letters* **464**, 138–142.

34 Gustafsson, M., Palmblad, M., Curstedt, T., Johansson, J., Schürch, S. (2000) Palmitoylation of a pulmonary surfactant protein C analogue affects the surface associated lipid reservoir and film stability. *Biochimica et Biophysica Acta* **1466**, 169–178.

35 Gustafsson, M., Griffiths, W.J., Furusjö, E., Johansson, J. (2001) The palmitoyl groups of lung surfactant protein C reduce unfolding into a fibrillogenic intermediate. *Journal of Molecular Biology* **310**, 937–950.

36 Häfner, D., Germann, P.-G., Hauschke, D. (1998) Effects of rSP-C surfactant on oxygenation and histology in a rat-lung-lavage model of acute lung injury. *American Journal of Respiratory and Critical Care Medicine* **158**, 270–278.

37 Håkansson, K., Reid, K.B.M. (2000) Collectin structure: a review. *Protein Science* **9**, 1607–1617.

38 Håkansson, K., Lim, N.K., Hoppe, H.J., Reid, K.B. (1999) Crystal structure of the trimeric alpha-helical coiled-coil and the three lectin domains of human lung surfactant protein D. *Structure Folding and Design* **7**, 255–264.

39 Halliday, H.L. and Speer, C.P. (1995) Strategies for surfactant therapy in established neonatal respiratory distress syndrome. In Robertson, B., Taeusch, H.W. (eds), *Surfactant Therapy for Lung Disease*. New York: Marcel Dekker, 443–459.

40 Hallman, M. (1992) Antenatal diagnosis of lung maturity. In Robertson, B., van Golde, L.M.G., Batenburg, J.J. (eds), *Pulmonary Surfactant: From Molecular Biology to Clinical Practice*. Amsterdam: Elsevier Science Publishers, 425–458.

41 Hallman, M., Merritt, T.A., Pohjavuori, M., Gluck, L. (1986) Effect of surfactant substitution on lung effluent phospholipids in respiratory distress syndrome: evaluation of surfactant phospholipid turnover, pool size, and the relationship to severity of respiratory failure. *Pediatric Research* **20**, 1228–1235.

42 Hallman, M., Paananen, R., Glumoff, V. *et al.* (2001) Surfactant proteins SP-A and SP-D are expressed in the upper airway and may protect against infections. *Biology of the Neonate* **80**, 36–37.

43 Hawgood, S., Derrick, M., Poulain, F. (1998) Structure and properties of surfactant protein B. *Biochimica et Biophysica Acta* **1408**, 150–160.

44 Hills, B.A. (1988) *The Biology of Surfactant*. Cambridge: Cambridge University Press.

45 Hoppe, H.-J., Reid, K.B.M. (1994) Trimeric C-type lectin domains in host defence. *Structure* **2**, 1129–1133.

46 Hummler, E., Barker, P., Gatzy, J. *et al.* (1996) Early death due to defective neonatal lung liquid clearance in αENaC-deficient mice. *Nature Genetics* **12**, 325–328.

47 Jacobs, H., Jobe, A., Ikegami, M., Conaway, D. (1983) The significance of reutilization of surfactant phosphatidylcholine. *Journal of Biological Chemistry* **258**, 4156–4165.

48 Jacobs, H.C., Ikegami, M., Jobe, A.H., Berry, D.D., Jones, S. (1985) Reutilitation of surfactant phosphatidylcholine in adult rabbits. *Biochimica et Biophysica Acta* **837**, 77–84.

49 Jobe, A., Ikegami, M. (1987) Surfactant for the treatment of respiratory distress syndrome. *American Review of Respiratory Disease* **136**, 1256–1275.

50 Johansson, J., Curstedt, T. (1997) Molecular structures and interactions of pulmonary surfactant components. *European Journal of Biochemistry* **244**, 675–693.

51 Johansson, J., Nilsson, G., Strömberg, R., Robertson, B., Jörnvall, H., Curstedt, T. (1995) Secondary structure and biophysical activity of synthetic analogues of the pulmonary surfactant polypeptide SP-C. *Biochemical Journal* **307**, 535–541.

52 Johansson, J., Szyperski, T., Wüthrich, K. (1995) Pulmonary surfactant-associated polypeptide SP-C in lipid micelles: CD studies of intact SP-C and NMR secondary structure determination of depalmitoyl-SP-C (1-17). *Federation of European Biochemical Societies Letters* **362**, 261–265.

53 Kallberg, Y., Gustafsson, M., Persson, B., Thyberg, J., Johansson, J. (2001) Prediction of amyloid fibril-forming proteins. *Journal of Biological Chemistry* **276**, 12945–12950.

54 Keough, K.M.W. (1992) Physical chemistry of pulmonary surfactant in the terminal air spaces. In Robertson, B., van Golde, L.M.G., Batenburg J.J. (eds), *Pulmonary Surfactant: From Molecular Biology to Clinical Practice*. Amsterdam: Elsevier Science Publishers, 109–164.

55 Kervinen, J., Tobin, G.J., Costa, J., Waugh, D.S., Wlodawer, A., Zdanov, A. (1999) Crystal structure of plant aspartic proteinase prophytepsin: inactivation and vacuolar targeting. *European Molecular Biology Organization Journal* **18**, 3947–3955.

56 Kobayashi, T., Shido, A., Nitta, K., Inui, S., Ganzuka, M., Robertson, B. (1990) The critical concentration of surfactant in fetal lung liquid at birth. *Respiration Physiology* **80**, 181–192.

57 Kobayashi, T., Nitta, K., Takahashi, R., Kurashima, K., Robertson, B., Suzuki, Y. (1991) Activity of pulmonary surfactant after blocking the associated proteins SP-A and SP-B. *Journal of Applied Physiology* **71**, 530–536.

58 Korfhagen, T.R., Levine, A.M., Whitsett, J.A. (1998) Surfactant protein A (SP-A) gene targeted mice. *Biochemica and Biophysica Acta* **1408**, 296–302.

59 Korfhagen, T.R., Sheftelyevich, V., Burhans, M.S. *et al.* (1998) Surfactant protein-D regulates surfactant phospholipid homeostasis in vivo. *Journal of Biological Chemistry* **273**, 28438–28443.

60 Kovacs, H., Mark, A.E., Johansson, J., van Gunsteren, W.F. (1995) The effect of environment on the stability of an integral membrane helix: Molecular dynamics simulations of surfactant protein C in chloroform, methanol and water. *Journal of Molecular Biology* **247**, 808–822.

61 Kramer, A., Wintergalen, A., Sieber, M., Galla, H.J., Amrein, M., Guckenberger, R. (2000) Distribution of the surfactant-associated protein C within a lung surfactant model film investigated by near-field optical microscopy. *Biophysical Journal* **78**, 458–465.

62 Kramer, B.W., Jobe, A.H., Bachurski, C. J., Ikegami, M. (2001) Surfactant protein A recruits neutrophils into the lungs of ventilated preterm lambs. *American Journal of Respiratory and Critical Care Medicine* **163**, 158–165.

63 Krol, S., Ross, M., Sieber, M., Künneke, S., Galla, H.J., Janshoff, A. (2000) Formation of three-dimensional protein-lipid aggregates in monolayer films induced by surfactant protein B. *Biophysical Journal* **79**, 904–918.

64 Kuroki, Y., Akino, T. (1991) Pulmonary surfactant protein A (SP-A) specifically binds dipalmitoylphosphatidylcholine. *Journal of Biological Chemistry* **266**, 3068–3073.

65 Kuroki, Y., Shiratori, M., Ogasawara, Y., Tsuzuki, T., Akino, T. (1991) Characterization of pulmonary surfactant protein D: its copurification with lipids. *Biochimica et Biophysica Acta* **1086**, 185–190.

66 Lam, B.D.D., Yeung, C.Y. (1999) Surfactant lavage for meconium aspiration syndrome: a pilot study. *Pediatrics* **103**, 1014–1018.

67 LeVine, A.M., Bruno, M.D., Huelsman, K.M., Ross, G.F., Whitsett, J.A., Korfhagen, T.R. (1997) Surfactant protein A-deficient mice are susceptible to group B streptococcal infection. *Journal of Immunology* **158**, 4336–4340.

68 Liepinsh, E., Andersson, M., Ruysschaert, J.M., Otting, G. (1997) Saposin fold revealed by the NMR structure of NK-lysin. *Nature Structure Biology* **4**, 793–795.

69 Liggins, G.C., Howie, R.N. (1972) A controlled trial of antepartum glucocorticoid treatment for prevention of the respiratory distress syndrome in premature infants. *Pediatrics* **50**, 515–525.

70 Lipp, M.M., Lee, K.Y.C., Zasadzinski, J.A., Waring, A.J. (1996) Phase and morphology changes in lipid monolayers induced by SP-B protein and its amino-terminal peptide. *Science* **273**, 1196–1199.

71 Mason, R.J., Voelker, D.R. (1998) Regulatory mechanisms of surfactant secretion. *Biochimica et Biophysica Acta* **1408**, 226–240.

72 Moses, D., Holm, B.A., Spitale, P., Liu, M.Y., Enhorning, G. (1991) Inhibition of pulmonary surfactant function by meconium. *American Journal of Obstetrics and Gynecology* **164**, 477–481.

73 Nakamura, H., Tonosaki, A., Washioka, H., Takahashi, K., Yasui, S. (1985) Monomolecular surface film and tubular myelin figures of the pulmonary surfactant in hamster lung. *Cell and Tissue Research* **241**, 523–528.

74 Nogee, L.M., de Mello, D.E., Dehner, L.P., Colten, H.R. (1993) Deficiency of pulmonary surfactant protein B in congenital alveolar proteinosis. *New England Journal of Medicine* **328**, 406–410.

75 Nogee, L.M., Dunbar, A.E., Wert, S.E., Askin, F., Hamvas, A., Whitsett, J.A. (2001) A mutation in the surfactant protein C gene associated with familial interstitial lung disease. *New England Journal of Medicine* **344**, 573–579.

76 O'Brodovich, H., Hannam, V., Seear, M., Mullen, J.B.M. (1990) Amiloride impairs lung water clearance in newborn guinea pigs. *Journal of Applied Physiology* **68**, 1758–1762.

77 Ogasawara, Y., Kuroki, Y., Akino, T. (1992) Pulmonary surfactant protein D specifically binds to phosphatidylinositol. *Journal of Biological Chemistry* **267**, 21244–21249.

78 Oosterlaken-Dijksterhuis, M.A., Haagsman, H.P., van Golde, L.M.G., Demel, R.A. (1991) Characterization of lipid insertion into monomolecular layers mediated by lung surfactant proteins SP-B and SP-C. *Biochemistry* **30**, 10965–10971.

79 Oosterlaken-Dijksterhuis, M.A., Haagsman, H.P., van Golde, L.M.G., Demel, R.A. (1991) Interaction of lipic vesicles with monomolecular layers containing lung surfactant proteins SP-B or SP-C. *Biochemistry* **30**, 8276–8281.

80 Oosterlaken-Dijksterhuis, M.A., van Eijk, M., van Golde, L.M.G., Haagsman, H.P. (1991) Surfactant protein composition of lamellar bodies isolated from rat lung. *Biochemical Journal* **274**, 115–199.

81 Oosterlaken-Dijksterhuis, M.A., van Eijk, M., van Golde, L.M.G., Haagsman, H.P. (1992) Lipid mixing is mediated by the hydrophobic surfactant protein SP-B but not by SP-C. *Biochimica et Biophysica Acta* **1110**, 45–50.

82 Osanai, K., Mason, R.J., Voelker, D.R. (1998) Trafficking of newly synthesized surfactant protein A in isolated rat alveolar type II cells. *American Journal of Respiratory Cell and Molecular Biology* **19**, 929–935.

83 Oviedo, J.M., Casals, C., Pérez-Gil, J. (2001) Pulmonary surfactant protein SP-B is significantly more immunoreactive in anionic than in zwitterionic bilayers. *Federation of European Biochemical Societies Letters* **494**, 236–240.

84 Pastrana, B., Mautone, A.J., Mendelsohn, R. (1991) Fourier transform infrared studies of secondary structure and orientation of pulmonary surfactant SP-C and its effect on the dynamic surface properties of phospholipids. *Biochemistry* **30**, 10058–10064.

85 Pastrana-Rios, B., Flach, C.R., Brauner, J.W., Mautone, A.J., Mendelsohn, R. (1994) A direct test of the 'squeeze-out' hypothesis of lung surfactant function. *Biochemistry* **33**, 5121–5127.

86 Pattle, R.E. (1955) Properties, function and origin of the alveolar lining layer. *Nature* **175**, 1125–1126.

87 Pérez-Gil, J., Keough, K.M.W. (1998) Interfacial properties of surfactant proteins. *Biochimica et Biophysica Acta* **1408**, 203–217.

88 Pérez-Gil, J., Casals, C., Marsh, D. (1995) Interactions of hydrophobic lung surfactant proteins SP-B and SP-C with dipalmitoylphosphatidylcholine and dipalmitoylphoshatidylglycerol bilayers studied by electron spin resonance spectroscopy. *Biochemistry* **34**, 3964–3971.

89 Persson, A.B., Gibbons, B.J., Shoemaker, J.D., Moxley, M.A., Longmore, W.J. (1992) The major glycolipid recognized by SP-D in surfactant is phosphatidylinositol. *Biochemistry* **31**, 12183–12189.

90 Pfenninger, J., Tschaeppeler, H., Wagner, B.P., Weber, J., Zimmerman, A. (1991) The paradox of adult respiratory distress syndrome in neonates. *Pediatric Pulmonology* **10**, 18–24.

91 Pitkänen, O., O'Brodovich, H. (1999) Development of lung epithelial ion transport: implications for neonatal lung disease. In Gaultier, C., Bourbon, J.R., Post, M. (eds), *Lung Development*. Oxford: Oxford University Press, 255–281.

92 Possmayer, F. (1988) A proposed nomenclature for pulmonary surfactant-associated proteins. *American Review of Respiratory Disease* **138**, 990–998.

93 Possmayer, F., Nag, K., Rodriquez, K., Qanbar, R., Schürch, S. (2001) Surface activity in vitro: role of surfactant proteins. *Comparative Biochemistry and Physiology Part A* **129**, 201–220.

94 Poulain, F.R., Allen, L., Williams, M.C., Hamilton, R.L., Hawgood, S. (1992) Effects of surfactant apolipoproteins on liposome structure: implications for tubular myelin formation. *American Journal of Physiology* **262**, L730–L739.

95 Putman, E., Creuwels, L.A.J.M., van Golde, L.M.G., Haagsman, H.P. (1996) Surface properties, morphology and

protein composition of pulmonary surfactant subtypes. *Biochemical Journal* **320**, 599–605.

96 Putz, G., Goerke, J., Taeusch, H.W., Clements, J.A. (1994) Comparison of captive and pulsating bubble surfactometers with use of lung surfactants. *Journal of Applied Physiology* **76**, 1425–1431.

97 Qanbar, R., Cheng, S., Possmayer, F., Schürch, S. (1996) Role of the palmitoylation of surfactant-associated protein C in surfactant film formation and stability. *American Journal of Physiology* **271**, L572–L580.

98 Rauprich, P., Möller, O., Walter, G., Herting, E., Robertson, B. (2000) Influence of modified natural or synthetic surfactant preparations on growth of bacteria causing infections in the neonatal period. *Clinical and Diagnostic Laboratory Immunology* **7**, 817–822.

99 Robertson, B., Kobayashi, T., Ganzuka, M., Grossmann, G., Li, W.Z., Suzuki, Y. (1991) Experimental neonatal respiratory failure induced by a monoclonal antibody to the hydrophobic surfactant-associated protein SP-B. *Pediatric Research* **30**, 239–243.

100 Robertson, B., Johansson J., Curstedt, T. (2000) Synthetic surfactants to treat neonatal lung disease. *Molecular Medicine Today* **6**, 119–124.

101 Rooney, S.A. (2001) Regulation of surfactant secretion. *Comparative Biochemistry and Physiology Part A* **129**, 233–243.

102 Scarpelli, E.M. (1998) The alveolar surface network: a new anatomy and its physiological significance. *Anatomical Record* **251**, 491–527.

103 Schürch, S. (1982) Surface tension at low lung volumes: dependence on time and alveolar size. *Respiration Physiology* **48**, 339–355.

104 Schürch, S., Bachofen, H. (1995) Biophysical aspects in the design of a therapeutic surfactant. In Robertson, B., Taeusch, H.W. (eds), *Surfactant Therapy for Lung Disease.* New York: Marcel Dekker, 3–32.

105 Schürch, S., Goerke, J., Clements, J.A. (1978) Direct determination of volume- and time-dependence of alveolar surface tension in excised lungs. *Proceedings of the National Academy of Sciences of the United States of America* **75**, 3417–3421.

106 Schürch, S., Bachofen, H., Goerke, J., Possmayer, F. (1989) A captive bubble method reproduces the in situ behavior of lung surfactant monolayers. *Journal of Applied Physiology* **67**, 2389–2396.

107 Schürch, S., Possmayer, F., Cheng, S., Cockshutt, A.M. (1992) Pulmonary SP-A enhances adsorption and appears to induce surface sorting of lipid extract surfactant. *American Journal of Physiology* **263**, L210–L218.

108 Schürch, S., Schürch, D., Curstedt, T., Robertson, B. (1994) Surface activity of lipid extract surfactant in relation to film area compression and collapse. *Journal of Applied Physiology* **77**, 974–986.

109 Schürch, S., Quanbar, R., Bachofen, H., Possmayer, F. (1995) The surface-associated surfactant reservoir in the alveolar lining. *Biology of the Neonate* **67**, 61–76.

110 Song, G.-W., Sun, B., Curstedt, T., Grossmann, G., Robertson, B. (1992) Effect of amiloride and surfactant on lung liquid clearance in newborn rabbits. *Respiration Physiology* **88**, 233–246.

111 Sun, B., Curstedt, T., Robertson, B. (1993) Surfactant inhibition in experimental meconium aspiration. *Acta Paediatrica* **82**, 182–189.

112 Sun, B., Curstedt, T., Lindgren, G. *et al.* (1997) Biophysical and physiological properties of a modified porcine surfactant enriched with surfactant protein A. *European Respiratory Journal* **10**, 1967–1974.

113 Suzuki, Y., Fujita, Y., Kogishi, K. (1989) Reconstitution of tubular myelin from synthetic lipids and proteins associated with pig pulmonary surfactant. *American Review of Respiratory Disease* **140**, 75–81.

114 Szyperski, T., Vandenbussche, G., Curstedt, T., Ruysschaert, J.-M., Wüthrich, K., Johansson, J. (1998) Pulmonary surfactant-associated polypeptide C in a mixed organic solvent transforms from a monomeric α-helical state into insoluble β-sheet aggregates. *Protein Science* **7**, 2533–2540.

115 Taeusch, H.W. (2000) Treatment of acute (adult) respiratory distress syndrome. The holy grail of surfactant therapy. *Biology of the Neonate* **77**, 2–8.

116 Taneva, S.G., Keough, K.M.W. (1994) Dynamic surface properties of pulmonary surfactant proteins SP-B and SP-C and their mixtures with dipalmitoylphosphatidylcholine. *Biochemistry* **33**, 14660–14670.

117 Tino, M.J., Wright, J.R. (1998) Interactions of surfactant protein A with epithelial cells and phagocytes. *Biochimica et Biophysica Acta* **1408**, 241–263.

118 Vandenbussche, G., Clercx, A., Clercx, M. *et al.* (1992) Structure and orientation of the surfactant-associated protein C in a lipid bilayer. *European Journal of Biochemistry* **203**, 201–209.

119 Vandenbussche, G., Clercx, A., Clercx, M. *et al.* (1992) Secondary structure and orientation of the surfactant protein SP-B in a lipid environment. A Fourier transform infrared spectroscopy study. *Biochemistry* **31**, 9169–9176.

120 Veldhuizen, E.J., Haagsman, H.P. (2000) Role of pulmonary surfactant components in surface film formation and dynamics. *Biochimica et Biophysica Acta* **1467**, 255–270.

121 Veldhuizen, E.J., Batenburg, J.J., Vandenbussche, G., Putz, G., van Golde, L.M.G., Haagsman, H.P. (1999) Production of surfactant protein C in the baculovirus expression system: the information required for correct folding and palmitoylation of SP-C is contained within the mature sequence. *Biochimica et Biophysica Acta* **1416**, 295–308.

122 von Nahmen, A., Schenk, M., Sieber, M., Amrein, M. (1997) The structure of a model pulmonary surfactant as revealed by scanning force microscopy. *Biophysical Journal* **72**, 463–469.

123 von Neergaard, K. (1929) Neue Auffassungen über einen Grundbegriff der Atemmechanik: die Retraktionskraft der Lunge, abhängig von der Oberflächenspannung in den Alveolen. *Zeitschrift für die Gesamte Experimentelle Medizin* **66**, 373–394.

124 Voorhout, W.F., Veenendaal, T., Haagsman, H.P., Verkleij, A.J., van Golde, L.M.G., Geuze, H.J. (1991) Surfactant protein A is localized at the corners of the pulmonary tubular myelin lattice. *Journal of Histochemistry and Cytochemistry* **39**, 1331–1336.

125 Vorbroker, D.K., Profitt, S.A., Nogee, L.M., Whitsett, J.A. (1995) Aberrant processing of surfactant protein C in hereditary SP-B deficiency. *American Journal of Physiology* **268**, L647–L656.

126 Walters, D.V. (1992) The role of pulmonary surfactant in transepithelial movement of liquid. In Robertson, B., van Golde, L.M.G., Batenburg, J.J. (eds), *Pulmonary Surfactant: From Molecular Biology to Clinical Practice.* Amsterdam: Elsevier Science Publishers, 193–213.

127 Wang, Z., Gurel, O., Baatz, J.E., Notter, R.H. (1996) Acylation of pulmonary surfactant protein-C is required for its optimal surface active interactions with phospholipids. *Journal of Biological Chemistry* **271**, 19104–19109.

128 Wang, Y., Griffiths, W.J., Curstedt, T., Johansson, J. (1999) Porcine pulmonary surfactant preparations contain the antibacterial peptide prophenin and a C-terminal

18-residue fragment thereof. *Federation of European Biochemical Societies Letters* **460**, 257–262.

129 Williams, M.C., Hawgood, S., Hamilton, R.L. (1991) Changes in lipid structure produced by surfactant proteins SP-A, SP-B and SP-C. *American Journal of Respiratory Cell and Molecular Biology* **5**, 41–50.

130 Yu, H., Possmayer, F. (1990) Role of bovine pulmonary surfactant-associated proteins in the surface-active property of phospholipid mixtures. *Biochimica et Biophysica Acta* **1046**, 233–241.

131 Zaltash, S., Palmblad, M., Curstedt, T., Johansson, J., Persson, B. (2000) Pulmonary surfactant protein B: a structural model and a functional analogue. *Biochimica et Biophysica Acta* **1466**, 179–186.

132 Zaltash, S., Griffiths, W.J., Beck, D., Duan, C.-X., Weaver, T.E., Johansson, J. (2001) Membrane activity of (Cys48Ser) lung surfactant protein B increases with dimerization. *Biological Chemistry* **382**, 933–939.

3

Lung liquid

DAFYDD V WALTERS

As pregnancy advances, the fetal lung faces a vital and an increasingly pressing problem. At the end of gestation it has to be able to adapt to air breathing within a few minutes of birth or the infant dies. Yet the lung has to develop and grow in a liquid environment right up to the point of delivery. All mammals, birds and reptiles are faced with the same problem – they all have to take a first breath and clear their lungs of liquid to establish adequate pulmonary gas exchange. This chapter deals with some of the physiological processes that enable the lung to make this dramatic and life-dependent adaptation at birth.

LUNG GROWTH AND FETAL LUNG LIQUID

The lung needs to be of adequate size and of sufficient histological and structural maturity at term to sustain independent gas exchange. It forms initially from an outgrowth of the foregut and even in the earliest sections the little pouch has a lumen that is liquid filled. The epithelium, which creates the wall of the outgrowth, invades the surrounding mesoderm and the cross-talk between the mesoderm and the epithelium determines the place and rate of epithelial growth in three-dimensional space. Growth continues from what is assumed to be a nidus of cells (the capital cells) at the end of each blind sac right through gestation and, indeed, until body growth ceases in adolescence (Chapter 1).

Epithelial permeability

The fetal lung epithelium secretes liquid of unique composition from as early in gestation as it has been possible to measure[1,57] (Table 3.1). Like all secretory epithelia, back-diffusion of the transported molecules must be prevented

Table 3.1 *Selected solute composition of fetal lung liquid, fetal plasma and amniotic fluid in the sheep*

	Na$^+$	K$^+$	Cl$^-$	HCO$_3^-$	Protein
Plasma	150	4.8	107	24	4.09
Lung liquid	150	6.3	157	2.8	0.03
Amniotic liquid	113	7.6	87	19	0.10

Units are mM/kg water except for protein which is in g/dl. Note that lung liquid cannot be formed by mixing plasma and amniotic liquid. Data from Adamson et al.[1]

or at least retarded, otherwise the secretion is 'short circuited' and ineffective. The developing lung is no exception and throughout gestation and into postnatal life, the pulmonary epithelium is the major barrier to solute diffusion between the lung lumen and the blood space. Functionally, it behaves as if it contains small pores of only 0.65 nanometres (nm) in radius. For comparison, the effective molecular radius of sucrose is 0.51 nm, of inulin is 1.39 nm and of albumin is 3.5 nm and a red cell is 7000 nm in diameter. The consequence is that molecules even of the size of sucrose are severely restricted in their diffusion across the pulmonary epithelium. The pulmonary endothelium is very leaky in comparison, effectively containing pores of 11–15 nm.[53]

Secretory and other transport mechanisms

The secretory force underlying fetal lung liquid secretion is the secondary active transport of chloride ions from the interstitial space into the lung lumen. There is no evidence that cystic fibrosis transmembrane regulator (CFTR) is involved in this process. Sodium ions and water follow passively, probably via a paracellular route, down electrical and osmotic gradients. This important characteristic of the fetal lung was discovered by comparing the experimentally measured rates of one-way fluxes of various ionic species across the epithelium with those predicted from measurement of the passive forces acting on those ions. The predicted passive fluxes were calculated from the Ussing Flux Ratio equation – the relevant forces being chemical activity (concentration) gradient and electrical potential difference across the epithelium. The lumen of the fetal lung is always negative compared to interstitium by about 5 mV. Olver and Strang[56] demonstrated that chloride ions were transported 'uphill', against the passive forces, into the lung lumen, whereas sodium was passively distributed. Subsequently, the presence of a Na/K:2Cl co-transporter on the basolateral aspect of the epithelium was demonstrated by inhibition of secretion by loop diuretics, frusemide and bumetanide.[17,69] The gradient across the fetal epithelium for hydrogen ion (lumen acid) increases with gestation and is about 1 pH unit at term.[57] The active process responsible (still unknown) persists into the postnatal lung.[49] Transport of glucose out of the lung by a sodium–glucose co-transporter in both fetuses and postnatal animals keeps the lumen free of glucose – an important feature discouraging infection.[6,10,46] Liquid can be moved out of the lung lumen by this means but it is difficult to estimate its relevance when lung liquid normally contains no glucose.

Fetal lung liquid secretion, lung growth and fetal breathing movements

Rates of fetal lung liquid secretion can be remarkable: term animals can secrete up to 5 ml/kg body weight which, if extrapolated to humans, means the average baby at term weighing 3.5 kg produces about 18 ml/h or over 400 ml/day.[15] The liquid flows upwards out of the larynx either to be swallowed or to pass out into the amniotic cavity. The contribution of fetal lung liquid to daily turnover of amniotic liquid is about one-third to one-half. The fast rate of lung liquid production is important because as it meets resistance to flow in the upper airway, it generates a pressure of a centimetre or so of water in the lumen of the lung in excess of that in the amniotic cavity. This small pressure seems to be vital for lung growth for if it is abolished in any way, hypoplastic lungs result. The liquid distributes the small distending pressure all over the lung internal surface and it seems that this is a stimulus for growth. If the lung liquid volume is artificially reduced over several days, lung growth slows, but if liquid volume is increased, the lungs grow more.[48] For example, if a tracheotomy-type fistula is made during fetal life which abolishes the pressure drop between lumen and amniotic cavity, the lungs do not grow.[32,33] Furthermore, displacement of lung liquid by bowel in the pleural space as occurs in diaphragmatic hernia, whether naturally or experimentally produced, also impedes lung growth.[59,60]

The effect of fetal breathing movements (FBM) on lung growth is not easily explained. No liquid is drawn into the lung from the amniotic fluid during each fetal 'breath': the 'tidal volumes' are much less than the anatomical dead space because the resistance to flow of liquid is so high compared to gas.[27] Nevertheless, the background net flow of liquid out of the lung is greater during episodes of fetal breathing than during apnea, because the larynx is more relaxed and thus provides less resistance to liquid outflow.[37,38] Paradoxically, maneuvers which abolish FBM (phrenic nerve ablation, high cervical transection, tetrodotoxin exposure) result in lung hypoplasia, an effect explained, at least in one theory, by prolonged abolition of diaphragmatic contraction allowing unopposed lung tissue recoil to slowly reduce lung liquid volume.[36] Thus, fetal lung liquid can be regarded as a malleable internal dynamic template which stimulates lung growth and around which the fetal lung develops.

Experiments on reversing hypoplastic lungs in animal models in which the outflow of the lung is temporarily blocked to stimulate lung growth have produced complex results. The lungs are abnormal after these interventions, although they may be the correct size and initially appear to function normally. It appears as if surfactant production is depressed but lung tissue compliance is increased by changes in collagen and elastic tissue content and altered alveolar structure.[26,59,60] This has potentially serious long-term implications for infants born after such fetal surgery (p. 491). The long-term clinical outcome of such experimental intervention is unknown, as the numbers performed so far are tiny and follow-up is short. It must be remembered, however, that the underlying condition is often fatal and the temptation to intervene surgically can be great.

LABOR, BIRTH AND LUNG LIQUID

Newborn infants do not secrete lung liquid, although sometimes at the resuscitation of a baby born by elective cesarean section, one would be forgiven for thinking otherwise. Something, therefore, has to stop the secretion. Almost all our understanding of this process comes from animal work on several different species and it is assumed that humans are no different. Indeed, what observational and anecdotal evidence that does exist in humans supports the assumption that the same processes apply across the animal kingdom.

Lung liquid absorption

Experiments in fetal lambs (the preferred species for such studies for many reasons including size, convenience and similar lung pathology to humans) demonstrated that during early labor, fetal lung liquid secretion slowed and by late labor it sometimes stopped altogether. By the time the fetus was proceeding down the birth canal, the liquid in the lung was being absorbed by the lung epithelium. The conditions of the experiments were such that, once born, the fetus was maintained as a fetus with an intact placental circulation and not breathing so that observations of lung liquid volume could continue for a variable time after birth. The robust sheep placental circulation is another characteristic of the species that was vital to these experiments. Lung liquid was absorbed at very rapid rates after birth, sufficiently fast to clear the lung lumen of liquid completely within 1–3 hours[15] (Figure 3.1).

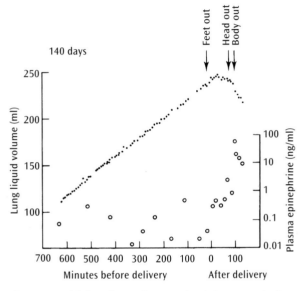

Figure 3.1 *This is a dramatic example of the reversal of fetal lung liquid formation at the time of birth. Lung liquid volume is on the y-axis and time on the x-axis. Zero time is at delivery of the fetus. Fetal lung liquid volume is measured by the indicator dilution technique in a chronically catheterized fetal lamb preparation and each point is calculated from one sample of lung liquid. A positive slope (increasing volume) indicates secretion and a negative slope, absorption of lung liquid. In this particular case, secretion continued until birth was imminent. After birth, the fetus was kept as an exteriorized fetus with an intact umbilical circulation. The decline in lung liquid volume indicates absorption across the pulmonary epithelium. The constraints of the experiment were such that the liquid could not be forced up through the larynx but could only diminish in volume by being absorbed across the pulmonary epithelium. The reversal of flow coincides with a rise in fetal epinephrine concentration of over 50-fold (note the log scale for epinephrine). A further series of experiments was able to demonstrate that the absorption of lung liquid could be accounted for totally by the rise in fetal epinephrine concentration. Data from Brown et al.[15]*

Several studies have explored where the liquid goes. Newborn rabbit pups were humanely killed at various times around delivery and their lungs were rapidly frozen. Low-power sections of the frozen lungs showed that liquid quickly accumulated in the interstitial and perivascular spaces after birth and that the volume of the interstitial space was maximal at about 1 hour.[13] The liquid is cleared more slowly thereafter by the lung lymphatics and via the circulation, so that by 6 hours all liquid has been removed from the lung.[14,52] Hydrostatic pressure in the interstitial space rises from near zero before air breathing to a maximum of $+6\,cmH_2O$ at 1–3 hours before falling to below atmospheric pressure at 6 hours after birth where it stays throughout life, unless pathology intervenes.[47]

These observations indicate that at birth a force is at work sufficiently powerful to clear the lungs rapidly of liquid against a hydrostatic pressure of at least $6\,cmH_2O$.

Labor and epinephrine

There is an enormous outpouring of fetal catecholamines during the process of birth (Figure 3.1 and Table 3.2). Several series of experiments proved that epinephrine was the agent responsible for liquid absorption during labor and that its rise in concentration was not merely a temporally associated phenomenon.[15] Dose–response curves correlating fetal blood epinephrine concentrations to rates of lung liquid secretion or absorption from experiments in fetuses not undergoing labor demonstrated that all the absorption observed in labor could be accounted for by the spontaneous, endogenously derived, rise in fetal blood epinephrine, which occurs as a response to the stress of being born. Epinephrine is cleared from fetal blood by the placenta – umbilical arterial levels are always higher than umbilical venous samples so the source of epinephrine is fetal, not maternal. Other experiments demonstrated

Table 3.2 *Pooled data from fetal sheep undergoing labor and delivery to demonstrate the timing of the onset of lung liquid absorption and the rise in fetal plasma catecholamines*

	Minutes before delivery			Minutes after delivery
	900–150	150–50	50–0	0–50
J_v (ml/h)	7.1	−2.2	−15.2	−28.7
Epinephrine (ng/ml)	0.09	0.52	6.82	7.17
Norepinephrine (ng/ml)	1.71	3.81	12.14	9.10

J_v is secretion or absorption rate, the latter indicated by a negative sign. Time zero is time of delivery. Data adapted from Brown et al.[15]

that the effect of epinephrine was mediated through β-adrenergic receptors since α-adrenergic agents had only a small effect on lung liquid secretion and the effect of epinephrine could be blocked by propranolol.[71]

The mature fetal lung is very sensitive to epinephrine and blood concentrations required to just stop secretion in the sheep fetus are very low, indeed so low that similar values are difficult to achieve in postnatal life. Concentrations of epinephrine and norepinephrine have been measured in samples of scalp blood in babies undergoing normal labor and in cord blood of those born by cesarean section (Table 3.3).[43,44] Catecholamines seem to rise earlier in humans than in sheep and even in early labor epinephrine concentrations are in excess of those required to stop secretion in fetal sheep and would be sufficient to cause rapid lung liquid absorption. The different shapes of the fetuses in the two species and differences in their presenting parts may explain the difference in timing. Lambs 'dive' out, feet first, and the widest diameter presented to the birth canal is the shoulder width. In humans, the head is the widest part and engages early. Consequently, epinephrine concentrations in human fetuses are much higher and high levels are present for longer than in sheep, suggesting that infants should have cleared their lung lumens of liquid well before they take their first breath. Infants born by cesarean section can have high epinephrine concentrations in cord blood also, but it should be noted that in elective cesarean sections, the epinephrine concentration has been elevated probably for only a brief time, a minute or two – insufficient time for the epinephrine to have had a chance to clear much liquid from the lung lumen. It is known that infants born by elective cesarean section have a higher incidence of lung disease, including transient tachypnea, than those born vaginally or by emergency cesarean section[30] (p. 273) and that lung function measurements in the first few hours after birth correlate with route of delivery and with catecholamine concentration. Generally, the more exposure to labor and the higher the catecholamines, the better the lung function.[31]

Table 3.3 *Catecholamine concentrations in human fetal blood during and after birth*

	Epinephrine (ng/ml)	Norepinephrine (ng/ml)
Cervix dilation		
3–5 cm	0.37	1.21
6–8 cm	0.49	1.76
9–10 cm	1.03	2.91
Cord (arterial)	1.60	10.56
Breech cord (arterial)	2.57	24.00
12 h postpartum (arterial)	0.41	0.79

In the sheep fetus, the concentration of epinephrine needed to stop lung liquid secretion is only 0.029 ng/ml.[15] Data in the table are derived from Lagercrantz *et al.*[44]

Mechanism of absorption

Amiloride, a diuretic, placed in the fetal lung lumen completely inhibits the action of epinephrine infused into fetuses not undergoing labor (Figure 3.2) and also blocks the absorption of lung liquid at birth.[54,58] Amiloride blocks sodium channels but specifically the epithelial sodium channel (ENaC). Fetal lung liquid absorption induced by epinephrine and labor is mediated by the activation or opening of sodium channels on the apical surface of the pulmonary epithelium (Figure 3.3). Subsequently, ENaC was cloned and final vindication of the proposed mechanism of lung liquid absorption was demonstrated in 'knockout' mice experiments.[40] Mice, bred to be homozygous for the null condition of the gene coding for one of the protein subunits of the channel (the alpha subunit),

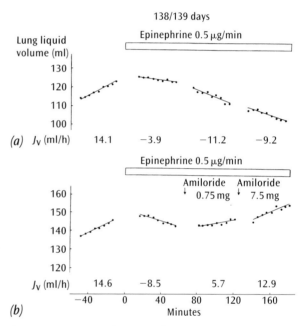

Figure 3.2 *Two experiments performed on consecutive days showing the effect of epinephrine (adrenaline) in producing absorption of lung liquid in a mature fetal lamb and the inhibitory effect of amiloride on the epinephrine action. Lung liquid volume was measured with an impermeant tracer technique and each point is calculated from one sample. The lines are the calculated regression lines and their slopes (J_v) give secretion (positive values) or absorption rates (negative values), which are given below each slope in ml/h. (a) Epinephrine was infused at 0.5 μg/min for 3 hours. Its effect of producing absorption was rapid and increased by the second hour but then stabilized. (b) Epinephrine was infused as on the previous day but amiloride was added to the lung liquid at the times indicated by the arrows to give concentrations of 2×10^{-5} M and 2×10^{-4} M. The latter concentration of amiloride effectively totally blocked the action of epinephrine. From similar experiments the K_I of amiloride in this system was determined to be 4×10^{-6} M. Data from Olver et al.[58]*

all die shortly after birth from respiratory failure. The lungs of these mice remain liquid filled 12 hours after birth (Figure 3.4).

Analogs of cAMP (cyclic adenosine monophosphate) have been shown to have very similar effects to those of epinephrine on fetal lungs, which is not surprising since the intracellular mediator of β-adrenergic receptors is usually cAMP.[72] The latter compound is believed to work through protein kinase A (PKA) and it is noteworthy that ENaC has PKA-binding sites in its sequence and is activated by serine proteases of which PKA is one. Confirming this theoretical sequence for the activation mechanism in the whole lung rather than in cells has not been completed, although the β-adrenergic receptor and cAMP steps seem certain.

It should be stated that the cells responsible for fetal lung liquid secretion have not been identified. Isolated cells used for experiments are usually distal epithelial cells and type II pneumocytes. They are able to absorb sodium and liquid but they seem unable to mimic the secretion seen in the whole fetal lung even when they are of fetal origin. It is not known whether the cells which secrete liquid in the fetus are the same ones which transform into absorptive ones under the action of epinephrine or whether completely different cell types are responsible. It is noteworthy that both the secretory and absorptive processes are driven by Na/K ATPase on the basolateral surface of the epithelial cells.

Maturation of the response to epinephrine: thyroid hormones and cortisol

The response of the fetal lung to epinephrine is very dependent on fetal maturity. Gestation in the sheep is 147 days and epinephrine produces lung liquid absorption only after about 130 days; before that time it only slows secretion and in very immature fetuses (<125 days) it does little to lung liquid formation.[15,71] Many hormones rise or fall over the latter part of gestation but, since it was already known that thyroid hormones and cortisol had maturing effects on lung histology, these hormones were studied first.[66] The concentrations of both hormones

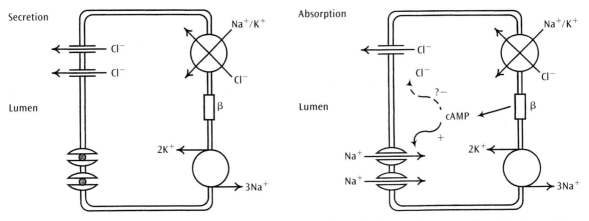

Figure 3.3 *A diagram representing some of the secretory and absorptive mechanisms acting across the epithelium of the lung.* **Secretion** *predominates in the fetus. Chloride ions enter the epithelial cell on the basolateral surface by Na/K:2Cl co-transport which can be inhibited by bumetanide and frusemide. The driving force for entry is the Na^+ gradient generated by Na/K ATPase located on the basolateral surface of the cells. The Cl^- then passes through a Cl^- channel in the apical membrane of the cell down a large electrical gradient. Sodium ions and water follow passively through paracellular routes. The osmotic force underlying secretion is thus the secondary active movement of chloride ions from the interstitium into the lumen.* **Absorption** *predominates in the postnatal, air-breathing lung. At birth epinephrine stimulates β-adrenergic receptors which generate intracellular cAMP which in turn activates Na sodium channels (ENaC) in the apical membrane. cAMP normally produces its effects via protein kinase A, a serine protease which is known to activate ENaC channels. Sodium ions enter the cell through the activated or opened channels down a steep electrochemical gradient and then they are rapidly extruded by Na/K ATPase into the interstitium. Water and other ions follow passively and any remaining Cl^- secretion is presumably overwhelmed. Not shown are other factors which may aid lung liquid absorption. Cyclic AMP is also generated by ADH (arginine vasopressin) acting on V_2 receptors and also by glucagon; the concentration of both these hormones rise in fetal blood during birth. ENaC can be stimulated directly by apical G-proteins and fatty acids. Lung expansion can stimulate ENaC by stretch. Somatostatin might inhibit the chloride channels during birth. Factors whose roles and mechanisms are even less well defined include atrial natriuretic factor, dopamine, serotonin and nitric oxide/cGMP.[19,22,23,25] CNG 1 channels can act as sodium channels but they appear in the lung epithelium in postnatal life. Sodium–glucose co-transport, which is certainly present in the fetal lung, is not shown because its role in the net movement of liquid out of the lung under physiological conditions has not been established.*

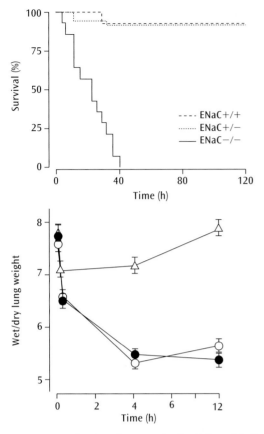

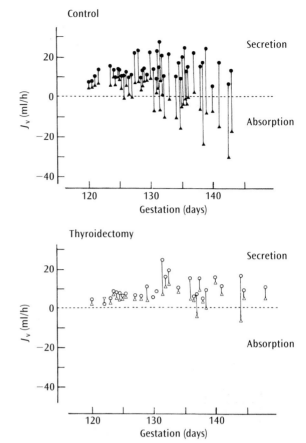

Figure 3.4 *Data showing the central role of the epithelial sodium channel (ENaC) to clearance of lung liquid at birth and to survival. Upper panel: survival of newborn mice born to parents who are heterozygotes for non-functioning ENaC. Offspring with normal ENaC (+/+) and heterozygotes for ENaC (+/−) have normal survival. Those who are homozygous for the non-functioning α-subunit of ENaC (−/−) all die by 40 hours of age. Lower panel: Wet:dry weight ratios of the lungs of a subgroup of a similar population of offspring shown in the upper panel sacrificed at various times after birth. Newborn mice with non-functioning ENaC (triangles) cannot clear their lung liquid and die a respiratory death while those with functioning ENaC, normal (+/+) and heterozygotes (+/−) clear their lungs of liquid normally. Figures from Hummler et al.[40]*

Figure 3.5 *Data showing the effect of fetal thyroidectomy on the development of the response of the fetal lung to infused epinephrine in sheep. Lung liquid secretion or absorption rates obtained from measurement over an hour are plotted on the y-axis; values above the dotted line indicate secretion, values below, absorption. Gestation is on the x-axis: term in sheep is 147 days. Circles are resting secretion rate and triangles the secretion or absorption rate in the presence of a standard infusion of epinephrine (0.5 μg/min) given to each fetus on each occasion. Vertical lines join the pairs of observations from one experiment, i.e. control (resting) secretion rate and the response to epinephrine. Upper panel: normal development of the epinephrine response in a group of fetuses. Note the small effect of epinephrine early in gestation but the universal absorption after about 137 days. Lower panel: thyroidectomy before 120 days of gestation abolishes the development of the response to epinephrine in the latter part of gestation. Other experiments demonstrated that the response to epinephrine would develop in thyroidectomized fetuses if thyroid hormone was infused from shortly after removal of the thyroid gland. Data from experiments described in Barker et al.[5]*

in fetal blood rise in late gestation at the time that the epinephrine effect appears. Thyroidectomy in immature fetuses prevents the fetal lung from developing a response to epinephrine (Figure 3.5) but replacing thyroid hormone by infusions of T4 or T3 in thyroidectomized fetuses allows normal maturation to take place.[5,7] These observations seemed to prove the central role of thyroid hormone in maturing this mechanism. Maturity, however, could not be accelerated by administering thyroid hormone early – indicating that some other factor was controlling the action of T3 on the lung. This factor turned out to be cortisol, which rose towards the end of

gestation from endogenous sources. Both hormones are necessary for maturation of the normal response of the fetal lung to epinephrine (Table 3.4).[8]

The effect of the endogenous hormones, T3 and cortisol, on the fetal lung is reversible in less than 24 hours and

Table 3.4 *The synergistic effect of T3 and cortisol in maturing the epinephrine response on fetal lung liquid*

	116 days		119 days	
	J_{vc}	J_{ve}	J_{vc}	J_{ve}
T3 group	7.2	4.0	9.2	5.9
Cortisol group	6.0	4.8	9.8	5.9
T3 and cortisol	4.6	2.8	6.6	−12.3

All values are ml/min. The negative value indicates absorption. Three sheep fetuses in each of the above groups (9 fetuses in total) were surgically prepared with indwelling catheters early in gestation. At 116 days resting lung liquid secretion rate was measured by the impermeant tracer technique over one hour. Epinephrine was then infused for one hour at 0.5 μg/min and secretion rate measured once more. After the experiment at 116 days, each fetus was infused with one of three possible solutions: (1) T3 at 30 μg/day; (2) cortisol at 10 mg/day; or (3) T3 and cortisol at the same doses together for 3 days. Resting (control) secretion rate (J_{vc}) and secretion rate during epinephrine infusion (J_{ve}) were measured once more. Each value in the table is the mean of 3 experiments (animals). Only when both hormones had been infused together did epinephrine produce absorption of lung liquid, demonstrating the synergistic effect of these two hormones. Data adapted from Barker *et al.*[8]

this is an important point to remember if they are used clinically.[8] Their onset of action is fast. Specific experiments to test the timing exactly showed that infusions of both hormones together (and they are effective only together, that is, their action is synergistic) allowed the epinephrine effect to mature within 2–4 hours, even in extremely immature fetuses (Figure 3.6). Protein synthesis inhibitors can block this maturing action.[8] Analogs of cAMP mimic the epinephrine effect even to the extent of also being absolutely dependent on the maturation of the fetal lung by thyroid hormone and cortisol.[5,72] The latter finding indicates that the hormones, thyroid and cortisol, produce their maturational effect at a rate-limiting point in the epithelial cell which is 'distal' to the production of cAMP and not by any effect on the β-adrenergic receptor. The rate-limiting step could be an expression of ENaC itself and there is evidence for this,[55,68] but it could still be up-regulation of one or more of a multitude of other regulatory proteins involved in ENaC function or activation.

Since thyroid hormones do not cross the placenta to any measurable extent, artificially elevating the blood levels of thyroid hormones in the human fetus is difficult in comparison to treating the fetus with glucocorticoids. Thyrotropin-releasing hormone (TRH) is one intervention that has been used, since it crosses the placenta and increases, at least temporarily, blood levels of fetal thyroid hormones. It must be remembered, however, that the effects of thyroid hormones on the fetal lung are reversible within 24 hours,[8] that the fetus has metabolic pathways to protect itself from elevated thyroid hormone levels,[21,39] and that the fetal hypothalamic/pituitary/thyroid axis may become exhausted by over-stimulation.

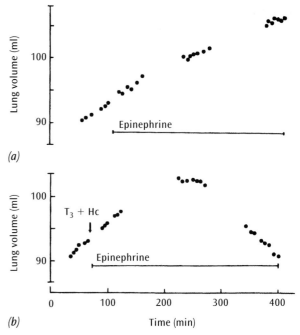

(a)

(b)

Figure 3.6 *Demonstration of the speed of action of triiodothyronine and cortisol in maturing the epinephrine response. Experiments were performed on consecutive days in an immature chronically catheterized sheep fetus of 116/117 days of gestation. Lung liquid volume was determined by the impermeant tracer technique. Each volume point is calculated from one sample and plotted on the y-axis. Experimental time is on the x-axis. Increasing lung liquid volume indicates secretion and declining volume, absorption. Regression lines have not been drawn. Upper panel: an i.v. infusion of epinephrine at 0.5 μg/min for 5 hours had a small effect on resting lung liquid secretion but absorption was not produced. Lower panel: the experiment was repeated on the following day but on this occasion 30 μg of T_3 and 2 mg of cortisol were injected at the start of the epinephrine (adrenaline) infusion. Cortisol was also infused at a rate of 10 mg/day after the initial bolus. Cessation of a liquid secretion occurred during the third hour and absorption began in the fourth hour. The starting secretion rate was about 4 ml/h and the final absorption rate was −5 ml/h. Infusions of epinephrine alone on consecutive days would not produce an enhanced response like this on the second exposure. Administration of T3 or cortisol alone would not have resulted in an absorptive response to epinephrine. Data from Barker et al.[8]*

Some of these possibilities might explain the disappointing, and some claim deleterious, effects seen in some clinical trials of TRH, particularly in babies born 48 hours or more after TRH administration (p. 257).[24]

Infants born prematurely have not been exposed to the maturing effects of slowly rising thyroid hormone and cortisol levels in the latter part of gestation, so their lungs are in no state to respond to epinephrine even if it is secreted in sufficient quantities. Thyroid hormone concentrations in the blood of premature infants are very low, the normal postnatal surge does not occur and blood concentrations remain low for weeks postnatally.[11] Low thyroid hormone levels are correlated with poor clinical outcome, but a causal relationship between thyroid hormone concentrations and respiratory morbidity has not been proven yet.

OXYGEN

From experiments on whole fetal/newborn animals as well as on isolated fetal distal lung epithelial (FDLE) cells, there is no doubt that exposure to postnatal oxygen tensions (tensions greater than 100 mmHg compared to 20 mmHg in the fetus) increases sodium transport across the pulmonary epithelium and also stimulates expression of the α-ENaC subunit.[2,4,62,63] Interestingly, these two effects are temporally dissociated with functional changes in sodium transport occurring before the increases in transcription are observed at 24–48 hours. The transcriptional effects appear to be mediated via NFκB, which has been described in other systems as an oxygen-sensitive regulator of gene expression.[35] The presence of hormones, thyroid and cortisol, to prime the tissue are not essential for the oxygen effect on isolated FDLE cells, but this does not seem to be the case in the whole lung in newborn animals.[2]

Oxygen does not have an effect on transcription rates of the β- and γ-ENaC subunits but they appear not to be necessary for producing effective sodium-conducting channels. Expression of the β- and γ-subunits increases slowly from late in gestation and into postnatal life without birth seeming to affect them, whereas the α-ENaC subunit expression falls following the surge associated with birth.[2]

Birth up-regulates the activity of Na-K ATPase, the sodium pump on the basolateral surface of the epithelium;[12] this may be due to exposure to postnatal oxygen tensions.[12,64] This could explain the increased sodium conductance of FDLE cells after oxygen exposure, but cannot explain on its own the reversal of net liquid movement seen at birth since the crucial and rate-limiting step for absorption of lung liquid is activation of apical sodium channels.

The effect of oxygen on lung liquid absorption obviously occurs too late to prepare the lung for air breathing, but the effect it has on increasing sodium conductance could be of benefit in increasing liquid clearance from the lung lumen in the few hours after birth. Whether the increased amount of ENaC protein present in the lung after birth, on its own, is sufficient to explain the continued and persisting absorption of liquid out of the lumen which characterizes the air-filled lung until death, is a moot point. There are sufficient sodium channels present in the mature

fetal lung to clear all the liquid that is present, but they need to be activated. It is likely, therefore, that intracellular mechanisms which activate the sodium channel permanently need to be present in the postnatal lung in addition to adequate numbers of sodium channels; these mechanisms remain to be discovered. The effect of oxygen on the sodium transport system in the immature lung remains unexplored.

OTHER STIMULI AND MECHANISMS OF ABSORPTION

ADH

ADH or arginine vasopressin rises markedly at delivery, which is not surprising since it is one of the 'stress hormones'. Like β-adrenergic stimulation its intracellular messenger is cAMP and it, too, has been shown to slow fetal lung liquid secretion independently, although its action does not appear to be as strong as that of epinephrine. Its action also is matured by thyroid hormone and cortisol, which suggests a common intracellular pathway for epinephrine and ADH, which is probably the production of intracellular cAMP.[16,18,70]

Stretch

Stretch of the epithelium appears to increase lung liquid absorption in at least three ways. It was shown decades ago that air breathing causes a temporary and seemingly well controlled increase in the permeability of the mature lung epithelium, thus short-circuiting any secretory ion transport. The increase in permeability lasts for about 12 hours, after which there is reversion towards the low permeability that characterizes the fetal lung epithelium.[28] The interaction of this process with sodium absorption is unknown. Stretch of the immature, surfactant-deficient, epithelium merely causes damage and leakage. Stretch, even by liquid in the mature fetal lung, also recruits ENaC to the apical surface of the epithelial cells as shown by the blocking of the absorption induced by stretch by amiloride.[50] Distension of the fetal lung, well within physiological limits, releases a diffusible substance as yet identified which inhibits chloride ion secretion rather than stimulating sodium absorption. It is neither somatostatin (see below) nor a catecholamine.[50,51]

Somatostatin and glucagon

Two other hormones, somatostatin and glucagon, have been shown to affect fetal lung liquid formation in the guinea pig. Somatostatin slows secretion and glucagon can induce absorption. Both hormones rise in concentration in blood at birth, but the development of their responses during gestation has not been studied.[20,61]

Other factors

Modulation of ion transport locally has been described for fatty acids, purinergic agonists and by agents binding directly to G-proteins on the apical surface of epithelial cells.[3,34,63] Factors whose roles and mechanisms are even less well defined include atrial natriuretic factor, dopamine, serotonin and nitric oxide/cGMP (cyclic guanosine monophosphate).[19,22,23,25] The physiological role of these mechanisms in lung liquid movement, if any, during fetal life or at birth has not been defined.

POSTNATAL MATURATION

The postnatal lung is capable of absorbing large amounts of sodium and liquid throughout life if they are presented to it.[9,45,65] Normally there is obviously little net movement of liquid across the postnatal pulmonary epithelium, but this mechanism, which develops in late gestation and is activated during labor, is essential for maintaining the relatively liquid-free lung lumen necessary for normal breathing. The volume of postnatal lung liquid is about 0.34 ml/kg body weight, which is one-hundredth of that in the fetus. It is spread very thinly over the internal surface of the lung and has an average thickness of only 0.15 μm. In an average adult human, its volume is only about 20–25 ml in total.[67] In adult animals the absorptive mechanism can continue to remove liquid until it concentrates protein in the lumen of the lung to generate an oncotic pressure of at least 100 cmH$_2$O resisting absorption.[45] How the tiny volume of postnatal lung liquid is produced and maintained in spite of this force is unknown.

It would be wrong to assume that lung physiological development ceases at birth. Although the sensitivity of the lung epithelium to epinephrine increases to a maximum at the end of gestation in sheep, after birth the sensitivity wanes. In neonatal lambs, epinephrine is able to increase the ability of the lung to absorb liquid above the normal resting rate, but with increasing postnatal age epinephrine has a declining effect. Equally, amiloride, which in neonatal lambs produces secretion of lung liquid, even in animals that have been breathing air for up to 2 weeks, has less effect with age, so that after 6 weeks of age it cannot block lung liquid absorption.[65] This change may be explained by the appearance of another channel, examined so far in sheep and in rats, which allows the passage of sodium. It is a cyclic nucleotide gated channel (probably CNG1), which is a non-selective cation channel.[41,42] Thus, in mature adult lungs both

ENaC and CNG1 channels are present simultaneously and both channels need to be blocked to prevent absorption of liquid from the lungs. Little work has been done on CNG1 in humans, but it is present in human airway epithelium (personal observation, E Baker). Its functional importance and postnatal ontogeny have not been properly defined yet.

Some experiments have indicated that chloride ion movement through CFTR is involved in absorbing liquid from the postnatal lung lumen in lung edema, but interestingly only that fraction which is stimulated by β-adrenergic agents.[29] How this mechanism interacts with lung liquid sodium absorption and whether it changes with development are unknown.

The results that underlie what has been described above have come from a variety of experiments on whole animals (including humans), isolated organs, isolated cells, primary cell cultures, immortal cell lines, membrane vesicles and molecular biological analyses. Extrapolating results from one to the other should be done cautiously. The ultimate test is whether postulated mechanisms hold in whole animals where tissues and systems are fully integrated.

REFERENCES

1 Adamson, T.M., Boyd, R.D.H., Platt, H.S., Strang, L.B. (1969) Composition of alveolar liquid in the fetal lamb. *Journal of Physiology* 204, 159–168.
2 Baines, D.L., Folkesson, H.G., Norlin, A. *et al.* (2000) The influence of mode of delivery, hormonal status and postnatal O$_2$ environment on epithelial sodium channel (EnaC) expression in perinatal guinea-pig lung. *Journal of Physiology* 522, 147–157.
3 Baines, D.L., MacGregor, G.G., Kemp, P.J. (2001) Fatty acid modulation and sequence identity of fetal guinea pig alveolar type II cell amiloride-sensitive Na+ channel. *Biochemical and Biophysical Research Communications* 288, 727–735.
4 Baines, D.L., Ramminger, S.J., Collett, A. *et al.* (2001) Oxygen-evoked Na+ transport in rat fetal distal lung epithelial cells. *Journal of Physiology* 532, 105–113.
5 Barker, P.M., Brown, M.J., Ramsden, C.A. *et al.* (1988) The effect of thyroidectomy in the fetal sheep on lung liquid reabsorption induced by adrenaline or cyclic AMP. *Journal of Physiology* 407, 373–383.
6 Barker, P.M., Boyd, C.A.R., Ramsden, C.A. *et al.* (1989) Pulmonary glucose transport in the fetal sheep. *Journal of Physiology* 409, 15–27.
7 Barker, P.M., Strang, L.B., Walters, D.V. (1990) The role of thyroid hormones in maturation of the adrenaline-sensitive lung liquid reabsorptive mechanism in fetal sheep. *Journal of Physiology* 422, 473–485.
8 Barker, P.M., Walters, D.V., Markiewicz, M., Strang, L.B. (1991) Development of the lung liquid reabsorptive mechanism in fetal sheep: synergism of triiodothyronine and hydrocortisone. *Journal of Physiology* 433, 435–449.
9 Basset, G., Crone, C., Saumon, G. (1987) Significance of active ion transport in transalveolar water absorption: a study in isolated rat lung. *Journal of Physiology* 384, 311–324.

10 Basset, G., Crone, C., Saumon, G. (1987) Fluid absorption by rat lung in situ: pathways for sodium entry in the luminal membrane of alveolar epithelium. *Journal of Physiology* **384**, 325–345.

11 Biswas, S., Buffery, J., Enoch. H. *et al.* (2002) A longitudinal assessment of thyroid hormone concentrations in preterm infants less than 30 weeks gestation during the first two weeks of life and their relationship to outcome. *Pediatrics* **109**, 222–227.

12 Bland, R.D., Boyd, C.A.R. (1986) Cation transport in lung epithelial cells derived from fetal, newborn and adult rabbits. *Journal of Applied Physiology* **61**, 507–515.

13 Bland, R.D., McMillan, D.D., Bressack, M.A., Dong, L. (1980) Clearance of liquid from the lungs of newborn rabbits. *Journal of Applied Physiology* **49**, 171–177.

14 Bland, R.D., Hansen T.N., Haberkern C.N. *et al.* (1982) Lung fluid balance in lambs before and after birth. *Journal of Applied Physiology* **53**, 992–1004.

15 Brown, M.J., Olver, R.E., Ramsden, C.A. *et al.* (1983) Effects of adrenaline and of spontaneous labour on the secretion and absorption of lung liquid in the fetal lamb. *Journal of Physiology* **344**, 137–152.

16 Cassin, S., Perks, A.M. (1993) Amiloride inhibits arginine vasopressin-induced decrease in fetal lung liquid secretion. *Journal of Applied Physiology* **75**, 1925–1929.

17 Cassin, S., Gausse, G., Perks, A.M. (1986) The effects of bumetanide and furosemide in lung liquid secretion in fetal sheep. *Proceedings of the Society of Experimental Biology and Medicine* **181**, 427–431.

18 Cassin, S., DeMarco, V., Perks, A.M. *et al.* (1994) Regulation of lung liquid secretion in immature fetal sheep: hormonal interaction. *Journal of Applied Physiology* **77**, 1445–1450.

19 Castro, R., Ervin, M.G., Ross, M.G. *et al.* (1989) Ovine fetal lung liquid response to atrial natriuretic factor. *Journal of Obstetrics and Gynecology* **161**, 1337–1343.

20 Choo, N., Liu, A.L., Perks, A.M. (2000) Effects of glucagon on in vitro liquid production by lungs from fetal guinea pigs. *Archives of Diseases of Childhood (Fetal Neonatal edition)* **83**, F28–F34.

21 Chopra, I.J., Solomon, D.H., Chopra, U. *et al.* (1978) Pathways of metabolism of thyroid hormones. *Recent Progress in Hormone Research* **34**, 521–567.

22 Chua, B.A., Perks, A.M. (1998) The effect of dopamine on lung liquid production by *in vitro* lungs from fetal guinea pigs. *Journal of Physiology* **513**, 283–294.

23 Chua, B.A., Perks, A.M. (1999) The pulmonary neuroendocrine system and drainage of the fetal lung: effects of serotonin. *General and Comparative Endocrinology* **113**, 374–387.

24 Crowther, C.A., Alfirevic, Z., Haslam, R.R. (2000) Prenatal thyrotropin-releasing hormone for preterm birth. *Cochrane Database Systematic Reviews* CD000019.

25 Cummings, J.J. (1997) Nitric oxide decreases lung liquid production in fetal lambs. *Journal of Applied Physiology* **83**, 1538–1544.

26 Davey, M.G., Hooper, S.B., Cock, M.L., Harding, R. (2001) Stimulation of lung growth in fetuses with lung hypoplasia leads to altered postnatal lung structure in sheep. *Pediatric Pulmonology* **32**, 267–276.

27 Dickson, K.A., Maloney, J.E., Berger, P.J. (1987) State-related changes in lung liquid secretion and tracheal flow rate in fetal lambs. *Journal of Applied Physiology* **62**, 34–38.

28 Egan, E.A., Olver, R.E., Strang, L.B. (1975) Changes in non-electrolyte permeability of alveoli and the absorption of lung liquid at the start of breathing in the lamb. *Journal of Physiology* **244**, 161–179.

29 Fang, X., Fukuda, N., Barbry, P., Sartori, C., Verkman, A.S., Matthay, M.A. (2002) Novel role for CFTR in fluid absorption from the distal airspaces of the lung. *Journal of General Physiology* **119**, 199–207.

30 Faxelius, G., Bremme, K., Largercrantz, H. (1982) An old problem revisited – hyaline membrane disease and caesarean section. *European Journal of Pediatrics* **139**, 121–124.

31 Faxelius, G., Hagnevik, K., Lagercrantz, H. *et al.* (1983) Catecholamine surge and lung function after delivery. *Archives of Diseases of Childhood* **58**, 262–266.

32 Fewell, J.E., Hislop, A.A., Kitterman, J.A., Johnson, P. (1983) Effect of tracheostomy on lung development in fetal lambs. *Journal of Applied Physiology* **55**, 1103–1108.

33 Fisk, N.M., Parkes, M.J., Moore, P.J. *et al.* (1992) Mimicking low amniotic pressure by chronic pharyngeal drainage does not impair lung development in fetal sheep. *American Journal of Obstetrics and Gynaecology* **166**, 991–996.

34 Gambling, L., Olver, R.E., Baines, D.L. (1999) Perinatal PTX-sensitive G-protein expression and regulation of conductive 22 Na^+ transport in lung apical membrane vesicles. *Biochimica et Biophysica Acta* **1450**, 468–479.

35 Haddad, J.J., Collett, A., Land S.C., *et al.* (2001) NF-κB blockade reduces the O_2-evoked rise in Na^+ conductance in fetal cells. *Biochemical and Biophysics Research Communications* **281**, 987–992.

36 Harding, R. (1994) Fetal breathing: relation to postnatal breathing and lung development. In Hanson M.A., Spencer J.A.D., Rodeck C.H., Walters, D.V.W. (eds), *Fetus and Neonate, Physiology and Clinical Applications. Vol. 2 Breathing*. Cambridge: Cambridge University Press, 63–84.

37 Harding, R., Bocking, S., Sigger J.N. (1986) Influence of upper respiratory tract on liquid flow to and from fetal lungs. *Journal of Applied Physiology* **61**, 68–74.

38 Harding, R., Bocking, S., Sigger, J.N. (1986) Upper airway resistances in fetal sheep: the influence of breathing activity. *Journal of Applied Physiology* **60**, 160–165.

39 Hume, R., Richard, K., Kaptein, E. *et al.* (2001) Thyroid hormone metabolism and the developing human lung. *Biology of the Neonate* **80** (Suppl 1), 18–21.

40 Hummler, E., Barker, P., Gatzy, J. *et al.* (1996) Early death due to defective neonatal lung liquid clearance in α-ENaC-deficient mice. *Nature Genetics* **12**, 325–328.

41 Junor, R.W.J., Benjamin, A., Alexandrou, D., Gruggino, S., Walters, D.V. (1999) A novel role for cyclic nucleotide gated channels in lung liquid homeostasis in sheep. *Journal of Physiology* **520**, 255–260.

42 Kemp, P.J., Kim, K.J., Borok, Z., Crandell, E.D. (2001) Re-evaluating the Na conductance of adult rat alveolar type II pneumocytes: evidence for the involvement of cGMP-activated cation channels. *Journal of Physiology* **536**, 693–701.

43 Lagercrantz, H., Bistoletti, P. (1977) Catecholamine release in the newborn infant at birth. *Pediatric Research* **8**, 889–989.

44 Lagercrantz, H., Bistoletti, P., Nylund, L. (1983) Sympathoadrenal activity in the fetus during delivery and birth. In Stern, L. (ed.), *Intensive Care of the Newborn 3*. New York: Mason Press, 1–12.

45 Matthay, M.A., Landolt, C.C., Staub, C.C. (1982) Differential liquid and protein clearance from the alveoli of anesthetized sheep. *Journal of Applied Physiology (Respirat. Environ. Exercise Physiology)* **53**, 96–104.

46 Meguer, J., King, L., Philips, B., Baker, E. (2001) Factors affecting glucose concentrations in human nasal secretions. *European Respiratory Journal* **18**, 366s.

47 Miserocchi, G., Poskurica, B.H., del Fabbro, M. (1994) Pulmonary interstitial pressure in anesthetized paralyzed

new-born rabbits. *Journal of Applied Physiology* **77**, 2260–2268.

48 Moessinger, A.C., Harding, R.D., Adamson, T.M. *et al.* (1990) Role of lung liquid volume in growth and maturation of the fetal sheep lung. *Journal of Clinical Investigation* **86**, 1270–1277.

49 Neilson, D. (1986) Electrolyte composition of pulmonary alveolar subphase in anaesthetized rabbits. *Journal of Applied Physiology* **60**, 972–979.

50 Nelson, P.G., Perks, A.M. (1996) Effects of lung expansion on lung liquid production *in vitro* by lungs from fetal guinea pigs. I Basic studies and the effects of amiloride and propranolol. *Reproduction, Fertility and Development* **8**, 335–346.

51 Nelson, P.G., Perks, A.M. (1996) Effects of lung expansion on lung liquid production *in vitro* by lungs from fetal guinea pigs. II Evidence for an inhibitory factor. *Reproduction, Fertility and Development* **8**, 347–354.

52 Normand, I.C.S., Reynolds, E.O., Strang, L.B. (1970) Passage of macromolecules between alveolar and interstitial spaces in foetal and newly ventilated lungs of the lamb. *Journal of Physiology* **210**, 151–164.

53 Normand, I.C.S., Olver, R.E., Reynolds, E.O.R. *et al.* (1971) Permeability of lung capillaries and alveoli to non-electrolytes in the fetal lamb. *Journal of Physiology* **219**, 303–330.

54 O'Brodovich, H., Hannam, V., Seear, M., Mullen, J.B. (1990) Amiloride impairs lung water clearance in newborn guinea pigs. *Journal of Applied Physiology* **68**, 1758–1762.

55 O'Brodovich, H., Canessa, C., Ueda, J. *et al.* (1993) Expression of the Na channel in the developing rat lung. *American Journal of Physiology* **265**, 491–496.

56 Olver, R.E., Strang, L.B. (1974) Ion flux across the pulmonary epithelium and the secretion of lung liquid in the fetal lamb. *Journal of Physiology* **241**, 327–357.

57 Olver, R.E., Schneeberger, E.E., Walters, D.V. (1981) Epithelial solute permeability, ion transport and tight junction morphology in the developing lung of the fetal lamb. *Journal of Physiology* **315**, 395–412.

58 Olver, R.E., Ramsden, C.A., Strang, L.B., Walters, D.V. (1986) The role of amiloride blockable sodium transport in adrenaline induced lung liquid reabsorption in the fetal lamb. *Journal of Physiology.* **376**, 321–340.

59 O'Toole, S.J., Sharma, A., Karamanoukian H.L. *et al.* (1996) Tracheal ligation does not correct the surfactant deficiency associated with congenital diaphragmatic hernia. *Journal of Pediatric Surgery* **31**, 545–550.

60 O'Toole, S.J., Karamanoukian, H.L., Morin III, F.C. *et al.* (1997) Surfactant decreases pulmonary vascular resistance and increases pulmonary blood flow in the fetal lamb model

of congenital diaphragmatic hernia. *Journal of Paediatric Surgery* **31**, 507–511.

61 Perks, A.M., Kwok, Y.N., McIntosh, C.H.S. *et al.* (1992) Changes in somatostatin-like immunoreactivity in lungs from perinatal guinea pigs, and the effects of somatostatin-14 on lung liquid production. *Journal of Developmental Physiology* **18**, 151–159.

62 Pitkanen, O., Tanswell, A.K., Downey, G., O'Brodovich, H. (1996) Increased PO_2 alters the bioelectric properties of fetal distal lung epithelium. *American Journal of Physiology* **270**, L1060–L1066.

63 Ramminger, S.J., Collett, A., Baines, D.L. *et al.* (1999) P2Y2 receptor-mediated inhibition of ion transport in distal lung epithelial cells. *British Journal of Pharmacology* **128**, 293–300.

64 Ramminger, S.J., Baines, D.L., Olver, R.E., Wilson, S.M. (2000) The effects of PO_2 upon transepithelial ion transport in fetal rat distal lung epithelial cells. *Journal of Physiology* **524**, 539–547.

65 Ramsden, C.A., Markiewicz, M., Walters, D.V. *et al.* (1992) Liquid flow across the epithelium of the artificially perfused lung of fetal and postnatal sheep. *Journal of Physiology* **448**, 579–597.

66 Smith, B.T., Sabry, K. (1983) Glucocorticoid-thyroid synergism in lung maturation: a mechanism involving epithelial–mesenchymal interaction. *Proceedings of the National Academy of Science of the United States of America* **80**, 1951–1954.

67 Stephens, R.H., Benjamin, A.R., Walters, D.V. (1996) Volume and protein concentration of epithelial lining liquid in perfused *in situ* postnatal sheep lungs. *Journal of Physiology* **80**, 1911–1920.

68 Tchepichev, S., Ueda, J., Canessa, C. *et al.* (1995) Lung epithelial Na channel subunits are differentially regulated during development and by steroids. *American Journal of Physiology* **269**, 805–812.

69 Thom, J., Perks, A.M. (1990) The effects of furosemide and bumetanide on lung liquid production by *in vitro* lungs from fetal guinea pigs. *Canadian Journal of Physiology, Pharmacology* **68**, 1131–1135.

70 Wallace, M.J., Hooper, S.B., Harding, R. (1990) Regulation of lung liquid secretion by arginine vasopressin in fetal sheep. *American Journal of Physiology* **258**, R104–R111.

71 Walters, D.V., Olver, R.E. (1978) The role of catecholamines in lung liquid absorption at birth. *Pediatric Research* **12**, 239–242.

72 Walters, D.V., Ramsden, C.A., Olver, R.E. (1990) Dibutyryl cAMP induces a gestation-dependent absorption of fetal lung liquid. *Journal of Applied Physiology* **68**, 2054–2059.

4

Control of breathing

ANTHONY D MILNER, HUGO LAGERCRANTZ AND RONNY WICKSTROM

The first observation that the respiratory rhythm is generated in the brainstem was made by Galen, who observed that gladiators injured below the neck continued to breathe. The existence of a 'noeud vitale' in the medulla was proposed by Flourens in 1840. The conventional view on the control of respiration is that a respiratory rhythm is generated in a respiratory center in the brainstem and driven by carbon dioxide (CO_2) and hypoxia. This view is not entirely correct, particularly not in the fetus and the neonate. Although there is a respiratory rhythm generator in the medulla, respiration is governed by a number of regulating mechanisms hierarchically arranged to generate respiratory activity and the magnitude and pattern of breathing movements in accordance with metabolic and other demands.[100]

Fetal breathing movements are driven by activity in the reticular system during rapid eye movement (REM) sleep rather than by CO_2.[20] Hypoxia inhibits breathing both in the fetus and the preterm infant. Sucking, babbling, talking and singing override the CO_2 drive, the autonomic respiratory rhythm generator and pulmonary reflexes. Although the respiratory rhythm generator is essential, the magnitude of breathing is mainly controlled by behavior during the awake state and by the reticular firing during REM sleep. Thus only during quiet sleep is respiration regular and mainly determined by the CO_2 drive.

The respiratory rhythm generator
(Figure 4.1)

A number of neurons in the cortex, amygdala and cerebellum can fire in phase with respiratory movements. Only one structure, however, can generate a respiratory rhythm *in vitro*: the so-called pre-Bötzinger complex. Bilateral destruction of this cell structure results in an ataxic

breathing pattern with markedly altered blood gases and pH, and pathological responses to challenges such as hyperoxia, hypoxia and anesthesia.[37] This loose complex of respiratory neurons lies within the ventrolateral region

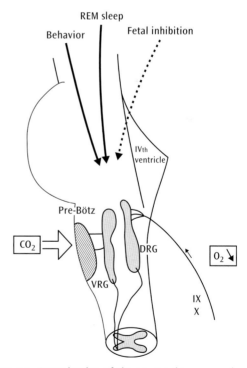

Figure 4.1 *Organization of the neuronal groups and drive mechanisms controlling respiration. The CO_2 drive is mediated by the central chemoreceptive area at the ventral surface. The hypoxic drive is mediated via the cranial nerves IX and X, which terminate at the dorsal respiratory group (DRG). The respiratory rhythm generator is assumed to be generated in the pre-Bötzinger complex (Pre-Bötz) of the ventral respiratory group (VRG).*

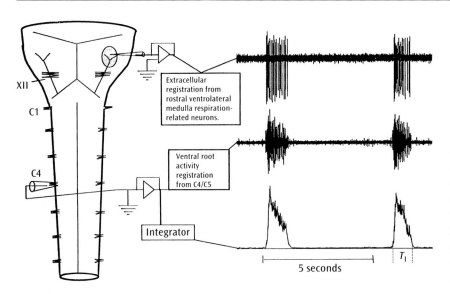

Figure 4.2 *Brainstem–spinal cord preparation. Respiratory activity can be recorded from the C4/C5 ventral roots and respiration-related activity from respiratory-related neurons in an en bloc brainstem–spinal cord preparation. (From the academic thesis by Eric Herlenius, 1999.)*

of the brainstem just caudal to the retrofacial nucleus and is localized above the Bötzinger complex, where the respiratory rhythm was first assumed to be generated. (Bötzinger refers to a Rhine wine, which was consumed at a respiratory meeting when these structures were discussed in German!) This respiratory activity can be recorded in isolated *en bloc* brainstem–spinal cord preparations or even in brain slices.[84] Respiratory activity can be monitored at C4/C5 ventral roots, and respiration-related activity in the ventrolateral medulla (VLM) using extracellular, conventional whole-cell or perforated patch clamp methods (Figure 4.2).

The respiratory rhythm has been assumed to be generated by pacemaker cells resembling those in the heart. There is a class of glutaminergic neurons within the pre-Bötzinger complex, which can generate this activity. Glutamate seems to be essential for sharpening the central pattern generator acting via α-amino-3-hydroxyl-5-methyl-4-isoxazole-proprionate (AMPA) and *N*-methyl-D-aspartate (NMDA) receptors. There are also subpopulations of neurons expressing opioid and substance P receptors in these structures.[36] Substance P is one of the most abundant neuropeptides in the respiratory kernels and it has been found to stimulate breathing.[103]

The respiratory rhythm oscillates in three neural phases: inspiration, post-inspiration and expiration.[84] The respiratory rhythm generator also produces sighs and gasps. All these three patterns may involve the same neural circuits. If slices are deprived of oxygen, the eupneic and sighing patterns are abolished and gasping triggered. Thus sighing and gasping can be produced by simply altering the cellular environment of the pre-Bötzinger complex *in vitro* and presumably also *in vivo*.[27]

Fetal breathing movements

A slow respiratory rhythm is present already at the E16 level of development in the rat and inhibition of this

activity by pontine structures evident at E18. The respiratory pattern recorded in the isolated brainstem becomes more regular during development, but there is no major change at birth.[48] Although the respiratory neural network is relatively mature at birth compared with many other neural systems,[84] the respiratory pattern is very irregular, probably due to incomplete neuronal interconnection and integration of signals. The membrane potential, however, is lower in neonatal preparations due to lower expression of persistent K$^+$ channels.

Fetal breathing movements have been studied extensively in the fetal sheep. These movements can be detected at an early stage. In the beginning they are irregular but continuous. Closer to birth, breathing becomes interrupted by prolonged apnea. This seems to be related to the maturation of the brain and the development of sleep states. Thus fetal breathing movements occur mainly during electrocortical low-voltage activity (active sleep) and not during high voltage (quiet sleep). During these apneic periods it is difficult to elicit breathing movements even by pinching the fetal lamb. This suggests that there is an active inhibition of fetal breathing movements. If the brainstem is transected at a mid-collicular level, breathing movements become continuous.[20]

Fetal breathing movements are probably also suppressed by humoral factors including endogenous opioids,[72] prostaglandins and adenosine. Prostaglandin antagonists, for example, indomethacin, produce continuous fetal breathing[87] and adenosine eliminates REM sleep and fetal breathing movements.[58] Adenosine is a metabolite of adenosine triphosphate (ATP) and its levels are increased during hypoxia. Adenosine also acts as an inhibitory neuromodulator, decreasing neural activity including respiratory neurons.[48] This effect is more pronounced during the pre- and perinatal periods in brainstem preparations from rat[58] and suggests that adenosine inhibits the fetal respiratory drive tonically via A1-receptors.

Fetal breathing can be stimulated by CO_2 only during active sleep (low-voltage electrocorticogram) while the

CO_2 has no effect on apnea during quiet sleep (high voltage). Hypoxia inhibits fetal breathing. This hypoxic inhibition of fetal breathing can be removed by mid-collicular transection of the brainstem of the fetal sheep.[20] Attempts to exactly localize the area from where this inhibition originates have been unsuccessful, but there is some suggestion that it may originate from the nucleus ruber.

Transition at birth (p. 59)

During parturition fetal breathing movements seem to be completely inhibited, although gasps may occur. Meconium, however, is usually not aspirated until after birth (Chapter 23), which explains why vigorous suction of the infant when the head is in the vulva seems to be effective. Only during severe asphyxia may gasps be triggered, leading to severe meconium aspiration.

Respiratory control after birth

THE FOREBRAIN DRIVE

There is a parallel voluntary and autonomic control of respiration particularly in the human. Stimulation of the primary motor cortex excites diaphragm activity and this neuronal pathway has been found to be oligosynaptic and fast-conducting.[32] Walking can produce an increased respiratory activity before changes of blood gases are found.[100] During sucking, breathing receives lower priority.[100] It is possible that the increasing voluntary control and development of babbling and speaking may suppress the more automatic breathing of the infant. This may be one reason why 2–4 months is a critical period with regard to the sudden infant death syndrome.

The breathing pattern during the awake state is fairly irregular and influenced by sensory input. If an infant is exposed to harmonic music, for example Mozart or Chopin, the breathing pattern looks more regular than if the infant listens to the more disharmonic music of Stravinsky.[60]

The forebrain drive seems to be nearly sufficient to maintain the $PaCO_2$ within normal limits. This is demonstrated in children with congenital hypoventilation syndrome (Ondine's curse), who completely lack a CO_2 drive and yet have normal blood gases when awake or in REM sleep.[35]

THE CO$_2$ DRIVE

The neural mechanisms regulating breathing receive continuous and rapid feedback from the partial pressure of CO_2 (PCO_2), as well as pH, in the blood. This feedback is believed to originate mainly from central chemoreceptors in the brainstem. Since the PCO_2 value represents a balance between the metabolic production of CO_2 by body tissues and the amount of ventilation of the alveolar space, the CO_2-sensitive chemoreceptors ensure that the alveolar ventilation is adequate to match the metabolism.

Even small changes in cerebrospinal fluid (CSF) pH alter respiration in the adult animal, producing a linear inverse relationship between CSF pH and alveolar ventilation.[28] This is in contrast to the relationship between the partial pressure of oxygen (PO_2) and ventilation, as changes in PO_2 above 70 mmHg (still keeping saturation high) only have minor effects on respiration. Hence, in contrast to PO_2, which is not an important chemical signal for respiratory control until it reaches levels associated with desaturation, PCO_2 provides key feedback for the control of normal breathing.

The response to inhalation of CO_2 is already present on the day after birth in rats and, during the first postnatal week, there is even a tendency to a decreased CO_2 response (R Wickström et al., unpublished observations). Thereafter, the ventilatory response increases due to increased tidal volumes. In older animals, hypercapnia appears to also increase the respiratory frequency.[1,4,7] It is thus apparent that, although present in the newborn rat, the sensitivity to CO_2 undergoes maturation in the postnatal period, leading to an increased ventilatory response. This maturation appears to have two phases, the first taking place during the second week in the newborn rat and being secondary to increased tidal volumes. This increase can also be due to a maturation of respiratory muscles, and/or a stiffer chest wall, rather than reflecting a change in CO_2 sensitivity per se. The second phase of maturation occurs during the third postnatal week in the rat and is entirely due to increased respiratory frequency in response to CO_2. Apart from signalling in response to changes in CO_2/pH, the central chemoreceptors also provide a tonic drive to the system that may be of importance for a regular breathing pattern.

THE CENTRAL CHEMORECEPTORS

The nature and function of the central chemoreceptors has recently been reviewed.[73] The exact nature of these chemoreceptors, however, remains unknown. Consequently, studying the development of these neurons has proved difficult due to the lack of definition of a structured organization of the chemosensory system at a cellular level. Using the expression of the immediate early gene c-fos, or its protein product Fos, as a marker of neuronal activation has, however, been useful in the study of these neurons. It appears that the main areas activated by hypercapnia in the adult rat, are also activated in the newborn[6] (R Wickström et al., unpublished observations). Some structures, such as the locus ceruleus of the pons, however, do not display c-fos expression in the newborn rat. Whether this truly reflects an absence of activation or that these neurons are activated without c-fos expression remains to be studied. It should also be noted that this method only identifies activated neurons and that inhibited neurons cannot be identified by c-fos expression. Hence, studies so far provide no definite information on the location at which the maturation of the CO_2

response occurs, but it may be speculated that areas that are activated in the adult rat are responsible for the increase in ventilatory frequency seen in older animals. This kind of geographical specificity among chemosensitive neurons has been proposed as one possible answer to the question as to why there is such a widespread distribution of chemosensitive neurons.[73]

As it is not known if CO_2 sensitivity represents either an intrinsic cell membrane property, an effect on synaptic transmission or cell pH regulation, it is difficult to study the mechanism underlying the maturation of the ventilatory response on a cellular level. *In vitro* studies in several of the chemosensitive areas of the brainstem of the adult rat have shown depolarization as a result of hypercapnia. This effect has been attributed to an intrinsic membrane property, possibly involving a potassium channel. Other types of H^--sensitive membrane channels are also putative mediators of this response. The development of these in the newborn period, as well as their effect on respiration, remains to be studied. Two neurotransmitter systems, acetylcholine and glutamate, have also been studied in relation to respiration, and both systems display a correlation to CO_2 sensitivity. It cannot be concluded, however, that this effect is indeed on chemosensitive neurons as they may also be synaptically

connected neurons affecting the chemosensitive neurons. Recent findings also indicate that ATP may mediate the CO_2 response, as it is blocked by ionophoretic application of purinergic P_2 receptor antagonists.[96] Thus, all these hypotheses concerning the mechanism of chemoreception are tenable and can also possibly differ between chemoreceptor locations. Studies of the mechanism underlying the maturation of the CO_2 response will be greatly facilitated when there has been further identification of CO_2-sensitive neurons.

THE PERIPHERAL CHEMORECEPTOR DRIVE

The peripheral chemoreceptors were earlier believed to be silent in the fetus and then activated at birth, playing a major role for the onset of air breathing. This idea, however, was rejected when it was found that carotid-denervated fetal sheep did not start to breathe later than sham-operated controls. In fact, the peripheral chemoreceptors were found to be tonically active in the fetal sheep.[8] The threshold to trigger firing of the sinus nerve, however, is set at a lower PO_2 level (Figure 4.3). They are probably adapted to the low PO_2 level *in utero*.

After birth, the peripheral chemoreceptors reset to a higher PO_2 level. This resetting occurs in 2–3 days in the

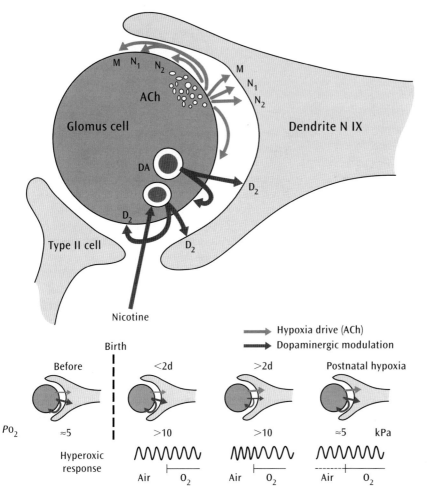

Figure 4.3 *Overview of the peripheral chemoreceptors. Acetylcholine is assumed to excite the sinus nerve (IX), while dopamine has a more modulatory role (modified after Donelly[23]). In the bottom panel the inhibitory effect of dopamine in the fetus and the newborn is demonstrated. This inhibition decreases after birth, but can be retained during postnatal hypoxia. The ventilatory response to hyperoxia is shown below.*

newborn lamb[8] and 1–2 days in the newborn rat.[25] If the rise in PO_2 is prevented by birthing in an environment with a low PO_2 similar to the intrauterine condition, this re-setting does not occur.[24] This resetting occurs also in human babies, which was tested by the so called Dejours test, that is, the infant was allowed to breathe pure oxygen, any decrease of breathing noted being an index of chemoreceptor drive. Newborn infants did not react to the pure oxygen, but after about 2 days, their minute ventilation decreased by about 10 percent.[49] Preterm infants who had chronic lung disease (CLD) were often found not to react to this hyperoxic test, until several weeks of oxygen treatment. Thus their resetting seemed to be delayed, compared with preterm infants without CLD who often responded with an approximately 20 percent decrease in their minute ventilation.[53]

The exact mechanism for this resetting of the peripheral chemoreceptors is not clear, but dopamine seems to play an important role.[23] Dopamine is one of the major neurotransmitters in the carotid bodies, which inhibits the transduction of the hypoxic drive. In the newborn rat the dopamine levels are relatively high in the first hours after birth. The turnover is also high immediately after delivery. Subsequently, the dopamine concentration increases, whereas turnover decreases, suggesting that very little dopamine is released. These changes in dopamine turnover occur at the same period of time as the appearance of the peripheral chemoreceptor reflex (Figure 4.3). Rat pups born and reared in a hypoxic environment for 2 days were found to sustain a low peripheral chemoreceptor response related to a relatively high dopamine turnover in the carotid bodies. Furthermore, infants who have died of the sudden infant death syndrome have sometimes been found to have very high levels of dopamine in their carotid bodies, according to postmortem analyses.

The setting of the sensitivity of the peripheral chemoreceptors may occur during a critical window. Infants born at high altitude in the Andes were found to have a blunted hypoxic ventilatory response as adults.[90]

Mitchell and colleagues have found that rats exposed to hyperoxia during the first month after birth had impaired hypoxic ventilatory responses as adults.[16] Exposure to hypoxia during fetal life causes long-term changes of monoamine turnover in the carotid bodies as well as in monoaminergic nuclei in the brainstem related to respiratory control.[76]

RESPIRATORY CONTROL REFLEXES

The pattern of breathing in the neonatal period is more susceptible to influence from respiratory reflexes than in the older child or adult. These reflexes arise from stretch receptors in the airways, the chest wall or upper airway.

The Hering–Breuer reflexes

In 1868, Hering and Breuer described the results of a series of investigations on dogs and rabbits which, although hardly meeting the demands of the clinical statistician, have stood the test of time.[98] The source of the Hering–Breuer reflexes remains incompletely described. The Hering–Breuer inflation reflex generates from stretch receptors within the airways and has an afferent path lying within the vagi. The receptors for the deflationary reflex appear also to lie within the lungs, as it is generated by reduction in lung volume, as occurs following the creation of a pneumothorax.[98] It is probable that the Hering–Breuer expiratory reflex and Head's paradoxical reflex have a similar origin.

HERING–BREUER INFLATION REFLEX (HBIR)

Hering and Breuer documented that inflation of the lung induced apnea, that is, a cessation of respiratory effort. The reflex has been extensively studied in the neonatal period, where its effect appears more pronounced than in later life.[17] A variety of methods have been used to provoke the reflex; these include lung inflation resulting from the application of continuous positive airways pressure (CPAP)[39] or mechanical ventilation[40] (Figure 4.4). The reflex can also be demonstrated by an increase in the expiratory time following airway occlusion at end inspiration or an increase in the duration of inspiration with

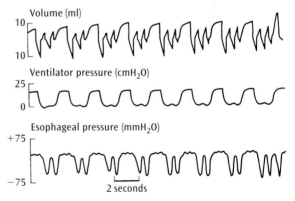

Figure 4.4 *Stimulation of the Hering–Breuer inflation reflex by positive pressure inflation. The figure is read from left to right. In between ventilator inflations the baby breathes well as demonstrated by the narrow negative deflections in the esophageal trace. During each positive pressure inflation there is a temporary inhibition of spontaneous inspiration as evidenced by the esophageal pressure trace remaining at a constant positive value during the ventilator breath. Reprinted from* Early Human Development, **8**, *Greenough, A., Morley, C.J., Davis, J.A., Respiratory reflexes in ventilated premature babies, 65–75, 1983, with permission from Elsevier Science.*

airway occlusion at end expiration. In the latter situation, the inspiratory effort during the occlusion produces no volume change, thus the stretch receptors are not stimulated, hence inspiration is prolonged.

The inflation reflex is increased in patients with non-compliant lungs[38] and those on theophylline.[97] Caffeine therapy, unlike theophylline, led to the fall in the strength of the HB_IR in a group of preterm babies, possibly as a result of increased compliance.[61]

In the newborn period, the reflex can be provoked within the tidal volume range, airway occlusion at end inspiration consistently delaying the onset of the next inspiratory effort by at least 40 percent. It has been claimed that there is an inspiratory volume of approximately 4 ml/kg above functional residual capacity (FRC) which has to be exceeded before activation of the HB_IR occurs and that the strength is greatly increased when occlusion is carried out at the peak of sighs. However, the investigators assumed that the brief apnea after a sigh was due to the HB_IR, rather than changes in arterial blood gases.[78] A more recent study has shown that the reflex is active from the FRC and is maximal after an inspiration of approximately 4 ml/kg above FRC (Figure 4.5).[45]

The claim that the HB_IR leads to a relatively shallow and fast pattern of breathing in the neonatal period has been challenged by Gagliardi and Rusconi,[31] who considered that the established relationship between the strength of the HB_IR and the respiratory rate of newborn infants was biased on the grounds that the HB_IR is normally expressed as a percentage increase in inspiratory time after occlusion. As a result, a stronger HB_IR was inevitable if the respiratory rate was high and inspiratory time short. A recent study, however, has shown that there remains a significant relationship between the strength of the HB_IR and respiratory rate when inspiratory time during occlusion is used rather than percentage increase,[45] as studied by Gagliardi and Rusconi.[31] In older patients,[15,39]

however, the magnitude of inspiration is only shortened if the tidal volume is increased above a certain critical threshold. In cats, the duration and magnitude of lung inflation determines the expiratory time.[57]

The effect of maturation on the strength of the reflex is controversial, although this may reflect the variety of techniques used to provoke the reflex (see above). Some authors[30,95] have suggested that there is no relationship with increasing gestational age, particularly amongst patients with non-compliant lungs.[13] Others[55,74] have reported the reflex to be stronger in the preterm compared to the term infant. Kirkpatrick[55] suggested the reflex decreased more markedly with intrauterine as compared to extrauterine maturation. By contrast, Bodegard et al.[9] found the reflex to be weak in infants up to 28 weeks of gestation, but then to increase in strength up to a peak at 36–38 weeks of gestation. Immediately after birth, postnatal age does not seem to affect the reflex, with no change being reported over the first 4 weeks after birth amongst immature infants with stiff lungs,[13] nor in term infants studied at 2 days and 6 weeks of age.[79] There was apparently a decline in the strength of the reflex by 32 percent over the first year after birth.[80] One study[92] has found that at 15 weeks postnatal age, the decay in the strength of the HB_IR was significantly greater in term than preterm infants. When the preterm infants were studied at 4 months post-term, however, the differences between the two groups disappeared. The reflex can, however, be provoked, if a suitable stimulus is used, in children[39] and adults.[15]

Babies born at high altitude have a modified HB_IR response, with an augmented prolongation of inspiration on occlusion, but reduced effect on expiration. This pattern was associated with a deeper but slower pattern of breathing.[71]

THE HERING–BREUER EXPIRATORY REFLEX

Hering and Breuer also noted that if the animals' lungs were kept inflated, prolonged expiratory muscle contraction was stimulated. This reflex would not seem to have any relevance to tidal respiration, but it may be equivalent to the active expiration which is seen in both term and preterm babies who are receiving ventilatory support with relatively long inspiratory times (Figure 4.6) (p. 156).[40,43]

HERING–BREUER DEFLATION REFLEX

Hering and Breuer noted that if the lung was rapidly deflated, either by attaching the endotracheal tube to a suction source or by creating a pneumothorax, a strong and prolonged inspiratory response was generated. This reflex can also be stimulated by an unusually vigorous expiratory effort causing lung volume to decrease below the end expiratory level. Hering and Breuer considered

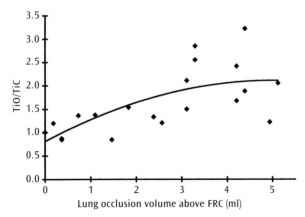

Figure 4.5 *Effect of volume of occlusion on the strength of the Hering–Breuer inflation reflex in a healthy newborn infant. The reflex is maximally stimulated at volumes of 4 ml/kg above FRC.*

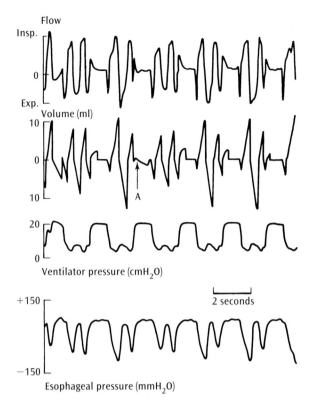

Flow
Insp.
0
Exp.

Volume (ml)
10
0
10
A

Ventilator pressure (cmH$_2$O)
20
0

2 seconds

+150

−150

Esophageal pressure (mmH$_2$O)

Figure 4.6 *The Hering–Breuer expiratory reflex. During each ventilator inflation the infant's spontaneous inspiratory activity is inhibited but, despite positive pressure inflation continuing, the infant is able to halt further gas flow into his chest during the last part of ventilator inflation or, as at point A, can actually cause gas to flow out of his chest. Reprinted from* Early Human Development, 9, Greenough, A., Morley, C.J., Davis, J.A., *Provoked augmented inspirations in ventilated premature infants, 111–117, 1984, with permission from Elsevier Science.*

the reflex might have an important role in the maintenance of the FRC. Recent studies[44,64] have shown it is certainly present in the newborn period, as reduction of lung volume by inflating a jacket with a rigid outer wall surrounding the infant's chest and abdomen produces a rapid and exaggerated inspiratory response (Figure 4.7).[64] The strength of this reflex is increased if the lung volume reduction is rapid, the jacket inflation pressure is raised and if the maneuver is commenced close to FRC rather than end inspiration.[44]

HEAD'S PARADOXICAL REFLEX

Hering and Breuer noted a further reflex response, but it was thought at the time to be an artifact. This response was active inspiration in response to inflation; in humans, this has subsequently been termed 'the inspiratory augmenting reflex' or 'provoked augmented inspiration'. The reflex was defined more extensively by Head,[46]

who noted that when vagal conduction was first blocked, a rapid inflation provoked a stronger and more sustained contraction of the diaphragm. This reflex has an important role in ensuring that infants who require resuscitation and are receiving inadequate inflation pressures, either via a face mask or endotracheal tube, obtain sufficient lung expansion to establish an FRC and overcome their relative asphyxia. It may be the underlying mechanism of the first breath and sighing. This response is also seen during intermittent positive pressure ventilation (Figure 4.8).[41] Its function appears to be to increase lung compliance and reopen partially collapsed alveole in the immediate perinatal period; outside that time period it has rarely been demonstrated.[17,41] An inverse relationship between the sensitivity of the reflex and lung compliance has been demonstrated.[83] The frequency of augmented breaths increases with increasing levels of hypercapnia and particularly hypoxia.[14]

The intercostal phrenic inhibitory reflex

Rapid distortion of the chest wall can result in short inspiratory efforts. This response is usually seen during REM sleep,[56] but is inhibited by an increase in FRC resulting from the application of CPAP. CPAP probably eliminates the reflex by improving chest wall stability.[65] Infants born at term have a prolonged inspiratory response to end expiratory airway occlusion, whereas the premature infants show a less marked response.[33,65] Intrinsic upper airway or imposed external airway obstruction[99] can induce apnea in preterm babies, particularly those having spontaneous apnoeic episodes. It has been postulated that this also represents a reflex response generated by distortion of the rib cage.[10] This has led to the suggestion that mixed apnea is caused by a respiratory effort against an obstructed upper airway, inducing chest wall deformity and hence the central apnea component.[99] This hypothesis is not supported by Riggato's group,[51] who found that airway closure and cessation of respiratory breaths occurred before the onset of respiratory efforts in preterm infants with mixed apnea.

Irritant reflexes

Inhalation of toxic gases can cause a change in the frequency and depth of respiration. The response, however, is variable dependent on the maturity of the patient. The reflex involves small myelinated vagal fibers, which are reduced in number in very premature infants. The fibers arise from subepithelial chemoreceptors located in the trachea, bronchi and bronchioles and are designed to detect delicate insults to the epithelial surface. The receptors are poorly developed in premature infants and their activity abolished in REM sleep.[29]

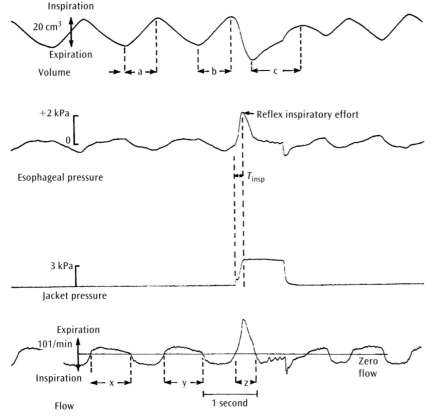

Figure 4.7 *The Hering–Breuer deflation reflex. Trace of tidal volume, esophageal pressure, external compression pressure (jacket pressure) and tidal flow before, during and after compression of the chest wall. The compression is accompanied by a brief rise in esophageal pressure, rapidly followed by a rapid and marked fall, indicating an inspiratory effort. This inspiratory effort (c) is prolonged compared to previous inspirations (a + b). Expiration (z) is shortened compared to previous unstimulated breaths (x + y).*

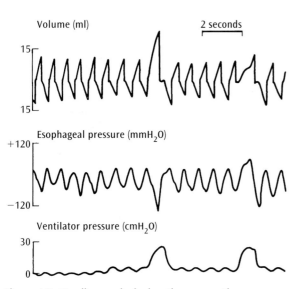

Figure 4.8 *Head's paradoxical or the augmenting inspiratory reflex. The positive pressure inflation in the center of the ventilator pressure recording provokes the augmented inspiration, as demonstrated by the large negative deflection in the esophageal pressure trace compared to that experienced during spontaneous inspiration between ventilator inflations. Reprinted from Early Human Development, **8**, Greenough, A., Morley, C.J., Davis, J.A., Respiratory reflexes in ventilated premature babies, 65–75, 1983, with permission from Elsevier Science.*

Upper airway chemoreflexes

Introduction of small quantities of water into the pharynx of term and preterm babies induces apnea, which has both central and obstructive features.[94] The region most sensitive to water appears to be in the interarytenoid notch.[77] This area is stimulated just before the fluid enters the larynx. The response probably has an important protective function for the upper airway. Apnea is seen far more commonly if water, rather than saline, is used.[19] The ability of the 'sensors' to distinguish between species-specific and other milks has not been demonstrated in man, but there are structures in the lining epithelium which are histologically very similar to taste buds.[50] It is not known how long these reflex responses persist, but one group found that ultrasonically nebulized distilled water was capable of inducing episodes of apnea in infants as old as 3 months of age (C O'Callaghan and AD Milner, unpublished data). Interestingly, this apneic response to water within the upper airway appears to be greater when the infant is in the prone rather than supine position,[52] providing another possible mechanism to explain why the sudden infant death syndrome is associated with sleeping prone. There also appears to be CO_2 sensors within the respiratory tract, possibly in the upper airway. Inhalation of high (76 percent) concentrations of CO_2 resulted in apnea in preterm infants.[3]

THE CHEST WALL AND RESPIRATORY MUSCLES

The chest wall

The ribs of the neonate are relatively elastic, in the paralyzed state the compliance of the chest wall is high, often exceeding 25 ml/cmH$_2$O. The stability of the chest wall is helped by the relatively horizontal positioning of the ribs, which tend to splint the thoracic cage open.[75] The upper ribs are shorter than the lower ones, giving a triangular shape to the thoracic cage in comparison to the dome shape seen in the adults (Figure 4.9).[21] This configuration limits the extent to which the outward (bucket handle) movement of the ribs can contribute to tidal exchange.

Although the chest wall is very compliant, it is relatively stable, as the intercostal muscles' main function appears to be to provide chest wall rigidity rather than expansion on inspiration. Measurements of chest wall compliance during spontaneous breathing, assessed by examining the proportion of transthoracic pressure conducted to the oesophagus during either positive end expiratory pressure[86] or continuous negative external pressure,[69] have demonstrated that approximately 50 percent of the applied pressure is transmitted. Those data indicate that the functional compliance of the chest wall is close to that of the lung,

which must be the case if gross paradoxical movement of the chest wall is to be avoided. In REM sleep, when respiratory muscle tone is reduced, paradox does occur,[18] and it is also a striking feature in term or preterm babies who have respiratory disease and are unable to compensate for their reduced lung compliance.[102]

Respiratory muscles

THE DIAPHRAGM

Respiratory exchange is largely brought about by the diaphragm which, in the neonate, lies more horizontally than in the adult. The area of diaphragm in contact with the chest wall is relatively small,[21] which reduces the ability of the diaphragm to increase the circumference of the lower thorax. Despite this, inspiratory pressures in excess of 120 cmH$_2$O have been recorded during the onset of respiration[101] and during crying in the immediate neonatal period.[22,88]

ACCESSORY MUSCLES

These are well developed. The external and internal oblique and the rectus and transversus abdominalis have been shown to generate positive intrathoracic and interabdominal pressures in excess of 100 cmH$_2$O in the

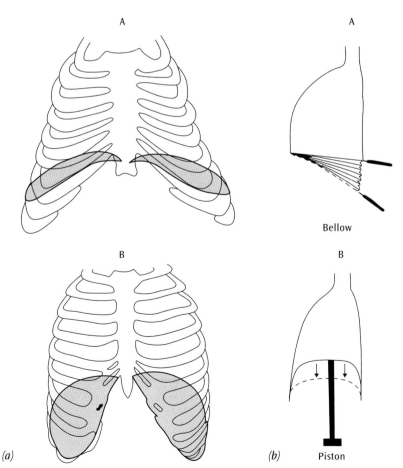

(a)   (b)

Figure 4.9 (a) The chest wall of the infant (A) has a triangular shape compared to that of the adult (B). (b) Ventilation in the infant is due to a bellows-like action (A) compared to the piston effect of the diaphragm in the adult (B). (Reproduced with kind permission from H Devlieger[21])

immediate neonatal period.[101] Such levels are not too dissimilar to the maximum pressures which can be generated in the adult. The scalene and sternomastoid muscles, which have an important role in aiding inspiration in early childhood and adult life, may, in the neonatal period, further stabilize the chest wall and thus aid inspiratory exchange.

RESPIRATORY MUSCLE STRUCTURE AND FUNCTION

The respiratory muscle fibers can be divided into two groups. The first group (type I) generate peak tension relatively slowly, but are very resistant to fatigue;[11] these are also known as the slow twitch fibers. The type II fibres[11] generate peak tensions much faster (fast twitch) and have been subdivided into type IIa and IIb according to their staining responses to NADH-tetrazolium reductase.[67] The main difference between the IIa and IIb fibers is that the latter type fatigue rapidly. The diaphragm of preterm babies contains approximately 10 percent of type I fibers,[54] which rises to 25 percent at term and subsequently to 55 percent in childhood. The constituents of the neonatal respiratory muscles, particularly the diaphragm mean that they are more prone to fatigue than later in life. There are two additional muscle fiber types, 2c and 2h, which occur only in the fetus and newborn infant.[67] It is thought that these muscle fibers also have a limited ability to withstand fatigue.

EFFECT OF SLEEP STATE

Tonic activity of the respiratory muscles is abolished in REM sleep;[63] this may cause chest wall distortion. In the preterm infant, this may lead to a reduction in tidal volume and reductions in saturation.[66,70] Sleep state also influences the post-inspiratory activity of the diaphragm, which is important as a braking mechanism to maintain lung volume and in the control of expiratory time. In addition, upper airway resistance is affected by sleep state. The abductor muscles, the thyroarytenoid, lateral cricoarytenoid and intra-arytenoid have a phasic expiratory activity during quiet sleep, which is lost in REM sleep.

Maintenance of the patency of the upper airway

In the newborn period, the upper airway is a very compliant structure. Maintenance of the airway is dependent on the complex interaction of upper airway muscles which function in conjunction with the diaphragm and chest wall muscles. If the function of these muscles is interrupted, for example by paralysis, the small negative pressure swings associated with inspiration are sufficient to cause collapse first of the oropharynx and then of the laryngeal orifice.[81] Electrical stimulation tests[85] have shown that the most important muscles in maintaining patency of the oropharynx are the genioglossus, geniohyoid, sternohyoid, sternothyroid and pharohyoid muscles. Electromyograph studies[12,82] found that these muscles interact during inspiration to counteract the negative pressure being generated by the downward movement of the diaphragm. In addition, the vocal cords tend to retract during inspiration, effectively reducing the inspiratory resistance. On expiration, the pharyngeal supporting muscles tend to relax, but the structure is then supported by the positive pressure within the lumen. In contrast to inspiration, there is active contraction of the laryngeal muscles, particularly in early expiration which, in combination with the relatively late relaxation of the inspiratory muscles, reduces the rate of flow early in expiration.[26] Those phasic changes are modified by CO_2 levels, as inhaling CO_2 reduces both the inspiratory and expiratory resistances in preterm infants.[68] In situations in which the FRC is reduced, for example respiratory distress syndrome (RDS), pneumonia or heart failure, this pattern is exaggerated so that the airway is almost completely occluded during expiration. Air is then driven out through the small residual orifice by the contraction of the abdominal muscles, producing the characteristic grunting form of respiration.

The effects of the chest wall and respiratory muscles on the FRC

The FRC in the neonatal period is approximately 25 ml/kg body weight when measured by a gas dilution technique[34] and 30 ml/kg when measured plethysmographically.[91] Those values are close to those seen in adults when related to body mass and, although measurements are limited in number,[89] they appear to represent a similar proportion of the total lung capacity. It has been claimed[47] that the FRC is largely maintained by respiratory muscle tone and that in REM sleep, when respiratory muscle tone is reduced, the FRC, as measured by total body plethysmograph, decreases by up to 60 percent.[47] Those data, however, were only from six individuals and subsequent studies on both term[93] and preterm babies[5] have failed to show any significant change in lung volume when there is a change from quiet to active sleep. There are, however, two factors that appear to be important in maintenance of the FRC. First, the residual volume, the volume at which all airways are closed and all remaining alveolar gas is trapped, is relatively close to the FRC in the neonatal period and tends to fall relative to the FRC as the infant grows. This has been demonstrated using the forced partial expiratory flow volume curve technique by the limited ability of an externally applied pressure to produce more than a few milliliters of expiratory reserve volume.[62] Second, the relationship between the time constant, that is, the product of the resistance and the compliance (see p. 117), and the infant's respiratory rate is important. The time constant in health is relatively unchanged throughout life, being between 0.22 and 0.4 seconds. The newborn respiratory rate, however, is high, tending to be between 40 and 60 breaths per minute. Under such conditions, there is insufficient time for the lung to deflate to the FRC, as determined by the balance of elastic forces produced by the lung on the one hand and the chest wall and respiratory muscles on the other. This produces a dynamic elevation of the FRC.[59] It may be that the increased respiratory rate occurring in REM sleep helps compensate for the reduction in intercostal muscle tone and so prevents a fall in FRC.[93] The FRC is unaffected by the body position of the full-term infant.[2]

REFERENCES

1 Abu-Shaweesh, J.M., Dreshaj, I.A., Thomas, A.J. *et al.* (1999) Changes in respiratory timing induced by hypercapnia in maturing rats. *Journal of Applied Physiology* **87**, 484–490.

2 Aiton, N.R., Fox, G.F., Alexander, J. *et al.* (1996) The influence of sleeping position on functional residual capacity and effective pulmonary blood flow in healthy neonates. *Pediatric Pulmonology* **22**, 342–347.

3 Alvaro, R.E., Weintraub, Z., Kwiatkowski, K. *et al.* (1992) A respiratory sensory reflex in response to CO_2 inhibits breathing in preterm infants. *Journal of Applied Physiology* **73**, 1558–1563.

4 Bamford, O.S., Schuen, J.N., Carroll, J.L. (1996) Effect of nicotine exposure on postnatal ventilatory responses to hypoxia and hypercapnia. *Respiration Physiology* **106**, 1–11.

5 Beardsmore, C.S., MacFadyen, U.M., Moosavi, S.S. *et al.* (1989) Measurement of lung volumes during active and quiet sleep in infants. *Pediatric Pulmonology* **7**, 71–77.

6 Belegu, R., Hadziefendic, S., Dreshaj, I.A. *et al.* (1999) CO_2-induced c-*fos* expression in medullary neurons during early development. *Respiration Physiology* **117**, 13–28.

7 Berquin, P., Bodineau, L., Gros, F., Larnicol, N. (2000) Brainstem and hypothalamic areas involved in respiratory chemoreflexes: a Fos study in adult rats. *Brain Research* **857**, 30–40.

8 Blanco, C.E., Dawes, G.S., Hanson, M.A., McCooke, H.B. (1984) The response to hypxoia of arterial chemoreceptors in fetal sheep and newborn lambs. *Journal of Physiology* **351**, 25–37.

9 Bodegard, G., Schwieler, G.H., Skoglund, S., Zetterstrom, R. (1969) Control of respiration in newborn babies. I. The development of the Hering Breuer inflation reflex. *Acta Paediatrica Scandinavica* **58**, 567–571.

10 Bryan, A.C., Bryan, M.H. (1978) Control of respiration in the newborn. *Clinics in Perinatology* **7**, 269–281.

11 Burke, R.E., Levine, D.N., Tsairis, P., Zajac, F.E. (1973) Physiologic types and histochemical profiles in motor units of the cat gastrocnemius. *Journal of Physiology* **234**, 723–748.

12 Carlo, W.A., Martin, R.J., Bruce, E.N. *et al.* (1983) Alae nasi activation (nasal flaring) decreases nasal resistance in preterm infants. *Pediatrics* **72**, 338–343.

13 Chan, V., Greenough, A. (1992) Lung function and the Hering Breuer reflex in the neonatal period. *Early Human Development* **28**, 111–118.

14 Cherniack, N.S., von Euler, C., Glogowska, M., Homma, J. (1981) Characteristics and rate of occurrence of spontaneous and provoked augmented breaths. *Acta Paediatrica Scandinavica* **111**, 349–360.

15 Clark, F.J., von Euler, C. (1972) On the regulation of depth and rate of breathing. *Journal of Physiology* **222**, 267–295.

16 Couser, R.J., Ferrara, B., Wright, G.B. *et al.* (1996) Prophylactic indomethacin therapy in the first 24 hours of life for the prevention of patent ductus arteriosus in preterm infants treated prophylactically in the delivery room. *Journal of Pediatrics* **128**, 631–637.

17 Cross, K.W., Klaus, M., Tooley, W.H., Weiser, K. (1960) The response of the newborn baby to inflation of the lungs. *Journal of Physiology* **151**, 551–565.

18 Davi, M., Sankaran, K., MacCallum, M. *et al.* (1979) Effect of sleep state on chest distortion and on the ventilatory response to CO_2. *Pediatric Research* **13**, 982–986.

19 Davies, A.M., Koenig, J.S., Thach, B.T. (1988) Upper airway chemoreflex responses to saline and water in preterm infants. *Journal of Applied Physiology* **64**, 1412–1420.

20 Dawes, G.S. (1984) The central control of fetal breathing and skeletal muscle movements. *Journal of Physiology* **346**, 1–18.

21 Devlieger, H. (1987) MD thesis, Université Catholique de Louvain, Louvain, pp. 136–140.

22 Dimitriou, G., Greenough, A., Dyke, H., Rafferty, G.F. (2000) Maximal airway pressures during crying in healthy preterm and term infants. *Early Human Development* **57**, 149–156.

23 Donnelly, D.F. (2000) Developmental aspects of oxygen sensing by the carotid body. *Journal of Applied Physiology* **88**, 2296–2301.

24 Eden, G.J., Hanson, M.A. (1987) Effects of chronic hypoxia from birth on the ventilatory response to acute hypoxia in the newborn rat. *Journal of Physiology* **392**, 11–19.

25 Eden, G.J., Hanson, M.A. (1987) Maturation of the respiratory response to acute hypoxia in the newborn rat. *Journal of Physiology* **392**, 1–9.

26 England, S.J., Stogren, H.A.F. (1986) Influence of the upper airway on breathing pattern and expiratory time constant in dog pups. *Respiratory Physiology* **66**, 181–192.

27 Feldman, J.L., Gray, P.A. (2000) Sighs and gasps in a dish. *Nature Neuroscience* **3**, 531–532.

28 Fencl, V., Miller, T.B., Pappenheimer, J.R. (1966) Studies on the respiratory response to disturbances of acid–base balance, with deductions concerning the ionic composition of cerebral interstitial fluid. *American Journal of Physiology* **210**, 459–472.

29 Fleming, P.J., Bryan, A.C., Bryan, M.H. (1978) Functional immaturity of pulmonary irritant receptors and apnea in newborn preterm infants. *Pediatrics* **61**, 515–518.

30 Frantz, I.D., Alder, S.M., Abroms, I.F., Thach, B.T. (1976) Respiratory response to airway occlusion in infants: sleep state and maturation. *Journal of Applied Physiologus* **41**, 634–635.

31 Gagliardi, L., Rusconi, F. (1995) Hering–Breuer reflex and respiratory rate: a biased association. *Journal of Applied Physiology* **78**, 1575–1578.

32 Gandevia, S.C., Rothwell, J.C. (1987) Activation of the human diaphragm from the motor cortex. *Journal of Physiology* **384**, 109–118.

33 Gerhardt, T., Bancalari, E. (1984) Apnea of prematurity: II. Respiratory reflexes. *Pediatrics* **74**, 63–66.

34 Geubelle, F., Francotte, M., Beyer, M. *et al.* (1977) Functional residual capacity and thoracic gas volume in normoxic and hyperoxic newborn infants. *Acta Paediatrica Belgica* **30**, 221–225.

35 Gozal, D., Gaultier, C. (1997) Proceedings from the first international symposium on the congenital central

hypoventilation syndrome in New Orleans (1996) *Pediatric Pulmonology* **23**, 133–168.

36 Gray, P.A., Rekling, J.C., Bocchiaro, C.M., Feldman, J.L. (1999) Modulation of respiratory frequency by peptidergic input to rhythmogenic neurons in the preBotzinger complex. *Science* **286**, 1566–1568.

37 Gray, P.A., Janczewski, W.A., Mellen, N. *et al.* (2001) Normal breathing requires preBotzinger complex neurokinin-1 receptor-expressing neurons. *Nature Neuroscience* **4**, 927–930.

38 Greenough, A. (1988) The premature infant's respiratory response to mechanical ventilation. *Early Human Development* **17**, 1–5.

39 Greenough, A., Pool, J. (1991) Hering–Breuer reflex in young asthmatic children. *Pediatric Pulmonology* **11**, 345–349.

40 Greenough, A., Morley, C.J., Davis, J.A. (1983) Respiratory reflexes in ventilated premature babies. *Early Human Development* **8**, 65–75.

41 Greenough, A., Morley, C.J., Davis, J.A. (1984) Provoked augmented inspirations in ventilated premature infants. *Early Human Development* **9**, 111–117.

42 Greenough, A., Wood, S., Morley, C.J., Davis, J.A. (1984) Pancuronium prevents pneumothoraces in ventilated premature babies who actively expire against positive pressure inflation. *Lancet* **i**, 1–3.

43 Greenough, A., Morley, C., Johnson, P. (1985) An active expiratory reflex in preterm ventilated infants. In Jones, C.T., Nathanielsz, P.W. (eds), *The Physiological Development of the Foetus and Newborn*. London: Academic Press, 259–263.

44 Hannam, S., Ingram, D.M., Rabe-Hesketh, S., Milner, A.D. (2001) Characterisation of the Hering–Breuer deflation reflex in the human neonate. *Respiration Physiology* **124**, 51–64.

45 Hassan, A., Gossage, J., Ingram, D. *et al.* (2001) Volume of activation of the Hering–Breuer inflation reflex in the newborn infant. *Journal of Applied Physiology* **90**, 763–769.

46 Head, H. (1889) On the regulation of respiration. *Journal of Physiology* **10**, 1–70.

47 Henderson-Smart, D.J., Read, D.J. (1979) Reduced lung volume during behavioral active sleep in the newborn. *Journal of Applied Physiology* **46**, 1081–1085.

48 Herlenius, E., Åden, U., Tang, L.Q., Lagercrantz, H. (2002) Perinatal respiratory control and its modulation by adenosine and caffeine in the rat. *Pediatric Research* **51**, 4–12.

49 Hertzberg, T., Lagercrantz, H. (1987) Postnatal sensitivity of the peripheral chemoreceptors in newborn infants. *Archives of Disease in Childhood* **62**, 1238–1241.

50 Ide, C., Munger, B.L. (1980) The cytologic composition of primate laryngeal chemosensory corpuscles. *American Journal of Anatomy* **158**, 193–209.

51 Idiong, N., Lemke, R.P., Lin, Y.J. *et al.* (1998) Airway closure during mixed apneas in preterm infants: is respiratory effort necessary? *Journal of Pediatrics* **134**, 796–798.

52 Jeffery, H.E., Megevand, A., Page, M. (1999) Why the prone position is a risk factor for sudden infant death syndrome. *Pediatrics* **104**, 263–269.

53 Katz-Salamon, M., Lagercrantz, H. (1994) Hypoxic ventilatory defence in very preterm infants: attenuation after long term oxygen treatment. *Archives of Disease in Childhood* **70**, F90–F95.

54 Keens, T.G., Bryan, A.C., Levison, H., Ianuzzo, C.D. (1978) Developmental pattern of muscle fiber types in human ventilatory muscles. *Journal of Applied Physiology* **44**, 909–913.

55 Kirkpatrick, S.M.L., Olinsky, A., Bryan, M.H., Bryan, A.C. (1976) Effect of premature delivery on the maturation of the Hering–Breuer inspiratory inhibitor reflex in human infants. *Journal of Pediatrics* **88**, 1011–1014.

56 Knill, R., Bryan, A.C. (1976) An intercostal-phrenic inhibitory reflex in human newborn infants. *Journal of Applied Physiology* **40**, 352–356.

57 Knox, C.K. (1973) Characteristics of inflation and deflation reflexes during expiration in the cat. *Journal of Neurophysiology* **36**, 284–295.

58 Koos, B.J., Maeda, T., Jan, C. (2001) Adenosine A(1) and A(2A) receptors modulate sleep state and breathing in fetal sheep. *Journal of Applied Physiology* **91**, 343–350.

59 Kosch, P.C., Stark, A.R. (1984) Dynamic maintenance of end-expiratory lung volume in full-term infants. *Journal of Applied Physiology* **57**, 1126–1133.

60 Lagercrantz, H., Milerad, J., Walker, D.W. (1991) Control of ventilation in the neonate. In Crystal, R.G., West, J.B. *et al.* (eds), *The Lung: Scientific Foundations*. New York: Raven Press, 1711–1722.

61 Laubscher, B., Greenough, A. (1998) Comparative effects of theophylline and caffeine on respiratory function of preterm infants. *Early Human Development* **50**, 185–192.

62 Le Souef, P.N., Hughes, D.M., Landau, L.I. (1986) Effect of compression pressure on forced expiratory flow in infants. *Journal of Applied Physiology* **61**, 1639–1646.

63 Lopes, J., Muller, N.L., Bryan, M.H. *et al.* (1981) Importance of inspiratory muscle tone in maintenance of FRC in the newborn. *Journal of Applied Physiology* **51**, 830–834.

64 Marsh, M., Fox, G., Hoskyns, E.W. *et al.* (1994) The Hering–Breuer deflationary reflex in the newborn infant. *Pediatric Pulmonology* **18**, 163–169.

65 Martin, R.J., Nearman, H.S., Katona, P.G., Klaus, M.H. (1977) The effect of a low continuous positive airway pressure on the reflex control of respiration in the preterm infant. *Journal of Pediatrics* **90**, 976–981.

66 Martin, R.J., Hernell, N., Rubin, D., Fanaroff, A. (1979) Effect of supine and prone positions on arterial oxygen tension in the preterm infant. *Pediatrics* **63**, 528–531.

67 Maxwell, L.C., McCarter, R.J.M., Kuehl, T.J., Robotham, J.L. (1983) Development of histochemical and functional properties of baboon respiratory muscles. *Journal of Applied Physiology* **54**, 551–561.

68 Miller, M.J., DiFiore, J.M., Strohl, K.P. *et al.* (1991) Effects of CO_2 rebreathing on pulmonary mechanics in premature infants. *Journal of Applied Physiology* **20**, 2582–2586.

69 Milner, A.D., Saunders, R.A., Hopkin, I.E. (1977) Effects of continuous distending pressure on lung volumes and lung mechanics in the immediate neonatal period. *Biology of the Neonate* **31**, 111–115.

70 Mortola, J.P., Saetta, M., Fox, G. *et al.* (1985) Mechanical aspects of chest wall distortion. *Journal of Applied Physiology* **59**, 295–304.

71 Mortola, J.P., Trippenbach, T., Rezzonico, R. *et al.* (1995) Hering–Breuer reflexes in high-altitude infants. *Clinical Science* **88**, 345–350.

72 Moss, I.R., Inman, J.G. (1989) Neurochemicals and respiratory control during development. *Journal of Applied Physiology* **67**, 1–13.

73 Nattie, E. (1999) CO_2, brainstem chemoreceptors and breathing. *Progress in Neurobiology* **59**, 299–331.

74 Olinsky, A., Bryan, M.H., Bryan, A.C. (1974) Influence of lung inflation on respiratory control in neonates. *Journal of Applied Physiology* **36**, 426–429.

75 Openshaw, P., Edwards, S., Helms, P. (1984) Changes in ribcage geometry during childhood. *Thorax* **39**, 624–627.

76 Peyronnet, J., Roux, J.C., Geloen, A. *et al.* (2000) Prenatal hypoxia impairs the postnatal development of neural and functional chemoafferent pathway in rat. *Journal of Physiology* **524**, 525–537.

77 Pickens, D.L., Schefft, G.L., Thach, B.T. (1989) Pharyngeal fluid clearance and aspiration preventive mechanisms in sleeping infants. *Journal of Applied Physiology* **66**, 1164–1171.

78 Rabbette, P.S., Stocks, J. (1998) Influence of volume dependency and timing of airway occlusions on the Hering–Breuer reflex in infants. *Journal of Applied Physiology* **85**, 2033–2039.

79 Rabbette, P.S., Costeloe, K.L., Stocks, J. (1991) Persistence of the Hering–Breuer reflex beyond the neonatal period. *Journal of Applied Physiology* **71**, 474–480.

80 Rabbette, P.S., Dezateux, C.A., Fletcher, M.E., Stocks, J. (1991) The Hering–Breuer reflex declines during the first year of life. *European Respiratory Journal* **4**, 533S.

81 Reed, R., Roberts, J.L., Thach, B.T. (1985) Factors influencing regional patency and configuration of the upper airway in human infants. *Journal of Applied Physiology* **58**, 635–644.

82 Remmers, J.E., deGroot, W.J., Sauerland, E.K. et al. (1978) Pathogenesis of upper airway occlusion during sleep. *Journal of Applied Physiology* **44**, 931–938.

83 Reynold, L.B. (1962) Characteristics of an inspiration augmenting reflex in anaesthetized cats. *Journal of Applied Physiology* **17**, 683–688.

84 Richter, D.W., Spyer, K.M. (2001) Studying rhythmogenesis of breathing: comparison of *in vivo* and *in vitro* models. *Trends in Neurosciences* **24**, 464–472.

85 Roberts, J.L., Reed, W.R., Thach, B.T. (1984) Pharyngeal airway stabilizing function of the sternohyoid and sternothyroid muscles of the rabbit. *Journal of Applied Physiology* **57**, 1790–1795.

86 Saunders, R.A., Milner, A.D., Hopkin, I.E. (1976) The effect of CPAP on lung mechanics and lung volumes in the neonatal period. *Biology of the Neonate* **29**, 171–183.

87 Savich, R.D., Guerra, F.A., Lee, C.-C.H., Kitterman, J.A. (1995) Effect of inhibition of prostaglandin synthesis on breathing movements and pulmonary blood flow in fetal sheep. *Journal of Applied Physiology* **78**, 531–538.

88 Shardonofsky, F.R., Perez-Chada, D., Carmuega, E., Milic-Emili, J. (1989) Airway pressures during crying in healthy infants. *Pediatric Pulmonology* **6**, 14–18.

89 Shulman, D.L., Goodman, A., Bar-Yishay, E., Godfrey, S. (1989) Comparison of the single breath and volume recruitment techniques in the treatment of total respiratory

90 Sorensen, S.C., Severinghaus, J.W. (1968) Respiratory sensitivity to acute hypoxia in man born at sea level living at high altitude. *Journal of Applied Physiology* **25**, 211–216.

91 Stocks, J., Godfrey, S. (1977) Specific airway conductance in relation to post-conceptional age during infancy. *Journal of Applied Physiology* **43**, 144–154.

92 Stocks, J., Dezateux, C., Hoo, A.F. et al. (1996) Delayed maturation of Hering–Breuer inflation reflex activity in preterm infants. *American Journal of Respiratory and Critical Care Medicine* **154**, 1411–1417.

93 Stokes, G.M., Milner, A.D., Newball, E.A. *et al.* (1989) Do lung volumes change with sleep state in the neonate? *European Journal of Pediatrics* **148**, 360–364.

94 Storey, A.T., Johnson, P. (1975) Laryngeal water receptors initiating apnea in the lamb. *Experimental Neurology* **47**, 42–55.

95 Thach, B.T., Frantz, I.D., Adler, S.M. *et al.* (1975) Vagal influence on inspiratory duration in premature infants as a function of postnatal age and gestational age. *Federation Proceedings* **34**, 358–363.

96 Thomas, T., Spyer, K.M. (2000) ATP as a mediator of mammalian central CO_2 chemoreception. *Journal of Physiology* **523**, 441–447.

97 Trippenbach, T., Zinman, R., Milic Emili, J. (1980) Caffeine effect on breathing pattern and vagal reflexes in newborn rabbits. *Respiration Physiology* **40**, 211–215.

98 Ullmann, E.T. (1970) In *Breathing: Hering–Breuer Centenary Symposium*. London: Churchill, 357–394.

99 Upton, C.J., Milner, A.D., Stokes, G.M. (1992) Response to external obstruction in preterm infants with apnea. *Pediatric Pulmonology* **14**, 233–238.

100 von Euler, C. (1983) On the central pattern generator for the basic breathing rhythmicity. *Journal of Applied Physiology: Respiratory* **55**, 1647–1659.

101 Vyas, H., Field, D., Hopkin, I.E., Milner, A.D. (1986) Determinants of the first inspiratory volume and functional residual capacity at birth. *Pediatric Pulmonology* **2**, 189–193.

102 Warren, R.H., Horan, S.M., Robertson, P.K. (1997) Chest wall motion in preterm infants using respiratory inductive plethysmography. *European Respiratory Journal* **10**, 2295–2300.

103 Yamamoto, M., Lagercrantz, H., von Euler, C. (1981) Effects of substance P and TRH on ventilation and pattern of breathing in newborn rabbits. *Acta Physiologica Scandinavica* **113**, 541–543.

compliance in anesthetized infants and children. *Anesthesiology* **70**, 921–927.

5

Development of the immune system

SUSAN LEECH

Stem cells	50	Innate immunity	55
Adaptive immunity	50	References	57

The immune system, as other systems, follows an orderly pattern of development following conception and continues to develop after birth. Immaturity of host defense mechanisms makes neonates susceptible to a wide variety of microbial pathogens. The more premature the infant, the greater the risk, as they have a less well-developed immune system and a greater need for invasive intensive care. Once infected, neonates become rapidly and seriously ill.

STEM CELLS

The cells of the immune system are derived from pleuripotential hematopoietic stem cells. They are first found in the blood islands of the yolk sac. During embryogenesis they migrate to the fetal liver, omentum, spleen and ultimately the bone marrow, which is the major repository of stem cells in adult life. Hematopoietic stem cells enter one of two major differentiation pathways. One generates the T and B lymphocytes of the adaptive immune system, following migration to the thymus or bone marrow, respectively. The second pathway generates the effector cells of the innate immune system: phagocytes (polymorphonuclear leukocytes, monocytes and macrophages), antigen-presenting cells (dendritic cells, Langerhans cells) and inflammatory cells (mast cells, basophils and eosinophils). Each step in the developmental process that generates the immune system is genetically controlled. All major cell lineages of the immune system are present by the onset of the second trimester.

ADAPTIVE IMMUNITY

Thymus development

The thymus is derived from three primitive germ layers. The endoderm of the third pharyngeal pouch forms the medullary epithelium. The ectoderm of the third branchial cleft forms the cortical epithelium. Mesenchymal elements, of neural crest origin, form the fibrous capsule, stroma and vessels (Figure 5.1).[4] These elements migrate caudally between 7 and 10 weeks of gestation, to the anterior mediastinum. By 12 weeks of gestation, a clear separation between the peripheral thymic cortex and central medulla is apparent. Different stages of T-cell development occur in different regions of the thymus. Thymic cellularity increases dramatically during the last trimester and continues to increase in cellularity after birth, until about 10 years of age. It then involutes, the cortex and medulla being replaced by fat. Mature CD4 and CD8 thymocytes are spared during involution whilst the immature, double-positive, cortical thymocytes are lost.

T-cell development

From 7 weeks of gestation, T-cell precursors enter the thymus. Primitive cells containing cytoplasmic CD3 can be detected in the prethymic mesenchyme and fetal liver at 8 weeks. By 12 weeks, T cells express a T-cell receptor. By 14 weeks of gestation, development of the T cell can be tracked as it passes through the thymus. The subcapsular region contains immature type 1 thymocytes, large blast cells that proliferate vigorously. The cells then pass to the

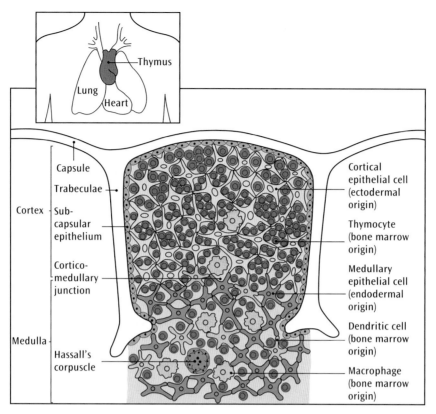

Figure 5.1 *The cellular organization of the thymus. The thymus, which lies in the midline of the body, above the heart, is made up from several lobules, each of which contains discrete cortical (outer) and medullary (central) regions. The cortex consists of immature thymocytes, branched cortical epithelial cells, with which the immature cortical thymocytes are closely associated, and scattered macrophages involved in clearing apoptotic thymocytes. The medulla consists of mature thymocytes, and medullary epithelial cells, along with macrophages and dendritic cells of bone marrow origin. Hassall's corpuscles found in the human thymus are probably also sites of cell destruction. The thymocytes in the outer cortical cell layer are proliferating immature cells, while the deeper cortical thymocytes are mainly cells undergoing thymic selection. The photograph shows the equivalent section of a human thymus, stained with hematoxylin and eosin. Photograph courtesy of CJ Howe. Reproduced with permission from Janeway and Travers.[22]*

cortex, where most T-cell development takes place. Smaller thymocytes, which express CD3, CD4 and CD8, and are termed 'double-positive' are found in the cortex. At this stage, positive and negative selection shapes the T-cell repertoire. T cells capable of recognizing molecules of the major histocompatibility complex (MHC) present on the thymic cortical epithelial cells (and therefore capable of recognizing antigen presented by self-MHC) are positively selected. This is followed by negative selection, mediated by bone marrow derived macrophages in the cortex and medulla and dendritic cells at the corticomedullary junction, which remove strongly self-reactive T cells. As a result of this 'thymic education', the T-cell repertoire is determined and 99 percent of T-cell precursors are eliminated by apoptosis (Figure 5.2). Finally, the T cell ends up in the medulla where one of the CD4 or CD8 glycoproteins is lost. The mature T cell is released into the circulation and traffics to other tissues. By 14 weeks of gestation, mature CD4 and CD8 T cells are found in the fetal liver and spleen.[2]

DEVELOPMENT OF THE T-CELL RECEPTOR

T-cell receptor diversity is generated from a small set of genes by DNA rearrangement. The recombinase activating gene enzymes create functional T-cell receptor genes by a looping-out mechanism. The splicing sites are imprecise and subject to the addition of random nucleotides by the enzyme terminal deoxynucleotidyltransferase (tTdT), which appears at 18 weeks of gestation. Beforehand, from 8 to 18 weeks of gestation, the fetal thymus demonstrates reduced diversity of sequences. By mid-gestation, the T-cell receptor repertoire is more varied.[41]

T-CELL FUNCTION

From 12 weeks of gestation, the early T-cell receptors are able to respond to foreign antigens presented by MHC. From mid-gestation to birth, fetal T cells probably have identical capabilities to neonatal T cells. Fetal thymocytes can recognize foreign cells and are capable of

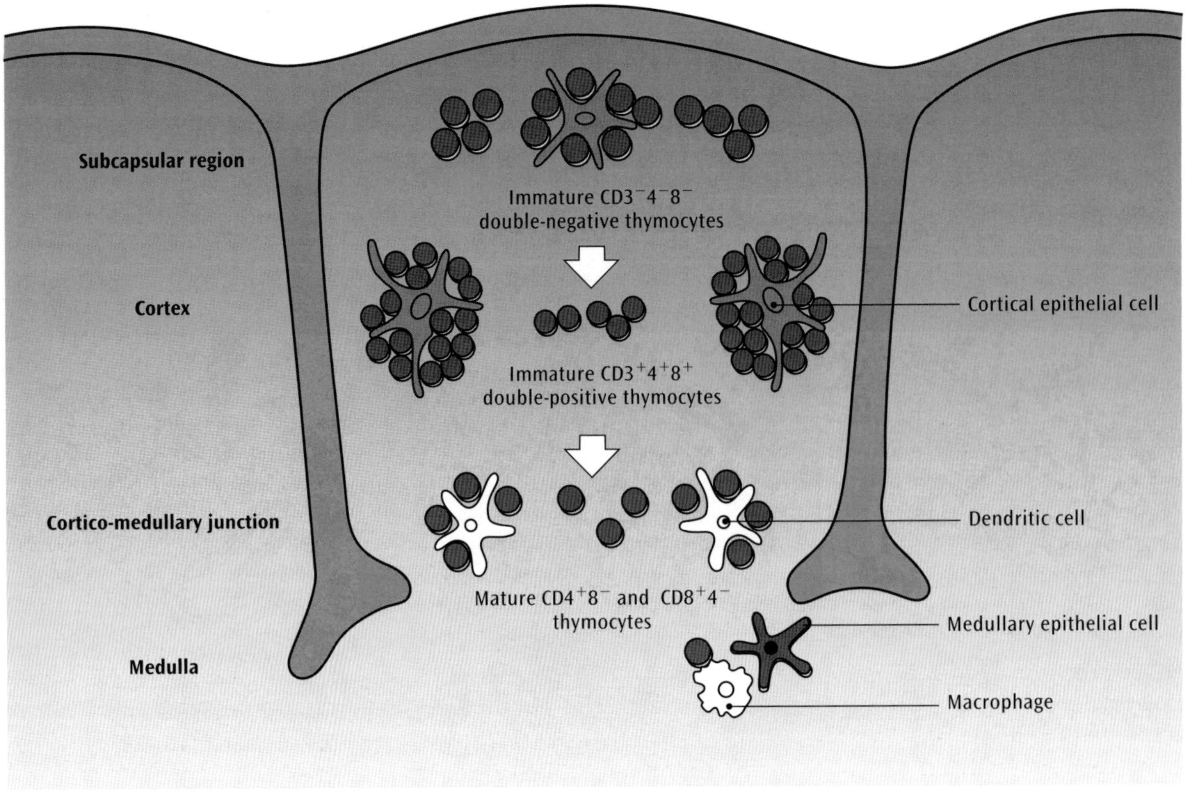

Figure 5.2 *Thymocytes of different developmental stages are found in distinct parts of the thymus. The earliest cells to enter the thymus are found in the subcapsular region of the cortex. As these cells proliferate and mature into double-positive thymocytes, they migrate deeper into the thymic cortex. Finally, the medulla contains only mature single-positive T cells, which eventually leave the thymus and enter the bloodstream. Reproduced with permission from Janeway and Travers.[22]*

causing graft-versus-host disease if transplanted into an immunodeficient recipient. Premature infants can therefore reject a transplant, demonstrate normal responses to *in vitro* tests of lymphocyte function and demonstrate lack of sequelae to neonatal thymectomy. T-cell function in the fetus and neonate, however, is impaired compared with that in adults. Diminished functions include T-cell-mediated lymphokine production, cytotoxicity, delayed-type hypersensitivity and help for B-cell differentiation. The lack of memory T cells may account for many of these differences. Limitations in T-cell numbers and in the available repertoire of T-cell receptors do not play a major role in the diminished immune responses by the neonate, although they may do so in the fetus before mid-gestation. Following neonatal infection, the acquisition of detectable T-dependent antigen-specific responses is delayed.

CYTOKINE PRODUCTION

Neonatal T cells produce quantities of IL-2, TNF-α and TNF-β similar to those made by adult cells, but make little or no IFN-γ, IL-3, IL-4, IL-5, IL-6 or GM-CSF.[13] The ability of T cells to synthesize cytokines is linked to their

degree of activation. The lack of antigen-driven post-thymic differentiation and absence of memory cells contributes to deficiencies in neonatal helper function.

EXPRESSION OF CD45 RO AND CD45 RA

There are two isoforms of transmembrane tyrosine phosphatase, CD45 present on T cells. CD45 changes from RA to RO after exposure to antigen, as the cell function changes from a naïve to memory cell. CD45 RA cells account for 90 percent of neonatal CD4 cells. CD45 RO cells constitute 50 percent of adult but only 5 percent of neonatal T cells.[21] The large number of neonatal CD45 RA T-cell population actively suppresses the helper function of CD45 RO cells.

B-cell development

B-cell development also occurs in discontinuous steps. The first stage involves the generation of a large, diverse repertoire of B-cell clones expressing unique antigen receptors from a relatively small number of stem cell precursors, analogous to intrathymic T-cell development. The generation of diverse immunoglobulin gene sequences occurs in a manner similar to that described for the T-cell receptor. B-cell development occurs in the omentum and liver in early fetal life and bone marrow as it becomes the hematopoietic organ.[5]

PROGENITOR B CELLS, PRE-B AND IMMATURE B CELLS

Progenitor B cells (pro-B) are the earliest recognizable cell of the B-cell lineage (Figure 5.3). They are the earliest hematopoietic cells which have surface expression of the pan-B marker CD19 and a membrane complex composed of surrogate light chain (ΨL) and a presumed surrogate heavy chain. They divide and have begun to rearrange the immunoglobulin heavy chain genes. Production of the heavy chain of the IgM molecule, μ, in the cell cytoplasm signals successful gene rearrangement and marks transition from pro-B to pre-B cell. Pre-B cells have lost CD34, express CD19 and bear cytoplasmic μ in the form of a ΨL/μ complex. Pre-B cells are present in the fetal liver and omentum by 8 weeks of gestation and in the fetal bone marrow by 13 weeks of gestation.[37] After 30 weeks of gestation, pre-B cells are only found in bone marrow where they make up less than 5 percent of the cell population. Rearrangement of light chain genes occurs after heavy chain rearrangement. Synthesis of intact light chain permits efficient assembly and transfer of monomeric IgM molecules to the cell surface. The expression of cell surface immunoglobulin marks the transition from pre-B to immature B cells. The B lymphocyte

also expresses pan-B differentiation markers CD19 and CD20. Cells expressing surface IgM are detectable from 10 weeks of gestation and B cells can be identified in the circulation by 11 weeks of gestation. Fetal B cells express IgM without IgD, unlike adult IgM-positive B cells, which also express surface IgD. Engagement of surface IgM at this stage of B-cell development delivers a tolerogenic intracellular signal, as opposed to one which leads to B-cell activation. Antigen exposure *in utero* may therefore induce specific tolerance rather than an antibody response.

GENERATION OF DIVERSITY

The fetal repertoire of expressed variable region genes is restricted and conserved. The genes expressed are scattered throughout the locus. There is less junctional diversity at splice sites between the V-D-J gene segments in fetal heavy chains than in neonatal heavy chains, reflecting delay in expression of tTdT. The neonatal repertoire contains a broader spectrum of V, D and J genes, somatic mutations and larger CDR3 regions.[29] An inevitable consequence of the generation of diversity is the production of self-reactive clones which are removed from the circulation by negative selection and clonal deletion.

ISOTYPE SWITCHING

The second stage of B-cell differentiation occurs after antigen binding and depends on signals from activated

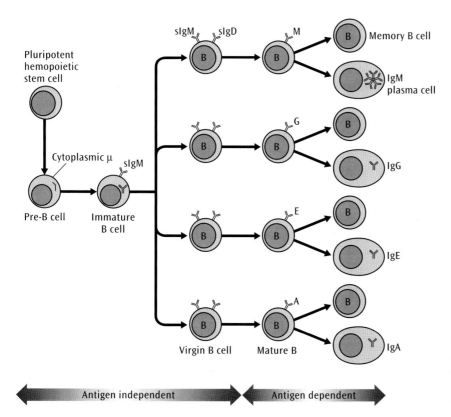

Figure 5.3 *The life cycle of the B cell in relation to antigen. Note how much B-cell development is antigen-dependent. Reproduced with permission from Peakman et al.[32]*

T cells. B cells, thus stimulated, proliferate and differentiate to form memory cells or antibody-secreting plasma cells. All antibody-secreting cells originate from precursors that express membrane IgM, by isotype switching. IgM is expressed first, because the Cμ gene (which codes for IgM) is closest to the V-D-J genes. Expression of isotypes which lie downstream of Cμ occurs by switch recombination. This is T-cell dependent and directed by the cytokine environment, for example IL-4 promotes class switching to IgE.[33] Lymphocytes expressing other immunoglobulin classes begin to appear in low frequency at 10–12 weeks of gestation. IgG-positive cells can be found by 10 weeks and cells bearing IgD and IgA develop slightly later. The number of B lymphocytes increases rapidly from 12 to 15 weeks of gestation. By 15 weeks of gestation, the proportion of immunoglobulin-bearing cells in blood, spleen and lymph nodes is the same as that found in adults. In the fetus and neonate, expression of IgA or IgG occurs exclusively on immature B cells that also express IgM with or without IgD.[17] Adult B cells expressing IgG or IgA express only the single isotype.

B cells, diffusely distributed in lymph nodes at 16–17 weeks of gestation, express CD21 [complement receptor 2 and Epstein–Barr virus (EBV) receptor] and IgD. The organization of primary follicles around follicular dendritic cells from 17 weeks onwards is associated with expression of CD5 on B cells. The development of splenic follicles follows the same pattern but occurs a few weeks later.[5]

B-1 POPULATION

B-1 cells express the surface glycoprotein CD5, they have a unique ontogeny, phenotype and adult tissue distribution.[25] The antibody repertoire of B-1 cells is also unique, using a small set of V-region immunoglobulin genes to produce polyreactive antibodies. Antibody production by B-1 cells is T-cell independent and largely of the IgM isotype, with little or no IgD, and encodes reactivity against autoantigens and idiotypes. B-1 cells develop before conventional B cells and are the predominant B cell throughout fetal and early neonatal life. They are derived from hematopoietic stem cells in the fetal liver and omentum.[37] After birth, a transitional population of B-1a cells are produced, which have a more diverse repertoire, before mature, conventional B cells are produced. In the adult, B-1 cells are sparse, but present in the blood and follicular mantle zones of the spleen, in the small B-cell population in the thymus and in the peritoneal and pleural cavities. The omentum continues to be the primary site for the development of B-1 cells.[37]

IMMUNOGLOBULIN PRODUCTION

The fetus and newborn have reduced capacity to produce either IgG or IgA antibodies to protein antigens or antibodies of any class to carbohydrate antigens. There is a long gap between the development of B lymphocytes bearing IgG or IgA isotypes late in the first trimester, and adult serum concentrations of these antibodies in middle to late childhood. B lymphocytes of newborn babies can synthesize and express these isotypes on their membranes but cannot differentiate into secretory plasma cells. Functional studies comparing *in vitro* responses of neonatal T and B cells with those of adult cells implicate both T and B cells in the impaired capacity to produce IgG and IgA. Neonatal T cells provide poor helper function and are active suppressers.[38] Neonatal B cells require higher concentrations of IL-2 and IL-4 or IL-6 than adult B cells to undergo differentiation into plasma cells. Neonatal T cells produce sufficient IL-2 to drive T-cell proliferation, but do not provide the additional cytokines required to support optimal B-cell differentiation.

PLACENTAL TRANSFER OF IMMUNOGLOBULIN

Placental IgG transport begins at 3 months of gestation. Only IgG is transferred across the placenta from mother to infant. The Fc portion of the IgG heavy chain has a special determinant that allows active transfer. The rate of maternal–fetal transfer is a function of maternal and fetal IgG levels and of the age of the placenta. Premature infants at birth have low serum levels of IgG in inverse proportion to the gestational age. The other immunoglobulins (IgM, A, D and E) are not transferred across the placenta, with the result that certain antibodies present in the maternal circulation are absent in the infant (Figure 5.4).

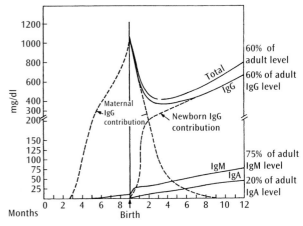

Figure 5.4 *Immunoglobulin (IgG, IgM and IgA) levels in the fetus and infant in the first year of life. The IgG of the fetus and newborn infant is solely of maternal origin. The maternal IgG disappears by the age of 9 months, by which time endogenous synthesis of IgG by the infant is well established. The IgM and IgA of the neonate are entirely endogenously synthesized, for maternal IgM and IgA do not cross the placenta. Reproduced with permission from Stiehm.[40]*

IgG

The term newborn synthesizes little immunoglobulin at birth but receives adult levels of IgG due to active transplacental transport from the mother. By term, the IgG level in the infant is slightly greater (110 percent) than the IgG level in the mother. Maternal IgG antibodies passively protect the infant from many infections for the first 6 months of life. After birth, the IgG level in the infant decreases due to normal catabolism of maternal IgG and the delay in the infant's own IgG synthesis. During this physiological hypogammaglobulinemia, the IgG level generally falls to a nadir of 300–500 ng/dl by 4 months. IgG synthesis the slowly increases and 60 percent of the adult IgG level of 1200 ng/dl is attained by 1 year. Adult levels are reached by 10 years. Levels of IgG are higher in post-mature infants than in term infants. In infants with Down's syndrome, IgG levels are decreased at birth, averaging 80 percent of the maternal concentrations. Premature infants, because of their lower cord IgG levels, have a more prolonged and severe physiological hypogammaglobulinemia and are more susceptible to neonatal infections.

IgM

IgM does not cross the placenta. There is some *in utero* synthesis and it is present in infants with a mean level of 10 ng/dl. IgM is the chief immunoglobulin synthesized by the newborn infant. Within a week of birth, IgM synthesis accelerates, stimulated by bacterial flora of the recently colonized gastrointestinal tract. Premature infants, regardless of gestational age, demonstrate a similarly accelerated IgM synthesis immediately after birth. IgM levels reach 50 percent of adult values by 6 months and 80 percent by 1 year.

IgA, IgD AND IgE

IgA, IgD and IgE neither cross the placenta, nor are synthesized in significant quantities by the newborn. Cord levels are extremely low and rise slowly in the first year, achieving 10–25 percent of adult levels by 12 months of age. IgA is occasionally elevated in post-mature infants, above 5 ng/dl in 5 percent. Adult levels are achieved by 15 years of age.

SECRETORY IgM AND IgA

sIgA and sIgM antibodies have been found in the saliva during the first few days after birth. sIgM antibodies predominate in the secretions of infants. As the synthesis and transport of sIgA antibodies into the saliva increases during the first 1–3 months of age, levels of the sIgM antibodies decrease in parallel, suggesting competition for the same transfer mechanism or replacement of the local IgM-producing cells by IgA producers. Adult concentrations of salivary sIgA antibodies develop from 6 months onwards.

INNATE IMMUNITY

Mononuclear cells

Macrophages are the first detectable element of the immune system. Primitive macrophages appear in the yolk sac from 4 weeks of gestation.[24] The early appearance of macrophages may be critical for normal embryogenesis, since tissue-specific ablation of macrophages in transgenic mice results in abnormalities in the development of these tissues. Later in gestation, when the fetal liver is the predominant site of hematopoiesis, first macrophages and then monocytes are produced.[24] After birth, hematopoiesis occurs in the bone marrow. In marrow, the monoblast, the mononuclear phagocyte precursor cell, differentiates to the promonocyte and subsequently to the mature, circulating monocyte.[10] The monoblast is a small, round cell that actively incorporates thymidine, is esterase and peroxidase negative, contains lysozyme and has complement and IgG receptors. The promonocyte contains specific monocyte enzymes, has complement and IgG receptors, and is capable of phagocytosis. The promonocyte divides several times before differentiating into the monocyte, and moving into the circulation. Blood monocytes circulate for 1–4 days, then migrate into the tissues. Some of the circulating blood monocytes bind to blood vessel walls and this marginating pool represents approximately 75 percent of the total intravascular monocyte pool. Resident tissue macrophages are replaced from the blood monocyte pool at a constant rate and exist both as fixed and free macrophages. Free macrophages are found in the pleural, synovial, peritoneal and alveolar spaces and in inflammatory sites. The less motile fixed tissue macrophages are present in the splenic sinusoids, in the liver as Kupffer cells, in reticulum cells of the bone marrow, in the lamina propria of the gastrointestinal tract, in specific sites in lymph nodes, in bone as osteoclasts and as microglia in the CNS.

Neutrophils

GRANULOCYTE DIFFERENTIATION

Neutrophil precursors appear later than macrophages. Neutrophils arise from bone marrow stem cells through a series of differentiation steps in which they lose their pleuripotency and commit to granulocyte differentiation. The last of the progenitor pool differentiate into committed myeloid cells of the neutrophil proliferative pool: myeloblasts, promyelocytes and myelocytes.

GRANULE DEVELOPMENT

The early promyelocyte is the first differentiation step to contain nucleated granules. The late promyelocyte is characterized by primary or azurophilic cytoplasmic granules containing hydrolases, proteases, lysosome and myeloperoxidase. With further differentiation, at the myelocytic stage, there is a loss of the deep blue appearance of the granules and a neutrophilic character is acquired, caused by an increase in secondary or specific granules. Specific granules of the neutrophil myelocyte contain lactoferrin and vitamin B12-binding protein; in the mature cell they outnumber the azurophilic granules by two to one. The neutrophil granules are generated in the Golgi complex and bud off from the endoplasmic reticulum. Early stages of neutrophil development are characterized by the presence of mitochondria; later stages are marked by a proliferation of glycogen with few mitochondria. This change represents a shift from aerobic metabolism to glycolysis as the major source of cell energy.

DEVELOPMENT OF MEMBRANE RECEPTORS

Early myeloid differentiation is characterized by the loss of CD34, the transient appearance and disappearance of HLA-DR on progenitor cells and the appearance of CD13 (aminopeptidase N) and CD38 (NAD glycohydrolase) on the myeloblast. Once they begin to differentiate, promyelocytes acquire complement receptors, CR3. Fcγ receptors appear at the metamelocyte stage.[15] These membrane adherence proteins are critical for chemotaxis and phagocytosis and their acquisition parallels development of these functions. Other factors play a role, as chemotaxis is reduced in early band forms compared to segmented forms.[6] Immature neutrophils are more rigid, because of altered actin polymerization, and have delayed microbial ingestion, compared to mature cells. Other surface receptors include erythrocyte and human granulocyte antigens. The granulocyte-specific antigens are polymorphic and responsible for immature neutropenias and febrile transfusion reactions.[3] Surface glycoprotein patterns change with maturation and this affects certain cell functions. Excessive N-acetylneuraminic acid on immature cells has been associated with a high negative surface charge with inhibition of adhesion and cell–cell interactions. Mature neutrophils are detected at 14–16 weeks of gestation.[8]

GRANULOCYTE FUNCTION

The bone marrow neutrophil storage pool of premature and term infants is considerably smaller than that of adults. Bacterial infection of the neonate may lead to rapid exhaustion of the storage pool and neutropenia.[14] It is uncertain at what age the infant storage pool achieves normal adult size. Neonatal neutrophils function poorly compared to those of older children and adults.[20] Most studies of neonatal granulocyte function have been performed on cord blood, containing both immature neutrophils (released under the stress of birth) and mature neutrophils exposed to cytokines associated with delivery, placental separation, acidosis and progesterone. Drugs used in delivery, such as anesthetics and antibiotics, may also alter the function of neonatal neutrophils.[16,27] Controversy, therefore, exists over which of the newborn neutrophil functions are abnormal. Chemotaxis and adherence related functions are decreased and chemotactic function does not reach adult levels until after 5 years of age.[28] Neonatal abnormalities in diapedesis-related functions include decreased expression of adherence proteins,[36] abnormal deformability, adherence, aggregation and actin polymerization[26,31] Cord blood neutrophils from elective cesarean sections have normal nitroblue tetrazolium reduction, oxygen consumption and hexose monophosphate shunt activity.[16] Unlike neutrophils from normal newborns, neutrophils from stressed or premature neonates have decreased oxidative responses and microbial killing activity.[11] This may explain the increased number of immature forms that accompany the neonate's response to stress. Phagocytosis is normal or supernormal.[19] Neutrophil lactoferrin levels are reduced in neonates and a high neutrophil turnover leads to decreased primary granule (myeloperoxidase-containing) content.[9]

Dendritic cells

Dendritic cells serve as accessory cells in initiation of primary immune responses. Dendritic cells have been identified as early as week 6 in the yolk sac.[23] By 12 weeks of gestation, they are present in the thymus, lymph nodes, spleen and non-lymphoid organs, where they occupy sites distinct from those of macrophages.[23] In the full-term newborn, dendritic cells can be cultured *in vitro* from cord blood hematopoietic progenitor cells.[35] Mononuclear phagocytes and dendritic cells have a common precursor.[34] In adults, dendritic cells are derived from bone marrow hematopoietic progenitor cells.[34] The kinetics of dendritic cell production are unclear. Some investigators propose heterogeneity in dendritic cell turnover, with rapidly and slowly dividing populations of cells in spleen and skin.[39] Most dendritic cells do not leave the organ they enter and are presumed to die *in situ*.[39]

Complement

Complement synthesis by fetal tissues occurs from 5.5 weeks of gestation. Complement proteins do not cross the placenta. C3, C4 and most other components are detectable in fetal serum by 10 weeks. Levels increase progressively with gestational age, reaching about 50–75 percent of maternal levels at term. As complement levels in the maternal circulation rise during pregnancy, this corresponds to 60–80 percent of normal adult levels. Levels of C8 and C9 are lower and may reach only 10 percent of the maternal concentration at term. C1 esterase inhibitor is present in adult concentrations from 28 weeks of gestation. Preterm and low-birth-weight infants have lower complement levels than term babies, but by 3 months of age, most complement levels are within the normal adult range. Relatively low levels of C3, Factor B and other components may be responsible for the decreased opsonic activity of neonatal serum and contribute to the increased susceptibility to infection. Lack of the febrile response and leukocytosis accompanying infection in some babies may also be related to the low complement component levels. Besides low complement levels, phagocytosis may be further compromised by the partial deficiency of the complement receptor, CR3, on the neonatal neutrophil which results in decreased adherence and complement-dependent phagocytosis when the cells are activated.[1]

Antigen processing and presentation

Fetal tissues express class 1 and class II MHC molecules at 12 weeks of gestation.[30] By this time, all the major 'professional' antigen-presenting cells (macrophages, B cells, Langerhan cells, dendritic cells) are present and their expression of class II MHC molecules is comparable with that in the adult.[12] At term, the fraction of blood monocytes from neonates that express HLA-DR, DP and DQ antigens is similar to that in adults,[12,18] although a subset expresses less HLA-DR.[18] Monocytes from newborns can present soluble and particulate antigens to maternal T cells as effectively as maternal monocytes, a response that is class II MHC restricted.[7] Fetal tissues are frequently vigorously rejected after transplantation into non-MHC-matched hosts. This indicates that the level of surface MHC expression on fetal tissues is sufficient to initiate an allogenic response by the host in which the foreign cells are killed by cytotoxic T cells and that antigen presentation by class I MHC for the generation of cytotoxic T cells is intact.

REFERENCES

1 Abughali, N., Berger, M., Tosi, M.F. (1994) Deficient total cell content of CR3 (CD11b) in neonatal neutrophils. *Blood* **83**, 1086–1092.

2 Asma, G.E., Van den Bergh, R.L., Vossen, J.M. (1983) Use of monoclonal antibodies in a study of the development of T lymphocytes in the human fetus. *Clinical Experimental Immunology* **53**, 429–436.

3 Billett, J.N., Caren, L.D. (1985) Human granulocyte antigens: current status and biological significance. *Experimental Biology Medicine* **178**, 12–23.

4 Bockman, D.E., Kirby, M.L. (1984) Dependence of thymus development on derivatives of the neural crest. *Science* **223**, 498–500.

5 Bofill, M., Janossy, G., Janossa, M. *et al.* (1985) Human B cell development. II. Subpopulations in the human fetus. *Journal of Immunology* **134**, 1531–1538.

6 Boner, A., Zeligs, B.J., Bellanti, J.A. (1982) Chemotactic responses of various differentiational stages of neutrophils from human cord and adult blood. *Infection and Immunity* **35**, 921–928.

7 Chilmonczyk, B.A., Levin, M.J., McDuffy, R., Hayward, A.R. (1985) Characterization of the human newborn response to herpesvirus antigen. *Journal of Immunology* **134**, 4184–4188.

8 Christensen, R.D. (1989) Hematopoiesis in the fetus and neonate. *Pediatric Research* **26**, 531–535.

9 Christensen, R.D., Rothstein, G. (1985) Neutrophil myeloperoxidase concentration: changes with development and during bacterial infection. *Pediatric Research* **19**, 1278–1282.

10 Douglas, S.D., Musson, R.A. (1986) Phagocytic defects – monocytes/macrophages. *Clinical Immunology and Immunopathology* **40**, 62–68.

11 Driscoll, M.S., Thomas, V.L., Ramamurthy, R.S., Casto, D.T. (1990) Longitudinal evaluation of polymorphonuclear leukocyte chemiluminescence in premature infants. *Journal of Pediatrics* **116**, 429–434.

12 Edwards, J.A., Jones, D.B., Evans, P.R., Smith, J.L. (1985) Differential expression of HLA class II antigens on human fetal and adult lymphocytes and macrophages. *Immunology* **55**, 489–500.

13 Ehlers, S., Smith, K.A. (1991) Differentiation of T cell lymphokine gene expression: the in vitro acquisition of T cell memory. *Journal of Experimental Medicine* **173**, 25–36.

14 Erdman, S.H., Christensen, R.D., Bradley, P.P., Rothstein, G. (1982) Supply and release of storage neutrophils. A developmental study. *Biology of the Neonate* **41**, 132–137.

15 Fleit, H.B., Wright, S.D., Durie, C.J., Valinsky, J.E., Unkeless, J.C. (1984) Ontogeny of Fc receptors and complement receptor (CR3) during human myeloid differentiation. *Journal of Clinical Investigation* **73**, 516–525.

16 Frazier, J.P., Cleary, T.G., Pickering, L.K., Kohl, S., Ross, P.J. (1982) Leukocyte function in healthy neonates following vaginal and cesarean section deliveries. *Journal of Pediatrics* **101**, 269–272.

17 Gandini, M., Kubagawa, H., Gathings, W.E., Lawton, A.R. (1981) Expression of three immunoglobulin isotypes by individual B cells during development: implications for heavy chain switching. *American Journal of Reproductive Immunology* **1**, 161–163.

18 Glover, D.M., Brownstein, D., Burchett, S., Larsen, A., Wilson, C.B. (1987) Expression of HLA class II antigens and secretion of interleukin-1 by monocytes and macrophages from adults and neonates. *Immunology* **61**, 195–201.

19 Harris, M.C., Stroobant, J., Cody, C.S., Douglas, S.D., Polin, R.A. (1983) Phagocytosis of group B streptococcus by neutrophils from newborn infants. *Pediatric Research* **17**, 358–361.

20 Hill, H.R. (1987) Biochemical, structural, and functional abnormalities of polymorphonuclear leukocytes in the neonate. *Pediatric Research* **22**, 375–382.

21 Janeway, C.A. Jr (1992) The T cell receptor as a multicomponent signalling machine: CD4/CD8 coreceptors and CD45 in T cell activation. *Annual Review of Immunology* **10**, 645–674.

22 Janeway, C.A. Jr, Travers, P. (1996) The thymus and the development of T lymphocytes. In *Immunobiology, the Immune System in Health and Disease*, 2nd edn. Edinburgh: Churchill Livingstone, 6.4.

23 Janossy, G., Bofill, M., Poulter, L.W. *et al.* (1986) Separate ontogeny of two macrophage-like accessory cell populations in the human fetus. *Journal of Immunology* **136**, 4354–4361.

24 Kelemen, E., Janossa, M. (1980) Macrophages are the first differentiated blood cells formed in human embryonic liver. *Experimental Hematology* **8**, 996–1000.

25 Kipps, T.J. (1989) The CD5 B cell. *Advances in Immunology* **47**, 117–185.

26 Krause, P.J., Maderazo, E.G., Scroggs, M. (1982) Abnormalities of neutrophil adherence in newborns. *Pediatrics* **69**, 184–187.

27 Krumholz, W., Demel, C., Jung, S., Meuthen, G., Hempelmann, G. (1993) The influence of intravenous anaesthetics on polymorphonuclear leukocyte function. *Canadian Journal of Anaesthesia* **40**, 770–774.

28 Mohandes, A.E., Touraine, J.L., Osman, M., Salle, B. (1982) Neutrophil chemotaxis in infants of diabetic mothers and in preterms at birth. *Journal of Clinical Laboratory Immunology* **8**, 117–120.

29 Mortari, F., Wang, J.Y., Schroeder, H.W. Jr (1993) Human cord blood antibody repertoire. Mixed population of VH gene segments and CDR3 distribution in the expressed C alpha and C gamma repertoires. *Journal of Immunology* **150**, 1348–1357.

30 Oliver, A.M., Sewell, H.F., Abramovich, D.R., Thomson, A.W. (1989) The distribution and differential expression of MHC class II antigens (HLA-DR, DP, and DQ) in human fetal adrenal, pancreas, thyroid, and gut. *Transplantation Proceedings* **21**, 651–652.

31 Olson, T.A., Ruymann, F.B., Cook, B.A., Burgess, D.P., Henson, S.A., Thomas, P.J. (1983) Newborn polymorphonuclear leukocyte aggregation: a study of physical properties and ultrastructure using chemotactic peptides. *Pediatric Research* **17**, 993–997.

32 Peakman, M., Vergani, D. (1997) *Basic and Clinical Immunology*. Edinburgh: Churchill Livingstone, 74.

33 Purkerson, J., Isakson, P. (1992) A two-signal model for regulation of immunoglobulin isotype switching. *FASEB Journal* **6**, 3245–3252.

34 Reid, C.D., Fryer, P.R., Clifford, C., Kirk, A., Tikerpae, J., Knight, S.C. (1990) Identification of hematopoietic progenitors of macrophages and dendritic Langerhans cells (DL-CFU) in human bone marrow and peripheral blood. *Blood* **76**, 1139–1149.

35 Santiago-Schwarz, F., Belilos, E., Diamond, B., Carsons, S.E. (1992) TNF in combination with GM-CSF enhances the differentiation of neonatal cord blood stem cells into dendritic cells and macrophages. *Journal of Leukocyte Biology* **52**, 274–281.

36 Smith, J.B., Campbell, D.E., Ludomirsky, A. *et al.* (1990) Expression of the complement receptors CR1 and CR3 and the type III Fc gamma receptor on neutrophils from newborn infants and from fetuses with Rh disease. *Pediatric Research* **28**, 120–126.

37 Solvason, N., Kearney, J.F. (1992) The human fetal omentum: a site of B cell generation. *Journal of Experimental Medicine* **175**, 397–404.

38 Splawski, J.B., Jelinek, D.F., Lipsky, P.E. (1991) Delineation of the functional capacity of human neonatal lymphocytes. *Journal of Clinical Investigation* **87**, 545–553.

39 Steinman, R.M. (1991) The dendritic cell system and its role in immunogenicity. *Annual Review of Immunology* **9**, 271–296.

40 Stiehm, R. (1996) *Immunologic Disorders in Infants and Children*, 4th edn. London: W.B. Saunders, 67.

41 Vandekerckhove, B.A., Baccala, R., Jones, D., Kono, D.H., Theofilopoulos, A.N., Roncarolo, M.G. (1992) Thymic selection of the human T cell receptor V beta repertoire in SCID-hu mice. *Journal of Experimental Medicine* **176**, 1619–1624.

6

Adaptation at birth

ANTHONY D MILNER with contributions from HUGO LAGERCRANTZ

THE ONSET OF BREATHING

Before the onset of labor the respiratory system is fluid-filled (Chapter 3) and receives less than 10 percent of the cardiac output.[59] Recent studies using three-dimensional ultrasound techniques have shown that the fetal fluid FRC at term is close to the functional residual capacity (FRC) of the neonate after adaptation.[5] Although there is great variability, the median time for the onset of respiratory effort is in the region of 10 seconds,[64] some infants commencing respiratory efforts immediately the thorax is released from the birth canal.

Stimuli for the first breath

Although the fetus makes intermittent respiratory efforts from 10 to 11 weeks of gestation,[10] these are usually absent immediately before and during labor. The factors responsible for the onset of breathing can be divided into intrinsic and extrinsic influences.

INTRINSIC FACTORS

Occlusion of the umbilical cord of the fetal lamb elicits gasping movements. Birth is also associated with the removal of respiratory inhibitory mechanisms including prostaglandins and adenosine. Unlike the fetus who is mainly asleep, the newly born infant is usually awake. This is probably related to the enormous surge of catecholamines at birth (p. 28). Even though most of the catecholamines do not pass the blood–brain barrier, there is probably a parallel activation of the cerebral noradrenergic system mainly originating from the locus ceruleus. The norepinephrine (noradrenaline) turnover is increased about two- to threefold in the newborn rat.[40] It may be a little contradictory as norepinephrine inhibits

the inspiration at a brainstem level. It is probable it is involved in an off-switch mechanism of the inspiratory drive. At birth, however, the global stimulation of the forebrain drive probably overrides the more local effects.[7] In addition, there is a switching on of genes encoding for neurotransmitters involved in respiratory control. For example, the expression of mRNA encoding for preprotachykinin A – the precursor of substance P – is increased about fourfold in the dorsal respiratory group of the newborn rabbit. This increased expression was only seen in newborn rabbits that had started to breathe.[63] Increased expression of mRNA for the SP precursor has also been observed in the newborn rat.[69] SP neurons seem to play an important role in the respiratory rhythm generation.

Activation of the CO_2 drive is also probably important to allow the control system to respond to metabolic demands. The central chemoreceptor areas seem to be activated at birth, as indicated by the expression of immediate early genes, such as c-*fos*. It is possible that skin cooling is involved in this activation.[33] The peripheral chemoreceptors were previously believed to be activated at birth and trigger the first breaths. Peripheral chemoreceptor integrity, however, is not critical to this response, as denervation of the carotid chemoreceptors did not prevent the onset of respiration[37] and severe hypoxia, a PaO_2 of 1.2 kPa (9.0 mmHg), stimulated inspiratory gasps even after total peripheral chemodenervation.[9] The carotid bodies are set at a lower PO_2 level and actually become silent at birth. If the baby is severely asphyxiated, it is possible that the peripheral chemoreceptors are activated, stimulating gasps. The peripheral chemoreceptor drive, however, is to some extent overridden by central hypoxic depression.

EXTRINSIC FACTORS

Cooling is probably the most important influence. Applying cool air to the snout of a term lamb induces breathing[46] and skin cooling results in respiratory activity in fetal lambs.[53] By contrast, nursing newborn lambs in warm water induces apnea[56] and the onset of respiration is delayed in the human neonate who is born directly into warm water. Painful stimuli such as the flicking of feet often stimulates the onset of respiratory efforts, both in animals[55] and the human newborn, a feature which has been made use of by countless generations of obstetricians and midwives. The role of audiovisual, proprioceptive and touch stimuli remains poorly defined but may well be important, possibly by recruiting central neurons and increasing central arousal.[18] The relationship of arousal to the onset of regular respiration has been investigated in newborn lambs.[35,36] Careful observation of the human neonate has shown that the infant is born hypotonic, but then develops tone often making movements associated with arousal before commencing breathing.[64]

The first breath

The first studies of the pressure/volume changes associated with the first breath were carried out by Karlberg and colleagues.[39] They used a water-filled catheter to measure intrathoracic pressure and a reverse plethysmograph to measure tidal exchange. After 97 attempts, data were obtained on 11 infants. The time to the first breath varied between 6 and 93 seconds and all but three infants took more than 20 seconds. The inspiratory volume varied from 12 to 67 ml and the inspiratory pressure ranged from 3 to 72 cmH$_2$O.

'OPENING PRESSURE PHENOMENON'

In five of Karlberg's infants[39] there was an apparent opening pressure phenomenon, that is, the intrathoracic pressure fell by more than 20 cmH$_2$O before any volume change occurred. In the remaining six, however, a variety of patterns were seen; either there was no opening pressure phenomenon, that is, volume entered the lung at the same time as pressure fell, or the first movement was expiratory and associated with a positive intrathoracic pressure. Milner and Saunders,[48] using very similar techniques except that intrathoracic pressure was measured by an esophageal balloon mounted on a catheter, were able to obtain data on 24 healthy newborn infants. They also found a range of inspiratory pressures were associated with the first breath, but five infants apparently expanded their lungs with pressures less than 20 cmH$_2$O and the 'opening pressure phenomenon' noted by Karlberg was rarely seen. An inspiratory volume of 40 ml was documented, a similar value to that noted previously.[39]

Karlberg et al.[39] considered the 'opening pressure' to be a normal requirement, as during the first breath an air–water interface forms within the alveoli and air only enters the isolated collapsed lung once a critical pressure, usually above 20 cmH$_2$O, is exceeded.[4] Karlberg[39] put forward three possible mechanisms whereby lung expansion occurred without an opening pressure having been exceeded. These were: first, by outward recoil of the chest wall as it escaped from the birth canal; second, by frog breathing, whereby the baby manages to force air down into his lungs by contraction of the buccal muscles; and third, by the capillary erection.[38] Jaykka[38] had suggested that distention of the lung capillaries, as the pulmonary vascular resistance fell, had a supporting effect on the walls of the 'crumpled sack-like alveoli'. There have been no observations in man to support the concept of frog breathing and, although there has been some recent interest in the capillary erectile theory, this effect is only likely to occur when the lungs have been expanded and the relative fetal hypoxia relieved. In an attempt to explore the role of chest wall recoil, further measurements were made commencing after delivery of the head but while the chest and abdomen remained in the birth canal. This proved to be a relatively simple procedure with a high success rate and in excess of 100 measurements were carried out using this approach.[61,64,65] It was confirmed that during delivery the chest and abdomen are exposed to very high pressures often exceeding 250 cmH$_2$O and that the intrathoracic pressure falls to atmospheric as the chest and abdomen escape from the birth canal. On no occasion, however, was any chest wall recoil effect observed (Figure 6.1). This is not surprising, however, as the chest wall of the neonate is a relatively compliant structure, very dependent on muscle tone to achieve its normal configuration. Immediately at birth the infant is almost always hypotonic, tone returning just before the onset of the first breath. These further measurements confirmed that an 'opening pressure' phenomenon was rarely seen. The lack of an opening pressure at the onset of inspiration was predictable as, immediately at birth, the air–water interface is not at the terminal bronchioles but in the pharynx.

INSPIRATORY PRESSURE

A number of the measurements by both Karlberg's and Milner's group had suggested that some infants expanded their lungs at birth with pressures of less than 20 cmH$_2$O. Some of the measurements, however, might have been artifactual as it has been well demonstrated that unless the pressure-sensing device lies in the lower third of the esophagus, intrathoracic pressure changes can be underestimated. It was obviously not possible in the short time available during the infant's birth to be sure that the balloon or water-filled catheter was correctly placed. To overcome that problem, a further series of measurements were made using a catheter onto which two micropressure transducers were mounted 5 cm apart. Attempts were made to position the catheter with the distal transducer in the stomach as evidenced by positive

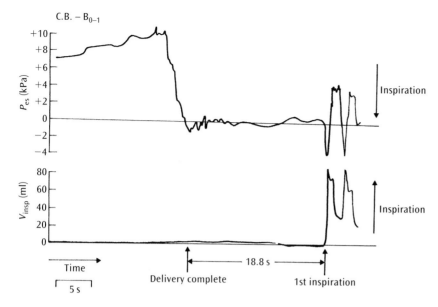

Figure 6.1 *Thoracic pressure and volume changes from soon after the delivery of the head up until the second breath had occurred. The thorax is initially compressed by pressures of up to 110 cmH₂O (10.5 kPa). There is no change in thoracic volume until the first active inspiration.*

Table 6.1 *Definitive first breath*

	PI (cmH₂O)	PE (cmH₂O)	VI (ml)	FRC (ml)	Squeeze (cmH₂O)
Mean	−52.3	71.3	37.7	15.1	145
Range	−28 to −105	18–115	6.5–69	0–32	88–264
Median	−38.6	72	36.5	15.2	128

pressure measurements. Such a position for the distal transducer would ensure that the more proximal transducer lay in the lower third of the esophagus, this would be confirmed by negative pressure recordings. Satisfactory stomach and esophageal pressure changes associated with the first breath were collected from 24 of 50 vaginal deliveries.[65] Although the inspiratory volume (mean 37.7 ml, range 6.5–69 ml) was very similar to that documented previously,[48] the mean inspiratory pressure was 52.3 cmH₂O (median 38.6 cmH₂O, range 28–105 cmH₂O) (Table 6.1). These data argue that the pressures of less than 20 cmH₂O found in previous studies[39,64] were indeed artifactual and almost certainly the result of incorrect placement of the esophageal pressure measuring device.

EXPIRATORY PRESSURE

The first expiration is almost always active and pressures ranging from 18 to 115 cmH₂O can be generated (Figure 6.1).[65] This pressure change, representing the first cry, is often prolonged, compared to the first inspiration. It may be important both in aiding ventilation distribution and helping clear further fluid from the lungs.

FORMATION OF FRC

Initial data on the formation of the FRC obtained by cineradiography studies on healthy newborn babies[31] indicated that there was often evidence of aeration after the first breath, whereas only seven of the 11 infants in

Karlberg's study[39] had established an FRC. Three subsequent studies[48,61,64] have confirmed an FRC is formed in more than 95 percent of infants, with values of 18 ml and 15.1 ml and a range of 1–32 ml. Although no direct relationship between the magnitude of the first inspiratory pressure and the FRC was demonstrated, there was a significant relationship between the product of the inspiratory pressure and inspiratory time and both the inspiratory volume and the formation of an FRC. Plethysmographic studies[11] showed that by 2 hours the FRC increased to a mean of 32.2 ml/kg, that is, in excess of 110 ml for a 3.5 kg baby. No significant further change occurred over the subsequent 48 hours.

The effects of delivery by cesarean section without and with labor

Delivery by elective cesarean section is associated with first breaths of similar inspiratory pressure and volume as occurred following vaginal delivery.[64] Those data were obtained from 12 term infants; an esophageal pressure transducer system was passed through the baby's mouth as soon as the infant's head was delivered through the uterine incision and a face mask pneumotachograph applied to the infant's face before the chest and trunk were delivered through the uterine incision. The mean chest wall compression recorded was 72.7 cmH₂O (range 18–113 cmH₂O), but this was applied for less than 10 seconds. The mean inspiratory pressure was 40 cmH₂O and inspiratory volume 33.4 ml. In only five of the 11 infants in whom these data could be obtained was an FRC achieved, the mean value was 10.8 ml. Measurements by total body plethysmograph revealed that at 2–6 hours, the FRC was only 21.6 ml/kg in babies born by cesarean section compared to 32.2 ml/kg in vaginally delivered babies. At 42–54 hours the FRC in the former group had risen to 30.4 ml/kg.[49] The failure of infants born by cesarean section to form an FRC has been recognized for many years. Flagg[29] wrote that 'cesarean section in which compression of the chest had not taken place leaves the child's respiratory tract filled with fluid, much of which is inhaled'.

Infants born by emergency cesarean section had an FRC at 2–6 hours of 28.3 ml, that is, intermediate between vaginally and elective cesarean section delivered infants. Their FRC rose to 35.5 ml by 18–30 hours, identical to the vaginally delivered babies.[11] These data suggest that both exposure to labor with the associated high catecholamine levels and passage down the birth canal aid in the formation of the FRC. Studies of crying vital capacity, the volume of air expelled during a vigorous induced cry, have demonstrated this also to be significantly lower in the infants born by cesarean section rather than by vaginal delivery.[14]

In conflict with these findings are studies by Mortola and colleagues,[51] who found that the FRC after the first breath after cesarean section was similar to that after vaginal delivery. Sandberg et al.[60] were unable to show any significant effect of mode of delivery on FRC measured at 2 and 26 hours of age using a nitrogen washout technique, but did find that thoracic gas volume (TGV) measured by body plethysmography was significantly lower in the cesarean section infants at 26 hours. Lodrup-Carlsen and Carlsen[44] were also unable to detect any effect of mode of delivery on respiratory system compliance or resistance in the first 4 days of life.

Prenatal epinephrine (adrenaline) infusions, however, led to improvements in postnatal blood gases in lambs born by cesarean section[6] and in a randomized controlled trial terbutaline given intravenously to the mother for 2 hours prior to elective cesarean section led to significant improvements in lung compliance and resistance in the babies compared to controls given only saline.[22]

In view of these conflicting results, a further series of postnatal lung volume measurements were carried out using both gas dilution (argon) and total body plethysmography.[41] Twenty infants were studied, 10 of whom were born by elective cesarean section. Although the reduction in TGV at 4–6 hours of age in the cesarean sectioned infants compared to those born vaginally failed to reach significance (23.1 vs 26.7 ml/kg, $P = 0.08$); only infants born by cesarean section had a significant increase in TGV between 4–6 and 24 hours. There was no significant difference in the results of the gas dilution FRC measurements between infants born by different modes of delivery (Figure 6.2). The differences between this study and the one carried out in 1981 by Boon and colleagues[11] may be due to improvements in obstetric anesthesia but continue to support the concept that failure of exposure to high levels of catecholamines during labor and delivery by cesarean section does place the newly born infant at a disadvantage.

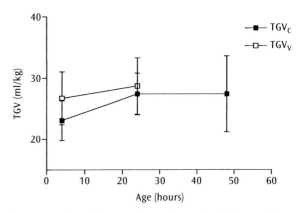

Figure 6.2 *Thoracic gas volume changes in the hours after birth in babies born by normal vaginal delivery (TGV$_V$) and after elective cesarean section delivery (TGV$_c$) (mean ±1 SD). Only in the infants born by cesarean section is there a significant increase in TGV between 4 and 24 hours (from Lee et al.[41]).*

Air trapping in the immediate neonatal period

A number of studies[32,52] have suggested that the resting lung volume (FRC) in the neonatal period when measured by gas dilution techniques is at least 30 percent lower than values obtained using a total body plethysmograph. One possible explanation for the differences is that the gas dilution techniques are usually performed under hyperoxic conditions, possibly leading to atelectasis, while the plethysmographic measurements have all been carried out while the infants are breathing air. This explanation, however, was not substantiated, as the results were similar when the measurements when repeated in either air or in 100 percent oxygen.[11] The gas dilution technique, unlike the plethysmographic method, only measures the volume of gas in direct contact with the central airways, thus an alternative hypothesis is that there is a significant amount of trapped gas in the lung immediately after birth.[62] It is likely, although unproven, that the trapped gas may be due to fluid within the small airways.[62] No studies have been carried out to assess the duration of this 'trapped gas' but measurements carried out on asymptomatic preterm babies over the age of 6 months have shown that the gas dilution FRC is then often within 10 percent of the plethysmographic lung volume.

CARDIOVASCULAR ADAPTATION AT BIRTH

During fetal life the lungs do not gas exchange and are bypassed by the circulation. In late gestation, 40 percent of the cardiac output goes to the placenta where gas exchange does take place. Two vascular shunts, the ductus venosus on the venous side of the circulation and the ductus arteriosus on the arterial side of the circulation, facilitate oxygenated blood avoiding the liver and lungs, respectively.

Closure of the ductus venosus

Blood from the umbilical vein can pass via the ductus venosus directly to the inferior vena cava (IVC); approximately 50 percent of the umbilical venous blood takes that route in the fetal lamb. After birth there is a large drop in blood flow through the ductus venosus, as 95 percent of the blood previously came via the umbilical vein.[21] Within hours of birth, this change is associated with functional closure of the ductus venosus occurring by retraction and inlet narrowing.[47] In the human, however, the ductus venosus can potentially reopen for days,[66] permanent obliteration by proliferation of connective tissue filling the lumen only being complete by 20 days.[47] It is unlikely that this is brought about by changes in prostaglandin levels.[1]

Closure of the ductus arteriosus

The ductus arteriosus connects the pulmonary artery to the descending aorta. It is made up of smooth muscle and patency in the fetus is maintained by both circulating and locally produced prostaglandins (PGE_2 and PGI_2). Constriction of the ductus begins soon after the onset of breathing and is complete in humans by 15 hours.[15] This is partly due to the increase in the oxygen tension of the blood perfusing the ductus. The sensitivity of the ductus to oxygen develops in the last trimester of pregnancy.[15] Ductal closure is also mediated by reduction in prostaglandin levels due to an increased catabolism of PGE_2 by the lung at higher gestational ages[16] and a higher rate of clearance with elevation of pulmonary blood flow at birth. The sensitivity of the ductus to PGE_2 and PGI_2 also decreases. In addition, ductal closure is facilitated by the decrease in pulmonary artery pressure.[17]

Changes in pulmonary blood flow and pulmonary vascular resistance

Before birth the pulmonary vascular resistance is higher than systemic and this results in an 80–90 percent right-to-left shunt.[59] The fetal pulmonary vessels are chemoreactive from mid-gestation and their sensitivity increases with advancing gestational age.[57] Hypoxia and acidosis increase constriction, whereas oxygen, acetylcholine and bradykinin stimulate dilation. At birth, the pulmonary vascular resistance falls rapidly to approximately 10 percent of fetal values and pulmonary blood flow increases tenfold.[43] There are two mechanisms: relief of hypoxia[58] and lung expansion.[13] Although perfusion of unventilated lungs by oxygenated blood and lung expansion with oxygenated liquids can cause vasodilation,[20,50] a response

also occurs following lung expansion with both air and 100 percent nitrogen. The mechanical effect results from the creation of surface forces at the gas–liquid interface within the alveoli; this physically expands small blood vessels and decreases perivascular pressure.[68] In addition, repeated expansion of the lung[42,43] stimulates the pulmonary production of prostaglandins. The pulmonary vasodilation occurs in two stages, a rapid component due to mechanical vasodilation and a slow one effected by elevation of prostaglandin levels. The pulmonary artery pressure falls from about 60 mmHg at birth to 30 mmHg by 24 hours of age.[23] The fall in pulmonary vascular resistance is associated with an increase in pulmonary blood flow.[28] Measurements using the argon, freon re-breathing method[19] have shown that the effective pulmonary blood flow, that is, the blood flow in contact with the alveoli, rises from 78 ml/kg/min at between 2 and 6 hours to 160 ml/kg/min at 72 hours of age in healthy full-term babies. Color and quantitative Doppler echocardiography studies in the first 24 hours after birth have facilitated documentation of differences in the rate of cardiac output, left pulmonary artery flow, aortopulmonary pressure difference, ductal flow and ductal flow characteristics between infants with and without respiratory distress.[68] In healthy infants, the majority of changes had occurred by 8 hours after birth, although there was some degree of right-to-left ductal shunting even up to 12 hours after birth. In infants with respiratory failure, however, there was a significant delay in ductal closure and a high incidence of persistent pulmonary hypertension (Figure 6.3).

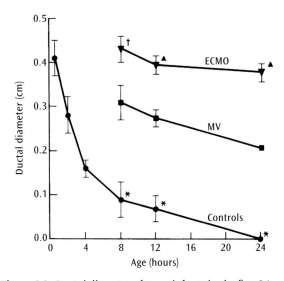

Figure 6.3 *Ductal diameter of term infants in the first 24 hours of life.* ●, *controls;* ■, *mechanical ventilation (MV);* ▼, *ventilated infants qualifying for ECMO (ECMO);* *, *controls versus MV and ECMO infants (P < 0.001);* †, *ECMO versus MV infants (P < 0.025);* ▲, *ECMO versus MV infants (P < 0.001).* *(Reproduced from Walther* et al. *1993)*

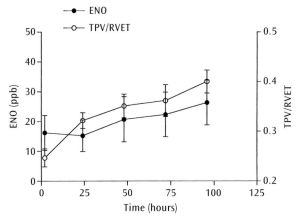

Figure 6.4 *Pulmonary vascular resistance as measured by the ratio of time to peak ejection velocity to right ventricular systolic ejection time (TPV/RVET) and mean expired nitric oxide concentration (ENO) in the hours after birth (mean ±1 SE). Over the first 24 hours there is an increase in the TPV/RVET but no change in the ENO. Subsequently both the ENO and the ratio increase with time (from Aiton, 1998).*

An important factor in the adaptation process is the balance between endogenous nitric oxide (NO), a smooth muscle relaxant and endothelin-1, an endothelium-derived contracting factor (p. 376). NO plasma metabolites (nitrites and nitrates) were found to be low at birth, but rose over the subsequent hours and days, while endothelin-1 fell with age.[25,26] The same group have shown that the ratio of NO metabolites to ET-1 was inversely related to the pulmonary artery pressure measured by pulsed Doppler.[27] Biban and colleagues[8] were unable to show any significant change in expired NO levels over the first 48 hours of age and no correlation between expired NO and plasma NO metabolites. However, Aiton and colleagues[3] found that, although the expired NO levels did not alter over the first 24 hours of age, there was then a significant and progressive increase. The pulmonary circulation, as assessed by pulmonary artery pressure (pulsed Doppler) and effective pulmonary blood flow measurements, increased progressively from birth. These changes were related to the expired NO levels, but only after 24 hours of age (Figure 6.4). These findings suggest that endogenous NO is not responsible for the initial drop in pulmonary vascular resistance, but is important subsequently.

Closure of the foramen ovale

At birth the left atrial pressure rises due to the increase in pulmonary blood flow, while at the same time the right atrial pressure falls due to cessation of the circulation from the placenta. This alteration in pressures occurs within the first few breaths and is associated with functional closure of the foramen ovale.[66] Permanent closure, which is brought about by fixation of the valve to the interatrial septum, can take months.

Changes in cardiac output

Cardiac output is highest 1 hour after birth; the increase, however, is short lived, lasting only for 4 hours.[68] This increase is dependent on the prenatal influence of thyroid hormone.[12] Cardiac output stabilizes by 24 hours of age.[2] The cardiac output of the full-term infant on the first day is relatively greater than that of older children and adults.[24] The high cardiac output of the newborn is due to a greater heart rate. The cardiac output is higher following vaginal delivery than cesarean section and in prematurely born children corrected for body weight.[30,67]

GASEOUS EXCHANGE AND BLOOD GASES AT BIRTH

Gaseous exchange in healthy term and preterm infants has been investigated by collection of expired gases over 15 second intervals from immediately after birth.[54] The mean oxygen uptake rose from 7 ml/kg/min at 15 seconds to nearly 12 ml/kg/min at 2 minutes, then fell back to 8 ml/kg/min by 5 minutes. Carbon dioxide elimination closely mimicked these changes rising from 6.5 ml/kg/min at 15 seconds to 10 ml/kg/min by 2 minutes. Infants born by cesarean section had a much slower rise in CO_2 excretion, remaining below 6 ml/kg/min for the first 90 seconds, but then rising to 8–9 ml/kg/min by 4 minutes of age. Interestingly, the preterm infants showed a very similar pattern of CO_2 excretion rate changes to the term infants delivered by cesarean section. The CO_2 excretion patterns are of particular interest, as they are affected by changes in both pulmonary blood flow and ventilation.

Improvements in arterial oxygenation in the minutes after delivery have been documented by oximetry. Arterial saturation rose from 61 percent at 1 minute to in excess of 85 percent by 5 minutes of age in 32 full-term infants born by vaginal delivery.[34] In 44 infants born by cesarean section, however, the initial saturation was significantly lower at 48 percent at 1 minute, but rose to greater than 85 percent by 7 minutes of age. A subsequent study[45] found that in infants born cesarean section the saturation, as measured by an oximeter mounted on the right hand, rose from 20 percent at 1 minute to over 90 percent by 4 minutes, while the saturation as measured on the right foot was initially less than 10 and took over 10 minutes to rise to above 90 percent. These data indicate the presence of right-to-left shunting at ductal level over the first few minutes of life.

REFERENCES

1 Adeagbo, A.S.O., Coceani, F., Olley, P.M. (1982) The response of the lamb ductus venosus to prostaglandins and inhibitors of prostaglandin and thromboxane synthesis. *Circulation Research* **51**, 580–586.

2 Agata, Y., Hirashi, S., Oguchi, K. *et al.* (1991) Changes in left ventricular output from fetal to early neonatal life. *Journal of Pediatrics* **119**, 441–445.

3 Aiton, N.R. (1998) The role of nitric oxide in cardiorespiratory adaptation at birth. MD Thesis, University of London.

4 Avery, M.E., Frank, N.R., Gribetz, I. (1959) The inflationary force produced by pulmonary vascular distension in excised lungs. The possible relation of this force to that needed to expand the lungs at birth. *Journal of Clinical Investigation* **38**, 456–461.

5 Bahmaie, A., Hughes, S.W., Clark, T.H. *et al.* (2000) Serial fetal lung volume measurement using three-dimensional ultrasound. *Ultrasound in Obstetrics and Gynecology* **16**, 154–158.

6 Berger, P.J., Kyriakides, M.A., Smolich, J.J. *et al.* (2000) Influence of prenatal adrenaline infusion on arterial blood gases after caesarean delivery in the lamb. *Journal of Physiology* **527**, 377–385.

7 Bianchi, A.L., Denavit-Saubie, M., Champagnat, J. (1995) Central control of breathing in mammals: neuronal circuitry, membrane properties, and neurotransmitters. *Physiological Reviews* **75**, 1–45.

8 Biban, P., Zangardim, T., Baraldi, E. *et al.* (2001) Mixed exhaled nitric oxide and plasma nitrites and nitrates in newborn infants. *Life Sciences* **68**, 2789–2797.

9 Biscoe, T.J., Purves, M.J. (1967) Carotid body chemoreceptor activity in the newborn lamb. *Journal of Physiology* **190**, 443–454.

10 Boddy, K., Robinson, J.S. (1971) External method for detection of fetal breathing *in utero*. *Lancet* **2**, 1231–1233.

11 Boon, A.W., Milner, A.D., Hopkin, I.E. (1981) Lung volumes and lung mechanics in babies born vaginally and by elective and emergency lower segmental caesarean section. *Journal of Pediatrics* **98**, 812–815.

12 Breall, J.A., Rudolph, A.M., Heymann, M.A. (1984) Role of thyroid hormone in postnatal circulatory and metabolic adjustments. *Journal of Clinical Investigation* **73**, 1418–1424.

13 Cassin, S., Dawes, G.S., Mott, J.C. *et al.* (1964) The vascular resistance of the total and newly ventilated lung of the lamb. *Journal of Physiology* **171**, 61–79.

14 Chiswick, M.L., Milner, R.D.G. (1976) Crying vital capacity measurement of neonatal lung function. *Archives of Disease in Childhood* **51**, 22–27.

15 Clyman, R.I. (1987) Ductus arteriosus: current theories of prenatal and postnatal regulation. *Seminars in Perinatology* **11**, 64–71.

16 Clyman, R.I., Mauray, F., Heymann, M.A., Roman, C. (1981) Effect of gestational age on pulmonary metabolism of prostaglandin E1 and E2. *Prostaglandins* **21**, 505–513.

17 Clyman, R.I., Mauray, F., Heymann, M.A., Roman, C. (1989) Influence of increased pulmonary vascular pressures on the closure of the ductus arteriosus in newborn lambs. *Pediatric Research* **25**, 136–142.

18 Condorelli, S., Scarpelli, E.M. (1975) Somatic-respiratory reflex and onset of regular breathing movements in the lamb foetus in utero. *Pediatric Research* **9**, 879–884.

19 Cotton, E.K., Cogswell, J.J., Cropp, G.J.A. (1971) Measurement of effective pulmonary blood flow in the normal newborn human infants. *Pediatrics* **47**, 520–528.

20 Dawes, G.S. 1968: *Foetal and Neonatal Physiology*. Chicago: Year Book Medical Publishers.

21 Edelstone, D.I., Rudolph, A.M., Heymann, M.A. (1978) Liver and ductus venosus blood flows in fetal lambs in utero. *Circulation Research* **42**, 426–433.

22 Eisler, G., Hjertberg, R., Lagercrantz, H. (1999) Randomised controlled trial of effect of terbutaline before elective caesarean section on postnatal respiration and glucose homeostasis. *Archives of Disease in Childhood Fetal and Neonatal Edition* **80**, F88–F92.

23 Emmanouilides, G.C., Moss, A.J., Duffie, E.R., Adams, F.H. (1964) Pulmonary arterial pressure changes in human newborn infants from birth to three days of age. *Journal of Pediatrics* **65**, 327–333.

24 Emmanouilides, G.C., Moss, A.J., Monset-Couchard, M. *et al.* (1970) Cardiac output in newborn infants. *Biology of the Neonate* **15**, 186–197.

25 Endo, A., Shimada, M., Ayusawa, M. *et al.* (1996) Nitric oxide and endothelin 1 during postnatal life. *Biology of the Neonate* **70**, 15–20.

26 Endo, A., Ayusawa, M., Minaot, M. *et al.* (1997) Endothelium-derived relaxing and contracting factors during the early neonatal period. *Acta Paediatrica* **86**, 834–836.

27 Endo, A., Ayusawa, M., Minato, M. *et al.* (2000) Physiologic significance of nitric oxide and endothelin-1 in circulatory adaptation. *Pediatrics International* **42**, 26–30.

28 Evans, N.J., Archer, L.N.J. (1990) Postnatal circulatory adaptation in healthy term and preterm neonates. *Archives of Disease in Childhood* **65**, 24–26.

29 Flagg, P.J. (1928) The treatment of asphyxia in the newborn. *Journal of the American Medical Association* **91**, 788–791.

30 Gessner, I., Krovetz, L.J., Benson, R.W. *et al.* (1965) Hemodynamic adaptations in the newborn infant. *Pediatrics* **36**, 752–762.

31 Geubelle, F., Karlberg, P., Koch, G. *et al.* (1959) L'aeration du poumon chez le nouveau-né. *Biologia Neonatorum* **1**, 169–174.

32 Geubelle, F., Francotte, M., Beyer, M. *et al.* (1977) Functional residual capacity and thoracic gas volume in normoxic and hyperoxic newborn infants. *Acta Paediatrica Belgica* **30**, 221–225.

33 Gluckman, P.D., Gunn, T.R., Johnston, B.M. (1983) The effect of cooling on breathing and shivering unanaesthetized fetal lambs in utero. *Journal of Physiology* **343**, 495–506.

34 Harris, A.P., Sendak, M.J., Donham, R.T. (1986) Changes in arterial oxygen saturation immediately after birth in the human neonate. *Journal of Pediatrics* **109**, 117–119.

35 Hasan, S.J., Rigaux, A. (1991) The effects of lung distention, oxygenation and gestational age on fetal behaviour and breathing movements in sheep. *Pediatric Research* **30**, 193–201.

36 Hasan, S.J., Rigaux, A. (1992) Effect of bilateral vagotomy on oxygenation, arousal and healthy movements in fetal sheep. *Journal of Applied Physiology* **73**, 1402–1412.

37 Jansen, A.H., Ioffe, S., Russell, B.J., Chernick, V. (1981) Effect of carotid chemoreceptor denervation on breathing in utero and after birth. *Journal of Applied Physiology* **51**, 630–633.

38 Jaykka, S. (1954) A new theory concerning the mechanism of initiation of respiration in the newborn. *Acta Paediatric Scandinavica* **43**, 339–344.

39 Karlberg, P., Cherry, R.B., Escardo, F.E., *et al.* (1962) Respiratory studies in newborn infants II. Pulmonary mechanics of breathing in the first minutes of life, including the onset of respiration. *Acta Paediatrica Scandinavica* **51**, 121–136.

40 Lagercrantz, H., Pequignot, J., Pequignot, J.M., Peyrin, L. (1992) The first breaths of air stimulate noradrenaline turnover in the brain of the newborn rat. *Acta Physiologica Scandinavica* **144**, 433–438.

41 Lee, S., Hassan, A., Ingram, D., Milner, A.D. (1999) Effects of different modes of delivery on lung volumes of newborn infants. *Pediatric Pulmonology* **27**, 318–321.

42 Leffler, C.W., Hessler, J.R., Terragno, N.A. (1980) Ventilation induced release of prostaglandin-like material from fetal lungs. *American Journal of Physiology* **238**, H282–H286.

43 Leffler, C.W., Hessler, J.R., Green, R.S. (1984) The onset of breathing at birth stimulates pulmonary vascular prostacyclin synthesis. *Pediatric Research* **18**, 938–942.

44 Lodrup-Carlsen, K.C., Carlsen, K.H. (1993) Lung function in awake healthy infants: the first five days of life. *European Respiratory Journal* **6**, 1496–1500.

45 Meier-Stauss, P., Bucher, H.U., Hurlimann, R. *et al.* (1990) Pulse oximetry used for documenting oxygen saturation and right to left shunting immediately after birth. *European Journal of Pediatrics* **149**, 851–855.

46 Merlet, C., Hoerter, J., Devilleneuve, C., Tchobroutsky, C. (1970) Mise en evidence de movements respiratoires chez le foetus d'agneau in utero au cours du dernier mois de la gestation. *Comptes Rendus de l'Academie des Sciences (Paris)* **270**, 2462–2246.

47 Meyer, W.W., Lind, J. (1966) The ductus venosus and the mechanisms of its closure. *Archives of Disease in Childhood* **41**, 597–605.

48 Milner, A.D., Saunders, R.A. (1977) Pressure and volume changes during the first breath of human neonates. *Archives of Disease in Childhood* **52**, 918–924.

49 Milner, A.D., Saunders, R.A., Hopkin, I.E. (1978) Effects of delivery by caesarian section on lung mechanics and lung volume in human neonates. *Archives of Disease in Childhood* **53**, 545–548.

50 Morin, F.C.I., Egan, E.A., Ferguson, W., Lundgren, C.E.G. (1988) Development of pulmonary vascular response to oxygen. *American Journal of Physiology* **254**, H542–H546.

51 Mortola, J.P., Fisher, J.T., Smith, J.B. *et al.* (1982) Onset of respiration in infants delivered by cesarean section. *Journal of Applied Physiology* **52**, 716–724.

52 Nelson, N.M., Prod'hom, S., Cherry, R.B. *et al.* (1963) Pulmonary function in the newborn infant. V. Trapped gas in the normal infant's lung. *Journal of Clinical Investigation* **42**, 1850–1857.

53 Olver, T.K.J. (1963) *Neonatal Respiratory Adaptation*. Public Health Services Publication 1432. US Department of Health Education and Welfare. Bethesda, MD, p. 117

54 Palme-Kilander, C., Tunell, R., Chiwei, Y. (1993) Pulmonary gas exchange immediately after birth in spontaneous breathing fetus. *Archives of Disease in Childhood* **68**, 6–10.

55 Pronin, L.A. (1966) Respiratory movements in utero and establishment of respiratory centre function in rabbit foetuses. *Federation Proceedings* **Supp 25**, 236–238.

56 Purves, M.J. (1974) Onset of respiration at birth. *Archives of Disease in Childhood* **49**, 333–343.

57 Rudolph, A.M. (1977) Fetal and neonatal pulmonary circulation. *American Review of Respiratory Disease* **115**, 11–18.

58 Rudolph, A.M. (1979) Fetal and neonatal pulmonary circulation. *Annual Review of Physiology* **41**, 383–395.

59 Rudolph, A.M., Heymann, M.A. (1967) The circulation of the fetus *in utero*. Methods for studying distribution of blood flow, cardiac output and organ blood flow. *Circulation Research* **21**, 163–169.

60 Sandberg, K., Sjoqvist, B.A., Hjalmarson, O., Olsson, T. (1986) Effects of delivery by caesarean section on lung function in health newborn infants. *Acta Paediatrica Scandinavica* **75**, 470–476.

61 Saunders, R.A., Milner, A.D. (1978) Pulmonary pressure/volume relationships during the last phase of delivery and their first postnatal breaths in human subjects. *Journal of Pediatrics* **93**, 667–673.

62 Scarpelli, E.M. (1978) Intrapulmonary foam at birth. An adaptional phenomenon. *Pediatric Research* **12**, 1070–1076.

63 Srinivasan, M., Yamamoto, Y., Persson, H., Lagercrantz, H. (1991) Birth-related activation of preprotachykinin-A mRNA in the respiratory neural structures of the rabbit. *Pediatric Research* **29**, 369–371.

64 Vyas, H., Milner, A.D., Hopkin, I.E. (1981) Comparison of intrathoracic pressure and volume changes during the spontaneous onset of respiration in babies born by caesarean section and by vaginal delivery. *Journal of Pediatrics* **99**, 787–791.

65 Vyas, H., Field, D., Hopkin, I.E., Milner, A.D. (1986) Determinants of the first inspiratory volume and functional residual capacity at birth. *Pediatric Pulmonology* **2**, 189–193.

66 Walsh, S.Z., Myer, W.W., Lind, J. 1974: *The Human Fetal and Neonatal Circulation*. Springfield, IL: Charles C Thomas.

67 Walther, F.J., Siassi, B., Ramadan, N. *et al.* (1985) Pulsed doppler determinations of cardiac output in neonates: normal standards for clinical use. *Pediatrics* **76**, 829–833.

68 Walther, F.J., Benders, M.J., Leighton, J.O. (1993) Early changes in the neonatal circulatory transition. *Journal of Pediatrics* **123**, 625–632.

69 Wickstrom, H.R., Holgert, H., Hokfelt, T., Lagercrantz, H. (1999) Birth-related expression of *c-fos*, *c-jun* and substance P mRNAs in the rat brainstem and pia mater: possible relationship to changes in central chemosensitivity. *Developmental Brain Research* **112**, 255–266.

PART 2

Antenatal and postnatal investigation

7

Clinical assessment

ANNE GREENOUGH, with contributions from NRC ROBERTON

Although the infant's main problem is in their respiratory system, it is obviously important to observe and examine the whole infant. This is not only to assess their general status and need for supportive therapy, but also to detect abnormal signs that could suggest or help to confirm the diagnosis of the respiratory problem. For example, Potter's facies and/or contractures can be seen in infants with pulmonary hypoplasia (Chapter 32), meconium staining in infants with meconium aspiration syndrome (Chapter 23), the presence of petechiae could indicate congenital infection with pneumonia (Chapter 21) and an abnormal posture is suggestive of a neuromuscular disorder (Chapter 36). Similarly, on examination, the finding of hepatosplenomegaly might indicate congenital infection. It is important, however, to distinguish an enlarged liver and spleen from organs which have been pushed down by the diaphragm in a tension pneumothorax (p. 312); in the latter scenario there may also be a color change above and below the diaphragm. The great vessels can be 'nipped' as they go through the diaphragm distorted by a tension pneumothorax; as a consequence the bottom half of the body is very pale and the top half cyanosed. The adequacy of the infant's perfusion should be assessed. This is particularly important in infants with persistent pulmonary hypertension of the newborn (PPHN) (p. 9). The rate of capillary refill after blanching the skin should be determined;[9] delayed refill suggests that the infant is hypovolemic.

A thorough examination of the respiratory system is essential to facilitate the diagnostic process and to monitor progress and the response to treatment.

OBSERVATION

The infant's chest should be inspected to assess the shape, which will be abnormal in conditions such as asphyxiating thoracic dystrophy (p. 506). It is also to determine the ratio of the infant's chest to abdomen; this will be reduced in infants with pulmonary hypoplasia (p. 455).

Color

It is important to determine whether the infant is centrally cyanosed and this is detected by looking at the central mucosal surface. This, however, can be difficult, depending on the infant's pigmentation. In addition, healthy infants can show acrocyanosis for several days after delivery; this can particularly be a problem if they are polycythemic or have suffered facial traumatic cyanosis at delivery.

Chest wall movement

Key to effective resuscitation is to ensure that the infant's chest is being inflated; the same rule applies during conventional ventilation. Sufficient peak inflating pressure should be used during conventional ventilation to ensure there is visible chest wall expansion, then the appropriateness of the settings checked by analysis of an arterial blood gas sample. During high-frequency oscillation (HFO), smaller tidal volumes are used[2] and in HFO-supported infants the observation which should be made is whether the chest wall is 'bouncing', that is, the oscillatory amplitude is adequate (p. 175). A gradual reduction in bounce without any change in the oscillator settings may indicate that the endotracheal tube is blocking and suction is required, whereas a sudden change may occur if there is endotracheal displacement or the development of a large air leak. The respective timings of inspiration and expiration can be determined by observation of the chest wall movement. Expiration is longer than inspiration,[8] but if very prolonged this has implications for choice of therapy and ventilator settings.

INFANT VENTILATOR INTERACTION

The spontaneous respiratory efforts of infants interact with positive pressure inflations in a variety of patterns (p. 159).[5] One of these patterns, active expiration, precedes the development of an air leak. This can be detected by observing the infant's respiratory efforts during ventilation, by noting the timing of each inflation to the direction of the chest wall movement.[4] Instead of the infant's chest moving upwards with each inflation, if the infant is actively expiring then the chest moves downwards. The optimal interaction is synchrony, that is, inflation and inspiration coincide, if the infant is completely synchronous then it should not be possible to detect the infant's respiratory efforts from ventilator inflations. If the infant's respiratory efforts are distinct from ventilator inflations, ventilator rate and inflation time manipulation (see below) should be reviewed. In addition, it should be investigated whether there are unwanted stimuli to the infant's respiratory efforts, for example, has the infant developed a respiratory acidosis or is the level of sedation/analgesia inadequate.

Rate

A respiratory rate greater than 60 breaths/min is considered abnormal, although there is considerable variation in the respiratory rate of healthy neonates. A persistently elevated respiratory rate may be the only sign of mild pulmonary hypoplasia.[1] A raised respiratory rate may not only be the consequence of lung disease, but can also be found, for example, in infants with heart failure (p. 387) or CNS disorders. Observation of the infant's respiratory rate is important in choosing a ventilator rate most likely to promote synchrony (p. 159). The ventilator rate must be above, but close to, the infant's respiratory rate.[6] During synchronized intermittent positive pressure ventilation (SIPPV), it is important to observe whether the triggered breath rate exceeds the back-up rate; if the two are similar, this indicates that use of SIPPV is inappropriate for the infant at that time. Explanations include that the infant remains sedated from medications used during conventional ventilation (p. 208) or an inappropriate triggering system is being used.[3] Some infants have poor respiratory efforts because of their prematurity and administration of a methylxanthine can improve the success of SIPPV.

Dyspnea

The signs of dyspnea include sternal retraction and intercostals recession and are the manifestation of diaphragmatic contractions trying to expand non-compliant lungs. The sternal retraction is directly due to the diaphragmatic traction on it and the recession is caused by the hypotonic intercostals being pulled inwards by the negative intrathoracic pressure during inspiration. In addition, infants may have suprasternal in-drawing and flaring of the alae nasae. They may also exhibit see-saw respiration, that is, abdominal expansion occurs at the same time as sternal recession, the expansion of the abdomen resulting from the downward movement of the diaphragm.

Dyspnea in association with worsening blood gases is an indication for increasing the infant's level of support. During SIPPV, if an infant is making obvious respiratory efforts prior to each positive pressure inflation, then the trigger delay is too long. Under such circumstances, an insufficient amount of the infant's respiratory effort is supported by positive pressure and the infant may develop a metabolic acidosis or become so exhausted that they fail to trigger the ventilator and become dependent on the back-up rate (see above).

TRANSILLUMINATION

Transilluminating the infant's chest with a fiberoptic bright light can detect collections of intrapleural air.[7] In the absence of an air leak, there is only a 0.5–1.0 cm halo of light around the probe. If there is a large tension pneumothorax in a very immature infant, then the whole of the hemithorax will 'light up'. The technique works less well in mature infants, as they have thicker chest walls and severe pulmonary interstitial emphysema (PIE) or lobar emphysema may be mistaken for a pneumothorax. Thus, unless the infant's condition is very poor, a rapidly obtained chest radiograph is the better method of diagnosing the presence and type of an air leak. It also has the advantage, that if an air leak is present, then the radiographer is on hand to perform further radiography of the infant to check the position of the chest drain tip.

LISTENING

Infants with RDS grunt. The infant keeps his vocal cords abducted throughout most of the expiratory cycle, but at the end of expiration the laryngeal adductors relax and the grunt is the explosive exhalation that follows. It is important to remember, however, that grunting is not pathognomonic of RDS, but is heard in infants with other conditions in which there is a low lung volume (p. 252).

Stridor can be a transient noise following overvigorous resuscitation or, if prolonged, a sign of a congenital anomaly or a worrying complication of intubation (p. 438).

Auscultation

It is important to ensure that there is bilateral symmetrical air entry. The commonest reason for asymmetrical air entry is a misplaced endotracheal tube down the right main bronchus. After intubating an infant, it is therefore important to observe good chest wall expansion (p. 154) and then to listen to both sides of the chest. If the air entry is poorer on the right, then the endotracheal tube should be slightly withdrawn and the quality of air entry reassessed. If the endotracheal tube has mistakenly been placed in the esophagus, the 'sound' of inflation can be transmitted from the abdomen, so hearing inflations in the chest does not guarantee appropriate endotracheal tube placement. It is, therefore, important to assess chest wall expansion (see above) and to determine the infant's response to the intubation from continuous monitoring. Not surprisingly, sick, prematurely born infants are frequently intolerant of malplaced endotracheal tubes. If the sound of inflation is louder over the abdomen than the chest, the diagnosis is clear. Care should be taken to listen for murmurs which could indicate that the infant's cyanosis is due to congenital heart disease (p. 387) or that a ventilated, prematurely born infant's worsening respiratory status is explained by a large patent ductus arteriosus.

Added sounds may be present, but are often nonspecific. For example, crepitations can occur in infants with heart failure or pneumonia. Wheezing is uncommon, but can occur in older infants with chronic lung disease and may then indicate that treatment with bronchodilators might be useful (p. 412). Rarely, bowel sounds are heard in the chest and indicate the presence of a congenital diaphragmatic hernia.

PALPATION

Displacement of the mediastinum, for example by a large pneumothorax, can be detected by deviation of the trachea and an abnormal position of the apex beat. For obvious reasons, these abnormal signs are difficult to elicit in a very small, prematurely born infant. Infants with massive air leaks may have subcutaneous emphysema (p. 311), giving the characteristic crackly feeling in the skin. When palpating the infant's chest, it is important to note whether there is chest wall edema; if this is severe it will greatly reduce the infant's respiratory system compliance and higher peak pressures will be needed to adequately inflate the infant's chest.

PERCUSSION

Areas of dullness can be detected by percussion and indicate consolidation or a large effusion. The percussion note is resonant over the hemithorax, if a large pneumothorax is present.

REFERENCES

1   Aiton, N.R., Fox, G.F., Hannam, S. *et al.* (1996) Pulmonary hypoplasia presenting as persistent tachypnoea in the first few months of life. *British Medical Journal* **312**, 1149–1150.

2   Dimitriou, G., Greenough, A., Kavvadia, V., Laubscher, B., Milner, A.D. (1998) Volume delivery during high frequency oscillation. *Archives of Disease in Childhood* **78**, 148–150.

3   Dimitriou, G., Greenough, A., Cherian, S. (2001) Comparison of airway pressure and airflow triggering systems using a single type of neonatal ventilator. *Acta Paediatrica* **159**, 289–292.

4   Greenough, A., Greenall, F. (1988) Observation of spontaneous respiratory interaction with artificial ventilation. *Archives of Disease in Childhood* **63**, 168–171.

5   Greenough, A., Morley, C., Davis, J. (1983) Interaction of spontaneous respiration with ventilation in preterm babies. *Journal of Pediatrics* **103**, 769–773.

6   Greenough, A., Greenall, F., Gamsu, H.R. (1987) Synchronous respiration – which ventilator rate is best? *Acta Paediatrica Scandinavica* **76**, 713–718.

7   Kuhns, L.R., Benarek, F.J., Wyman, M.L. *et al.* (1975) Diagnosis of pneumothorax or pneumomediastinum in the neonate by transillumination. *Pediatrics* **56**, 355–360.

8   South, M., Morley, C.J. (1986) Spontaneous respiratory tracing in intubated infants with RDS. *Early Human Development* **14**, 147–148.

9   Strozik, K.S., Pieper, C.H., Roller, J. (1997) Capillary refilling time in newborn babies: normal values. *Archives of Disease in Childhood* **76**, F193–F196.

Microbiology

AMANDA FIFE

Neonatal respiratory infection remains an important cause of morbidity and mortality. While the incidence of infection in otherwise healthy full-term neonates is estimated to be 1 percent or less, it is at least 10 percent in infants requiring intensive care.[10] Pneumonia in the neonatal period frequently presents as part of disseminated multisystem infection. Acquisition may occur by: transplacental transfer of an infecting agent *in utero*: as a result of ascending infection; aspiration of vaginal and perineal organisms during birth and postnatal contact with family members, healthcare workers and colonized medical devices or equipment. Bloodstream infections from distant sources may spread to the lungs and aspiration of oropharyngeal contents may occur. Classification of neonatal respiratory infections by route of acquisition is useful for understanding their pathogenesis and epidemiology, but less helpful when considering the nature and timing of the clinical presentation. For example, perinatally acquired infections such as *Chlamydia trachomatis* may not present for several weeks. Neonates are uniquely predisposed to respiratory infection because of immature lung function and cellular and humoral immune responses (Chapter 5), problems exacerbated by prematurity. The need for intravascular access, invasive procedures and mechanical ventilation further compromises the integrity of fragile neonatal skin and respiratory defenses by providing portals of entry via which colonizing organisms may establish systemic infection. The reduced respiratory reserve in infants with chronic lung disease renders them susceptible to deterioration in the face of superadded infection.[36]

INVESTIGATION

Clinical features of pneumonia in the neonate are often non-specific, at least in the early stages. The microbiological investigation of pneumonia is therefore part of a 'septic screen'. One of the main problems facing clinicians is the lack of sensitive and specific rapid tests for identifying many infecting agents. When results of cultures become available, they have to be interpreted retrospectively in the light of the patient's condition when the specimens were collected and subsequent clinical progress. It can be impossible to distinguish between colonizing and infecting organisms from specimens from non-sterile sites. Given the non-specific presentation of many infective episodes in hospitalized neonates and the delay inherent in standard microbiological investigations, other laboratory indices are used as markers of infection, although they are not specific for pneumonia. No individual test or combination of tests, however, has sufficient sensitivity or specificity to exclude infection at the time the neonate clinically deteriorates.

Blood culture

The utility of blood culture in the diagnosis of early onset neonatal pneumonia was shown by Webber *et al.*,[34] who found that 46 percent of infants had positive blood cultures, although the rate was less (17 percent) for infants with late-onset pneumonia. These rates compare favorably with the less than 16 percent blood culture positive rate found in adults with community-acquired pneumonia.[6]

Blood for culture should ideally be collected by venepuncture of a peripheral vein after skin disinfection. The skin should be allowed to dry to give the agent time to kill vegetative bacteria. The sensitivity of blood culture increases with the volume of blood cultured. Sometimes, lack of venous access makes it necessary to collect blood cultures from indwelling intravascular lines. Cultures positive for organisms that are both common contaminants and common causes of infection, such as coagulase-negative staphylococci, can be difficult to interpret, especially if the signs of infection are equivocal. Most blood cultures will become positive in the first 24–48 hours, but organisms such as *Candida* species may take longer to grow. One study noted that in four of 34 candidemic neonates, the initial blood culture had taken more than 4 days to become positive.[2] Recovery of organisms is also affected by antibiotic treatment. Cultures should be repeated if there is any doubt about the significance of an organism or if the patient continues to show signs of sepsis despite negative blood cultures and empirical antibiotic treatment.

Automated continuously monitored blood culture systems (which detect carbon dioxide produced by microbial metabolism) are available in many microbiology laboratories. Early systems required radioactive culture media, but have been superseded by systems utilizing non-radiometric methods such as colorimetry or fluorescence. The absolute concentration of carbon dioxide in inoculated blood culture bottles and changes in carbon dioxide levels over time are monitored approximately every 20 minutes. When a specimen exceeds the threshold level, the system alerts laboratory staff, who then perform a Gram's stain and culture. The advantages over manual methods are more rapid growth detection and a reduced chance of contaminating bottles by repeated subculture. Manufacturers supply a variety of media including bottles suitable for pediatric use. The latter are formulated to provide optimal blood-broth dilution for recovery of organisms from small volumes of blood (which may be as small as 0.5 ml in a neonate, although 1 ml should be the minimum volume). Modern systems compare with the Isolator tube method in their sensitivity for the detection of fungi.[8,12] Manual methods are still in use in laboratories in areas of the world where the capital and maintenance costs of automated systems are prohibitive.

Respiratory tract specimens

The problems of interpreting culture results of specimens obtained from the neonatal respiratory tract are well recognized. Sherman *et al.*[27,28] suggested that Gram's stain and culture of tracheal secretions obtained within 12 hours of birth was helpful in the diagnosis of early onset bacteremia and pneumonia, although the sensitivity was limited. Several studies have shown that beyond the first day after birth, culture of tracheal secretions is neither sensitive nor specific for identifying the cause of sepsis in infants requiring intensive care. A large study assessing the utility of surface cultures in predicting the cause of systemic sepsis found that endotracheal secretions obtained on the day of blood culture had 59 percent sensitivity and 74 percent specificity and

the sensitivity of routine surveillance cultures was only 26 percent.[13] Slagle *et al.*[29] found that routine tracheal cultures predicted the cause of late onset bacteremia in only 19 percent of cases. Another prospective study, which specifically examined pneumonia, found that respiratory cultures predicted the cause of bacteremia in only one case of seven episodes of bacteremic late-onset infection, and would have led to inappropriate antibiotic therapy in four cases.[34]

The problems of diagnosing ventilator-associated pneumonia in adults have led to the controversial use of quantitative cultures of lower respiratory tract specimens collected bronchoscopically. Fagon *et al.*[14] demonstrated a good correlation between histological pneumonia and the results of quantitative culture and also showed improved outcome for invasively investigated patients compared with those who received standard care.[15] Due to the technical difficulties and risks inherent in obtaining good quality lower respiratory tract specimens in very small infants, there are few published data about the use of quantitative cultures in ventilated neonates. Ruderman *et al.*[23] examined quantitative cultures of tracheal aspirates in infants more than 24 hours old who required intubation; they found that greater than 10^5 organisms/ml in the aspirate was 100 percent specific and 75 percent sensitive for the diagnosis of clinical pneumonia. The study, however, was small and the results were less encouraging for infants who were already intubated at the time the diagnosis was suspected. The results of bacterial respiratory tract cultures after the first few hours of life are insufficiently predictive of the cause of sepsis to guide antibiotic treatment.

If pertussis is suspected clinically, the investigation of choice is culture. A calcium alginate swab of the posterior nasopharynx or a fresh nasopharyngeal aspirate is suitable. The samples should be cultured as soon as possible after collection.

Chlamydia trachomatis pneumonia can be diagnosed by inoculation of nasopharyngeal secretions into tissue culture and demonstration of intracytoplasmic inclusions.[25] The sensitivity of culture is highly dependent on technical expertise and is only offered by specialist laboratories. Although highly sensitive, automated DNA amplification methods are not suitable for nasopharyngeal specimens. Interpretation of direct fluorescent antibody stains of infected material is subjective and requires considerable expertise.[30] The most reliable way to diagnose the infection is serologically.

Viruses such as respiratory syncytial virus (RSV), influenza and parainfluenza can be cultured from nasopharyngeal aspirates. Several sensitive and specific rapid techniques are available, including detection of virus-infected cells by immunofluorescence or enzyme immunoassay and amplification of virus-specific sequences in clinical material by polymerase chain reaction.[3,33]

Specimens from other sites

CEREBROSPINAL FLUID

Cerebrospinal fluid (CSF) should always be collected as part of a septic screen unless there are clear contraindications or the site of infection is clinically obvious. Bacteremic pneumonia may spread hematogenously to the meninges. If viral infection is suspected, CSF should be submitted for virus culture and, if appropriate, for polymerase chain reaction (PCR)-based viral nucleic acid detection (enteroviruses, herpes simplex virus).

URINE

Culture of urine for cytomegalovirus (CMV) should be performed in the case of suspected congenital infection and conventional culture should be carried out in cases of late-onset sepsis.

SURFACE SITES

The use of surface cultures to predict both early- and late-onset infections has been discredited. Evans et al.[13] showed that the overall sensitivity, specificity and positive predictive value of surface cultures for sepsis were, at best, 56, 82 and 7.5 percent, respectively. Thompson et al.[31] found that the ear canal, but not other sites, was always positive in cases of group B streptococcal (GBS) sepsis and Dobson et al.[11] found no cases of early-onset sepsis which were missed by culturing the ear canal and throat only. The ear canal may contain infected residual amniotic fluid. In Dobson's study, late-onset sepsis rates did not change after all surface cultures (except for a weekly endotracheal sample for infection control surveillance) ceased. The costs and work involved in collecting and processing multiple superficial specimens are not justified in terms of diagnostic yield. Surface cultures should be performed for specific clinical reasons only, such as the diagnosis of skin sepsis or viral culture of possible herpetic lesions. Throat swabs in viral transport medium should be submitted if mucosal lesions suggestive of herpes simplex are present or enterovirus or adenovirus infection is suspected (a stool sample should also be sent).

STOOL SAMPLES

Enterovirus and adenovirus can be isolated from stool samples. Caution is required, however, in the interpretation of positive isolates for adenovirus, as only some subtypes will cause diarrhea. *Listeria monocytogenes* can be isolated from the first meconium passed by an infected infant (p. 287).

Hematological indices

The total white cell count is subject to wide normal variation and is influenced by many non-infective factors. Neutrophil counts are more helpful and a low absolute neutrophil count accompanied by an elevated ratio of immature forms:total neutrophil count (I:T ratio) of more than 0.2 is highly suggestive of infection.[7,10] Thrombocytopenia is seen in about 50 percent of neonates who have proven bacterial sepsis but this may not be detected until the clinical manifestations are obvious.[7] It is also non-specific and is seen in ventilated infants who do not have infection.[1] Eosinophilia in the setting of pneumonia suggests *Chlamydia trachomatis* infection.[26]

C-Reactive protein

Elevated levels of C-reactive protein (CRP) in serum have not been found to be helpful in the early diagnosis of infection. Mathers and Pohlandt[20] showed that a rise in CRP lagged behind the appearance of an abnormal I:T ratio in infected infants and others have demonstrated a delay between the appearance of signs and a rise in the CRP.[21] Serial measurements appear more useful than single determinations as persistently normal CRP levels during and after an episode of suspected sepsis make it very unlikely that infection is genuinely present.[21]

Indirect and non-culture methods

Antigen detection tests for the detection of GBS antigen in body fluids, including urine, have been used as rapid diagnostic methods. Commercial kits, using antibody-coated latex beads, are available. Doubt has been cast on their usefulness as screening test in infants with risk factors for GBS sepsis.[24,35] Williamson and colleagues[35] found that, although sensitive, the test had a false-positive rate of 30 percent and a specificity of only 70 percent using a case definition which included positive surface swabs in an appropriate clinical setting. The Food and Drug Administration in the USA does not recommend urinary antigen testing.[4]

Serological tests

These are sometimes used to diagnose infections for which no other suitable technique exists. Determinations of changing titers of antibody, however, can be difficult to interpret in the presence of maternal antibody. The demonstration of disease-specific IgM is helpful in a number of situations. Anti-rubella IgM confirms the diagnosis in neonates suspected of having congenital rubella. Most infants with chlamydial pneumonia will have high levels of anti-chlamydial IgM.[26] Cord blood IgM has not been reliable for diagnosing congenital syphilis, but postnatal IgM positivity is useful, as is the demonstration of falling rapid plasma reagent (RPR) or Venereal Disease Research Laboratory (VDRL) titers over time, although the most useful guide is the mother's status at delivery.[32] Identification of maternal IgG by immunofluorescence is useful to confirm previous varicella infection and thus immunity, when there is a history of recent exposure. The presence of CMV-specific IgM in a single maternal sample,

Table 8.1 *Guide to antimicrobial treatment*

Organism	Antimicrobial
Group B streptococcus (plus groups A, G streptococci, *Streptococcus pneumoniae**)	Benzylpenicillin and aminoglycoside (gentamicin)
Enterococci	Ampicillin/amoxicillin and gentamicin
Escherichia coli	Third-generation cephalosporin and aminoglycoside (cefotaxime or ceftriaxone)
Listeria monocytogenes	Ampicillin/amoxicillin and gentamicin
Haemophilus species	Third-generation cephalosporin or ampicillin (if sensitive) and gentamicin
Coagulase-negative staphylococci and MRSA	Vancomycin
Methicillin sensitive *Staphylococcus aureus*	Flucloxacillin
Multi-resistant *Klebsiella, Enterobacter*	Carbapenem** (meropenem or imipenem) and aminoglycoside (amikacin)
Pseudomonas aeruginosa	Ceftazidime or carbapenem and aminoglycoside
Candida species	Amphotericin B
Herpes simplex/varicella zoster	Aciclovir
Respiratory syncytial virus	Ribavirin

* Increasing incidence world wide of infection caused by pneumococci highly resistant to penicillin, although it is not known if this will emerge as a problem in the neonatal population. Third-generation cephalosporin and vancomycin may be necessary for resistant pneumococci.

MRSA, Methicillin-resistant *Staphylococcus aureus*.

** Carbapenems do not have a UK license for babies <3 months but have been used successfully in this group.

however, can be misleading. It can indicate a recent infection but, as IgM can persist for up to 16 weeks, it may reflect a preconceptional maternal infection.[18] Active infection is indicated by seroconversion of two separate maternal blood samples, otherwise it is not possible to distinguish between primary and secondary maternal infection.[5]

ANTIBIOTIC TREATMENT

Synergism between aminoglycosides and β-lactams is observed *in vitro* for many organisms including GBS, Enterobacteriaceae and *Listeria* and *in vivo* for several animal models of infection.[17] It is tempting to use antibiotics that cover all eventualities for early-onset sepsis (such as ampicillin/cefotaxime/gentamicin). This approach, however, has been associated with the emergence of resistant organisms in intensive care.[9] The alternative is to use benzylpenicillin and gentamicin unless there are specific clinical or microbiological indications to do otherwise (Table 8.1). Empirical treatment of nosocomial infection is subject to conditions within individual units and policies should be devised in consultation with the medical microbiologist.

PREVENTION AND INFECTION CONTROL

Education about and adherence to good infection control practice by all staff is vital in the prevention of nosocomial infection. Thorough hand-washing alone is an effective intervention[22] and measures such as isolation and cohort nursing can help to control outbreaks. The importance of maintaining correct staffing levels for workload is illustrated by Isaacs *et al.*,[19] who showed that aminoglycoside use was less important than workload indicators in the spread of gentamicin-resistant Gram-negative bacilli in their unit. Although environmental reservoirs are unusual sources of infection, the importance of good maintenance and cleaning of equipment has been shown by Garland.[16] Efforts should be made to limit the exposure of at-risk infants to community-acquired infections. Staff are reluctant to take time off for apparently trivial illnesses, but should be excluded from high-risk areas until they have recovered. Parents and siblings of patients are to be encouraged to spend time with their baby but they should be educated about the potential risks of community-acquired infection and asked not to visit if they have symptoms.

REFERENCES

1 Ballin, A., Koren, G., Kohelet, D. *et al.* (1987) Reduction in platelet count induced by mechanical ventilation in newborn infants. *Journal of Pediatrics* **111**, 445–449.

2 Benjamin, D.K., Ross, K., McKinney, R.E. *et al.* (2000) When to suspect fungal infections in neonates: a clinical comparison of *Candida albicans* and *Candida parapsilosis* fungemia with coagulase-negative staphylococcal bacteremia. *Pediatrics* **106**, 712–718.

3 Breese Hall, C., McCarthy, C.A. (2000) Respiratory syncytial virus. In Mandell, G.L., Bennett, J.E., Dolin, R. (eds), *Mandell, Douglas and Bennett's Principles and Practice of Infectious Diseases*, 5th edition. Philadelphia: Churchill Livingstone, 1782–1800.

4 Burlington, D.B. (1997) Risks of devices for direct detection of group B streptococcal antigen. FDA Safety Alert.

5 Cederqvist, L.L., Abdel-Latiff, N., Meyer, J., Doctor, L. (1986) Fetal and maternal humoral immune response to cytomegalovirus infection. *Obstetrics and Gynecology* **24**, 214–216.

6 Chalasani, N.P., Valdecanas, M.A.L., Gopal, A.K. *et al.* (1995) Clinical utility of blood cultures in adult patients with community-acquired pneumonia without defined underlying risks. *Chest* **108**, 932–936.

7 Clifford Robinson, N.R. (1995) Pneumonia. In Greenough, A., Milner, A. (eds), *Neonatal Respiratory Disorders*, first edition. London: Arnold, 286–312.

8 Cockerill, F.R. III, Reed, G.S., Hughes, J.G. *et al.* (1997) Clinical comparison of BACTEC 9240 Plus Aerobic/F Resin bottles and the Isolator aerobic culture system for detection of bloodstream infections. *Journal of Clinical Microbiology* **35**, 1469–1472.

9 De Man, P., Verhoeven, B.A., Verbrugh, H.A. *et al.* (2000) An antibiotic policy to prevent emergence of resistant Gram negative bacilli. *Lancet* **355**, 973–978.

10 Dennehy, P.H. (1987) Respiratory infections in the newborn. *Clinics in Perinatology* **14**, 667–682.

11 Dobson, S.R.M., Isaacs, D., Wilkinson, A.R., Hope, P.L. (1992) Reduced use of surface cultures for suspected neonatal sepsis and surveillance. *Archives of Disease in Childhood* **67**, 44–47.

12 Engler, H.D., Fahle, G.A., Gill, V.J. (1996) Clinical evaluation of the BacT/Alert and isolator aerobic blood culture systems. *American Journal of Clinical Pathology* **105**, 774–781.

13 Evans, M.E., Schaffner, W., Federspiel, C.F. *et al.* (1988) Sensitivity, specificity and predictive value of body surface cultures in a neonatal intensive care unit. *Journal of the American Medical Association* **259**, 248–252.

14 Fagon, J.-Y., Chastre, J., Domart, Y. *et al.* (1984) Nosocomial pneumonia in patients receiving continuous mechanical ventilation: prospective analysis of 52 episodes with use of a protected specimen brush and quantitative culture techniques. *American Review of Respiratory Disease* **139**, 877–884.

15 Fagon, J.-Y., Chastre, J., Wolff, M. *et al.* (2000) Invasive and non-invasive strategies for the management of suspected ventilator-associated pneumonia. A randomised trial. *Annals of Internal Medicine* **18**, 621–630.

16 Garland, S.M., Mackay, S., Tabrizi, S., Jacobs, S. (1996) *Pseudomonas aeruginosa* outbreak associated with a contaminated blood-gas analyser in a neonatal intensive care unit. *Journal of Hospital Infection* **33**, 145–151.

17 Gilbert, D. (2000) Aminoglycosides. In Mandell, G.L., Bennett, J.E., Dolin, R. (eds), *Mandell, Douglas and Bennett's Principles and Practice of Infectious Diseases*, 5th edition. Philadelphia: Churchill Livingstone, 307–336.

18 Griffiths, P.D., Stagno, S., Pass, R.F. *et al.* (1982) Infection with cytomegalovirus during pregnancy: specific IgM antibodies as a marker of recent primary infection. *Journal of Infectious Disease* **145**, 647–653.

19 Isaacs, D., Catterson, J., Hope, P.L. (1988) Factors affecting colonisation with gentamicin resistant Gram negative organisms in the neonatal unit. *Archives of Disease in Childhood* **63**, 533–535.

20 Mathers, N.J., Pohlandt, F. (1987) Diagnostic audit of C-reactive protein in neonatal infection. *European Journal of Pediatrics* **146**, 147–151.

21 Pourcyrous, M., Bada, H.S., Korones, S.B. *et al.* (1993) Significance of C-reactive protein responses in neonatal infection and other disorders. *Pediatrics* **92**, 431–435.

22 Royle, J., Halasz, S., Eagles, G. *et al.* (1999) Outbreak of extended spectrum beta lactamase producing *Klebsiella pneumoniae* in a neonatal unit. *Archives of Disease in Childhood Fetal and Neonatal Edition* **80**, F64–F68.

23 Ruderman, J.W., Srugo, I., Morgan, M.A. (1994) Pneumonia in the intensive care unit: diagnosis by quantitative bacterial tracheal cultures. *Journal of Perinatology* **14**, 182–186.

24 Sanchez, P.J., Siegel, J.D., Cushion, N.B., Threlkeld, N. (1990) Significance of a positive urine group B streptococcal latex agglutination test in neonates. *Journal of Pediatrics* **116**, 601–606.

25 Schacter, J., Grossmann, M., Holt, J. *et al.* (1979) Infection with *Chlamydia trachomatis:* involvement of multiple anatomic sites in neonates. *Journal of Infectious Diseases* **139**, 232–234.

26 Schacter, J., Ridgeway, G.L., Collier, L. (1998) Chlamydial diseases. In Collier, L., Balows, A., Sussman, M. (eds), *Topley and Wilson's Microbiology and Microbial Infections, Volume 3, Bacterial Infections*, 9th edition. London: Arnold.

27 Sherman, M.P., Goetzman, B.W., Ahlfors, C.E. *et al.* (1980) Tracheal aspiration and its clinical correlates in the diagnosis of congenital pneumonia. *Pediatrics* **65**, 258–263.

28 Sherman, M.P., Chance, K.H., Goetzman, B.W. (1984) Gram's stains of tracheal secretions predict neonatal bacteremia. *American Journal of Disease in Childhood* **138**, 848–850.

29 Slagle, T.A., Bifano, E.M., Wolf, J.W., Gross, S.J. (1989) Routine endotracheal cultures for the prediction of sepsis in ventilated babies. *Archives of Disease in Childhood* **64**, 34–38.

30 Stamm, W.E. (1988) Diagnosis of *Chlamydia trachomatis* genitourinary infections. *Annals of Internal Medicine* **108**, 710–717.

31 Thompson, P.J., Greenough, A., Nicolaides, K.H., Philpott-Howard, J. (1992) Congenital bacterial sepsis in preterm infants. *Journal of Medical Microbiology* **36**, 117–120.

32 Tramont, E.C. (2000) *Treponema pallidum* (syphilis). In Mandell, G.L., Bennett, J.E., Dolin, R. (eds), *Mandell, Douglas and Bennett's Principles and Practice of Infectious Diseases*, 5th edition. Philadelphia: Churchill Livingstone, 2474–2490.

33 Treanor, J.J. (2000) Influenza virus. In Mandell, G.L., Bennett, J.E., Dolin, R. (eds), *Mandell, Douglas and Bennett's Principles and Practice of Infectious Diseases*, 5th edition. Philadelphia: Churchill Livingstone, 1823–1848.

34 Webber, S., Wilkinson, A.R., Lindsell, D. *et al.* (1990) Neonatal pneumonia. *Archives of Disease in Childhood* **65**, 207–211.

35 Williamson, M., Fraser, S.H., Tilse, M. (1995) Failure of the urinary group B streptococcal antigen test as a screen for neonatal sepsis. *Archives of Disease in Childhood* **73**, 109–111.

36 Yuksel, B., Greenough, A. (1992) Acute deterioration in neonatal chronic lung disease. *European Journal of Pediatrics* **151**, 697–700.

9

Immunology

SUSAN LEECH

IMMUNOGLOBULINS

IgG is actively transported across the placenta. Healthy neonates have IgG and IgG subclass values similar to those in their mothers, but have little or no detectable IgM and IgA. Following birth, there is a diminution in the concentration of IgG, reflecting the loss of maternally derived IgG and the gradual accumulation of IgG synthesized by the infant. The physiological low point is normally reached at 3–4 months. In infants born prematurely, the nadir will be proportionately lower, because of the diminished amount of IgG received from the mother and values may remain less than those of term infants throughout the first year after birth. The values in premature infants are lower than those of term infants until 10 months of age. Concentrations of IgM and IgA are also characteristically low at this age, rising gradually thereafter. Quantitative immunoglobulin determination of levels of IgG, IgM, IgA, IgE and IgD (the last not usually performed routinely) may be performed by laser nephelometry, radioimmunoassay or enzyme-linked immunosorbent assays. Levels must be compared with age-matched controls (Table 9.1).[11]

IgG subclasses

After birth, synthesis of IgG_1 and IgG_4 occurs early and rapidly. Normal circulating amounts of IgG_3 are not achieved until 10 years of age, and IgG_2 until 12 years of age. Reliable determinations of IgG subclasses should be done in laboratories performing these on a regular basis. Levels must be compared with age-matched controls (Table 9.2).[14]

Table 9.1 *Normal ranges for immunoglobulin levels in UK Caucasians: these are expressed as 5th–95th centile ranges*

Age		IgM (g/l)	IgG (g/l)	IgA (g/l)
Cord		0.02–0.0	5.2–18.0	<0.02
Weeks	0–2	0.05–0.2	5.0–17.0	0.01–0.08
	2–6	0.08–0.4	3.9–13.0	0.02–0.15
	6–12	0.15–0.7	2.1–7.7	0.05–0.4
Months	3–6	0.2–1.0	2.4–8.7	0.10–0.5
	6–9	0.4–1.6	3.0–9.0	0.15–0.7
	9–12	0.6–2.1	3.0–10.9	0.20–0.7
Years	1–2	0.5–2.2	3.1–13.8	0.3–1.2
	2–3	0.5–2.2	3.7–15.8	0.3–1.3
	3–6	0.5–2.0	4.9–16.1	0.4–2.0
	6–9	0.5–1.8	5.4–16.1	0.5–2.4
	9–12	0.5–1.8	5.4–16.1	0.7–2.5
	12–15	0.5–1.9	5.4–16.1	0.8–2.8
	15–45	0.5–1.9	5.4–16.1	0.8–2.8
	>45	0.5–2.0	5.3–16.5	0.8–4.0

Note that adult levels of IgM are reached by about 1 year of age. IgG levels, high at birth since they are maternal antibodies transmitted across the placenta, decrease up to about 9–12 months and then increase as *de novo* IgG becomes apparent. IgA levels continue to increase throughout life. Reproduced with permission from Playfair and Lydyard.[11]

IgM

IgM does not cross the placenta. There is some *in utero* synthesis, which accelerates rapidly after birth in response to bacterial colonization of the gastrointestinal tract (Table 9.1).[11]

In congenital infection, cord blood IgM levels are increased, usually to levels exceeding 20 mg/dl.[17] In 1–3

Table 9.2 *Serum immunoglobulin levels (mg/ml)*

Age (years)	No. of subjects	IgG	IgG$_1$	IgG$_2$	IgG$_3$	IgG$_4$
0–1	22	4.2 (2.5–6.9)	3.4 (1.9–6.2)	0.59 (0.3–1.4)	0.39 (0.09–0.62)	0.19 (0.06–0.13)
1–2	42	4.7 (2.7–8.1)	4.1 (2.3–7.1)	0.68 (0.3–1.7)	0.34 (0.11–0.98)	0.13 (0.04–0.43)
2–3	36	5.4 (3.0–9.8)	4.8 (2.8–8.3)	0.98 (0.4–2.4)	0.28 (0.06–1.3)	0.18 (0.03–1.2)
3–4	52	6.0 (4.0–9.1)	5.3 (3.5–7.9)	1.2 (0.5–2.6)	0.30 (0.09–0.98)	0.32 (0.05–1.8)
4–6	31	6.6 (4.4–10.0)	5.4 (3.6–8.1)	1.4 (0.6–3.1)	0.39 (0.09–1.6)	0.39 (0.09–1.6)
6–8	24	8.9 (5.6–14.0)	5.6 (2.8–11.2)	1.5 (0.3–6.3)	0.48 (0.4–2.5)	0.81 (0.11–6.2)
8–10	21	10.0 (5.3–19)	6.9 (2.8–17.4)	2.1 (0.8–5.5)	0.85 (0.22–3.2)	0.42 (0.1–1.7)
10–13	33	9.1 (5.0–16.6)	5.9 (2.7–12.9)	2.4 (1.1–5.5)	0.58 (0.13–2.5)	0.6 (0.07–5.3)
13–16	19	9.1 (5.8–14.5)	5.4 (2.8–10.2)	2.1 (0.6–7.9)	0.58 (0.14–2.4)	0.6 (0.11–3.3)

Geometric means are presented for each Ig at every age. The normal bounds, given in parentheses, are obtained by taking the mean logarithm ± twice the SD of the logarithms then taking the antilogs of the results. Reproduced with permission from Schur *et al.*[14]

percent of all infants, cord blood IgM is elevated. Although it is not always possible to identify an infection, these infants should be watched carefully and regarded as a high-risk group. In infants with congenital rubella, toxoplasmosis, CMV and syphilis, IgM levels are usually, but not invariably, raised. In infants with CMV, IgA levels may also be elevated.

Elevated IgM in cord blood also occurs as a result of leakage from mother to fetus, resulting in a false-positive IgM test for congenital infection. Maternal to fetal leakage is responsible for 5–10 percent of instances of elevated IgM and should be suspected if the cord blood IgA exceeds the cord IgM, as maternal IgA is higher than IgM. It can be confirmed by a repeat assay of infant IgM and IgA levels. Maternally derived IgM and IgA decrease after 3–4 days because of their short half-lives. By contrast, levels of IgM and IgA synthesized by the infant increase or are maintained.

LYMPHOCYTE COUNTS

T cells constitute 70 percent or more of peripheral blood lymphocytes; therefore lymphopenia usually indicates T-cell depletion. In the presence of a low lymphocyte count (less than 2.8×10^9/l), immunoglobulin levels and lymphocyte surface marker analysis should be performed as the first step in the investigation of immunodeficiency. Neither antenatal administration of glucocorticoids, to prevent RDS, nor hydrocortisone administered on the first day after birth[6] affects the lymphocyte count or immunoglobulin production by the neonate.[5,13]

Enumeration of T- and B-cell numbers

Estimation of peripheral blood B- and T-cell numbers is usually done by flow cytometry of cells stained with monoclonal antibodies. Total numbers of T cells are measured by staining for CD3 and T-cell subsets can be measured by staining for CD4 and CD8. The membrane antigens used to delineate B cells are CD19 or CD20. Normal values vary with age (Table 9.3).[3] B-cell quantitation in immunodeficiency is rarely indicated if the immunoglobulin levels are normal. If numbers of B cells are low, pre-B cells can be evaluated by staining bone marrow cells for cytoplasmic μ chains in the absence of light chain staining. Plasma cells are measured by routine histological staining.

ASSESSMENT OF CELLULAR IMMUNITY

Healthy term neonates lack detectable delayed cutaneous hypersensitivity responses and *in vitro* proliferative responses to antigens. Cellular immunity may be evaluated by determining the ability of the patient's lymphocytes to proliferate *in vitro* by mitogens [phytohemagglutinin (PHA), concanavalin A], allogenic cells or monoclonal antibodies. The proliferative response is assayed after 3–7 days by ^{3}H- or ^{14}C-labeled thymidine incorporation followed by DNA extraction or cell precipitation onto filter paper and subsequent liquid scintillation counting. Data on unstimulated and stimulated cultures should be compared. The stimulation index (ratio of counts to unstimulated controls) of PHA-activated lymphocytes

Table 9.3 *Absolute size of lymphocyte subpopulations in blood*

Lymphocyte subpopulations	Age groups									
	Neonatal	1 week–2 months	2–5 months	5–9 months	9–15 months	15–24 months	2–5 years	5–10 years	10–16 years	Adults
N	20	13	46	105	70	33	33	35	23	51
Lymphocytes	4.8 (0.7–7.3)	6.7 (3.5–13.1)	5.9 (3.7–9.6)	6.0 (3.8–9.9)	5.5 (2.6–10.4)	5.6 (2.7–11.9)	3.3 (1.7–6.9)	2.8 (1.1–5.9)	2.2 (1.0–5.3)	1.8 (1.0–2.8)
$CD19^+$ B	0.6 (0.04–1.1)	1.0 (0.6–1.9)	1.3 (0.6–3.0)	1.3 (0.7–2.5)	1.4 (0.6–2.7)	1.3 (0.6–3.1)	0.8 (0.2–2.1)	0.5 (0.2–1.6)	0.3 (0.2–0.6)	0.2 (0.1–0.5)
$CD3^+$ T lymphocytes	2.8 (0.6–5.0)	4.6 (2.3–7.0)	3.6 (2.3–6.5)	3.8 (2.4–6.9)	3.4 (1.6–6.7)	3.5 (1.4–8.0)	2.3 (0.9–4.5)	1.9 (0.7–4.2)	1.5 (0.8–3.5)	1.2 (0.7–2.1)
$CD3^+/CD4^+$ T lymphocytes	1.9 (0.4–3.5)	3.5 (1.7–5.3)	2.5 (1.5–5.0)	2.8 (1.4–5.1)	2.3 (1.0–4.6)	2.2 (0.9–5.5)	1.3 (0.5–2.4)	1.0 (0.3–2.0)	0.8 (0.4–2.1)	0.7 (0.3–1.4)
$CD3^+/CD8^+$ T lymphocytes	1.1 (0.2–1.9)	1.0 (0.4–1.7)	1.0 (0.5–1.6)	1.1 (0.6–2.2)	1.1 (0.4–2.1)	1.2 (0.4–2.3)	0.8 (0.3–1.6)	0.8 (0.3–1.8)	0.4 (0.2–1.2)	0.4 (0.2–0.9)
$CD3^+/HLA\text{-}DR^+$ T lymphocytes	0.09 (0.03–0.4)	0.3 (0.03–3.4)	0.2 (0.07–0.5)	0.2 (0.07–0.5)	0.2 (0.1–0.6)	0.3 (0.1–0.7)	0.2 (0.08–0.4)	0.2 (0.05–0.7)	0.06 (0.02–0.2)	0.09 (0.03–0.2)
$CD3^-/CD16\text{–}56^+$ NK cells	1.0 (0.1–1.9)	0.5 (0.2–1.4)	0.3 (0.1–1.3)	0.3 (0.1–1.0)	0.4 (0.2–1.2)	0.4 (0.1–1.4)	0.4 (0.1–1.0)	0.3 (0.09–0.9)	0.3 (0.07–1.2)	0.3 (0.09–0.6)

Absolute counts ($\times 10^9$/l): median and percentiles (5th–95th percentiles).

should be at least 20–100. Using PHA at varying dilutions may identify patients with partial immune defects. Normal term neonates lack detectable *in vitro* proliferative responses to bacterial antigens, which only develop following antigen exposure, but do proliferate in response to bacterial superantigens. Lymphocyte proliferation may also be measured by the appearance of the IL-2 receptor (CD28) using flow cytometry.

NEUTROPHIL FUNCTION TESTS

The principal disorders of neutrophil function are chronic granulomatous disease and leukocyte adhesion defect type one. Chronic granulomatous disease may be detected by testing for defects in the neutrophil respiratory burst, using nitro blue tetrazolium reduction or flow cytometric detection of hydrogen peroxide production. Leukocyte adhesion defect type one, where delayed separation of the umbilical cord beyond 10 days may be a feature, can be detected by testing for expression of the β_2-integrin, CD18, by flow cytometry.

C-REACTIVE PROTEIN

C-reactive protein (CRP) is a member of the pentraxin family, which acts as a non-specific opsonin for bacteria. It is produced by the liver during acute infection due to bacteria and fungi. Viral infection does not lead to a large rise in CRP levels. It is the most useful marker of the acute phase response, rising within hours of an inflammatory stimulus and having a circulatory half-life of about 8 hours. It does not cross the placenta, but serum concentrations in the fetus and neonate are similar to those in adults[1] and increase in response to infection or inflammation in a similar way.[16] The normal range in the neonatal period may differ from that normally quoted in adults (<4 mg/l), as levels are found above the 'normal' range without evidence of disease.

COMPLEMENT

Fetal complement synthesis commences at 6 weeks of gestation and is not transferred across the placenta. There is much variability in reports of levels in neonates and the levels of some components are within the adult range. Overall, the abundance and activity of the alternative pathway are diminished relative to those in the classical pathway. A marked deficiency of C9 is associated with poor killing of Gram-negative bacteria with neonatal serum. Preterm neonates have diminished activity of both classical and alternative pathways. Birthweight has no effect on complement activity.[10] After birth, the concentration of most complement components increases, approaching adult values by 6–18 months of age (Table 9.4).[8]

Table 9.4 *Summary of published complement levels in neonates**

Complement component	Mean percentage of adult levels	
	Term neonate	Preterm neonate
CH_{50}	56–90 (5)**	45–71 (4)
AP_{50}	49–65 (4)	40–55 (3)
C1q	61–90 (4)	27–58 (3)
C4	60–100 (5)	42–91 (4)
C2	76–100 (3)	67–96 (2)
C3	60–100 (5)	39–78 (4)
C5	73–75 (2)	67 (1)
C6	47–56 (2)	36 (1)
C7	67–92 (2)	72 (1)
C8	20–36 (2)	29 (1)
C9	<20–52 (3)	<20–41 (2)
B	35–64 (4)	36–50 (4)
P	33–71 (6)	16–65 (3)
H	61 (1)	–
C3bi	55 (1)	–

Reproduced with permission from Remmington and Klein.[12]
*Number of studies.
Data are derived from the review of Johnston, R.B., Stroud, R.M. (1977) Complement and host defense against infection. *Journal of Pediatrics* **90, 169–179; from Notarangelo, Chirico, Chiara, *et al.*[10] from Davis, C.A., Vallota, E.H., Forristal, J. (1979) Serum complement levels in infancy: age-related changes. *Pediatric Research* **13**, 1043–1046; from Lassiter, H.A., Watson, S.W., Seifring, M.L., Tanner, J.E. (1992) Complement factor 9 deficiency in serum of human neonates. *Journal of Infectious Diseases* **166**, 53–57; from Wolach, B., Dolfin, T., Regev, R. *et al.* (1997) The development of the complement system after 28 weeks' gestation. *Acta Paediatrica* **86**, 523–527; from Zilow, G., Bruessau, J., Hauck, W., Zilow, E.P. (1994) Quantitation of complement component C9 deficiency in term and preterm neonates. *Clinical and Experimental Immunology* **97**, 52–59.

NEONATAL IMMUNODEFICIENCY

Primary immunodeficiency

RECOGNITION OF PRIMARY IMMUNODEFICIENCY IN THE NEONATE

Several syndromes have characteristic clinical findings permitting early diagnosis, for example, the thrombocytopenia of Wiskott–Aldrich syndrome, the hypocalcemia, facies and congenital heart disease of DiGeorge and the skeletal dwarfing in cartilage-hair hypoplasia. Elevated IgE is present in hyperimmunoglobulin E syndrome and hypereosinophilia in patients with Omenn's syndrome. Patients with leukocyte adhesion defect may have omphalitis and delayed separation of the umbilical cord. Patients with severe combined immunodeficiency (SCID) may present with severe mucocutaneous candidiasis, protracted diarrhea, *Pneumocystis carinii* pneumonia, severe eczema and lymphopenia. A family history of immunodeficiency or early unexplained death is also suggestive. Chronic granulomatous disease may present in the neonatal period and should be considered in the term infant with severe bacterial infections with oxidase-positive bacteria or fungi. Primary immunodeficiency should be considered in all infants presenting with unusually severe, recalcitrant or recurrent infections, particularly if they have no other risk factors. Early aggressive antimicrobial therapy, isolation and early referral to a specialist center improve the prognosis.

INVESTIGATION OF SUSPECTED IMMUNODEFICIENCY

Healthy term neonates lack delayed-type hypersensitivity responses to antigens and have IgG passively transferred from their mother. Other immunoglobulin classes are very low. Therefore, common screening tests for immunodeficiency in older children are unhelpful. Useful tests include:

- chest radiograph for thymus size;
- total lymphocyte count, which should raise concern if the count is less than 2.8×10^9/l;
- enumeration of T, B and NK cells;
- lymphocyte proliferative responses;
- staining for CD11a, CD11b and CD18;
- neutrophil function tests.

Secondary immunodeficiency: HIV

Most children acquire HIV vertically. As a consequence of acquisition of infection at a time of immunological immaturity and an increased number of susceptible target cells, the pace of HIV disease progression in children is accelerated. Vertically infected children exhibit a bimodal pattern of disease progression.[2,4,9] About 10–25 percent develop profound immunosuppression, *Pneumocystis carinii* pneumonia, severe encephalopathy, organomegaly and multiple opportunistic infections in the first few months after birth.[4,9] HIV should always be included in the differential diagnosis of neonates who appear to have SCID. Without treatment, few of these children survive more than 2 years.[15]

USE OF SPECIFIC IMMUNOGLOBULIN FOR NEONATAL RESPIRATORY DISEASE

Cytomegalovirus (CMV) infection (p. 297)

Hyperimmune plasma and globulin have been used with some success as prophylaxis for primary CMV in immunosuppressed patients. A humanized monoclonal antibody is now available and may be more efficacious. It is unlikely that passive immunization will be beneficial in the treatment of congenital CMV identified weeks or months after an *in utero* infection. It may, however, be a means of preventing primary CMV infection and disease in perinatally infected or transfusion-acquired infections in prematurely born infants. There are, however, no results from randomized controlled studies.[7]

Respiratory syncytial virus (RSV) (p. 294)

RSV infections are frequently acquired by infants during the first weeks after birth and can be nosocomially acquired on a neonatal unit. A number of studies have demonstrated the benefits of administering RSV intravenous immune globulin (RSVIVIG) to infants at high risk of severe disease.[19] An RSV monoclonal antibody, Palivizumab, is now available. In a large randomized trial,[18] administration of Palivizumab was demonstrated to reduce hospitalization for RSV infection in high-risk infants by 55 percent. Palivizumab is given intramuscularly and appears to have fewer side-effects than RSVIVIG. There are no randomized trials assessing the efficacy of Palivizumab in preventing nosocomial infection on a neonatal intensive care unit.

REFERENCES

1 Ainbender, E., Cabatu, E.E., Guzman, D.M., Sweet, A.Y. (1982) Serum C-reactive protein and problems of newborn infants. *Journal of Pediatrics* **101**, 438–440.

2 Auger, I., Thomas, P., Degruttola, V. *et al.* (1988) Incubation periods for pediatric aids patients. *Nature* **336**, 575–577.

3 Comans-Bitter, W.M., de Groot, R., van den, Beemd, R. *et al.* (1997) Immunophenotyping of blood lymphocytes in childhood. Reference values for lymphocyte subpopulations. *Journal of Pediatrics* **130**, 388–393.

4 Duliege, A.M., Messiah, A., Blanche, S., Tardieu, M., Griscelli, C., Spira, A. (1992) Natural-history of human-immunodeficiency-virus type-1 infection in children – prognostic value of laboratory tests on the bimodal progression of the disease. *Pediatric Infectious Disease Journal* **11**, 630–635.

5 Gleicher, N., Siegel, I., Cederqvist, L.L. (1981) Do glucocorticosteroids affect the fetal immune system? *American Journal of Reproductive Immunology* **1**, 184–185.

6 Gunn, T., Reece, E.R., Metrakos, K., Colle, E. (1981) Depressed T cells following neonatal steroid treatment. *Pediatrics* **67**, 61–67.

7 Hamilton, A.A., Manuel, D.M., Grundy, J.E. *et al.* (1997) A humanised antibody against cytomegalovirus (CMV) gpUL75 (gH) for prophylaxis or treatment of CMV infections. *Journal of Infectious Diseases* **176**, 59–68.

8 Lewis, D.B., Wilson, C.B. (2001) Developmental immunology and role of host defenses in fetal and neonatal susceptibility to infection. In Remington, J.S., Klein, J.O. (eds), *Infectious Diseases of the Fetus and Newborn*, 5th edn. Philadelphia: W.B. Saunders, 25–138.

9 Mayaux, M.J., Burgard, M., Teglas, J.P. *et al.* (1996) Neonatal characteristics in rapidly progressive perinatally acquired HIV-1 disease. *Journal of the American Medical Association* **275**, 606–610.

10 Notarangelo, L.D., Chirico, G., Chiara, A. *et al.* (1984) Activity of classical and alternative pathways of complement in preterm and small for gestational age infants. *Pediatric Research* **18**, 281–285.

11 Playfair, J.H.L., Lydyard, P.M. (1995) Changes in circulating lymphocyte populations and serum immunoglobulin levels with age. In Playfair, J.H.L., Lydyard, P.M. (eds), *Medical Immunology for Students.* Edinburgh: Churchill Livingstone, 100.

12 Remmington, J.S., Klein, J.O. (2001) *Infectious Diseases of the Fetus and Newborn Infant*, 5th edn. Philadelphia: W.B. Saunders, 88.

13 Ryhanen, P., Kauppila, A., Koivisto, M. (1980) Unaltered neonatal cell-mediated immunity after prenatal dexamethasone treatment. *Obstetrics and Gynecology* **56**, 182–185.

14 Schur, P.H., Rosen, F., Norman, M.E. (1979) Immunoglobulin subclasses in normal children. *Pediatric Research* **13**, 181–183.

15 Scott, G.B., Hutto, C., Makuch, R.W. *et al.* (1989) Survival in children with perinatally acquired human immunodeficiency virus type-1 infection. *New England Journal of Medicine* **321**, 1791–1796.

16 Squire, E., Favara, B., Todd, J. (1979) Diagnosis of neonatal bacterial infection: hematologic and pathologic findings in fatal and nonfatal cases. *Pediatrics* **64**, 60–64.

17 Stiehm, E.R., Fudenberg, H.H. (1966) Serum levels of immune globulins in health and disease: a survey. *Pediatrics* **37**, 715–727.

18 The Impact-RSV Study Group (1998) Palivizumab, a humanized respiratory syncytial virus monoclonal antibody, reduces hospitalization from respiratory syncytial virus infection in high risk infants. *Pediatrics* **102**, 531–537.

19 The PREVENT Study Group (1997) Reduction of respiratory syncytial virus hospitalization among premature infants and infants with bronchopulmonary dysplasia using respiratory syncytial virus immune globulin prophylaxis. *Pediatrics* **99**, 93–99.

10

Histopathology

DI RUSHTON, with contributions from S GOULD

Pathological changes in the lung are of critical importance in determining survival and, while in those countries with advanced neonatal care facilities the classical features may be modified by the effects of treatment, they are still the major cause of morbidity and mortality, particularly in prematurely born neonates.[53] The embryology and developmental physiology of the respiratory tract has been discussed in earlier chapters. In this section, morphological effects of disturbance in development and physiological adaptation, as well as the deleterious effects of therapy and acquired disease on the lung, are outlined.

CONGENITAL MALFORMATIONS

There are a large number of individual malformations of the respiratory tract, generally classified by their anatomical location.

Nasal and oral malformations

Disturbances of nasal development affecting the external nares are most commonly seen in association with abnormalities of cerebral development; in the most extreme form the nose is replaced with a blind-ended proboscis.[20] The most common posterior nasal defect is choanal atresia, which may be unilateral or bilateral, isolated, or form part of a malformation syndrome.[21] Cleft palate is the commonest abnormality of the respiratory tract and may occur in isolation or with cleft lip. Isolated cleft palate differs from cleft lip whether alone or in combination with cleft palate in that the latter is twice as common in males. Cleft lip occurs twice as commonly on the left side[55] and not infrequently presents as part of a multiple malformation syndrome, for example trisomy 13. Clefting syndromes,

of which there are more than 350, may be dominant, recessive or X-linked as well as sporadic.[21]

Laryngeal malformations (p. 438)

Laryngeal atresia has been classified anatomically into three subgroups,[43] depending on whether the glottis, infraglottic region or both the supra- and infraglottic regions are involved.[29] The anomaly is thought to arise as a result of failure of re-canalization between the eighth and tenth weeks of gestation. The more extensive lesions are usually inconsistent with survival. Obstruction of normal lung fluid drainage may result in voluminous heavy lungs (p. 9). Many affected infants have additional malformations. Laryngeal stenoses are usually sited below the vocal cords and consist of cartilage, fibrous tissue and mucous glandular elements in various proportions. Laryngeal stenosis may also follow prolonged intubation and is typically subglottic in distribution (p. 443).[23] Laryngeal clefts[56] rarely are anterior and they are the result of failure of fusion of the thyroid cartilage. Posterior clefting is more common and is due to a failure of formation of the septum dividing the trachea and esophagus. The lesion is most frequently small, but may on occasion involve the full length of the trachea to the carina. Clefts involving only the larynx are commonly seen in association with tracheoesophageal fistula. Cystic lesions[9,15] are not uncommon in the laryngeal, pharyngeal and epiglottic regions and may be developmental in origin or be due to sequestrated and distended mucous glands.

Tracheal malformations

Atresia of the trachea is seen in association with tracheoesophageal fistula, the commonest congenital

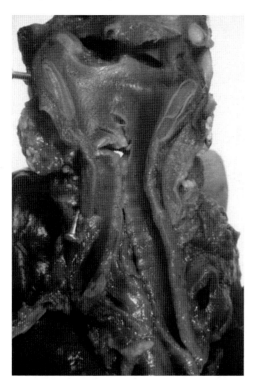

Figure 10.1 *Absence of trachea. The two main bronchi can be seen arising from the lower end of the larynx.*

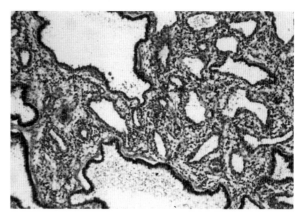

Figure 10.2 *Congenital cystic adenomatoid lung type 2. Cystic spaces lined by bronchiolar type epithelium devoid of cartilage. No normal lung is present. H&E × 100.*

abnormality of the trachea, but may be an isolated finding. It may be associated with multiple malformations. Tracheal stenosis may involve a single segment or several segments resulting in a funnel-like configuration.[4] The latter is common in association with anomalies of the left pulmonary artery. Anomalies of tracheal cartilage are present in some forms of skeletal dysplasia. Tracheal webs and tracheomalacia occur as in the larynx.[44] Tracheal agenesis (Figure 10.1) is very rare.[22]

Lung malformations

Pulmonary agenesis may very rarely be bilateral, but is usually unilateral.[6,31] There is a spectrum of abnormalities from complete absence of the lung and bronchus through to nodules of dysplastic lung tissue attached by a rudimentary bronchus. Agenesis is commonly associated with other congenital abnormalities (p. 449). Bronchial abnormalities may be extrapulmonary, for example, isomerism where both lungs are identical, or intrapulmonary, for example, atresia and stenosis. The former is frequently associated with abnormalities of the heart,[28] while the latter may be associated with other forms of cystic lung disease such as adenomatoid malformation. Stenotic lesions usually arise from extrinsic pressure. Bronchogenic cysts[41] occur within the chest, neck and occasionally within the abdomen. They do not communicate with the bronchial tree and their walls contain

tissue elements normally found in the bronchus in varying proportions.

Pulmonary sequestrations[45] are masses of abnormally developed lung tissue which do not communicate with the bronchial tree and are supplied by an aberrant systemic artery usually from the aorta either above or below the diaphragm. Such lesions may be intrapulmonary, typically in the left lower lobe, or extrapulmonary, within the thorax or upper abdomen.[10] The extrapulmonary lesions may show histological features of adenomatoid lung.[13] Some may communicate with the esophagus or stomach. Congenital cystic adenomatoid malformation of the lung (CCAM) is now frequently diagnosed antenatally. Some forms are incompatible with life, while others may be discovered incidentally on chest radiographs. Macroscopically the affected lung may appear solid and/or cystic. Pathologically, five types of lesion are recognized (p. 466) (Figure 10.2).[47] Congenital lobar emphysema results from localized overdistention of the lung after birth with compression of adjacent tissues leading to respiratory distress. The degree of hyperinflation may be such as to lead to death as a result of mediastinal shift. It may result from abnormal development of cartilage within the affected bronchus,[76] but external compression or partial intrinsic obstruction of an airway leading to a 'ball valve' effect could produce the same effect. Some cases may follow inflammatory lung disease.

Lung hypoplasia[30,38] is a relatively common disorder; up to a 15 percent incidence at perinatal autopsies has been suggested. It is not difficult for the pathologist to make the diagnosis (Figure 10.3). The lung to body weight ratio is commonly used to identify cases, the ratio varying from less than 0.015 below 28 weeks of gestation to 0.012 above that gestational age[54] These figures are, however, not an absolute indicator, as they may be influenced by other pathology occurring in the lungs. Lungs should always be in excess of 1.2 percent of the body weight.[2]

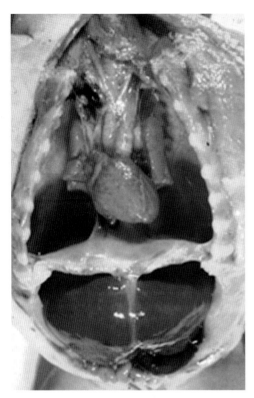

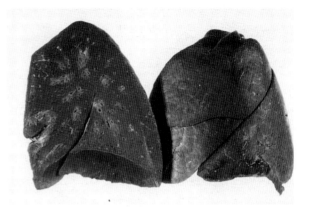

Figure 10.4 *Hyaline membrane disease. The lungs are rigid and airless retaining their shape. The cut surface appears solid.*

Figure 10.3 *Pulmonary hypoplasia. Tiny lungs on either side of the mediastinum. Hydrops fetalis with bilateral pleural effusions.*

While it is possible to use histomorphometric techniques to confirm lung hypoplasia, these are not routine laboratory procedures.

Pulmonary lymphangiectasia[8] may be an isolated abnormality or part of a more generalized disorder of the lymphatic system. It is rarely the result of a failure of normal communication between the lymphatics in the lungs and the thoracic duct, but more commonly it is secondary to cardiac malformations. It is frequently associated with pleural effusions.[19,42] The lymphatics on the surface of the lungs are very prominent, giving the appearance of Moroccan leather, a term used to describe these findings. Microscopically, there is a varying degree of lymphatic dilatation throughout the lung.

Pulmonary vascular anomalies

Arterial anomalies may occur as part of more complex cardiac malformations, be part of certain more generalized syndromes or confined to lung malformations.[3] An aberrant origin of the left artery from the right side can result in compression of the trachea and present as respiratory distress.[5] Other malformations include absence of the proximal part of the pulmonary artery, pulmonary arterial hypoplasia and segmental stenosis of the arteries. Arteriovenous fistulae may occur as developmental

anomalies or as the result of trauma. Anomalous venous return, both partial and complete, and stenosis of the pulmonary veins occur (p. 391).

NEONATAL LUNG DISEASE

Pulmonary immaturity

The classical lung lesion of prematurity is hyaline membrane disease (HMD),[40] a pathologically descriptive term of the microscopic appearances of the affected lung. While often used interchangeably with the clinical manifestation of the disease idiopathic respiratory distress syndrome (RDS), the terms are not strictly identical since hyaline membranes are found in other clinical situations and respiratory distress may occur in the absence of hyaline membranes. The macroscopic appearance of uncomplicated RDS is virtually pathognomonic, the lungs being of firm consistency evidenced by their retention of their intrathoracic shape on removal from the chest (Figure 10.4). Typically of a dark plum color, sometimes with prominent surface lymphatics, the cut surfaces are airless and congested, the lungs sinking when placed in fixative. The major airways are empty or contain lung fluid.

The microscopic appearances depend on the stage of evolution of the disease. The membranes, bands of eosinophilic material lining the dilated distal respiratory bronchioles (Figure 10. 5), form 12–24 hours after delivery (they do not form before birth and are not seen in stillbirths) and vary in extent and thickness. The more distal airways are collapsed. Although described as hyaline, the membranes contain cellular debris derived from alveolar lining cells and blood constituents that have leaked from abnormally permeable capillaries. The lung is typically uniformly collapsed and airless but congested. Those airways lined by membranes may also contain edema fluid

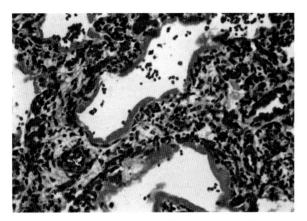

Figure 10.5 *Hyaline membrane disease. The membranes can be seen lining dilated alveolar ducts. H&E × 250.*

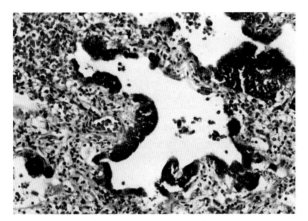

Figure 10.6 *Blue hyaline membranes. The membranes are much darker in color due to colonization with group B streptococci. H&E × 250.*

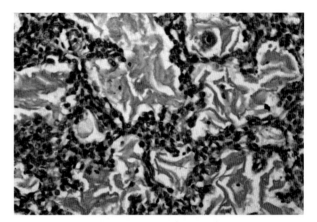

Figure 10.7 *Meconium aspiration. The alveoli are distended by aspirated squamous cells. H&E × 250.*

(or uncleared lung fluid) and desquamated lining cells from the respiratory tract. Not uncommonly there are also aspirated fetal squames in the airways. While the membranes are classically eosinophilic, they may have a greenish color if the neonate was jaundiced,[16] due to the protein in the membrane binding bilirubin, while a bluish color (Figure 10. 6) is seen in the presence of some infections, particularly group B streptococcal infection due to the large numbers of organisms within the membranes. In infants surviving the initial phase of the disease, there is progressive healing and repair of the lung,[7] a process often modified by the effects of treatment. The surface epithelium of the damaged airways re-establishes itself by growing over the membrane, which is simultaneously being removed by macrophages. Histological resolution in untreated cases occurs at about 1 week. If the response was insufficient at this time, death usually followed. Today, in many centers, this course of events is modified by the use of exogenous surfactant[24] and sophisticated ventilatory techniques, but long-term complications of neonatal respiratory support are still of major concern to

neonatologists. It is, however, of note that there do not appear to be any significant iatrogenic complications following the introduction of exogenous surfactant.[48]

Surfactant protein anomalies

Genetic disorders affecting surfactant proteins[34] are associated with neonatal respiratory distress and familial lung disease.[37] Pathologically, the alveoli are filled with proteinaceous material and resemble those seen in adult pulmonary alveolar proteinosis.[18] Electron microscopical investigations have identified another form of congenital surfactant defect.[51]

Intrauterine and birth asphyxia

The pathological manifestations of acute intrauterine asphyxia are classically seen in association with placental abruption. The baby is cyanosed and has frequently passed and aspirated and/or swallowed meconium. There may be petechial hemorrhages in the skin. The skin creases may contain meconium-stained vernix and after more prolonged exposure to meconium the finger and toenails may be stained green. The lungs are heavy, airless and cyanotic. There may be large numbers of subpleural petechial hemorrhages, which may become confluent. The airways are filled with fluid, which is often blood stained and/or contains meconium. Occasionally white specks are seen beneath the pleura, which on microscopy are found to consist of plugs of fetal squames (Figure 10. 7). Meconium is also frequently seen in the esophagus, the stomach, which may be distended with amniotic fluid, and sometimes in the upper small intestines. Microscopy shows the terminal airways to be filled with proteinaceous fluid, meconium and varying numbers of squames. Hemorrhages may fill groups of alveoli or be diffusely distributed through the aspirated material. Evidence of inflammation is unusual, although, because the passage of meconium and its aspiration are not confined to hypoxic insults, overwhelming infections such as group B streptococcal disease may produce a combined picture of aspiration and infection (p. 283).

In the asphyxiated neonate, hypoxic damage to the surfactant-producing cells (which may also be damaged by the aspirated material) may contribute to the development of hyaline membranes.[14,35] Inflammatory changes may be secondary to concomitant aspiration of organisms or due to chemical damage to the lungs. Uneven aeration of the lungs and trapping of air behind aspirated material may lead to interstitial emphysema and pneumothorax. Where the aspirated material is confined to the larger airways, lavage and suction may be effective, but once material has reached alveoli removal is more difficult and depends to a great extent on the normal mechanisms for the clearing of foreign material. In survivors squames may be found in the lungs several weeks after delivery. In a small proportion of infants that have aspirated meconium, there are in addition to the features described above abnormalities of the pulmonary arteries and arterioles, which are clinically associated with persistent pulmonary hypertension.[36] The exact mechanism leading to these changes is debatable, but chronic intrauterine hypoxia has been suggested as a factor. Such changes also challenge the view that the passage of meconium occurs shortly before birth.[49] Chronic intrauterine meconium aspiration may result in lung infarction and rupture.[25] There is hypertrophy of the medial muscle in the pre- and intra-acinar pulmonary arteries and muscularization of the precapillary vessels.

Pulmonary hemorrhage

Minor pulmonary hemorrhages can be found in the majority of postmortem lungs in the neonatal period and may reflect at least in part, the mechanisms of death rather than indicate causation.[12,52] In a few infants, the bleeding may be massive, the infants appearing to have drowned in their own blood.[17,50] At autopsy all areas of the lungs are filled with red cells (Figure 10.8).

INFECTION

Transplacental infections

These include viral infections such as cytomegalovirus (Figure 10.9), rubella, herpes simplex, varicella and enteroviruses. Other organisms include *Listeria monocytogenes*, *Toxoplasma gondii*, *Treponema pallidum* and *Mycobacterium tuberculosis*. All these infections are generalized in nature and while they may present diagnostic problems during life, many show characteristic pathological changes at autopsy.

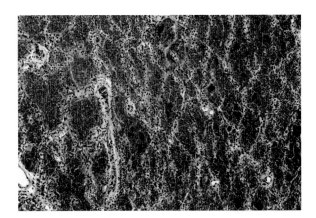

Figure 10.8 *Massive pulmonary hemorrhage. Every airspace is packed with red cells. H&E × 100.*

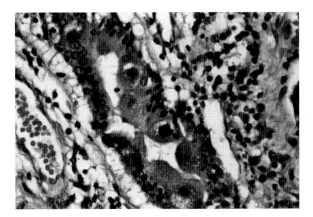

Figure 10.9 *Cytomegalovirus pneumonia. The bronchial epithelial cells contain characteristic nuclear inclusions. H&E × 400.*

Intra- and postpartum infections

Pathologically early lethal infections may show little evidence of a cellular response, which if present is frequently patchy in distribution. Edema and hemorrhage may be prominent and, because of damage to surfactant-producing cells, hyaline membranes may be evident. These membranes tend to be coarser and less regular both in outline and distribution than those seen in RDS. They may be colonized by bacteria. In infants surviving for longer periods, an acute bronchopneumonia can develop which, depending on the organism involved, may lead to abscess formation and, rarely, empyema. If there is infection with Gram-negative organisms, particularly *Proteus* and *Pseudomonas*, initially there may be a sparse cellular response, hemorrhage and widespread edema containing vast numbers of organisms which may also be present within the walls of blood vessels. The latter may lead to local thrombus formation in the pulmonary circulation. While definitive identification of the causative organism in the living neonate is normally dependent on culture,

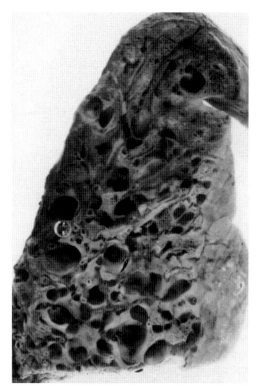

Figure 10.10 *Pulmonary interstitial emphysema.*

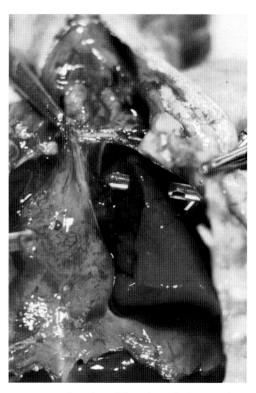

Figure 10.11 *Perforation of lung by a drainage tube.*

histological techniques may also provide specific answers after death, particularly since the advent of immuno-histochemical and molecular techniques.

Pulmonary interstitial emphysema (PIE) and pneumothorax

Inspired gases escaping from the respiratory tree may enter the interstitial tissues of the lungs (Figure 10.10), typically the interlobular and interlobar fissures, the pulmonary lymphatics and on occasion the pulmonary vessels, usually the pulmonary veins. Small, clinically undetectable leakages are commonly identified in neonatal lungs at autopsy and are almost invariably seen in the presence of pneumothorax in the absence of clinical PIE. Extensive involvement results in a 'Swiss cheese' pattern on the cut surfaces of affected lung. This may be associated with subpleural emphysematous bullae, which rupture, leading to pneumothorax. Escaping gas may also spread widely in the mediastinum, involve the pericardium and extrathoracic organs and cavities. If the infant survives, much, if not all the escaped gas will be resorbed or lost following drainage but occasionally it becomes loculated as encysted interstitial emphysema,[11] a condition sometimes mistaken for some forms of congenital cystic lung in surgically excised specimens. Encysted interstitial emphysema usually has no microscopically identifiable lining, but often the wall of the cyst contains scattered multinucleate giant cells.

CHEST DRAINAGE

The usual indication for chest drainage is pneumothorax, although pleural effusions and chylothorax may also require aspiration. Occasionally blood or pus may necessitate removal. Drainage may only require the introduction of a needle into the chest, but in more severe cases the use of a trochar and drainage tubes is necessary. Both techniques carry the risk of puncture of the lung, resulting in air leaks, bronchopleural fistula or hemorrhage. Rarely, other intrathoracic structures such as major blood vessels or the heart may be injured and occasionally intra-abdominal organs such as the liver may be punctured. Longer-term drainage by tube may introduce infection and changes in the plasticity of drainage tubes, leading to increased rigidity and puncture or transfixion of the lung (Figure 10.11).

Bronchopulmonary dysplasia (BPD)

The evolution of BPD has been detailed by Anderson and Engel[1] and can be divided into three phases. First, there is an acute phase, which lasts up to 2 weeks, which combines an exudative necrotizing reaction with an early healing response. The changes are usually added to those of the preceding RDS. Epithelial changes occur in the bronchi and bronchioles. The nuclei of the ciliated respiratory epithelium migrate to the luminal surface and are extruded

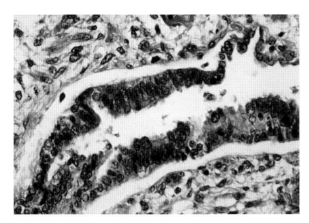

Figure 10.12 *Early metaplastic change in bronchial epithelium due to oxygen toxicity. H&E × 400.*

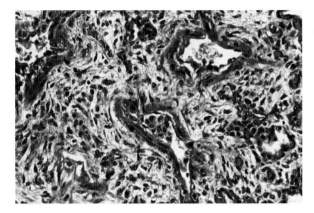

Figure 10.13 *Bronchopulmonary dysplasia. Most of the airspaces are obliterated by fibrous tissue. Those present are lined by abnormal pneumocytes containing bizarre nuclei. H&E × 400.*

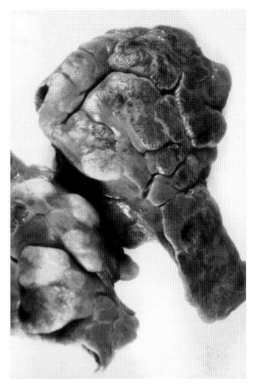

Figure 10.14 *Bronchopulmonary dysplasia. The lungs are distorted with an exaggerated lobular pattern. The irregular surface reflects areas of collapsed and hyperinflated lung.*

and the damaged lining is replaced by metaplastic squamous epithelium (Figure 10.12). There is diffuse alveolar damage and necrosis of bronchioles. Healing results in obliteration of the damaged airways together with interstitial fibrosis. While at this stage some of these changes may be reversible, the fibrosis and obliterative lesions are unlikely to resolve, although they may not progress once the respiratory support is withdrawn. Both, however, are significant in that lung growth is impaired, a feature which may have long-term sequelae. Next follows a subacute phase which continues until about the end of the first month after the onset of the BPD and is associated with progressive fibrosis, particularly around alveolar ducts. Perialveolar fibrosis and smooth muscle proliferation occur (Figure 10.13). Lesions in the alveolar ducts result in both collapse and hyperdistention of more distal airways, accentuating the lobular architecture of the lungs (Figure 10.14). Type 2 pneumocytes repopulate the damaged alveoli and often contain bizarre nuclei. Finally, there is a chronic phase, which may continue for months after the onset of the BPD and is associated with progressive

fibrosis, further smooth muscle proliferation and the development of 'honeycomb' lung. There are also changes in the pulmonary vessels resulting in pulmonary hypertension and eventually right heart failure may ensue. Destructive obliterative lesions are, however, absent. Squamous metaplasia frequently persists throughout this phase. Pathologically, a variant form of chronic lung disease in very small preterm infants dying some months after delivery has been described and is characterized by adjacent areas of hyperdistended and collapsed lung parenchyma (p. 402).[32,46]

NEONATAL LUNG CYTOLOGY

The normal source of lung cytology specimens in the neonate is bronchial lavage fluid, although occasionally pleural aspirates may require examination. Apart from the identification of evidence of infection (recognition of specific organisms, identification of inflammatory cells), lavage fluid may be used: to identify yellow hyaline membrane disease,[16] to investigate RDS and bronchopulmonary dysplasia,[33] experimentally to manage the meconium aspiration syndrome[27] and to seek evidence of aspiration into the lungs by demonstrating the presence of lipid-laden macrophages in lavage samples.[26]

PLACENTAL EXAMINATION

Placenta examination is important for both stillborn and liveborn infants, indeed all placentae of infants admitted to the neonatal unit should be subjected to pathological examination. In the context of neonatal respiratory disease, the most common placental pathology of significance is chorioamnionitis, which indicates the presence of ascending infection and may be associated with an early-onset pneumonia. The infection is sometimes macroscopically obvious, but unless the chorioamnionitis is due to *Candida*, microscopy and histology is usually non specific. *Listeria monocytogenes* infection can generate a characteristic villitis.

REFERENCES

1 Anderson, W.R., Engel, R.R. (1983) Cardiopulmonary sequelae of reparative stages of bronchopulmonary dysplasia. *Archives of Pathology and Laboratory Medicine* **107**, 603–608.

2 Askenazi, S.S., Perlman, M. (1979) Pulmonary hypoplasia: lung weight and radial alveolar count as criteria of diagnosis. *Archives of Disease in Childhood* **54**, 614–618.

3 Becker, A.E., Anderson, R.H. (1981) *Pathology of Congenital Heart Disease*. London: Butterworths.

4 Benjamin, P., Pitkin, J., Cohen, D. (1981) Congenital tracheal stenosis. *Annals of Otology, Rhinology and Laryngology* **90**, 364–371.

5 Berdon, W.E., Baker, D.H. (1972) Vascular anomalies and the infant lung: rings, slings and other things. *Seminars in Roentgenology* **7**, 39–64.

6 Booth, J.B., Berry, C.L. (1967) Unilateral pulmonary agenesis. *Archives of Disease in Childhood* **42**, 361–374.

7 Boss, J.H., Craig, J.M. (1962) Reparative phenomena in lungs of neonates with hyaline membranes. *Pediatrics* **29**, 890–898.

8 Bouchard, S., Di Lorenzo, M., Youssef, S. *et al.* (2000) Pulmonary lymphangiectasia revisited. *Journal of Pediatric Surgery* **35**, 796–800.

9 Canty, T.G., Hendren, W.H. (1975) Upper airway obstruction from foregut cysts of the hypopharynx. *Journal of Pediatric Surgery* **10**, 807–812.

10 Carpentieri, D.F., Guttenberg, M., Quinn, T.M., Adzick, N.S. (2000) Subdiaphragmatic pulmonary sequestration: a case report with review of the literature. *Journal of Perinatology* **20**, 60–62.

11 Cohen, M.C., Drut, R.M., Drut, R. (1999) Solitary unilocular cyst of the lung with features of persistent interstitial pulmonary emphysema: report of four cases. *Pediatric and Developmental Pathology* **2**, 531–536.

12 Cole, V.A., Normand, I.C.S., Reynolds, E.O.R. (1973) Pathogenesis of hemorrhagic pulmonary edema and massive pulmonary hemorrhage in the newborn. *Pediatrics* **51**, 175–187.

13 Conran, R.M., Stocker, J.T. (1999) Extralobar sequestration with frequently associated congenital cystic adenomatoid malformation, type 2: report of 50 cases. *Pediatric and Developmental Pathology* **2**, 454–463.

14 Dargaville, P.A., South, M., McDougall, P.N. (2001) Surfactant and surfactant inhibitors in meconium aspiration syndrome. *Journal of Pediatrics* **138**, 113–115.

15 Desanto, L.W., Devine, K.D., Weiland, L.H. (1970) Cysts of the larynx – classification. *Laryngoscope* **80**, 145–176.

16 Doshi, N., Klionsky, B., Kanbour, A. (1983) Yellow hyaline membrane disease in neonates: clinical diagnosis by tracheal aspiration cytology. *Pediatric Pathology* **1**, 193–198.

17 Fedrick, J., Butler, N.R. (1971) Certain causes of neonatal death. IV. Massive pulmonary haemorrhage. *Biology of the Neonate* **18**, 243–262.

18 de la Fuente, A.A., Voorhout, W.F., de Mello, D.E. (1997) Congenital alveolar proteinosis in the Netherlands: a report of five cases with immunohistochemical and genetic studies on surfactant apoproteins. *Pediatric Pathology and Laboratory Medicine* **17**, 221–231.

19 Gardner, T.W., Domm, A.C., Brock, C.E., Pruitt, A.W. (1983) Congenital pulmonary lymphangiectasis. A case complicated by chylothorax. *Clinical Pediatrics* **22**, 75–78.

20 Gifford, G.H., Swanson, L., MacCollum, D.W. (1972) Congenital absence of the nose and anterior nasopharynx. *Plastic and Reconstructive Surgery* **50**, 5–12.

21 Gorlin, R.J., Cohen, M.M., Levin, L.S. (1997) *Syndromes of the Head and Neck*, 3rd edn. New York: Oxford University Press.

22 Gould, S.J (2001) Chapter 17. In Keeling, J. (ed.), *Fetal and Neonatal Pathology*, 3rd edn. London: Springer, 447–448.

23 Gould, S.J., Howard, S. (1985) The histopathology of the larynx in the neonate following endotracheal intubation. *Journal of Pathology* **146**, 301–311.

24 Halliday, H.L. (1996) Where are we now with prenatal steroids and postnatal surfactant. *Biology of the Neonate* **69**, 186–187.

25 Kearney, M.S. (1999) Chronic intrauterine meconium aspiration causes fetal lung infarcts, lung rupture and meconium embolism. *Pediatric and Developmental Pathology* **2**, 544–551.

26 Knauer-Fischer, S., Ratjen, F. (1999) Lipid-laden macrophages in bronchoalveolar lavage fluid as a marker for pulmonary aspiration. *Pediatric Pulmonology* **27**, 419–422.

27 Lam, B.C., Yeung, C.Y., Fu, K.H. *et al.* (2000) Surfactant tracheobronchial lavage for the management of a rabbit model of meconium aspiration syndrome. *Biology of the Neonate* **78**, 129–138.

28 Landing, B.H. (1984) Five syndromes (malformation complexes) of pulmonary symmetry, congenital heart disease and multiple spleens. *Pediatric Pathology* **2**, 125–151.

29 Landing, B.H., Dixon, L.G. (1979) Congenital malformations and genetic disorders of the respiratory tract (larynx, trachea, bronchi and lungs). *American Review of Respiratory Diseases* **120**, 151–185.

30 Langston, C. (1989) Prenatal lung growth and pulmonary hypoplasia. In Stocker J T (ed.), *Pediatric Pulmonary Disease*. New York: Hemisphere, 1–92.

31 Maltz, D.L., Nadas, A.S. (1968) Agenesis of the lung: presentation of eight new cases and review of the literature. *Pediatrics* **42**, 175–188.

32 McKay, C.A., Faulkner, C.S., Edwards, W.H. (1985) Unusual pulmonary reaction to respiratory therapy in a premature newborn. *Human Pathology* **16**, 629–631.

33 Merritt, T.A., Puccia, J.M., Stuard, I.D. (1981) Cytologic evaluation of pulmonary effluent in neonates with respiratory distress syndrome and bronchopulmonary dysplasia. *Acta Cytologica* **25**, 631–639.

34 Mildenberger, E., de Mello, D.E., Lin, Z. *et al.* (2001) Focal congenital alveolar proteinosis associated with abnormal surfactant protein B messenger RNA. *Chest* **119**, 645–647.

35 Moses, D., Holm, B.A., Spitale, P. *et al.* (1991) Inhibition of pulmonary surfactant by meconium. *American Journal of Obstetrics and Gynecology* **164**, 477–481.

36 Murphy, J.D., Vawter, G.F., Reid, L.M. (1984) Pulmonary vascular disease in fatal meconium aspiration. *Journal of Pediatrics* **104**, 758–762.

37 Nogee, L.M., Dunbar, A.E., Wertz, S.E. *et al.* (2001) A mutation in the surfactant protein C gene associated with familial interstitial lung disease. *New England Journal of Medicine* **344**, 573–579.

38 Porter, H.J. (1999) Pulmonary hypoplasia. *Archives of Disease in Childhood Fetal and Neonatal Edition* **81**, 81–83.

39 Powell, H.C., Eliott, J.L. (1977) Congenital lobar emphysema. *Virchows Archives A* **374**, 197–203.

40 Rosan, S.C. (1975) Hyaline membrane disease and a related spectrum of neonatal pneumonopathies. *Perspectives in Pediatric Pathology* **2**, 15–60.

41 Sayler, D.C., Sayler, W.R., Eggleston, J.C. (1977) Benign developmental cysts of the mediastinum. *Archives of Pathology and Laboratory Medicine* **101**, 136–139.

42 Shannon, M.P., Grantmyre, E.B., Reid, W.D., Wotherspoon, A.S. (1974) Congenital pulmonary lymphangiectasis. Report of two cases. *Pediatric Radiology* **2**, 235–240.

43 Smith, I.I., Bain, A.D. (1977) Congenital atresia of the larynx. A review of nine cases. *Annals of Otology, Rhinology and Laryngology* **86**, 338–349.

44 Solomons, L.B., Prescott, C.A.J. (1987) Laryngomalacia: a review and the surgical management of severe cases. *International Journal of Pediatric Otology, Rhinology and Laryngology* **13**, 31–39.

45 Stocker, J.T. (1986) Sequestrations of the lung. *Seminars in Diagnostic Pathology* **3**, 106–121.

46 Stocker, J.T. (1986) Pathologic features of long standing healed bronchopulmonary dysplasia: a study of 28 3 to 40 month old infants. *Human Pathology* **16**, 943–961.

47 Stocker, J.T., Madewell, J.E., Drake, R.M. (1977) Congenital adenomatoid malformation of the lung: classification and morphological spectrum. *Human Pathology* **8**, 155–171.

48 Thornton, C.M., Halliday, H.L., O'Hara, M.D. (1994) Surfactant replacement therapy in preterm neonates: a comparison of postmortem pulmonary histology in treated and untreated infants. *Pediatric Pathology* **14**, 945–953.

49 Thureen, P.J., Hall, D.M., Hoffenberg, A., Tyson, R.W. (1997) Fatal meconium aspiration in spite of appropriate perinatal airway management: pulmonary and placental evidence of prenatal disease. *American Journal of Obstetrics and Gynecology* **176**, 967–975.

50 Trompeter, R., Yu, V.Y.H., Aynsley-Green, A., Roberton, N.R.C. (1975) Massive pulmonary haemorrhage in the newborn infant. *Archives of Disease in Childhood* **50**, 123–127.

51 Tryka, A.F., Wertz, S.E., Mazursky, J.E. *et al.* (2000) Absence of lamellar bodies with accumulation of dense bodies characterizes a novel form of congenital surfactant defect. *Pediatric and Developmental Pathology* **3**, 335–345.

52 Wigglesworth, J.S. (1977) Pathology of neonatal respiratory distress. *Proceedings of the Royal Society of Medicine* **70**, 861–863.

53 Wigglesworth, J.S., Desai, R. (1982) Is fetal respiratory function a major determinant of perinatal survival? *Lancet* **1**, 264–267.

54 Wigglesworth, J.S., Desai, R., Guerrini, P. (1981) Fetal lung hypoplasia: biochemical and structural variations and their possible significance. *Archives of Disease in Childhood* **56**, 606–615.

55 Wyszynski, D.F., Beaty, T.H., Maestri, N.E. (1996) Genetics of nonsyndromic oral clefts revisited. *Cleft Palate-Craniofacial Journal* **33**, 406–417.

56 Zaw-Tum, H.I.A. (1988) Development of laryngeal atresias and clefts. *Annals of Otology, Rhinology and Laryngology* **97**, 353–358.

Antenatal imaging and therapy

KYPROS H NICOLAIDES with contributions by ANNE GREENOUGH

TECHNIQUES

Ultrasound

Ultrasound is the principal diagnostic tool for the prenatal detection of congenital abnormalities. It allows examination of the external and internal anatomy of the fetus and the detection of major malformations, as well as more subtle ones, which may be markers of chromosomal defects or genetic syndromes. Furthermore, ultrasonography plays a central role in enhancing the safety and effectiveness of invasive diagnostic and therapeutic procedures.

THREE-DIMENSIONAL (3-D) ULTRASOUND

Three-dimensional (3-D) ultrasound enables imaging in three orthogonal planes and may provide better assessment, than 2-D conventional ultrasound, of the site and extent of an abnormality. An ultrasound sweep through the area of interest allows the acquisition of a volume, which can subsequently be rotated into standard anatomical planes. The images can be reconstructed and modified to permit display of different structures within the same data set. The technique has potential application in cases of congenital diaphragmatic hernia and congenital cystic adenomatoid malformation by allowing 3-D assessment of both the pathological process and fetal lung volume. It may prove to be beneficial in assessment in cases where fetal surgery is an option. Reference ranges for fetal lung growth have been established from lung volume measurements using an ultrasound-based 3-D system;[1] such results may be useful in the prediction of pulmonary hypoplasia. Three-dimensional reconstruction of power Doppler images may facilitate appreciation of vascular anatomy, for example, in cases of pulmonary sequestration with systemic vascular supply. Presently, however, 3-D ultrasound is often limited by technical considerations, particularly artifact caused by fetal movement, loss of information when the fetus is pressed against the uterine wall or placenta, or lack of amniotic fluid around the region of interest.

COLOR DOPPLER

Color flow mapping allows visualization of pulmonary arteries and veins from the heart into the peripheral pulmonary segments. In suspected diaphragmatic hernia, visualization of liver vessels in the thorax can confirm the diagnosis. In bronchopulmonary sequestration, the diagnosis can be made by the demonstration of the feeding artery arising directly from the descending aorta. Color Doppler has been found to be useful in the diagnosis of the very rare condition of unilateral lung agenesis. Some cardiac defects, such as pulmonary valve atresia with ventricular septum defect, are associated with multiple aortopulmonary collateral arteries, which may complicate the neonatal course. There are contradictory reports on the potential value of Doppler assessment of the pulmonary vessels in the prediction of pulmonary hypoplasia and pulmonary hypertension.

FETAL MAGNETIC RESONANCE IMAGING

During the last decade there has been increasing interest in MRI for the evaluation of sonographically detected fetal abnormalities. Detailed imaging was previously prevented by fetal movement artifact, but single-shot rapid acquisition sequences have now partly overcome this problem. These ultrafast techniques with subsecond images capture 'snapshot' views of the fetus. Currently, fetal MRI is mainly used in the investigation of cerebral abnormalities suspected from ultrasound. There is also potential value in assessing lung maturation and the volume of normal lung. The normal fetal lung on T2-weighted images at 16–24 weeks of gestation is homogeneous and has moderate signal density. Maturation of the lungs is associated with increased production of alveolar fluid; this is associated with an increased T2 signal and a decreased T1 signal.[9] Fetal MRI also has potential to assess pulmonary abnormalities, for example, congenital cystic adenomatoid malformation (CCAM) or pulmonary sequestration. The appearance of a CCAM on fetal MRI is variable, depending on whether the lesion is micro- or macrocystic. Microcystic lesions are high in signal density compared to normal lung.[8] Pulmonary sequestrations on antenatal MRI may appear as wedge-shaped areas of very high homogeneous signal density on T2-weighted images.[8] MRI may be useful with regard to prediction of outcome in fetuses with congenital diaphragmatic hernia (CDH). It can be used to locate the position of the liver (p. 488); on T2-weighted images the liver is high in signal density. In addition, both the right and left lungs can be visualized with MRI and the lung volumes obtained.[9]

Echoplanar imaging (EPI)

This is a rapid MRI method of assessing organ volumes. Imaging studies can take less than 5 minutes and no sedation may be required.[12] Variations in lung volumes can be assessed by EPI MR imaging.[6,7] Lung volumes have been demonstrated to increase from 21 ml at 23 weeks of gestation to a maximum of 94 ml at term.[2] In infants following CDH repair, EPI demonstrated low lung volume in the ipsilateral lung of left-sided CDH infants.[12]

FETAL KARYOTYPING

Fetal karyotyping is essential in the assessment of fetuses with diaphragmatic hernia, because about 50 percent have chromosomal abnormalities. This can be done by chorionic villous sampling at 11–15 weeks of gestation or amniocentesis after 15 weeks of gestation.

Amniocentesis

A needle is introduced through the maternal abdomen and directed into the amniotic cavity under continuous ultrasound guidance. Fluid (10 ml) is aspirated and used for cytogenetic analysis. The risk of miscarriage from amniocentesis is about 1 percent. Amniocentesis is also associated with an increased risk of respiratory distress syndrome and pneumonia in neonates. In addition, some studies have reported an association with increased incidence of talipes and dislocation of the hip. Amniocentesis is best performed after 16 weeks of gestation. In the late 1980s, early amniocentesis at 10–14 weeks of gestation was introduced. However, several randomized studies in the 1990s demonstrated that this procedure is associated with a high risk of miscarriage and a high incidence of talipes equinovarus.

Chorionic villus sampling

Chorionic villus sampling was first attempted in the late 1960s by hysteroscopy, but the technique was associated with low success in both sampling and karyotyping and was abandoned in favor of amniocentesis. In the 1970s, the desire for early diagnosis led to the revival of chorionic villus sampling, which was initially carried out by aspiration via a cannula that was introduced 'blindly' into the uterus through the cervix. Subsequently, ultrasound guidance was used for the transcervical or transabdominal insertion of a variety of cannulas or biopsy forceps. Several randomized studies have examined the rate of fetal loss following first-trimester chorionic villus sampling compared to that of amniocentesis at 16 weeks of gestation. The results demonstrated that, in centers experienced in both procedures, fetal loss is no greater after first-trimester chorionic villus sampling compared to second-trimester amniocentesis. In the early 1990s, severe transverse limb abnormalities, micrognathia and microglossia were reported in some pregnancies that had undergone chorionic villus sampling at less than 10 weeks of gestation. Possible mechanisms by which early sampling may lead to limb defects include hypoperfusion, embolization or release of vasoactive substances, and all these mechanisms are related to trauma. It is therefore imperative that chorionic villus sampling is performed only after 11 weeks of gestation by appropriately trained operators.

INTERVENTIONS

Pleural-amniotic shunting

Pleural effusions or pulmonary cysts can be drained into the amniotic cavity through a double pigtail silastic catheter. The catheter, with external and internal diameters of 0.21 and 0.15 mm, has radio-opaque stainless steel inserts at each end and lateral holes around the coil. Ultrasound scanning is used to obtain a transverse section of the fetal thorax. With the transducer in one hand, held parallel to the intended course of the cannula, the

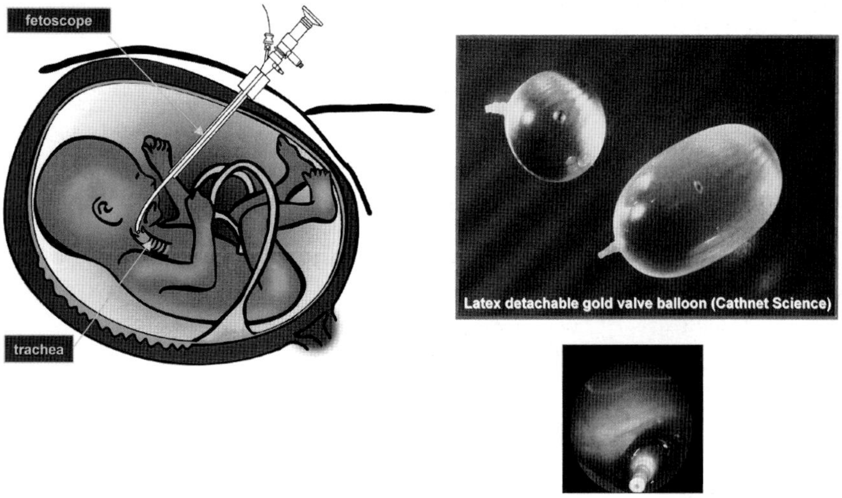

Figure 11.1 *Fetal endotracheal occlusion. On the left is a diagrammatic representation of insertion of a balloon in the trachea. On the right is a picture of the balloons (upper picture) and a view through a fetoscope of the balloon* in situ *in the trachea (lower picture).*

chosen site of entry on the maternal abdomen is cleaned with antiseptic solution and local anaesthetic is infiltrated down to the myometrium. Under ultrasound guidance, a metal cannula with a trocar (external diameter 3 mm, length 15 cm) is introduced transabdominally into the amniotic cavity and inserted through the fetal chest wall, in the mid-thoracic region, into the effusion or cyst. The trocar is removed and the catheter inserted into the cannula. A short introducer rod is then used to deposit half of the catheter into the effusion or cyst. Subsequently, the cannula is gradually removed into the amniotic cavity where the other half of the catheter is pushed by a longer introducer. If drainage of the contralateral lung is also needed, the appropriate fetal position is achieved by rotation of the fetal body using the tip of the cannula. After insertion of the shunt, serial ultrasound scans are performed at weekly intervals to determine if the effusions reaccumulate, in which case another shunt may be inserted. After delivery the chest drains are immediately clamped and removed to avoid development of pneumothorax.

Laser ablation of blood vessels

This technique is used to ablate the blood supply to large and rapidly expanding solid tumors, such as adenomatoid malformation or sequestration. Detailed ultrasound examination, including color flow mapping, is first performed to identify blood vessels within the tumor. The appropriate site of entry on the maternal abdomen is chosen to avoid injury to the placenta or fetus and to allow access to the intrathoracic tumor. The chosen site of entry on the maternal abdomen is cleaned with antiseptic solution and local anesthetic is infiltrated down to the myometrium. Under ultrasound guidance, an 18 gauge cannula is introduced into the amniotic cavity and inserted through the fetal chest wall into the tumor.

A 400 μm diameter Nd:YAG laser fiber is then passed down the cannula. Color flow mapping is used to visualize the blood supply to the tumor. The laser fiber is placed adjacent to the vessel, which is to be coagulated. The total procedure usually takes 10 minutes to complete. Serial ultrasound scans are performed at weekly intervals to demonstrate shrinkage of the tumor and return of the mediastinum to its normal position.

Fetal endotracheal occlusion by a balloon

Congenital diaphragmatic hernia with intrathoracic liver and a lung area to head circumference ratio of <1 is associated with high neonatal mortality due to pulmonary hypoplasia and hypertension (p. 493). Experimental tracheal occlusion may overcome these complications (p. 492).[4,5] Preliminary data from the application of the technique in human fetuses suggest that tracheal occlusion at 26–28 weeks of gestation may reverse pulmonary hypoplasia. The mother is first given general anesthesia and the fetus is then injected with pancuronium for immobilization and atropine to block a vasovagal response. The injection is given into the fetal thigh through a 20 gauge needle introduced through the maternal abdomen and guided by ultrasound. A Teflon cannula with trocar (external diameter 3 mm) is inserted into the amniotic cavity through the maternal abdomen and directed towards the fetal mouth. The trocar is then replaced by a curved metal sheath (external diameter 3 mm) loaded with a fetoscope (external diameter 1.2 mm) and a vascular occlusion catheter with a latex balloon (Figure 11.1). A combination of ultrasonographic and direct vision is used to introduce the fetoscope into the fetal mouth in the midline above the tongue and past the uvula into the nasopharynx and larynx (Figure 11.2). The vascular occlusion catheter with the balloon is then passed through the vocal cords, the balloon is inflated with saline (1 ml) and

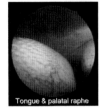
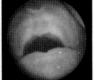
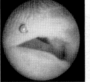
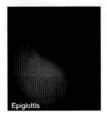
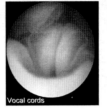
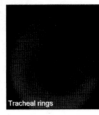
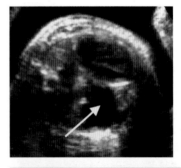

Figure 11.2 *Fetal endotracheal occlusion. Views through the fetoscope – the upper pictures are of the fetal face, the lower pictures are of the tongue, epiglottis, vocal cords and tracheal rings seen as the fetoscope moves down the upper respiratory tract.*

deposited into the fetal trachea below the vocal cords. The total procedure usually takes 10–15 minutes to complete. Delivery is by cesarean section; the fetal head is delivered and while the baby is still attached to the umbilical cord, intubation and removal of the balloon is undertaken through a bronchoscope.[3,10]

EXAMPLES OF CONDITIONS SUSCEPTIBLE TO ANTENATAL DIAGNOSIS AND INTERVENTION

Diaphragmatic hernia

Herniation of the abdominal viscera into the thorax usually occurs at about 10–12 weeks of gestation, when the intestines return to the abdominal cavity from the umbilical cord. At least in some cases, however, intrathoracic herniation of viscera may be delayed until the second or third trimester of pregnancy. In about 50 percent of affected fetuses, however, there are associated chromosomal abnormalities (mainly trisomy 18, trisomy 13 and Pallister–Killian syndrome – mosaicism for tetrasomy 12p), other defects (mainly craniospinal defects, including spina bifida, hydrocephaly and the otherwise rare anencephaly, and cardiac abnormalities) and genetic syndromes (such as Fryns syndrome, de Lange syndrome and Marfan syndrome).

DIAGNOSIS

Prenatally, the diaphragm is imaged by ultrasonography as an echo-free space between the thorax and abdomen. Diaphragmatic hernia can be diagnosed by the ultrasonographic demonstration of stomach and intestines (90 percent of the cases) or liver (50 percent) in the thorax and the associated mediastinal shift to the opposite side. Herniated abdominal contents, associated with a left-sided diaphragmatic hernia, are easy to demonstrate because the echo-free fluid-filled stomach and small

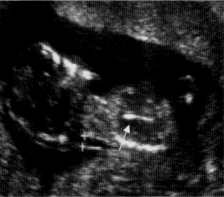

Figure 11.3 *Congenital diaphragmatic hernia. Ultrasound pictures demonstrating the appearance of a congenital diaphragmatic hernia (indicated by arrows).*

bowel contrast dramatically with the more echogenic fetal lung (Figure 11.3). By contrast, a right-sided hernia is more difficult to identify because the echogenicity of the fetal liver is similar to that of the lung, and visualization of the gall bladder in the right side of the fetal chest may be the only way of making the diagnosis. Polyhydramnios (usually occurring after 25 weeks of gestation) is found in about 75 percent of cases and this may be the consequence of impaired fetal swallowing due to compression of the esophagus by the herniated abdominal organs. The main differential diagnosis is from cystic lung disease, such as cystic adenomatoid malformation or mediastinal

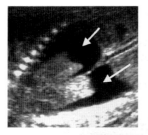
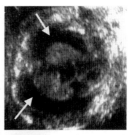
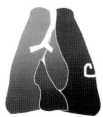
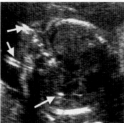

Figure 11.4 *Bilateral pleural effusions. On the left are diagrammatic representations of insertion of the shunt (upper picture) and the shunt in situ (lower picture). On the right are pictures (middle and right upper) of ultrasound scans showing bilateral pleural effusions (indicated by the arrows) and bilateral pleuroamniotic shunts (indicated by the arrows) in situ (lower picture).*

cystic processes, e.g. neuroenteric cysts, bronchogenic cysts and thymic cysts. In these cases, a fluid-filled structure causing mediastinal shift may be present within the chest. However, in contrast to diaphragmatic hernia, the upper abdominal anatomy is normal.

Antenatal prediction of pulmonary hypoplasia remains one of the challenges of prenatal diagnosis because this would be vital in both counseling parents and also in selecting those cases that may benefit from prenatal surgery. Poor prognostic signs are, first, increased nuchal translucency thickness at 10–14 weeks of gestation, second, intrathoracic herniation of abdominal viscera before 20 weeks of gestation, and, third, severe mediastinal compression suggested by an abnormal ratio in the size of the cardiac ventricles, a low lung area to head circumference ratio and the development of polyhydramnios.

FETAL THERAPY

Although isolated diaphragmatic hernia is an anatomically simple defect, which is easily correctable by postnatal surgery, the mortality rate is about 50 percent. The main cause of death is hypoxemia due to pulmonary hypoplasia and hypertension, resulting from the abnormal development of the pulmonary vascular bed. Extensive animal studies have suggested that pulmonary hypoplasia and hypertension are reversible by intrauterine surgery. In a few cases of diaphragmatic hernia, hysterotomy and fetal surgery have been carried out, but this intervention has now been abandoned in favor of minimally invasive surgery. Animal studies have demonstrated that obstruction of the trachea results in expansion of the fetal lungs by retained pulmonary secretions. Endoscopic occlusion of the fetal trachea has initially been carried out by clipping the trachea but a less traumatic approach is the endotracheal insertion of a balloon. The usefulness of this technique is under investigation.

Pleural effusion (p. 355)

Fetal pleural effusions may be unilateral or bilateral, may be an isolated finding or they may occur in association with generalized edema and ascites. Chromosomal abnormalities, mainly trisomy 21, are found in about 5 percent of cases with apparently isolated pleural effusions.

FETAL THERAPY

Isolated pleural effusions in the fetus may either resolve spontaneously or they can be treated effectively after birth. Nevertheless, in some cases, severe and chronic compression of the fetal lungs can result in pulmonary hypoplasia and neonatal death. In others, mediastinal compression leads to the development of hydrops and polyhydramnios, which are associated with a high risk of premature delivery and perinatal death. Attempts at prenatal therapy by repeated thoracocenteses for drainage of pleural effusions have been generally unsuccessful in reversing the hydropic state, because the fluid reaccumulates within 24–48 hours of drainage. A better approach is chronic drainage by the insertion of thoracoamniotic shunts (Figure 11.4).[11] This is useful for both diagnosis and treatment. First, the diagnosis of an underlying cardiac abnormality or other intrathoracic lesion may become apparent only after effective decompression and return of the mediastinum to its normal position. Second, it can reverse fetal hydrops, resolve polyhydramnios and thereby reduce the risk of preterm delivery, and may prevent pulmonary hypoplasia. Third, it may be useful in the prenatal diagnosis of pulmonary hypoplasia because, in such cases, the lungs often fail to expand after shunting. Furthermore, it may help to distinguish between hydrops due to primary accumulation of pleural effusions, in which case the ascites and skin edema may resolve after shunting, and other causes of hydrops such as infection, in which drainage of the

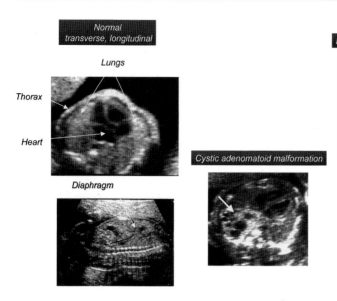

Figure 11.5 *Cystic adenomatoid malformation of the lung and pulmonary sequestration. The ultrasound scans on the left show the appearance of the normal lung in transverse (above) and longitudinal (below) section. The middle picture is a transverse scan showing a cystic adenomatoid malformation (indicated by the arrow). On the right is a picture of transverse scan showing an extralobar sequestration (indicated by the arrow).*

effusions does not prevent worsening of the hydrops. Survival after thoracoamniotic shunting is more than 90 percent in fetuses with isolated pleural effusions and about 50 percent in those with hydrops.

Cystic adenomatoid malformation

Cystic adenomatoid malformation may be bilateral, involving all lung tissue, but in the majority of cases it is confined to a single lung or lobe. The lesions are either macrocystic (cysts of at least 5 mm in diameter) or microcystic (cysts less than 5 mm in diameter). In 85 percent of cases, the lesion is unilateral with equal frequency in the right and left lungs and equal frequency in the microcystic and macrocystic types. In about 10 percent of cases, there are other abnormalities, mainly cardiac and renal.

DIAGNOSIS

Prenatal diagnosis is based on the ultrasonographic demonstration of a hyperechogenic pulmonary tumor which is cystic (CAM type 1), mixed (CAM type 2), or solid – microcystic (CAM type 3) (Figure 11.5). Microcystic disease results in uniform hyperechogenicity of the affected lung tissue. In macrocystic disease, single or multiple cystic spaces may be seen within the thorax. Both microcystic and macrocystic disease may be associated with deviation of the mediastinum. When there is compression of the heart and major blood vessels in the thorax, fetal hydrops develops. Polyhydramnios is a common feature and this may be a consequence of decreased fetal swallowing of amniotic fluid due to esophageal compression, or increased fluid production by the abnormal lung tissue. Prognostic features for poor outcome include major lung compression causing pulmonary hypoplasia, polyhydramnios and development of hydrops fetalis irrespective of the type of the lesion.

FETAL THERAPY

Large intrathoracic cysts causing major mediastinal shift can be treated effectively by the insertion of thoracoamniotic shunts. In the case of large solid tumors resulting in hydrops, intrauterine surgery involving hysterotomy and excision of the tumor has been reported. A less invasive approach is ultrasound-guided laser ablation of the blood supply to the tumor.

Extralobar pulmonary sequestration

This condition is classically divided into intralobar (about 75 percent) and extralobar (about 25 percent), but the difference (which is based on the presence or absence of a separate pleural covering from the normal lung) cannot be accurately determined with prenatal ultrasound (Figure 11.5).

DIAGNOSIS

The sequestrated portion of the lung appears as a homogeneous, brightly echogenic mass in the lower lobes of the lungs or in the upper abdomen (infradiaphragmatic sequestration). The diagnosis is confirmed by color Doppler demonstration that the vascular supply of the sequestered lobe arises from the abdominal aorta. A large lung sequestration may act as an arteriovenous fistula and cause high-output heart failure and hydrops.

Laryngeal obstruction

On ultrasound examination, voluminous lungs may be detected (Figure 11.6).

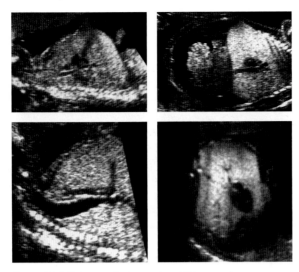

Figure 11.6 *Laryngeal obstruction. Ultrasound appearances of laryngeal obstruction – note the dilated trachea above the obstruction and the voluminous lungs.*

REFERENCES

1   Bahmaie, A., Hughes, S.W., Clark, T. *et al.* (2000) Serial fetal lung volume measurement using three-dimensional ultrasound. *Ultrasound in Obstetrics and Gynecology* **16**, 154–158.

2   Baker, P.N., Johnson, I.R., Gowland, P.A., Freeman, A., Adams, V., Mansfield, P. (1994) Estimation of fetal lung volume using echo-planar magnetic resonance imaging. *Obstetrics and Gynecology* **83**, 951–954.

3   Bouchard, S., Johnson, M.P., Flake, A.W. *et al.* (2002) The EXIT procedure: experience and outcome in 31 cases. *Journal of Pediatric Surgery* **37**, 418–426.

4   Deprest, J.A., Evrard, V.A., Van Ballaer, P.P. *et al.* (1998) Tracheoscopic endoluminal plugging using an inflatable device in the fetal lamb model. *European Journal of Obstetrics, Gynecology and Reproductive Biology* **81**, 165–169.

5   Deprest, J.A., Evrard, V.A., Verbeken, E.K. *et al.* (2000) Tracheal side effects of endoscopic balloon tracheal occlusion in the fetal lamb model. *European Journal of Obstetrics, Gynecology and Reproductive Biology* **92**, 119–126.

6   Duncan, K., Gowland, P., Freeman, A. *et al.* (1999) The changes in magnetic resonance properties of the fetal lungs: a first result and potential tool for non-invasive *in utero* demonstration of fetal lung maturation. *British Journal of Obstetrics and Gynaecology* **106**, 122–125.

7   Duncan, K.R., Gowland, P.A., Moore, R.J., Baker, P.N., Johnson, I.R. (1999) Assessment of fetal lung growth in utero with echo-planar MR imaging. *Radiology* **210**, 197–200.

8   Hubbard, A., Adzick, N., Crombelholme, T. *et al.* (1999) Congenital chest lesions. Diagnosis and characterization with prenatal imaging. *Radiology* **212**, 43–48.

9   Hubbard, A.M., States, L.J. (2001) Fetal magnetic resonance imaging. *Topics in Magnetic Resonance Imaging* **12**, 93–103.

10 Mychaliska, G.B., Bealer, J.F., Graf, J.L., Rosen, M.A., Adzick, N.S., Harrison, M.R. (1997) Operating on placental support: the ex utero intrapartum treatment procedure. *Journal of Pediatric Surgery* **32**(2), 227–230; discussion 230–231.

11 Nicolaides, K.H., Blott, M., Greenough, A. (1987) Chronic drainage of fetal pulmonary cyst. *Lancet* **1**, 618.

12 O'Callaghan, C., Chapman, B., Coxon, R. *et al.* (1988) Evaluation of infants by echo planar imaging after repair of diaphragmatic hernia. *Archives of Disease in Childhood* **63**, 186–189.

Neonatal imaging

JOHN KARANI

In the last decade there has been continued development in the diagnostic imaging techniques of computerized tomography (CT), magnetic resonance imaging (MRI) and ultrasound (US). All are now achieving speeds of data acquisition resulting in enhanced resolution of the thorax. CT can now define lung anatomy and pathological processes within the lung to the level of the secondary pulmonary lobule. Despite this, the standard portable chest radiograph remains the diagnostic fulcrum of the radiological investigation of neonatal lung disorders. Harnessing the newer techniques with the chest radiograph for an accurate diagnosis in the neonate requires an understanding not only of their appropriate clinical indications, but also the limitations that may alter their diagnostic utility. In this chapter, the basic physical principles of the techniques and their radiological interpretation according to recognized disease classifications are described.

CHEST RADIOGRAPH

General principles

Standard chest radiographs are taken in the supine position using an anterior-posterior projection with a film focus distance of 1 m and the neonate gently breathing, that is, avoiding the extremes of the respiratory cycle. Whether taken portably or within the radiology department, attention to detail in technique is essential. Poor positioning of the infant[12] and overlying monitoring equipment can produce appearances and artifacts, which often result in misinterpretation or 'overdiagnosis' of a normal radiograph. The onus to avoid such problems lies with the radiographer, but guidance from the pediatric radiologist and assistance from neonatal practitioners are core elements. When assessing the chest radiograph, it is essential not only to carefully view the appearance of the lungs, but also the bony structures (p. 505) and the structures visible outside the thorax (Figure 11.7a and b).

Interpretation of the chest radiograph requires an understanding of normal anatomy, the variance in appearance with gestational age and the normal variants that may simulate pathology. In addition, it is important to correlate the objective radiological signs with the clinical diagnosis. Assessment of the radiological signs requires consistent descriptive terminology. Only by use of the same radiological language will there be clear understanding of the relationship of pathology to radiology. There is agreement as to the appearance of 'perihilar haziness', 'interstitial shadowing' and 'cystic change' and their relationship to gauging the severity of chronic lung disease (CLD). The definition of 'mottled' and 'fluffy shadows' is less clear. Adopting rigid terminology facilitates the use of scoring systems, which correlate with physiological parameters and can then act as predictors of prognosis (p. 408).[6]

Normal anatomy

In the newborn, the bifurcation of the trachea lies at the level of the third thoracic vertebra, but during inspiration it elongates, dilates and moves anteriorly in a caudal direction. This appearance may be increased by any degree of rotation. Interpretation of tracheal deviation should take account of such normal physiological variation and the phase of respiration. The position of the individual lobes is established in the early weeks of life, although the

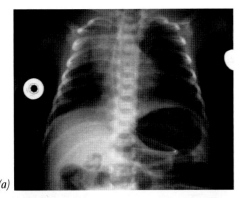

(a)

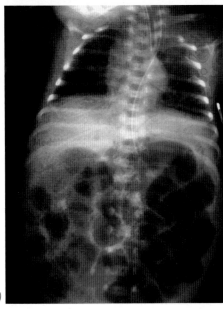

(b)

Figure 11.7 *(a) Chest radiograph of a small-for-dates 30-week gestation infant who had an acute deterioration. The chest radiograph revealed right upper lobe collapse, but also intraluminal gas in the abdomen in the right upper quadrant. (b) The infant required intubation and ventilation and the abdominal radiograph taken one hour after the first radiograph demonstrated extensive necrotizing enterocolitis.*

relative size, shape and position of the fissures are variable. None of the finer components of the lobules, namely the individual alveoli, lobes or septa, are usually visible, but may become apparent as an abnormal sign with the development of interstitial lung disease. Hilar shadows are composite, representing pulmonary vasculature, proximal bronchi, peribronchial connective tissue and lymphatics. A variation in hilar size is well recognized. The phase of respiration, the radiographic projection, as well as developmental variants, may influence hilar size, narrowing the window between abnormal and normal. 'Normal' pleura is invisible radiologically, so that demonstration of any pleural reflection indicates a pathological process. On the radiograph, however, it might not be possible to distinguish between fluid, particularly if it is

encysted or adjacent to the mediastinum, and an area of solid pleura other than by ultrasound or CT examination. The mediastinum is prominent in neonates on the antero-posterior (AP) projection and may be further exaggerated by a lordotic projection, expiration or a 'normal', but prominent thymus gland. The normal thymus may be difficult to distinguish from pathological abnormalities, but should be identifiable in the first day after birth even in a neonate with respiratory distress and usually does not displace normal mediastinal structures. Rapid enlargement of the thymus, termed thymic rebound, may occur following a period of neonatal stress and may mimic mediastinal disease.

In neonatal lung disorders, the interpretation of the chest radiograph allows the diagnosis of three broad categories of disease: abnormalities of aeration, circulation and development (Table 11.1).

ABNORMAL AERATION

Air in the alveoli and, to a lesser extent, the bronchial tree provides a natural radiolucency to contrast with the soft tissue density of the mediastinum and bony density of the thoracic cage. Any process which affects alveolar aeration by producing transudation of fluid into the small alveoli with atelectasis (RDS), increased interstitial and alveolar exudates (congenital pneumonia) or increased alveolar fluid (transient tachypnea of the newborn, cardiac failure, pulmonary hemorrhage) results in increased lung opacity, air bronchograms and altered lung expansion. It is an important radiological principle that, although alveolar 'filling' can be detected radiologically, the exact diagnosis can only be established in connection with clinical data. For example, instilled exogenous surfactant will also fill the alveoli, maintaining patency of the terminal bronchioles and this pattern of diffuse opacification with air bronchograms will mimic retained lung fluid or aspiration and may seem at odds with an improving respiratory status in the baby. Hypoventilation will result in the false observation of reduced lung volume even in the presence of normal lung structure and volume. Abnormalities of the thoracic musculature, diaphragmatic paralysis and developmental or acquired disorders of the central nervous system, which limit thoracic excursion, are recognized causes. All orders of the lung structure are underaerated from the central airways to the alveoli, however, and, therefore, air bronchograms and variable alveoli aeration tend not to be a feature. The distribution of this trapped air may be alveolar, lobular, segmental, lobar or affect one or both lungs in a varying distribution dependent on the underlying pathological process. If it involves a single lung or both lungs symmetrically, then this is an indication of air trapping consequent to large airways obstruction or secondary to an iatrogenic cause of 'overventilation'. If confined to more distal airways, then areas of hyperinflation and atelectasis generally coexist. Such changes are

Table 11.1 *Radiological features of specific disorders*

Respiratory distress syndrome (Chapter 19)
- Normal to decreased aeration
- Patent terminal airways surrounded by airless alveoli results in diffuse opacification
- Proximal air bronchograms

Transient tachypnea of the newborn (Chapter 20)
- Overaeration of lung fields with flattening of diaphragms
- Diffuse opacification with air bronchograms
- Interstitial fluid in the fissures and other reflections of the pleura
- Clearance may be asymmetrical with or delayed in the perihilar zones
- Overaeration may persist as fluid clears within 48 hours

Meconium aspiration (Chapter 23)
- Overaeration of lung fields with focal areas of air trapping
- Areas of segmental consolidation
- Pulmonary edema with small effusions and septal lines may occur
- PPHN, barotrauma or bacterial infection may complicate initial radiological signs

Congenital pneumonia (Chapter 21)
- Specific infections, such as GBS, may mimic RDS
- Segmental infiltrates or lobar consolidation
- Normal lung volumes or focal overaeration occur

Persistent pulmonary hypertension (Chapter 26)
- Normal lung volumes and aeration
- Pulmonary oligemia

Pulmonary venous obstruction and pulmonary edema (Chapter 27)
- Diffuse opacification with air bronchograms and interstitial pulmonary edema
- Hypoplastic left heart syndrome, total anomalous pulmonary venous return with obstruction of the anomalous vein and the non-cardiogenic causes of pulmonary edema are all associated with these non-specific chest radiograph signs. The differential diagnosis includes pulmonary lymphangiectasia

Chronic lung disease (Chapter 29)
- Diffuse opacification with zonal or total lung involvement
- Hyperinflation with cystic changes
- Interstitial changes of compressed lung and fibrosis adjacent to areas of emphysema and cyst formation

characteristic of prolonged ventilation for RDS, meconium aspiration syndrome and pneumonia. Chronic lung disease results in destruction of alveoli, producing areas of focal emphysema appearing radiologically as cystic change. These cysts can enlarge in size, compressing adjacent lung parenchyma and producing a mixed pattern of aeration.

Determining the anatomical location of intrathoracic air can be a radiological challenge, as there are often differing clinical implications. Pneumothorax and pneumomediastinum produce a well-recognized appearance

(p. 313). Differentiating interstitial air from overdistended alveoli, however, is often difficult. Classically interstitial air is seen in a subpleural location, along the lines of the fissures in a perihilar, perivascular distribution. Both interstitial air and overdistended alveoli may vary with the degree of lung inflation, but usually cysts are clearly marginated and constant in anatomical site.

Abnormalities of the circulation

The diagnosis of circulatory disturbances secondary to congenital cardiac abnormalities is no longer the province of the chest radiograph, but rather than of echocardiography. Recognition of pulmonary oligemia or plethora, abnormalities of the vascular pedicle or coexistent skeletal features of a syndrome, however, may be helpful in suggesting a non-pulmonary diagnosis in a hypoxic neonate.

Cardiac failure leads to stasis of blood in the pulmonary vessels and accumulation of fluid in the alveoli and interstitium. Engorgement results in enlargement of vascular markings both centrally at the hilar and in the lung periphery (p. 388). Non-cardiogenic transfusion reactions, uremia and intracerebral trauma produce the same patterns and cannot be differentiated other than by clinical correlation. The diagnosis of left heart failure in association with the hypertension of CLD is often difficult because the distribution of the fluid is atypical. The characteristic perihilar 'bat's wing' appearance is absent and replaced by a pattern of segmental consolidation mirroring infection. A response to diuretics demonstrated on an early interval film may be the only radiological sign by which the diagnosis may be made.

Abnormalities of development

Many developmental abnormalities will have been diagnosed by antenatal ultrasound (p. 92) and the postnatal radiological findings at birth are often confirmatory and may provide a baseline for management. Careful evaluation on the radiograph of the extent and pattern of involvement in a bone dysplasia may allow a definitive diagnosis to be made and the outcome predicted.

The early diagnosis of esophageal atresia with or without tracheoesophageal fistula is reliant on the correct radiological interpretation. In more than 85 percent of infants with esophageal atresia there is communication of the trachea or one of the primary bronchi with the inferior esophageal segment. Aspiration from the blind upper esophageal pouch into the larynx and main bronchi results in consolidation and atelectasis. More problematical is the tracheoesophageal fistula without atresia. Recurrent widespread pneumonia associated with abdominal distention can occur. Investigation is directed at identification of the fistula by videofluoroscopy. It is important to recognize that opening of the fistula may be intermittent and more than one study may be necessary to make the diagnosis.

Intrapulmonary developmental abnormalities such as lung cysts, cystic adenomatoid malformations and pulmonary sequestration may be diagnosed on the chest radiograph (p. 465). The characteristic features may be modified by antenatal intervention; for example, placement of transthoracic drains may produce a pleural reaction or pneumothorax and alter the appearance of the cyst at birth by decompression. Awareness of these factors will help to prevent erroneous diagnoses.

Indications

Clearly, any infant who has had an acute deterioration in respiratory status should have a chest radiograph. A policy of routinely obtaining daily chest radiographs in mechanically ventilated, very low birthweight infants during the acute stage of their illness can also be helpful as it yields new information with regard for patient care. In one study,[7] new abnormalities were demonstrated in 50 percent of chest radiographs examined. Differences in the chest radiograph appearance can also document responses to therapy.[2,13,14] The chest radiograph appearance can also be predictive of chronic oxygen dependency[8] and the development of chronic respiratory problems at follow-up.[15] It has, however, been questioned whether the chest radiograph appearance is reliable for the prediction of bronchopulmonary dysplasia (BPD).[9] The lung area can be assessed from the chest radiograph and using computer-assisted analysis the lung area so derived correlates closely with lung volume.[3] The chest radiograph lung area has been used to predict the likely success of extubation,[1] outcome in infants with congenital diaphragmatic hernia (CDH)[4] and facilitate optimization of oxygenation on transfer to high-frequency oscillation (HFO).[5]

ULTRASOUND

Principles

Ultrasound is now established as a contributory method to our understanding of anatomical relations and to image soft tissue pathology. Quantitation of movement using the Doppler techniques allows studies of blood flow. There is no conclusive evidence that when ultrasound is used at diagnostic levels of intensity, tissue damage results. Recent advances have resulted in the development of small, mobile machines with a high-resolution capability, invaluable to neonatal units. Its efficacy, however, remains dependent on the interpretive skills and level of expertise of the operator; for example, ultrasound is subject to many artifactual signals which complicate interpretation.

Physical principles

Ultrasound is a high-frequency mechanical vibration produced by a transducer made of a piezoelectric material, which changes thickness as a voltage is applied to it. Ceramic materials, in particular lead zirconate (Pbt) derive their piezoelectric properties from their possession of a large charged atom loosely held in a complex crystal. When pulsed it produces a resonant frequency for transmission. The piezoelectric effect is symmetrical, so a returning ultrasound wave is converted into an electrical signal for analysis. The principle of image production is dependent on the interaction of the ultrasound wave with tissue by conduction, attenuation and reflection. In basic terms, reflection of a sound wave occurs when it crosses an interface of two tissues of differing elasticities. Some of the incident energy fails to cross and returns as an echo. The echo intensity depends on the degree of change of the elasticity of the interfacing tissues. The greater the differential in elasticity, the greater the reflection with production of acoustic 'shadowing'. Visceral gas and bone, which are markedly different in their elasticity from surrounding soft tissue, are impenetrable windows to ultrasound. The Doppler principle is the basis of blood flow assessment. It depends on a shift in frequency of a wave when the source moves relative to the receiver. The shift in frequency is proportional to the velocity of the blood, so measurements are directional and quantitative.

Indications (Table 11.2) and limitations

Established applications of ultrasound are in obstetrics and examination of the abdomen, cardiovascular system and neonatal brain. The inability of high-frequency sound waves to cross tissue–gas or tissue–bone interfaces has limited its applications to the thorax. Fluid-filled lungs antenatally become air-filled at birth so its impact in structural lung disorders is largely lost at birth. Real-time

Table 11.2 *Indications for ultrasound in the neonate*

- Diagnosing pleural disease, the presence of fluid, and its anatomical site
- Confirming renal agenesis in the presence of pulmonary hypoplasia
- Diagnosing congenital heart disease as a cause of an acute respiratory presentation
- Evaluating intracranial complications in seriously ill neonates
- Assessment of the hepatobiliary system when liver function abnormalities develop
- Guidance for drainage procedures or central venous line placement

scanning, however, could facilitate the placement of catheters and drainage catheters into areas of potential pathology.

COMPUTERIZED TOMOGRAPHY

General principles

Computerized tomography provides an important adjunct to the chest radiograph in the assessment of structural lung disorders.[10] Advances in technology are now directed at faster scanning times with improved spatial resolution. Such developments enhance the potential role of CT in pediatrics, although controlling irradiation must remain a fundamental aim.

Physical principles

Computerized tomography uses ionizing radiation to produce a cross-sectional image of the patient. Optimal direction of the beam results in detection of fine differences of attenuation so that soft tissues, fat, air and bone can be more clearly distinguished. The scanner consists of a moving table coupled with a gantry, which contains an array of detectors receiving the variably attenuated beam from differing sections of the patient. Multidetector scanners detect and analyze a 'slice' in milliseconds so that cardiac and respiratory movement does not degrade the image and resolution is enhanced.

The CT image is displayed on a video monitor and consists of a matrix of picture elements (pixels) representing the linear attenuation values at that level. The attenuation values of the emergent beam are expressed as CT numbers. The scale of Hounsfield units (HU) relates the attenuation value of tissues to that of water on a scale of $+1000$ to -1000. Bone and soft tissue have higher attenuation levels than water and are expressed as positive numbers, whilst fat and air are expressed as negative numbers. The CT number for air is $-1000\,HU$, for soft tissue $+40$ to $+60\,HU$ and for fat -60 to $-100\,HU$.

Iodinated contrast agents injection allows demonstration of vascular anatomy and distinguishes a mass from normal vascular structures in the mediastinum, for example. Following the early intravascular phase, contrast rapidly enters the extravascular space by diffusion. Parenchymal enhancement may be a key factor in differentiating normal from abnormal tissue by their differing vascularity. The liver and kidney provide the best examples of this phenomenon. Tumors within these organs alter blood flow and therefore appear of differing attenuation to the normal surrounding parenchyma.

High-resolution computed tomography (HRCT) has further advanced our understanding of lung structure and its alteration in disease. There are two key differences between conventional CT and HRCT; first, the beam collimation/slice thickness is narrower (1–3 mm), improving spatial resolution. Second, a specialized algorithm is used to construct the data in HRCT, accentuating the natural density differences between the aerated lung and the interstitium, improving the conspicuity of vessels, small bronchi and interlobular septa. In a typical HRCT examination, images are interspaced at a gap of 10–20 mm and hence the lungs are sampled at certain levels, minimizing the radiation exposure to the patient. Subtle changes in lung density with areas of decreased attenuation, particularly in the expiratory phase, termed mosaic perfusion, are characteristic of small airways disease. In addition, interstitial processes produce radiological signs that may be pathognomonic of their etiology.

Although this technique is of limited utility in acute respiratory distress, its sensitivity in diagnosing small or large airways disease in later life as a sequel of these neonatal respiratory disorders is predictable and may form a further method of scoring severity of disease and predicting prognosis.

Indications (Table 11.3) and limitations

Computerized tomography scanners cannot be used at the cotside. Transfer of ventilated, hemodynamically unstable neonates to the radiology department presents logistical problems. Although these can be overcome, the indication for the examination and influence of the result on management has to be critically examined. Often high-quality images can only be produced under general anesthesia, which may be undesirable in a neonate with chronic lung disease. The examination must be tailored to the clinical problem. The radiologist conducting the examination must therefore have a clear idea of the question to be answered. Lesions in infants with CLD with chronic pulmonary dysfunction are visualized better on CT scan than on chest radiograph

Table 11.3 *Indications for CT examination*

- Determination of anatomical sites of areas of cystic change (congenital or acquired) and whether single or multiple lobar involvement is present
- Identification of the extent of small and large airways disease in CLD
- Evaluation of mediastinal masses and their relationship to normal vascular structures
- Evaluation of pleural disease (in conjunction with ultrasound)
- Assessing intra-abdominal masses, which may be limiting diaphragmatic movement. Ultrasound is the initial technique of choice, but evaluation of the retroperitoneum may be superior with CT, although often they produce complementary images

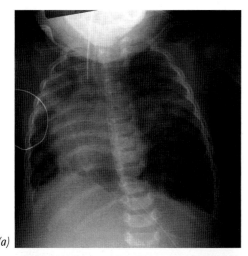

(a)

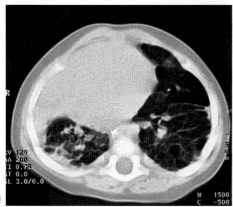

(b)

Figure 11.8 *(a) Chest radiograph demonstrating changes of BPD (p. 407) and right upper lobe collapse. (b) CT scan of the same infant. The right upper lobe collapse is obvious; the mediastinal shift, subpleural cysts and areas of emphysema are much more prominent on the CT scan than the chest radiograph.*

(Figure 11.8a and b). Common findings in such prematurely born infants include multifocal areas of hyperaeration, linear and triangular subpleural opacities, but not bronchiectasis.[11]

MAGNETIC RESONANCE IMAGING

General principles

Magnetic resonance imaging is a non-invasive technique, which avoids ionizing radiation and appears without hazard. Complex physical principles are employed, but the basis of the technique is the use of radiofrequency waves in a magnetic field to produce cross-sectional images by portraying the distribution of hydrogen nuclei and their motion in water and lipids. All scanners are constructed from a large magnet in which are situated gradient coils, to receive or transmit the signal. MRI is based on the principle that when a uniform magnetic field is applied to the hydrogen nuclei (or protons) within tissue they align with

the magnetic field in a movement known as precession. After this disturbance, the magnetization returns to equilibrium. This changing magnetic field induces a small voltage in a receiver coil surrounding the patient. The pattern of relaxation to equilibrium is the basic parameter for analysis. Many parameters, which are beyond the scope of this text, may be analyzed for image production, but the most commonly used are proton density, longitudinal relaxation time (T1) and transverse relaxation time (T2). Proton density parallels electron density of radiographs, fluid having a high proton density followed in diminishing order by soft tissue, liver, gray matter, white matter, cartilage, cortical bone and air. Conditions resulting in edema produce increased proton density. A decrease occurs in fibrosis and if calcification develops. Individual tissues have characteristic T1 and T2 measurements according to the strength of the applied field.

Edema similarly results in an increase in both T1 and T2. Paramagnetic particles, of which hemosiderin is the most common endogenous product, or gadolinium diethylene triamine pentaacetic acid (DTPA) injected as a contrast agent, decrease T1 and T2.

Clinical indications and limitations

More specific tissue characterization, multiplanar images and quantitative measurement of flow are the inherent advantages of MRI over CT. Like CT, MRI is not portable and clear clinical indications must be sought. Motion and respiratory artifact place potential limits on resolution, but these are being addressed by fast scan times coupled with cardiac and respiratory gating.

Many of its clinical indications mirror those of CT, but most observers recognize its advantage in neuroimaging, particularly for white matter disease and also within the musculoskeletal system. To date no clear advantage has been found in the thorax for structural lung abnormalities and there is a limiting physical principle of lung tissue susceptibility on MR that suggests CT will remain pre-eminent. Imaging of congenital heart defects is now established, but echocardiography remains the baseline investigation of choice. Magnetic resonance angiography (MRA) displays vascular anatomy non-invasively and is based on the principle of protons in flowing blood producing a high signal against a background of little or no signal from stationary tissues. Consequently the requirement for invasive vascular procedures other than as a prelude to intervention is receding.

NUCLEAR MEDICINE

General principles

Radioactive gases (xenon or krypton) are used to assess regional ventilation. When these are inhaled while technetium-labelled particles or macro-aggregated albumin or human serum albumin is injected, ventilation and perfusion matching in the lung can be evaluated.

Indications and limitations

Regional lung function may be assessed in children with chest wall deformities with serial studies. Unilateral pulmonary hypoplasia, lobar emphysema, cystic adenomatoid malformation and pulmonary sequestration produce ventilation/perfusion-matching defects. In acquired disturbances of aeration, classically chronic lung disease of prematurity, abnormal areas of ventilation, which are areas of focal emphysema, may be demonstrated. It is not uncommon for areas abnormal on the chest radiograph to have relatively normal ventilation. The 'functional' study therefore provides important information for management when matched with the structural imaging techniques.

REFERENCES

1 Dimitriou, G., Greenough, A. (2000) Computer assisted analysis of the chest radiograph lung area and prediction of failure of extubation from mechanical ventilation in preterm neonates. *British Journal of Radiology* **73**, 156–159.

2 Dimitriou, G., Greenough, A., Giffin, F.J., Karani, J. (1995) The appearance of early chest radiographs and the response to surfactant replacement therapy. *British Journal of Radiology* **68**, 1177–1180.

3 Dimitriou, G., Greenough, A., Kavvadia, V., Shute, M., Karani, J. (1999) A radiographic method for assessing lung area in neonates. *British Journal of Radiology* **72**, 335–338.

4 Dimitriou, G., Greenough, A., Davenport, M., Nicolaides, K. (2000) Prediction of outcome by computer assisted analysis of lung area on the chest radiograph of infants with congenital diaphragmatic hernia. *Journal of Pediatric Surgery* **35**, 489–493.

5 Dimitriou, G., Greenough, A., Alvares, B.R., Shute, M., Karani, J., Peacock, J. (2001) Chest radiograph lung area and oxygenation optimisation on transfer to HFO. *British Journal of Intensive Care* **11**: 78–82.

6 Greenough, A., Kavvadia, V., Johnson, A., Calvert, S., Peacock, J., Karani, J. (1999) A simple chest radiograph score to predict chronic lung disease in prematurely born infants. *British Journal of Radiology* **72**, 530–533.

7 Greenough, A., Dimitriou, G., Alvares, B.R., Karani, J. (2001) Routine daily chest radiographs in ventilated, very low birthweight infants. *European Journal of Pediatrics* **160**, 147–149.

8 Maconchie, I., Greenough, A., Yuksel, B., Page, A., Karani, J. (1991) A chest radiograph scoring system to predict chronic oxygen dependency in low birthweight infants. *Early Human Development* **26**, 37–43.

9 Moya, M.P., Bisset, G.S., Auten, R.L., Miller, C., Hollingworth, C., Frush, D.F. (2001) Reliability of CXR for the diagnosis of bronchopulmonary dysplasia. *Pediatric Radiology* **31**, 339–342.

10 Newman, B., Kuhn, J.P., Kramer, S.S., Carcillo, J.A. (2001) Congenital surfactant protein B deficiency – emphasis on imaging. *Pediatr Radiol* **31**, 327–331.

11 Oppenheim, C., Marmou-Mani, T., Sayegh, N., de Blic, J., Scheinmann, P., Lallemand, D. (1994) Bronchopulmonary dysplasia: value of CT in identifying pulmonary sequelae. *American Journal of Roentgenology* **163**, 169–172.

12 Rost, J.R., Frush, D.P., Auten, R.L. (1999) Effect of neck position on endotracheal tube location in low birthweight infants. *Pediatric Pulmonology* **27**, 199–202.

13 Schrod, L., Neuhaus, T., Horwitz, A.E., Speer, C.P. (2001) The effect of dexamethasone on respirator dependent very low birthweight infants is best predicted by chest X-ray. *Pediatric Radiology* **31**, 332–338.

14 Soll, R.F., Horbar, J.F., Grissom, N.T. *et al.* (1991) Radiographic findings associated with surfactant treatment. *American Journal of Perinatology* **8**, 114–118.

15 Thomas, M.R., Greenough, A., Johnson, A. *et al.* Frequent wheeze at follow-up of very preterm infants – which factors are predictive? *Archives of Disease in Childhood* (in press).

Neonatal bronchoscopy

JACQUES DE BLIC

In the last 20 years, bronchoscopy, especially flexible bronchoscopy, has emerged as an important diagnostic tool for pulmonary pediatricians.[8,29,38] Technical improvements have led to the development of small instruments that are now suitable for use in neonates, even those born prematurely.[37] Bronchoscopy, however, is still underutilized, particularly for infants on neonatal intensive care units (NICUs).

TECHNIQUES

Initially, rigid bronchoscopy was the only form of direct airways visualization possible in neonates and some units still use this technique. Examination is usually performed under general anesthesia. The sizes of bronchoscopes used for neonates are 2.5 mm and 3 mm. A rod lens telescope passed through the rigid bronchocope allows a very high optical resolution. The internal diameter of rigid bronchoscopes allows the insertion of instruments and operative manipulation (for example, excision of granulation tissue). Rigid bronchoscopy also appears better for examination of the posterior aspect of the larynx and tracheoesophageal fistulae (TOF).[3,22] Small flexible bronchoscopes (FBs) were developed 20 years ago. Three sorts of FB are currently available for neonates:

- The standard pediatric FB (BF 3C40 Olympus corporation, FB-10V Pentax corporation) is 3.5 mm in outside diameter and has a suction channel 1.2 mm in diameter.
- The 'slim' FB, recently available on the market (BFXP40 Olympus Corporation), is 2.7 mm in outside diameter and still has a suction channel 1.2 mm in diameter. More therapeutic maneuvers, such as aspiration of

mucous plugs, and satisfactory bronchoalveolar lavage may be possible in the intubated newborn.[5]
- More extensive miniaturization of FBs has led to 'ultrathin' FBs. Models currently available (2.2 mm BFN20 Olympus Corporation, 2.2 mm ENT 30F Machida) have a directed tip but no suction channel. Some models have neither distal flexion nor suction capability. These later instruments are useful for limited purposes, primarily to verify the patency and possibly the position of endotracheal or tracheostomy tubes.

In mature, spontaneously ventilating and stable neonates, the procedure may be performed on an out-patient basis. Heart rate and oxygen saturation must be continuously monitored in all patients during the procedure. As in older children, a combination of intravenous sedation (midazolam, 75 µg/kg), and topical analgesia [2 percent lidocaine (lignocaine) sprayed on the vocal cords] is used commonly. Deep sedation, however, has the advantage that the airway is constantly monitored by an anesthesist. The bronchoscope can be inserted pernasally, through a laryngeal mask[21] or through the tracheostomy port. In infants of weight less than 3 kg, the 3.5 mm FB will usually nearly totally obstruct the airways and a 2.7 mm FB is preferred. Adequate oxygenation can be obtained by preoxygenation with 100 percent oxygen, but adequate ventilation will not be achieved if a 3.5 mm FB is used. Supplementary oxygen during the procedure may be given by nasal prongs or via a facial mask. If a 2.2 mm FB bronchoscope is used, the upper airways should be carefully suctioned, as the instrument has no operator channel.

In ventilated neonates, new 'slim' and 'ultrathin' FBs are sufficiently small to pass through a no. 3 (also a 3.5 mm which is preferred) endotracheal tube (ET) and a 2.5 ET tube, so that extubation is no longer necessary for airway exploration (Figure 12.1). The cross-section of

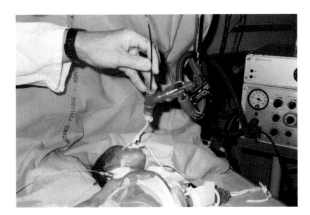

Figure 12.1 *Passage of a flexible bronchoscope in a ventilated infant.*

Table 12.1 *Main complications of bronchoscopy in neonates*

Hypoxia
Apnea
Hypercapnia
Bradycardia
Pulmonary hemorrhage
Infection
Pneumothorax
Transient rise in systolic blood pressure
Intracranial hemorrhage
Hypothermia

the 2.2 mm diameter BFN20 is approximately one-third that of the pediatric FB ($3.8 \, mm^2$ versus $10 \, mm^2$), thus allowing sufficient spontaneous ventilation, even in low birthweight newborns. All FBs are performed after pre-oxygenation in order to obtain oxygen saturation greater than 90 percent. Except for supplementary oxygen changes, ventilator settings remain unchanged during the procedure. Analgesia with narcotic agents such as fentanyl is commonly used, but sedation is rarely administered. The FB is passed through a double swivel bronchoscopic adaptor located between the ET tube or the tracheostomy and the ventilator. The adaptor is specially fitted with a cleft to accommodate the FB and thus allows uninterrupted mechanical ventilation and oxygen delivery. As the time the bronchoscope is below the glottis is limited to no more than 30–40 seconds,[38] video recording of the procedure is necessary for a further and closer assessment of the findings.

Tolerance

Due to the small airways of neonates, the risk of complications of bronchoscopy is greater than in older children (Table 12.1). Hypoxemia and transient bradycardia are common and indicate the need to remove the bronchoscope from the airway and to deliver oxygen by mask. Cohn *et al.*[6] noted complications during 4 of 129 procedures (3 percent) using a 3.5 mm FB in infants with bronchopulmonary dysplasia (BPD). Three suffered moderate complications (bradycardia, mild nasopharyngeal bleeding, transient stridor) and one a severe complication (respiratory distress).

Ultrathin FBs are better tolerated and the studies using 2.2 mm FBs highlighted that, after preoxygenation, no serious adverse cardiovascular effects occurred. Shinwell reported no severe changes in oxygen saturation or arterial blood gases; transient hypoxemia (SaO_2 always greater than 82 percent) and bradycardia occurred during procedures, but resolved spontaneously in less than 1 minute.[34] In the study of Schellhase,[33] transient hypoxemia occurred in 5 of 21 procedures and the lowest SaO_2 noted was 82 percent. Transient bradycardia occurred in 4 of the 21 procedures; the lowest heart rate noted was 60 beats/min. Tolerance of the patients in our series was quite similar.[10] Unexplained rises in systolic blood pressure of more than 10 mmHg occurred in 8 of 21 infants and lasted for up to 1 hour in three infants, but this was without any clinical manifestation.[33]

Clearly, to be well tolerated, flexible bronchoscopy in the neonate requires certain precautions. The procedure must be done in an intensive care unit, rapidly, under cardiac and oximetry monitoring and by an experienced pediatric bronchoscopist. Flexible bronchoscopy in neonates requires competent well-trained operators, using a videosystem.[29]

Rigid or flexible bronchoscopy?

Most bronchoscopists who regularly use both rigid and flexible bronchoscopes believe that most of the data yielded by rigid bronchoscopy may also be obtained by flexible bronchoscopy even in neonates.[38] The choice is often as much a matter of individual preference as of the instruments available. The advantages of FB over rigid bronchoscopy include that they may be used as a bedside technique, FB can be done under local anesthesia and thus allows visualization of airway dynamics, and diagnosis of tracheomalacia and bronchomalacia and FB can be performed in an intubated patient. Conversely, in low birthweight neonates, FB obstructs the proximal airway more than rigid bronchoscopy. In addition, rigid bronchoscopy allows a better examination if there is suspicion of an H-type TOF or posterior laryngeal problems and rigid bronchoscopy is irreplaceable when operative manipulations are necessary (p. 442).

INDICATIONS AND RESULTS OF BRONCHOSCOPY

The indications for bronchoscopy in neonates and long-term intubated premature infants can be based

Table 12.2 *Main indications for flexible bronchoscopy in neonates*

Persistent atelectasis/hyperinflation
Unexplained episodes of cyanosis
Unexplained respiratory distress
Failure to extubate
Assessment and diagnosis of stridor
Acute atelectasis
Assessment of lung malformation
Assessment of unexplained pulmonary hemorrhage
Difficult intubation
Position of endotracheal tube
Interstitial pneumonitis

Table 12.3 *Indications for 201 flexible bronchoscopies at the Necker Enfants Malades Hospital*

Indication	Number
Persistent atelectasis/hyperinflation	77
Unexplained episodes of cyanosis	23
Unexplained respiratory distress	20
Control of previously diagnosed stenosis or granuloma	16
Stridor	14
Acute atelectasis	15
Interstitial pneumonitis	11
Pulmonary interstitial emphysema	10
Assessment of lung malformation	8
Miscellaneous	7

Table 12.4 *Findings on 201 FBs in 171 infants (one or more findings may be observed during the same flexible bronchoscopy)*

Finding	Number
Normal flexible bronchoscopy	58
Important inflammation and mucous secretions	36
Stenosis	23
trachea	9
right main stem bronchus	2
bronchus intermedius	11
left main stem bronchus	2
Granuloma	14
trachea	6
right bronchi	8
left bronchi	3
Malacia	27
trachea	20
bronchomalacia	14
Proximal airway compression	13
Tracheobronchial abnormality (tracheal bronchus, fistula, lung hypoplasia)	16
Blood-tinged aspiration	7
Laryngomalacia	3
Foreign body	1
Isolation of RSV in BAL	3

upon clinical signs and/or radiological abnormalities (Table 12.2).[24,31,35] At the Necker Enfants Malades Hospital we performed 201 bronchoscopies in infants between January 1982 and January 1992 (Tables 12.3 and 12.4). One hundred and nineteen infants were intubated at the time of examination. The main indications for FB were unexplained episodes of respiratory distress or cyanosis and persistent atelectasis/hyperinflation, and bronchoscopy was done to search for airway obstruction.

Congenital malformations affecting the tracheobronchial tree

ESOPHAGEAL ATRESIA AND TRACHEOESOPHAGEAL FISTULA

Rigid bronchoscopy under general anesthesia should be considered in neonates suspected of an H-type TOF.[22,23,31] Bronchoscopy is helpful in the diagnosis of TOF and evaluation of associated congenital anomalies in the tracheobronchial tree and position of the aortic arch, which decides the side of the thoracotomy. Instillation of 10 percent diluted methylene blue into the upper esophagus may assist in detection of the TOF when blue fluid can be seen coming from the fistula tract.

CONGENITAL OBSTRUCTION OF THE AIRWAY

Laryngomalacia with an elongated or floppy epiglottis is the major cause of benign congenital stridor. In a neonate with an inspiratory and/or expiratory component stridor, however, airway obstruction is highly likely and endoscopy is required. Indeed, an endoscopic examination of the entire respiratory tract remains the most effective way to establish an accurate diagnosis. Wood and Postma found that nearly 15 percent of young patients with stridor had a significant lesion below the glottis level, although a plausible explanation for the stridor was also seen at the glottis or above.[38] Numerous intrinsic or extrinsic congenital malformations may be considered.

ANOMALIES OF THE TRACHEOBRONCHIAL TREE

A wide variety of tracheal or bronchial anomalies may be explored by endoscopy:[30] these include congenital tracheal stenosis with concentric circular cartilagous rings, bronchial stenosis, esophageal bronchus, unilateral hypoplastic or agenetic lung.

Vascular anomalies

Anterior compression of the intrathoracic trachea due to the innominate artery is the commonest vascular lesion obstructing the airway. Bronchoscopy visualizes the tracheal compression about 1–2 cm above the carina.[13]

Surgical correction should be restricted for patients with severe symptoms (p. 393). An aberrant right subclavian artery is also a frequent finding but in general does not cause respiratory symptoms. When such an anomaly is discovered by barium esophagogram, endoscopy shows usually a small and non-significant, posterior pulsatile compression which is not associated with any malacia. With rigid bronchoscopy (but not with FB), compression of the pulsatile bulge by the tip of the bronchoscope induces the loss of the radial pulse. In a very small number of cases, an aberrant right subclavian artery is responsible for a significant tracheal compression and needs surgical repair. By contrast, complete vascular rings, whatever the type, usually show more severe compression.[2,16] The residual tracheal lumen has a triangular or a comma shape. In these cases an important malacia is frequently associated, which may mask the vascular compression. Finally, compression may be due to a pulmonary artery sling, which is often associated with tracheal stenosis.

EXTRINSIC COMPRESSION DUE TO BRONCHOGENIC CYST, HEMANGIOMA, TERATOMA

Bronchoscopy is an important diagnostic tool in such cases in association with other examinations such as computed tomography.

CONGENITAL HEART DISEASE

Some severe congenital cardiac disorders (agenesis of the pulmonary valves, an important left-to-right shunt and mitral insufficiency) are associated with enlargement of large vessels which may cause compression of proximal airways.[27] Significant airway compression by a large vessel may explain pulmonary chest radiograph abnormalities.[10]

Bronchoscopy in mechanically ventilated neonates

FREQUENCY

The true incidence of proximal airways injury due to mechanical ventilation is unknown, as systematic examination has rarely been performed, except in the prospective study performed by Schellhase.[33] Using a 2.2 mm FB, they performed 21 serial bronchoscopies in eight conventionally ventilated premature infants (mean birthweight 1.239 kg). FB was done within 24–36 hours of admission, then 3–5 days, 10–12 days and finally at 4 weeks of age. Mucosal changes were classified as normal, mild, moderate and severe according to the degree of erythema, edema, the character and amount of secretions and the presence of areas of hemorrhage and ulcerations. Obstructive changes were classified according to whether there were pseudomembranes, granulations,

stenosis and malacia. The authors found that during the first days after birth, moderate to severe distal tracheal mucosal injury, but not obstructive injury, occurred frequently. Mucosal injury appeared to improve during the first month after birth, while mild obstructive injury began during the second week after birth. No definitive conclusions can be drawn, but one can speculate that moderate to severe distal tracheal mucosal injury may be an important risk factor for the development of later obstructive injury. Two other prospective studies have yielded conflicting results.[7,14] In da Silva's series,[7] less than 5 percent of the 227 intubated neonates developed respiratory stridor after extubation. Four underwent bronchoscopy, mild subglottic stenosis was observed in one and granulation tissue in three patients. By contrast, in Downing's series,[14] flexible bronchoscopy identified airway abnormalities in 27.3 percent of the 117 preterm infants who were intubated for 7 days or more. The abnormalities included subglottic stenosis and/or tracheomalacia.

OBSTRUCTIVE LESIONS

In an intubated neonate, persistent lung atelectasis, localized hyperinflation, unexplained acute respiratory failure and unexplained attacks of cyanosis constitute well-accepted indications for urgent bronchoscopy. A high frequency of mechanical or dynamic obstruction of the airway may be found. Furthermore, FB may disclose significant, but clinically unsuspected airway disease. Important localized inflammation, stenosis and granuloma formation represent the most frequent lesions observed.[10,14,26,28] In addition, FB can demonstrate inflammatory phenomena which are associated with long-term ventilation. Irregular and asymmetric stenoses, associated with mucosal inflammation located at the distal section of the trachea and on the right side (main stem and bronchus intermedius) can be seen; these are the target of the suction catheter during suctioning. In another study of 129 flexible bronchoscopies in 47 patients with BPD,[6] mechanical obstruction of proximal airways was also frequently seen. The patients had a mean age of 17 months, but had required mechanical ventilation and/or supplemental oxygen for at least the first 30 days after birth. The indications for endoscopy were usually the evaluation of previous subglottic stenosis and tracheostomy. FB, however, frequently disclosed unexpected tracheal and bronchial lesions including granuloma in 34 percent of cases, important inflammation or edema in 25 percent of cases and tracheal (with or without bronchial) stenosis in 36 percent of the infants.

In our study of 37 FBs performed in 33 infants on the neonatal unit and using a 2.2 mm FB,[10] 28 procedures were performed via endotracheal tube or tracheostomy. When searching for airway obstruction in the presence of persistent radiological abnormalities in mechanically ventilated infants (particularly in cases of BPD and cardiothoracic malformations), we found that in 80 percent of the cases, an ultrathin FB examination demonstrated intrinsic abnormalities (granuloma, inflammatory stenosis), malformation (tracheal bronchus), severe extrinsic compression, or severe tracheo- and/or bronchomalacia. These airway anomalies can exist concurrently and their correct diagnosis is of paramount importance in influencing management decisions. In the presence of inflammatory lesions, granuloma or tracheobronchial stenosis, due to prolonged ventilation and repeated suctioning, the suction catheter should not be passed beyond the end of the endotracheal tube. Probably, more extended use of ultrathin FB in NICUs will confirm the high frequency of such lesions even in neonates and infants without abnormal chest radiograph.

MALACIA

Excessive expiratory collapse of the trachea or the main stem bronchus is a well known cause of stridor, chronic productive cough, recurrent pneumonia and cyanosis in neonates. Primary tracheomalacia and bronchomalacia, due to an inherent weakness of the cartilaginous walls of the tracheobronchial tree, are rare and may be localized or diffuse. Localized secondary malacia is observed following correction of esophageal atresia and when there is any extrinsic pressure due to vascular anomalies or a bronchogenic cyst. FB allows the evaluation of the degree and extent of the narrowing. FB without general anesthesia is the best instrument to diagnose bronchomalacia and tracheomalacia because it allows a dynamic view of both the upper and the lower airways. In the long term, intubated neonates and especially in those with bronchopulmonary dysplasia, FB may reveal tracheomalacia and bronchomalacia in up to 30–50 percent of cases.

SPECIFIC USE OF THE FLEXIBLE BRONCHOSCOPE

Evaluation of ET position and patency
Initially, the main indication of FBs and especially ultrathin FBs in intubated neonates was to check the position or patency of the ET.[17,18,36] Flexible bronchoscopy with ultrathin FBs is a rapid and effective method for ensuring appropriate tube position and patency when, in acute circumstances, there is the question as to whether the ET has been dislodged or may be blocked with mucus.

Difficult intubation
Using the FB as a rigid guidewire for the ET helps to achieve difficult intubation in selected patients.[4,19] Ultrathin FB was successfully used to intubate 23 neonates with craniofacial malformations such as Goldenhar, Larsen and Pierre Robin syndromes and other disorders that prevented adequate visualization of the larynx.[19]

Acquired subglottic stenosis and tracheostomy
Acquired subglottic stenosis may occur in neonates and infants who require prolonged intubation. Post-extubation

stridor lasting more than 24 hours is an indication for bronchoscopy.[7] Bronchoscopy may be performed with a rigid bronchoscope, but a flexible bronchoscope is more useful to study the dynamics and the anatomy of the lower airway. Only with a rigid bronchoscope, however, can granulation tissue be removed if needed.

BRONCHOALVEOLAR LAVAGE IN THE NEONATES

In contrast to older infants, non-bronchoscopic techniques in intubated newborn infants are used to obtain bronchoalveolar lavage (BAL) fluid.[11] Two aliquots of 1 ml/kg of physiological saline at room temperature are instilled and re-aspirated. The availability of 'slim' bronchoscopes incorporating a suction channel will, however, probably expand the use of BAL in neonates. There are no data regarding the yield of BAL in infectious diseases of neonates, but BAL may disclose infectious agents such as *Chlamydia trachomatis*, *Mycobacterium tuberculosis*, *Pneumocystis carinii*, respiratory syncytial virus (RSV) and cytomegalovirus (CMV). Neonatal manifestations of non-infectious interstitial pneumonia are uncommon.[12]

THERAPEUTIC BRONCHOSCOPY

Atelectasis
Rigid and flexible (with a suction channel) bronchoscopes are useful to treat acute actelectasis. Atelectasis is frequently observed post-extubation and/or post-thoracic surgery. Only the few cases of atelectasis persisting for several days despite chest physiotherapy require FB. Removal of mucous plugs, or sometimes instillation and re-aspiration of physiological saline into the atelectatic lobe, allows re-aeration and improvement of respiratory status.[20,34] In such acute atelectasis, FB reveals fewer anatomical changes, but it is much more effective than when used in persistent atelectasis.

Pulmonary interstitial emphysema (PIE)
Bronchoalveolar lavage has been proposed for medical management of severe chronic PIE.[9] Distal bronchoalveolar lavages were performed with small volume of saline and in six of nine infants so treated, the PIE resolved in less than 24 hours. Resolution of the PIE was accompanied by clinical improvement, allowing extubation. Distal lavage may have affected the PIE by removing bronchiolar obstruction due to fibrinous exudate, or alveolar debris. Use of this technique has not been examined in a randomized controlled trial (p. 422).

Necrotizing tracheobronchitis
Necrotizing tracheobronchitis is a rare complication of mechanical (including high-frequency) ventilation (p. 171). Sloughing of the respiratory epithelium occludes the proximal airways. Diagnosis relies upon bronchoscopy, which reveals extensive plugging of the distal trachea and main stem bronchi. Endoscopic removal of obstructing debris is essential to improve outcome.[25,32]

Stenosis

Endoscopic treatment of acquired tracheal or bronchial stenosis and of obstructive granuloma may be necessary. Endoscopic excision with biopsy forceps, bouginage or balloon dilatation[15] during rigid bronchoscopy is the most often used but flexible bronchoscopy and argon laser techniques have been evaluated.[1]

REFERENCES

1 Azizkhan, R., Lacey, S., Wood, R. (1990) Acquired symptomatic bronchial stenosis in infants: successful management using argon laser. *Journal of Pediatric Surgery* **25**, 19–24.

2 Backer, C., Ilbawi, M., Idriss, F., De Leon, S. (1989) Vascular anomalies causing tracheoesophageal compression. *Journal of Thoracic and Cardovascular Surgery* **97**, 725–731.

3 Benjamin, B. (1980) Endoscopy in congenital tracheal anomalies. *Journal of Pediatric Surgery* **15**, 164–171.

4 Biban, P., Rugolotto, S., Zoppi, G. (2000) Fiberoptic endotracheal intubation through an ultra-thin bronchoscope with suction channel in a newborn with difficult airway. *Anesthesia and Analgesia* **90**, 1007.

5 Chedevergne, F., Jugie, M., Le Bourgeois, M. *et al.* (2000) Value of a new 2.7 mm flexible bronchoscope in infants. Presented to the European Respiratory Society meeting, Florence, Italy 2000 (abstract no. 3359).

6 Cohn, R., Kercsmar, C., Dearborn, D. (1988) Safety and efficacy of flexible bronchoscopy in children with bronchopulmonary dysplasia. *American Journal of Diseases of Children* **142**, 1225–1228.

7 da Silva, O., Stevens, D. (1999) Complications of airway management in very low birth weight infants. *Biology of the Neonate* **75**, 40–45.

8 de Blic, J., Scheinmann, P. (1992) Fibreoptic bronchoscopy in infants. *Archives of Disease in Childhood* **67**, 159–161.

9 de Blic, J., Scheinmann, P., Paupe, J. (1984) Successful treatment of persistent neonatal interstitial emphysema by flexible bronchoscopy. *Lancet* **2**, 1389–1390.

10 de Blic, J., Delacourt, C., Scheinmann, P. (1991) Ultrathin flexible bronchoscopy in neonatal intensive care units. *Archives of Disease in Childhood* **66**, 1383–1385.

11 de Blic, J., Midulla, F., Barbato, A. *et al.* (2000) Bronchoalveolar lavage in children. ERS Task Force on bronchoalveolar lavage in children. *European Respiratory Journal* **15**, 17–34.

12 de la Fuente, A.A., Voorhout, W.F., deMello, D.E. (1997) Congenital alveolar proteinosis in the Netherlands: a report of five cases with immunohistochemical and genetic studies on surfactant apoproteins. *Pediatric Pathology and Laboratory Medicine* **17**, 221–231.

13 Dohlemann, C., Hauser, M., Nicolai, T., Kreuzer, E. (1995) Innominate artery enlargement in congenital arteriovenous fistula with subsequent tracheal compression and stridor. *Pediatric Cardiology* **16**, 287–290.

14 Downing, G.J., Kilbride, H.W. (1995) Evaluation of airway complications in high-risk preterm infants: application of flexible fiberoptic airway endoscopy. *Pediatrics* **95**, 567–572.

15 Elkerbout, S.C., van Lingen, R.A., Gerritsen, J., Roorda, R.J. (1993) Endoscopic balloon dilatation of acquired airway stenosis in newborn infants: a promising treatment. *Archives of Disease in Childhood* **68**, 37–40.

16 Erwin, E.A., Gerber, M.E., Cotton, R.T. (1997) Vascular compression of the airway: indications for and results of surgical management. *International Journal of Pediatric Otorhinolaryngology* **40**, 155–162.

17 Fan, L.L., Sparks, L.M., Dulinski, J.P. (1986) Applications of an ultrathin flexible bronchoscope for neonatal and pediatric airway problems. *Chest* **89**, 673–676.

18 Finer, N.N., Etches, P.C. (1989) Fibreoptic bronchoscopy in the neonate. *Pediatric Pulmonology* **7**, 116–120.

19 Finer, N.N., Muzyka, D. (1992) Flexible endoscopic intubation of the neonate. *Pediatric Pulmonology* **12**, 48–51.

20 Hasegawa, S., Hitomi, S., Murakawa, M., Mori, K. (1996) Development of an ultrathin fiberscope with a built-in channel for bronchoscopy in infants. *Chest* **110**, 1543–1546.

21 Hinton, A.E., O'Connell, J.M., van Besouw, J.P., Wyatt, M.E. (1997) Neonatal and paediatric fibre-optic laryngoscopy and bronchoscopy using the laryngeal mask airway. *Journal of Laryngology and Otology* **111**, 349–353.

22 Karnak, I., Senocak, M.E., Hicsonmez, A., Buyukpamukcu, N. (1997) The diagnosis and treatment of H-type tracheoesophageal fistula. *Journal of Pediatric Surgery* **32**, 1670–1674.

23 Kosloske, A.M., Jewell, P.F., Cartwright, K.C. (1988) Crucial bronchoscopic findings in esophageal atresia and tracheoesophageal fistula. *Journal of Pediatric Surgery* **23**, 466–470.

24 Lindahl, H., Rintala, R., Malinen, L. *et al.* (1992) Bronchoscopy during the first month of life. *Journal of Pediatric Surgery* **27**, 548–550.

25 Metlay, L.A., Macpherson, T.A., Doshi, N., Milley, J.R. (1987) Necrotizing tracheobronchitis in intubated newborns: a complication of assisted ventilation. *Pediatric Pathology* **7**, 575–584.

26 Miller, R.W., Woo, P., Kellman, R.K., Slagle, T.S. (1987) Tracheobronchial abnormalities in infants with bronchopulmonary dysplasia. *Journal of Pediatrics* **111**, 779–782.

27 Monrigal, J.P., Granry, J.C. (1996) Excision of bronchogenic cysts in children using an ultrathin fibreoptic bronchoscope. *Canadian Journal of Anaesthesia* **43**, 694–696.

28 Myer, C.M., Thompson, R.F. (1988) Flexible fiberoptic bronchoscopy in the neonatal intensive care unit. *International Journal of Pediatric Otorhinolaryngology* **15**, 143–147.

29 Nicolai, T. (2001) Pediatric bronchoscopy. *Pediatric Pulmonology* **31**, 150–164.

30 Nose, K., Kamata, S., Sawai, T. *et al.* (2000) Airway anomalies in patients with congenital diaphragmatic hernia. *Journal of Pediatric Surgery* **35**, 1562–1565.

31 Prinja, N., Manoukian, J.J. (1998) Neonatal/infant rigid bronchoscopy. *Journal of Otolaryngology* **27**, 31–36.

32 Sauer, P.J., vd Schans, E.J., Lafeber, H.N. (1986) Bronchoscopic treatment of necrotizing tracheo-bronchitis in a newborn. *European Journal of Pediatrics* **144**, 596–597.

33 Schellhase, D.E. (1990) Routine fiberoptic bronchoscopy in intubated neonates? *American Journal of Diseases of Children* **144**, 746–747.

34 Shinwell, E.S. (1992) Ultrathin fiberoptic bronchoscopy for airway toilet in neonatal pulmonary atelectasis. *Pediatric Pulmonology* **13**, 48–49.

35 Ungkanont, K., Friedman, E.M., Sulek, M. (1998) A retrospective analysis of airway endoscopy in patients less than 1-month-old. *Laryngoscope* **108**, 1724–1728.

36 Vigneswaran, R., Whitfield, J.M. (1981) The use of a new ultra-thin fiberoptic bronchoscope to determine endotracheal tube position in the sick newborn infant. *Chest* **80**, 174–177.

37 Wood, R. (1985) Clinical applications of ultrathin flexible bronchoscopes. *Pediatric Pulmonology* **1**, 244–248.

38 Wood, R., Postma, D. (1988) Endoscopy of the airway in infants and children. *Journal of Pediatrics* **112**, 1–6.

13

Measurement of lung function

ANTHONY D MILNER AND GERRARD F RAFFERTY

Techniques are now available which now make it possible to obtain a comprehensive picture of the lung function of a neonate.[28,70] In the past, the results obtained were highly influenced by the characteristics of the equipment used and the methods of data collection and analysis, so that it was difficult to compare the results from different laboratories. This problem has to some extent been resolved by the European Respiratory Society and the American Thoracic Society's task force on standards for infant respiratory function testing which has provided guidelines for specifications.[36,37]

Despite these problems, infant lung function tests have provided very important information on the normal physiology of the neonatal lung, the process of adaptation in the perinatal period,[112] and how these processes are adversely affected by neonatal pulmonary pathology. They have also been useful in the evaluation of new therapies, in the development of management strategies and in the prediction of outcome.[42] Their role as diagnostic tools is not so clearly defined, although the introduction of less invasive techniques is likely to lead to their increased use in optimizing therapy for individual babies. The aim of this chapter is to provide information on the techniques available, their clinical role, research potential and limitations.

VOLUME MEASUREMENTS

The volumes which can be measured are divided into those generated by respiratory muscle activity, which are defined as 'dynamic', and those resulting from the structural limits of the respiratory system and by the recoil characteristics of the lung and chest wall which are defined as 'static'.

Dynamic volume measurements

The measurement of tidal volume alone is of limited value in the spontaneously breathing baby, although an indication of the breathing pattern is helpful in identifying those with recurrent apnea. This requirement can be met by semi-quantitative systems such as impedance plethysmography,[8] in which the resistance to a small electrical current between electrodes placed on either side of the chest is measured; as the baby breathes in, the resistance increases. Respiration can also be monitored by attaching a movement sensor such as a pressure capsule (Graseby Dynamics)[1] or pressure sensor to the abdominal skin. The problems associated with and limitations of these devices are discussed elsewhere (p. 164).

INDUCTANCE PLETHYSMOGRAPHY

A system has been developed commercially whereby tidal exchange can be measured by changes in the area within coils surrounding both the chest and the abdomen; it makes use of the currents induced by changes in strength of the magnetic field.[26] The coils consist of copper wire which surround the chest and the abdomen in a zig-zag manner; the total width of each coil is approximately 2 cm (Figure 13.1). They are mounted on cotton strips, which can be held in place by self-retaining material such as Velcro. During quiet sleep when the chest and the abdomen are moving synchronously, the chest and the abdominal signal can be summed to provide an index of the depth as well as the rate of respiration. In adults it has proved possible to achieve a reasonably accurate calibration of the system by simultaneously measuring volume change at the mouth with a device such as the spirometer while, for several breaths, keeping the abdominal wall as still as possible and then further measurements while

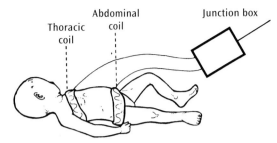

Figure 13.1 *Inductance plethysmograph for measuring changes in abdominal and chest wall circumference.*

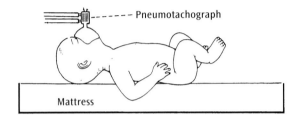

Figure 13.2 *Pneumotachograph system. The flow is measured as the calibrated pressure drop across a small resistance under conditions of laminar flow.*

moving the chest wall as little as possible.[18] This allows the two coils to be calibrated independently and the summed signal quantified. This is obviously impossible in the neonatal period. Claims have been made, however, that the chest and abdominal coils can be calibrated by comparing the output from the two coils with volume changes at the mouth. This is done over a range of breathing patterns, during which the phase relationships between the chest and the abdomen have changed, and essentially uses the quadratic equation approach.[81,106] Although this would appear to be an attractive option, our own experience and that of others has indicated that, over relatively short periods, particularly in the presence of lung disease, poor accuracy is achieved.[38]

PNEUMOTACHOGRAPH

A pneumotachograph, which can be attached to a face mask (Figure 13.2) or endotracheal tube, ensures that the flow across a relatively low resistance is laminar, i.e. smooth and not turbulent. These laminar flow conditions can be achieved either by having a relatively wide diameter at the point at which the resistance is inserted so that the speed of the gas molecules is reduced or by conducting the flow through a number of cylindrical tubes. Under these circumstances, the pressure change across the resistance is directly related to the flow. The flow is derived by measuring the pressure drop across the resistance using a differential pressure transducer and calibrating the pressure drop against a rotameter. The signal can then be converted to volume by feeding it through an electronic device (an integrator), which integrates flow against time.

Problems with pneumotachography

Although simple in concept, there are a number of problems associated with the use of pneumotachographs.[43] First, the pressure drop across the device depends on the viscosity of the individual gases. These differ considerably so that the device should always be calibrated using the mixture inspired by the subject. The differences in constitution of the gas between inspiration and expiration also have effects but, fortunately, the overall effect is small, introducing an error of approximately 1 percent. A second problem is that the small resistance within the pneumotachograph, whether this be a metal gauze or system of tubes, tends to be at a lower temperature to that of the expired air, so that water condenses out on expiration. This will increase the resistance further, giving artifactually high flow and hence volume readings. This is usually overcome by heating the pneumotachograph, but it must be remembered that the viscosity of the gas increases with temperature and therefore the calibration should only be carried out once the pneumotachograph has been left on sufficiently to warm up to the operational temperature. A further problem results from drift in the volume trace. This may arise from the differential pressure transducer, but even more so from the integrator itself so that it may be difficult to achieve a stable volume signal for more than 1–2 minutes. One approach has been to ensure that the integrator re-zeroes at the beginning and end of each inspiration. Further problems can arise if the pneumotachograph is inserted into a ventilator circuit or patient manifold. If the tubes leading from the pneumotachograph to the differential pressure transducer are not identical or if, indeed, the two sides of the pressure transducer have different volumes, time constant inequalities will be introduced so that the ventilator pressures will be conducted to the two sides of the differential pressure transducer diaphragm at different rates. Finally, even under conditions of perfect laminar flow, no pneumotachograph has a totally linear relationship between flow and pressure drop across the internal resistance so that a microprocessor will be needed if highly accurate flow and volume recordings are to be achieved.[33] This is rarely needed in clinical practice. It is obviously also important to ensure that the flow limit at which laminar conditions break down and turbulence takes over as specified by the manufacturers, are not exceeded during measurements.

THERMISTORS

Thermistors work on the principle that the electrical resistance of a heated wire varies with temperature.[40] As the cooling effect of a flow of air over the thermistor is directly related to the rate of flow, the device can be calibrated against a rotameter in the same way as a pneumotachograph. The cooling effect of a gas is related to its specific heat and so, as with the pneumotachograph, it is

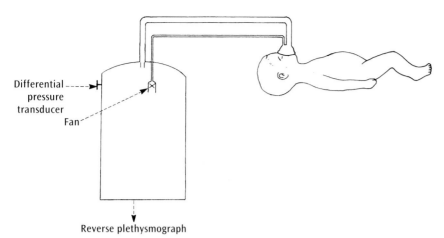

Figure 13.3 *Reverse plethysmograph system with fan-assisted circulation to reduce the effects of hypercapnia and hypoxia.*

necessary to use an appropriate gas for calibration purposes.

Unlike the pneumotachograph, a single thermistor is unable to determine flow direction. This can be overcome by mounting two thermistors in the flow stream, one of which is shaded from either the inspiratory or expiratory flow by a baffle. The output from the thermistor can be fed to an integrator to derive a volume trace.

REVERSE PLETHYSMOGRAPH

The reverse plethysmograph consists of a rigid container which is at least 1000 times greater than the tidal volume to be measured.[72] This will ensure that the pressure changes within the circuit remain less than 1 cmH$_2$O. The container is attached to a face mask by two tubes with a circulating pump to limit rebreathing (Figure 13.3). Once the face mask has been placed over the infant's mouth and nose, the tidal exchange produces small pressure changes within the chamber which can be measured by a suitable pressure transducer. The system can then be calibrated against a syringe to provide an accurate measurement of tidal exchange. Reverse plethysmography has the major advantage that the volume trace is considerably more stable than an integrator-based technique, providing the environmental conditions remains reasonably constant, as changes in temperature will lead to expansion or contraction of the pressure of the gas within the system. Dramatic baseline shifts will, therefore, occur if the reservoir is exposed to direct sunlight.

As the reverse plethysmograph is a pressure system, errors can be introduced due to the adiabatic effect. Compression of a gas generates heat so that under perfect thermal insulation conditions the pressure change in an air-containing system will be 30 percent higher than that predicted from Boyle's law ($P_1V_1 = P_2V_2$). This effect depends on the specific heat of different gases so that the pressure change will be 40 percent higher if the gas is helium, rather than air and 20 percent if the system is filled with carbon dioxide (CO$_2$). Pressure changes

within a chamber will, however, follow Boyle's law if heat conduction is perfect so that the temperature of the gases remains constant, that is, the conditions are isothermal. In practice, systems such as reverse plethysmographs function somewhere between the adiabatic and the isothermal conditions. To limit error, calibration should be carried out by injecting and withdrawing volumes at the infant's own respiratory rate. While the reverse plethysmograph has the major advantage of long-term stability, it can only be used in spontaneously breathing infants.

SPIROMETER

Water-filled and dry spirometers are now available for use in the neonatal period. These should be lightweight and have internal volumes of less than 500 ml in order to have appropriate sensitivity. A CO$_2$-absorbing circuit and facility for bleeding in oxygen is necessary if measurements are to be continued for more than 1–2 minutes.

TRUNK PLETHYSMOGRAPH

This device was used extensively by Cross[19] and consists of a chamber which encompasses the infant's body. The initial device had an inflatable rubber ring to produce an air seal around the infant's face. This technique has the advantage that there is no added respiratory dead space and no facial stimulation from the face mask.[115] An alternative approach is to immerse the infant totally within an airtight container, but to use a face mask which is connected both to a bias flow and to atmosphere through the side of the chamber. Under both these circumstances the changes in lung volume produced by the baby produce alterations in pressure within the plethysmograph which can be calibrated against a syringe. This system has very good long-term stability, but is prone to adiabatic errors so that calibration should be carried out at the infant's respiratory rate. This problem can also be avoided by measuring the thoracic volume change by a spirometer connected to the plethysmography.[115]

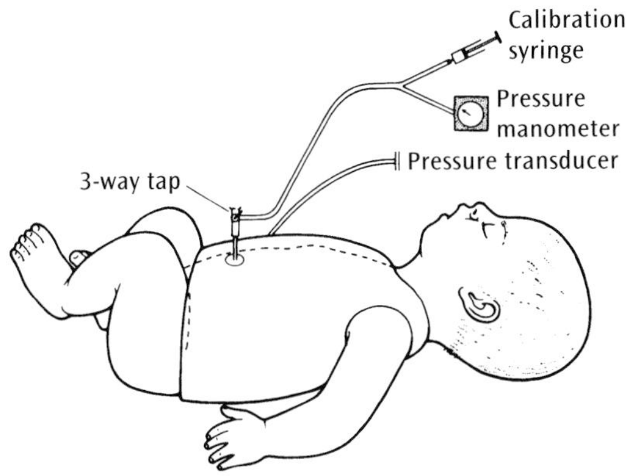

Figure 13.4 *Jacket plethysmograph.*

JACKET PLETHYSMOGRAPH

An alternative approach has been to encompass the infant's chest and abdomen in a soft rubber jacket which is inflated to a pressure of 2–4 cmH$_2$O. Pressure changes within the jacket resulting from tidal breathing are then measured (Figure 13.4).[47] These changes are in the region of 1–2 mmH$_2$O and so have no measurable effect on the breathing pattern. Calibration is achieved by injecting and withdrawing known volumes of air from the jacket and measuring the change in end tidal baseline. This system has the advantage that it has very good long-term stability. It can be used on babies breathing spontaneously or requiring respiratory support, but can lead to over-heating if used for prolonged periods.

BAROMETRIC PLETHYSMOGRAPH

A further and ingenious method for measuring tidal exchange has been to nurse infants in an airtight container which is kept at a constant temperature some degrees below that of the infant.[35] As the infant breathes out, the expired air, which is saturated with water vapor at 37°C, will cool and shrink, leading to a fall in chamber pressure. The reverse happens on inspiration. This provides a very non-invasive method for monitoring tidal exchange over prolonged periods.

Clinical and research applications

MEASUREMENTS ON SPONTANEOUSLY BREATHING BABIES

Measurements of tidal breathing are of limited value in the neonatal period. Semi-quantitative devices such as the impedance, inductance and abdominal pressure sensors are adequate for the identification of central and mixed apnea, but respiratory rate and tidal volumes are so variable in the neonatal period that these measurements are otherwise of little diagnostic value.[19] Attempts have been made to use the degree of variability of breathing pattern to identify sleep state using a breath-by-breath

variability of greater than 10 percent as an indication of rapid eye movement (REM) sleep. The correlation, however, between this relatively simplistic form of sleep staging and that achieved by full electromyograph (EMG) and electro-oculograph (EOG) monitoring is poor.[84] An alternative approach has been to use the phase relationship between the chest and abdominal movement as a sleep staging device. Again, although there is a tendency for 'out-of-phase' breathing to be associated with REM sleep, the correlation with other methods of sleep staging is poor.[104]

There has recently been considerable interest in the flow pattern during tidal breathing, in particular the relationship between the time to reach peak expiratory flow and total expiratory flow time (t_{PTEF}/t_E).[66] It has been claimed that, when this measurement is carried out in early infancy, it can identify at least some of the infants who are likely to develop respiratory symptoms later.[118] It was also found to be significantly reduced in a group of infants born to mothers who smoked during pregnancy.[102] More recent work has suggested that this technique is poorly reproducible in the immediate neonatal period but further work is needed.[63,74] The technique also has a relatively poor sensitivity and specificity as an indicator of abnormal lung function. Its main role is in large epidemiological studies, rather than assessing lung function in the individual infant. This measurement can be obtained using pneumotachographs or thermistors, which measure flow directly, but can also be derived from techniques which primarily measure volume, such as reverse plethysmographs, spirometers, trunk plethysmographs and uncalibrated inductance plethysmographs, by using a differentiator to derive flow from volume.[102] Measurements obtained from trunk plethysmograph and inductance techniques are likely to differ from those using face masks due to the phase shift between tidal flow at the mouth and movement of the chest wall.[47]

Currently it is unclear why a low t_{PTEF}/t_E value should be associated with abnormal lung mechanics. Dezateux and colleagues[21] found a weak correlation between t_{PTEF}/t_E and functional residual capacity but no significant relationship between t_{PTEF}/t_E and specific conductance, a value derived by relating the reciprocal of resistance to lung volume. Surprisingly, the t_{PTEF}/t_E appears to be more closely related to results of measurements of compliance rather than to those of airway resistance.[96]

MEASUREMENT OF RESPIRATORY DRIVE AND RESPIRATORY RESERVE

Measurement of spontaneous breathing patterns have, however, been very useful in determining the sensitivity of the peripheral and central chemoreceptors. The peripheral chemoreceptors can be assessed by measuring the increase in tidal exchange following a short, sometimes single breath, exposure to increased ambient CO$_2$.[91] More

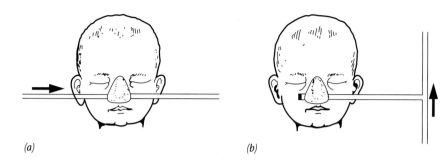

Figure 13.5 *Tube breathing technique. (a) Basal breathing is first recorded using a zero dead space system. (b) Dead space of 2.2 or 4.4 ml/kg body weight is then added using a 4 mm bore tube as a 'snorkel tube'.*

prolonged exposure to an increased CO_2 environment will provide an assessment of the sensitivity of both the central and peripheral chemoreceptors. This response will be damped in the presence of lung damage, but can then be used to provide a measure of respiratory reserve. The sensitivity of peripheral chemoreceptors has also been assessed by examining the response to either a single breath of 100 percent oxygen, which normally produces a transient depression of respiration, or to breath-by-breath alterations in the inspired oxygen concentration.[109] A more prolonged exposure to hypoxia produces an initial stimulation followed by a depression of respiration in the immediate neonatal period.[92] Unfortunately, these methods of assessing chemoreceptor sensitivity are poorly reproducible, making it difficult to identify those with partial sensitivity deficiency.

An alternative approach has been to measure basal breathing using a face mask with a bias flow, thereby eliminating any dead space.[111] A known dead space, in the form of a tube with an internal diameter of 4 mm and an internal volume of two anatomical dead spaces (4.4 ml/kg), is then introduced (Figure 13.5). Healthy term infants produce an increase in minute volume of approximately 150 percent and which is within 10 percent of the increase predicted from the size of the added dead space, after allowing for changes in respiratory rate.[111] Information on the rate of response of the chemoreceptor control system can be obtained by making continuous breath-by-breath measurements from the time of the application of the dead space to the formation of new steady state. Each breath is then expressed as a minute volume rate by multiplying the tidal volume by 60 and dividing by the total breath time in seconds. These values are then plotted against the times of each breath. The most useful measurement is the time constant, which is the time in seconds for 63 percent of the increase in minute ventilation produced by the added dead space to occur.[111]

MEASUREMENTS DURING VENTILATION

Devices such as pneumotachographs have allowed assessment of the effects of different ventilation strategies on tidal exchange in the neonatal intensive care unit. When used in this way, it is important to ensure that the pneumotachograph is not adversely affecting ventilation by increasing the dead space to any clinically significant extent. This can be avoided by using pneumotachographs with very small dead spaces. Alternatively, a bias flow can be driven or sucked across the device through a high resistance to ensure that errors are not introduced due to variation in the bias flow with the ventilator pressure cycles.[31] These measurements have provided important information on the effects of rate and inspiratory time on tidal exchange and also the effects of different levels of positive end expiratory pressure (PEEP) on tidal volume. It is important that devices such as the impedance technique should be used in a direct current (DC) mode for this purpose as under alternating current (AC) conditions, the signal will inevitably drift back to a preset zero on disconnection from the ventilator, so that changes in end tidal volume will be lost.

Volume measurements have also been used to identify situations in which alveolar PEEP is occurring and increasingly, commercially available neonatal ventilators have facilities for monitoring both tidal volume and tidal flow (p. 229). It is claimed (p. 231) that these measurements can help identify situations in which endotracheal obstruction is occurring and when there has been a sudden change in lung compliance, for example, the occurrence of a pneumothorax or pulmonary interstitial emphysema (p. 230).

Measurement of tidal exchange and airway opening pressure

Simultaneous measurements of airway pressure and tidal volume can provide very useful information on the mechanical characteristics of the respiratory system.

MEASUREMENTS ON SPONTANEOUSLY BREATHING BABIES – SINGLE BREATH LUNG MECHANICS

Single breath lung mechanics can be used to obtain information on both the compliance of the respiratory system, that is the volume change produced by one unit of pressure, and resistance, which is the pressure generated by one unit of flow. Stopping the egress of air from a face mask and pneumotachograph system at the top of a

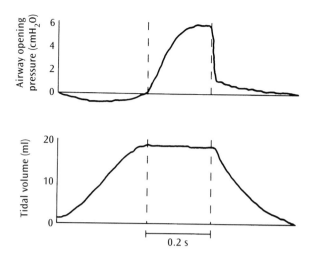

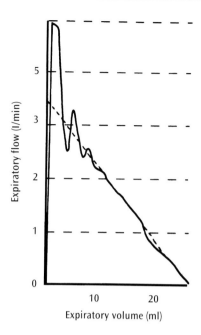

Figure 13.6 *Trace of tidal volume and face mask pressure before and after a period of occlusion.*

Figure 13.7 *Flow–volume trace after release of occlusion. The time constant is measured from the straight part of the slope of the flow–volume curve.*

breath for 0.2–0.4 seconds will induce a brief apnea via the Hering–Breuer reflex.[80] Under these circumstances, the elastic recoil of the respiratory system can be measured by the pressure within the face mask using a suitable pressure transducer (Figure 13.6). Relief of the obstruction will then result in the expired gases passing out through the pneumotachograph passively, that is, in the absence of respiratory muscle activity. Under these conditions, both flow and volume will fall exponentially once the flow has reached a peak, providing the mechanical characteristics of the lungs remain unchanged. Under these circumstances the time constant, that is the time for 63 percent of the tidal volume to leave the lung, can be measured either from the volume trace or from the slope of the plot of expiratory volume against expiratory flow (Figure 13.7).[60] This latter approach is preferable as deviation from a straight line towards the end of tidal expiration indicates that expiration is no longer passive. In addition, extrapolation of the flow volume slope to zero flow will provide a measure of the true functional residual capacity (FRC). This is important as newborn babies tend to start inspiration before full passive expiration has occurred,[54] leading to dynamic elevation of the FRC. This corrected volume can then be used in the calculation of total respiratory system compliance, i.e. $\Delta V/\Delta P$. As the time constant is equal to the compliance multiplied by the resistance, it is also possible to obtain a measure of the overall respiratory system resistance. These resistance measurements are up to 100 percent higher than values obtained using total body plethysmography.[27] Compliance measurements obtained using the single breath technique are not always satisfactory. It is sometimes difficult to induce the Hering–Breuer response and achieve a satisfactory plateau and the relationship between the respiratory flow and volume is sometimes totally non-linear.[27,39]

Alternative methods for measuring total respiratory system compliance are by repeated brief occlusion during expiration and measuring the compliance from the volume above FRC and the mouth pressure during periods of occlusion.[45] Alternatively, the egress from the pneumotachograph can be connected to different levels of continuous positive airway pressure (CPAP), e.g. 5, 10 and 15 cmH$_2$O, and then plot the expiratory volumes on releasing this pressure against the levels of CPAP. A further method now is the weighted spirometer technique.[108] Baseline tidal breathing is measured using a water-filled spirometer (Figure 13.8). A suitable weight, sufficient to increase the pressure within the spirometer circuit by 2–3 cmH$_2$O, is placed on top of the spirometer base. Total respiratory system compliance is then calculated by dividing the resultant increase in FRC as measured by the changes in end tidal baseline by the change pressure within the circuit.

CLINICAL AND RESEARCH APPLICATIONS

Single breath lung mechanics have become extremely popular due to the relatively non-invasive nature of the investigation and the availability of computer systems which can perform the analyses. They have been used to assess the response to bronchodilator drugs, particularly in those with chronic lung disease (p. 412) and increasingly to measure lung mechanics in babies developing respiratory distress syndrome (RDS) in an attempt to identify those who are likely to require surfactant supplementation. Considerable care is needed, however, in

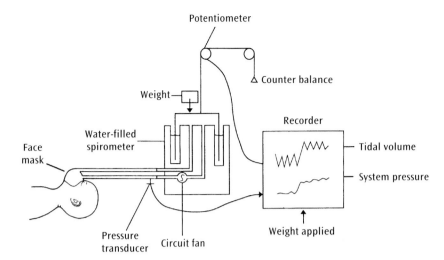

Figure 13.8 *Diagram of equipment needed to measure total respiratory system compliance using the weighted spirometer system.*

performing these measurements and in the identification of acceptable traces.

Measurements during ventilation

The information gained by measuring tidal exchange during respiratory support using a pneumotachograph or thermistor device can be considerably increased by simultaneously measuring the airway pressure. It is then easy to obtain a measure of the respiratory system compliance by dividing the tidal exchange by the ventilator inflation pressure. Studies have shown that even low levels of PEEP, for example 2–3 cmH$_2$O, can significantly reduce the compliance of the lung.[32] A more accurate measure of the lung compliance can be obtained if the expired gases are vented to ambient pressure at the end of an inflation.[5,114] Under these circumstances, it is also possible using the technique as described above to measure the time constant of the lung and thus the resistance of the respiratory system with the endotracheal tube *in situ*. The resistance of the respiratory system including endotracheal tube and work of breathing can be obtained by using the airway opening pressure swings and tidal volumes to produce pressure–flow and pressure–volume loops (p. 232).

An alternative approach has been to use a ventilator which produces constant flow during inflation.[105] Under these circumstances the respiratory system compliance can be obtained by dividing the slope of the inspiratory volume trace by the slope of the airway opening pressure (Figure 13.9). In addition, the resistance can be calculated by extrapolating the pressure volume slope back to zero volume. The resistance can then be calculated by dividing the residual pressure by the flow rate during inspiration. These different techniques produce similar results for compliance, but not for resistance.[65]

Measurements of compliance (lung stiffness) are being increasingly used to document progress during ventilatory support and response to therapies such as surfactant administration (p. 249). The measurements

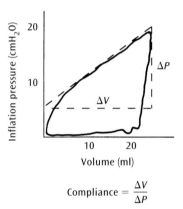

$$\text{Compliance} = \frac{\Delta V}{\Delta P}$$

Figure 13.9 *Trace of pressure volume–loop during inflation at a constant flow rate. The compliance is calculated from the slope of the inspiratory part of the trace ($\Delta V/\Delta P$) and the resistance by dividing the pressure at the zero volume pressure intercept by the constant flow.*

have also taught us a great deal about optimizing mechanical ventilation (p. 157).

Simultaneous measurements of tidal exchange and intrathoracic pressure

Considerable information can be obtained on the mechanical characteristics of the lungs by simultaneously measuring tidal exchange and the pressures generated intrathoracically by the infant. These measurements are achieved by using one of a number of techniques to record pressure changes in the lower third of the esophagus. One method is to pass a thin-walled balloon mounted on a 6 FG (French gauge) catheter through the nose or mouth until it reaches the stomach and then slowly withdraw it until negative pressures are recorded during inspiration.[12] Placing the balloon too high will inevitably result in an under-recording of the true pressure change. For optimal function, the esophageal balloon will need to be nearly empty of air, as otherwise the elastic properties of the balloon will adversely affect the recordings.[12] Alternatively, a water-filled catheter of at least a 6 FG diameter,[10] or a micropressure transducer mounted on a catheter of similar dimensions can be used. Again it is important to ensure that the functioning part, that is the micropressure transducer or the open end of the water-filled catheter, lie in the lower third of the esophagus by first entering the stomach and then withdrawing slowly. It is essential to ensure that no air bubbles develop in the water-filled catheter system. This is best achieved by perfusing the system with water at a rate of 1–2 ml/h. There are also micropressure transducers mounted on 5 or 6 FG catheters which can be passed either via the mouth or the nose so that the device lies in the lower third of the esophagus.[113]

Information on lung mechanics can then be obtained by simultaneously using one of these devices and measuring the volume change at the mouth by a pneumotachograph or thermistor integrator system, spirometer or reverse plethysmograph. A measure of lung stiffness, the dynamic compliance can be calculated by dividing the tidal volume by the esophageal pressure difference between the beginning and end of inspiration (Figure 13.10a).[55] In health this will approximate closely to measurements of static compliance providing the respiratory rate is below 60 breaths/min. Under conditions where the baby is breathing faster or there is airways obstruction present, the dynamic compliance will give a lower value than the static compliance.

The total pulmonary resistance can also be calculated using these techniques.[55] For this, the midpoints of inspiration and expiration are selected (Figure 13.10b). It is assumed that at these points the lungs are at the same degree of distention so that none of the pressure difference (Figure 13.10b) is due to elastic recoil but represents the pressure needed to drive the air up and down the airways against airflow resistance. This is therefore measured by dividing the pressure gradients between the mid-volume points by the simultaneous difference in flow.

Finally, the work of breathing can be measured by constructing pressure–volume loops. The area within the loop then represents the work necessary to overcome the resistive forces and the quadrangular area to the left of the pressure–volume loop, that necessary to overcome the elastic recoil of the lung (Figure 13.11).[103] In practice this measurement is of limited value. If, for example, the baby opts to breathe at half the rate but twice the tidal volume, his work of breathing per breath will be effectively quadrupled and the work of breathing per minute therefore doubled, although there has been no change in the mechanical characteristics of the lungs. All these techniques are dependent on accurate measurements of esophageal pressure and an assumption that this pressure closely follows the mean intrapleural pressure changes.

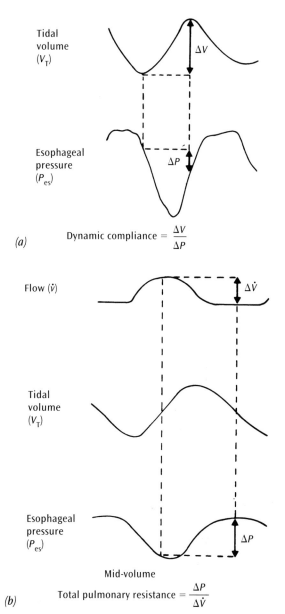

(a)

Dynamic compliance $= \dfrac{\Delta V}{\Delta P}$

(b)

Total pulmonary resistance $= \dfrac{\Delta P}{\Delta \dot{V}}$

Figure 13.10 *(a) Volume and esophageal pressure trace during spontaneous breathing. The dynamic compliance is calculated by dividing the tidal volume ($\Delta \dot{V}$) by the pressure gradient between the beginning and end of inspiration (ΔP). (b) Flow, volume and pressure trace during tidal breathing. The total pulmonary resistance is calculated by dividing the pressure gradient between mid-inspiration and mid-expiration (ΔP) by the simultaneous flow difference (ΔV).*

CLINICAL AND RESEARCH APPLICATIONS

These techniques have been used extensively to assess the effects of pulmonary adaptation at birth and neonatal pulmonary pathology on lung function.[18] Unfortunately, they are less reliable when the lung disease is severe, particularly when accompanied by chest wall recession.[59] Under these circumstances, esophageal pressure measurements may underestimate the true mean pressure changes by as much as 50 percent. Attempts have been made to validate the measurements by comparing esophageal and mouth pressure swings during respiratory efforts against an obstructed external airway[73] and only accepting results when these are within 10 percent of each other.

Although this will identify some infants in whom the esophageal pressure device is reading inappropriately, a satisfactory correlation does not guarantee that the system is functioning well as respiratory efforts against an obstruction are likely to eliminate variations in pressure throughout the thoracic cavity.

Forced partial expiratory flow–volume loops (FPEFVL)

This technique has gained considerable popularity since it was introduced in 1982.[107] The infant's chest and abdomen (and often arms) are enclosed in an inflatable jacket of relatively low volume whose outer wall is relatively rigid (Figure 13.12). The jacket is connected to a pressure reservoir by a three-way tap and can be rapidly inflated with pressures of between 20 and 80 cmH$_2$O, inducing a rapid passive expiration. The expired flow and volume are measured using a face mask and pneumotachograph system. The technique involves measuring quiet tidal breathing while displaying tidal flow and tidal volume. At the top of a breath the jacket is inflated by the air within the pressure reservoir and the resultant expiratory flow–volume trace used for analysis. Although the peak expiratory flow can be measured, this is poorly reproducible. The measurement used most frequently has been the maximum flow at FRC (V_{max} FRC) determining the FRC from the previous breaths (Figure 13.13). The measurements are relatively reproducible in individual infants, although the scatter of results from healthy infants is very wide. One of the problems is that in the neonatal period, there is dynamic elevation of the FRC, that is, the infant commences to breathe in before the lung volume has fallen to the true FRC. If the single breath technique is used to correct for this (p. 116), more reproducible results can be obtained and the scatter of results from healthy control

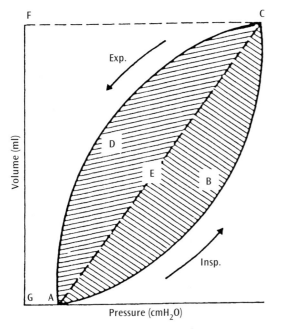

Figure 13.11 *Pressure–volume curve during spontaneous breathing. The area within the loop (ABCDA) represents the resistive work of breathing, the area to the left of the compliance line (AEC), the elastic work of breathing.*

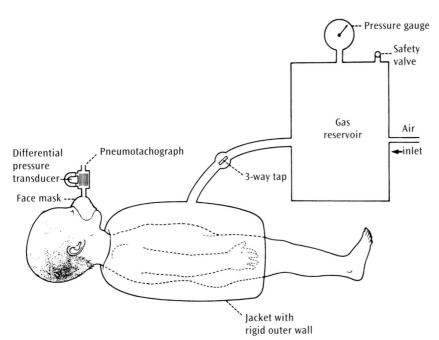

Figure 13.12 *Diagram of system for generating and measuring the forced partial expiratory flow–volume loop.*

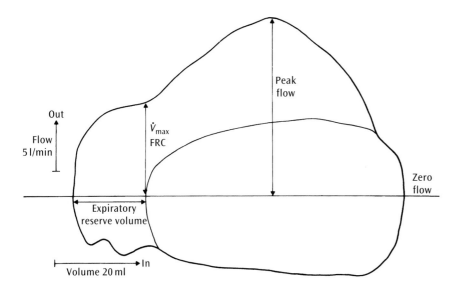

Figure 13.13 *Flow–volume curve during measurement of the forced partial expiratory flow–volume loop. The inner loop is generated during quiet breathing, the outer loop by the external squeeze.*

infants is also reduced.[48] It has been assumed that flow limitation has been achieved, that is, raising the jacket pressure further will not significantly increase V_{max} FRC. There remains, however, controversy as to the optimal jacket pressure, some investigators considering that a range of pressures should be used for each measurement.[61] More recent studies have found that pressures of $60\,cmH_2O$ are adequate at any rate in healthy infants.[89] There is also increasing evidence that inflating the jacket induces the Hering–Breuer deflationary reflex, that is, it stimulates the infant to make an inspiratory effort.[46,51] There remains some dispute whether the infant's inspiratory efforts do significantly alter the flow at FRC or only affect the flow trace beyond the FRC point. Recently, recommendations have been published by the ERS/ATS task force on infant respiratory function on the apparatus to be used and the most appropriate methods and analysis for this technique.[101]

THE RAISED VOLUME RAPID THORACOABDOMINAL COMPRESSION TECHNIQUE

A modification of the FEPFVL is now gaining popularity. In this modification, the infant's lung volume is raised close to total lung capacity (TLC) by pressurizing the face mask to $20–25\,cmH_2O$ immediately before inflating the jacket.[9,16,30] This technique allows the construction of time–volume and flow–volume curves, comparable with those produced in older children. The $FEV_{0.5}$ (forced expiratory volume in half a second) is used rather than the $FEV_{1.0}$ or $FEV_{0.75}$ as the next inspiration usually commences within 0.75 seconds.

An alternative approach only applicable to paralyzed and ventilated infants is to measure the expiratory flow–volume curve produced by connecting the airway opening to a negative pressure source.[76] The expiratory flow is recorded using a pneumotachograph. This technique has the advantage that the flow–volume curve cannot be distorted by the infant's inspiratory efforts, and so it results in higher V_{max} FRC values than the FEPFVL technique.

STATIC LUNG VOLUME MEASUREMENTS

None of the techniques described so far provides any indication of the size of the lung or whether the lung is hyperinflated. This is of considerable importance as lung volume and airway resistance measurements are inversely correlated. In addition, it is obviously important to be able to identify those babies who have small lungs, whether this be due to pulmonary hypoplasia or abnormalities of the chest wall such as asphyxiating thoracic dystrophy (p. 506). The techniques available for carrying out these measurements are dependent either on gas dilution or on plethysmography.

Gas dilution techniques

MEASUREMENTS IN SPONTANEOUSLY BREATHING BABIES

The standard technique has been to use a face mask/tap device to connect the infant to a circuit consisting of a spirometer, fan and CO_2 absorber (Figure 13.14).[14] The total circuit, including the spirometer, should have a volume which does not exceed the anticipated lung volume by more than 200–300 percent. Before commencing the measurement, a marker gas is added to the circuit. This gas has to be highly insoluble in water and readily diffusible; for these reasons, helium is often used. The concentration of the marker gas is measured using either a

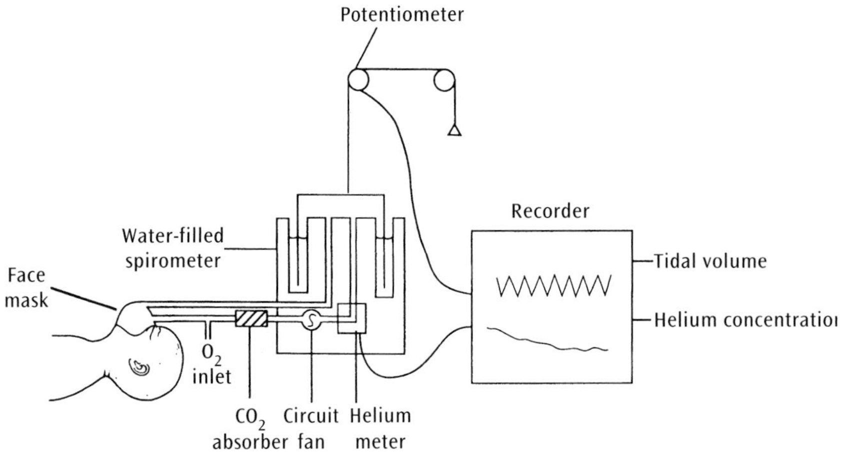

Potentiometer

Recorder

Face mask

Water-filled spirometer

O_2 inlet

CO_2 absorber | Circuit fan | Helium meter

Tidal volume

Helium concentration

Figure 13.14 *Diagram of the system used to measure the function residual capacity using the helium closed circuit technique.*

catherometer or mass spectrometer. The infant is then connected to the circuit by the turn of the tap, aiming to achieve this at end expiration. As, however, the infant's tidal volume will be measured by an electronic output from the spirometer, correction can subsequently be made if the infant is connected at a point above FRC. Oxygen then has to be added to the circuit to compensate for oxygen consumption, usually at a rate of 6ml/kg body weight.[50] Measurements are continued until the concentration of the tracer gas has stabilized, i.e. has been diluted into the volume consisting of the face mask and infant's respiratory tract. By knowing the initial volume and the fall in concentration of the tracer gas it is then possible to calculate the infant's FRC. This technique has proved easy to apply with a coefficient of variation of less than 4 percent.[14] An alternative approach has been to replace the circuit with a 'bag in a bottle device' (Figure 13.15).[2,79] The bag is then partially filled with a known volume of gas consisting of 25–30 percent oxygen and 5–10 percent of the tracer gas which is usually either helium or argon. The infant is connected to the system, again by turning a tap. If a pneumotachograph is mounted into the wall of the bottle, it is again possible to make corrections for commencing the test above FRC. Equilibration usually takes place within 30–40 seconds but small errors will be introduced as CO_2 will accumulate and oxygen taken up during the period of measurement. These errors are partly due to the fact that the respiratory quotient is likely to be α, 1 but, in addition, the CO_2 concentration in the bag rises more slowly than the corresponding fall in oxygen due to the buffering effect of the body for CO_2. The tracer gas is usually monitored, again using either a mass spectrometer or a catherometer.

EFFECTIVE PULMONARY BLOOD FLOW

One of the main advantages of the bag in the bottle technique is that it provides a means whereby effective pulmonary blood flow can be measured simultaneously. To

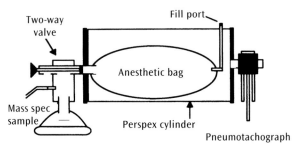

Two-way valve

Fill port

Anesthetic bag

Mass spec sample

Perspex cylinder

Pneumotachograph

Figure 13.15 *Diagram of the bag in the bottle system.*

do this, a second tracer gas, either freon or acetylene, is added to the system. These gases are highly soluble in water and so, unlike helium or argon, their concentrations will continue to fall due to conduction away from the lungs by the blood flow through the pulmonary capillaries. One approach is to measure the rate of disappearance of the argon or acetylene once equilibration has been achieved for the other marker gas (argon or helium). This may, however, introduce errors due to the recirculation of blood. An alternative is to express the end expiratory concentration of the soluble gas as a percentage of the insoluble marker gas on a breath-by-breath basis.[5] This will produce a straight line relationship when plotted semi-logarithmically. Computer programs are now available which allow rapid calculation of the results so that this is now a relatively simple technique to apply.

NITROGEN WASHOUT TECHNIQUE

Lung volume can also be measured by changing the inspired gas over to 100 percent at end expiration and sampling the expired gases using either a nitrogen meter or mass spectrometer. The procedure continues until the nitrogen concentration falls to 2 percent.[49,100] If the expired gases are collected in either a bag or spirometer, the amount of nitrogen washed from the lungs can be determined by measuring this volume and its nitrogen concentration. By knowing the pre-test and final nitrogen

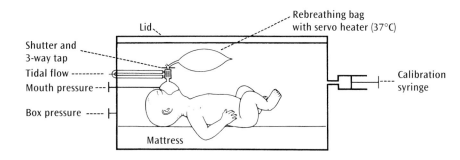

Figure 13.16 *Diagram of total body plethysmograph for measuring thoracic gas volume and airways resistance.*

concentration of the baby's lungs, it is then possible to calculate the FRC. This technique will become progressively less accurate at higher inspired oxygen concentrations, and is not practicable when the fraction of inspired oxygen (FiO_2) exceeds 0.6.

Measurement during ventilation

GAS DILUTION TECHNIQUES

It is obviously not possible to obtain measurements of lung volume of infants on ventilators using the spirometer circuit technique. It has, however, proved relatively easy to use the bag in the bottle method.[5,22,90] The technique is identical to that used for spontaneously breathing babies except that facilities must be made to ensure that, as the infant is connected to the bag in the bottle system, mechanical ventilation is continued to the bottle, rather than to the infant. Thus, for 30–40 seconds the infant will be ventilated using the gases contained within the bag. Under these circumstances it will be necessary to ensure that the oxygen concentration within the bag is at least as high as that provided by the ventilator so that the infant will not become desaturated. One potential problem is any leak around the endotracheal tube. This may be prevented by applying gentle pressure with two fingers over the trachea, but it is still necessary to examine the gas concentration traces carefully subsequently for evidence of leak, for example, failure to reach equilibration within 20–30 seconds. It has also proved possible to add either freon or acetylene to the bag in the bottle device so that effective pulmonary blood flow can be measured simultaneously using the techniques described above.[5,15]

NITROGEN WASHOUT

Techniques have also been devised whereby the nitrogen washout technique can be applied to infants receiving ventilatory support.[100] The technique is essentially the same as that described above whereby the inspired gas is changed over to 100 percent and the expired gases collected until the end tidal nitrogen level is less than 2 percent. Alternatively the nitrogen in the expiratory

limb can be integrated against flow in order to determine the amount of nitrogen washed out.

PLETHYSMOGRAPHIC METHOD[24,25]

For these measurements the baby must be nursed within an airtight, preferably transparent container (Figure 13.16). Facilities must be available for holding a face mask incorporating a shutter system and a pneumotachograph firmly, but gently, over the infant's mouth and nose in order to achieve an airtight seal.[85] The pressure within the face mask proximal to the shutter and the pressure within the chamber of the plethysmograph are monitored continuously using pressure transducers of appropriate sensitivity. Measurements are obtained by closing the shutter for three to four breaths. Usually the infant will continue to make regular respiratory efforts without waking up. The change in volume of the respiratory system due to compression and decompression of the alveolar gas is calculated from the changes in pressure within the plethysmograph chamber, which can be calibrated to read volume by measuring the pressure changes within the chamber during periods in which air is injected into and withdrawn from the chamber with a syringe. These injections should be carried out at approximately the same rate as the infant's respiratory effort to avoid errors due to the adiabatic effect (see above). During the period of occlusion, the pressure within the respiratory system can be measured from pressure changes in the face mask as there is essentially no flow of air in the airways. From these two measurements the total volume of the respiratory system plus the volume within the face mask and tube leading to the face mask pressure transducer can be calculated according to Boyle's law using the formula $V = P_A \times \Delta V / \Delta P_M$ where V is the volume to be measured, P_A is atmospheric pressure minus water vapor pressure (47 mmHg), ΔV is the change in volume of the thorax during breathing movements against the obstruction and ΔP_M is the simultaneous change in pressure within the face mask. Measurements made at end expiration often overestimate the true lung volume.[13] This error appears to arise as a result of small airway closure in babies with airways obstruction so that the pressure swings within the face mask underestimate the true intrathoracic pressure changes. This error can be limited by closing the shutter instead at full inspiration and then subtracting both the tidal volume and the dead space of the face mask and tubing to obtain a more accurate FRC. It is now possible to use computer software to carry out the analysis. This has the advantage that any drift in the pressure signals can be compensated for.[110]

CLINICAL AND RESEARCH APPLICATIONS

The techniques can be useful to identify those infants with a raised respiratory rate who have a degree of pulmonary hypoplasia[3] and for documenting progress in those who have had congenital abnormalities such as diaphragmatic hernia or cystic adenomatoid malformations. The research applications of these measurements have been very considerable. Plethysmographic measurements have been made to investigate the adaptation of the lung in the immediate neonatal period, showing that babies born vaginally tend to establish a stable FRC within 2–3 hours while those who have been born by cesarean section take up to 48 hours.[14,58] This delay in reaching a normal degree of aeration is due to delay in fluid clearance from the lung.

Measurements made by gas dilution techniques tend to be significantly lower than those determined by plethysmography.[69,117] The reasons for this are probably due to poor ventilation distribution, exacerbated in the immediate neonatal period by fluid within the airways.[14] In healthy infants, the ratio between the FRC by gas dilution and FRC by plethysmography is approximately 0.93 after the first day after birth.[117] Measurements obtained during respiratory support for RDS have shown that there is a very striking reduction in lung volume, often as low as 5–7 ml/kg body weight.[5,90] These techniques have allowed us to explore the mechanism of action of treatments such as surfactant therapy and demonstrated that the improvements in blood gases following surfactant are accompanied by the FRC often increasing by up to 100 percent.[5] Studies have also shown that there is an improvement in effective pulmonary blood flow, indicating a reduction in the right-to-left shunt through poorly or unventilated areas.[71] Lung volume measurements have also provided useful information on the effects of surgical intervention on infants with diaphragmatic hernias and congenital lung cysts.[53]

MEASUREMENT OF AIRWAYS RESISTANCE

Total body plethysmography allows us to obtain a measurement of the airways resistance as distinct from total pulmonary or total respiratory resistance.[13,85] Although when breathing in the total body plethysmograph, the infant's tidal volume is taken from and returns to the air within the chamber, pressure changes do occur during the respiratory cycle. These swings are due to changes in alveolar pressure, which fall below atmospheric on inspiration, rising to above atmospheric during expiration. It is possible to measure these pressure swings by knowing the lung volume and calibrating the chamber pressure swings against a syringe as described above. Resistance is calculated by dividing these pressure changes by the simultaneous flow changes as measured by the pneumotachograph. The formula used for the calculation is $R_{aw} = \Delta P_M / \Delta V_1 \times \Delta V_2 / \Delta V$, where ΔP_M and ΔV_1 are changes in mouth pressure and thoracic volume during periods of occlusion and ΔV_2 and ΔV are derived from the changes in chamber pressure and simultaneous flow during spontaneous breathing. It is necessary to correct these values for the dead space of the equipment and also to subtract the resistance of the face mask and pneumotachograph. Computer software is now used to calculate the resistance from the thoracic gas volume (TGV) and the plethysmograph pressure and tidal flow loops. High digital sampling rates permit the construction of 'best-fit' regression lines. A recent study has shown that optimal results are obtained if this technique is used over the first 50 percent of the rise portion of the inspiratory flow, although any part of the inspiratory or expiratory flow trace can be selected.[110]

Clinical and research applications

Plethysmographic measurements of airways resistance can be used to assess the response to therapy in individual babies although, particularly in the neonatal period, this information can more easily be obtained using esophageal balloons or by single breath lung mechanics. Airways resistance measurements have been used extensively in evaluating the effects of therapy. It is also possible to compensate for the changes in resistance values produced by alteration in the resting FRC. This is achieved by calculating the reciprocal of the resistance (the conductance) and dividing this by the lung volume to give the specific conductance. This measurement in health remains virtually constant throughout life at 0.2–0.4.

ASSESSMENT OF RESPIRATORY MUSCLE FUNCTION

Diaphragm function

There are a number of techniques which can be used to assess diaphragmatic function in neonates including pressure measurements, diaphragmatic movements, phrenic nerve stimulation, EMG recording and thoracoabdominal motion.

Real-time ultrasonography has been used to record axial movement of the right hemidiaphragm.[20,56] Although it may be of clinical value in assessing diaphragm, rib cage or abdominal wall defects, it is limited in that it does not provide a quantitative measure of diaphragmatic function. In hemidiaphragm paralysis, an elevated diaphragm may be visible on chest radiography; however, with substantial bilateral diaphragm weakness the chest radiograph may show elevated hemidiaphragms which can appear relatively normal.[57] Similarly, a cephalad movement of the diaphragm is commonly observed on fluoroscopy during inspiratory maneuvers, but this test has the disadvantages of a significant false-positive rate[4] and also provides little information concerning the degree of diaphragm weakness. Also, accurate diagnosis using real-time ultrasound and fluoroscopy can often be difficult when patients are receiving continuous positive pressure ventilation.[44,67] Transcutaneous electrical stimulation of the phrenic nerve during fluoroscopy or real-time ultrasound (sonoscopy) of the diaphragm allows more precise functional evaluation than fluoroscopy and/or sonoscopy alone.[68]

EMG activity of the diaphragm can be recorded via surface and/or esophageal electrodes. However, due to the insertion of the diaphragm, the signal from surface electrodes can be contaminated by the EMG activity of other muscles. Analysis of the EMG power spectrum allows a number of variables to be derived, such as peak amplitude,[64,78] high:low frequency ratio[64,78] and centroid frequency[17] and it has been suggested that a fall in high frequency and a rise in low-frequency power is associated with diaphragmatic fatigue in preterm infants.[64,78] EMG provides a measure of the electrical activity but not force production by the diaphragm and there is evidence to suggest that power spectrum analysis may not be a reliable measure of low-frequency muscle fatigue.[77] EMG activity of the intercostal[64] and abdominal muscles has also been recorded in infants.[83] Clinically, recording respiratory muscle EMG activity is particularly useful during a sleep study.[82]

Uncalibrated respiratory inductive plethysmography has been used to indirectly evaluate diaphragm function. The uncalibrated signals from the ribcage and abdomen are used to provide a measure of the relative magnitude and timing of thoracic and abdominal movement. The phase angle derived from an x-y plot of the ribcage versus abdominal movements gives an index of thoraco-abdominal asynchrony.[6,7,41,99] Changes in thoracoabdominal asynchrony reflect the changes in lung mechanics induced by bronchodilators and hence may be a useful indicator of respiratory muscle function in lung disease.[6] Procedures which are thought to reduce the work of breathing such as prone positioning,[116] continuous positive airway pressure[62] and abdominal loading,[34] all improve thoracoabdominal synchrony. As with EMG recordings, inductive plethysmography only gives an indirect measure of global respiratory muscle function and will not provide a direct measure of diaphragm force production.

Scott et al.[95] has used a technique involving measurements of transdiaphragmatic pressure (P_{di}) to assess diaphragmatic function in infants. They measured maximal P_{di} during crying in 38 infants ranging from 8 to 21 months postconceptional age. There was a significant positive correlation between maximal P_{di} and postconceptional age, suggesting a developmental pattern of increasing maximal transdiaphragmatic pressure in infants during crying. Chest wall distortion, however, can influence esophageal pressure measurement[59] and the accuracy should be checked by comparison to mouth pressure during occlusion.[12]

Phrenic nerve stimulation in the neck allows diaphragm function to be assessed directly.[86] Electrical stimulation of the phrenic nerves is generally performed transcutaneously using bipolar electrodes. Precise electrode placement is essential if supramaximal stimulation is to be achieved, which often requires repeated stimulations that are painful due to the high stimulus voltage needed to overcome the resistance of the skin. This has limited the extent to which this technique is applied in clinical studies. Electrical stimulation has been used primarily to measure phrenic nerve latency.[52,75,93,94] Values for normal phrenic nerve latency are 6–8 ms at birth, increasing to about 5 ms at 1 year of age, despite an increase in conduction distance.[52] The increase in nerve conduction velocity is dependent on the physical properties of the nerve, such that with growth the size of the nerve fibers and the degree of myelination increases. The overall variability of the phrenic nerve latency with transcutaneous electrical stimulation is approximately ±1 ms; differences greater than this between measurements are likely to reflect a real change in phrenic nerve function.[94]

Many of the problems associated with electrical stimulation can be overcome by magnetic stimulation. Discharging a magnetic coil creates a pulsed magnetic field, which causes current to flow in the nerve and the muscle to contract.[11] Using a 90 mm double, circular stimulating coil placed over the phrenic nerves on the anterolateral aspect of the neck, supramaximal unilateral and bilateral phrenic nerve stimulation can be achieved in infants and children (Figure 13.17).[87,88] Diaphragm force is assessed as transdiaphragmatic pressure obtained from balloons positioned in the mid-esophagus and stomach (Figure 13.18). Magnetic stimulation provides an ideal, effort-independent technique to assess diaphragm contractility in neonates and children as it is both technically easy to perform and painless. Painful stimuli would arouse the patient and possibly prevent reproducible measurements of TwP_{di} due to twitch potentiation from crying. As the stimulating currents are produced in situ, their intensities can be very low, possibly explaining the absence of pain when using magnetic stimulation.[11] Magnetic stimulation is able to stimulate underlying nervous tissue without contact with or pressure on the overlying skin and could therefore be useful

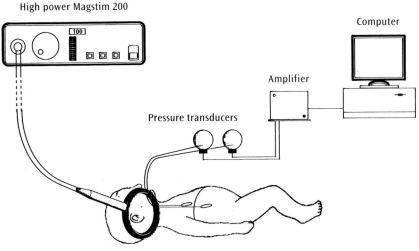

High power Magstim 200

Computer

Pressure transducers

Amplifier

90 mm Double circular coil

Figure 13.17 *Diagrammatic representation of the apparatus used with the magnetic coil positioned for unilateral magnetic stimulation of the phrenic nerve.*

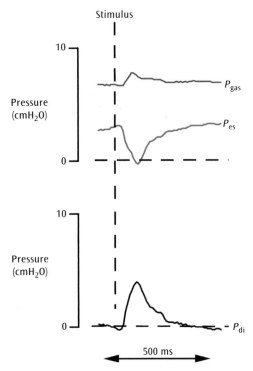

Figure 13.18 *Representative diaphragm force response following unilateral anterior magnetic phrenic nerve stimulation. Esophageal and gastric pressure are shown in the upper trace and the resulting transdiaphragmatic pressure has been transposed and shown in the lower trace.*

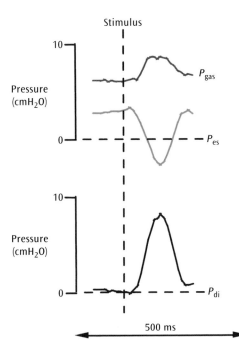

Figure 13.19 *Representative diaphragm force response following bilateral anterior magnetic phrenic nerve stimulation. Esophageal and gastric pressure are shown in the upper trace and the resulting transdiaphragmatic pressure has been transposed and shown in the lower trace.*

when contact is painful or access is limited, for example, due to vascular catheters. Furthermore, the stimulating coils are easy to position and compared to electrical stimulation require less precise positioning. The technique can be used to stimulate just one (Figure 13.18) or both phrenic nerves simultaneously (Figure 13.19). The stimulus does not irritate the skin and it is non-thermal. To date no side-effects of single, repeated magnetic stimulation, whether used transcortically or peripherally, have been reported.[11,29]

Measurement of maximal static inspiratory (P_{IMAX}) and expiratory (P_{EMAX}) pressure

Measurement of P_{IMAX} and P_{EMAX} obtained by occluding the airway during crying provides a good, reproducible estimate of the respiratory muscle strength in both healthy infants[97] and in infants with muscle weakness.[98] In contrast to Shardonofsky et al.,[97] who suggested that the measurement was independent of age, sex and anthropometrics, Dimitriou et al.[23] demonstrated that both P_{IMAX} and P_{EMAX} were significantly higher in term than in preterm infants and positively correlated with increasing gestational and postconceptional age. Maturation at the time of measurement should therefore be taken into account when interpreting the results of tests of respiratory muscle strength.

REFERENCES

1 Abraham, N.G., Stebbens, V.A., Samuels, M.P., Southall, D.P. (1990) Investigation of cyanotic/apneic episodes and sleep related upper airway obstruction by long term non-invasive bedside recordings. *Pediatric Pulmonology* **8**, 259–262.

2 Aiton, N.R., Fox, G.F., Alexander, J. et al. (1996) The influence of sleeping position on functional residual capacity and effective pulmonary blood flow in healthy neonates. *Pediatric Pulmonology* **22**, 342–347.

3 Aiton, N.R., Fox, G.F., Hannam, S. et al. (1996) Pulmonary hypoplasia presenting as persistent tachypnoea in the first few months of life. *British Medical Journal* **312**, 1149–1150.

4 Alexander, C. (1966) Diaphragm movements and the diagnosis of diaphragmatic paralysis. *Clinical Radiology* **17**, 79–83.

5 Alexander, J., Milner, A.D. (1995) Lung volume and pulmonary blood flow measurements following exogenous surfactant. *European Journal of Pediatrics* **154**, 392–397.

6 Allen, J.L., Wolfson, M.R., McDowell, K., Shaffer, T.H. (1990) Thoracoabdominal asynchrony in infants with airflow obstruction. *American Review of Respiratory Disease* **141**, 337–342.

7 Allen, J.L., Greenspan, J.S., Deoras, K.S. et al. (1991) Interaction between chest wall motion and lung mechanics in normal infants and infants with bronchopulmonary dysplasia. *Pediatric Pulmonology* **11**, 37–43.

8 Allison, R.D., Holmes, E.L., Nyboer, J. (1964) Volumetric dynamics of respiration as measured by electrical impedance plethysmography. *Journal of Applied Physiology* **19**, 166–173.

9 Anonymous. (2000) The raised volume rapid thoracoabdominal compression technique. The Joint American Thoracic Society/European Respiratory Society Working Group on Infant Lung Function. *American Journal of Respiratory and Critical Care Medicine* **161**, 1760–1762.

10 Asher, M.I., Coates, A.L., Collinge, J.M., Milic-Emili, J. (1982) Management of esophageal pressure in neonates. *Journal of Applied Physiology* **52**, 491–494.

11 Barker, A., Freeston, I., Jalinous, R., Jarrett, J. (1987) Magnetic stimulation of the human brain and peripheral nervous system: an introduction and the results of an initial clinical evaluation. *Neurosurgery* **20**, 100–109.

12 Beardsmore, C., Helms, P., Stocks, J. et al. (1980) Improved esophageal balloon technique for use in infants. *Journal of Applied Physiology* **49**, 735–742.

13 Beardsmore, C.S., Stocks, J., Silverman, M. (1982) Problems in the measurement of thoracic gas volume in infancy. *Journal of Applied Physiology* **52**, 995–999.

14 Boon, A.W., Ward-McQuaid, J.M.C., Milner, A.D., Hopkin, I.E. (1981) Thoracic gas volume, helium functional residual capacity and airtrapping in the first six hours of life. The effect of oxygen administration. *Early Human Development* **5**, 157–166.

15 Bose, C.L., Lawson, E.E., Green, A. et al. (1986) Measurement of cardiopulmonary function in ventilated neonates with respiratory distress syndrome using rebreathing methodology. *Pediatric Research* **20**, 316–320.

16 Castile, R.G., Filbrun, D., Flucke, R. et al. (2000) Adult-type pulmonary function tests in infants without respiratory distress. *Pediatric Pulmonology* **30**, 215–227.

17 Chambille, B., Vardon, G., Monrigal, J.P. et al. (1989) Technique of on-line analysis of diaphragmatic electromyogram activity in the newborn. *European Respiratory Journal* **2**, 883–886.

18 Cohn, M.A., Wagson, H., Beisshant, R. et al. (1978) A Transducer for Non-invasive Monitoring of Respiration. International Symposium on Ambulatory Monitoring. New York/London: Academic Press.

19 Cross, K.W. (1949) The respiratory rate and ventilation in the newborn baby. *Journal of Applied Physiology* **109**, 459–473.

20 Devlieger, H., Daniels, H., Marchal, G. et al. (1991) The diaphragm of the newborn infant: anatomical and ultrasonographic studies. *Journal of Developmental Physiology* **16**, 321–329.

21 Dezateux, C.A., Stocks, J., Dundas, I. et al. (1994) The relationship between t_{PTEF}:t_E and specific airway conductance in infancy. *Pediatric Pulmonology* **18**, 299–307.

22 Dimitriou, G., Greenough, A. (1995) Measurement of lung volume and optimal oxygenation during high frequency oscillation. *Archives of Disease in Childhood Fetal and Neonatal Edition* **72**, F180–F183.

23 Dimitriou, G., Greenough, A., Dyke, H., Rafferty, G.F. (2000) Maximal airway pressures during crying in healthy preterm and term infants. *Early Human Development* **57**, 149–156.

24 DuBois, A.B., Botelho, S.Y., Bedell, B.N. et al. (1956) A rapid plethysmographic method for measuring thoracic gas volume: a comparison with a nitrogen washout method for measuring functional residual capacity in normal subjects. *Journal of Clinical Investigation* **35**, 322–326.

25 DuBois, A.B., Botelho, S.Y., Comroe, J.H. (1956) A new method for measuring airway resistance in man using a body plethysmograph: values in normal subjects and in patients with respiratory disease. *Journal of Clinical Investigation* **35**, 327–332.

26 Duffty, P., Spriet, L., Bryan, M.H., Bryan, A.C. (1981) Respiratory induction plethysmography (Respitrace): an evaluation of its use in the infant. *American Review of Respiratory Disease* **123**, 542–546.

27 Dundas, I., Dezateux, C.A., Fletcher, M.E. et al. (1995) Comparison of single-breath and plethysmographic measurements of resistance in infancy. *American Journal of Respiratory and Critical Care Medicine* **151**, 1451–1458.

28 England, S.J. (1988) Current techniques for assessing pulmonary function in the newborn and infant: advantages and limitations. *Pediatric Pulmonology* **4**, 48–53.

29 Eyre, J.A., Flecknell, P.A., Kenyon, B.R. et al. (1990) Acute effects of electromagnetic stimulation of the brain on cortical activity, cortical blood flow, blood pressure and heart rate in the cat: an evaluation of safety. *Journal of Neurology, Neurosurgery and Psychiatry* **53**, 507–513.

30 Feher, A., Castile, R., Kilsing, J. et al. (1996) Flow limitation in normal infants: a new method for forced expiratory maneuvers from raised lung volumes. *Journal of Applied Physiology* **80**, 2019–2025.

31 Field, D., Milner, A.D., Hopkin, I.E. (1984) High and conventional rates of positive pressure ventilation. *Archives of Disease in Childhood* **59**, 1151–1154.

32 Field, D., Milner, A.D., Hopkin, I.E. (1985) Effects of positive end expiratory pressure during ventilation of the preterm infant. *Archives of Disease in Childhood* **60**, 843–847.

33 Finucane, K.E., Egan, B.A., Dawson, S.V. (1972) Linearity and frequency response of pneumotachographs. *Journal of Applied Physiology* **32**, 121–126.

34 Fleming, P.J., Muller, N.L., Bryan, H., Bryan, A.C. (1979) The effects of abdominal loading on rib cage distortion in premature infants. *Pediatrics* **64**, 425–428.

35 Fleming, P.J., Levine, M.R., Long, A.M., Cleave, J.P. (1988) Postneonatal development of respiratory oscillators. *Annals of the New York Academy of Sciences* **533**, 305–313.

36 Frey, U., Stocks, J., Coates, A. *et al.* (2000) Specifications for equipment used for infant pulmonary function testing. ERS/ATS Task Force on Standards for Infant Respiratory Function Testing. European Respiratory Society/American Thoracic Society. *European Respiratory Journal* **16**, 731–740.

37 Frey, U., Stocks, J., Sly, P., Bates, J. (2000) Specification for signal processing and data handling used for infant pulmonary function testing. ERS/ATS Task Force on Standards for Infant Respiratory Function Testing. European Respiratory Society/American Thoracic Society. *European Respiratory Journal* **16**, 1016–1022.

38 Gagliardi, L., Rusconi, F., Aston, H., Silverman, M. (1996) Occlusion maneuver to detect the relative contribution of the rib cage and abdomen to tidal volume using respiratory inductive plethysmography in infants. *Pediatric Pulmonology* **21**, 132–137.

39 Gappa, M., Colin, A.A., Goetz, I., Stocks, J. (2001) ERS/ATS Task Force on Standards for Infant Respiratory Function Testing. European Respiratory Society/American Thoracic Society. Passive respiratory mechanics: the occlusion techniques. *European Respiratory Journal* **17**, 141–148.

40 Godal, A., Belenky, D.A., Standaert, T.A. *et al.* (1976) Application of the hot-wire anemometer to respiratory measurements in small animals. *Journal of Applied Physiology* **40**, 275–277.

41 Goldman, M.D., Pagani, M., Trang, H.T. *et al.* (1993) Asynchronous chest wall movements during non-rapid eye movement and rapid eye movement sleep in children with bronchopulmonary dysplasia. *American Review of Respiratory Diseases* **147**, 1175–1184.

42 Greenough, A., Naik, S., Itakura, Y. *et al.* (1998) Perinatal lung function measurements and prediction of respiratory problems in infancy. *Physiological Measurement* **19**, 421–426.

43 Grenvik, A., Hedstrand, U., Sjogren, H. (1966) Problems in pneumotachography. *Acta Anaesthesiologica Scandinavica* **10**, 147–155.

44 Gurakar, A., Hassanein, T., van Thiel, D.H. (1995) Right diaphragmatic paralysis following orthotopic liver transplantation. *Journal of the Oklahoma State Medical Association* **88**, 149–153.

45 Guslits, B.G., Wilkie, R.A., England, S.J., Bryan, A.C. (1987) Comparison of methods of measurement of compliance of the respiratory system in children. *American Review of Respiratory Disease* **136**, 727–729.

46 Hannam, S., Ingram, D.M., Rabe-Hesketh, S., Milner, A.D. (2001) Characterisation of the Hering-Breuer deflation reflex in the human neonate. *Respiration Physiology* **124**, 51–64.

47 Helms, P., Taylor, B.W., Milner, A.D., Hatch, D.J. (1982) Critical assessment of jacket plethysmograph for use in young children. *Journal of Applied Physiology* **52**, 267–273.

48 Henschen, M., Stocks, J. (1999) Asessment of airway function using partial expiratory flow–volume curves. *American Journal of Respiratory and Critical Care Medicine* **159**, 480–486.

49 Hentschel, R., Suska, A., Volbracht, A. *et al.* (1997) Modification of the open circuit N2 washout technique for measurement of functional residual capacity in premature infants. *Pediatric Pulmonology* **23**, 434–441.

50 Hey, E.N. (1969) The relation between environmental temperature and oxygen consumption in the newborn baby. *Journal of Physiology* **200**, 589–603.

51 Hoskyns, E.W., Milner, A.D., Hopkins, I.E. (1987) Validity of forced expiration volume loops in neonates. *Archives of Disease in Childhood* **62**, 895–900.

52 Imai, T., Shizukawa, H., Imaizumi, H. *et al.* (2000) Phrenic nerve conduction in infancy and early childhood. *Muscle and Nerve* **23**, 915–918.

53 Kavvadia, V., Greenough, A., Laubscher, B. *et al.* (1997) Perioperative assessment of respiratory compliance and lung volume in infants with congenital diaphragmatic hernia: prediction of outcome. *Journal of Pediatric Surgery* **32**, 1665–1669.

54 Kosch, P.C., Stark, A.R. (1984) Dynamic maintenance of end-expiratory lung volume in full-term infants. *Journal of Applied Physiology* **57**, 1126–1133.

55 Krieger, I. (1963) Studies on mechanics of respiration in infancy. *American Journal of Diseases of Children* **105**, 439–448.

56 Laing, I.A., Teele, R.L., Stark, A.R. (1988) Diaphragmatic movements in newborn infants. *Journal of Pediatrics* **112**, 638–643.

57 Laroche, C.M., Carroll, N., Moxham, J., Green, M. (1988) Clinical significance of severe isolated diaphragm weakness. *American Review of Respiratory Disease* **138**, 862–866.

58 Lee, S., Hassan, A., Ingram, D., Milner, A.D. (1999) Effects of different modes of delivery on lung volumes of newborn infants. *Pediatric Pulmonology* **27**, 318–321.

59 LeSouef, P.N., Lopes, J.M., England, S.J. *et al.* (1983) Influence of chest wall distortion on esophageal pressure. *Journal of Applied Physiology* **55**, 353–358.

60 LeSouef, P.N., England, S.J., Bryan, A.C. (1984) Passive respiratory mechanics in newborns and children. *American Review of Respiratory Disease* **129**, 552–556.

61 LeSouef, P.N., Hughes, D.M., Landau, L.I. (1986) Effect of compression pressure on forced expiratory flow in infants. *Journal of Applied Physiology* **61**, 1639–1646.

62 Locke, R., Greenspan, J.S., Shaffer, T.H. *et al.* (1991) Effect of nasal CPAP on thoracoabdominal motion in neonates with respiratory insufficiency. *Pediatric Pulmonology* **11**, 259–264.

63 Lodrup Carlsen, K.C., Samuelsen, S.O., Botten, G., Calsen, K.H. (1993) *Lung Function in 448 Healthy Norwegian Infants.* Oslo: European Paediatric Respiratory Society.

64 Lopes, J.M., Muller, N.L., Bryan, M.H., Bryan, A.C. (1981) Synergistic behavior of inspiratory muscles after diaphragmatic fatigue in the newborn. *Journal of Applied Physiology* **51**, 547–551.

65 Manczur, T., Greenough, A., Rafferty, G.F. *et al.* (2000) Measurement of respiratory mechanics in the pediatric intensive care unit: a comparison of techniques during pressure- and volume-limited ventilation. *Pediatric Pulmonology* **30**, 265–267.

66 Martinez, F.D., Morgan, W.J., Wright, A.L. *et al.* (1988) Diminished lung function as a predisposing factor for wheezing respiratory illness in infants. *New England Journal of Medicine* **319**, 1112–1117.

67 McAlister, V.C., Grant, D.R., Roy, A. *et al.* (1993) Right phrenic nerve injury in orthotopic liver transplantation. *Transplantation* **55**, 826–830.

68 McCauley, R.G., Labib, K.B. (1984) Diaphragmatic paralysis evaluated by phrenic nerve stimulation during fluoroscopy or real-time ultrasound. *Radiology* **153**, 33–36.

69 McCoy, K.S., Castile, R.G., Allen, E.D. *et al.* (1995) Functional residual capacity (FRC) measurements by plethysmography and helium dilution in normal infants. *Pediatric Pulmonology* **19**, 282–290.

70 Milner, A.D. (1990) Lung function testing in infancy: personal experience. *Archives of Disease in Childhood* **65**, 548–552.

71 Milner, A.D. (1993) How does exogenous surfactant work? *Archives of Disease in Childhood* **68**, 253–254.

72 Milner, A.D., Saunders, R.A. (1977) Pressure and volume changes during the first breath of human neonates. *Archives of Disease in Childhood* **52**, 918–924.

73 Milner, A.D., Saunders, R.A., Hopkin, I.E. (1978) Relationship of intra-oesophageal pressure to mouth pressure during the measurement of thoracic gas volume in the newborn. *Biology of the Neonate* **33**, 314–319.

74 Milner, A.D., Marsh, M.J., Ingram, D.M. *et al.* (1999) Effects of smoking in pregnancy on neonatal lung function. *Archives of Disease in Childhood Fetal and Neonatal Edition* **80**, F8–F14.

75 Moosa, A. (1981) Phrenic nerve conduction in children. *Developmental Medicine and Child Neurology* **23**, 434–448.

76 Mortola, J.P., Saetta, M. (1987) Measurements of respiratory mechanics in the newborn: a simple approach. *Pediatric Pulmonology* **3**, 123–130.

77 Moxham, J., Edwards, R.H., Aubier, M. *et al.* (1982) Changes in EMG power spectrum (high-to-low ratio) with force fatigue in humans. *Journal of Applied Physiology* **53**, 1094–1099.

78 Muller, N., Gulston, G., Cade, D. *et al.* (1979) Diaphragmatic muscle fatigue in the newborn. *Journal of Applied Physiology* **46**, 688–695.

79 Nelson, N.M., Prod'hom, S., Cherry, R.B. *et al.* (1963) Pulmonary function in the newborn infant. V. Trapped gas in the normal infant's lung. *Journal of Clinical Investigation* **42**, 1850–1857.

80 Olinsky, A., Bryan, A.C., Bryan, M.H. (1976) A simple method of measuring total respiratory system compliance in newborn infants. *South African Medical Journal* **50**, 128–130.

81 Poole, K.A., Thompson, J.R., Hallinan, H.M., Beardsmore, C.S. (2000) Respiratory inductance plethysmography in healthy infants: a comparison of three calibration methods. *European Respiratory Journal* **16**, 1084–1090.

82 Praud, J.P., D'Allest, A.M., Nedelcoux, H. *et al.* (1989) Sleep-related abdominal muscle behavior during partial or complete obstructed breathing in prepubertal children. *Pediatric Research* **26**, 347–350.

83 Praud, J.P., Egreteau, L., Benlabed, M. *et al.* (1991) Abdominal muscle activity during CO_2 rebreathing in sleeping neonates. *Journal of Applied Physiology* **70**, 1344–1350.

84 Prechtl, H.V. (1974) The behavioral status of the newborn infant (a review). *Brain Research* **76**, 185–212.

85 Radford, M. (1974) Measurement of airway resistance and thoracic gas volume in infancy. *Archives of Disease in Childhood* **49**, 611–615.

86 Rafferty, G.F., Greenough, A., Dimitriou, G. *et al.* (1999) Assessment of neonatal diaphragmatic paralysis using magnetic phrenic nerve stimulation. *Pediatric Pulmonology* **27**, 224–226.

87 Rafferty, G.F., Greenough, A., Dimitriou, G. *et al.* (2000) Assessment of neonatal diaphragm function using magnetic stimulation of the phrenic nerves. *American Journal of Respiratory and Critical Care Medicine* **162**, 2337–2340.

88 Rafferty, G.F., Greenough, A., Manczur, T.I. *et al.* (in press) Magnetic phrenic nerve stimulation to assess diaphragm function in children following liver transplantation. *Pediatric Critical Care Medicine* (in press).

89 Ratjen, F., Grasemann, H., Wolstein, R., Wiesemann, H.G. (1998) Isovolume pressure/flow curves of rapid thoracoabdominal compressions in infants without respiratory disease. *Pediatric Pulmonology* **26**, 197–203.

90 Richardson, P., Bose, C.L., Carlstrom, J.R. (1986) The functional residual capacity of infants with respiratory distress syndrome. *Acta Paediatrica Scandinavica* **75**, 267–271.

91 Rigatto, H., Brady, J.B., Verduzco, R.T. (1975) Chemoreceptor reflexes in preterm infants I. The effect of gestational and postnatal age on the ventilatory response to inhalation of 100% and 15% oxygen. *Pediatrics* **55**, 604–613.

92 Rigatto, H., Brady, J.B., Verduzco, R.T. (1975) Chemoreceptor reflexes in preterm infants II. Effect of gestation and postnatal age on the ventilatory response to inhaled carbon dioxide. *Pediatrics* **55**, 614–628.

93 Ross Russell, R.I., Helps, B.A., Dicks Mireaux, C.M., Helms, P.J. (1993) Early assessment of diaphragmatic dysfunction in children in the ITU: chest radiology and phrenic nerve stimulation. *European Respiratory Journal* **6**, 1336–1339.

94 Ross Russell, R.I., Helps, B.A., Elliot, M.J., Helms, P.J. (1993) Phrenic nerve stimulation at the bedside in children equipment and validation. *European Journal of Pediatrics* **6**, 1332–1335.

95 Scott, C.B., Nickerson, B.G., Sargent, C.W. *et al.* (1983) Developmental pattern of maximal transdiaphragmatic pressure in infants during crying. *Pediatric Research* **17**, 707–709.

96 Seddon, P.C., Davis, G.M., Coates, A.L. (1996) Do tidal expiratory flow patterns reflect lung mechanics in infants? *American Journal of Respiratory and Critical Care Medicine* **153**, 1248–1252.

97 Shardonofsky, F.R., Perez-Chada, D., Carmuega, E., Milic-Emili, J. (1989) Airway pressures during crying in healthy infants. *Pediatric Pulmonology* **6**, 14–18.

98 Shardonofsky, F.R., Perez-Chada, D., Milic-Emili, J. (1991) Airway pressures during crying: an index of respiratory muscle strength in infants with neuromuscular disease. *Pediatric Pulmonology* **10**, 172–177.

99 Sivan, Y., Deakers, T.W., Newth, C.J.L. (1990) Thoracoabdominal asynchrony in acute upper airway obstruction in small children. *American Review of Respiratory Disease* **142**, 540–544.

100 Sjoqvist, B.A., Sandberg, K., Hjalmars, W.O., Olsson, T. (1983) Assessment of lung volumes in newborn infants by computer assisted plethysmographic N2 washout methods. Goteborg, Sweden: Laboratory of Medical Electronics, Chambers University of Technology, 4:83.

101 Sly, P.D., Tepper, R., Henschen, M. *et al.* (2000) Tidal forced expirations. ERS/ATS Task Force on Standards for Infant Respiratory Function Testing. European Respiratory Society/American Thoracic Society. *European Respiratory Journal* **16**, 741–748.

102 Stick, S.M., Buiton, P.R., Gurrin, L. *et al.* (1996) Effects of maternal smoking during pregnancy and a family history of asthma on respiratory function in newborn infants. *Lancet* **348**, 1060–1064.

103 Stokes, G.M., Hodges, I.G.C., Henry, R.L. *et al.* (1983) Nebulised therapy in acute severe bronchiolitis in infancy. *Archives of Disease in Childhood* **58**, 279–283.

104 Stokes, G.M., Milner, A.D., Upton, C.J. (1992) Is thoraco-abdominal phase relationship an indicator of sleep state? *European Journal of Pediatrics* **151**, 526–527.

105 Storme, L., Riou, Y., Leclerc, F. *et al.* (1992) Respiratory mechanics in mechanically ventilated newborns: a comparison between passive inflation and occlusion methods. *Pediatric Pulmonology* **12**, 203–212.

106 Tabachnik, E., Muller, N., Toye, B., Levison, H. (1981) Measurement of ventilation in children using the respiratory inductance plethysmograph. *Journal of Pediatrics* **99**, 895–899.

107 Taussig, L.M., Landau, L.I., Godfrey, S., Arad, I. (1982) Determinants of forced expiratory flows in newborn infants. *Journal of Applied Physiology* **53**, 1220–1227.

108 Tepper, R.S., Pagtakhan, R.D., Taussig, L.M. (1984) Non-invasive determination of total respiratory compliance in infants by the weighted spirometer method. *American Review of Respiratory Disease* **139**, 461–466.

109 Thomas, D.A., Poole, K., McArdle, E.K. *et al.* (1996) Peripheral chemoresponses of infants measured by a minimally invasive method utilizing two-breath alternations in FiO$_2$. *European Respiratory Journal* **9**, 1261–1268.

110 Thomas, M., Greenough, A., Blowes, R. *et al.* (2002) Airway resistance estimation in very premature infants by best-fit analysis. *Physiological Measurement* **23**, 279–285.

111 Upton, C., Stokes, G.M., Wilson, A.J., Milner, A.D. (1990) Dynamic response to tube breathing during the first 10 days of life. *Pediatric Pulmonology* **9**, 72–79.

112 Vyas, H., Milner, A.D., Hopkin, I.E. (1981) Intrathoracic pressure and volume changes during the spontaneous onset of respiration in babies born by Cesarean section and by vaginal delivery. *Journal of Pediatrics* **99**, 787–791.

113 Vyas, H., Field, D., Hopkin, I.E., Milner, A.D. (1986) Determinants of the first inspiratory volume and functional residual capacity at birth. *Pediatric Pulmonology* **2**, 189–193.

114 Wilkie, R.A., Bryan, M.H., Tarnow-Mordi, W.O. (1994) Static respiratory compliance in the newborn. II: Its potential for improving the selection of infants for early surfactant treatment. *Archives of Disease in Childhood* **70**, F16–F18.

115 Wilson, S.J., O'Brien, C., Harris, M.A., Masters, I.B. (1998) Measuring tidal volume and functional residual capacity change in sleeping infants using a volume displacement plethysmograph. *European Respiratory Journal* **12**, 1186–1190.

116 Wolfson, M.R., Greenspan, J.S., Deoras, K.S. *et al.* (1992) Effect of position on the mechanical interaction between the rib cage and abdomen in preterm infants. *Journal of Applied Physiology* **72**, 1032–1038.

117 Yüksel, B., Greenough, A. (1995) Functional residual capacity to thoracic gas volume (FRC:TGV) ratio in healthy neonates. *Respiratory Medicine* **89**, 429–433.

118 Yüksel, B., Greenough, A., Giffin, F.J., Nicolaides, K.H. (1996) Tidal breathing parameters in the first week of life and subsequent cough and wheeze. *Thorax* **51**, 815–818.

PART 3

Clinical management of the neonate with respiratory problems

14

Resuscitation at birth

ANTHONY D MILNER

HISTORY

Although the importance of providing appropriate facilities for all newborn babies has only been generally appreciated over the last 40 years, a recommendation that every accoucheur should carry along with him to every labor a tracheal pipe, a little tube of silver designed to pass down the trachea, was first made by Blundell, an obstetrician at Guy's Hospital in 1834.[28] He recommended that the fourth finger of the left hand be slid down 'the roof of the tongue and into the rim of the glottis and then, using the tube with the right hand, insert the tube'. The lungs were then to be inflated from the operator's own lungs. Although not in regular use since then, this was re-described in 1941 by Russ and Strong,[96] and recently by neonatologists from Washington.[51] In 1842, Evanson and Maunsell recommended the use of oropharyngeal suction followed by mouth-to-mouth resuscitation.[32] This was very much against the recommendation of the Royal Humane Society,[95] which deprecated the use of mouth-to-mouth resuscitation on the grounds that 'stale' air was unlikely to be of value in resuscitation. In 1889, Doe and Braun described the use of a box ventilator, a rather clumsy precursor of the tank ventilators which were used extensively for the treatment of poliomyelitis victims.[24] In the 1920s, a paper published in the *Journal of the American Medical Association* recommended the use of T-piece face mask resuscitation (see below).[54] The main claim for the introduction of neonatal resuscitation must be ascribed, however, to Flagg who, in 1928, advocated intubation and intermittent positive pressure ventilation (IPPV).[39]

An alternative approach recommended by Blaikley and Gibberd of Queen Charlotte's and Guy's Hospitals, London in 1935 was that of intubation and high level continuous positive airways pressure.[10] Despite this, there remained interest in other forms of resuscitation including gastric oxygen[2] and hyperbaric oxygen.[64] Although these approaches did have some advocates who were perhaps having problems coming to terms with the skills of intubation and ventilation, interest in them has now disappeared!

EFFECTS OF ASPHYXIA ON THE NEWBORN

It is well established that the neonatal primate,[23] including the human,[103] can survive acute total asphyxia for up to 20 minutes without suffering any neurological sequelae. This is because the neonatal brain has the ability to metabolize lactate and ketones. Unfortunately, this information is of little use in deciding when resuscitation should be commenced, as isolated acute total asphyxia is rare, the majority of babies failing to breathe at birth because of a combination of acute and chronic partial asphyxia.

The first marker often noticed by the mother of chronic partial asphyxia is a cessation of general motor activity. The response to this form of asphyxia in the human infant just before delivery has been well documented by fetal monitoring and cordocentesis. The fetal heart initially responds to hypoxia by an increase in heart rate, usually to above 160 beats/min (bpm). As the fetal heart is relatively poor in sacromeres, the fetus may improve cardiac output only by a rise in heart rate rather than by an increase in stroke volume. With persisting hypoxia, the beat-to-beat variation in heart beat disappears due to loss of ability of the heart to respond to the vagus. As the asphyxia persists with fall in pH, CO_2 retention and relative hypoxia [often to levels of below 2.5 kPa (18.8 mmHg)], late decelerations are seen, that is the bradycardia occurring in association with uterine contractions and due to head compression which persists into the non-contractile interval. Unfortunately, monitoring of the fetal heart rate during labor has failed to be as sensitive and specific an indicator of significant fetal asphyxia as was initially hoped,[89] and certainly will not identify all cases of moderate or even severe asphyxia.[81]

What is increasingly apparent is that hours or even days before the onset of labor, the fetus can suffer an asphyxial or hypoxic insult and then apparently make a total recovery, breathing spontaneously at birth, even though the baby has extensive brain damage which is not apparent for weeks or even months.[105,106]

Although all the metabolic processes of the newborn can be adversely affected by the hypoxia, hypoperfusion and metabolic acidosis associated with perinatal asphyxia, some organs are more susceptible than others.

Central nervous system

Asphyxial effects on the brain include cerebral edema and selective neuronal necrosis, which may affect the cortex generally, but also often involves Sonnen's section of the hippocampus, the cerebellar cortex, thalamus and brainstem.[40] In preterm infants, periventricular leukomalacia and intraventricular hemorrhage can occur. In the full-term baby, those severely affected will show features of hypoxic ischemic encephalopathy ranging from a state of hyperreactivity through transient fits to unresponsive unconsciousness and opisthotonos, resulting either in death or severe global impairment.[98] It is now well established that although the primary asphyxial insult can result in irreversible brain damage, there is then a therapeutic window lasting for up to 48 hours followed by a secondary energy failure with further neuronal necrosis and apoptosis.[60,70] This secondary damage results from a number of biochemical insults including calcium overload and generation of oxygen free radicals during the reperfusion period.[27,37] This raises the exciting possibility that long-term neurological deficit may be reduced by early therapeutic intervention. Approaches under investigation include the use of calcium channel blockers,[8] oxygen free radical scavengers and inhibitors[7,112] and, perhaps the most encouraging, total body[5] or selective head cooling.[6]

Cardiovascular system

Myocardial depression is common after a severe ischemic insult, resulting in hypotension, cardiac failure and necrosis

of cardiac muscle. Tricuspid regurgitation occurs secondary to cardiac dilatation and stretching of the tricuspid valve ring.[15] In a recently published study, more than 80 percent of 43 infants with severe perinatal asphyxia had ECG and/or biochemical evidence of myocardial ischemia and 24 had cardiovascular symptoms.[107] As a result of these changes, plasma expanders should be used with caution; fortunately, however, the myocardium does often respond to inotropes.

Renal system

Acute renal failure is common after neonatal asphyxia often due to acute tubular necrosis, and associated with myoglobinemia.[74] Fortunately, in all except those with severe ischemic damage, the kidneys usually recover within days; this is often accompanied by a diuresis.

Gastrointestinal

Occasionally resuscitation may be accompanied by either esophageal or gastric perforation (see below). A worrying complication of acute asphyxia in full-term babies is necrotizing enterocolitis,[97] often presenting within hours of delivery. This may be very extensive and lead to the early demise of the infant.

Respiratory system

It is well established that neonatal asphyxia in the preterm baby worsens respiratory distress syndrome (RDS).[109] In addition, severe asphyxia can cause extensive damage to the alveolar epithelium and the underlying capillary bed, leading to acute respiratory distress syndrome (ARDS) (p. 396).[33] Perinatal asphyxia is also associated with an increased incidence of pulmonary hemorrhage,[35] probably due to a combination of capillary damage and poor left ventricular function. Ischemic insult at the time of birth also inhibits the process whereby the pulmonary artery pressure falls, leading to persistent pulmonary hypertension of the newborn (Chapter 26).

Metabolic effects

Neonatal hypoxic insults interfere with the baby's ability to metabolize brown adipose tissue so that hypothermia is likely to occur unless the baby is nursed in an appropriately warm environment.[101] Both asphyxia and cold stress can produce hypoglycemia, which may compound any cerebral damage that is occurring. Although the liver is relatively resistant to hypoxic damage, clotting factor deficiencies are common and respond poorly to vitamin K.[50]

RESUSCITATION FACILITIES FOR USE IN THE LABOR SUITE

Thus, although the unstressed neonate is relatively resistant to hypoxic damage, the first priority in the provision of neonatal care must be to ensure that adequate resuscitation facilities are available for all deliveries and that deliveries likely to be associated with severe hypoxia are attended by staff capable of providing the full range of advanced life support techniques.

Facilities for neonatal resuscitation are most easily provided by a commercially available resuscitation trolley. The component parts (Table 14.1) are as follows:

- A cushioned shelf on which to lie the baby. This is usually tiltable. There is no evidence to suggest that babies have any respiratory advantage nursed head down compared to flat.[83] It is, however, most important that the personnel who use the resuscitation system are comfortable.
- An overhead radiant heat source with an output of approximately 300 W and designed to perform within the performance regulations specified by the relevant International Standards, that is the maximum irradiance level at any point on the mattress does not exceed 100 mW/cm^2 in the total infrared spectrum. Although overhead radiant heaters can often be used both in standard and servo-control mode, only the standard mode is suitable for neonatal resuscitation. In addition to the overhead radiant heater, there should be

Table 14.1 *Resuscitation equipment*

Padded shelf/resuscitation trolley
Towels
Overhead heater
Overhead light oxygen supply
Wall/cylinder oxygen supply
Clock (second/minute)
Stethoscope
Airway pressure manometer and pressure relief valve
Face mask
Oropharyngeal airways 00+0
Bag (500 ml) and mask or T-piece face mask system
T-piece device for endotracheal tubes if not integral
Suction catheters (sized 5, 8, 10 FG)
Variable suction source 100–200 mmHg
Mechanical and/or manual suction with double trap
Two laryngoscopes with spare blades
Endotracheal tubes 2, 2.5, 3, 3.5 and 4 mm
Introducer for endotracheal tubes
Umbilical artery/vein catheterization set
2, 10 and 20 ml syringes with needles
Cord clamps
ECG and transcutaneous oxygen saturation monitor

Note: capnometers are a strongly recommended optional extra.

protective sides to the resuscitation platform to reduce convective and evaporative water losses.
- A stop clock. This should record minutes and seconds. Some systems include preset alarms to provide an audible indication of the passage of time.
- Gas supplies. Standard resuscitation trolleys have two oxygen inputs which can be operated either from a wall supply or from cylinders stored on the back of the trolley. One output which incorporates a relatively high pressure relief valve (40–50 cmH$_2$O) provides an oxygen supply either to a soft funnel or loosely fitting face mask designed so that pressure cannot accumulate. This oxygen supply can also be used to raise the oxygen concentration within bag and mask systems. The second oxygen output has a variable pressure control, usually set at 25–30 cmH$_2$O. This output is used for face mask T-piece or T-piece endotracheal resuscitation. Both oxygen outlets require flow meters which can deliver up to 10 l/min. Anxieties about possible damage from the generation of oxygen free radicals in the reperfusion period and evidence that most term babies can be resuscitated using room air[99] (p. 139) has led to a consumer demand for gas-mixing facilities so that the oxygen concentration used for resuscitation can be limited to clinical requirements. If piped compressed air is not available in the labor suite, compressed air cylinders will be required.
- Suction system. This is either provided by connection to a wall source or from a Venturi system mounted on the trolley. This will provide suction for the upper airway (FG 8 and 10) and to clear an endotracheal tube (sized 2 or 3 FG). For routine use, the pressure should be limited to 100 mmHg, but it should be possible to increase to 200 mmHg for clearing thick secretions from the upper airway.
- Face mask resuscitation system. If a self-filling bag and mask system is selected, this should have a volume of at least 500 ml (see below). Ideally the face mask should be round with a pneumatic rim in order to obtain the optimum face seal.[86] Some neonatologists prefer an anesthetic rebreathing bag and mask system in which the escape vent from the bag is controlled by the physician's fourth and fifth fingers while squeezing the bag with the other fingers.[111] Alternatively, a simple T-piece connector can be attached to the face mask, a system which requires very little training and leaves one hand free (see below).[62] This system must be attached to the oxygen output with the variable pressure control.
- A selection of appropriately sized oropharyngeal airways, sizes 00 and 000.
- At least two laryngoscopes. Most neonatologists prefer the straight-bladed varieties such as the Wisconsin, Magill or the Oxford Infant type.
- A selection of endotracheal tubes and connectors for use either with resuscitation bags or T-piece systems. Most neonatologists find oral tubes easier to pass in

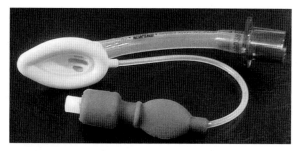

Figure 14.1 *Laryngeal mask.*

Table 14.2 *Drugs which should be available on the resuscitation trolley*

Sodium bicarbonate 4.2 percent or 8.4 percent, 10 ml ampoules
THAM 7 percent, 10 ml ampoules
Normal saline, 10 ml ampoules
Dextrose 10 percent, 10 ml ampoules
Naloxone 0.04 mg/ml, 2 ml ampoules
Vitamin K, 1 mg ampoule
Epinephrine 1 in 10 000, 5 ml ampoules

Also immediately available
Normal saline, 100 ml bottles
O-negative blood

Table 14.3 *High-risk deliveries*

Type of delivery	Post-term (≥44 weeks)
High forceps	Small for dates
Ventouse	Rhesus isoimmunization
Cesarean section under	Hydramnios and
general anesthetic	oligohydramnios
	Abnormal baby
Fetal conditions	
Fetal distress	*Maternal conditions*
Reduced fetal movement	Antepartum hemorrhage
Abnormal presentation	Severe pregnancy-
Prolapsed cord	induced hypertension
Meconium staining	Heavy sedation
of liquor	Drug addiction
Multiple pregnancy	Diabetes mellitus
Pre-term (<34 weeks)	Chronic illness

Table 14.4 *Apgar score*

	Score		
Clinical failure	**0**	**1**	**2**
Heart	0	<100	>100
Respiration	Absent	Gasping or irregular	Regular
Muscle tone	Limp	Diminished	Normal
Response to pharyngeal catheter	Nil	Grimace	Cough
Colour of trunk	White	Blue	Pink

the emergency situation. In very small babies, however, the laryngoscope blade and oral tube may block the view of the larynx. The shouldered tubes have the advantage that they are stiffer and therefore easier to pass. Introducers are often used to facilitate intubation. If nasoendotracheal intubation is preferred, it is necessary to ensure that there are at least two Magill forceps on the trolley. Laryngeal mask airways should be available for use when endotracheal intubation has failed. These are passed 'blind' and form a seal around the entrance to the larynx (Figure 14.1).

- Additional items include nasogastric tubes size 6 and 8, syringes, needles, specimen bottles, intravenous cannulae, and intraosseous needles,[30] adhesive tape, scissors and a stethoscope.
- Surgical packs. Packs should be available for immediate cannulation of the umbilical vessels and also for the draining of pneumothorax.
- Two additional facilities useful for all but the briefest of resuscitation are ECG and saturation monitoring devices.
- Certain drugs should be immediately available on the trolley (Table 14.2).

LABOR WARD MANAGEMENT OF TERM BABIES

It has been estimated that approximately 70 percent of infants requiring some resuscitation can be identified

prior to delivery.[48,87,91] This identifiable group involves up to 40 percent of all deliveries (Table 14.3). The remaining 30 percent of infants requiring intubation are totally unexpected, underlying the importance of ensuring there is at least one person available capable of providing basic resuscitation to the baby at all deliveries, while a second person skilled in advanced resuscitation can be summoned within 5–10 minutes. In total, approximately 10 percent of all infants are given some form of resuscitation and approximately 2 percent require intubation.[17,48,83] Approximately 1 percent of infants born at term will require intubation; this figure rises to more than 60 percent for babies born at less than 28 weeks of gestation.

Assessment at birth

The initial stage of assessment is, while drying excess water off the baby, to look very briefly for gross congenital abnormalities as their presence may influence the resuscitation steps to be taken.

THE APGAR SCORE

Although the Apgar score[3] is routinely used to assess the overall condition of the baby at 1 and 5 minutes (Table 14.4), its main role is to identify those infants who are at risk of developing long-term neurological problems.[84] The components of the Apgar score which will influence whether active resuscitation is to be undertaken are the baby's color, respiratory activity and heart rate. Cord blood gas measurements are also often carried out, but the results of these will not be available for several minutes and so are not very useful in the acute management of the infant, but, like the Apgar score, provide useful prognostic information which may influence the subsequent management of the infant. There are also some data indicating that the absence of a metabolic acidosis with perinatal asphyxia may be indicative of a failure of adaptation to the hypoxia and be associated with a worse outcome.[36]

The procedure to be followed once it is recognized that the newly born infant is failing to breathe spontaneously and adequately, has to a considerable extent been standardized by the consensus statement of the International Liaison Committee on Resuscitation (ILCOR) and American Heart Association/American Academy of Pediatrics (AHA/AAP) which published their guidelines in 2000.[85] These recommendations have been adopted by most developed countries. The working party identified that few resuscitation interventions had been subjected to randomized controlled trials. There have, however, been a number of small physiological studies on the effects of these interventions. The vast majority of infants will commence spontaneous respiration with a median time of less than 10 seconds.[100] At 1 minute, however, approximately 10 percent of infants will have failed to establish regular respiration.[17] In this latter group of patients who have a heart rate in excess of 80 bpm, the first step is to provide facial oxygen which probably acts by providing a cold stimulus to the face, and also to apply a tactile stimulation, for example, flicking the feet. If there is blood or debris around the baby's mouth, this can be sucked out. Routine oropharyngeal suction is not recommended and can, if applied too vigorously, inhibit the onset of respiratory effort.

Face mask resuscitation

If the infant fails to show an immediate response, but still has a heart rate in excess of 80 bpm, face mask resuscitation should be commenced. There are three possible approaches.

BAG AND MASK

There are a number of commercially available bag and mask systems. These comprise a face mask, a pressure-limiting device which may be either a spring-loaded valve or a leak system and a self-inflating bag to which oxygen can be added. Studies have shown that a round face mask with a pneumatic lip provides the optimal seal.[86] Most of the pressure-limiting devices can be overridden; for example, it is usually possible to hold the spring-loaded valve

closed with the tip of a finger to prevent leak from the system. When occluded in this way, it is possible to generate pressures up to 50–60 cmH$_2$O,[115] although in routine practice, a leak between the face and the mask usually limits the pressure to between 30 and 35 cmH$_2$O.

The volume of the self-inflating bag is of considerable importance. Studies on term babies have shown that the 250 ml bag devices rarely deliver tidal volumes in excess of the infant's anatomical dead space to babies requiring resuscitation at birth, with a mean of only 5.5 ml for the neonatal Laerdal.[38,116] Values at least twice that, however, were achieved using the pediatric Laerdal and the Ambu baby, which have reservoir volumes of 500 ml. The main reason for the failure of the neonatal device is that air escaped rapidly through the pressure-relief valve so that peak pressures tended to be lower and were maintained for less than 0.5 seconds. Although the inspiratory time is similar to that generated by babies commencing to breathe spontaneously at birth,[117] the product of pressure and inspiratory time is of critical importance and with 250 ml bag and mask systems is too low to produce an adequate tidal exchange. Satisfactory outcome from bag and mask resuscitation then depends on stimulating Head's paradoxical reflex in infants who have not suffered from severe asphyxia and who might well have commenced to breathe regularly without excessive interference (p. 43).[38]

If these systems are to be used effectively, it is essential to use one hand to support the chin and hold the face mask in place, while squeezing the bag between the fingers of the other hand at approximately 60/min.

One anxiety frequently expressed in the past was that the opening pressure of the esophagus might be lower than the pressure necessary to produce alveolar inflation. This could potentially lead to a situation in which a large gastric air bubble was created, splinting the diaphragm and impeding further attempts at resuscitation. A study, however,[115] measuring both the amount of pressure transmitted down the esophagus and also the volume of air in the stomach at the end of bag and mask resuscitation showed that this was not a problem when performing resuscitation at birth. It is obviously, however, of considerable clinical significance when resuscitating infants in the neonatal unit and beyond. The main reason for the difference appears to be that infants do not swallow until after the onset of spontaneous ventilation, a fact well documented by studying the onset of respiration.[82,100,117]

ANESTHETIC REBREATHING FACE MASK SYSTEM

An alternative to the bag and mask is to attach an anesthetic rebreathing bag attached to a round face mask and incorporate a spring-loaded blow-off valve between the rebreathing bag and the mask. Another approach is to control the leak from an open rebreathing bag by holding the escape tube between the fourth and fifth fingers while squeezing the bag between the thumb and the second and third fingers. This system will only be effective if there is a flow of gas of at least 6, and preferably, 10 l/min into the system to keep the anesthetic rebreathing bag distended. The system has the advantage that both the length of inspiration and the inspiratory pressure can be varied on a breath-to-breath basis while observing the movement of the chest wall. This technique does, however, require a considerable amount of training and again requires the use of both hands.

FACE MASK T-PIECE SYSTEM

An easier technique has been to use a round face mask with a pneumatic rim to which a T-piece device is attached.[62] This is connected to the pressure limited oxygen outlet on the resuscitation trolley. All that is then required is for the face mask to be lowered on to the baby's face while held between the thumb and third finger, while the egress of gas from the T-piece is occluded intermittently by the tip of the index finger. The advantages of this system are first, that this technique is very easy to use, requiring the minimum of training. Second, the length of the inspiratory time can be controlled so that, for the first few breaths, inspiration can be maintained for at least a second. One study has shown that this allows a significantly greater tidal exchange to occur even in babies with unexpanded lungs, similar to that achieved by standard endotracheal ventilation.[62] The third advantage is that only one hand is required so that the other hand can be used to listen to the chest with a stethoscope. This technique is now incorporated into a number of commercially available resuscitation systems, or as an add-on device (e.g. Neopuff).

Endotracheal intubation and ventilation

Although face mask resuscitation provides an excellent method for ensuring the onset of regular respiration in infants who are slow to breathe but have not suffered severe acute/chronic asphyxia, at least 1 percent of infants are unlikely to survive unless intubation and ventilation is commenced. This group comprises infants in whom face mask ventilation has failed to produce an improvement in saturation, or respiratory efforts within 15–30 seconds and those in whom the heart rate is either below 60 bpm at birth or falls, despite basic resuscitation.

Although the nasal route can be used for intubation in the labor suite, most neonatologists find orotracheal intubation easier and faster. For intubation the infant should be placed so that the head is close to the front of the resuscitation platform. It is important to have the head in the same plane as the body. The neck should be slightly extended and not twisted to either side. The laryngoscope is held in the left hand and passed over the center of the tongue, inserting it deeper into the infant's throat until the epiglottis comes into view. If the blade is then placed

over the epiglottis and slightly lifted, the vocal cords will come into view. If the baby is not hypotonic, the larynx may be held in an anterior position, making good visualization difficult. Under these circumstances the entrance to the larynx can be brought into view by pressing gently over the cricoid cartilage either with the fourth finger of the hand holding the laryngoscope, or with the help of an assistant. Sometimes in the rush to intubate, the blade of the laryngoscope is pushed too far so that the esophagus is entered. Under these circumstances the best approach is to slowly withdraw the blade. The larynx should then fall into view as the blade passes out of the esophagus. It is important, when passing the laryngoscope blade, to keep to the midline. This will not only aid visualization, but will also help ensure that the endotracheal tube is correctly passed.

During this process it is often necessary to suck out the upper airway in order to get a good view of the vocal cords. Once these have been visualized, the endotracheal tube can be passed. The optimal device is probably the shouldered oral endotracheal tube with integral T-piece as this is relatively stiff. Although not essential, introducers are a useful aid as they increase the stiffness further. Providing too small a tube has not been selected, the shoulder will usually ensure that the tube is not inserted too far. Alternatively, straight tubes can be used but it will then be necessary to resort to an introducer. This has the disadvantage that unless great care is taken to ensure that the introducer does not protrude out of the end of the endotracheal tube, tracheal perforation can occur. The policy is to use the largest tube that will fit comfortably down the trachea, that is a 3.5 mm tube for a full-term infant and a 3 mm for infants of birth weights of 1200–1500 g. For smaller infants it is often necessary to resort to 2.5 mm or even 2 mm tubes. It is, however, extremely difficult to maintain the patency of a 2 mm tube during subsequent ventilation. Once the endotracheal tube has been placed, the laryngoscope can be removed. Care must be taken to hold the tube firmly between the finger and thumb to ensure that it is not displaced from the trachea.

An alternative method of intubation, first demonstrated in adults by Vesalius in 1543 and in neonates by J Blundell in 1838,[28] is finger intubation. In this technique the index finger is passed along the tongue until the epiglottis is felt, the endotracheal tube is then advanced like a pencil held between the index finger and thumb of the other hand, using the other index finger as a guide. This was assessed in 37 infants requiring ventilation in the neonatal period and found to be always associated with successful intubation after a mean time of 7 seconds.[51]

Intubation can be particularly difficult in infants with congenital abnormalities of the upper airway. For these and for situations where the available staff have limited intubation skills, laryngeal masks should be available. These are passed blind, i.e. without the use of a laryngoscope.

OXYGEN CONCENTRATIONS

The current recommendation is that 100 percent oxygen should be used but that if this is not available positive pressure ventilation should be commenced using room air. This recommendation may well change as the results of more controlled trials become available. The reason for this is that there is increasing anxiety that at least some of the long-term neurological damage following birth asphyxia is caused by the toxic effects of oxygen free radicals generated particularly during the reperfusion period. Animal experiments have shown that asphyxiated newborn piglets respond as rapidly to resuscitation with air as with 100 percent oxygen[93] and with similar brain pathology at postmortem. A further study on piglets rendered hypoxic by induced pneumothoraces had a similar outcome except that the piglets receiving air had better neurological examination scores subsequently.[108] Three randomized controlled studies on newborn infants have been published. The first, carried out in India on 84 infants requiring resuscitation at birth, revealed no outcome difference between those receiving oxygen and those air.[92] Some of the infants in the air group were, however, given 100 percent oxygen as they were still cyanosed at 90 seconds. The second larger international study involved 609 infants.[99] In this study, the only significant outcome differences were that the onset of spontaneous breathing and of crying were significantly delayed in the infants receiving 100 percent. The failure rate, that is, persistence of cyanosis at 90 seconds, was similar in the two groups. This delay in the onset of spontaneous breathing was also found in the third randomized study from Spain.[113] This group also found evidence of persisting oxidative stress at 28 days in the oxygen-treated infants with higher erythrocyte superoxide dismutase and catalase levels. Interestingly, the respiratory depressant effect of 100 percent oxygen has been well documented in animal experiments[65] and to a lesser extent in healthy newborn infants.[1]

The current consensus is that air is probably as good as 100 percent oxygen for most asphyxiated term infants. It is likely that some infants will require supplementary oxygen, possibly an inspired oxygen concentration of 30 or 40 percent. There is no evidence that air reduces neurological damage in infants, although the number of infants studied is relatively small so that any benefit could be hidden by a type II error. This problem can only be overcome by a very large multicenter study involving thousands of asphyxiated infants.

Ventilatory support

Once the endotracheal tube has been passed, the lungs can be inflated using one of four techniques. These are: intermittent positive pressure using a T-piece and blow-off valve (T-piece/IPPV); self-inflating resuscitation bag with pre-set pressure control, ventilation using an anesthetic rebreathing bag or by connecting to a commercial infant ventilator.

T-PIECE/IPPV

This is achieved by either using an endotracheal tube which incorporates a T-piece or alternatively attaching a separate T-piece device. Oxygen is fed to the T-piece via tubing which incorporates a pressure-limiting device, usually in the form of a spring-loaded valve. A cheap alternative is to have a water column. The latter has two main disadvantages: first, unless the water is changed frequently there is a considerable risk of infection with organisms such as *Pseudomonas* and, second, water within the tube has an inertial effect so that high inflation pressures will initially be achieved.[57] These, however, are of short duration and are probably not important. If high flow rates are used, turbulence occurs at the lower end of the tube, where air escapes into the surrounding water and may generate higher pressures than anticipated.

Although infants often generate negative pressures in excess of $50\,cmH_2O$ in association with the first breath, an upper limit of $30\,cmH_2O$ for positive pressure resuscitation has been justified on the grounds that pressures in excess of this would be more likely to result in a pneumothorax. Data to substantiate this are very limited; Rosen and Laurence[94] subjected isolated newborn lungs to increasing pressure until they ruptured. This commonly occurred when pressures of $60\,cmH_2O$ were exceeded, but was rare at pressures below $35\,cmH_2O$. It is, however, an artificial situation as overdistention and rupture of lung units is more likely to occur in the isolated lung than in the intact respiratory system. Nevertheless, some newborn babies do not require pressures in excess of $20\,cmH_2O$ for the first breath and considerably lower pressures for subsequent lung inflation.

The current recommendations for the resuscitation of term infants are that an inflation pressure of $25–30\,cmH_2O$ should be used and that the infants should be ventilated at a rate of approximately 30/min with an I:E ratio of 1:1. Studies, however, have shown that this pattern of inflation rarely produces an inspiratory volume of greater than 20 ml (that is, half of that achieved by infants commencing to breathe spontaneously)[11] and that a functional residual capacity (FRC) is rarely formed. A more effective approach is to maintain the first inflation for at least 3 seconds (Figure 14.2). This has been shown to achieve tidal exchange similar to that seen in the spontaneously breathing infant and leads to the formation of an FRC within the first one to two breaths.[114] Subsequently, infants can be ventilated satisfactorily using a rate of 30/min and 1:1 I:E ratio. There have, however, been no controlled studies carried out to establish whether the early formation of an FRC alters outcome.

Although this provides a simple approach to resuscitation, it is obviously far from physiological. Studies on

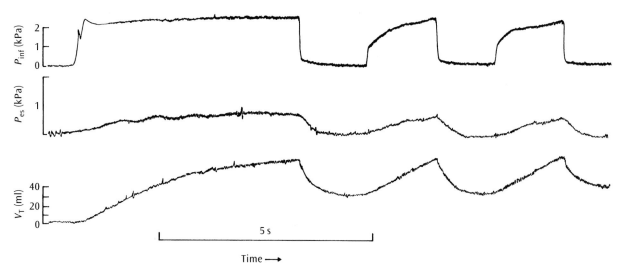

Figure 14.2 *The effect of prolonging the first inflation on inspiratory volume and FRC. Gas continues to enter the lungs for 4 seconds.*

babies breathing spontaneously have shown that some can inflate their lungs with pressures as low as $20\,cmH_2O$ while others generate pressures in excess of $80\,cmH_2O$. Hull[63] found that if full-term infants are resuscitated using a constant volume (40 ml), a similar pattern emerges, some infants' lungs expanding satisfactorily with airway pressures of less than $20\,cmH_2O$ whereas others required in excess of $40\,cmH_2O$.

SELF-INFLATING BAG

In many units resuscitation is achieved by connecting a self-inflating resuscitation bag to the endotracheal tube. As already stated, these bags tend to empty relatively rapidly through the pressure-relief valve, so that it is normal to squeeze the bag between the thumb and second and third fingers at a rate of approximately 60/min. Under these circumstances, pressures of $20–25\,cmH_2O$ will usually be generated.[38] Much higher pressures in excess of $60\,cmH_2O$ can be produced if the blow-off valve is occluded.[115] There are currently no data on the volumes delivered to babies during this form of resuscitation. The relatively high ventilatory rates often used may well lead to a degree of air trapping which may be of advantage in the formation of the initial FRC.

ANESTHETIC REBREATHING BAG

This is the pattern of resuscitation favored by anesthetists in which the leak from the bag is controlled by squeezing the egress between the fourth and fifth fingers. A relatively high flow of gas is required to keep the bag distended. Some systems do incorporate a pressure relief valve in addition. One study has shown that if the bag is squeezed sufficiently to produce visible chest wall movements, the pressures generated will be in the region of $50\,cmH_2O$ but sustained for less than 0.5 second.[111] This pattern is very similar to that generated by infants who commence to breathe spontaneously at birth.[117] Although this would seem to be the most physiological approach, it does require a considerable degree of skill and currently there are no controlled studies to show that one form of resuscitation is better than any other.

Complications of intubation and IPPV resuscitation

The commonest complication leading to ineffectual resuscitation is positioning the endotracheal tube within the esophagus. It should be possible to detect this immediately as part of the resuscitation process involves listening to both sides of the chest with a stethoscope immediately after commencing ventilation. If there is no air entry, despite reasonable inflation pressures, it is very likely that the endotracheal tube is misplaced and intubation should be repeated.

It is claimed that the use of in-line end tidal carbon dioxide detectors helps identify esophageal intubation more rapidly. In one study malposition was detected in a mean of 8.1 seconds (SD $\pm$ 2.0 seconds) compared to 39.7 seconds (SD $\pm$ 15.3 seconds) by clinical evaluation. However, in 10 percent of the infants who had been correctly intubated, no CO_2 was detected due to inadequate lung perfusion.[4]

Positioning the endotracheal tube down the esophagus has three other complications. These are esophageal or hypopharyngeal perforation,[44,110] which can lead to mediastinitis, perforation of the stomach and loss of the endotracheal tube down the esophagus.[13] These complications can prove fatal.

Tracheal perforation is usually associated with the use of introducers, but has been reported in their absence. This can lead to a massive mediastinal air leak, which has proved fatal on occasions. Ruptured stomach has also occurred as a complication of resuscitating babies with tracheo-esophageal fistulae.

A common problem, often experienced by those who are relatively inexperienced and select too narrow a tube, is selective intubation of the bronchi to the right middle and lower lobe. This will produce differential air entry on auscultation. If suspected, the stethoscope should be placed over the left lung and the endotracheal tube slowly withdrawn 1–2 cmH$_2$O while continuing to ventilate the baby. If the diagnosis is correct, air entry will spread to the left chest and the infant's condition will improve dramatically.

There are three other conditions which can produce differential air entry. The first is pneumothorax, which is said to occur in 1–2 percent of all infants breathing spontaneously (Chapter 22). Symptomatic pneumothoraces, which are usually of the tension variety even amongst infants requiring resuscitation, are relatively rare. If possible, the presence of a pneumothorax should be confirmed using either a cold light source or chest radiograph, but if the infant's condition is sufficiently critical, needling is an acceptable approach proceeding to insertion of a drain if free air is found (p. 418). An alternative diagnosis, which can also produce differential air entry, is diaphragmatic hernia. This is sometimes, but not always, associated with a scaphoid abdomen and can mimic the signs of a pneumothorax with displacement of the mediastinum although the side with reduced air entry will normally be dull to percussion due to the presence of the fluid-filled bowel. This picture can also be mimicked by cystic adenomatoid malformation (p. 466). Differential air entry with poor response to resuscitation is also seen in the presence of a pleural effusion. Pleural effusions may be bilateral (p. 355) and are then often associated with ascites, which can further limit the response to resuscitation due to splinting of the diaphragm. Diagnosis should obviously be suspected in any baby who has hydrops.[46] It may then be necessary to drain off both some of the pleural fluid and the ascitic fluid before adequate tidal exchange can be achieved.

External cardiac massage

This should be commenced in all infants in whom the heart rate is below 60 bpm and who do not improve within 30 seconds of the onset of adequate ventilatory support. This is best achieved by placing both hands round the chest so that the thumbs are over the lower part of the sternum and the fingertips close to the spine.[85,90] The sternum is then depressed by one-third of the diameter of the chest, which represents a depression of approximately 2 cm, at a rate of 100–120/min.[21] This form of cardiac massage is only possible if a second assistant is available to provide respiratory support. Alternatively, it is possible for a single person to provide both respiratory and cardiac support if external cardiac massage is provided

by depressing the sternum by the tips of the second and third finger. This, however, has been shown to be a less effective method for maintaining cardiac output.[21] A ratio of three compressions to one ventilation, with a rate of 120 'events' per minute, providing approximately 90 compressions per minute, is now recommended.[72] The pulse rate should be checked periodically, preferably the brachial or femoral and chest compressions discontinued once the heart rate exceeds 80 bpm.

Medication

If the baby's heart rate fails to improve on commencing external cardiac massage, 0.1–0.3 ml/kg of 1:10 000 epinephrine (adrenaline) can be injected down the endotracheal tube.[77,85] Although the blood supply through the lungs must be very small at this stage, this maneuver can lead to a rapid increase in heart rate or indeed return of the heart beat after a period of cardiac arrest. This dose may be revised as evidence from adults and stable infants have indicated that the endotracheal dose needs to be at least ten times the intravenous dose to have achieved the same serum levels.[71] This may, however, result in a large reservoir of epinephrine in the lungs which could produce a sustained and unwanted hypertension.[119]

If the endotracheal epinephrine fails to produce a response, the umbilical vein should be catheterized and a further dose of epinephrine (0.1–0.3 ml/kg of 1:10 000 strength) given by that route. The intraosseous route can be used as an alternative.[30] Inevitably, however, the baby will be severely acidotic by this stage and response to epinephrine may be poor or non-existent unless some attempt is made to correct this acidosis. This can be achieved by giving sodium bicarbonate but there are now concerns that this may not be in the infant's best interest. The induced metabolic alkalosis will result in a left shift of the oxygen dissociation curve, reducing the delivery of oxygen to the tissues. The CO$_2$ generated may diffuse rapidly across cell membranes in situations where the circulation is sluggish, leading to greater intracellular acidosis.[73] There is also some evidence that giving bicarbonate reduces cerebral blood flow,[80] and the large osmotic load may lead to intracranial hemorrhages in preterm infants if given too rapidly.[104] There are no randomized studies on the efficacy of bicarbonate in infants but in adults the use of bicarbonate during resuscitation has been abandoned as a result of studies showing either no benefit or higher mortality rates.[29,75] It is, however, worth stressing that in adults resuscitation is required for a primary cardiac arrest, while in newborn infants the arrest is secondary to hypoxia and acidosis.

The current recommendation is that bicarbonate should be restricted to those with prolonged arrest and in a dose of 1–2 mEq/kg of a 0.5 mEq/ml solution and given over at least 2 minutes.[85] Alternatively, tris-(hydroxymethyl)aminomethane (THAM) can be given. The main disadvantage of THAM is that it tends to suppress respiration and so may prolong the time to the onset of spontaneous respiration. Again, there are no controlled trials to support this approach.

NALOXONE

Naloxone is an opiate antagonist but, unlike its predecessor nalorphine, does not produce any respiratory depression. Nevertheless, the administration of naloxone should not be given until the infant is receiving adequate ventilatory support and then only if there is a good reason for assuming that the infant's respiratory depression has resulted from maternal opiate administration. The normal approach is to give 0.1 mg/kg intravenously or via the endotracheal tube.[85] The intramuscular route leads to a slower response. A further dose of 0.1 mg/kg may be required. This should not be given to the newborns of opiate-addicted mothers as it can then precipitate acute withdrawal symptoms.[45]

PLASMA EXPANDERS

Volume expanders are indicated if there is hypovolemia. The most likely cause is acute bleeding from the feto-maternal unit; this is suggested by pallor, which persists after oxygenation. The first-line volume expanders recommended are isotonic saline or Ringer's solution as there is evidence that saline is more effective than albumin[31] and that administration of albumin adversely affects outcome if given in the neonatal period.[19] Group O Rhesus negative blood is preferable if the hypotension is due to massive blood loss. The guidelines recommend that 10 ml/kg body weight should be given over 5–10 minutes and the response assessed.[85]

PHYSIOLOGICAL RESPONSE TO RESUSCITATION

The now classical studies of Dawes[22] on the response of newborn higher mammals to acute total asphyxia predicted that two types of response to resuscitation at birth would occur in the human neonate. Either the resuscitation would stimulate the onset of respiration so that spontaneous respiratory efforts occurred before the infant became pink, indicating that the infant was in primary apnea or, alternatively, the infant would make no response until intensive resuscitation had led to an improvement in both the infant's color and cardiac output, indicating that the infant was in secondary or terminal apnea. In practice, although the latter situation can certainly be seen in infants who have suffered severe asphyxia, the pattern of responses are very variable, suggesting that there is a continuum of asphyxia rather than a two-phase response.

The reason for this deviation from the animal model is almost certainly because the newborn at birth has usually suffered from subacute or chronic asphyxia rather than acute total asphyxia after delivery.

Three patterns of response were seen in association with the onset of resuscitation in a study confined to full-term babies fulfilling the requirements for intubation immediately after birth.[12] In 24 percent of the inflations, the infant remained apneic, not making any respiratory efforts as determined by the esophageal pressure monitoring device. On a further 27 percent of inflations, the infant was stimulated to make an inspiratory effort of their own, a pattern first documented by Hering and Breuer,[55] but defined more closely by Head in 1889 (p. 43).[53] This is obviously a very appropriate response, leading to a significant tidal exchange and often followed by the formation of an FRC. This reflex probably explains the successful outcome after face mask resuscitation using conventional systems which, as already discussed,[38] rarely produce sufficient tidal exchange to clear the dead space when the baby remains apneic. The third pattern was that of active expiration with pressures of 70 cmH$_2$O often being generated within the thorax and also present within the stomach due to contraction of the abdominal muscles (Figure 14.3). The pressures are often sufficiently large to prevent or at least greatly reduce the tidal volume. This response was commonly seen at the onset of resuscitation and on occasions followed by a period of apnea before the infant commenced with Head's paradoxical reflex responses. Although an FRC was sometimes formed as

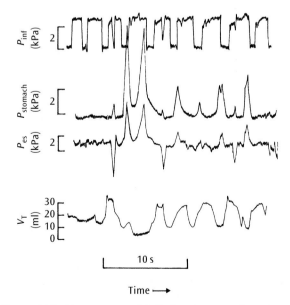

Figure 14.3 *Measurement of inflation, intragastric and intraesophageal pressures and tidal volume during resuscitation. The third inflation is associated with a Head's paradoxical reflex and the subsequent two breaths by active expiration (this is apparent on both the esophageal and intragastric traces).*

the result of passive ventilation, aeration more frequently accompanied the onset of respiratory efforts.

Pulmonary gas exchange has been measured during resuscitation of asphyxiated infants. Hull was able to measure oxygen consumption.[63] He found values as high as 11 ml/kg body weight over the first 2 minutes, but his technique was unable to differentiate between oxygen uptake in the blood and the volume that was being used to form the initial FRC. Palme-Kilander and Tunnell have measured the pulmonary gas exchange over 15-second intervals from the onset of resuscitation at birth.[88] In the majority of infants little or no carbon dioxide was detectable in the expired gases until the babies made their first inspiratory effort. This was particularly a feature of infants born very preterm and probably represents a failure of pulmonary vasodilatation to occur until the infants had made at least one inspiratory effort. This finding is of considerable interest and warrants further investigation.

Meconium aspiration syndrome (p. 334)

Meconium is present in the amniotic fluid of 12–15 percent of all babies at birth (Chapter 23). It is rare before 37 weeks but present in 30–50 percent of those in labor after 42 weeks.[120] In some infants, the passage of meconium is secondary to a hypoxic stress, in others it can be a physiological event associated with gastrointestinal maturation. Often the meconium staining is relatively thin and may have been present for some time. Only approximately 5 percent of those born through meconium will develop meconium aspiration syndrome (MAS).[18]

Amnioinfusion, which dilutes the meconium and may relieve pressure on the umbilical cord, can reduce the frequency of MAS,[59] but can lead to obstetric complications and so is still considered to be an experimental technique.

It has been claimed that the incidence of this condition can be significantly reduced by appropriate management in the labor suite (Chapter 23). As already stated, all labors complicated by the presence of thick meconium should be attended by a pediatrician skilled in intubation. The recommendation has been that the upper airway should be sucked out as soon as the head presents. This was based on an observational study using historical controls.[16] A more recent prospective observational study found that upper airway suction on the perineum had no effect on the incidence of MAS and was associated with an increased incidence of air leak.[34] Whether this form of intervention is useful is currently unclear.

It has also been recommended that direct laryngoscopy is carried out as soon as the infant is born. If meconium was visible below the larynx, the infant should immediately be intubated and as much meconium as possible sucked out.[43,47] This is best carried out by connecting the endotracheal tube to a suction source, occluding the opening and withdrawing the endotracheal tube. It may then be necessary to re-intubate the child and repeat the process until either no further meconium is recovered or the heart rate drops down to below 80 bpm. This approach was again based on observational studies using historical controls and was applied to all infants born through thick meconium. However, Linder and colleagues randomized otherwise healthy meconium-contaminated infants to either intubation and suction or conservative management.[78] None of the control infants developed MAS compared to 4 of the 300 intubated children. A recent large multicentered randomized trial involving more than 2000 vigorous but meconium-stained infants found that the incidence of MAS was higher in the intubated group although the differences failed to reach significance.[41]

As a result of these findings, the current recommendation is that elective intubation and suction should be reserved for meconium-contaminated infants who have absent or depressed respiration, a heart rate of less than 100 bpm or poor muscle tone.[85]

Attempts to prevent the baby breathing, by cricoid pressure, epiglottic blockage or applying chest wall squeeze, are not helpful and may be dangerous.[42] Chest wall squeeze will actually stimulate the baby to make inspiratory efforts as a result of the Hering–Breuer deflationary reflex.[52,63]

Diaphragmatic hernia (p. 487)

Due to the compressive effect of the presence of abdominal organs and associated pulmonary hypoplasia, infants with diaphragmatic hernias are often difficult to resuscitate so that staff skilled in intubation will need to be present at the delivery when the condition has been recognized antenatally. Face mask resuscitation using either T-piece pressure inflations or bag and mask systems are contraindicated as they are likely to lead to further distention of bowel within the thoracic cavity. These infants should be paralyzed in the labor suite to prevent swallowing. High pressures may be needed, sometimes exceeding 40 cmH$_2$O, despite the risk of creating a pneumothorax.

Upper airway obstruction and resuscitation

There is a further group of infants who make appropriate respiratory efforts soon after birth but fail to obtain any tidal exchange as a result of upper airway obstruction. In some, for example those with choanal atresia or the Pierre Robin syndrome, this situation can be rapidly remedied by passing an oropharyngeal airway. There are others who have major congenital abnormalities, including laryngeal webs and tracheal atresia, who will obviously fail to respond to this maneuver. Attempts can be made to achieve a temporary airway by inserting a wide bore needle directly into the trachea, or carrying out a tracheostomy, but these are usually unsuccessful.

PRETERM BABIES

It is now well established that limitation of asphyxia at birth can reduce the incidence of RDS and reduce mortality. One study showed that the mortality was reduced from 50 to 30 percent (Table 14.5, study A), when all infants compared to only 3 percent of infants less than 28 weeks were intubated in the labor suite.[25] In many units it is standard policy to intubate and ventilate all very immature babies, for example those less than 28 weeks gestation. If the distance between the labor suite and the neonatal unit is considerable this is a reasonable safety precaution. On the other hand, those babies who do start to breathe spontaneously immediately after birth and are vigorous, are likely to be difficult to intubate and will almost certainly have some degree of hypoxia as a result of the intubation exercise. For this reason, a policy of selective rather than elective intubation should be adopted (Table 14.5, study B).

There are, however, very few data available on how preterm infants should best be resuscitated. Hoskyns *et al.* found that using pressures of 25–30 cmH$_2$O maintained for up to 1 second using a T-piece endotracheal tube technique produced poor tidal exchange when compared to that achieved in full-term infants requiring resuscitation, rarely producing a tidal volume in excess of twice the anatomical dead space.[61] That group also examined the response of preterm infants to resuscitation using an anesthetic rebreathing bag approach with inflation pressures of up to 50 cmH$_2$O.[111] This provided more satisfactory tidal exchange. There are, however, considerable anxieties that the use of high pressures for the resuscitation of preterm infants will induce pulmonary interstitial emphysema. More worryingly is the animal-based evidence that the lung of the preterm mammal is very susceptible to damage from volutrauma in the first few minutes of life. Bjorklund and colleagues found that six inflations of 60 cmH$_2$O, each lasting for 5 seconds, given to preterm lambs before the administration of surfactant resulted in lower lung compliance for the next 4 hours and worse lung histology compared to matched controls.[9] In a more physiological study, the same group gave five sustained inflations which generated inflation volumes of 8, 16 and 32 ml/kg to preterm lambs.[67] They found dose-dependent lung damage but even those receiving only 8 ml/kg, similar to the volume generated by spontaneously breathing term infants, had worse lung mechanics than nonintubated controls. Giving surfactant immediately before the inflations had little beneficial effect,[67] although the surfactant was protective if the inflations were delayed for 15 minutes.[67,118]

Although the fact that these preterm animals were exposed to high inflation pressures, raising the possibility that the damage was caused by barotrauma, this is unlikely, as similar experiments on adult rats and infant rabbits have shown that the lung injury can be largely eliminated

Table 14.5 *Results of selective and elective resuscitation policies in preterm babies (<30 weeks)**

	Selective	Elective
Study A		
Number	96	69
Birthweight (kg)	1.025	1.018
Gestation (weeks)	28.5	28.9
Apgar 1	5	5
Survival (percent)	51	77
Intubated at birth (percent)	3	100
Intubated at 10 hours (percent)	37	100
Not intubated (percent)	60	–
Bronchopulmonary dysplasia (percent)	8	14
Retinopathy of prematurity (percent)	12	16
Study B		
Number	29	26
Birthweight (kg)	1.050	1.170
Gestation (weeks)	28.1	28.2
Apgar 1	5.1	6.6
Survival (percent)	76	76
Intubated at birth (percent)	62	100
Intubated (percent survival)	61	76
Not intubated (percent survival)	82	–
Mean 12 hour scores	3.32	3.28
Respiratory support (hours)	11.5	13.5

*(A) when only 3 percent of the selective group were intubated[25] and (B) where a more liberal policy was adopted (62 percent) (Field *et al.*[38], unpublished data). In only the first study was there an excess of mortality associated with the selective policy.

by restricting chest wall expansion with either rubber bands,[26] or plaster casts.[56] A further anxiety is that the use of high inflation volumes will result in hypocapnia, which is known to be causally related to the development of subsequent brain damage.[20,76]

One approach has been to commence the resuscitation of preterm babies with pressures as low as 16 cmH$_2$O and then increasing the pressure generated at the endotracheal tube opening until chest wall movement becomes apparent. Using this approach, a satisfactory short-term outcome was achieved with pressures that never exceeded 32 cmH$_2$O.[58] What remains unclear is whether even the use of the lowest effective inflation pressure will prevent lung damage at birth.

Use of CPAP in resuscitation

Upton and Milner found a close correlation between the failure to form an FRC during the first few inflations and the subsequent development of the respiratory distress

Table 14.6 *Relationship between the formation of an FRC during resuscitation of preterm babies and the subsequent development of RDS[111]*

	FRC	No FRC
Mild/no RDS	10	3
Severe RDS	2	7, $P < 0.02$

syndrome (Table 14.6).[111] This raises the possibility that the use of CPAP from the onset of resuscitation might have beneficial effects. It is also established that CPAP can conserve surfactant (Chapter 2).

It is now possible to provide CPAP using either the Neopuff-like device or a neonatal ventilator. There are currently no published studies on this.

Although more information is required, a pragmatic approach is to commence face mask resuscitation at 30 seconds, providing the infant's heart rate is satisfactory, and to proceed to intubation at 1 minute using inflation pressures of 15–20 cmH$_2$O but, if necessary, increasing this in order to obtain visible chest wall movement. The use of drugs in infants at the extremes of viability, i.e. less than 26 weeks, remains controversial.[69]

An alternative approach has been to use nasal cannulae to inflate the lungs using an initial pressure of 20–25 cmH$_2$O, sustained for 15–20 seconds, and then provide CPAP, with pressures of 4–6 cmH$_2$O in preterm infants.[79] This is very similar to the technique recommended by Blaikley and Gibberd in 1935![10] In a study on extremely low birth weight infants using historical controls, this led to a reduction in the need for intubation and IPPV in the labor suite from 84 percent to 40 percent.[79] Significantly fewer of those receiving nasal CPAP had a severe intraventricular hemorrhage (IVH) and/or BPD and the duration of hospitalization was shorter. This study is of interest but the technique does need to be assessed in a randomized control trial.

WITHDRAWAL OF RESUSCITATION

External cardiac massage should be ceased if there is no effective cardiac output within 15 minutes, despite adequate ventilation, correction of acidosis and treatment with epinephrine. Resuscitation should also be withdrawn if, by 20 minutes of age, the infant has not made at least some gasping movements, even in the presence of a good cardiac output, as the long-term outlook is likely to be appalling.[49,68,102] Those who have made some respiratory efforts should be transferred to the neonatal unit so that decisions on further management can be made after appropriate discussion with parents.

The indications for resuscitation at the extreme of viability present particular ethical problems. Most neonatologists would not attempt intubation or external cardiac massage in infants less than 24 weeks, except in response to parental pressure. Even at 24 weeks, many consider active resuscitation is not indicated if the infant is in poor condition, with low heart rate and little if any respiratory activity.[14]

REFERENCES

1 Aizad, T., Bodani, J., Cates, D. *et al.* (1984) Effect of a single breath of 100 percent oxygen on respiration in neonates during sleep. *Journal of Applied Physiology* **57**, 1531–1535.

2 Akerren, Y., Furstenberg, N. (1950) Gastro-intestinal administration of oxygen in treatment of asphyxia in the newborn. *Journal of Obstetrics and Gynecology* **57**, 205–213.

3 Apgar, V. (1953) A proposal for a new method of evaluation of the newborn infant. *Current Research in Anaesthesia and Analgesia* **32**, 260–267.

4 Aziz, H.F., Martin, J.B., Moore, J.J. (1999) The pediatric disposable end-tidal carbon dioxide detector role in endotracheal intubation in newborns. *Journal of Perinatology* **19**, 110–113.

5 Azzopardi, D., Robertson, N.J., Cowan, F.M. *et al.* (2000) Pilot study of treatment with whole body hypothermia for neonatal encephalopathy. *Pediatrics* **106**, 684–694.

6 Battin, M.R., Dezoete, J.A., Gunn, T.R. *et al.* (2001) Neurodevelopmental outcome of infants treated with head cooling and mild hypothermia after perinatal asphyxia. *Pediatrics* **107**, 480–484.

7 Berger, R., Garnier, Y. (1999) Pathophysiology of perinatal brain damage. *Brain Research Review* **30**, 107–134.

8 Berger, R., Lehmann, T., Karcher, J. *et al.* (1998) Low dose flunarizine protects the fetal brain from ischemic injury in sheep. *Pediatric Research* **44**, 277–282.

9 Bjorklund, L.J., Curstedt, T., Ingimarsson, J. *et al.* (1996) Lung injury caused by neonatal resuscitation of immature lambs – relation to volume of lung inflations. *Pediatric Research* **39**, 326A.

10 Blaikley, L.B., Gibberd, G.F. (1935) Asphyxia neonatorum. *Lancet* **1**, 736–739.

11 Boon, A.W., Milner, A.D., Hopkin, I.E. (1979) Lung expansion, tidal volume and formation of functional residual capacity during resuscitation of asphyxiated neonates. *Journal of Pediatrics* **95**, 1031–1036.

12 Boon, A.W., Milner, A.D., Hopkin, I.E. (1979) Physiological responses of the newborn to resuscitation. *Archives of Disease in Childhood* **54**, 492–498.

13 Bowen, A., Dominquez, R. (1981) Swallowed neonatal endotracheal tube. *Pediatric Radiology* **10**, 178–179.

14 Boyle, R.J., McIntosh, N. (2001) Ethical considerations in neonatal resuscitation: clinical and research issues. *Seminars in Neonatology* **6**, 261–269.

15 Cabal, L.A., Devaskar, U., Siassi, B. *et al.* (1980) Cardiogenic shock associated with perinatal asphyxia in term infants. *Journal of Pediatrics* **96**, 705–710.

16 Carlson, B.S., Losey, R.W., Bowes, W.W., Simmons, M.A. (1976) Combined obstetric and pediatric approach to prevent meconium aspiration syndrome. *American Journal of Obstetrics and Gynecology* **126**, 712–715.

17 Chamberlain, R., Chamberlain, G., Howlett, H., Claireaux, A. (1975) *British Births 1970 The First Week of Life*, Chapter 4. London: William Heinemann Medical Books Ltd.

18 Cleary, G.M., Wiswell, T.E. (1998) Meconium-stained amniotic fluid and the meconium aspiration syndrome: an update. *Pediatric Clinics of North America* **45**, 511–529.

19 Cochrane Injuries Group Albumin Reviewers. (1998) Human albumin administration in critically ill patients: systematic review of randomised controlled trials. *British Medical Journal* **317**, 235–240.

20 Dammann, O., Alled, E., Kubar, K.C. *et al.* (2001) Hypocarbia during the first 24 postnatal hours and white matter echolucencies in newborns ⩽28 weeks gestation. *Pediatric Research* **49**, 388–393.

21 David, R. (1988) Closed chest cardiac massage in the newborn infant. *Pediatrics* **71**, 552–554.

22 Dawes, G.S. (1968) *Fetal and Neonatal Physiology*. Chicago: Year Book Medical Publishers Inc.

23 Dawes, G.S., Hibbard, E., Windle, W.F. (1964) The effect of alkali and glucose infusion on permanent brain damage in rhesus monkeys asphyxiated at birth. *Journal of Pediatrics* **65**, 801–806.

24 Doe, O.W. (1889) Apparatus for resuscitating asphyxiated children. *Boston Medical and Surgical Journal* **120**, 9–10.

25 Drew, J. (1982) Immediate intubation at birth of very low birth weight infants: effect on survival. *American Journal of Diseases of Children* **136**, 207–210.

26 Dreyfuss, D., Soler, P., Basset, G., Saumon, G. (1988) High inflation pressure pulmonary edema. Respective effects of high airway pressure, high tidal volume and positive end-expiratory pressure. *American Review of Respiratory Disease* **137**, 1159–1164.

27 du Plessis, A.J., Johnston, M.V. (1997) Hypoxic-ischemic brain injury in the newborn. Cellular mechanisms and potential strategies for neuroprotection. *Clinics in Perinatology* **24**, 627–654.

28 Dunn, P.M. (1989) Perinatal lessons from the past: Dr James Blundell (1790–1878) and neonatal resuscitation. *Archives of Disease in Childhood* **64**, 494–495.

29 Dybvik, T., Strand, T., Steen, P.A. (1995) Buffer therapy during out-of-hospital cardiopulmonary resuscitation. *Resuscitation* **29**, 89–95.

30 Ellemunter, H., Simma, B., Trawoger, R., Maurer, H. (1999) Intraosseous lines in preterm and full term neonates. *Archives of Disease in Childhood Fetal and Neonatal Edition* **80**, F74–F75.

31 Emery, E.F., Greenough, A., Gamsu, H.R. (1992) Randomized controlled trial of colloid infusions in hypotensive preterm infants. *Archives of Disease in Childhood* **67**, 1185–1188.

32 Evanson, R.T., Maunsell, H. (1842) *Practical Treatise on the Management of Children*. Dublin: Fannin and Co.

33 Faix, R.G., Viscardi, R.M., DiPietro, M.A., Nicks, J.J. (1989) Adult respiratory distress syndrome in full-term newborns. *Pediatrics* **83**, 971–976.

34 Falciglia, H.S., Henderschott, C., Potter, P., Helmchen, R. (1992) Does DeLee suction at the perineum prevent meconium aspiration syndrome? *American Journal of Obstetrics and Gynecology* **167**, 1243–1249.

35 Fedrick, J., Butler, N.R. (1971) Certain causes of neonatal death, IV. Massive pulmonary haemorrhage. *Biology of the Neonate* **18**, 243–262.

36 Fee, S.C., Malee, K., Deddish, R. *et al.* (1990) Severe acidosis and subsequent neurologic status. *American Journal of Obstetrics and Gynecology* **162**, 802–806.

37 Fellman, V., Raivio, K.O. (1997) Reperfusion injury as the mechanism of brain damage after perinatal asphyxia. *Pediatric Research* **41**, 599–606.

38 Field, D.J., Milner, A.D., Hopkin, I.E. (1986) Efficacy of manual resuscitation at birth. *Archives of Disease in Childhood* **61**, 300–302.

39 Flagg, P.J. (1928) The treatment of asphyxia in the newborn. *Journal of the American Medical Association* **91**, 788–791.

40 Friede, R.L. (1975) *Developmental Neuropathology*. New York: Springer-Verlag.

41 Fuloria, M., Wiswell, T.E. (1999) Management of meconium-stained amniotic fluid. *Clinics in Perinatology* **26**, 659–668.

42 Fuloria, M., Wiswell, T.E. (2000) Managing meconium aspiration. *Contemporary Pediatrics* **17**, 125–143.

43 Gage, J.E., Taeusch, H.W., Treves, S., Caldicot, T. (1981) Suctioning of the upper airway meconium in newborn infants. *Journal of the American Medical Association* **246**, 2590–2592.

44 Galvis, A.G., Kelley, C.F. (1979) Hypopharynx perforation during infant resuscitation. *Journal of the American Medical Association* **242**, 1526–1527.

45 Gibbs, J., Newson, T., Williams, J., Davidson, D.C. (1989) Naloxone hazard in infants of opioid abusers. *Lancet* **ii**, 159–160.

46 Goldsmith, J.P., Chen, C. (1991) Ventilatory management case book. Resuscitation in hydrops fetalis. *Journal of Perinatology* **11**, 285–289.

47 Gregory, G.A., Gooding, C.A., Phibbs, R.H., Tooley, W.H. (1974) Meconium aspiration in infants: a prospective study. *Journal of Pediatrics* **85**, 848–852.

48 Gupta, J.M., Tizard, J.P.M. (1967) The sequence of events in neonatal apnoea. *Lancet* **1**, 55–59.

49 Haddad, B., Mercer, B.M., Livingston, J.C. *et al.* (2000) Outcome after successful resuscitation of babies born with Apgar scores of 0 at both 1 and 5 minutes. *American Journal of Obstetrics and Gynecology* **182**, 1210–1214.

50 Hambleton, G., Appleyard, W.J. (1973) Controlled trial of fresh frozen plasma in asphyxiated low birthweight infants. *Archives of Disease in Childhood* **48**, 31–35.

51 Hancock, P.H., Peterson, G. (1992) Finger intubation of the trachea in newborns. *Pediatrics* **89**, 325–327.

52 Hannam, S., Ingram, D.M., Rabe-Hesketh, S., Milner, A.D. (2001) Characterisation of the Hering-Breuer deflation reflex in the human neonate. *Respiration Physiology* **124**, 51–64.

53 Head, H. (1889) On the regulation of respiration. *Journal of Physiology* **10**, 1–70.

54 Henderson, Y. (1928) The prevention and treatment of asphyxia in the newborn. *Journal of the American Medical Association* **90**, 583–586.

55 Hering, E., Breuer, J. (1868) Die selbsteurung der Amnung durch den nevus vagus sitzber. *Sitzungsbericht der Kaiserlichen Akademie der Wissenschaften in Wien* **57**, 672–677.

56 Hernandez, L.A., Peevy, K.J., Moise, A.A., Parker, J.C. (1989) Chest wall restriction limits high airway pressure-induced lung injury in young rabbits. *Journal of Applied Physiology* **66**, 2364–2368.

57 Hey, E., Lenney, W. (1973) Safe resuscitation at birth. *Lancet* **2**, 103–104.

58 Hird, M.F., Greenough, A., Gamsu, H.R. (1991) Inflating pressures for effective resuscitation of preterm infants. *Early Human Development* **26**, 69–72.

59 Hofmeyr, G.J. (2000) Amnioinfusion for meconium-stained liquor. *Current Opinion in Obstetrics and Gynecology* **12**, 129–132.

60 Hope, P.L., Costello, A.M., Cady, E.B. *et al.* (1984) Cerebral energy metabolism studied with phosphorus NMR spectroscopy in normal and birth-asphyxiated infants. *Lancet* **2**, 366–370.

61 Hoskyns, E.W., Boon, A.W., Vyas, H. *et al.* (1987) Endotracheal resuscitation of preterm infants at birth. *Archives of Disease in Childhood* **62**, 663–667.

62 Hoskyns, E.W., Milner, A.D., Hopkin, I.E. (1987) A simple method of face mask resuscitation at birth. *Archives of Disease in Childhood* **62**, 376–379.

63 Hull, D. (1969) Lung expansion and ventilation during resuscitation of asphyxiated newborn infants. *Journal of Pediatrics* **75**, 47–58.

64 Hutchinson, J.H., Kerr, M.M., Williams, K.G., Hopkinson, W.I. (1963) Hyperbaric oxygen in the resuscitation of the newborn. *Lancet* **ii**, 1019–1022.

65 Hutchison, A.A. (1987) Recovery from hypopnea in preterm lambs: effects of breathing air or oxygen. *Pediatric Pulmonology* **3**, 317–323.

66 Ingimarsson, J., Bjorklund, L.J., Curstedt, T. *et al.* (1997) Preceding surfactant treatment does not protect against lung volutrauma at birth. *Pediatric Research* **41**, 255A.

67 Ingimarsson, J., Bjorklund, L.J., Curstedt, T. *et al.* (1998) Lung trauma from five moderately large manual inflations immediately after surfactant instillation in newborn immature lambs. *Pediatric Research* **43**, 286A.

68 Jain, L., Ferre, C., Vidyasagar, D. *et al.* (1991) Cardiopulmonary resuscitation of apparently stillborn infants: survival and long term outcome. *Journal of Pediatrics* **118**, 778–782.

69 Jankov, R.P., Asztalos, E.V., Skidmore, M.B. (2000) Favourable neurological outcomes following delivery room cardiopulmonary resuscitation of infants < or = 750 g at birth. *Journal of Paediatrics and Child Health* **36**, 19–22.

70 Johnston, M.V., Trescher, W.H., Taylor, G.A. (1995) Hypoxic and ischemic central nervous system disorders in infants and children. *Advances in Pediatrics* **42**, 1–45.

71 Jonmarker, C., Olsson, A.K., Jogi, P., Forsell, C. (1996) Hemodynamic effects of tracheal and intravenous adrenaline in infants with congenital heart anomalies. *Acta Anaesthesiologica Scandinavica* **40**, 927–931.

72 Kattwinkel, J., Niermeyer, S., Nadkarni, V. *et al.* (1999) Resuscitation of the newly born infant: an advisory statement from the Pediatric Working Group of the International Liaison Committee on Resuscitation. *Resuscitation* **40**, 71–88.

73 Kette, F., Weil, M.H., von Planta, M. *et al.* (1990) Buffer agents do not reverse intramyocardial acidosis during cardiac resuscitation. *Circulation* **81**, 1660–1666.

74 Kojima, T., Kobayashi, T., Matsuzaki, S. *et al.* (1985) Effects of perinatal asphyxia and myoglobinuria on development of acute neonatal renal failure. *Archives of Disease in Childhood* **60**, 908–912.

75 Levy, M.M. (1998) An evidence-based evaluation of the use of sodium bicarbonate during cardiopulmonary resuscitation. *Critical Care Clinics* **14**, 457–483.

76 Liao, S.L., Lai, S.H., Chou, Y.H., Kuo, C.Y. (2001) Effect of hypocapnia in the first three days of life on the subsequent development of periventricular leukomalacia in premature infants. *Acta Paediatrica Taiwanica* **42**, 90–93.

77 Lindemann, R. (1984) Resuscitation of the newborn. Endotracheal administration of epinephrine. *Acta Paediatrica Scandinavica* **73**, 210–212.

78 Linder, N., Aranda, J.V., Tsur, M.N. *et al.* (1988) Need for endotracheal intubation and suction in meconium-stained neonates. *Journal of Pediatrics* **112**, 613–615.

79 Lindner, W., Vossbeck, S., Hummler, H., Pohlandt, F. (1999) Delivery room management of extremely low birthweight infants: spontaneous breathing or intubation? *Pediatrics* **103**, 961–967.

80 Lou, H.C., Lassen, N.A., Friis-Hansen, B. (1978) Decreased cerebral blood flow after administration of sodium bicarbonate in the distressed newborn infant. *Acta Neurologica Scandinavica* **57**, 239–247.

81 Low, J.A., Pickersgill, H., Killen, H., Derrick, E.J. (2001) The prediction and prevention of intrapartum fetal asphyxia in term pregnancies. *American Journal of Obstetrics and Gynecology* **194**, 724–730.

82 Milner, A.D., Saunders, R.A. (1977) Pressure and volume changes during the first breath of human neonates. *Archives of Disease in Childhood* **52**, 918–924.

83 Milner, A.D., Vyas, M. (1985) Resuscitation of the newborn. In Milner, A.D., Martin, R.J. (eds), *Neonatal and Pediatric Respiratory Medicine*. London: Butterworths, 16.

84 Moster, D., Lie, R.T., Irgens, L.M. *et al.* (2001) The association of Apgar score with subsequent death and cerebral palsy: a population-based study in term infants. *Journal of Pediatrics* **138**, 791–792.

85 Niermeyer, S., Kattwinkel, J., Van Reempts, P. *et al.* (2000) International guidelines for neonatal resuscitation: an excerpt from the Guidelines 2000 for cardiopulmonary resuscitation and emergency cardiovascular care: International consensus on science. Contributors and Reviewers for the Neonatal Resuscitation Guidelines. *Pediatrics* **106**, E29.

86 Palme, C., Nystrom, B., Tunell, R. (1985) An evaluation of the efficiency of face masks in the resuscitation of newborn infants. *Lancet* **i**, 207–210.

87 Palme-Kilander, C. (1992) Methods of resuscitation in low Apgar score newborn infants – a national survey. *Acta Paediatrica* **81**, 739–744.

88 Palme-Kilander, C., Tunell, R. (1998) Pulmonary gas exchange during facemask ventilation immediately after birth. *Archives of Disease in Childhood* **68**, 11–16.

89 Parer, J.T., King, T. (2000) Fetal heart rate monitoring: is it salvageable? *American Journal of Obstetrics and Gynecology* **182**, 982–987.

90 Phillips, G.W., Zideman, D.A. (1986) Relationship of infant heart to sternum: its significance in cardiopulmonary resuscitation. *Lancet* **1**, 1024–1025.

91 Primhak, R.A., Herber, S.M., Whincup, G., Milner, R.D.G. (1984) Which deliveries require paediatricians in attendance? *British Medical Journal* **289**, 16–18.

92 Ramji, S., Ahuja, S., Thirupuram, S. *et al.* (1993) Resuscitation of asphyxic newborn infants with room air or 100 percent oxygen. *Pediatric Research* **34**, 809–812.

93 Rootwelt, T., Loberg, M., Moen, A. *et al.* (1992) Hypoxemia and reoxygenation with 21 percent or 100 percent oxygen in newborn pigs. Changes in blood pressure, base deficit and hypoxanthine and brain morphology. *Pediatric Research* **32**, 107–113.

94 Rosen, M., Laurence, K.M. (1965) Expansion pressure and rupture pressure in the newborn lung. *Lancet* **2**, 721–722.

95 Royal Humane Society Animal Report. 1812.

96 Russ, J.D., Strong, R.A. (1941) Resuscitation of the asphyxiated newborn infant. *American Journal of Diseases of Children* **61**, 1–12.

97 Ryder, R.W., Shelton, J.D., Guinan, M.E., The Committee on Necrotizing Enterocolitis. (1980) Necrotizing enterocolitis. A prospective multicenter investigation. *American Journal of Epidemiology* **112**, 113–124.

98 Sarmat, H.B., Sarmat, M.S. (1976) Neonatal encephalopathy following fetal distress. *Archives of Neurology* **33**, 696–705.

99 Saugstad, O.D., Rootwelt, T., Aalen, O. (1998) Resuscitation of asphyxiated newborn infants with room air or oxygen: an international controlled trial: the Resair 2 Study. *Pediatrics* **102**, e1.

100 Saunders, R.A., Milner, A.D. (1978) Pulmonary pressure/volume relationships during the last phase of delivery and their first postnatal breaths in human subjects. *Journal of Pediatrics* **93**, 667–673.

101 Scopes, J.W., Ahmed, I. (1966) Minimal rates of oxygen consumption in sick and premature newborn infants. *Archives of Disease in Childhood* **41**, 407–416.

102 Scott, H.M. (1976) Outcome of very severe birth asphyxia. *Archives of Disease in Childhood* **51**, 712–716.

103 Shelley, H.J. (1961) Glycogen reserves and their changes at birth and in anoxia. *British Medical Bulletin* **17**, 137–143.

104 Simmons, M.A., Adcock, E.W.I., Bard, H., Battaglia, F.C. (1974) Hypernatremia and intracranial hemorrhage in neonates. *New England Journal of Medicine* **291**, 6–10.

105 Skillman, C.A., Plessinger, M.A., Woods, J.R., Clark, K.E. (1985) Effect of graded reductions in uteroplacental blood flow in the fetal lamb. *American Journal of Physiology* **249H**, 1098–1105.

106 Stoddard, R.A., Clark, S.L., Minton, S.D. (1988) In utero ischemic injury: sonographic diagnosis and medicolegal implications. *American Journal of Obstetrics and Gynecology* **159**, 23–25.

107 Tapia-Rombo, C.A., Carpio-Hernandez, J.C., Salazar-Acuna, A.H. *et al.* (2000) Detection of transitory myocardial ischemia secondary to perinatal asphyxia. *Archives of Medical Research* **31**, 377–383.

108 Temesvari, P., Karg, E., Bodi, I. *et al.* (2001) Impaired early neurologic outcome in newborn piglets reoxygenated with 100 percent oxygen compared with room air after pneumothorax-induced asphyxia. *Pediatric Research* **49**, 812–819.

109 Thibeault, D.W., Hobel, C.J. (1974) The interrelationship of the foam stability test, immaturity and intrapartum complications in the respiratory distress syndrome. *American Journal of Obstetrics and Gynecology* **118**, 56–61.

110 Topsis, J., Kinas, H.Y., Kandall, S.R. (1989) Esophageal perforation – a complication of neonatal resuscitation. *Anesthesia and Analgesia* **69**, 532–534.

111 Upton, C., Milner, A.D. (1991) Endotracheal resuscitation of neonates using a rebreathing bag. *Archives of Disease in Childhood* **66**, 39–42.

112 van Bel, F., Shadid, M., Moison, R.M.W. *et al.* (1998) Effect of allopurinol on postasphyxial free radical formation, cerebral hemodymanics and electrical brain activity. *Pediatrics* **101**, 185–193.

113 Vento, M., Asensi, M., Sastre, J. *et al.* (2001) Resuscitation with room air instead of 100 percent oxygen prevents oxidative stress in moderately asphyxiated term neonates. *Pediatrics* **107**, 642–647.

114 Vyas, H., Milner, A.D., Hopkin, I.E., Boon, A.W. (1981) Physiological responses to prolonged and slow rise inflation. *Journal of Pediatrics* **99**, 635–639.

115 Vyas, H., Milner, A.D., Hopkin, I.E. (1983) Face mask resuscitation: does it lead to gastric distension? *Archives of Disease in Childhood* **58**, 373–375.

116 Vyas, H., Milner, A.D., Hopkin, I.E. (1984) Efficacy of face mask resuscitation at birth. *British Medical Journal* **289**, 1563–1565.

117 Vyas, H., Field, D., Milner, A.D., Hopkin, I.E. (1986) Determinants of the first inspiratory volume and functional residual capacity at birth. *Pediatric Pulmonology* **2**, 189–193.

118 Wada, K., Jobe, A.H., Ikegami, M. (1997) Tidal volume effects on surfactant treatment responses with the initiation of ventilation in preterm lambs. *Journal of Applied Physiology* **83**, 1054–1061.

119 Wenzel, V., Prengel, A.W., Linder, K.H. (2000) A strategy to improve endobronchial drug administration (editorial; comment). *Anesthesia and Analgesia* **91**, 255–256.

120 Wiswell, T.E. (2001) Handling the meconium-stained infant. *Seminars in Neonatology* **6**, 225–231.

15

Respiratory support

ANNE GREENOUGH, including 'Proportional Assist Ventilation' by ANDREAS SCHULZE and 'Liquid Ventilation' by THOMAS H. SHAFFER and MARLA R. WOLFSON

OXYGEN ADMINISTRATION

Techniques

HEADBOX

If the infant requires a very modest increase in the inspired oxygen concentration (≤25 percent), this can be achieved by administering the oxygen-rich inspired gas into the incubator. In practice, however, every time the incubator portholes are opened there will be a sudden drop in the oxygen concentration. If the infant requires an increased inspired oxygen fraction, >0.25, the oxygen should be given into a perspex box placed over the baby's head and shoulders (headbox). The oxygen concentration should be continuously monitored by an analyzer placed near the baby's mouth. The oxygen should be humidified.

NASAL CANNULAE

Nasal cannulae are frequently used to deliver supplementary oxygen to infants who have chronic lung disease (CLD). This may be administered via a purpose built double cannula system or an 8 FG feeding catheter cut to length, which is inserted 2–3 cm into one nostril. The advantages of administering oxygen via nasal cannula rather than into a headbox are that the infant has greater mobility and there is greater access to the infant. This improved access is particularly important for older infants in whom developmental stimulation must be considered (p. 413).

Nasal cannula gas flow can cause changes in respiration due in part to the generation of positive end expiratory pressure (PEEP).[275] Although nasal cannula with an outside diameter of 0.2 cm did not deliver pressure or alter thoracoabdominal motion, a 0.3 cm diameter cannula did deliver PEEP, at a magnitude which was related to the gas flow rate.[275] This could, on occasions, be put to advantage as use of the larger cannulae was associated with a reduction in thoracoabdominal motion asynchrony. It does, however, mean that changes in the systems used to deliver oxygen should be made with caution, as they could be associated with alterations in clinical status.

Complications

Administration of oxygen through a nasopharyngeal catheter has been associated with the development of subcutaneous emphysema and pneumoperitoneum via gastric rupture.[85] The latter complication can be prevented by avoiding excessive advancement of the catheter, correct fixation of the catheter to the nostril to prevent accidental displacement and restricting the flow rate.

PERCUTANEOUS

The skin of a very premature infant is extremely thin. As a consequence, oxygen can be absorbed through the skin if the baby is kept in a high oxygen environment. A mean increase in PaO_2 of 1.2 kPa is achieved when babies are nursed in 95 percent oxygen rather than air in their incubators.[64]

CONTINUOUS POSITIVE AIRWAYS PRESSURE (CPAP)

Techniques

CPAP was originally given via an endotracheal tube.[199,451] Later it was applied via a Gregory headbox or a face chamber. CPAP may also be delivered into a face mask,[8] via a tube into one nostril,[47] a pair of tubes inserted into both nostrils or a binasal tube.[5,242] These latter devices can be connected via a T-piece circuit to a standard neonatal ventilator or specific device.[35,52] Either system gives gas mixing, pressure setting and humidification facilities. Endotracheal CPAP can be delivered using an underwater seal. If bubbling is vigorous then infants may experience vibration of their chest at frequencies similar to those experienced during high-frequency oscillation ventilation (HFOV) (p. 172). In one small randomized crossover study involving infants ready for extubation,[267] 'bubble CPAP' was associated with a significant reduction in minute volume yet maintenance of gas exchange, suggesting the chest vibrations may have contributed to gas exchange.

The technique via which the CPAP is applied may alter its efficacy. Goldman et al.[170] reported an almost 100 percent increase in the work of breathing with nasal CPAP compared to face mask CPAP. This adverse effect was attributed to flow resistance within the nasal attachment. Further disadvantages of nasal CPAP systems are that there may be the leakage of breathing gas either from the attachment or through the patient's mouth.[259,294] This latter problem may be overcome in nose breathing babies who are said to shut the pharynx so that no air comes out through the mouth.[83] In view of the above limitations, alternative nasal CPAP delivery systems have been developed. One such system[295] consists of two separated jets which are directed towards the nasal openings and through which the humidified air oxygen mixture is delivered. It contains no mechanical valves and the expiratory limb is open to ambient air. A continuous flow rate of breathing gas of approximately 5–11 l/min generates a CPAP of 2–10 cmH_2O.

There have been few studies in which methods of CPAP delivery have been compared. Post-extubation, a binasal system [Infant Flow Driver (IFD), EME Ltd, Brighton UK] was not shown to have advantages over a single nasal prong and ventilator in a non-randomized study involving preterm infants.[245] Significant reductions in supplementary oxygen were only seen amongst those supported by the single prong system and four infants supported by the IFD became hyperoxic.[245] The IFD has been shown to deliver 2 percent more oxygen than a single nasal prong and ventilator system.[6] Comparison of continuous flow nasal CPAP via CPAP prongs, continuous flow nasal CPAP via modified nasal cannulae and variable flow nasal CPAP, however, demonstrated that lung recruitment was greater with the variable flow nasal CPAP system.[98] In addition, others demonstrated that the work of breathing was decreased by the variable flow nasal CPAP.[310] In infants with mild disease, the possibility of lung overdistention at CPAP levels greater than 6 cmH_2O with the variable flow device, however, was highlighted. The positive benefits of the variable flow device may be due to gas entrainment by the high velocity jet flows, the less variable CPAP level and better prong design. By contrast, gas flow continues towards the nares during exhalation when constant flow nCPAP is used and the patient must overcome this excessive flow, leading to increased expiratory work. Variable flow nCPAP may improve extubation success.[400]

Level of CPAP

Caution should be used regarding the level of pressure used, as if this is too high both circulatory and ventilatory function can be severely compromised. Relatively mature infants with respiratory distress syndrome (RDS) may need up to 6–8 cmH_2O of CPAP. Infants in the recovery stage of RDS, particularly those less than 28 weeks of gestation will often tolerate only 2–3 cmH_2O of CPAP, higher levels causing CO_2 retention. As such infants have relatively compliant lungs, the probable mechanism is via lung overdistention. It has been suggested that the most appropriate CPAP level may be indicated by results from esophageal balloon pressure measurements,[401] the optimal pressure being 1–2 cmH_2O lower than the pressure at which there is a sudden step up in the applied pressure sensed by the balloon. In practice, little applied pressure is transmitted in infants with stiff lungs,[180] but is transmitted in healthy infants.[292] CPAP was shown to reduce dynamic compliance by one-third in 12 healthy newborns; approximately 50 percent of the distending pressure was transmitted to their mediastinal structures[292] Pressures generated during bi- and oronasal CPAP are similarly delivered to the oropharynx, but neither mode resulted in pressure generation to the thorax.[315]

Clinical studies

Early studies[204,451] in relatively mature infants (mean gestation 33 weeks) with RDS demonstrated that endotracheal CPAP could improve oxygenation without adversely affecting $PaCO_2$ or blood pressure. The respiratory rate decreased resulting in a lowered minute ventilation. The reduction in respiratory rate is primarily due to a prolongation of expiratory time.[129] CPAP administration was also noted to stabilize the rib cage, reduce chest wall distortion during inspiration and consequently increase the efficiency of the diaphragm.[379] In infants with respiratory insufficiency, CPAP reduced the relative paradoxical motion of the rib cage, that is, prevented the rib cage collapsing inward instead of expanding outward early in inspiration – suggesting enhanced chest wall stability.[274] CPAP applied via a face mask in healthy premature infants reduced total pulmonary resistance; 60 percent of this change was due to a reduction in total supraglottic resistance. It is speculated that this may occur directly through mechanical splinting of the airway (see below).

APNEA

nCPAP abolishes obstructive and mixed apnea, but not central apnea (p. 431).[290] It may act by distending and maintaining the upper airway rather than by a direct effect on respiratory drive (p. 431).

EARLY nCPAP

Introduction of early nCPAP has been associated in non-randomized studies with a significant reduction in the requirement for intubation and ventilation[166,235,291,324] and the incidence of CLD.[17,243] A retrospective review of the outcome of 1625 infants cared for in eight centers highlighted that the center which instituted CPAP soon after birth had the lowest CLD incidence.[17] Other practices in that institution, however, differed from those in the other centers and included avoidance of both hyperventilation and use of muscle relaxants; in addition, permissive hypercapnia was practised. The timing of starting CPAP is debated. Although CPAP is started in the labor ward in some centers, in a randomized trial,[203] infants who received CPAP from birth were significantly worse at 48 hours than those who were given CPAP only when the PaO_2 was below 6 kPa in an FiO_2 of 0.50. The results of two randomized studies have indicated that if early CPAP is used surfactant should also be given[427] and surfactant administered early rather than once infants have developed moderate to severe disease.[428] A higher arterial to alveolar oxygen tension and reduced subsequent need for ventilation (43 versus 85 percent) was experienced when surfactant was given with CPAP compared to when CPAP was used alone.[427] Early rather than late surfactant administration was associated with fewer infants (21 percent versus 63 percent) requiring mechanical ventilation or dying within 7 days.[428] Clearly a large prospective randomized trial comparing use of early CPAP to intermittent positive pressure ventilation (IPPV) with long-term outcomes is needed. Clinicians using early CPAP, however, have felt it would be difficult to get acceptance for such a study, as the so-called soft approach has been linked in certain centers to a major emphasis on early parental involvement in the practical case of babies.[278] Nevertheless, a randomized trial has been performed to compare the efficacy of early nCPAP with prophylactic surfactant early nCPAP with or without rescue surfactant, early mechanical ventilation with prophylactic surfactant and conventional management (defined as ventilation with or without rescue surfactant).[415] The time to wean was significantly shorter in infants randomized to early nCPAP with or without rescue surfactant compared to early nCPAP with prophylactic surfactant. No other significant differences between the four groups, however, were noted, but only 237 infants were recruited into the trial.

EXTUBATION

Different conclusions have been drawn from at least eight randomized trials assessing whether CPAP facilitates extubation. Meta-analysis of the results of those trials, which included in total 569 infants, demonstrated use of nCPAP reduced the need for increased respiratory support (relative risk 0.57, 95 percent CI 0.43–0.73). The need for re-intubation, however, was not significantly reduced (relative risk 0.89, 95 percent CI 0.68–1.17). Nasal CPAP did not significantly influence the intraventricular hemorrhage rate, reported in four studies (relative risk 1.0, 95 percent CI 0.55–1.82) nor of oxygen dependency at 28 days reported in six studies (relative risk 1.0, 95 percent CI 0.8, 1.25).[117] Adverse effects were commented on in very few of the trials. It should be noted that in the trials which were systematically reviewed, CPAP was delivered by a variety of methods which may have influenced the results. An earlier meta-analysis had demonstrated nCPAP reduced oxygen dependency at 28 days.[106] Two trials subsequently reported, however, demonstrated a trend for use of nCPAP to increase oxygen dependency. That result reversal, as further small studies were added to the meta-analysis, stresses the superiority of information obtained from one large well-designed multicenter randomized trial.

UPPER AIRWAYS OBSTRUCTION

CPAP is of value in infants with upper airways obstruction, as occurs in infants with Pierre Robin syndrome or in infants with stridor due to a congenital abnormality or laryngeal damage following ventilation. In these situations the tip of the nasopharyngeal CPAP tube should pass through the posterior choanae into the upper pharynx.[207]

Adverse effects

Face mask CPAP is associated with the highest rate of complications of any of the CPAP techniques.[198] The face mask must be tightly applied to prevent gas leaks, and to achieve and maintain the desired CPAP level. Unfortunately, this requires tight strapping around the baby's head which can cause distortion, pressure necrosis and intracerebral or cerebellar hemorrhage.[311] Use of a naso-gastric tube is contraindicated as this will break the seal of the face mask. Stomach distention can occur and, of course, there is limited access to the baby's nose and mouth. CPAP applied via the nose can result in inflammation or pressure erosion of the septum by the prong(s) although pressure lesions of the nasal septum have been described following use of the Argyle's silastic binasal tube.[242] Use of short prongs held in place with straps which pass around the head has also been associated with cosmetic deformities.[345] In 6 months, nasal trauma was documented in seven infants (a 20 percent complication rate in the VLBW infants so supported); this included columella nasi necrosis, which occurred within 3 days, flaring of the nostrils which worsened within the duration of CPAP and snubbing of the nose which persisted after prolonged use of CPAP.[345] The trauma resulted from the shape of the prong, which was reported not to be anatomical[345] and the base not allowing for projection of the columella beyond the alar rim. The prongs were perpendicular to the base, not converging as the baby's nasal passages do and the base of the prongs were closest together where the columella was widest. It was suggested that a curved design with tapering prongs would be more suitable.[345] Other recommendations to avoid nasal trauma include ensuring appropriate fit of the prongs, tying the hats to the prongs more horizontally to prevent upward pull on the nose and supporting the weight of the tubing. In addition, the nose should be rested for half an hour every 4–6 hours,[345] although such a policy may be impractical in a CPAP-dependent infant.

Rhodes et al.[339] claimed CPAP reduced both pneumothorax and BPD, but pneumothoraces do occur on CPAP,[242] 10 percent of infants so treated developing air leaks in an early series.[204] Bilateral pneumothoraces in association with extensive vascular embolus have been described, albeit rarely.[444] Application of CPAP can also result in gaseous distension of the bowel and, although this has not been associated with necrotizing enterocolitis (NEC) or bowel obstruction, it can necessitate withholding of feeds.

VENTILATORY MODES DELIVERED BY NASAL PRONGS

Nasal prong IPPV

Nasal prong IPPV (nIPPV) has been used as an alternative strategy to nCPAP to provide ventilatory support in VLBW infants and to reduce apnea.[271,297,350] In apneic infants it may improve the patency of the upper airway by creating intermittently elevated pharyngeal pressures, and by intermittent inflation of the pharynx it could activate respiratory drive.[298] A high frequency of sighs in preterm infants receiving nIPPV for prevention of apneic

spells has been observed.[271] nIPPV has not always been helpful in the post-extubation period,[350] perhaps because of poor transmission of gases through the airways in asynchronous infants.[298] nIPPV is more effective when the ventilator rate is adjusted to be similar to the patient's spontaneous rate.[297] Meta-analysis of two trials comparing nIPPV and nCPAP in apneic infants demonstrated no difference between the groups with regard to their carbon dioxide levels after 4–6 hours of support.[270] No data were given in either trial on gastrointestinal complications; this is surprising as, in an earlier study,[155] a 30-fold increased risk of developing gastric or intestinal perforation was reported in infants treated with cyclic ventilation by nasal prongs rather than ventilation via an endotracheal tube.

Nasal prong SIMV/SIPPV

Thoracoabdominal asynchrony, which occurs because of the negative intrapleural pressure changes transmitted to the highly compliant chest wall of a preterm infant, has been suggested to be more effectively reduced by nSIMV rather than nCPAP, perhaps by better stabilization of the chest wall.[253] In a randomized trial involving 41 infants,[150] respiratory failure developing post-extubation was significantly lower amongst infants supported by nSIMV rather than nCPAP (5 percent versus 37 percent), but a variety of definitions of respiratory failure were used. The ventilator used was triggered from outward movements of the abdomen detected by an abdominal pressure capsule (Graseby Dynamics Inc, Herts, UK). Others have used a commercial time-cycled pressure-limited neonatal ventilator (MOG 2000, Gineviri), which detects the inspiratory effort of the infant by means of a hot wire anemometer flow sensor. The Ginevri MOG 2000 is supplied by an electronic device that analyses the signal coming from the flow sensor. The continuous component of the flow signal due to leaks from the mouth and the nostrils is eliminated while the variation of the signal deriving from the patient's inspiration is used to trigger the ventilator.[298] Using this device, nSIPPV compared to nCPAP was associated with a significant reduction in the patient's respiratory efforts,[298] which perhaps explains the lower rate of respiratory failure in the nSIPPV group of the randomized study.[150] Nevertheless, very few patients were studied and whether nSIPPV using such a system will be feasible in all preterm infants remains untested. Relatively few side-effects of nSIPPV/SIMV have been reported and include non-significant abdominal distention and self-resolving epistaxis. Nevertheless, the small number of infants included in randomized trials and the important theoretical adverse consequences of administration of high inspiratory pressures at the level of the nasopharynx highlight that an appropriately sized study with long-term outcomes should be undertaken.

Nasal prong HFOV (nHFOV)

Use of nHFOV has been associated with a reduction in carbon dioxide levels in infants with a moderate respiratory acidosis on nCPAP,[423] even in those born as early as 24 weeks of gestational age.[223] In one series, however, five of 21 infants supported by nHFOV had to be intubated after a median of 6.5 hours, because of carbon dioxide retention and a high oxygen requirement.[423] Further studies, which include a randomized comparator group, are required to determine the merits of this nasal ventilatory mode.

CONTINUOUS NEGATIVE EXTRATHORACIC PRESSURE (CNEP)

Intermittent negative pressure ventilation for neonates was first introduced in the 1960s. CNEP was later delivered by a modification of the Ohio Air Shields Isolette.[429] Its primary application was for larger infants (birthweight 1500 g and gestational age 32 weeks) with uncomplicated RDS in whom it reduced morbidity and mortality.[18,395] It was suggested that CNEP was likely to be useful for infants with conditions characterized by a reduced tidal volume and functional residual capacity (FRC).[81] Complications, however, limited its acceptability and until the late 1980s positive pressure ventilation was the mainstay of neonatal respiratory support.

Techniques

To apply CNEP using the Air Shields Isolette, the Isolette was first warmed and the infant's torso placed inside the negative pressure chamber. The infant's head was then delivered through the iris-type diaphragm into the head chamber; all lines, wires and tubing being passed through the side portholes. When the diaphragm, side portholes and end door were closed, this isolated the infant's torso in an airtight negative pressure chamber. The built-in vacuum pump then generated a CNEP of between 4 and 10 cmH_2O. At the initiation of CNEP, the ventilatory pressures sometimes remained constant or were reduced by an amount equal to the applied negative pressure.[100] Samuels and Southall[353] developed a CNEP system chamber, consisting of a perspex lid hinged to one side of an aluminum base with a rubber seal around its edge. The neck seal was achieved using a rectangular sheet of latex, in which a hole was cut with an area about two-thirds of the neck. The elasticity of the neck seal allowed it to be stretched over the infant's head. Problems with the seal were further avoided by putting a double thickness elasticated tubular stockinette around the infant's neck. Three sizes of chambers were available depending on the infant's weight and accommodated those less than 4 kg, 3–8 kg

or 5–20 kg. The smallest neonatal chamber was used on a modified incubator base, which provides circulation of warmed air, servocontrolled to the ambient air temperature within the chamber. CNEP of between −6 and −10 cmH_2O can be instituted over several seconds. In patients already receiving positive pressure ventilation the peak and end expiratory pressures are reduced by the magnitude of the negative pressure used. To remove the patients from the chamber, the negative pressure was tailed off slowly over 5–15 minutes to avoid a sudden fall in lung volume. Full nursing care and physiotherapy can be performed while the negative pressure was maintained for the sickest patients.[353] After extubation, Samuels and Southall kept their patients in the CNEP chamber for a minimum of 24 hours and, as their condition improved, increasingly longer times were spent out of the chamber. Treatment was discontinued when no change was noted in the inspired oxygen concentration with or without CNEP.

Clinical studies

CONTINUOUS NEGATIVE EXTRATHORACIC PRESSURE

Outerbridge et al.[308] described use of CNEP (4–8 cmH_2O) in 14 infants with severe RDS. On transfer to CNEP their PaO_2 rose significantly by a mean of 23 mmHg and their alveolar-arterial oxygen differene ($AaDO_2$) fell by a mean of 34.8 mmHg; the least impressive results were obtained in infants with meconium aspiration syndrome. Only four infants, however, could be supported throughout their illness by CNEP only. Eight of the remaining 10 survived, but additional use of conventional respiratory management was required. No complications were experienced, in particular no hypothermia, but it should be noted the infants were relatively mature, being between 30 and 37 weeks of gestational age.

In a randomized trial,[354] infants from 4 hours of age received either standard neonatal intensive care or CNEP (−4 to −6 cmH_2O) applied within a purpose-designed neonatal incubator. Two hundred and forty-four patients [mean gestational age (GA) 30.4 ± 3.5 weeks] were recruited. Use of CNEP was associated with a lower duration of oxygen therapy (18.3 versus 33.6 days). There were, however, trends towards an increase in mortality and cranial ultrasound abnormalities in the CNEP group, although these did not reach statistical significance.[354]

CNEP AND INTERMITTENT MANDATORY VENTILATION (IMV)

CNEP together with IMV improved oxygenation in infants with persistent pulmonary hypertension of the newborn (PPHN) whose $AaDO_2$ was sufficiently high to qualify them for extracorporeal membrane oxygenation (ECMO).

Sills et al.[383] reported five such infants survived without pulmonary or neurological complications. In 12 preterm infants with severe pulmonary interstitial emphysema (PIE), oxygenation also improved on introduction of CNEP. The infants were started on CNEP when they failed to achieve a PaO_2 of 50 mmHg in an FiO_2 of 1.0. Only six infants, however, ultimately survived, but in four of six survivors there was radiographic resolution of the PIE.[101] Cvetnic et al.[102] subsequently reported their experience of CNEP with IMV in 37 infants with a variety of diagnoses including PIE, RDS, PPHN and meconium aspiration syndrome. All had failed to achieve a PaO_2 of 50 mmHg on IMV alone. No significant change in pH or $PaCO_2$ occurred. Although all the infants experienced an improvement in oxygenation on transfer to CNEP, the response was best in the 'non-meconium aspiration syndrome' PPHN group. It was possible over the subsequent 72 hours of ventilation to maintain oxygenation despite a reduction in mean airway pressure (MAP). Samuels and Southall[353] reported use of CNEP with or without IMV in a group of 88 infants and young children suffering from a variety of diagnoses, which included BPD and RDS. In 75 infants it was possible to reduce the inspired oxygen concentration by a median of 15 percent (range 4–40 percent) 2 hours after starting treatment. In 29 infants $PaCO_2$ was measured, in 21 there was an improvement and in only eight an increase. CNEP support was required from between 2 and 236 days. The final outcome, however, was variable; extubation was facilitated in 28 patients, but 34 died.

Adverse effects

Early attempts at CNEP were poorly tolerated by infants of birthweight less than 1000 g. There were technical limitations in securing the infant within the device and hypothermia resulted from convective heat loss around the head and neck. Another concern was impedance of venous return from the head resulting in intraventricular hemorrhage (IVH). Postmortem data, however, failed to demonstrate a significant difference in the incidence of IVH in infants treated with CNEP, no ventilation or positive pressure ventilation.[273,385,397] A study of 10 patients aged between 2 and 36 months of age, seven of whom had BPD, demonstrated no significant changes in heart rate, oxygen saturation, transcutaneous carbon dioxide or cardiac output on commencing CNEP.[331] In acute lung injury induced by saline lavage, CNEP has been shown to have similar effects to equivalent levels of PEEP on dynamic lung compliance, lung resistance, end expiratory lung volume, blood gases, pulmonary and systemic vascular resistance and cardiac output.[130] CNEP has not been shown to have an adverse effect on respiratory function when given at less than 6 cmH_2O. In prematurely born infants studied when breathing room air, application of CNEP resulted in a reduction in respiratory rate, due to a prolongation of expiratory time. Compliance improved in the infants with low baseline values but not in those with normal lung function; there were no consistent changes in respiratory system resistance.[153]

INTUBATION

The infant should be lying flat with the neck only slightly extended; it is unnecessary to incline the infant to the horizontal as on a resuscitaire. A straight bladed laryngoscope with a C cross-section should be used, as the top of the 'C' prevents the soft tissues falling onto the bottom part of the blade, obscuring the view of the larynx. The tip of the blade is placed in the cavity between the back of the tongue and the anterior surface of the epiglottis (vallecula); it is then tilted upwards; this both keeps the tongue out of the way and pulls the larynx forwards. If the larynx fails to come into view, gentle pressure should be put over the cricoid cartilage. During nasal intubation, the process is similar except that the tube should be placed in the nostril and advanced until the tip can be seen in the back of the pharynx with the laryngoscope in place. The tip is then grasped by Magill's forceps and the tube inserted through the cords. Whether the infant is intubated orally or nasally, the tube should be positioned through the vocal cords when they are abducted in inspiration. The tip should lie 0.5–1.0 cm proximal to the carina. This positioning allows for flexion or extension of the infant's head and avoids intubation of either bronchus (p. 321).

Some authorities recommend intubation should only be performed immediately after the infant has received atropine and pancuronium.[248] During intubation, catecholamine levels increase,[269,382] and this can be associated with elevation of blood pressure and intracranial pressure.[333] Prior treatment with pancuronium and atropine significantly reduced the rise in catecholamine levels and so may avoid some of the adverse effects of intubation.[248] The disadvantage of paralyzing an infant prior to intubation is that the infant is then without respiratory effort and intubation may not be successfully accomplished. We, therefore, prefer to sedate infants for a non-emergency tube change (p. 208). 'Elective' changing of an endotracheal tube is unnecessary providing adequate humidification and suction is practised (p. 263) and should be avoided because of the complications of intubation. The signal for an endotracheal tube change is the signs of obstruction.

Endotracheal tube shape and size

Cuffed tubes are not used in neonates, but 'hi-lo' tubes (p. 170) are needed with some types of jet ventilation. There has been considerable debate regarding whether straight or shouldered endotracheal tubes should be used.

Shouldered tubes may be easier to fixate because of their greater relative width at the mouth, but it has been claimed that they are more likely to cause subglottic stenosis. In a retrospective review of the incidence of subglottic stenosis in the four metropolitan regions, there was no significant difference in the incidence of subglottic stenosis between neonatal intensive care units which used straight or shouldered endotracheal tubes (Rivers *et al.*, unpublished data). Nevertheless, impaction of the shouldered part of the endotracheal tube onto the cricoid ring could lead to pressure necrosis in the subglottic region.[262,329] Impaction of the endotracheal tube can be avoided if the tip of the endotracheal tube is positioned so that it lies at or above the level of the clavicles on the chest radiograph. It should be remembered, however, that neck position can affect the position of the tip of the endotracheal tube.[305,347] The endotracheal tube moves caudal with neck flexion and cephalad with neck extension; mean displacements 3.1 and 7.4 mm, respectively, in one series of low birthweight infants[347] and 1.8 and 3.5 cm in a series of term infants.[305]

Although it is common practice to ventilate children and adults with a leak between the endotracheal tube and tracheal wall, in neonates, particularly in the acute stage of the illness, this is not done. This would require use of a small tube and if an endotracheal tube is employed with an internal diameter less than 2.5 mm, suction is impossible. In addition, if a leak is present, it is not possible to achieve pressures greater than 25–30 cmH$_2$O which are necessary to ventilate very stiff lungs. This means at least a 3.0 mm tube is needed and in a very small baby this can only be accommodated without a leak. After a period of ventilation, tracheal dilation can occur,[41] then an even larger tube will be necessary. A further reason to use a 'large' tube is that inspiratory and expiratory resistances are significantly affected by tube size. The calculated mean difference in expiratory resistance between endotracheal tubes of 2.5 and 3.5 mm internal diameter was 93 cmH$_2$O/l/s.[135] The resistance of the endotracheal tube adds to the inspiratory work of breathing. Additional work is a function of the tube's size, each 1 mm decrease in diameter leading to a 67–100 percent increase in work when measured in endotracheal tubes used to support adults.[137] Measurement of resistance of straight endotracheal tubes, internal diameters (IDs) between 2.5 and 6 mm and shouldered (Coles) tubes, ID/outside diameter (OD) between 2.5/4 and 3.5/4 mm, demonstrated resistance increased as endotracheal tube diameter decreased. At flows of 5 l/min the resistance of the 6 mm ID endotracheal tube was 4.6 cmH$_2$O/l/s and for the 2.5 mm ID endotracheal tube was 92 cmH$_2$O/l/s. Shortening an endotracheal tube to a length appropriate for patient use (for example a 4.0 mm ID from 20.7 to 11.3 cm) reduced its resistance on average by 22 percent. The resistance of a Coles tube was approximately 50 percent lower than that of a straight tube with an ID corresponding to the narrow part of the shouldered tube.[282] The additional work of breathing can be overcome by sufficient amount of pressure support.

Oral or nasal intubation

Nasal endotracheal tubes, once in place, can be fixed rigidly to the baby's face, which might reduce the incidence of subglottic stenosis.[262] Nasal intubation, however, has been suggested to be a risk factor for bacteremia[123] and can lead to ulceration and excoriation of the nostrils. At follow-up, notches in the alae of the nose and damage to the nasal septum have been described in infants who had undergone nasal intubation.[149] Oral tubes are generally thought easier to insert, but can be harder to stabilize. Infants may suck and swallow on an oral endotracheal tube. At follow-up, high palatal arches, narrow pressure-induced grooves or clefts in the palate,[279] and damage to the alveolar ridge leading to dentition problems have been described.[149]

Methods of securing endotracheal tubes in neonates

A variety of methods have been used to secure endotracheal tubes. These include use of adhesive tape which is stuck round the endotracheal tube and the infant's upper lip or an H-shaped piece of zinc oxide tape to stabilize the tube. Purpose-made devices include a flange which is tied or sewn to the endotracheal tube and then the flange tied on either side of a bonnet. A Logan bow (or nucal device) can be used;[55] an adhesive head sling is employed to anchor the device and an oral endotracheal tube. In one series,[432] the average accidental extubation rate was six times greater with conventional strapping compared to using a Logan bow in infants weighing 0.5–1.0 kg. Purpose-made devices, however, do have disadvantages; extreme care needs to be taken in very sick immature infants to avoid pressure necrosis injuries if a bonnet ligature and flange system is used.[175] If such a system is used, dental rolls should be placed just in front of the ears under the ligatures to relieve any pressure on the ears.

Complications of prolonged intubation

The presence of an endotracheal tube within hours causes changes in the tracheal mucosa which include deciliation, necrosis and desquamation.[157] Not surprisingly, once extubated, infants can develop hoarseness and stridor. Serious damage to the larynx and trachea is, however, uncommon (p. 443). Nasal intubation can lead to ulceration and excoriation of the nostrils. Oral intubation may result in dentition problems and a long narrow pressure-induced groove or even cleft in the palate.[279] Inappropriate positioning of the endotracheal tube, for example in the right main bronchus, is frequently associated with lobar collapse, even persisting post-extubation. In addition, to avoid such a complication it is important to minimize tube movement associated with head movement and positioning.

Indications for positive pressure ventilation

The development of expertise in mechanical ventilation of the newborn has allowed less rigorous indications for intubation and positive pressure ventilation.[337] Nowadays, many extremely low birthweight (ELBW) infants, who do not initially have regular respiratory activity, will be intubated and ventilated immediately in the labor suite (Table 15.1). The importance of establishing control over respiration in such infants, who are at particular risk of intracerebral hemorrhage, has been emphasized.[341] There are no randomized trials, however, to demonstrate such a policy improves outcome and certain authorities argue for a less aggressive approach (see p. 144).

Once on the neonatal unit, an infant who suddenly collapses with apnea and does not respond promptly to bag and mask resuscitation should be intubated and ventilated. Any infant who develops recurrent minor apneas or whose respiratory status deteriorates merits intubation. The level at which this is undertaken does, however, depend on the degree of immaturity of the infant (Table 15.1), their postnatal age and underlying disease. Some infants are intubated and ventilated to manage their underlying condition, for example, hypoxic ischemia encephalopathy (see p. 519), severe pulmonary hypertension, sepsis, congenital diaphragmatic hernia (see p. 487) and massive pulmonary hemorrhage.

Table 15.1 *Criteria for intubation and positive pressure ventilation*

Absolute
Major apnea with failure to respond promptly to bag and mask resuscitation

Relative
ELBW infants <28 weeks gestational age in the labor suite
Recurrent minor apnea unresponsive to CPAP and methylxanthines
Deteriorating respiratory status
  PaO_2 ≤50 mmHg in FiO_2 0.6
    ≤32 weeks gestation
  PaO_2 ≤50 mmHg in FiO_2 0.8
    >32 weeks gestation
  pH <7.25, $PaCO_2$ >50 mmHg
    ≤32 weeks gestation
  pH <7.2, $PaCO_2$ >60 mmHg
    >32 weeks gestation
Cerebral edema due to hypoxic ischaemic encephalopathy

PRESSURE-LIMITED TIME-CONTROLLED VENTILATION

In this form of ventilation a constant flow of gas is delivered to the infant, distending the lung for a preset inspiratory time to a predetermined pressure [peak inflating pressure (PIP)]. During expiration, the gas flow continues to deliver PEEP. The amount of gas which enters the lungs is determined by the peak pressure set on the ventilator blow-off valve and by the gas flow rate, which should always be large enough to ensure the PIP is reached in the available time. The higher the flow rate, the squarer the airway pressure waveform. Once the PIP has been reached, the pressure-limiting valve is opened and this prevents any further rise in pressure. The higher the pressure set the greater the volume of gas which enters the lungs, although, if the infant has non-compliant lungs, the leak around the endotracheal tube becomes more critical at higher pressures.

Ventilator performance

As rate is increased there is a change in the airway pressure waveform shape,[49] with loss of the positive pressure plateau (Figure 15.1). In addition, inadvertent PEEP can develop, particularly if flow is increased to maintain pressure as rate is elevated. This impairment of function occurs in ventilators which do not incorporate assisted expiratory valves, but this is rare in modern ventilators. Inadvertent PEEP can occur in any situation in which the alveolar pressure is higher than the proximal airway pressure and complete exhalation cannot take place.[21] This raises the MAP which may improve oxygenation, but has the disadvantage that it is likely to cause carbon dioxide retention. Inadvertent PEEP can be difficult to measure. The simplest technique is to occlude the endotracheal tube at end expiration and measure the equilibration pressure distal to the occlusion.[318,351] If there is gas trapping, then the measured pressure will be greater than the 'dialled in' PEEP. When gas trapping occurs there may also be a reduction in compliance.[386] In such a situation compliance then can be improved by increasing the expiratory time.[386]

Several studies have demonstrated neonatal ventilators differ in their performance and monitoring reliability.[111,239] Comparison of four ventilators (Babylog 8000, BP 2001, Sechrist IV 100B and InfantStar) demonstrated flow dependence of pressure for all ventilators tested, except the Babylog 8000. All either under- or overestimated the PIP and/or PEEP depending on the ventilator assessed. There are several explanations. Observer-related reading errors can occur if the pressure monitoring device consists of a mechanical pressure transducer read by visual observation. Second, no mechanical procedure is possible other than a zero adjustment. Third, the ventilator measured its pressure at a distance from the endotracheal tube.[239] The inspired oxygen concentration was also under-estimated, but less than 5 percent even at $FiO_2 > 0.3$. These data argue strongly for regular checking of the equipment reliability.[239]

Neonatal respiration monitors (p. 229)

Several of the ventilators currently available incorporate or have 'add-on' respiratory function monitors. Given that lung function tests (LFTs) have not only been used to predict extubation success (p. 229), but also outcome,

and to assess disease severity (p. 230) and the efficacy of interventions (p. 229), such monitors seem highly desirable. It is important, however, to be aware that such measurements have been performed in the context of research studies with carefully validated equipment. Data generated from respiration monitors must be accurate throughout the range of conditions experienced on a neonatal intensive care unit (NICU) if they are to be clinically useful. The clinician must ensure the device gives similar results regardless of, for example, the level of humidity of the inspired gas or the inspired oxygen concentration. Such information may not be available from

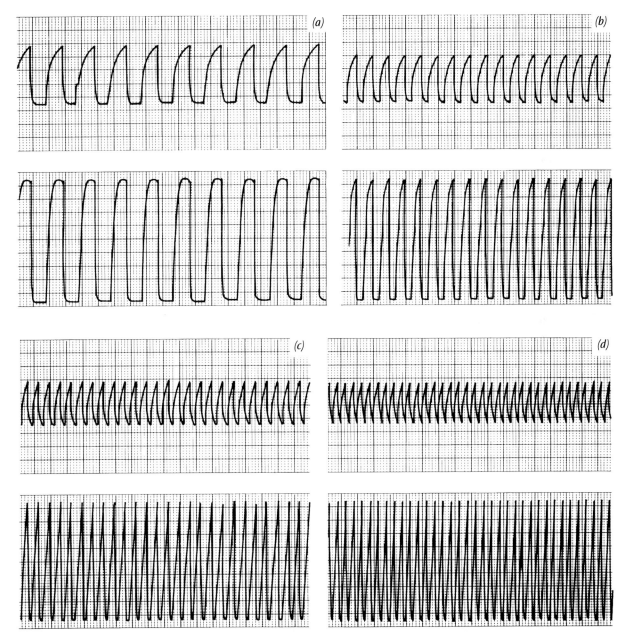

Figure 15.1 *Changes in airway pressure waveform and delivered volume as frequency increases. In each of the four recordings, the upper trace is the volume trace (inflation upwards, deflation downwards) and the lower trace is the airway pressure recording. Picture ventilator rate: (a) 30/min; (b) 60/min; (c) 90/min; (d) 120/min.*

the manufacturer and detailed testing reveals impaired performance in the clinical setting.[121] Some ventilators measure expired tidal volumes without compensation for the compliance of the ventilator circuit or for uncontrolled variations in the circuit set-up, for example the addition of an in-line suction device.[60] A significant discrepancy was demonstrated between ventilator-determined tidal volume and a pneumotachometer placed at the endotracheal tube-derived volume; the latter, therefore, is the recommended method.

HUMIDIFICATION

British Standards[53] recommend that the minimal acceptable humidity is 33 mg/l inspired gas. The American National Standards Institute felt that the minimum level of 10 mg/l was the lowest acceptable humidity level necessary to minimize mucosal damage to the upper airway. In addition, that level will provide approximately 50 percent relative humidity at 72°F ambient conditions;[79] this is three-quarters of that attained with normal breathing without intubation. There are a variety of humidifiers and heated circuits commercially available, but many do not meet the British Standards.[403] Problems with appropriate humidification may increase the pneumothorax rate.[403]

Peak inflating pressure (PIP)

A PIP sufficient to cause visible chest wall expansion must be used. This is usually about 18–20 cmH$_2$O, unless the infant has very stiff lungs. Once this is achieved, subsequent changes in pressure are determined by monitoring the arterial blood gases. High PIPs cause barotrauma and are significantly related to the development of pneumothoraces; thus the lowest PIP compatible with acceptable blood gases should be employed. Many now advocate permissive hypercapnia, that is, minimizing the peak pressures and allowing the carbon dioxide level to rise. This policy follows from the observations that low $PaCO_2$ levels appeared to be associated with an increased incidence of CLD (p. 9). A multicenter historical cohort analysis of 235 infants with birthweight between 750 and 1000 g revealed that a $PaCO_2$ of less than 40 mmHg at 48 or 96 hours after birth was the best predictor of CLD.[258] In a subsequent study, in those infants in whom the lowest $PaCO_2$ level was 29 mmHg or less, the odds for CLD were five to six times those of infants whose lowest $PaCO_2$ was 40 mmHg or more.[156] Numerous researchers have reported a significant relationship between hypocapnia, the development of periventricular leukomalacia (PVL) and adverse neurodevelopmental outcome. Thus, hypocapnia cannot now be advocated as a treatment for pulmonary hypertension (p. 380); indeed hypocapnia resulting from hyperventilation in PPHN has been associated with increased sensorineural hearing loss[210] and low psychomotor developmental test scores.[136] Wung et al. have advocated

allowing $PaCO_2$ levels up to 60 mmHg,[446] but there are no data from randomized studies to support such an approach.

Positive end expiratory pressure (PEEP)

PEEP holds open the peripheral airways between positive pressure inflations. Early studies demonstrated addition of PEEP during ventilation improved oxygenation.[211] PEEP conserves surfactant by reducing the shearing forces present when inspiration starts from atmospheric pressure in partially collapsed alveoli.[448] Preliminary concerns which suggested that this maneuver might increase pneumothorax have not been confirmed.[36] Too high a level of PEEP, however, does cause alveolar overdistension and carbon dioxide retention.[379] The optimum level of PEEP varies with the type of lung disease suffered by the infant. Although infants with RDS treated with surfactant may not tolerate levels greater than 3 cmH$_2$O, those with type I CLD have improved blood gases at 6 cmH$_2$O.[192] Increased PEEP may elevate CVP as a result of increased intrathoracic pressures obstructing venous return from the inferior and superior vena cavae. It may also decrease cardiac output and mean arterial pressure, thus reducing cerebral perfusion. In patients with non-compliant lungs, however, there is less transmission of airway pressure to the vasculature and hence less increased CVP.[285] In neurosurgical patients with normal intracranial pressure and no severe lung disease, PEEP levels of 5 cmH$_2$O did not significantly alter intracranial pressure. Higher levels of PEEP (10–15 cmH$_2$O) increased intracranial pressure, but did not affect cerebral perfusion.[285] Nevertheless, in preterm newborns, use of PEEP levels greater than 6 cmH$_2$O needs to be carefully evaluated.

Mean airway pressure (MAP)

MAP is a measure, approximately, of the average airway pressure applied throughout the cycle. It can be calculated from a variety of formulae:

$T_I/(T_I + T_E) \times$ PIP $+ (I - T_I)/(T_I + T_E) \times$ PEEP (Dillard[109])
PEEP $+ [($PIP $-$ PEEP$) \times T_I]/(T_I + T_E)$ (Field et al.[138])

where T_I is inspiratory time and T_E is expiratory time.

Both these formulae assume a square wave inflating pressure and thus will overestimate MAP in many cases. In practice most ventilators now have a MAP display or at least an 'add-on' monitor which measures MAP. In several studies,[48,211] MAP was shown to have a good correlation with oxygenation At a critical level, however, determined by the infant's lung function, further elevation of MAP does not improve oxygenation and indeed may cause impairment. MAP is not the sole determinant of oxygenation in spontaneously breathing ventilated infants, as during weaning similar PaO_2 levels were achieved despite use of two MAP levels.[189,190]

MAP can be elevated by increasing the inspiratory time, PEEP, PIP or some combination of the three. Thus, if elevation of MAP is required to improve oxygenation, this can be achieved by measures which may cause less barotrauma than elevation of PIP. There are, however, restrictions; prolongation of T_I beyond a critical duration stimulates active expiration and too high a PEEP can impair lung function. Field *et al.*[141] demonstrated that among preterm infants with a mean gestational age of 30 weeks, the use of a reverse inspiratory:expiratory (I:E) ratio was a less efficient method of improving oxygenation than raising PEEP to cause the same increase in MAP. Raising the PEEP level is a more effective method of improving lung volume and hence oxygenation, than either prolonging the inflation time or raising the peak inflating pressure.

Ventilator rate

Early studies demonstrated 'slow' rates of 30–40 breaths/min (bpm) which incorporated a long inspiratory time were more effective than fast rates in oxygenating the infant and reducing the incidence of BPD.[46,211,338] The disadvantage of such a strategy was, however, a pneumothorax rate of up to 50 percent. This adverse effect may have resulted from longer inspiratory times used at slower rates.[402] Since those early studies,[211,338] there have been improvements in ventilator performance. The newer ventilators are less likely to develop inadvertent PEEP at fast rates and more capable of maintaining their waveform.[177] Those changes may explain why, in the 1990s, fast rates were reintroduced with success. Improvements in oxygenation were noted at 120 bpm compared to 30 bpm.[188] The higher rate, when a ventilator without an assisted expiratory valve was used, resulted in improved CO_2 elimination. Both randomized and non-randomized studies have shown that ventilation at 60 bpm or more compared to 30 bpm can reduce the incidence of pneumothoraces.[10,44,183,208,325] In 237 infants with moderately severe RDS, rates of 60 bpm versus 40 bpm or less were associated with a lower pneumothorax rate (18 percent versus 33 percent, odds ratio 0.5, 95 percent CI 0.3 to 0.8).[10] Those studies, however, preceded routine use of antenatal corticosteroids and postnatal surfactant. Whether rates of 60 bpm or more compared to slower rates are still associated with a lower pneumothorax rate remains to be tested in a large randomized trial.

Ventilator rate has an important influence on the infant's respiratory efforts. At rates of 30–40 bpm, infants are rarely apneic and tend to breathe in one of four distinct interactions.[182] These interactions include the Hering–Breuer reflex, provoked augmented inspiration, synchrony and active expiration. The latter interaction is statistically significantly related to the development of a pneumothorax (p. 312).[184] As ventilator rate is increased, active expiration becomes less common and synchrony more frequent.[140] Provocation of respiratory reflexes is more common in infants with non-compliant lungs. Thus, in surfactant-treated infants, manipulation of the ventilator rate to avoid active expiration may be less necessary. The changes in respiratory interaction with increasing ventilator rate are related to the spontaneous respiratory rates of infants with RDS. In the first 48 hours of life, respiratory rate in infants with RDS appears to be inversely related to gestational age: infants of gestational age 32 weeks have a respiratory rate of approximately 70 bpm, whereas those of 26–28 weeks breathe at 100 bpm.[186] Thus, using fast ventilator rates more closely mimics such frequencies and hence provokes synchronous respiration (Figure 15.2). Those guidelines regarding ventilator rate, however, only apply to infants with RDS who are capable of making spontaneous respiratory efforts. Once an infant is paralyzed, ventilator rate should be reduced to approximately 60 bpm. This applies particularly to relatively mature infants (greater than 32 weeks of gestation) in whom, when paralyzed, rates $\geq$60 bpm are associated with gas trapping.[217] In addition, increasing ventilator rate beyond 60 bpm does not confer any advantage to infants ventilated beyond the first week after birth. Such infants, if fully ventilated, rarely show active expiration[221] and thus there is no need to increase the rate to prevent pneumothorax by that mechanism. Elevation of rate above 60 bpm does not improve blood gases in that group.[73]

Inspiratory and expiratory times

An I:E ratio of 1:1.2 to 1:1.5 is frequently used initially during ventilation of infants with acute RDS as this mimics the I:E ratio of spontaneous respiration.[393] It has been suggested that using a T_I of 0.31 seconds and a T_E of 0.42 seconds, being the average T_I and T_E found in one series would frequently provoke synchrony.[393] It may, however, not be necessary to be so precise, as in a subsequent study, a ventilator rate close to, but slightly higher than the infant's predicted respiratory rate was more successful in capturing the infant's respiration.[221] Using a longer T_I has the theoretical advantage that, as it increases MAP, it may improve oxygenation. It has the real risk, however, that it will stimulate active expiration.[140] It is our practice, therefore, only to increase T_I beyond 0.4 seconds in a paralyzed infant who has poor oxygenation and in whom we wish to avoid further increases in PIP or PEEP. Rarely, in infants with severe RDS, particularly those more mature than 32 weeks of gestation, a reverse ratio of 1.5:1 to 2:1 may be useful. If such a ratio is employed, then rate should be decreased to 30 or 40 bpm to avoid gas trapping.

In infants ventilated beyond the first week after birth, an I:E ratio of 1:1 is probably the most useful.[72] Comparison

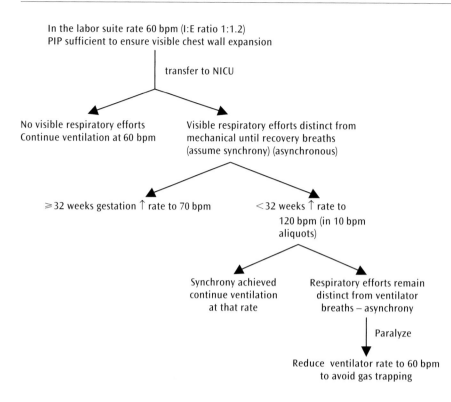

In the labor suite rate 60 bpm (I:E ratio 1:1.2)
PIP sufficient to ensure visible chest wall expansion

transfer to NICU

No visible respiratory efforts
Continue ventilation at 60 bpm

Visible respiratory efforts distinct from
mechanical until recovery breaths
(assume synchrony) (asynchronous)

≥32 weeks gestation ↑ rate to 70 bpm

<32 weeks ↑ rate to
120 bpm (in 10 bpm
aliquots)

Synchrony achieved
continue ventilation
at that rate

Respiratory efforts remain
distinct from ventilator
breaths – asynchrony

Paralyze

Reduce ventilator rate to 60 bpm
to avoid gas trapping

Figure 15.2 *Choosing a ventilator rate for infants with RDS. Synchrony, no respiratory efforts distinct from positive pressure inflation.*

was made of arterial blood gases in infants ventilated in the second and also the third week of life at I:E ratios of 1:1, 1:2 and 1:3 at ventilator rates of 30 and 60 bpm. Differences in blood gases were relatively small at the different settings, but those which were statistically significant suggested the optimum settings were a ventilator rate of 60 bpm and an I:E ratio of 1:1. In older infants ventilated at approximately 7 weeks of age, a $T_I \geq 0.6$ seconds compared to 0.4 seconds increased the effectiveness of mechanical ventilation as determined by measurements of tidal volume, dynamic compliance and alveolar ventilation.[171] There was, however, no further significant improvement on prolonging T_I to 0.8 seconds.

Flow rates

There are few published data on the effect of flow rates on ventilation outcome. As a consequence, NICUs arbitrarily usually chose flow rates of between 6 and 10 l/min. It should be noted that some ventilators have a fixed flow rate (SLE 2000). Increasing the flow rate is necessary to maintain waveform at fast rates in some ventilators[177] and in most if a combination of high peak pressures and fast ventilator rates are used.

Ventilator settings for RDS

Protocols have been developed for ventilator settings at the initiation of positive pressure support (Figure 15.2).[179] Once the infant is in synchrony, alteration in ventilator

Table 15.2 *Change in ventilator settings to be made in response to abnormal blood gases*

Blood gas abnormality		Change in ventilator settings
PaO_2	$PaCO_2$	
Too low	Too high	↑PIP
Too low	Acceptable	↑FiO_2 first, then ↑MAP but by ↑PEEP or↑ T_I, (*not* by ↑PIP)
Too low	Too low	Overventilation – confirmed by chest radiograph appearance ↓PIP
Acceptable	Too high	↑rate ↓PEEP
Acceptable	Too low	↓rate (↑PEEP in infants with extensive chest excursion)
Too high	Acceptable	↓FiO_2
Too high	Too low	↓PIP

settings is according to changes in blood gases (Table 15.2). Some infants will remain asynchronous despite manipulation of ventilator rate and inspiratory time and to prevent pneumothorax some action needs to be taken. This may be to paralyze the infant with a neuromuscular blocking agent (p. 316) or, in certain infants, to use a patient triggered ventilator (p. 315). Ventilator settings for respiratory failure, other than due to RDS is discussed in the relevant chapters.

WEANING AND EXTUBATION (FIGURE 15.3)

The longer an infant is ventilated the greater the risks of nosocomial infection, barotrauma and tracheal injury.

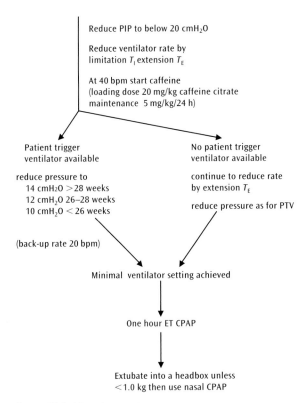

Reduce PIP to below 20 cmH$_2$O

Reduce ventilator rate by limitation T_I extension T_E

At 40 bpm start caffeine (loading dose 20 mg/kg caffeine citrate maintenance 5 mg/kg/24 h)

Patient trigger ventilator available

reduce pressure to
14 cmH$_2$O >28 weeks
12 cmH$_2$O 26–28 weeks
10 cmH$_2$O <26 weeks

(back-up rate 20 bpm)

No patient trigger ventilator available

continue to reduce rate by extension T_E

reduce pressure as for PTV

Minimal ventilator setting achieved

One hour ET CPAP

Extubate into a headbox unless <1.0 kg then use nasal CPAP

Figure 15.3 *Weaning strategy.*

Table 15.3 *'Weaning' therapies*

Drug	Dosage	Side-effects
Theophylline	4 mg/kg/day in two divided doses	Tachycardia Agitation Gastrointestinal upset
Caffeine	Loading dose 20 mg/kg caffeine citrate (equivalent to 10 mg/kg caffeine base). Maintenance 5 mg/kg caffeine citrate every 24 hours	Increased left ventricular output and blood pressure (Walther et al.[435])
Doxapram	2–2.5 mg/kg/hour infusion [half life 5–13 hours (Burnard et al.[56])]	Convulsions Hypertension

It is thus essential to wean infants as soon as their respiratory status allows. It is our policy, if there is no evidence of a respiratory acidosis and blood gases have been maintained for 4–6 hours, to start reducing respiratory support irrespective of the stage of the infant's illness. PIP should be reduced in preference to rate until the PIP is less than 20 cmH$_2$O. PIP is reduced if blood gases are maintained or the PaO_2 is high in association with a low $PaCO_2$, but if the $PaCO_2$ is within the normal range the FiO_2 is reduced in preference (Table 15.3). If the infant has been receiving a pulmonary vasodilator, we reduce the FiO_2 to 0.6 before stopping the vasodilator. Once the PIP is below 20 cmH$_2$O then we start to reduce rate, particularly if the $PaCO_2$ is low, but PaO_2 not elevated. We do not reduce the ventilator rate below 20 bpm except in exceptional circumstances. Rate may be reduced by turning down the frequency and maintaining the I:E ratio or keeping T_I constant and reducing rate by lengthening T_E. The former has the advantage of maintaining MAP, whereas the latter weaning method is associated with a lower rate of active expiration.[187] In a randomized trial,[190] limitation of T_I and prolongation of T_E was associated with a shorter duration of weaning, but no increased incidence of complications such as pneumothorax or reventilation. During weaning frequent changes in the inspired oxygen concentration may be required. Clinically an arterial blood gas is usually obtained 20–30 minutes after the inspired oxygen concentration has been

altered. Data from adults, however, suggest that 10 minutes is sufficient for equilibration after a 0.20 change in the inspired oxygen fraction.[58]

An alternative method of weaning is to maintain the infant on the rate received during the acute stage of their illness (≥60 bpm) and gradually reduce PIP to very low levels (8–10 cmH$_2$O). This has the theoretical advantage that the infant will stay synchronous but, as they recover from RDS their compliance is likely to increase, which may be associated with a slowing of their spontaneous respiratory rate.

Whichever method of weaning is chosen, it is important not to expose the infant to a prolonged period on endotracheal CPAP. It is our practice to keep the infants for less than 1 hour on endotracheal CPAP to ensure they have satisfactory blood gases. If after that time there has been no development of a respiratory acidosis, then the infant is extubated into a headbox. It is also important to choose the optimum level of endotracheal CPAP prior to extubation.[37] Oxygenation and FRC on 2 cmH$_2$O endotracheal CPAP did not differ significantly from that achieved post-extubation, but in both situations oxygenation and FRC were significantly higher than that achieved at 0 cmH$_2$O endotracheal CPAP.[37]

Extubation should only be performed if there is a high chance of success. It is important, therefore, before it is attempted, to ensure the infant is not anemic, gastric feeds are stopped for at least 4 hours and the stomach emptied. Very immature infants (birthweight less than 1.0 kg) may fail extubation despite all these precautions, a normal chest radiograph appearance and acceptable blood gases on minimal respiratory support. If, on more than two occasions, such infants require reintubation, our practice is to wait for some days and achieve appropriate weight gain (p. 216) prior to reattempting extubation.

LUNG MECHANICS AND PREDICTION OF SUCCESSFUL WEANING

Weaning is accomplished during the recovery stage of the respiratory illness when lung compliance is likely to be improving; it thus might be expected that measurement of lung mechanics would be useful to predict successful weaning. To date, however, experience has been mixed. Balsan et al.[19] found a compliance less than 0.5 ml/cmH$_2$O was usually associated with unsuccessful weaning, whereas Veness-Meehan et al.[426] found no such correlation. More recently,[246] the results of lung function tests (compliance, functional residual capacity, tidal volume and respiratory rate) made before and after extubation were compared to the ventilator settings recorded immediately prior to extubation with regard to their ability to predict extubation success in mechanically ventilated, prematurely born infants. An FRC of less than 26 ml/kg post-extubation had the highest predictive value in predicting extubation failure and performed better than commonly used clinical indices, that is, ventilator settings. In preterm infants weighing less than 2000 g, a spontaneously generated minute ventilation at least 50 percent of the mechanically generated minute ventilation predicted readiness for extubation in 86 percent of the 35 patients studied.[439]

THERAPEUTIC AGENTS (TABLE 15.3)

Weaning duration can be shortened by administration of a methylxanthine.[185] Methylxanthines enhance respiratory effort by stimulating the respiratory center,[104,228] intercostal muscles and diaphragm.[16] They also act directly on the lungs and airways, improving compliance[105,185] and decreasing airway resistance. Theophylline also stimulates the surfactant pathway. It can be given intravenously or orally. Even in unfed preterm infants therapeutic levels can be reached within 6 hours of oral administration.[131] Prospective controlled trials[128,185] have demonstrated that theophylline aids the weaning process either by reducing the duration of weaning[185,205] or reducing the need for reintubation.[430] These advantageous effects seem limited to babies less than 30 days old.[346] Use of theophylline is associated with side-effects which include tachycardia, gastrointestinal upset including vomiting, hyperglycemia and diuresis. Such side-effects appear to be dose related and thus levels must be regularly checked. A further disadvantage of theophylline is that it needs to be administered three times a day. Other studies have shown that caffeine (Table 15.3), which is given once a day, has a lower toxicity level with fewer side-effects[228] and seems equally effective as theophylline.[388] In a blinded randomized trial of 45 infants, the mean time from study entry to extubation in both 23 theophylline-treated and 22 caffeine-treated infants was 2.7 days. Three infants in both groups developed respiratory failure necessitating reintubation.[388] It remains to be appropriately tested whether extubation of the present population of very immature ventilated infants is facilitated by administration of methylxanthines.

Doxapram may be an option in infants who appear resistant to methylxanthines and in whom no cause for weaning failure can be found. Eight infants who continued to have apnea despite treatment with aminophylline responded to the administration of doxapram with complete cessation of the apnea. In another study,[25] doxapram increased minute ventilation and tidal volume and also reduced the apnea rate. The long-term effects of doxapram on apnea, however, may be incomplete and not sustained beyond the first week of treatment.[316] There are, however, few published data, it is often difficult to frequently monitor levels and this medication has numerous side-effects.

Problems following extubation

Copious secretions (bronchorrhea) may occur, particularly in infants ventilated for longer than 1 week.[289] Such infants are at high risk of lobar collapse post-extubation.[447] Regular physiotherapy and suction is of proven benefit in such patients (Chapter 18).[143] As physiotherapy is not always well tolerated, it is essential to identify high-risk patients; this can be achieved by a post-extubation chest radiograph. Tracheal problems may declare themselves post-extubation. Stridor with respiratory compromise may develop, then nebulized epinephrine (adrenaline) and systemic steroids, 0.5 mg/kg can be used, although there is no convincing evidence that this is helpful.[405] In infants who have previously failed extubation because of stridor, steroids should be started prior to extubation.

VOLUME-SET TIME-LIMITED VENTILATORS

This type of ventilator delivers a preset volume to the infant. This is done irrespective of the pressure necessary to achieve that volume, and thus a major disadvantage is that very high pressures may be used in an infant with non-compliant lungs. The delivered volume is determined by the inflation time, flow, pressure limit and patient compliance and resistance. Volume-controlled ventilators end inspiration after a preset tidal volume has been delivered. Total inspiration is determined by tidal volume and the inspiratory flow settings. It is difficult in a small baby to determine the volume that should be preset; in such patients the volume change due to gas compression becomes more critical as does loss around the endotracheal tube. If the volume delivered during pressure-set ventilation is measured in a series of babies at a time when they all have blood gases within the acceptable therapeutic range, there is great interindividual variation (Figure 15.4). This would suggest that extrapolating from the expected tidal volume related to body weight, as

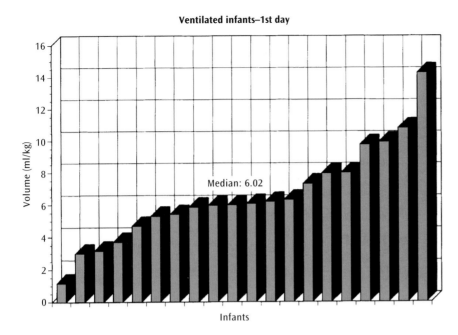

Ventilated infants–1st day

Median: 6.02

Volume (ml/kg)

Infants

Figure 15.4 *Histogram depicting inflating volumes in 20 infants, all less than 24 hours of age (individual data demonstrated by histogram bars). Although the median volume is 6.02 ml/kg, there is considerable variation.*

is done in pediatric and adult intensive care units, would not necessarily give optimum ventilation in a neonate. Volume guarantee (VG) ventilation may be a better option (p. 167).

Clinical studies

Early attempts at volume-controlled ventilation (VCV) failed because of technological limitations in both ventilator design and monitoring as well as a belief that this form of ventilation was associated with a high incidence of air leak and chronic lung disease.[22] In the early 1990s, VCV again became available following improvements in ventilator design. Initially it was used as a rescue modality with dramatic improvements in oxygenation in a small number of patients. This was suggested to be due to more consistent delivery of tidal volume and minute ventilation, improving lung volume stabilization and decreasing ventilation-perfusion mismatch.[22] Several randomized trials of VCV versus patient-controlled ventilation (PCV) have now been performed and suggest VCV may have advantages. In one,[322] VCV use was associated with less hypotension and serious intracranial hemorrhage (ICH) and, in another,[389] a shorter duration of ventilation. Limitations of study design of both trials, however, mean that it remains unclear if VCV should be the preferred option. PVC in the first study was not delivered by a comparable ventilator.[322] In the second study,[389] the ventilator settings were manipulated so that volume delivery was similar by the two modes, making it difficult to understand how such a significant difference in outcome occurred. In addition, the airway pressure waveforms in both modes lacked a positive pressure plateau[193] and this has been assumed to be important in facilitating gas

exchange. Thus, a large randomized trial comparing the effect of VCV to standard PCV on long-term outcomes is required.

PATIENT-TRIGGERED VENTILATION (PTV)

PTV was reintroduced in the neonatal nursery in 1986.[286] During PTV, positive pressure inflations are delivered in response to the infant's spontaneous respiratory efforts. The number of inflations and shape of the airway pressure waveform (magnitude of PIP and T_I) are dependent on the triggered mode used (p. 165). Theoretically, during PTV, the infant should always breathe in synchrony with the ventilator; this may be the explanation for the lower epinephrine concentrations noted in infants on PTV compared to those on conventional mechanical ventilation (CMV).[330] In addition, the contribution of the infant's respiratory effort to the transpulmonary pressure should enable a reduction in peak pressure, thus decreasing the incidence of chronic lung disease. Unfortunately, to date these theoretic advantages have not been confirmed. During PTV, the infant's respiratory efforts are sensed by the 'triggering device'. If the respiratory effort exceeds the critical trigger level, then the signal is fed back into the ventilator and a positive pressure inflation is delivered to the infant. A number of ventilators and triggering devices capable of delivering PTV are available.

Triggering devices

A variety of devices have been used to detect the infant's respiratory efforts. In an early ventilator modified to deliver PTV (SLE 250), respiratory effort was detected by abdominal movements using the pneumatic capsule of the MR10 respiration monitor.[286] The pneumatic capsule was taped onto the patient's abdominal wall in the subxiphisternal position. Unfortunately, that device had a long trigger delay.[66,219] The signal was then fed into the manual breath control of the SLE 250 ventilator. The pneumatic capsule system has been used with other ventilators, but without the electronics of the MR10 respiration monitor the trigger delay is much shorter. An esophageal balloon to sense pleural pressure changes[180] was also used as a triggering device.[178] Unfortunately, the balloon was not suitable for long-term use, as its presence in the esophagus stimulated peristaltic activity interfering with the detection of the infant's respiratory effort.

Impedance pneumotachograph has also been used.[431] The signal obtained from the output of a standard cardiopulmonary monitor is used to trigger the exhalation solenoid of a conventional neonatal respirator. Placement of the monitor electrodes was modified to obtain a transthoracic impedance respiratory waveform; this was usually best achieved by placing the electrodes in the anterior axillary line on the right and the posterior axillary line on the left. The timing of the start of inflation could theoretically be varied during inspiration and inflation was terminated at the onset of active expiration. A mandatory minimum expiratory time of 0.2 seconds was incorporated to prevent build up of intrathoracic pressure due to repetitive respirations or autotriggering. The device is triggered only with the onset of spontaneous inspiration and provides synchronized assisted ventilation for infants (SAVI).

Triggering devices also use signals from the airway. Changes in airflow may be detected using either a pneumotachograph[293] or a thermistor[220] mounted in the patient's manifold of the ventilator circuit. A variable area differential pressure flow transducer has also been used to detect changes in gas flow (Ventilator Flow Synchronizer, VFS, Bird Products Corporation). The flow signal triggers an otherwise time-cycled pressure-limited ventilator. Changes in airway pressure can be sensed by a pressure transducer connected by non-compliant tubing to a point on the patient manifold just proximal to the endotracheal tube.[66] In other systems (SLE 2000) the pressure transducer is sited within the ventilator but detection of the infant's respiratory efforts is improved by putting a resistor in the inspiratory limb of the ventilator circuit near the patient's manifold. This necessitates an increased respiratory effort at the beginning of inspiration.[192]

PERFORMANCE

The performance of the triggering device can be judged by a number of criteria, as follows.

Liability to autotriggering

This means that positive pressure inflations are triggered artifactually. One cause is the to and fro movement of excessive condensation in the ventilation circuit, resulting in flow or pressure changes. Autotriggering is most likely to occur if the triggering device is set at maximum sensitivity. A large leak around the endotracheal tube may also result in autotriggering, as there are detectable flows in expiration, even at low PEEP levels, which can reach the trigger threshold of a flow-triggered ventilator.[230] Comparison of three flow-triggered ventilators (Draeger Babylog 8000, BearCub and VIP Bird) demonstrated the BearCub had the highest autotriggering rate.[38] The BearCub triggering system, however, was less susceptible to autotriggering than an impedance triggering system (SAVI, Sechrist Industries, Anaheim CA, USA).[230]

Sensitivity

This is the percentage of the infant's respiratory efforts triggering positive pressure inflations. A high sensitivity is optimum as this means the majority or preferably all of the infant's respiratory efforts in SIPPV mode will be supported by positive pressure inflations.

Trigger delay/response time

This is the time from the onset of inspiration to the commencement of positive pressure inflation. The trigger delay should be as short as possible to ensure the beginning of inflation occurs early in inspiration, thus the majority of the infant's breath is positive pressure inflated. In addition, if the trigger delay is very short, the inflation time does not have to be reduced to prevent inflation extending into expiration (asynchrony). If the trigger delay is long, then unless pressure support ventilation (PSV) is used (p. 167) inflation must be shortened to prevent asynchrony. Reducing the inflation time can impair volume delivery,[139] even using the new generation of neonatal ventilators (p. 156).[118] The trigger delay consists of two components: first, the time taken for the infant's respiratory efforts to exceed the critical trigger level; and second, the response time or systems delay of the ventilator. Ideally the systems delay time should not exceed 10 percent of the total inflation time, a systems delay of 36 ms permits a maximum ventilator rate of 83 bpm.[133] An early study demonstrated that a long trigger delay was significantly related to poor outcome of SIPPV;[221] that is, infants could not be supported on SIPPV throughout their ventilatory career and/or developed a pneumothorax.

Comparison of performance of triggering devices

Numerous studies have been undertaken both in infants and preclinical models to compare the performance of the triggering devices. Much of that literature, however, is redundant as it precedes the latest developments to the ventilators and their triggering devices. Currently available systems usually have a trigger delay of less than 100 ms. Assessment, however, has usually been undertaken in relatively mature infants with or recovering from RDS. The infant's respiratory function is likely to be an important determinant of the performance of a triggering system.

For example, a flow triggering will perform very differently in an infant with non-compliant, low volume lungs due to RDS than in an infant who has a high airways resistance due to meconium aspiration syndrome. There are insufficient data available to confidently conclude that the triggering systems will function sufficiently well in all neonatal clinical scenarios. All of the devices' performance will be influenced by the infant's gestational age.[68,218] Poor respiratory activity, as indicated by a weak Hering–Breuer reflex, further results in a long trigger delay.[77] In addition, the performance of certain types of triggering devices are further compromised in prematurely born infants because chest wall distortion occurs because of their compliant rib cage. The chest wall distortion results in a negative impedance signal during the beginning of inspiration and, if a large phase shift results, ventilator inflations will be triggered after the end of spontaneous inspiration. A major criticism of studies purporting to assess triggering device performance is that the triggering devices were examined with different ventilators. Thus any differences detected could be due to the performance of the trigger device, the ventilator, or a combination of the trigger device and ventilator and marked differences in performance of ventilators currently available have been noted.[111] Use of a single ventilator type[118] has allowed appropriate comparison of two triggering systems. That comparison demonstrated that an airflow rather than an airway pressure trigger performed better in very immature infants. The airflow trigger had a shorter trigger delay and lower rate of asynchrony but in some patients both systems had unacceptably long trigger delays (p. 164).

Synchronized intermittent positive pressure ventilation (SIPPV) and synchronized intermittent mandatory ventilation (SIMV)

SIPPV was the first trigger mode to be made available in the 1980s and, as a consequence, PTV and SIPPV have been used interchangeably to indicate triggered ventilation. SIPPV has also been called assist control (A/C). During SIPPV, any number of positive pressure inflations can be triggered, providing that the inspiratory effort exceeds the critical trigger level. During SIMV only a preset number of inflations can be triggered regardless of the frequency of the inspiratory efforts. Thus, if the infant breathes at 80 bpm, but the triggered ventilator rate is present at 40 bpm, a maximum of 40 triggered inflations can be delivered to the infant.

TRANSFER TO SIPPV OR SIMV

On transfer to SIPPV or SIMV, the PIP, PEEP and FiO_2 should initially be left unchanged and subsequently modified according to the arterial blood gas estimations.[293] The inflation time, however, may need shortening. An inflation time greater than 0.4 seconds is associated with a reduced minute volume as the baby's spontaneous breathing rate is slowed, presumably via the Hering-Breuer reflex.[422] A long inflation time is also more likely to result in inflation extending into expiration, provoking active expiration.[176] Shortening inflation time below 0.2 seconds is, however, not beneficial as this is likely to reduce the tidal exchange.[139] The optimal inflation time is determined by observation of the baby's respiratory efforts while receiving CPAP for up to 1 minute.[293] The inflation time should be approximately equal to the spontaneous inspiratory time after deduction of the system delay. The inflation time is then reduced if necessary until the baby's respiratory efforts are indistinct from ventilator inflation.[293] To ensure continued support should the infant become apneic, a minimum ventilator back-up rate or expiratory time should be dialled in. This is usually selected in conventional mode prior to transferring the infant to PTV. The exact mechanism by which the back-up breath is given varies between ventilators. In certain ventilators, each minute is divided into a number of aliquots of time by the back-up rate. In each 'aliquot', if the infant does not trigger the ventilator in either the whole aliquot on the first half, then a back-up breath will be given. For example, if a back-up breath rate of 30 bpm is chosen, the ventilator will scan each 2-second period. The back-up rate is chosen according to the severity of the infant's illness and amount of support needed. If too fast a rate is chosen, for example greater than 60 bpm, this may not give an infant who is recovering from respiratory distress sufficient time to trigger the ventilator. In practice, we tend to start SIPPV with a back-up rate of 40 bpm for an infant during the acute stage of the illness and increase this to 60 bpm if the patient is having frequent apneas. Once recovery begins, as indicated by reduction in ventilator pressures, the back-up rate is gradually reduced.

Infants on SIPPV who, because of vigorous respiratory efforts, are hypocapnic despite reduction in the peak inflating pressure should be transferred to SIMV. This scenario usually occurs in mature infants with mild respiratory distress. The SIMV rate, however, should be maintained at least at 20 bpm (p. 161).

Clinical studies of SIPPV/SIMV

Initial experience suggested that blood gases improved in the majority of infants transferring from IPPV to triggered ventilation.[181,286,422] Those studies, however, were carried out for only a short time period and, as the infants usually received more support during the triggered modes, the results were not surprising. In subsequent studies, care was taken to ensure that the level of support provided was similar on all ventilation modes. Their results demonstrated that SIMV compared to IMV provided superior oxygenation, higher tidal volumes and lower asynchrony rates.[39] In addition, during SIMV infants achieved the same total minute ventilation with less inspiratory effort, as indicated by lower esophageal pressure swings.[229] A lower amplitude and duration of diaphragmatic EMG activity, also indicating lower inspiratory activity, has also been noted during SIMV. The lower work of breathing during SIMV may be due in part to the reduced asynchrony rate. Increased abdominal muscle activity when the infant is asynchronous can lead to a higher expiratory work of breathing.[92] Lower beat-to-beat blood pressure fluctuations[229] and cerebral blood flow velocity fluctuations[174] have been noted on SIPPV/SIMV.

COMPARISONS OF SIPPV TO SIMV

SIPPV and SIMV have rarely been directly compared. Volume-targeted SIPPV has been shown to result in more consistent tidal volumes at lower respiratory rates than either IMV or SIMV in preterm infants with RDS (p. 167).[300] Randomized trials performed in preterm infants recovering from RDS suggest that SIPPV may be the more advantageous weaning mode, but only when compared to reduction in the SIMV rate below 20 bpm (p. 161).

RANDOMIZED TRIALS COMPARING SIPPV/SIMV TO CMV

At least six randomized trials (Table 15.4) have been performed. The trials have differed with respect to sample size and whether SIMV or SIPPV was used. The majority of infants, however, had or were recovering from RDS. The same type of ventilator was not always used in each arm of a trial and this may have biased the results (p. 156).[111] Meta-analysis of the results of those studies demonstrated that the only significant difference in outcome between the ventilatory modes was that the duration of ventilation was significantly shorter in the SIPPV/SIMV supported infants (weighted mean difference of 31.9 hours, 95 percent CI 9.6–54.1).[195] There was no excess of adverse effects in any trial, but in the largest one,[30] amongst infants less than 28 weeks of gestation, there was a trend for more pneumothoraces in the SIPPV group (18.8 percent versus 11.8 percent). In addition,

more infants in the SIPPV group departed from the randomized mode of ventilation (27 percent versus 15 percent). In that study,[30] which was of a pragmatic design, a variety of ventilators were used which may have influenced the results (p. 156), but the majority of infants randomized to the SIPPV group were supported by a ventilator incorporating an airway pressure trigger. The poorer performance of the airway pressure trigger may have contributed to the unexpectedly non-positive SIPPV results.[118] Other limitations of the trial have been commented on.[126] Thus, although the trial has the merit of a large sample size, on its results alone, it cannot be confidently concluded that SIPPV/SIMV has no advantages for preterm infants with RDS. The results of the meta-analysis of the six trials, however, show no positive advantage other than a shorter duration of ventilation. Thus, triggered modes seem best reserved for infants recovering from RDS. In the one trial which exclusively recruited such infants, a significantly shorter duration of weaning was reported.[69]

In preterm infants recovering from RDS, the results of three randomized trials have suggested SIPPV rather than SIMV is the more efficacious weaning mode (Table 15.5). Although SIMV allows more flexible weaning than SIPPV as rate, pressure or both can be reduced, overall the duration of weaning tended to be shorter on SIPPV.[70,112] In three trials, weaning on SIPPV was by pressure reduction alone, as of course the infant controls the delivered ventilator rate. In three trials, weaning on SIMV differed; in one only rate was reduced with PIP kept constant, in another rate and PIP were decreased and in the third PIP reduced and rate decreased but only to 20 bpm. Only in the latter trial was the duration of weaning similar in the SIMV and SIPPV groups. Those results suggest that, even during weaning, a minimum number of the infant's breaths must be supported, otherwise the work of breathing to overcome the resistance of the endotracheal tube will be increased and consequently the duration of weaning prolonged. In support of that hypothesis is the finding

Table 15.4 *Results of meta-analysis of six randomized trials comparing SIPPV/SIMV to CMV (Greenough et al.[195])*

Outcome	Relative risk	95 percent CI
Air leaks	1.03	0.80, 1.34
Chronic oxygen dependency beyond:		
28 days	0.93	0.77, 1.14
36 weeks PCA	0.90	0.75, 1.08
Severe intracerebral hemorrhage	1.04	0.75, 1.44

Table 15.5 *Randomized trials comparing SIPPV to SIMV during respiratory distress recovery[38,70,112]*

	SIPPV	SIMV
SIMV weaning		
Rate reduction to 5 bpm	22 (4–339)	36 (8–647)
Rate reduction to 5 bpm and pressure reduction	24 (7–432)	50 (12–500)
Rate reduction to 20 bpm and pressure reduction	33 (4–912)	30 (7–408)

Results are expressed as median (range) duration of weaning. In all trials weaning during SIPPV was by pressure reduction alone. (Reproduced with permission from Bernstein *et al.*[38] NB: There were no statistically significant differences in any of the three trials with regard to the numbers of infants who required re-intubation.

that at low rates of ventilator support, oxygen consumption is increased.[349] As a consequence, it is our practice to usually wean preterm infants on SIPPV by pressure reduction down to low PIPs before extubation. The level of PIP is dependent on the infant's size and gestational age; for an infant of 32 weeks, extubation from $14\,cmH_2O$ can be attempted, but for a 24-week gestation infant, the PIP may be reduced even as far as $6–8\,cmH_2O$ if extubation is to be successful. The infants must, however, be able to cope with such low pressures at an $FiO_2 \leqslant 0.30$ if extubation is to be successful (p. 160). Some infants, particularly those delivered near or at term, can become hypocapnic on SIPPV during weaning; such infants we wean on IMV or SIMV, but we always maintain a minimum ventilator rate of 20 bpm prior to transfer to a short trial of endotracheal tube CPAP before extubation (p. 161).

VOLUME MONITORING DURING TRIGGERED VENTILATION

Certain ventilators providing triggered modes also allow tidal volume monitoring. Thus, the clinician may maintain the delivered volume within a predetermined range by adjusting the peak inflating pressure. In one study,[300] volume-targeted SIPPV was shown to produce more consistent tidal volumes than IMV or SIMV.

Volume guarantee (VG)

In this mode, the peak inspiratory pressure is servocontrolled so that the volume preset by the clinician is delivered during triggered ventilation (SIPPV, SIMV, PSV). Increased patient effort results in less applied pressure and vice versa. Using the Draeger Babylog 8000, adjustments are carried out from one breath to the next. The expired tidal volume is measured and compared with the desired volume and a new pressure plateau calculated for the next breath. The desired volume, however, will not be delivered if the preset peak pressure is too low or there is no positive pressure plateau. Several studies have shown that adequate gas exchange can be achieved at lower airway pressures during VG.[4,80,212] One explanation is that, during VG, the infant makes a greater contribution to the minute volume.[212] Those data are, however, from a short-term physiological study and the infant's ability to contribute to minute ventilation is likely to vary according to the stage of the respiratory illness. Nevertheless, results so far suggest VG may facilitate weaning; switching over to VG would allow the clinician to determine if the infant would tolerate lower airway pressures. During VG, there may be lower breath to breath variability in delivered volume,[4] but this is not a consistent finding.[80] Theoretically, breath-to-breath adjustment, particularly if the infant had periodic breathing, could lead to greater variability.

Pressure support ventilation (PSV)

During PSV, the patient's inspiratory efforts trigger a positive pressure inflation at a preset level but, in addition, the end of spontaneous inspiration also dictates termination of the inflation. For example, inflation is terminated when the inspiratory flow is reduced to 15 percent of the maximum inspiratory flow when the Draeger Babylog is used in PSV mode and if the termination sensitivity of the Bird VIP is used then inflation can be terminated between 5 and 25 percent of the maximum inspiratory flow. Employment of PSV can reduce the aysnchrony rate by decreasing the inflation time.[114] Amongst very immature infants, increasing termination sensitivity to maximum reduced the asynchrony rate almost to zero.[114] In that study, despite the reduction in inflation time, the tidal volume was maintained, perhaps by an increase in the infant's respiratory efforts. The infants were only examined for a short period and whether PSV with short inflation times would be tolerated throughout the infant's respiratory career needs to be examined. In addition, whether use of PSV will reduce the pneumothorax rate also requires testing.

During PSV, cardiac output has been noted to increase above that experienced during CMV.[201] The decrease in MAP resulting from the lower inspiratory: expiratory ratio during PSV may explain the higher cardiac output.

Proportional assist ventilation (PAV)

Patient-triggered ventilation modes typically synchronize one or two events of the ventilator cycle to certain points in the spontaneous respiratory cycle (start and end of inspiratory effort). Between these points in time, the applied ventilator pressure plateau and waveforms remain preset without adapting to the course of spontaneous breathing activity. The concept of 'respiratory mechanical unloading' and 'proportional assist ventilation' (RMU/PAV) is fundamentally different from this conventional perception of a ventilator being a 'pump' that releases 'bursts of air' when triggered. During RMU/PAV, the applied ventilator pressure is servocontrolled based on a continuous input from the patient. This input signal alone controls the instantaneous ventilator pressure continuously, virtually without a time lag. The input signal is the modified tidal volume and/or airflow signal of the patient's spontaneous breath. The ventilator becomes fully enslaved, allowing the patient to control timing, depth and the entire airflow contour of the breath. Applying such ventilator pressure waveforms proportionally enhances the effect of the respiratory muscle effort on ventilation. The clinician sets the 'gain' of this enhancement. The higher the 'gain', the less mechanical work of breathing needs to be performed by the patient.

ELASTIC LOADING AND ELASTIC UNLOADING

In the first model, the subject's lungs are connected through an endotracheal tube to a rigid box (Figure 15.5). Being connected to the box means a higher respiratory muscle workload during spontaneous breathing, because the pressure inside the box and at the endotracheal tube level decrease when volume is inspired into the lung. At any point in time during such loaded inspiration, the decrease in pressure is in proportion to the inspired volume, that is, there is a constant ratio between the change in pressure (pressure at the airway opening, P_{ao}) and the change in volume (V) throughout the respiratory cycle. The ratio P_{ao}/V is the elastance of the box and is a measure of the additional elastic workload imposed on spontaneous breathing when the subject breathes from the box. If the box is replaced by a ventilator which generates instantaneous pressure changes in the opposite direction, that is, an increase in P_{ao} in proportion to the inspired volume, the ventilator will support (unload rather than load) spontaneous breathing. The ratio P_{ao}/V is a measure of the ventilator's elastance which is 'negative' because the pressure moves in the opposite direction compared to the pressure behavior of a 'positive' elastance such as a container. This ventilatory modality has therefore been called 'negative ventilator elastance'[356] or 'elastic unloading'[326,363] or 'volume-proportional assist'. It specifically decreases the elastic work of breathing imposed on respiratory muscles during spontaneous breathing.

RESISTIVE LOADING AND RESISTIVE UNLOADING

In the second model resistive load symbolized by a narrow tube attached to the airway (Figure 15.6). At the attachment point, the pressure will decrease below baseline during inspiration and increase above baseline during expiration when the subject breathes spontaneously through the tube. There will be a constant ratio of change in pressure per unit of airflow. This ratio represents the resistance of the tube. In the resistance unloading mode, however, the ventilator generates pressure changes at the level of the endotracheal tube adaptor in the opposite direction so that P_{ao} increases during inspiration above baseline and decreases during expiration in proportion to the instantaneous flow of spontaneous breathing (flow-proportional assist). This is, therefore, a negative resistance and causes the opposite effect of resistive loading, i.e. unloading. Resistive unloading facilitates both inspiratory and expiratory airflow throughout the spontaneous respiratory cycle. It does not, however, initiate the cycle. The assist decreases and ceases as soon as the spontaneous flow decreases and stops. By adjusting the magnitude of change in ventilator pressure per unit of flow (in $cmH_2O/l/s$), the clinician determines the degree of relief of the resistive work of breathing.[362]

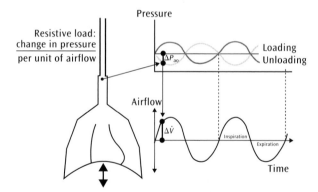

Figure 15.6 *Mechanical model of resistive loading and unloading. Resistive loading occurs during breathing through a tube such as an endotracheal tube. This causes the airway pressure at the level of the attachment to the airway (P_{ao}) to decrease below (inspiratory flow) and increase above (expiratory flow) the baseline (zero-flow) airway pressure. The P_{ao} changes in proportion to the respiratory airflow. If the tube is substituted for a flow-proportional assist device, the airway pressure contour is turned upside down in comparison with loading. It increases in proportion to the inspiratory airflow and thereby generates resistive unloading. The higher the ratio of change in pressure per unit of airflow is set by the clinician, the more assist is provided to the spontaneously breathing subject.*

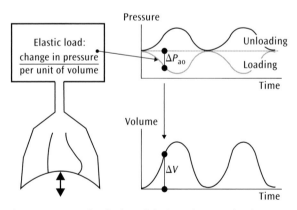

Figure 15.5 *Mechanical model of respiratory elastic loading and unloading. Elastic loading occurs during breathing out of and back into a sealed box. This causes the pressure at the airway opening (P_{ao}) to decrease in proportion to the inspired volume. If the box is substituted for a volume-proportional assist device, the airway pressure contour is turned upside down in comparison with loading so that the pressure increases in proportion to the inspired volume, thereby generating elastic unloading. The higher the ratio of increase in pressure per unit of inspired volume is set by the clinician, the more assist is provided to the spontaneously breathing subject.*

COMBINED RESISTIVE AND ELASTIC UNLOADING

During combined unloading, the applied ventilator pressure changes in proportion to both the volume and airflow of spontaneous breathing such that it is a weighted sum of the volume and the flow signal at any point in time.[364,369] Both elastic and resistive work of breathing are reduced. The clinician can set the gains of the two components independently. This makes it possible to tailor the ventilator pressure waveform to compensate for specific changes in lung compliance and airway resistance independently. The term 'proportional assist ventilation' specifically referred to applying the assist during inspiration only, but in proportion to both the tidal volume and airflow signal.[449,450] During full-cycle 'respiratory mechanical unloading', the airway pressure proportionally tracks the signals throughout the respiratory cycle.

APPLICATION

The clinician can specifically address the three main types of derangement in respiratory mechanics with RMU/PAV: decreased compliance, increased resistance, and decreased functional residual capacity (FRC). To apply this modality, three independent controls need to be set to address *the individual degree* of impairment in compliance, resistance, and FRC:

- The gain of elastic unloading (volume-proportional assist) relieves the elastic work of breathing for patients with 'stiff lungs'. This gain is adjusted on a continuous scale in cmH_2O/ml (applied ventilator pressure per unit of tidal volume).
- The gain of resistive unloading (flow-proportional assist) relieves the resistive work of breathing for patients with obstructive airway disease or those with a high-resistance endotracheal tube. This is adjusted in $cmH_2O/l/s$ (applied ventilator pressure per unit of airflow).
- The level of PEEP influences the FRC as it does during other conventional mechanical ventilation modalities.[364]

A simple way to initiate RMU/PAV in a clinical setting is to start with zero gains and let the patient briefly breathe without the assist at constant positive airway pressure (CPAP). The elastic unloading gain is then gradually increased to a level judged as 'appropriate' by clinical criteria such as reduction in chest wall distortion, tidal volume size, and regularity of breathing.[301,367] It is likely that smaller infants will need higher gains of elastic unloading (in absolute terms, that is, in cmH_2O/ml) as tidal volume and compliance relate to body weight. As a general rule, infants with a birthweight below 1000 g usually need about 1 cmH_2O/ml or more of elastic unloading gain while larger infants need less. The selected gain of resistive unloading should at least compensate for the resistance imposed by the endotracheal tube. This is about 20–30 $cmH_2O/l/s$ of resistive unloading for a 2.5 mm ID endotracheal tube. The required gain settings can also be calculated from measured or estimated pulmonary mechanics data.[360]

THEORETICAL PROBLEMS

If the applied unloading gains are excessive, in that they surpass lung elastic recoil and/or pulmonary resistance, a 'runaway' of the ventilator pressure may occur.[366] In such a situation, a small initial change in volume (airflow) triggers an increase in ventilator pressure, which then self-perpetuates through the positive feedback until the ventilator pressure reaches its set upper limit. At this point the inflation pressure is automatically aborted to the PEEP level where it will remain until the cycle repeats with the next onset of spontaneous inspiration. This will turn RMU/PAV into a modality similar to patient-triggered ventilation when airway pressure alternates between PEEP and PIP with each onset of a spontaneous respiratory effort. A similar ventilator pressure derangement may occur with a major endotracheal tube leak. The leakflow mimics inspiration and may cause the ventilator pressure to repeatedly rise to the set upper pressure limit. Ventilator software algorithms, however, can eliminate such leak effects up to a leak of about 30 percent of the tidal volume.[359] Ventilator software for RMU/PAV in infants must also reliably recognize hypoventilation and apnea and automatically initiate back-up ventilation.

CLINICAL STUDIES

While RMU has been extensively studied in small animals with and without lung injury,[231,327,366,367,369] there is only one published trial in preterm infants.[368] This study compared proportional assist to assist/control and to conventional mechanical ventilation in a crossover design involving 36 infants with birthweight between 600 and 1200 g who had mild to moderate acute respiratory illness. Short-term physiological outcome variables were evaluated. During proportional assist, the required mean airway pressures and transpulmonary pressures were lower at equivalent oxygen concentrations, equivalent pulmonary oxygen uptake and similar CO_2 removal rates. Under the strictly controlled conditions of the study, proportional assist appeared safe and at least as effective as the conventional modes. Infants on proportional assist typically showed a 'fast and shallow' respiratory pattern, with rates between about 50 and 80/min (Figure 15.7). Tidal volumes were usually smaller than 5 ml/kg. Proportional assist has not been formally evaluated as the initial and sole ventilatory modality in preterm infants with respiratory failure or in infants with other types of pulmonary or cardiac diseases. Investigations on RMU/PAV as a means for weaning from mechanical ventilation have also not been undertaken. Studies are underway to explore potential benefits of the application of RMU/PAV in

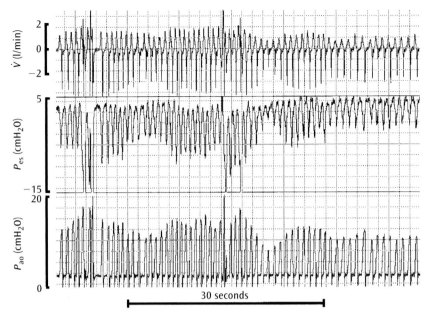

Figure 15.7 Tracings of airflow $\dot{V}$ and airway pressure (P_{ao}) as recorded between the Y-adaptor of the ventilator circuit and the endotracheal tube for a preterm infant on proportional assist ventilation. Inspiratory airflow is shown above and expiratory airflow below the zero-flow line. Note the characteristic fluctuations in peak inspiratory pressure in relation to the changes in esophageal pressure and flow. (From Schulze and Schaller[362] with permission.)

conjunction with other modalities such as SIMV and partial liquid ventilation.[232,412]

Future developments are likely to provide improved ventilator software for RMU/PAV in infants with adaptive algorithms to adjust back-up ventilation for apneic and hypoventilation episodes. The use of body surface signals to drive the ventilator in the RMU/PAV modes has a potential to avoid problems associated with endotracheal tube leaks and the additional dead space of the pneumotachograph.[370]

HIGH-FREQUENCY JET VENTILATION (HFJV)

HFJV was originally introduced to provide respiratory support during bronchoscopy in adults. In this technique, high-velocity bullets of gas are fired down into the airways from a small cannula mounted in the endotracheal tube.[151] The 'bullets' are fired at rates of 200–600 per minute and this entrains humidified gas down the endotracheal tube. The 'bullets' of high velocity gas stream down the center of the airway penetrating through the dead space gas, which simultaneously moves outward along the periphery of the airway.

Jet ventilators

Keszler and Durand have described jet ventilators in detail (see below).[249] The Bunnel Left Pulse HFJV is used in tandem with a conventional ventilator, the latter generates the PEEP. Short pulses of heated and humidified gas at high velocity are delivered to the upper airway through a narrow injector lumen in the Life Port adapter, which is a special 15 mm endotracheal tube adaptor. The 'tandem' conventional ventilator also provides IMV

breaths as required, usually at a rate of 2–10 bpm. The amplitude of the HFJV breaths is determined by the difference between the jet peak inspiratory pressure and the conventional PEEP.[249] The InfantStar has a microprocessor controlling a set of metered pneumatic valves; this device acts as a flow-controlled source to produce pressure oscillations in the patient circuit. It also contains a Venturi system on the exhalation valve to prevent inadvertent PEEP.[162] The InfantStar is a hybrid of HFJV and HFO and does not have a jet (Venturi) effect, which causes the pulses of gas produced by HFJV to stream down the center of the airway; there is no acceleration of the pulses of gas to a high velocity by passage through a narrow orifice.[249] Chakrabarti and Whitwam reported a valveless jet ventilator in which a single breathing tube was used; the respiratory gas was introduced near the patient's airway while a jet in the more distal part of the tube drove the respiratory gas into the patient's lungs.[65] The driving gas did not take part in gas exchange and there were no valves in the breathing system.

Jet ventilators may operate like constant-flow time-cycled ventilators and produce a triangular waveform; others are pressure servocontrolled with square waveforms. HFJV functions best over a relatively narrow range of inspiratory and expiratory times. If too short an inspiratory time is used, then a high pressure is necessary to compensate and provide an adequate tidal volume. An expiratory time below 170 ms is associated with gas trapping.

Ventilatory settings

The Life Pulse HFJV is usually started at a frequency of 7 Hz, the frequency altered according to the infant's time constant and an inspiratory time of 0.02 seconds.[249] The PEEP is increased to 6–8 cmH$_2$O to optimize lung volume.

Initially, the same PIP should be employed as used on CMV, but may require reduction within a few minutes if improved lung expansion results in better compliance. A background IMV rate of two to five breaths, inflation time 0.4–0.5 seconds is recommended, as these will act as intermittent sighs to open up the alveoli on inspiration.[249] Weaning, as on HFOV (p. 176), should initially be by decreasing the FiO_2, then the MAP – the philosophy being to maintain optimal lung volume at all times.

Clinical studies

Early rescue studies demonstrated that in infants with severe respiratory failure, HFJV could improve gas exchange in comparison with that attained on conventional ventilation.[50] It also appeared to have a role in stabilizing infants with diaphragmatic herniae. HFJV has been suggested to have advantages in infants with gross air leak. A decrease in the leak chest drains in infants with bronchopleural fistula has been noted[172] and similarly reduced flow through tracheoesophageal fistula with improved gas exchange[168] on transfer to HFJV. This advantage may be due to the very short inspiratory times that can be used during HFJV. A combination of helium and oxygen with HFJV may be useful in infants with severe respiratory failure.[416] Infants with abdominal distention may experience improved gas exchange on HFJV, as on HFO (p. 177). Randomized trials, however, have yielded conflicting results. Carlo et al.[62] randomized 42 infants with clinical and radiological evidence of severe RDS to receive either HFJV or conventional ventilation. There was no significant difference in the mortality (19 percent versus 24 percent), incidence of air leaks (48 percent versus 52 percent) or IVH (33 percent versus 43 percent) in the HFJV between the two groups. Carlo used a device that is not commercially available. By contrast, Keszler et al.[250] demonstrated HFJV was more useful than conventional ventilation in infants with RDS complicated by PIE. One hundred and forty-four infants were randomized to HFJV or rapid rate, conventional ventilation. Treatment success (defined as resolution of PIE for more than 24 hours and substantial radiological improvement of PIE and reduction of MAP to 40 percent less than pre-study levels was commoner in the HFJV (61 percent) than the conventional group (37 percent). There was a trend to a lower incidence of CLD in the HFJV group (67 percent versus 50 percent). Survival and the incidence of patent ductus arteriosus (PDA) and intraventricular hemorrhage (IVH) were similar in the two groups. In a multicenter randomized trial involving 130 patients,[252] HFJV use was associated with a reduction in the incidence of BPD at 36 weeks (20 percent versus 40 percent) and the need for home oxygen in premature infants with uncomplicated RDS, but no reduction in air leak. Increasing the PEEP by at least 1 cmH$_2$O from the pre-HFJV baseline and/or use of a PEEP level of at least 7 cmH$_2$O compared to a traditional HFJV strategy of low airway pressures or conventional ventilation was associated with better oxygenation. A trial involving 73 infants, mean gestational age 26.8 weeks, randomized to either early HFJV or conventional ventilation, however, was halted for safety reasons, as use of HFJV was associated with a significant increase in both severe ICH (22 percent CMV; 41 percent HFJV) and cystic PVL (6 percent CMV 31 percent HFJV).[440] There were no significant differences in the incidence of CLD between the groups (CMV 19 percent; HFJV 15 percent) or survival without CLD (CMV 69 percent, HFJV 57 percent).

In infants at near term or term with persistent pulmonary hypertension, although HFJV acutely improved oxygenation and ventilation, there were no significant differences in the duration of oxygen therapy, ventilation and hospitalization or differences in survival without use of ECMO, but only 24 infants were recruited into the study.[132] HFJV has been used in combination with surfactant replacement therapy to support infants with meconium aspiration syndrome, RDS or pneumonia. The infants all had severe respiratory failure despite surfactant treatment, that is MAP $\geq$ 12 cmH$_2$O, PIP $\geq$ 30 cm H$_2$O, arterial/alveolar oxygen (a/AO$_2$) ratio <0.1. One hour after being commenced on HFJV, there were significant improvements in PIP, MAP and the a/AO$_2$ ratio. This, however, was not sustained and further doses of surfactant were required. Twenty-five of the 28 infants survived, necrotizing tracheobronchitis (NTB) occurred in a premature infant who died. Meta-analysis of three randomized trials examining the elective use of HFJV compared to conventional ventilation demonstrated HFJV is associated with a reduction in CLD at 36 weeks PMA (RR 0.58, 0.34, 0.98).[40] In addition, there was a lower use of home oxygen (RR 0.24, 0.202, 0.79). Overall, there was a trend towards an increased risk of PVL, which was not significant.

Adverse effects

Use of HFJV has been associated with a high incidence of tracheal lesions; this is due to intraluminal tracheal pressure compromising mucosal and submucosal blood flow resulting in an ischemic lesion. Although NTB is not described by all who use HFJV,[61] in early series the prevalence ranges from 44 to 85 percent.[50,145] This was originally thought to be due to poor humidification. Animal experiments,[49] however, demonstrated that HFJV in comparison with conventional ventilation always produced the most tracheal lesions regardless of the level of humidity. Indeed, the severity of tracheal lesions was directly associated with the frequency used and the duration HFJV was employed. The lesions varied from inflammation and moderate erythema of the airway to severe erosion with total tracheal obstruction and are collectively termed NTB.[281] The lesions are also the consequence of the high-pressure bullets being aimed directly at the trachea, high mean pressure and the near constant intraluminal pressure. Subglottic stenosis and tracheal webs have been described after HFJV.[304] Gas trapping can be a feature of HFJV.[20] In a rabbit model, before and after meconium instillation, gas trapping was noted after HFJV but not HFO. HFJV may be a risk factor for the development of PVL, the possible mechanism being the production of hypocapnia in the first 3 days after birth.[441] Other randomized trials of HFJV, however, have found no significant differences in the incidence of PVL or ICH between HFJV and conventionally supported infants. The infants treated in Wiswell's study were more immature. A *post hoc* analysis of Keszler *et al.*'s trial suggested that ICH/PVL may be more likely when a low volume strategy was used.[252] In that study, 9 percent of the optimal volume subgroup had ICH/PVL compared to 33 percent in the low-pressure HFJV group and 28 percent in the conventional group. The low-pressure group had significantly lower carbon dioxide tensions in the first 24 hours.

HIGH-FREQUENCY FLOW INTERRUPTION (HFFI)

During HFFI, a high-pressure source of flow is interrupted. This can be done using a rotating ball valve (Emerson device).[148] The ball valve is rotated by a variable speed motor and interrupts the heated, humidified air–oxygen mixture. A valve at the distal end of the circuit controls the continuous distending pressure. Frequencies up to 20 Hz (1200/min) can be used. As with HFJV there is no active expiratory phase.

Clinical studies

HFFI has produced improvements in both blood gases and radiological appearance of infants with PIE.[148] Frantz *et al.*[148] were able to support infants with PIE on lower pressures using HFFI than conventional ventilation. HFFI may also be useful in the support of infants with meconium aspiration syndrome. This has been reported anecdotally[42] and in a comparative study in a piglet model the histological changes were less after HFFI than conventional ventilation. In a non-randomized study involving infants with PPHN,[238] the HFFI compared to the hyperventilation group required less vasopressor support, shorter mean time to extubation, shorter time for hospitalization and fewer infants with chronic lung disease. In a randomized trial comparing HIFI to CMV in premature infants weighing ≤1800 g and with RDS,[312] there were no significant differences in mortality, incidence of air leaks, pulmonary complications or blood gas analysis, but only 24 patients in total were examined.

Adverse effects

An increased incidence of tracheal necrosis has been reported in animals ventilated at a frequency of 10 Hz with a partially valved flow interruptor. Extremely high MAPs were used and this may be a factor in the pathogenesis of NTB.[108] In a piglet model, prior administration of hydrocortisone (2 mg/kg intravenously) reduced the severity of total airway injury following 8 hours of HFFI.[95]

HIGH-FREQUENCY OSCILLATION (HFO)

HFO is usually delivered at frequencies between 10 and 15 Hz (p. 173). In experimentally induced RDS, oxygenation can be improved by using sufficient pressure to prevent alveolar collapse and maintain lung distention. If oscillations, at least at a rate of 10 Hz (600 bpm), are applied on top of the mean airway pressure, then carbon dioxide elimination is ensured. At such frequencies, although the oscillatory pressures may be high, there is considerable dampening with less than a 25 percent pressure swing at the lower end of the endotracheal tube and perhaps 5 percent in the alveoli. HFO has been used to support neonates with severe respiratory failure (p. 176). Use of HFO can also reduce alveolar capillary leak and inhibit hyaline membrane formation.[202] Thus, it has been proposed that early use of HFO might reduce CLD; that hypothesis has now been tested in at least 10 randomized controlled trials.

Oscillator performance

A variety of techniques have been used to generate HFO. These include a sine wave pump or a diaphragm driven by a linear motor (SensorMedics). The Babylog produces pressure swings by a computer-controlled diaphragm oscillating in the exhalation block. During expiration, a jet Venturi system creates a negative pressure with respect to the chosen MAP. The software continually adjusts the inspiratory and expiratory times to ensure the inspiratory time is always shorter. The SLE creates a sinusoidal waveform by a jet rotating in the frequency range 3–20 Hz in the expiratory limb. The InfantStar has multiple solenoid inspiratory valves to create a rapid increase in flow in the arm of the circuit. The expiratory phase is favored by a Venturi system in the expiration valve creating subambient pressure in the exhalation arm of the circuit. The method by which HFO is generated influences the airway pressure waveform.[264] The oscillator, which has a diaphragm driven by a linear motor, delivers an asymmetrical and complex waveform, whereas the SLE

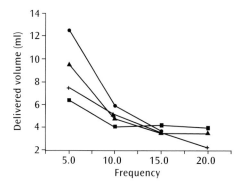

Figure 15.8 *Frequency dependence of delivered volume with the Draeger (X) the SLE (▲), SensorMedics (●) and InfantStar (■)*

has a more sinusoidal waveform. The method of generating HFO also influences performance as assessed by the volume delivered. Using apparently similar oscillatory settings, the SensorMedics delivered much greater volumes, particularly at low frequencies (Figure 15.8).[264] As frequency was increased the volume delivered by all oscillators falls (Figure 15.8).[264] A lab-based assessment of five oscillators,[206] the SensorMedics 3100A, Draeger Babylog 8000, Merran Humming V, InfantStar and InfantStar 950, demonstrated that at 15 Hz, confirmed variation in the delivered volume at 100 percent amplitude varied from 2.1 to 8.8 ml.[206] Again, generally the delivered volume decreased with increasing frequency. As the frequency is increased there is shorter time for diaphragm movement with the SensorMedics.[67,71,74] The impairment of oscillator performance with increasing frequencies has implications for carbon dioxide elimination during HFO (p. 174). The oscillators also vary with regard to whether they have a fixed inspiratory and expiratory ratio. The InfantStar has a fixed inspiratory time (18 ms), a range of frequencies is achieved by employing a variable valve-off time, this gives I:E ratios from 1:27 to 1:1.5. The SensorMedics oscillator has a variable inspiratory time and HFO can be achieved with I:E ratios of 1:1 or 1:2. Use of the shorter fractional inspiratory time was suggested to reduce the risk of gas trapping.[88] Measurements using a jacket plethysmograph, however, did not demonstrate any significant differences in lung volume as the fractional inspiratory time was increased from 30 to 50 percent.[7] Oscillators also vary with respect to the meaning of the displayed MAP.[206] Compared to the mean lung distending pressure measured during a brief occlusion maneuver (p. 156), the displayed mean airway pressure can either overestimate when the SensorMedics is used with 33 percent inspiratory fraction, be approximate with the InfantStar or underestimate with the Draeger.

HFO techniques

HFO is usually delivered on a background of a constant mean airway pressure. Certain oscillators (SensorMedics)

can only deliver HFO in this manner. HFO can, however, be delivered on a background of conventional ventilation. HFO can be delivered only during PEEP (Draeger) or on peak inflation (SLE) or throughout the conventional ventilatory cycle (SLE). There are disadvantages to the combined technique. The combination of conventional ventilation and HFO will produce the largest transpulmonary pressure swings, which could increase CLD (p. 402). To reduce the risk of gas trapping when HFO is used in combination with IMV, with the Babylog HFO is stopped for 100 ms before a mandatory IMV breath and then it does not resume for 50 ms afterwards to ensure adequate time for exhalation.

Manipulation of blood gases

OXYGENATION

During HFO, oxygenation is controlled by the inspired oxygen concentration and the MAP which controls lung volume. Oxygenation during HFO is independent of frequency and tidal volume,[357] except at very low values.[51] Two 'volume or pressure strategies' can be employed during HFO; low volume/low pressure[9] or high volume/high pressure.[88] The former strategy is used with the aim of reducing barotrauma and the latter to maintain lung volume above its closing pressure[54] and ensure lung recruitment. The high-volume strategy can improve pulmonary mechanics and is associated with a reduction in the inspired oxygen concentration and diminished structural injury.[202,284,288] HFO using a high- or low-volume strategy was compared to conventional ventilation in 20 surfactant-deficient lung-lavaged rabbits.[284] The high-volume strategy resulted in an FRC of 23.4 ml/kg compared to 7.8 and 4.3 ml/kg in the 'low-volume' HFO and conventional ventilation groups, respectively. Oxygenation was significantly better in the high-volume group, who also had significantly less hyaline membranes and severe airway epithelial damage. In both animals with diseased lungs[57] and sick newborns,[67] increasing MAP on transfer from conventional ventilation to HFO (high-volume strategy) improves oxygenation. Whereas transfer to HFO at the same MAP as used on conventional ventilation had a variable effect on oxygenation, increasing MAP by 2–5 cmH$_2$O improved oxygenation in the majority of infants with severe RDS.[67] The mean airway pressure necessary to optimize oxygenation during HFO is directly correlated with disease severity.[76] Infants with severe RDS with poor gas exchange on conventional ventilation frequently have very low lung volumes.[110] Not surprisingly, then, such infants require the largest changes in mean airway pressure to optimize their lung volume and hence oxygenation. Such a strategy, however, is not appropriate to the healthy lung, when alteration of MAP in modest amounts does not affect gas exchange,[97,241] but large increases cause deterioration in blood gases due to lung overdistention.[357] Similarly, in 'healthy' rabbits, an MAP level greater than 13 cmH_2O was not be tolerated for prolonged periods, due to cardiac depression.[357]

For any infant, there is an MAP level at which lung volume is optimum and hence so is oxygenation. Increasing MAP above that optimum level will impair oxygenation, as will reducing it below that level. The optimum MAP level will depend on the infant's disease severity and hence lung volume. Ideally, prior to transfer to HFO, the lung volume should be assessed and then the MAP increased accordingly.[110] Measurement of functional residual capacity using a helium gas dilution technique, however, is usually only available in the context of a research setting. An alternative approach is to use computer-assisted assessment of the lung area on the chest radiograph lung area;[119] using such a technique lung area was shown to correlate significantly with the change in MAP necessary to optimize oxygenation. In a piglet model, direct current coupled respiratory inductive plethysmography (RIP) (p. 112) has been shown to accurately detect lung overdistention during HFO;[436] whether such an approach in the clinical setting would be useful remains to be tested. Measurement of respiratory system compliance throughout lung volume optimization, however, has not proved useful.[240] Although CRS was inversely related to the optimal distending pressure, as we had noted previously,[76] CRS remains unchanged throughout lung volume optimization in infants with RDS.[240] In the absence of such measurement technique, the clinician should increase MAP in incremental steps, allowing sufficient time for lung volume to equilibrate. Measurement of lung volume using an inert gas (SF6) technique demonstrated that, in the majority of infants, lung volume equilibration occurred within 10 minutes of an MAP change, but in some infants up to 20 minutes was required.[410] In clinical practice, infants transferred to HFO should be continuously monitored by assessment of oxygen saturation or preferably by invasive arterial oxygen measurements. Changes in MAP should only occur when such continuous monitoring indicates that there are no further changes in oxygenation.

The relationship between the mean airway pressure displayed on any given oscillator and the mean alveolar pressure in the infant's lungs will vary with the device. In the SensorMedics at 30 percent inspiration the mean alveolar pressure is lower than displayed; the same is true for the InfantStar. For the Humming Bird and possibly other sine wave generators with an I:E ratio of 1:1, the displayed and actual pressures are about equal but, if using a Draeger Babylog 8000, the intrapulmonary pressures will be higher than the displayed pressure.[206] This has practical implications if a hospital has more than one type of oscillator. For example, a switch from a SensorMedics 3100A to a Draeger ventilator at a display pressure of 12 cmH_2O could result in a 5–8 cmH_2O abrupt increase in distending pressure.[206]

CARBON DIOXIDE ELIMINATION

Carbon dioxide elimination during HFO is usually independent of MAP.[414] Indeed, one of the desirable features of HFOV is independent control of $PaCO_2$ with amplitude adjustments and PaO_2 control with MAP adjustments.[206] This does not, however, occur with the Draeger at low MAP and high amplitude; if the MAP is then increased so is volume increased and hence CO_2 elimination. The explanation for this is that it avoids subjecting the airways to subatmospheric pressures and inducing flow limitation and traumatizing tissues. As a result, during the expiratory phase of the oscillatory cycle, the machine would pull out of the lungs only until the airway pressure became subatmospheric.[206] Carbon dioxide elimination is affected by the frequency and the delivered volume (squared).[97] The delivered volume is mainly influenced by the amplitude[113] and much less by frequency between 10 and 15 Hz, particularly in an infant with stiff lungs.[264] The inspiratory to expiratory ratio, as this also influences delivered volume, will also affect carbon dioxide elimination.[116]

Frequency

During HFO, the delivered volume might be expected to be greatest at the resonant frequency of the respiratory system. Phase analysis to determine the resonant frequency of infants with RDS demonstrated the resonant frequency remained remarkably constant in the early stages of the illness (within 2 Hz in eight babies and within 6 Hz in all 12 babies studied) despite larger changes in compliance (increases in compliance over the first 7 days varied from 27 to 129 percent).[268] In post mortem specimens of severe RDS the resonant frequency was found to be between 15 and 23 Hz,[127] and those data correlated with the relationship of maximum volume delivery to frequency in a clinical study of infants with RDS.[227] In that latter study, however, a piston oscillator, which delivered a constant volume regardless of frequency, was used, whereas the volume delivered by commercially available oscillators decreases as frequency is increased (p. 172).[264] Thus, in the clinical setting increasing frequency should result in improvements in delivered volume as the resonant frequency is approached but this is counterbalanced by impairment of oscillator performance. Hence, although increasing from 10 to 15 Hz resulted in a significant change in carbon dioxide elimination, the size of the change was small and not clinically significant.[76] Reducing the frequency below 10 Hz, particularly with the SensorMedics, results in a much greater volume delivery and hence can be a useful maneuver in term infants with severe respiratory acidosis.

I:E ratio

Pillow and colleagues measured the mean airway opening pressure at the alveolar pressure using the alveolar capsule technique in four adult rabbits receiving HFO.[320]

They found that at I:E ratios of 1:1, there was essentially no difference between the mean airway opening and mean alveolar pressure, supporting the claim that this I:E ratio is not associated with airtrapping.[7] They also showed that at I:E ratios of 1:2 the mean alveolar pressure was significantly reduced compared to the airway opening pressure and this reduction was directly related to the frequency of oscillation, the size of the endotracheal tube, the tidal volume and the difference between the inspiratory and expiratory flow rates. This difference could exceed 6 cmH$_2$O under clinical conditions. Their conclusion was that an I:E ratio of 1:1 was preferable, as the reduction in alveolar pressure was unpredictable and could change as ventilator settings and lung mechanics altered. Increasing the I:E ratio from 1:2 to 1:1 in the clinical setting has been shown to increase the delivered volume and hence carbon dioxide elimination.[116] In addition, if no compensatory changes in flow are made, MAP and oxygenation were higher at the 1:1 I:E ratio.[116] As such a maneuver has not been associated with gas trapping in infants,[7] except in very immature infants requiring MAP of less than 8 cmH$_2$O, our preferred starting I:E ratio is 1:1.

Mechanism of gas exchange

During certain forms of oscillation, the delivered volume is less than half the dead space and thus gas transport cannot be by convection. There is gas transport between gas exchanging units, as some alveoli will empty or fill faster than others (Pendelluft). Turbulence, due to high frequency fluctuations and augmented diffusion may also enhance gas exchange during HFO. Some alveoli close to the airways, however, are directly ventilated even at tidal volumes smaller than the dead space. In the clinical setting, Dimitriou *et al.*,[113] using recognized techniques of tidal volume measurement at very fast frequencies,[51,97] found that the delivered volume in a number of infants was at least 50 percent of the infant's estimated dead space;[261] thus conventional gas exchange can take place during HFO.

Clinical use of oscillation

TRANSFER FROM CONVENTIONAL VENTILATION (FIGURE 15.9)

Prior to transfer to HFO, it is important to ensure an appropriately sized endotracheal tube is being used and, if not, changed to a larger tube. Down the length of the endotracheal tube there is attenuation of the oscillatory amplitude signal. The degree of attenuation was greatest with smaller endotracheal tubes and lower oscillatory amplitudes. For all oscillators tested,[264] this amounted to between 35 and 45 percent attenuation. This attenuation resulted in a lower volume delivery; compared to a 2.5 mm endotracheal tube, the volumes delivered via a

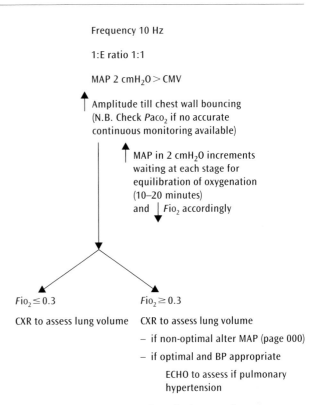

Frequency 10 Hz

1:E ratio 1:1

MAP 2 cmH$_2$O > CMV

↑ Amplitude till chest wall bouncing (N.B. Check $Paco_2$ if no accurate continuous monitoring available)

↑ MAP in 2 cmH$_2$O increments waiting at each stage for equilibration of oxygenation (10–20 minutes) and ↓ Fio_2 accordingly

$Fio_2 \leq 0.3$
CXR to assess lung volume

$Fio_2 \geq 0.3$
CXR to assess lung volume
 – if non-optimal alter MAP (page 000)
 – if optimal and BP appropriate
   ECHO to assess if pulmonary hypertension

Figure 15.9 *Oscillatory settings during transfer to rescue HFO (high-volume strategy).*

3.5 mm endotracheal tube were on average 20 percent higher.[264] A similar comparison during conventional ventilation results in only a 2.4 percent difference in the delivered volume. If a high-volume strategy is to be pursued, then a MAP at least 2 cmH$_2$O higher than that used during conventional ventilation should be used initially.[67] The MAP should then be increased in incremental stages, continuously monitoring oxygenation. The oscillatory amplitude is increased until the chest wall is 'bouncing'. It is important to ensure, prior to transfer, that the infant is normovolemic and normotensive. HFO aggravates hypotension due to hypovolemia and this must therefore be corrected if HFO is being considered. As oxygenation improves, the inspired oxygen concentration should be reduced, preferably down to 0.30, before the MAP level is decreased. Some infants initially show an improvement in oxygenation on transfer to HFO when MAP is increased, but then it is not possible to reduce the FiO_2 to the desired level. Such infants frequently have associated pulmonary hypertension and it is important to perform an echocardiographic examination. For affected infants, additional or alternative respiratory support should be used. If an inhaled pulmonary vasodilator is to be employed, it is essential lung volume is optimized (p. 184). If transfer to high-volume strategy HFO is contemplated, prior to transfer it is important to increase the PEEP and hence MAP level. Improvement in oxygenation in response to PEEP elevation indicates that a high-volume strategy HFO will improve gas exchange, whereas if there is no improvement in oxygenation, high-volume strategy HFO is unlikely to be helpful.

MANAGEMENT DURING HFO

It is essential to perform a chest radiograph soon after commencing HFO to ensure adequate lung expansion has occurred and there is no evidence of overexpansion. Once optimum lung volume has been established, it is important that lung volume is maintained. This has implications for nursing procedures, particularly regarding suction. Any procedure which requires the infant to be disconnected from the oscillator should be done as infrequently and as quickly as possible. It is preferable to use a closed system suctioning device (p. 237). Hand ventilation is a relatively ineffective method of volume recruitment.[54] Once reconnected to the oscillator, therefore, to attain an appropriate lung volume, stepwise increase in MAP above the predisconnection level might be necessary to restore oxygenation.

Routine paralysis is not necessary during HFO. In the HIFI trial only 17 percent of infants were paralyzed because of agitation or adverse respiratory efforts.[9] It had been suggested from animal studies that HFO induces apnea. In our own experience apnea is uncommon, although a significant reduction in respiratory rate does occur on transfer to HFO.[78] Continuance of respiratory efforts during HFO does not necessarily impair gas exchange in the majority of infants.[78]

Changes in oxygenation are, therefore, first counteracted by manipulation of MAP accompanied, if necessary, by performance of a chest radiograph to assess if the infant is over- or underinflated. Alternative causes of poor oxygenation should also be sought, that is, hypotension and anemia. Changes in $PaCO_2$ are controlled by alterations in the oscillatory amplitude; if the $PaCO_2$ has increased, the oscillatory amplitude should be elevated and vice versa. Only in cases of severe respiratory acidosis on high amplitudes, are frequencies less than 10 Hz required.

WEANING THE INFANT FROM HFO

It is important to maintain lung volume to optimize oxygenation, thus, as recovery from RDS begins, the inspired oxygen concentration should be turned down before altering the MAP level (p. 175). Once the inspired oxygen concentration has been reduced to 30 percent, the MAP is then reduced in 2 cmH_2O steps at a rate dictated by the blood gases. If weaning is performed too rapidly, atelectasis will occur and it is necessary to increase the MAP level above that at which the weaning process occurred to optimize respiratory status once more. Once the MAP level has been reduced to 8 cmH_2O there are two options for further weaning. One option is to extubate the infant directly from HFO. The second option is to change the infant to a short period of PTV prior to extubation; such a policy is facilitated by the machines that offer a choice of oscillation, triggered and conventional ventilation. A period on PTV can be useful to confirm that the infant has adequate respiratory drive to ensure successful extubation.

Clinical studies

Initial studies demonstrated that during HFO, compared to conventional ventilation, adequate gas exchange could often be achieved at lower pressures[147] and inspired oxygenation concentrations.[283] Other studies demonstrated that a high-volume strategy HFO could improve gas exchange in infants whose respiratory failure was poorly responsive to conventional ventilation despite use of surfactant as appropriate.[74] Comparison with non-randomized controls suggested that a policy of initiating HFO immediately after intubation and attempting early lung volume optimization before surfactant was administered in VLBW infants could shorten the need for respiratory support and significantly reduce the incidence of chronic lung disease at 36 weeks postconceptional age (PCA) (0 percent versus 34 percent).[340] The number of infants recruited into the study ($n = 71$) was small, but the results are in keeping with those from animal studies. HFO begun at birth has been shown to limit the development of alveolar proteinaceous edema in premature primates at risk of RDS.[234,288] In addition, results suggested that HFO might be a useful alternative to ECMO. In one series, 46 of 50 infants referred for ECMO were first tried on HFO and approximately half the infants were successfully maintained on HFO without recourse to ECMO.[63] There were no significant differences between the HFO and ECMO groups regarding mortality or hospital stay, but greater morbidity was experienced in the ECMO cohort.

PREDICTION OF OUTCOME

Transfer to HFO may fail to improve oxygenation. Results from anecdotal studies have shown that a lack of improvement in oxygenation within 6 hours of transfer is significantly associated with an increased risk of mortality[75,387] or survival with disability.[82] A low oxygen intake (OI) and $AaDO_2$ at the beginning of oscillation and no development of air leak syndromes have been associated with higher survival.[387]

SPECIFIC RESPIRATORY CONDITIONS

Meconium aspiration syndrome (MAS)

The effect of MAS on the lung varies according to the severity of the disease and age since birth (p. 338). When the disease has produced a very asymmetrical picture, HFO is less successful and this may explain the conflicting results from animal studies (p. 345). Randomized trials of term or near-term infants have included those with MAS, but also infants with other respiratory conditions;

no differences in major outcomes were found between those supported by HFO compared to those on CMV. The combination of HFO and inhaled nitric oxide (iNO) in MAS infants, however, has been shown to reduce ECMO requirement.[256] On current evidence, use of HFO in MAS should be restricted to rescue support, particularly in those infants with relatively symmetrical lung disease.

Severe abdominal distention

Infants with severe abdominal distention often have reduced lung volume and impaired diaphragmatic movement resulting in poor gas exchange on conventional ventilation. Recruitment of lung volume and improvement in gas exchange can be achieved in affected infants by use of high-volume strategy HFO.[144]

Air leak syndrome

Infants whose gas exchange deteriorates because of the development of a pneumothorax, clearly respond better to drainage of the pneumothorax rather than simply being transferred to HFO. Only when successful drainage has been accomplished, if gas exchange remains poor, should HFO be considered. In a prospective non-randomized study,[303] transfer of infants with PIE to HFOV at the same MAP resulted in improvements in gas exchange and no compromise to cardiac output (CO). Infants with PIE pose a difficult challenge and, as they have relatively compliant lungs,[303] easily suffer severe lung overdistention despite relatively modest increases in MAP which could compromise cerebral circulation. Transfer of infants with PIE to HFO, therefore, should be at the same MAP or lower than that used during CMV. Oxygenation should be improved by elevating the inspired oxygen concentration and arterial oxygen levels of 6–7 kPa (45–52.5 mmHg) accepted, providing this is not causing compromise, for example being associated with a metabolic acidosis.

RANDOMIZED TRIALS

Severe respiratory failure

Term neonates. There has been only one randomized trial comparing HFO and conventional ventilation in term or near-term infants with severe respiratory failure.[89] Treatment failure criteria were well defined and a greater proportion of the infants meeting those criteria in the CMV group could be rescued by HFO than vice versa (63 percent versus 13 percent, $P = 0.03$), that was despite significantly more of the HFO group meeting ECMO criteria at randomization (67 versus 40 percent, $P = 0.03$). There were, however, no significant differences in the longer-term outcomes of the two groups, for example requirement for ECMO (RR 2.05, 0.85–4.92), days on ventilator or in oxygenation or hospital.[89]

Preterm neonates. Similarly, there has only been one trial comparing HFO to conventional ventilation in preterm neonates with severe respiratory failure. The positive finding from that study was that use of HFO was associated with a reduction in new pulmonary air leak developing (RR 0.73, 0.55–0.96), the number of infants needed to be treated to prevent one infant having a pulmonary air leak was six (95 percent CI 3, 37). There was, however, no difference in the rate of PIE or gross pulmonary air leak, mortality or use of IPPV at 30 days between the two groups.[214] In addition, the rate of ICH of any grade was increased in infants treated with HFO (RR 1.77, 1.06–2.96). This means that for every six infants (95 percent CI 3.50) treated with HFO, one ICH would be caused.

Prophylactic trials

There have been at least 10 randomized trials in which infants have been randomized to HFOV or CMV in the first 24 hours. They have differed with respect to antenatal steroid and postnatal surfactant usage, the exact timing of randomization and the type of conventional ventilation and ventilator employed. Importantly, no lung recruitment strategy was used in the control groups of the majority of trials and this may have influenced the outcome, as pressure-controlled ventilation with sufficient level of PEEP and small driving pressure amplitudes is as effective as HFOV in maintaining optimal gas exchange, improving lung mechanics and preventing protein influx.[425] Meta-analysis[209] of the results of the six randomized trials[9,88,163,306,335,411] demonstrated HFO, particularly if a lung recruitment strategy was used, was associated with a reduction in CLD. No significant differences in mortality were noted, but there was a tendency towards an increase in ICH and air leak.[209] A subsequently reported randomized trial,[299] however, demonstrated that the only positive effect of HFO was that fewer of the HFO-supported infants required two or more doses of surfactant (30 percent versus 92 percent, odds ratio 0.27, 95 percent CI 0.16–0.44). There was, however, no significant difference in CLD and a greater proportion of the HFO group developed severe intraventricular hemorrhage (24 percent versus 14 percent); this trend was no longer significant when adjusted for differences in pregnancy-related hypertension between the two groups. In that study, surfactant therapy was given and all the researchers taking part were experienced in oscillation. Since the study, the OFHI oscillator used has been withdrawn from clinical service, which has led some to suggest its use may explain the poor results of Moriette's trial.[299] In bench studies, however, the OHFI oscillator has been shown to perform similarly to other oscillators.[239] An alternative explanation for the difference in Moriette's results compared to previous trials was that in the earlier studies there may have been less than optimal use of conventional ventilation. The UK Oscillation Study (UKOS), which recruited more than 800 infants, has recently been completed. All researchers who took part in the study were experienced in both conventional and oscillatory ventilation and there was a high usage of both antenatal steroids and postnatal surfactant. No statistically significant negative or positive results were demonstrated by that trial. Three different oscillators were used, but all have been shown to function similarly at the settings used in that trial.[264] It thus seems unlikely that the oscillator types resulted in the 'negative' results. A more plausible explanation is that the lack of effect reflected that the researchers were all experienced with both ventilatory modes. An interpretation of those data is that HFO and CMV are equally effective when started soon after birth, but it should be noted that the results were generated in the context of a randomized trial and all patients, regardless of allocation, do better in such a study (Hawthorne effect). There are continuing concerns about the adverse effects of HFO regarding intracerebral pathology, particularly in inexperienced hands; for that reason we no long use HFO 'prophylactically'.

ADVERSE EFFECTS

During high-volume strategy HFO, the constant mean airway pressure and intrathoracic volume could increase the risk of depressing organ blood flow and diuresis. In one series,[29] however, premature infants less than 30 weeks of gestational age randomized to HFO, despite being exposed to higher mean airway pressures, had similar reductions in extracellular volumes and onset of diuresis to those infants randomized to the conventional group. In the HIFI trial, HFO compared to conventional ventilation was associated with a significantly higher rate of grade 3 and 4 IVH and periventricular leukomalacia (PVL). This adverse effect was suggested to be due to the near-constant MAP used during HFO resulting in compromise of venous return, in turn leading to a rise in cerebral venous pressure and decrease in cerebral blood flow. The hypothesis was initially supported by studies in baboons,[108] but more recently HFO was not found to cause any adverse effects on central venous pressure, cardiac output or cerebral blood flow in the same animal model.[254] Interestingly, in the HIFI trial,[9] a 'low-volume, low-pressure' strategy was employed[54] and in two subsequent studies when a high-volume strategy was used, no such excess of cerebral pathology was noted.[88,306] Indeed, in the latter study, a reverse trend was noted with 9 percent PVL in the conventional group compared to 2 percent in the HFO group. The latter two studies recruited many fewer infants than the HIFI trial and thus a type II error cannot be discounted. A meta-analysis published in 1996 of randomized trials,[90] including the HIFI study, demonstrated trends towards an increase in all IVH and grade 3 and 4 IVH when HFO was used and a significant effect regarding PVL (OR 1.7, 95 percent CI 1.06, 2.74). Those trends, however, disappeared when the results of the HIFI trial were removed. One explanation[54] for the conflicting results regarding the incidence of IVH between

the studies[9,306] is population and/or management differences between centers involved in the trials. The incidence of IVH experienced in the HIFI trial overall was very much higher than that experienced by infants supported either conventionally or by HFO in the Japanese study.[306] In addition, the incidence of grade 3 and 4 IVH varied from 6 to 44 percent between centers in the HIFI trial; those differences were greater than that experienced between the HFO and conventional ventilation groups.[9] Subsequent meta-analyses[94] have failed to demonstrate a significant relationship of an increase in ICH and HFO. There remain, however, the concerning data of Moriette et al.[299] Criticisms levelled at the HIFI study, lack of experience of certain researchers in the trial and an inappropriate strategy did not occur in Moriette's study. Increased intracerebral pathology during HFO might occur as a result of lung overdistention or rapidly reduced carbon dioxide tensions. Large increases in mean airway pressure to optimize oxygenation could reduce venous return, increasing intracerebral blood volume and intracranial pressure with a consequent reduction in cerebral blood flow. Assessment of cerebral blood flow velocity (CBFV) using a continuous Doppler blood flow measurement technique,[247] however, revealed no change in CBFV as mean airway pressure was increased during volume optimization on HFO. In two individuals, however, large changes in CBFV occurred on transfer to HFO and these were associated with marked changes in carbon dioxide tensions. Those results emphasize that if HFO is to be used safely, continuous carbon dioxide monitoring should be employed.[247] Other possible adverse effects relate to the noise generated during HFO; this particularly applies to the SensorMedics oscillator. The maximum level of noise recommended by the US Environmental Protection Agency is 55 dB during waking hours and 45 dB during sleeping hours in the neighborhood, but 45 and 35 respectively in the hospital setting.[12]

FOLLOW-UP

Respiratory

Follow-up studies have usually demonstrated similar lung function in children who had been supported by HFO compared to those who had received conventional ventilation. Pulmonary mechanics measured serially up to 4 weeks of age in 43 infants who had been randomized to HFO or conventional ventilation revealed no significant difference in lung function between the groups, but the sample size was small. In addition, the incidence of BPD did not differ (57 percent in the HFO group; 50 percent in the conventional ventilation group).[1] In 53 infants lung function was measured prior to discharge;[161] although both groups had abnormal lung function, decreased lung compliance and elevated pulmonary resistance, there was no significant difference between infants treated conventionally or by HFO. Follow-up of children aged 8–9 years who were entered into the HIFI trial demonstrated a mildly obstructive pattern in the prematurely born children. More severe obstruction was seen in the children who had physician-diagnosed asthma or who had used bronchodilators in the past. The prevalence of abnormalities, however, was similar regarding the two forms of respiratory support.[319] Eighty-seven percent of infants who were originally assigned to receive treatment with HFO or CMV in the Provo trial have been examined at a mean age of 77 months. There were no differences in the frequency of hospitalization, pulmonary illness, asthma or disability. Unusually, in that study, patients randomized to treatment with CMV had worse lung function at follow-up, as evidenced by lower peak expiratory flows, increased residual lung volume and maldistribution of ventilation.[164]

Neurodevelopmental

No significant differences have been found in infants entered into prophylactic trials related to mode of ventilation. Bayley psychometric evaluations and central nervous system examinations were performed at 16–24 months in 77 percent of survivors from the HIFI trial. Cerebral palsy was diagnosed in 10 percent of the HFO and 11 percent of the conventional ventilation group. There was a significantly higher incidence of hydrocephaly (12 percent versus 6 percent, $P < 0.05$) and lower normal neurological status, Bayley score >83 (54 versus 65 percent, $P < 0.05$) in the HFO compared to the conventional ventilation group. No significant difference in respiratory status or growth was found between the groups.[9] Growth, verbal IQ and motor development were appropriate for age and did not differ between the two groups.[164] By contrast, in infants exposed to rescue HFO at 2 years of age compared to case controls matched for gestational age, the HFO infants had worse neurodevelopmental outcome, particularly if born at very early gestational ages.[120]

EXTRACORPOREAL MEMBRANE OXYGENATION (ECMO)

This is a form of cardiopulmonary bypass. Initially introduced for adults, it was abandoned when randomized trials failed to demonstrate it improved survival over that achieved by conventional therapy. Bartlett et al.[26] reactivated interest in this technique, but for use in neonates.

Technique

There are two forms of ECMO; venoarterial (VA), in which blood is taken from the right jugular vein and returned via the right common carotid artery, and venovenous (VV) in which blood is taken from the right jugular vein and returned usually through the femoral vein, although the umbilical vein has also been used. VA ECMO has the advantage that approximately 80 percent cardiopulmonary bypass is achieved and thus the level of respiratory support can be reduced, limiting further barotrauma. The disadvantage of VA is that there is the potential for clots or air to enter directly into the arterial circulation. In addition, in the smallest babies carotid artery reconstruction[99] following decannulation may be difficult and carotid artery ligation is not without risk.[372] During venovenous ECMO, cardiopulmonary bypass is not attained and thus the infant must have good myocardial function. In addition, femoral vein ligation following decannulation may result in leg edema. There have not been head-to-head trials of VA versus VV ECMO. Using data from the ELSO registry, however, a matched-pair analysis was undertaken which highlighted that there was a survival advantage for VV ECMO (91.5 percent versus 83.8 percent).[158]

ECMO CIRCUIT (FIGURE 15.10)

In both VA and VV ECMO, the venous blood is pumped to an oxygenator which has blood and gas compartments separated by semipermanent membranes where diffusion of oxygen and carbon dioxide occurs. Oxygen transfer is controlled by the membrane's surface area, pump flow and the degree of saturation of the 'venous' blood. Carbon dioxide elimination is adjusted by altering the flow rate; it is often necessary to add CO_2 to the blood returned to the infant. Prior to returning to the infant, the blood is passed through a heat exchanger, as heat is

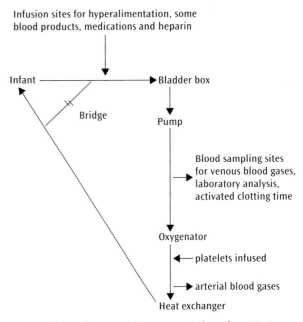

Figure 15.10 *Diagrammatic representation of an ECMO circuit.*

lost in the oxygenator due to its large surface area. It is obviously essential that the blood is pumped around the circuit at a rate compatible with the venous return; to ensure this there are a variety of devices which can be incorporated into the circuit. One such is a bladder box, which contains a sensor to detect collapse or overexpansion of the bladder; the sensor then controls the pump speed accordingly. Another device is a dual transducer, which measures pressures on both sides of the circuit. Centrifugal pumps provide simple and safe technology for transportation on ECMO. Non-occlusive pumps, centrifugal pumps or the assistence respiratoire extracorporelle (AREC) system which enables single needle VV ECMO, have been successfully used in ECMO for neonatal, cardiac and pediatric patients.[420]

It is possible to infuse and sample from various points in the circuit (Figure 15.10). Most infusions are administered prior to the bladder box, which functions as an air trap. Platelets, however, are infused after the oxygenator to reduce the risk of aggregation.

Management during ECMO

The largest cannulae possible should be used, 12 or 14 FG, as the catheter's diameter influences the flow rate that can be attained. Paralysis is necessary for the insertion of the cannula, but need not be maintained throughout the ECMO period. Continuous sedation should be administered, but problems with fentanyl have been experienced, including the development of tolerance and dependence.[13] Fully heparin-bonded circuits are not presently available. As a consequence, it is necessary to heparinize the infant and measure that an appropriate level is maintained by performing serial estimations of the activated clotting time (ACT). The infant's packed cell volume should be maintained at 40–45 percent by transfusion when necessary and platelet infusions are given to keep the platelet level above $75\,000\,mm^3$.[276] In critically ill patients maintained on ECMO, renal function is often inadequate. This is best dealt with by putting a hemodialysis unit in the circuit.

During ECMO, the PaO_2 is kept between 80 and $100\,mmHg$ and $PaCO_2$ 40 and $50\,mmHg$.[276] In VA ECMO, once cardiopulmonary bypass has been achieved, the level of respiratory support can be reduced. Atelectasis, however, can be a problem and high $(10–12\,cmH_2O)$ rather than low $(2–5\,cmH_2O)$ levels of PEEP are more successful in preventing a deterioration in lung function and in shortening the duration of ECMO.[251]

WEANING

This is achieved by gradually reducing the flow rate. When only a low flow rate is needed, then the circuit is clamped and blood diverted across one of the 'bypass'

bridges. If blood gases are maintained after a few hours, then the infant will be decannulated.

Eligibility for ECMO

ECMO facilities are limited and it is important to reserve ECMO for an infant who has a high chance of recovery within a short time. Conventional therapy is extremely successful in the majority of infants, even those with severe respiratory failure, and ECMO has complications (p. 182). It is therefore desirable to further restrict ECMO use to those infants who would respond poorly to conventional therapy. Previously an OI greater than 40 had been used as this had been associated historically with >90 percent mortality. In the UK ECMO trial, an OI of >40 was only associated with a 41 percent mortality, which may reflect adoption of newer techniques of respiratory support and that an OI of 40 is no longer an appropriate level on which to recommend institution of ECMO. Guidelines for ECMO use have been drawn up (Table 15.6). It has been estimated that between 1 in 3400 infants[280] to 1 in 4000 infants[421] in the UK require ECMO.

Clinical studies

MORTALITY

Up to January 2002, 18 546 neonates had been reported to the ELSO Registry as receiving ECMO worldwide; survival during ECMO was 86 percent in respiratory and 56 percent in cardiac cases. Survival to discharge was 78 percent and 39 percent, respectively. Infants from Europe reported to the Registry overall had 74 percent survival

Table 15.6 *ECMO eligibility*

- Birthweight > 2.0 kg
- Gestational age > 34 weeks (85 percent of infants in one series[86] with gestational age <35 weeks developed intracranial hemorrhage on ECMO)
- No bleeding disorder
- No congenital abnormality incompatible with quality life
- Disorders with short-term reversibility – usually interpreted as having received less than 10 days' aggressive mechanical ventilation
- A predicted mortality >80 percent (this is usually determined from historical controls)
  - $AaDO_2 \geqslant 610\,mmHg$ for 8 hours (associated with 79 percent mortality by Beck *et al.*[32])
  - $AaDO_2 > 620\,mmHg$ for 12 hours[260]
  - Oxygen index > 40*

$AaDO_2 = FiO_2 \times (760 - 47\,mmHg) - PaO_2 - PaCO_2$ where $760\,mmHg$ = atmospheric pressure and $47\,mmHg$ = water vapour pressure.
*Oxygen index = (mean airway pressure $\times FiO_2$)/ $(PaO_2$ (postductal) $\times 100$).

rate, more than 90 percent of MAS infants surviving but only 50 percent of CDH infants surviving. There is also a mortality related to transporting infants to a center for ECMO.[45] Factors influencing survival include the ECMO center's experience[417] and the infant's birthweight,[336] mortality being higher in infants of lower birthweight. In addition, the original diagnosis has an important influence on outcome.

CDH INFANTS

Poorer survival rates are reported for infants with CDH; this appears to be related to complications such as bleeding and renal failure.[263] In addition, the severity of pulmonary hypoplasia and pulmonary vasculature abnormality of some infants with CDH is such as to be incompatible with life despite ECMO. It is obviously desirable to detect such infants prior to embarking on ECMO. It has been suggested that such factors as failure to achieve satisfactory oxygenation (preductal $PaO_2 > 100\,mmHg$) on maximum therapy or a $PaCO_2 < 50\,mmHg$ can identify such individuals.[398] Initial assessment of PDA flow may help predict ECMO outcome,[173] with right-to-left PDA flow suggesting a worse outcome. Antenatal diagnosis and transfer of the mother prior to birth to an ECMO center did not improve the outcome of CDH infants.[45] The mode of ECMO in CDH also does not appear to influence survival.[122] Interrogation of the ELSO Registry for newborns with CDH treated with ECMO during a 10-year period demonstrated VA ECMO was utilized in 2257 and VV ECMO in 371. The pre-ECMO status of the two groups was similar, but there was greater use of surfactant and inotropes in the VV group. Survival rate was similar (58.4 percent for VV and 52.2 percent for VA), but VA ECMO was associated with more seizures (12.3 percent vs 6.7 percent) and cerebral infarction (10.5 percent vs 6.7 percent). Sixty-four treatments were converted from VV to VA.[122]

BPD INFANTS

Search of the ELSO Registry revealed the survival rate of ECMO-treated BPD infants was 78 percent.[213] Results from a single institution, however, highlighted a high rate of pulmonary prolonged ventilator dependence of many months and neurodevelopmental sequelae.[213]

TRISOMY 21

Between 1984 and 1999, 15 942 infants including 91 with trisomy 21 were placed on ECMO. The infants with trisomy 21 were over-represented in the ECMO infants compared to the general population, perhaps as a result of delayed extrauterine pulmonary vascular adaptation, as manifested in the high rate of primary persistent pulmonary hypertension as the primary diagnosis. The survival to discharge was lower in the trisomy 21 patients (65.9–75.6 percent) because of increased post-ECMO mortality.[394]

OTHER DIAGNOSES

In a series of three infants, ECMO was suggested to be beneficial in infants with therapy-resistant gastric rupture, all three infants surviving despite two having developed major hemorrhagic complications.[302] Use of ECMO to manage ventilation during tracheal repair of children with tracheal stenosis and obstruction may allow better visualization at the surgical site and obviates the need for indwelling endotracheal tubes and high-pressure ventilation.[93]

RANDOMIZED TRIALS

The first two trials recruited in total only 31 infants and their study designs were criticized.[27,307] The trial of Bartlett et al.[27] used a 'play the winner' analysis. This meant that after success or failure of the first patient's treatment, subsequent randomization was biased towards a successful outcome and away from a non-successful outcome. The first patient was randomized to conventional ventilation and died; the next 12 infants were randomized to ECMO and 11 survived. The trial was then terminated as the results were significant in favor of ECMO. In O'Rorke's study,[307] a maximum of four deaths were permitted in either arm of the trial. Four of 10 infants who received conventional ventilation died, but the nine who received ECMO survived. This trial was criticized as it was underpowered to differentiate meaningful differences in outcome between ECMO and conventional therapy. In a subsequent randomized trial,[11] infants were recruited who had an oxygenation index of at least 40 or an arterial partial pressure of carbon dioxide of 12 kPa (90 mmHg) for 3 hours or more. In addition, they had to be greater than 35 weeks of gestational age at birth, a birthweight of 2 kg, have received less than 10 days of high-pressure ventilation, be younger than 28 days of age and have no contraindication to ECMO, such as a previous cardiac arrest or intraventricular hemorrhage. Infants were randomized to receive conventional therapy in a tertiary center or be transferred to one of five ECMO centers in the UK. One hundred and eight infants with CDH, PPHN, MAS, sepsis, IRDS were randomized from 55 centers. Fifty-nine percent of infants randomized to receive ECMO survived, which was significantly greater than the 32 percent survival rate in the conventionally treated group. Subanalysis demonstrated survival was better in the ECMO infants in all diagnostic categories except CDH infants. Fourteen of 18 CDH infants supported by ECMO died and all 17 in the conventional arm died. Mortality among infants with a primary diagnosis other than CDH was 21 percent in the ECMO group compared with 49 percent in the conventional group (relative risk 0.43, 0.27–0.71) ($P = 0.0006$).[421]

Morbidity

ACUTE

Infants eligible for ECMO are critically ill and therefore already have considerable morbidity. Use of ECMO adds the risks of emboli, infarction and bleeding to these complications. The patients can also suffer from anemia, leukopenia and thrombocytopenia as a result of consumption of blood products at the oxygenator's membrane surface. Bleeding may be reduced by use of a fibrin sealant.[15] Some infants who are put on ECMO will have undiagnosed severe congenital cardiac abnormalities which have been masked by their respiratory failure.[309] Mechanical problems related to the circuit and pump failure appear to occur in up to 20 percent of cases.[134] The incidence of septic complications in neonates receiving ECMO does not appear to be influenced by feeding route; in 16 neonates enteral nutrition was well tolerated and not associated with side-effects.[437]

CHRONIC

Neurological, growth and chronic respiratory problems are reported in ECMO survivors.[28,373] These results, however, have to be interpreted with caution as the infants were extremely ill prior to commencing ECMO and their original illness may have been responsible for at least some of the morbidity. In one series of 103 survivors of ECMO, 31 percent required rehospitalization in the first year of life because of respiratory illness; 26 percent had abnormal growth and 20 percent had some form of handicap.[373] Follow-up of 67 children demonstrated abnormal neurodevelopmental outcome was significantly associated with cerebral infarction and the development of chronic lung disease.[225] Two-year follow-up of 57 infants treated with ECMO demonstrated survival rate was lower and morbidity higher in CDH compared to non-CDH infants.[236] Respiratory and gastrointestinal sequelae were commoner in the CDH group (p. 497).

Follow-up to 1 year of infants entered in the UK Collaborative Study demonstrated ECMO support had reduced the risk of death without a concomitant increase in severe disability. At 4 years of age, one in four survivors had evidence of impairment with or without disability; the ECMO group had higher survival rates.[34] Other non-randomized studies support the concept that use of ECMO in infants with severe respiratory failure does not increase the relative risk of neurodevelopmental handicap.[167,332]

Respiratory follow-up

In non-randomized comparisons, ECMO survivors have been demonstrated to have significantly less chronic lung disease, less chronic reactive airway disease and less frequent hospitalization.[434] Examination at 1 year of age of 77 surviving infants from the UK ECMO trial suggested that the ECMO-treated infants had slightly better lung function, with higher inspiratory conductance and V_{max} FRC.[31]

COST-EFFECTIVENESS OF ECMO

An economic evaluation of the UK ECMO trial estimated the cost of a day of ECMO to be £1813.[343] This meant a cost per additional survivor without severe disability at 1 year of approximately £51 222. Others have, however, pointed out that the average cost for an ECMO-treated infant is very similar to a conventionally treated infant.[371]

CHANGES IN ECMO REQUIREMENT

Introduction of new respiratory support modes for term or near-term infants has been associated with a reduction in the number of infants being referred for ECMO. In one center,[215] comparison of two time periods, surfactant, iNO and HFOV being available in the second, demonstrated the proportion of infants with severe respiratory failure who were treated with ECMO fell from 42.8 percent to 27.7 percent. In Europe in 1997, 158 ECMO runs for neonates were undertaken. This was the peak activity. This fell progressively to 97 runs in 2001. Review of 12 175 neonates reported to the ELSO registry over a 10-year period revealed that although there was no significant difference in the gestational age of infants being referred for ECMO the diagnoses had altered, CDH infants representing 26 percent rather than 18 percent and RDS 4 percent rather than 15 percent. The reduced number of RDS infants, again likely reflecting changes in the availability of other respiratory support techniques, for example, the use of surfactant, HFJV and iNO, increased from 0 percent in 1988 to 36 percent, 46 percent, and 24 percent, respectively, in 1997. Delay in institution of ECMO in infants with severe MAS, however, has been associated with significantly longer ECMO runs and post-ECMO ventilation.[165] In addition, an increased time to ECMO has been associated with a significant increase in mortality (mortality rate of 4.8 percent in the group who received ECMO within 24 hours of birth and 7.7 percent in the group who were put on ECMO after 96 hours).[165] There has also been a change in the type of ECMO used; VA ECMO remains the primary mode, but VV in one series increased from 1 percent to 32 percent. This was associated with the average duration of ECMO increasing from 161 to 238 hours and the average number of neonatal patients per center fell from a peak of 18 in 1991 to nine in 1997. The occurrence of intracranial hemorrhage and/or infarct remained constant at 16 percent.[347]

Inter-hospital transportation of patients on ECMO

Limiting the number of ECMO centers to ensure each has a critical number of patients each year to maintain experience will mean transportation of infants with severe respiratory failure to ECMO centers, often over long distances. Some infants will be too unstable to transport with conventional support. Such infants can be 'cannulated' by a mobile ECMO team at the referring hospital and transported on ECMO via either ground ambulance, helicopter or fixed wing vehicle. Review of the outcome of 29 patients including 15 neonates,[272] transported from between 4 and 1500 km demonstrated this can be achieved without patient complications and only two technical problems occurred – one ambulance compressor malfunctioned and one of two electric supply circuits malfunctioned during a helicopter transport.

NITRIC OXIDE (NO)

NO, a gas, has an extra electron, making it a free radical. It has a short half-life in oxygen, reacting to form nitrogen dioxide (NO_2), which then reacts with water to form first nitrous and then nitric acid. NO is present in the atmosphere at concentrations of 20–60 parts per billion (ppb) and in cigarette smoke at concentrations of up to 1000 parts per million (ppm) and is partially responsible for the effects of pollution. NO is an important modulator of vascular tone in the pulmonary circulation and regulates smooth muscle tone via changes in cyclic guanosine monophosphate (cGMP).

Physiology

In 1987, Ignarro *et al.* identified NO as the transmitter responsible for vascular tone, previously having been named as endothelial derived relaxing factor. NO is generated in the endothelial cells by the effects of NO synthetase on L-arginine, forming citrulline and NO. Newborns who suffer from pulmonary hypertension may have low arginine levels,[433] but this is not a universal finding.[244] NO diffuses into the smooth muscle cells, where it activates guanylate cyclase to increase intracellular guanosine 3,5-monophosphate (GMP) and produces relaxation of the smooth muscle. Infants with PHN have been reported to have increased levels of endothelin-1 (ET-1) and decreased cGMP, suggesting their L-arginine NO cGMP system is deranged.[84] NO reacts with hemoglobin to form methemoglobin. When NO is inhaled, it diffuses across the alveolar-capillary membrane and activates guanylate cyclase in the pulmonary arteriolar smooth muscle by binding to its heme component.[152] The resulting increase in cGMP causes smooth muscle relaxation[381] and vasodilation. Having caused pulmonary artery vasodilation, NO is essentially deactivated by tight binding to hemoglobin in the blood passing through the pulmonary circulation.

Delivery

iNO was originally supplied in a concentration of one part per thousand and fed into the ventilator circuit between the humidifier and manifold. Sampling ports on the inspiratory and expiratory limbs were used to measure the concentrations of NO and NO_2, respectively. Continuous monitoring of the inspired oxygen concentration between the mixing point and the patient was important to limit administration of non-diluted NO. Now, NO is produced as a drug to pharmaceutical standards and can be delivered accurately in 0.1 ppm increments. Comparison of continuous titration of NO using a rotameter into an HFO circuit at three sites (pre-humidifier, post-humidifier and after the bellows) to the INOvent system revealed the latter system was simple to use and delivered an accurate and precise NO concentration.[43]

NO has a very short duration of action and thus, if it is suddenly withdrawn, rapid rebound pulmonary vasoconstriction and hypoxemia can result. This has implications for nursing procedures, for example, suction and handbagging. In-line suction devices are, therefore, preferred and handbagging circuits should contain an additional iNO source. Units which use iNO must have the facilities to transport an infant on iNO or reliable access to a transport system that has that capability.

Monitoring

Certain of the adverse effects of iNO can be minimized by using low doses of NO and avoiding high levels of NO_2. Continuous and accurate monitoring of NO and NO_2 is essential. NO and NO_2 levels have been monitored using mass spectroscopy, infrared, chemiluminescence and electrochemical devices. Chemiluminescence devices are also used to measure atmospheric pollutants and capable of measuring very low NO levels, but the devices are expensive. Infrared systems can give falsely low values as they are sensitive to humidity. Electrochemical devices perform similarly to chemiluminescence systems.[287] Currently, in the USA and parts of Europe, NO and NO_2 monitoring is provided by the iNO delivery system (INOvent).

It has also been recommended that units who deliver iNO should have invasive monitoring, as it is important to ensure infants have adequate blood pressure. In addition, the ability to have chest radiographs on a 24-hour a day basis is essential to exclude other pathology and echocardiography should also be available. In an emergency situation, NO may be started prior to an ECHO, but this should be performed as soon as possible. If the response to NO is transitory, the ECHO should be organized as an emergency procedure. Infants who respond well to iNO should still have an ECHO within 6 hours of commencing it, as a positive response does not exclude congenital heart disease.

SCAVENGING

UK, US and other regulatory bodies suggest that it is not necessary to scavenge exhaust NO in a well-ventilated environment (8–12 air changes per hour). It is good practice to scavenge exhaust ventilator gas when iNO is administered in poorly ventilated surroundings. Environmental NO_2 levels should be monitored to reassure staff that environmental levels are insignificant and to assist in the detection of accidental macrocontamination.

Dosage studies

TERM INFANTS

Initial studies used high concentrations of NO.[342] NO administered at 80 ppm in 90 percent oxygen increased the postductal oxygen tensions from 5.2 to 15.4 kPa (39 to 115.5 mmHg) in seven term infants with PPHN, three of whom had meconium aspiration.[342] Once the NO was discontinued, hypoxemia recurred after 5 minutes. Subsequently, lower NO levels were used.[255] NO at 10 and 20 ppm also caused a rapid improvement in oxygenation in nine newborn infants with PPHN who fulfilled criteria for ECMO. The PaO_2 rose from 5.5 to 13.6 kPa after 15 minutes of treatment. Clinical improvement was maintained over the next 24 hours using only 6 ppm.[255] In two randomized trials, low doses (5 and 6 ppm) were shown to be equally as effective as higher doses (20 ppm).[102,445] In one study,[445] 6 ppm used continuously was equally as effective as 20 ppm for 4 hours followed by 6 ppm in reducing the likelihood of death or requirement for ECMO in term or near-term infants with PPHN. In a randomized placebo-controlled double-masked dose–response multicenter trial,[102] similar improvements in oxygenation were seen with 5, 20 or 80 ppm of iNO. Doses lower than 5 ppm of iNO, however, may not always be effective. In infants with PPHN, iNO at 2 ppm attenuated the rate of clinical deterioration, but did not acutely improve oxygenation or prevent clinical deterioration.[96] Using a very low dose (2 ppm) of iNO initially may alter the subsequent response to iNO. Administration of 20 ppm to infants initially treated with 0 ppm, but not 2 ppm, acutely improved oxygenation.[96] Those results suggest that initial treatment with a subtherapeutic dose of iNO may diminish the clinical response to higher doses and have adverse clinical sequelae.[96] We, therefore, start infants born at term on 5 ppm of iNO and then wean as rapidly as possible.

PRETERM INFANTS

Low levels of iNO have been demonstrated to improve oxygenation in infants born prematurely,[390,424] but are not always successful.[265] Similar changes in oxygenation were reported in response to 1, 5, 10 and 20 ppm in 11 infants with a median gestational age of 30 weeks[424] and in infants randomized to receive 5 or 20 ppm of iNO.[390] In infants with PIE or born at very early gestations (that is less than 28 weeks), however, 40 ppm may be necessary

to maximize oxygenation. In infants with PIE, the mechanical barrier resulting from dissection of the lung connective tissue by gas and the high interstitial water content of very immature infants might reduce diffusion, hence higher iNO levels are required to be effective. Infants with PIE who are so hypoxic that they require iNO frequently have a poor outcome.[115] Side-effects of iNO are increased at high level concentrations. We, therefore, start at 5 ppm of iNO, but then would increase the level in infants who had a poor response but pulmonary hypertension proven on echocardiograph examination. Treatment with PIE of infants with iNO should be individualized.

LUNG VOLUME RECRUITMENT

iNO acts very rapidly and improvements in oxygenation are experienced within at least 30 minutes. If no such effect occurs, then it is worth increasing the dose, particularly in a premature infant. Some have suggested a response in iNO might only be experienced after 12 hours, but the mechanism of such a response is unclear, particularly if the infant's condition had been optimized with regard to eliciting a response; based on current evidence, a response will always occur within 4 hours. iNO is unlikely to work in an infant with atelectatic lungs and should be given following lung recruitment by elevation of PEEP, transfer to high-volume strategy HFO or surfactant administration. The systemic blood pressure should also be appropriate and inotropes given if necessary.

DISCONTINUING A TRIAL OF iNO

It is important to be aware that rebound hypoxia can result from withdrawal in an infant who has had no initial response to iNO. This may result from increased degradation of cGMP via enhanced phosphodiesterase activity during NO administration. Such a process takes a certain amount of time and hence, if there is no initial response, we recommend stopping iNO after only a short trial.

WEANING

Once there has been improvement in oxygenation in response to iNO administration and the infant stabilized, then attempts should be made to reduce the iNO level. If the infant is left too long on relatively high levels of iNO and becomes tolerant, it may become impossible to wean the infant at all.[169] A randomized, double-blind placebo, double-marked dose–response trial was undertaken to identify the safest withdrawal process.[103] All the infants recruited had echocardiographic evidence of PPHN, none had had surfactant therapy or were on HFO or had pulmonary hypoplasia. Infants received 5, 20 or 80 ppm of iNO. The arterial oxygen levels decreased only at the final step of iNO withdrawal and on cessation from 1, 4, 16 ppm there was a dose-dependent related reduction in oxygenation. Reduction to 1 ppm before its discontinuation minimized the deterioration in oxygenation. Those results have been subsequently confirmed by review of the records of 505 prospectively collected iNO weaning attempts on 84 neonates with hypoxic respiratory failure.[391] In addition, prior surfactant treatment was highlighted as appearing to enhance the oxygenation reserve when weaning iNO. It is our practice, therefore, to wean the iNO at 1 ppm per hour to one ppm. On discontinuation of the iNO, we tolerate an increased supplementary oxygen requirement of 0.20, before restarting the iNO at 1 ppm and then repeating the withdrawal process some hours later. There is some evidence to suggest that increasing the FiO_2 by 0.1–0.2 immediately prior to cessation of iNO prevents or minimizes rebound hypoxemia. It has been shown in children receiving cardiac intensive care[314] that plasma ET-1 levels are increased by iNO and that the increased ET-1 levels might contribute to rebound pulmonary hypertension upon iNO withdrawal. Agents such as phosphodiesterase inhibitors and other vasodilators have not been proven in randomized trials to improve the outcome of iNO withdrawal. Babies who fail to wean from iNO should be carefully assessed. Prolonged iNO dependence has been associated with underlying lung abnormalities such as pulmonary hypoplasia[169] or alveolar capillary dysplasia.

Side-effects

NITROGEN DIOXIDE

NO_2 is rapidly formed from oxygen and NO. The rate of NO_2 formation is dependent on the concentration of oxygen and the square of the concentration of NO.[102] NO_2 reacts with the water within the lungs to form nitric and nitrous acid, which cause pulmonary toxicity. NO_2 levels of 25 ppm or more can cause histological changes in the lung. Lower levels of NO_2 can cause respiratory function abnormalities. Airway hyperreactivity resulted from continuous exposure to 1.5 ppm of NO_2 in healthy adult volunteers, but not from continuous exposure to 0.6 ppm continuously or 2 ppm intermittently.[146] It would then be predicted that infants exposed to iNO might have lung function abnormalities at follow-up; unfortunately this has rarely been assessed. No differences in lung function test results were found at 4–12 months between 14 infants who had received iNO and seven who had not, but only FRC and compliance were measured.[124] The Occupational Safety and Health Administration recommend NO_2 levels should be kept below 5 ppm.

METHEMOGLOBINEMIA

Eighty to ninety percent of iNO is absorbed into the bloodstream and reacts with hemoglobin to form methemoglobin. The development of methemoglobinemia is dependent on the dose of NO delivered and the level of methemoglobin reductase. Both partial and complete methemoglobin reductase deficiency is common in native American Indians[374] and levels are lower in neonates than older children. Use of low NO levels and careful monitoring to allow early detection of rising levels of methemoglobin reduces the likelihood of methemoglobinemia. Indeed, methemoglobinemia has not been reported to be an important problem in published clinical trials and fatal methemoglobinemia rarely documented. Methemoglobinemia can be treated with methylthionine[277] or methylene blue.[169]

SURFACTANT DYSFUNCTION

NO combines readily with superoxide to form peroxynitrite, an extremely strong oxidant. Peroxynitrite damages surfactant proteins and inhibits phosphatidylcholine synthesis by type II alveolar cells; its other toxic effects include oxidation of membrane lipids and DNA bases. Plasma 5-nitrotyrosine, a marker of peroxynitrite-mediated stress, however, was not increased in BPD infants treated with iNO.[23]

MUTAGENICITY

Exposure to NO significantly enhanced mutation in *Salmonella typhimurium* TA 1535; the effect was time- and dose-dependent.[14] NO_2 exposure is associated with chromosome aberrations, mainly of the chromatid type.[233]

BLEEDING PROBLEMS

iNO administration has been associated with an increased bleeding time in adults[226] and infants.[160] In adult volunteers, only exposure to 30 ppm of iNO increased the bleeding time, which reverted to normal 60 minutes after iNO discontinuation. The bleed time was doubled in neonates exposed to 40 ppm for 30 minutes.[160] Endogenous NO from endothelial cells suppresses platelet adhesion and activation. iNO can inhibit platelet aggregation, probably via inducing increased platelet cGMP dehydrogenase-dependent protein kinases;[296] the effect resolves after only a few minutes of discontinuing the iNO.[160] iNO may have less effect on platelet function *in vivo* because of the rapid scavenging effect of hemoglobin.

There is conflicting evidence with regard to whether iNO increases 'bleeding' complications. A high incidence of intracranial hemorrhage (ICH) has been noted in certain series.[317,424] Four of eight infants born following preterm premature rupture of the membranes (PPROM) developed ICH.[317] In the second series,[424] three infants had an ICH on their first cranial ultrasound examination only 60 minutes after exposure to iNO; four other infants subsequently developed ICH. Premature infants given iNO as 'rescue' treatment usually have severe illness and this may explain the association with a high ICH rate.

Table 15.7 *Randomized studies of iNO in preterm infants*

Reference	iNO %	Controls %
Death		
Subhedar et al.[399]	50	32
The Franco-Belgium Collaborative NO Trial Group[406]	27	35
Kinsella et al.[257]	48	53
Oxygen dependency at 36 weeks PCA		
Subhedar et al.[399]	50	64
The Franco-Belgium Collaborative NO Trial Group[406]	24	29
Kinsella et al.[257]	60	80
ICH		
The Franco-Belgium Collaborative NO Trial Group[406]	27	32
Kinsella et al.[257]	51	50

Sixty-four percent of infants born prior to 34 weeks and given iNO after a second dose of surfactant developed ICH or PVL, but the National Institute of Child Health and Human Development (NICHD) Neonatal Research Network reported intracranial abnormalities developed in a similar proportion of infants who had not received iNO. In preterm infants exposed to iNO 'prophylactically' in randomized trials (Table 15.7), no excess of ICH/PVL has been reported. Nevertheless, it seems prudent to avoid iNO therapy in infants with a low platelet count ($<100\,000$), a bleeding diathesis or more than a grade 1 ICH or at least withhold iNO until the bleeding problems had been corrected.

Clinical studies

TERM INFANTS

There are now many reports of iNO improving oxygenation in anecdotal series of term or near-term infants. Serial echocardiographic examinations have demonstrated that the incidence of residual pulmonary hypertension in infants who had severe hypoxemic respiratory failure and were treated with iNO is low.[418] The group at highest risk are those with structural heart disease. Not all term infants, however, respond to iNO. A poor response can be seen in infants with severe parenchymal disease, systemic hypotension, myocardial dysfunction and structural pulmonary abnormalities, including pulmonary hypoplasia,[169] congenital diaphragmatic hernia[381] and alveolar capillary dysplasia.[396] Although an initial response may be seen in infants with CDH, the effect may not be sustained, tachyphylaxis developing and ECMO becoming necessary.[381] Similarly, although an initial response

was seen to 80 ppm of iNO, all infants with alveolar capillary dysplasia so treated died.[396] A retrospective chart review demonstrated that the response to iNO was highly correlated with the baseline OI, infants with the highest OI having the largest change in OI.[313]

Prediction of outcome

A poor response to iNO is predictive of a poor outcome.[2,43,107,169] In one randomized trial,[107] 90 percent of infants whose OI remained above 40, despite iNO, either required ECMO or died; by contrast, improvement in oxygenation was sustained in 87 percent of infants whose OIs fell below 40. In a series of 25 near-term infants consecutively treated with iNO, the 11 infants with an initial and sustained response survived, compared to only one of two non-responders.[169]

Randomized trials

iNO versus placebo. Meta-analysis of the results of eight randomized trials[24,102,107,256,342,407,408,438] demonstrated iNO resulted in improved oxygenation (RR 0.63, 95 percent CI 0.54–0.74).[142] It also reduced the combined outcome of ECMO requirement or death (RR 0.72, 95 percent CI 0.60–0.87), the effect was due to a reduction in ECMO requirement (RR 0.69, 95 percent CI 0.60–0.87) (the relative risk of death was 1.03, 95 percent CI 0.62–1.72). Other positive benefits noted in non-CDH infants include fewer days of NICU stay and a reduced need for β-mimetics or steroids.[406] iNO given at 20 ppm for 24 hours followed by 5 ppm for no more than 5 hours has been reported to reduce oxygen dependency at 30 days (7 percent versus 20 percent).[91]

iNO and HFOV. The combined intervention of iNO and HFOV was more successful than either iNO or HFOV alone in rescuing infants with respiratory failure.[256] The response was disease-specific and infants with severe respiratory disease responded best to HFOV with iNO, whereas those without significant parenchymal lung disease responded better to iNO or HFO with iNO than HFO alone. There were no significant differences in outcome related to the method of respiratory support in the CDH infants.[256] In anecdotal series,[334] the combination iNO with HFOV compared to iNO with conventional ventilation was more successful in reducing the need for ECMO. The success of HFOV with iNO in the infants with severe disease is explained by HFOV recruiting and sustaining lung volume, HFOV then augmenting the response to iNO by decreasing intrapulmonary shunting and improving iNO delivery to the pulmonary circulation.

CDH infants. No significant long-term positive benefits have been reported in infants with CDH.[91,408] In one randomized trial,[408] death at less than 120 days of age or the need for ECMO occurred in 82 percent of control infants compared with 96 percent of iNO infants and death occurred in 43 percent of controls and 48 percent of iNO infants. Short-term improvements in oxygenation are seen in some CDH infants and may be of benefit in stabilizing infants for transport and initiation of ECMO.

Long-term outcome

Follow-up of infants at or near term entered into randomized trials have not demonstrated iNO to be associated with an increase in neurodevelopmental, behavioral or medical abnormalities at 2 years of age.[409] From the NINOS trial,[407] 29.6 percent of the control group and 34.5 percent of the iNO-treated group had at least one disability. CDH infants had similar outcomes, but a higher incidence of sensorineural hearing loss.[408]

PRETERM INFANTS

There are numerous reports of iNO improving oxygenation in prematurely born infants, including those with severe respiratory failure due to RDS,[424] prolonged rupture of the membranes,[317] developed[87] and established chronic lung disease.[23,413] iNO may act in CLD patients by a direct effect on the pulmonary vasculature, reducing vascular remodeling, bronchodilation and/or decreased inflammation. The rapidity of the response seen[23] suggests that the mechanism must at least in part be due to a direct effect on the pulmonary vasculature. The response in infants with CLD is variable; in one study iNO was less efficacious in infants with mild disease.[216] A response to iNO, however, does not guarantee a good outcome in CLD. In one series,[23] 10 of 16 CLD infants treated with iNO at between 1 and 7 months of age had an improvement in oxygenation which was sustained throughout the duration of treatment, which was between 8 and 90 days. Only four of the responders were weaned off mechanical ventilation. Whether iNO in infants with established CLD improves long-term outcome requires testing in a multi-center trial. CLD infants who become acutely hypoxic in response to an intercurrent infection can experience an improvement in oxygenation following iNO administration. It then does seem reasonable to give a short trial of iNO in such patients.

Randomized trials

There have been few randomized trials of iNO involving prematurely born infants;[257,399,406] none has demonstrated significant benefits (Table 15.7). Meta-analysis of three trials[257,399,406] demonstrated the odds ratio for iNO treatment regarding death were 0.97 (95 percent CK 0.54–1.70), and for ICH were 1.37 (95 percent CI 0.69– 2.74).[224] In one trial,[257] the iNO-treated infants required fewer days of ventilation (median 26 versus 37 days, $P < 0.05$).

Long-term outcome

No benefit regarding long-term survival or neurodevelopmental status was reported in one series but only 25 infants survived until discharge.[33]

Indications

TERM OR NEAR-TERM INFANTS

Infants at or near term should be considered for iNO if they have hypoxic respiratory failure, usually an OI greater than 25. Prior to starting iNO, ventilation should be optimized to produce adequate lung volume, cardiovascular status stabilized and an echocardiograph performed to exclude congenital heart disease as a cause of the hypoxia.

PRETERM INFANTS

There is insufficient evidence to recommend routine use of iNO in prematurely born infants and iNO should usually be administered within the context of a randomized trial. In exceptional circumstances, iNO should be given as a last resort for prematurely born infants with severe respiratory failure or in those with CLD who experience an acute hypoxic deterioration.

CONTRAINDICATIONS

Absolute contraindications are hypoxemia secondary to congenital heart disease, right ventricle-dependent circulation, severe left ventricle dysfunction, duct-dependent circulation and methemoglobinemia.

LIQUID VENTILATION

Liquid ventilation (LV) has been explored for over three decades as an alternative means of supporting pulmonary gas exchange while preserving lung structure and function in infants, children, and adults. Liquid breathing has not yet become clinically available, although physiological and experimental data are promising.

PERFLUOROCHEMICAL (PFC) LIQUIDS

Pure medical-grade perfluorochemical (PFC) liquids currently exist for LV purposes because these chemicals are already used in clinical medicine for different organ systems.[380] Liquid ventilation uses a PFC liquid to replace nitrogen gas as the carrier for oxygen and carbon dioxide. Physiological processes are supported by the combination of the physicochemical properties of the PFC liquid (Table 15.8) and the biophysical effects of the liquid on lung mechanics. Perfluorochemical instillation, with its relatively low surface tension, high respiratory gas solubility, and high spreading coefficients, replaces the gas–liquid interface with a liquid–liquid interface at the lung surface while supporting an adequate alveolar reservoir for pulmonary gas exchange.[375] High surface tension at the gas–liquid interface is eliminated, and interfacial

Table 15.8 *Factors relevant for maintenance of perfluorochemical (PFC) lung volume during partial liquid ventilation*

PFC physicochemical properties	Physiological factors
Vapor pressure	Alveolar ventilation
Density	Distribution of PFC liquid
Viscosity	Distribution of inspired gas
Spreading coefficient	Pathophysiology
Gas solubility	Pulmonary function
	Positioning
	PFC dosing
	Ventilation strategy
	Ventilation duration

tension is reduced. Pulmonary blood flow is more homogenous in the fluid-filled lung compared with the gas-filled lung because transmural pressures across the alveolar-capillary membrane are more evenly matched. For these reasons, LV appears to be a promising treatment for infants and children with respiratory distress and injured lungs.

LIQUID VENTILATION TECHNIQUES

Currently, LV techniques for the support of respiratory gas exchange in infants comprise PFC lavage, tidal liquid ventilation (TLV), and partial liquid ventilation (PLV). Non-gas exchange applications of PFC in the lung include pulmonary administration of pharmacological agents and gene products, as well as pulmonary imaging agents.[377] There is also exciting evidence which identifies that low-pressure PFC-induced mechanical distention without ventilation may accelerate lung growth without pathophysiological consequences in infants (p. 450).

PULMONARY LAVAGE

A variety of animal models with acute lung injury have been lavaged with perfluorochemical liquid. In preterm lambs, adequate gas exchange and acid–base balance can be maintained both during and after bilateral PFC lavage, thereby demonstrating the usefulness of bilateral PFC lavage as a means of alveolar debridement, particularly in aspiration syndromes of the newborn. In this regard, poor gas exchange, acidosis, and poor pulmonary compliance were present at birth and during gas ventilation (GV) of meconium-stained lambs. Improvements were noted during LV in PaO_2, $PaCO_2$, alveolar-arterial oxygen gradient, and pulmonary compliance; and pulmonary blood flow was more uniform.

In another study, it was shown that cats with severe acute lung injury demonstrated improved gas exchange and pulmonary compliance for approximately 1 hour after pulmonary lavage with oxygenated PFC. This improvement could be repeated during subsequent serial PFC lavages, in the face of a lung injury which caused 100 percent mortality in 4 hours in the untreated control group. Although this lavage technique has not been studied as a clinical investigation, clinical studies with partial liquid ventilation (PLV) have noted the need for pulmonary suctioning of alveolar debris due to the lavage effect of PFC liquid.

TOTAL LIQUID VENTILATION

Liquid ventilation, in its purest form, is the transport of respiratory gases solely in the dissolved form through tidal volume exchange of PFC liquid to and from the lung, thus TLV. All gas–liquid interfacial tension is eliminated, the lung is provided maximal protection from inflation pressures, lung volume is recruited, compliance is increased, and, thus, inflation pressures and pulmonary barotrauma are reduced (Figure 15.11). To initiate the TLV process, PFC fluid is instilled into the gas-filled lung while the thorax is gently manipulated to help remove resident gas volumes into the expiratory line. The gas–liquid interface at the alveolar surface is eliminated because gas is transported in its dissolved form, and there are no breath sounds. The liquid volumes in the lung and ventilator are controlled and monitored to ensure effective gas exchange. Tidal liquid ventilation is accomplished by cycling fluid from a reservoir to and from the lung by a mechanical ventilator. This ventilator has evolved over the years to include manually controlled flow-assist pneumatic systems, roller pumps with pneumatic/fluidic/electronic controls, gravity driven, and modified extracorporeal membrane oxygenation (ECMO) circuits. Different control strategies have been explored, including constant-pressure or constant-flow time-cycling, with pressure (system, airway, or alveolar) and/or volume (lung volume, tidal volume) limitation. The current approach emphasizes microprocessor-based feedback control. During inspiration, warmed and oxygenated PFC liquid is pumped from a fluid reservoir into the lung, and expiration is achieved by pumping liquid from the lung with passive assist of the lung recoil. The fluid is then filtered, circulated to a gas exchanger for desired levels of oxygenation and CO_2 'scrubbing' and then to the fluid reservoir. Condensing vapor in the expired gas conserves PFC fluid. The PFC lung volume is tightly controlled, maintaining global lung protection. Various animal studies across age, with and without lung injury, suggest that TLV maintains effective gas exchange and cardiovascular stability at lower ventilatory pressures and minimizes structural damage throughout the lung typically incurred as a result of gas ventilation.[443]

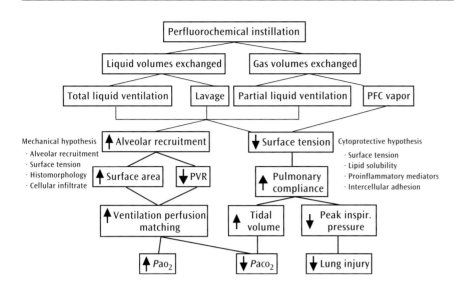

Figure 15.11 *Proposed mechanism of improved pulmonary function with less barotrauma during perfluorochemical ventilation. (Reproduced by kind permission from Shaffer and Wolfson.[376])*

PARTIAL LIQUID VENTILATION

Partial liquid ventilation is performed by filling and maintaining the lung with a predetermined volume of PFC liquid while mechanical gas ventilation is performed. Partial liquid ventilation is similar to TLV because it uses the alveolar recruitment capabilities of a low surface tension fluid to establish an adequate functional residual capacity in a surfactant-deficient or impaired lung. The PFC liquid is oxygenated, and CO_2 is exchanged in the lung through mechanical gas ventilation. The optimum PFC filling strategy and subsequent gas ventilation scheme are currently being investigated. A range of techniques has been explored, including instilling PFC liquid in the lungs for brief periods (3–5 minutes) rapidly instilling a bolus of up to 30 ml/kg of oxygenated PFC with the ventilator disconnected and slowly infusing oxygenated or room air equilibrated PFC in doses up to 30 ml/kg during continuous gas ventilation. A range of breathing frequencies has also been investigated in a variety of large and small animal preparations with acute respiratory distress syndrome (ARDS), aspiration syndromes, and lung hypoplasia due to congenital diaphragmatic hernia. Even though the technical aspect of instilling PFC liquid into the lungs with PLV appears straightforward to the intensive care clinician who is familiar with the gas ventilator, optimum ventilation of a partially filled lung introduces new clinical challenges. There are still many unknown factors with respect to the distribution of PFC fluid in the lung, including continual alteration in lung mechanics, evaporative loss of PFC, and, thus, changing volumes of gas and PFC liquid volumes. Studies that used analyzer systems designed to quantitate expired PFC vapor have shown that PFC liquid volume loss and evaporation rate from the lungs are influenced by many factors (Table 15.8) such as time, PFC vapor pressure and initial dose, ventilation strategy, lung pathophysiology, repositioning of the subject, body temperature, and the administration of supplemental PFC doses to the lungs.[442]

Maintenance of PFC lung volume during PLV has necessitated the development of adjunctive instrumentation to quantitate evaporative loss to optimize a protective ventilation strategy.

Clinical trials

In the initial clinical study, premature human infants who were near death at the time of treatment were enrolled.[196] A gravity-assisted approach was used with tidal volumes of liquid in brief cycles. The infants tolerated the procedure, showed improvement in several physiological parameters including lung compliance and gas exchange, and maintained some improvement after discontinuation of LV. This study used a form of TLV, but also reported a sustained benefit of gas ventilation with the residual PFC liquid-filled lung. Subsequent clinical protocols have used the PLV approach (Figure 15.12).

There have been several completed human studies of PLV using the PFC perflubron (LiquiVent, Alliance Pharmaceutical Corp., San Diego, CA, USA). A study by Leach et al.[266] reported 13 premature infants with severe respiratory distress syndrome (RDS) in whom conventional treatment had failed. This was not a randomized or blinded study. They treated the infants with PLV for up to 96 hours. The infants' lungs were filled with perflubron, and supplemental doses were given frequently, generally hourly. The arterial oxygen tension and dynamic compliance significantly increased, and the oxygenation index was reduced within 1 hour of initiation of PLV. Clinical improvement and survival in some infants who were not predicted to survive was noted. Pranikoff et al.[328] reported results from four patients with congenital diaphragmatic hernia who were managed on ECMO. In a phase I/II trial, PLV was performed with daily dosing for up to 6 days with improvements in gas exchange and pulmonary compliance. Greenspan et al.[197] presented six term infants with respiratory failure who showed no improvement

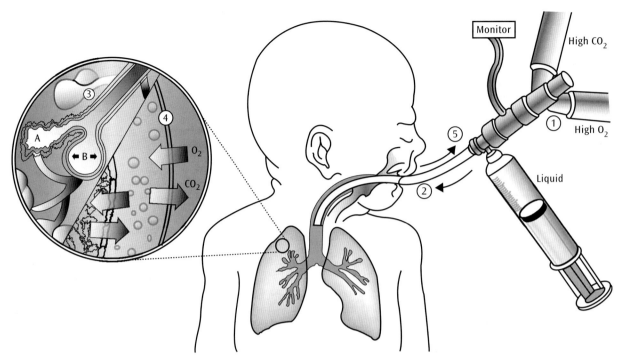

Figure 15.12 *Schematic of the clinical technique for partial liquid ventilation. (Reproduced with kind permission from Shaffer and Wolfson.[378])*

while receiving ECMO. The infants were treated with PLV with LiquiVent for up to 96 hours, with hourly dosing. Dynamic pulmonary compliance significantly increased, and lung volume was recruited.

The initial studies of PLV in neonates are encouraging and suggest this technique may be useful in neonates with severe RDS and ARDS. It has been observed and reported that the underlying pathophysiology influences the impact of LV. The response of the sick term infant to PLV is frequently more gradual than is typically observed in the preterm infant with RDS. The preterm infant often experiences improvement in lung compliance and gas exchange within hours of PLV initiation, most likely due to reduction in surface tension and volume recruitment. Debris removal, which takes time, is often required in the term infant on PLV to improve lung function.

Three studies have evaluated PLV in children. None of the studies used a control group. Hirschl *et al.*[222] treated seven pediatric patients with ARDS requiring ECMO. They found improvement in gas exchange and pulmonary compliance during PLV for 1–7 days. Gauger *et al.*[159] reported six pediatric patients with ARDS requiring extracorporeal life support. They treated the patients with LiquiVent PLV with daily dosing for 3–7 days and observed some improvement in gas exchange and pulmonary compliance over the 96 hours from the initial dose; all the patients survived. Toro-Figueroa *et al.*[419] presented results from 10 children with ARDS aged up to 17 years treated with PLV for up to 96 hours. Nine of the 10 patients tolerated initial dosing, and all nine experienced improvement in

gas exchange over the 48-hour treatment period. Lung function did not improve in these patients.

The initial phase I/II trials have indicated potential safety and efficacy of PLV, particularly in younger populations of sick patients. An understanding of the utility of this technique awaits the results of phase III trials. A large, randomized phase III PLV trial in adults with ARDS has been completed in North America and Europe using LiquiVent. Several LV trials in infants and children are currently under design in Europe.

LV technology has the potential to impact the clinical management of pulmonary pathophysiology including premature lung disease, aspiration syndromes, pneumonia, ARDS, and pulmonary hypoplasia. Documentation of efficacy in human disease is still required even though laboratory studies have been impressive. To date, more than 700 patients have been enrolled in LV studies with LiquiVent. Recent studies, unfortunately, have been limited to the adult population. Once safety and efficacy are proven in adults, it is hoped that drug approval and subsequent re-initiation of controlled studies in infants and children will be forthcoming.

HOME RESPIRATORY SUPPORT

Home oxygen

Discharging infants home on supplementary oxygen can facilitate early discharge.[59,125,321] Affected infants, however, may require many months of supplementary oxygen at home.[191] Maintaining adequate oxygen saturations by giving supplementary oxygen increases weight gain[200] and reduces pulmonary artery pressure,[384] airways resistance and the frequency of intermittent hypoxemic episodes.[323] Maintaining the oxygen saturation levels at least at 95 percent may also reduce the hospital readmission rate.[2,154] There is, however, no consensus regarding the minimum oxygen saturation level which should be maintained in prematurely born infants with CLD. A survey of neonatal units in the United Kingdom demonstrated that the oxygen saturation levels at which supplementary oxygen was discontinued varied from 85 to 93 percent.[392] The situations which would prevent discontinuation of supplementary oxygen also varied and included desaturations while feeding/sleeping or excercising (95 percent of responders), failure to gain weight (78 percent of responders), presence of pulmonary hypertension (62 percent of responders) and recent withdrawal of corticosteroids (52 percent of responders).[392]

Infants who should be considered for home oxygen therapy are those who have no ongoing medical needs, other than a requirement for supplementary oxygen to maintain an adequate oxygen saturation. Some centers consider infants for home oxygen who additionally require tube feeding. It is important to provide such infants and their parents appropriate healthcare professional support in the community. Such support should include access to a dietitian, as infants with chronic oxygen dependency are prone to failure to thrive, if adequate nutritional support is not provided.[355] It is important to be aware that infants who are receiving home oxygen are at high risk of ongoing morbidity. Comparison of infants with CLD who were or were not sent home in supplementary oxygen demonstrated that the former group required significantly more and longer admissions and more out-patient attendances.[194] Not surprisingly, the total cost of care was greater for the home oxygen infants; this reflected higher costs for hospital stay, total in-patient care and primary care drugs.

Oxygen for home use can be delivered from cylinders or concentrators; the former method is suitable if the oxygen requirement is low. Whichever method is chosen, small oxygen cylinders must be available, as these are necessary for transport purposes. At regular intervals the infants should be seen in the hospital and/or the community to have their progress and weight checked and their ongoing supplementary oxygen needs assessed. Once the PaO_2 is at least 55 mmHg after a period of room air with oxygen saturations of at least 93 percent, then the supplementary oxygen can be weaned. This process is greatly facilitated by use of an oxygen saturation monitor with a 'memory', which can be downloaded and subsequently analyzed. This form of monitoring is vital to provide adequate overnight assessment. Initially, the supplementary oxygen is weaned during the day; infants can continue to require supplementary oxygen at night for many months after supplementation has been discontinued during the day. When assessing a CLD infant's oxygen needs, it is important to examine the infant when sleeping supine, as in that posture the oxygen requirements are highest.

Early hospital discharge can result in savings in hospital costs.[321] Such savings, however, must be balanced against the costs of providing appropriate support in the community. In addition, home oxygen therapy can result in significant financial and emotional burdens for the family.

Home ventilation

A survey in the UK demonstrated that very few infants or children were receiving long-term ventilation at home. One hundred and forty-one children were identified; of these 33 were receiving continuous positive pressure ventilation by tracheostomy and 103 ventilation when asleep by a non-invasive mask ($n = 62$), tracheostomy ($n = 32$) or negative pressure ventilation ($n = 9$). Only six of the patients had BPD.[237]

A similar survey in Japan also demonstrated a small number of infants and children receiving home ventilation.[352] This reflects the enormous investment in equipment and community services, as well as education of parents, required to support a ventilated patient in the community. The infants usually require a tracheostomy, although this may not be necessary if curasse ventilation is employed. In one series,[358] the average duration of ventilation at home for BPD was 365 days.

REFERENCES

1 Abbasi, S., Bhutani, V.K., Spitzer, A.R., Fox, W.W. (1991) Pulmonary mechanics in preterm neonates with respiratory failure treated with high-frequency oscillatory ventilation compared with conventional mechanical ventilation. *Pediatrics* **87**, 487–493.

2 Abman, S.H., Accurso, F.J., Koops, B.L. (1984) Experience with home oxygen in the management of infants with bronchopulmonary dysplasia. *Clinical Pediatrics (Philadelphia)* **23**, 471–476.

3 Abman, S.H., Griebel, J.L., Parker, D.K. *et al.* (1994) Acute effects of inhaled nitric oxide in children with severe hypoxemic respiratory failure. *Journal of Pediatrics* **124**, 881–888.

4 Abubakar, K.M., Keszler, M. (2001) Patient–ventilator interactions in new modes of patient-triggered ventilation. *Pediatric Pulmonology* **32**, 71–75.

5 Agostino, R., Orzalesi, M., Nodari, S. *et al.* (1973) Continuous positive airway pressure (CPAP) by nasal cannula in the respiratory distress syndrome (RDS) of the newborn. *Pediatric Research* **7**, 50.

6 Ahluwahlia, J.S., White, D.K., Morley, C.J. (1998) Infant flow driver or single prong nasal continuous positive airway pressure: short term physiological effects. *Acta Paediatrica* **87**, 325–327.

7   Alexander, J., Blowes, R., Ingram, D., Milner, A.D. (1993) Determination of the resonant frequency of the respiratory system during high frequency oscillatory ventilation. *Early Human Development* **35**, 234.

8   Allen, L.P., Reynolds, E.O.R., Rivers, R.P.A. *et al.* (1977) Controlled trial of continuous positive airway pressure given by face mask for hyaline membrane disease. *Archives of Disease in Childhood* **52**, 373–378.

9   Anonymous (1989) High frequency oscillatory ventilation compared with conventional mechanical ventilation in the treatment of respiratory failure in preterm infants. The HIFI Study Group. *New England Journal of Medicine* **320**, 88–93.

10 Anonymous (1991) Multicentre randomised controlled trial of high against low frequency positive pressure ventilation. Oxford Region Controlled Trial of Artificial Ventilation (OCTAVE) Study Group. *Archives of Disease in Childhood* **66**, 770–775.

11 Anonymous (1996) UK collaborative randomized trial of neonatal extracorporeal membrane oxygenation. UK Collaborative ECMO Trial Group. *Lancet* **348**, 75–82.

12 Anonymous. (1997) Noise: a hazard for the fetus and newborn. American Academy of Pediatrics. Committee on Environmental Health. *Pediatrics* **100**, 724–727.

13 Arnold, J.H., Truog, R.D., Orav, E.J. *et al.* (1990) Tolerance and dependence in neonates sedated with fentanyl during extracorporeal membrane oxygenation. *Anesthesiology* **73**, 1136–1140.

14 Arroyo, P.L., Hatch-Pigott, V., Mower, H.F., Cooney, R.V. (1992) Mutagenicity of nitric oxide and its inhibition by antioxidants. *Mutation Research* **281**, 193–202.

15 Atkinson, J.B., Gomperts, E.D., Kang, R. *et al.* (1997) Prospective, randomized evaluation of the efficacy of fibrin sealant as a topical hemostatic agent at the cannulation site in neonates undergoing extracorporeal membrane oxygenation. *American Journal of Surgery* **173**, 479–484.

16 Aubier, D., Troyer, A., Sampson, M. *et al.* (1981) Aminophylline improves diaphragmatic contractility. *New England Journal of Medicine* **305**, 249–252.

17 Avery, M.E., Tooley, W.H., Keller, J.B. *et al.* (1987) Is chronic lung disease in low birth weight infants preventable? A survey of eight centers. *Pediatrics* **79**, 26–30.

18 Ballard, R.A., Kraybill, E.M., Hernandez, J. *et al.* (1973) Idiopathic respiratory distress syndrome. Treatment with continuous negative-pressure ventilation. *American Journal of Diseases of Children* **125**, 676–681.

19 Balsan, M.J., Jones, J.G., Watchko, J.F., Guthrie, R.D. (1990) Measurements of pulmonary mechanics prior to the elective extubation of neonates. *Pediatric Pulmonology* **9**, 238–243.

20 Bancalari, A., Gerhardt, T., Bancalari, E. *et al.* (1987) Gas trapping with high frequency ventilation: jet versus oscillatory ventilation. *Journal of Pediatrics* **110**, 617–625.

21 Bancalari, E. (1986) Inadvertent positive end expiratory pressure during mechanical ventilation. *Journal of Pediatrics* **108**, 567–569.

22 Bandy, K., Nicks, J.J., Donn, S.M. (1992) Volume controlled ventilation for severe neonatal respiratory failure. *Neonatal Intensive Care* **5**, 70–74.

23 Banks, B.A., Seri, I., Ischiropoulos, H. *et al.* (1999) Changes in oxygenation with inhaled nitric oxide in severe bronchopulmonary dysplasia. *Pediatrics* **103**, 610–618.

24 Barefield, E.S., Karle, V.A., Philips, J.B., Carlo, W.A. (1996) Inhaled nitric oxide in term infants with hypoxemic respiratory failure. *Journal of Pediatrics* **129**, 279–286.

25 Barrington, K.J., Finer, N.N., Peters, K.L., Barton, J. (1986) Physiologic effects of doxapram in idiopathic apnea of prematurity. *Journal of Pediatrics* **108**, 124–129.

26 Bartlett, R.H., Andrews, A.F., Toomasian, J.M. *et al.* (1982) ECMO for newborn respiratory failure, 45 cases. *Surgery* **92**, 425–433.

27 Bartlett, R.H., Roloff, D.W., Cornell, R.G. *et al.* (1985) Extracorporeal circulation in neonatal respiratory failure: a prospective randomized study. *Pediatrics* **76**, 479–487.

28 Bartlett, R.H., Gazzaniga, A.M., Toomasian, J.M. *et al.* (1986) Extracorporeal membrane oxygenation (ECMO) in neonatal respiratory failure: 100 cases. *Annals of Surgery* **204**, 236–244.

29 Bauer, K., Buschkamp, S., Marcinkowski, M. *et al.* (2000) Postnatal changes of extracellular volume, atrial natriuretic factor, and diuresis in a randomized controlled trial of high-frequency oscillatory ventilation versus intermittent positive-pressure ventilation in premature infants <30 weeks gestation. *Critical Care Medicine* **28**, 2064–2068.

30 Baumer, J.H. (2000) International randomized controlled trial of patient triggered ventilation in neonatal respiratory distress syndrome. *Archives of Disease in Childhood Fetal and Neonatal Edition* **82**, F5–F10.

31 Beardsmore, C., Dundas, I., Poole, K. *et al.* (2000) Respiratory function in survivors of the United Kingdom Extracorporeal Membrane Oxygenation Trial. *American Journal of Respiratory & Critical Care Medicine* **161**, 1129–1135.

32 Beck, R., Anderson, K.D., Pearson, G.D. *et al.* (1986) Criteria for extracorporeal membrane oxygenation in a population of infants with persistent pulmonary hypertension of the newborn. *Journal of Pediatrics* **21**, 297–302.

33 Bennett, A.J., Shaw, N.J., Gregg, J.E., Subhedar, N.V. (2001a) Neurodevelopmental outcome in high-risk preterm infants treated with inhaled nitric oxide. *Acta Paediatrica* **90**, 573–576.

34 Bennett, C.C., Johnson, A., Field, D.J. *et al.* (2001b) UK collaborative randomised trial of neonatal extracorporeal membrane oxygenation: follow-up to age 4 years. *Lancet* **357**, 1094–1096.

35 Benveniste, D., Berg, O., Pedersen, J.E.P. (1976) A technique for delivery of continuous positive pressure to the neonate. *Journal of Pediatrics* **88**, 1015–1019.

36 Berg, T.J., Pagtakhan, T.D., Reed, M.H. *et al.* (1975) Bronchopulmonary dysplasia and lung rupture in hyaline membrane disease: influence of continuous distending pressure. *Pediatrics* **55**, 51–53.

37 Berman, L.S., Fox, W.W., Raphaely, R.C., Downes, J.J. (1976) Optimum levels of CPAP for tracheal extubation of newborn infants. *Journal of Pediatrics* **89**, 109–112.

38 Bernstein, G., Cleary, J.P., Heldt, G.P. *et al.* (1993) Response time and reliability of three neonatal patient triggered ventilators. *American Review of Respiratory Disease* **148**, 358–364.

39 Bernstein, G., Heldt, G.P., Mannino, F.L. (1994) Increased and more consistent tidal volumes during synchronized intermittent mandatory ventilation in newborn infants. *American Journal of Respiratory and Critical Care Medicine* **150**, 1444–1448.

40 Bhuta, T., Henderson-Smart, D.J. (2002) Elective high frequency jet ventilation versus conventional ventilation for respiratory distress syndrome in preterm infants (Cochrane Review). In The Cochrane Library, Issue 1. Update Software, Oxford.

41 Bhutani, V.K., Ritchie, W.G., Schaffer, T.H. (1986) Acquired tracheomegaly in very preterm neonates. *American Journal of Diseases in Children* **140**, 449–452.

42 Biarrent, D., Steppe, M., Muller, F. *et al.* (1985) High frequency jet percussive ventilation in newborn and infants with damaged lung. *Acta Anaesthesiologica Belgica* **127**, 128–135.

43 Biban, P., Trevisanuto, D., Pettenazzo, A. *et al.* (1998) Inhaled nitric oxide in hypoxaemic newborns who are candidates for extracorporeal life support. *European Respiratory Journal* **11**, 371–376.

44 Bland, R.D., Kim, M.H., Light, M.J. (1980) High frequency mechanical ventilation in severe hyaline membrane disease: an alternative treatment? *Critical Care Medicine* **8**, 275–280.

45 Boedy, R.F., Howell, C.G., Kanto, W.P. (1990) Hidden mortality rate associated with extracorporeal membrane oxygenation. *Journal of Pediatrics* **117**, 462–464.

46 Boros, S.J., Campbell, K. (1980) A comparison of the effects of high frequency-low tidal volume and low frequency-high tidal volume mechanical ventilation. *Journal of Applied Physiology* **97**, 108–112.

47 Boros, S.J., Reynolds, J.W. (1975) Hyaline membrane disease treated with early nasal end expiratory pressure: one year's experience. *Pediatrics* **56**, 281–223.

48 Boros, S.J., Matalon, S.V., Ewald, R. *et al.* (1977) The effect of independent variations in inspiratory-expiratory ratio and end expiratory pressure during mechanical ventilation in hyaline membrane disease; the significance of mean airway pressure. *Journal of Pediatrics* **91**, 794–798.

49 Boros, S.J., Bing, D.R., Mammel, M.C. *et al.* (1984) Using conventional infant ventilators at unconventional rates. *Pediatrics* **74**, 487–492.

50 Boros, S.J., Mammel, M.C., Coleman, J.M. *et al.* (1985) Neonatal high frequency jet ventilation: four years' experience. *Pediatrics* **75**, 657–663.

51 Boynton, B.R., Hammond, M.D., Fredberg, J.J. *et al.* (1989) Gas exchange in healthy rabbits during high frequency oscillatory ventilation. *Journal of Applied Physiology* **66**, 1343–1351.

52 Brendstrup, A., Benveniste, D., Pedersen, J.E.P. (1975) The magnitude of air admixture with a jet device in paediatric anaesthesia. *British Journal of Anaesthesia* **47**, 1335–1337.

53 British Standards Institution. (1970) Specifications for humidifiers for use with breathing machines. *BS (4494)* London, 7.

54 Bryan, A.C., Froese, A.B. (1991) Reflections on the HIFI trial. *Pediatrics* **87**, 565–567.

55 Budd, R.A. (1982) The 'Logan bow' method for securing endotracheal tubes in neonates. *Critical Care Nurse* **2**, 27–28.

56 Burnard, E.D., Morre, R.G., Nichol, H. 1978: A trial of doxapram in the recurrent apnea of prematurity. In Stern, L., Oh, W., Friis-Hansen, B. (eds), *Intensive Care of the Newborn II.* New York: Masson, 143–148.

57 Byford, L.J., Finckler, J.H., Froese, A.B. (1988) Lung volume recruitment during high frequency oscillation in atelectasis-prone rabbits. *Journal of Applied Physiology* **64**, 1607–1614.

58 Cakar, N., Tuorul, M., Demirarslan, A. *et al.* (2001) Time required for partial pressure of arterial oxygen equilibration during mechanical ventilation after a step change in fractional inspired oxygen concentration. *Intensive Care Medicine* **27**, 655–659.

59 Campbell, N.A., Zarfin, Y., Perlman, M. (1984) Selective bronchial intubation for pulmonary emphysema. *Archives of Disease in Childhood* **59**, 890–892.

60 Cannon, M.L., Cornell, J., Tripp-Hamel, D.S. *et al.* (2000) Tidal volumes for ventilated infants should be determined with a pneumotachometer placed at the endotracheal tube. *American Journal of Respiratory & Critical Care Medicine* **162**, 2109–2112.

61 Carlo, W.A., Chatburn, R.L., Martin, R.J. (1987) Randomized trial of high frequency jet ventilation versus conventional ventilation in respiratory distress syndrome. *Journal of Pediatrics* **110**, 275–282.

62 Carlo, W.A., Siner, B., Chatburn, R.L. *et al.* (1990) Early randomized intervention with high frequency jet ventilation in respiratory distress syndrome. *Journal of Pediatrics* **117**, 765–770.

63 Carter, J.M., Gerstmann, D.R., Clark, R.H. *et al.* (1990) High frequency oscillatory ventilation and extracorporeal membrane oxygenation for the treatment of acute neonatal respiratory failure. *Pediatrics* **85**, 159–164.

64 Cartlidge, P.H., Rutter, N. (1988) Percutaneous oxygen delivery to the preterm infant. *Lancet* **i**, 315–317.

65 Chakrabarti, M.K., Whitwam, J.G. (1983) A new valveless all-purpose ventilator. Description and laboratory evaluation. *British Journal of Anaesthesia* **55**, 1005–1015.

66 Chan, V., Greenough, A. (1992) Evaluation of triggering systems for patient triggered ventilation for neonates ventilator-dependent beyond 10 days of age. *European Journal of Pediatrics* **151**, 842–845.

67 Chan, V., Greenough, A. (1993) Determinants of oxygenation during high frequency oscillation. *European Journal of Pediatrics* **152**, 350–353.

68 Chan, V., Greenough, A. (1993) Neonatal patient triggered ventilators. Performance in acute and chronic lung disease. *British Journal of Intensive Care* **3**, 216–219.

69 Chan, V., Greenough, A. (1993) Randomised controlled trial of weaning by patient triggered ventilation or conventional ventilation. *European Journal of Pediatrics* **152**, 51–54.

70 Chan, V., Greenough, A. (1994) Comparison of weaning by patient triggered ventilation or synchronous intermittent mandatory ventilation in preterm infants. *Acta Paediatrica* **83**, 335–337.

71 Chan, V., Greenough, A. (1994) The effect of frequency on carbon dioxide levels during high frequency oscillation. *Journal of Perinatal Medicine* **22**, 103–106.

72 Chan, V., Greenough, A. (1994) Inspiratory and expiratory times for infants ventilator-dependent beyond the first week of life. *Acta Paediatrica* **83**, 1022–1024.

73 Chan, V., Greenough, A., Hird, M.F. (1991) Comparison of different rates of artificial ventilation for preterm infants ventilated beyond the first week of life. *Early Human Development* **26**, 177–183.

74 Chan, V., Greenough, A., Milner, A.D. (1993) The effect of frequency and mean airway pressure on volume delivery during high frequency oscillation. *Pediatric Pulmonology* **15**, 183–186.

75 Chan, V., Greenough, A., Gamsu, H.R. (1994) High frequency oscillation for preterm infants with severe respiratory failure. *Archives of Disease in Childhood* **70**, F44–F46.

76 Chan, V., Greenough, A., Giffin, F. (1994) Disease severity and optimum mean airway pressure level on transfer to high frequency oscillation. *Pediatric Pulmonology* **17**, 178–182.

77 Chan, V., Greenough, A., Muramatsu, K. (1994) Influence of lung function and reflex activity on the success of patient triggered ventilation. *Early Human Development* **37**, 9–14.

78 Chan, V., Greenough, A., Dimitriou, G. (1995) High frequency oscillation, respiratory activity and changes in blood gases. *Early Human Development* **40**, 87–94.

79 Chatburn, R.L., Primiano, F.P. (1987) A rational basis for humidity therapy. *Respiratory Care* **32**, 249–254.

80 Cheema, I.U., Ahluwalia, J.S. (2001) Feasibility of tidal volume-guided ventilation in newborn infants: a randomized, crossover trial using the volume guarantee modality. *Pediatrics* **107**, 1323–1328.

81 Chernick, V. (1973) Continuous negative chest wall pressure therapy for hyaline membrane disease. *Pediatric Clinics of North America* **20**, 407–417.

82 Cheung, P.-Y., Prasertsom, W., Finer, N.N., Robertson, C.M.T. (1997) Rescue high frequency oscillatory ventilation for

preterm infants: neurodevelopmental outcome and its prediction. *Biology of the Neonate* **71**, 282–291.

83 Chilton, H.W., Brooks, J.G. (1979) Pharyngeal pressures in nasal CPAP. *Journal of Pediatrics* **94**, 808–810.

84 Christou, H., Adatia, I., van Marter, L.J. *et al.* (1997) Effect of inhaled nitric oxide on endothelin-1 and cyclic guanosine 5′-monophophate plasma concentrations in newborn infants with persistent pulmonary hypertension. *Journal of Pediatrics* **130**, 603–611.

85 Cigada, M., Gavazzi, A., Assi, E., Luccarelli, M. (2001) Gastric rupture after nasopharyngeal oxygen administration. *Intensive Care Medicine* **27**, 939.

86 Cilley, R.E., Zwischenberger, J.B., Andrews, A.F. *et al.* (1986) Intracranial haemorrhage during extracorporeal membrane oxygenation in neonates. *Pediatrics* **78**, 699–704.

87 Clark, P.L., Ekekezie, I.I., Kaftan, H.A. *et al.* (2002) Safety and efficacy of nitric oxide in chronic lung disease. *Archives of Disease in Childhood Fetal and Neonatal Edition* **86**, F41–F45.

88 Clark, R.H., Gerstman, D.R., Null, D.M., deLemos, R.A. (1992) Prospective randomized comparison of high frequency oscillatory and conventional ventilation in respiratory distress syndrome. *Pediatrics* **89**, 5–12.

89 Clark, R.H., Yoder, B.A., Sell, M.S. (1994) Prospective, randomized comparison of high frequency oscillation and conventional ventilation in candidates for extracorporeal membrane oxygenation. *Journal of Pediatrics* **124**, 447–454.

90 Clark, R.H., Dykes, F.D., Bachman, T.E., Ashurst, J.T. (1996) Intraventricular hemorrhage and high-frequency ventilation: a meta-analysis of prospective clinical trials. *Pediatrics* **98**, 1058–1061.

91 Clark, R.H., Kueser, T.J., Walker, M.W. *et al.* (2000) Low-dose nitric oxide therapy for persistent pulmonary hypertension of the newborn. *New England Journal of Medicine* **342**, 469–474.

92 Cleary, J.P., Bernstein, G., Mannino, F.L., Heldt, B.P. (1995) Improved oxygenation during synchronized intermittent mandatory ventilation in neonates with respiratory distress syndrome: a randomized, crossover study. *Journal of Pediatrics* **126**, 407–411.

93 Connolly, K.M., McGuirt, W.F.J. (2001) Elective extracorporeal membrane oxygenation: an improved perioperative technique in the treatment of tracheal obstruction. *Annals of Otology, Rhinology & Laryngology* **110**, 205–209.

94 Cools, F., Offringa, M. (1999) Meta-analysis of elective high frequency ventilation in preterm infants with respiratory distress syndrome. *Archives of Disease in Childhood Fetal and Neonatal Edition* **80**, F15–F20.

95 Cordero, L., Tallman, R.D., Qualman, S., Gardner, D. (1990) Necrotizing tracheobronchitis following high frequency ventilation: effect of hydrocortisone. *Pediatric Pathology* **10**, 663–670.

96 Cornfield, D.N., Maynard, R.C., de-Regnier, R.-A.O. *et al.* (1999) Randomized controlled trial of low dose inhaled nitric oxide in the treatment of term and near-term infants with respiratory failure and pulmonary hypertension. *Pediatrics* **104**, 1089–1094.

97 Courtney, S.D., Weber, K.R., Spohn, W.A. *et al.* (1990) Measurement of tidal volume using a pneumotachometer during high frequency oscillation. *Critical Care Medicine* **18**, 651–653.

98 Courtney, S.E., Pyon, K.H., Saslow, J.G. *et al.* (2001) Lung recruitment and breathing pattern during variable versus continuous flow nasal continuous positive airway pressure in premature infants: an evaluation of three devices. *Pediatrics* **107**, 304–308.

99 Crombleholme, T.M., Adzick, N.S., deLorimier, A.A. *et al.* (1990) Carotid artery reconstruction following extracorporeal membrane oxygenation. *American Journal of Diseases of Children* **144**, 872–874.

100 Cvetnic, W.G., Waffarn, F., Martin, J.M. (1989) Continuous negative pressure and intermittent mandatory ventilation in the management of pulmonary interstitial emphysema: a preliminary study. *Journal of Perinatology* **9**, 26–32.

101 Cvetnic, W.G., Cunningham, M.D., Sills, J.H., Gluck, L. (1990) Reintroduction of continuous negative pressure ventilation in neonates: two-year experience. *Pediatric Pulmonology* **8**, 245–253.

102 Davidson, D., Barefield, E.S., Kattwinkel, J. *et al.* (1998) Inhaled nitric oxide for the early treatment of persistent pulmonary hypertension of the term newborn: a randomized, double-masked, placebo-controlled, dose-response, multicenter study. *Pediatrics* **101**, 325–334.

103 Davidson, D., Barefield, E.S., Kattwinkel, J. *et al.* (1999) Safety of withdrawing inhaled nitric oxide therapy in persistent pulmonary hypertension of the newborn. *Pediatrics* **104**, 231–236.

104 Davis, J.M., Stafano, J.L., Butani, V.K. *et al.* (1986) Ventilatory response to caffeine in infants with bronchopulmonary dysplasia. *Pediatric Research* **20**, 202A.

105 Davis, J.M., Richter, S.E., Kendig, J.W., Notter, R.H. (1992) High frequency jet ventilation and surfactant treatment of newborns with severe respiratory failure. *Pediatric Pulmonology* **13**, 108–112.

106 Davis, P.G., Henderson-Smart, D.J. (1999) Nasal continuous positive airways pressure immediately after extubation for preventing morbidity in preterm infants (Cochrane Review). In *The Cochrane Library Issue 2* Oxford Update Software: The Cochrane Collaboration,

107 Day, R.W., Lynch, J.M., White, K.S., Ward, R.M. (1996) Acute response to inhaled nitric oxide in newborns with respiratory failure and pulmonary hypertension. *Pediatrics* **98**, 698–705.

108 deLemos, R.A., Gerstmann, D.R., Clark, R.H. *et al.* (1987) High frequency ventilation—the relationship between ventilator design and clinical strategy in the treatment of hyaline membrane disease and its complications: a brief review. *Pediatric Pulmonology* **3**, 370–372.

109 Dillard, R.G. (1980) Mean airway pressure calculation. *Journal of Pediatrics* **97**, 506–507.

110 Dimitriou, G., Greenough, A. (1995) Measurement of lung volume and optimal oxygenation during high frequency oscillation. *Archives of Disease in Childhood Fetal and Neonatal Edition* **72**, F180–F183.

111 Dimitriou, G., Greenough, A. (2000) Performance of neonatal ventilators. *British Journal of Intensive Care* **10**, 186–188.

112 Dimitriou, G., Greenough, A., Giffin, F., Chan, V. (1995) Synchronous intermittent mandatory ventilation modes compared with patient triggered ventilation during weaning. *Archives of Disease in Childhood* **72**, F188–F190.

113 Dimitriou, G., Greenough, A., Kavvadia, V. *et al.* (1998) Volume delivery during high frequency oscillation. *Archives of Disease in Childhood Fetal and Neonatal Edition* **78**, F148–F150.

114 Dimitriou, G., Greenough, A., Laubscher, B., Yamaguchi, N. (1998) Comparison of airway pressure triggered and airflow triggered ventilation in very immature infants. *Acta Paediatrica* **87**, 1256–1260.

115 Dimitriou, G., Greenough, A., Kavvadia, V. *et al.* (1999) Outcome predictors in nitric oxide treated preterm infants. *European Journal of Pediatrics* **158**, 589–591.

116 Dimitriou, G., Greenough, A., Kavvadia, V., Milner, A.D. (1999) Comparison of two inspiratory:expiratory ratios during high frequency oscillation. *European Journal of Pediatrics* **158**, 796–799.

117 Dimitriou, G., Greenough, A., Kavvadia, V. *et al.* (2000) Elective use of nasal continuous positive airway pressure following extubation of preterm infants – improves outcome? *European Journal of Pediatrics* **159**, 434–439.

118 Dimitriou, G., Greenough, A., Cherian, S. (2001) Comparison of airway pressure and airflow triggering systems using a single type of neonatal ventilator. *Acta Paediatrica* **90**, 445–447.

119 Dimitriou, G., Greenough, A., Alvares, B.R. *et al.* (2001) Chest radiograph lung area and oxygenation optimization on transfer to high frequency oscillation. *British Journal of Intensive Care* **11**, 78–82.

120 Dimitriou, G., Greenough, A., Broomfield, D., Morton, M. (2002) Rescue high frequency oscillation, hypocarbia and neurodevelopmental outcome in preterm infants. *Early Human Development* **66**, 133–141.

121 Dimitriou, G., Greenough, A., Sumi, K. (in press) Performance of a commercially available neonatal respiration monitor. *British Journal of Intensive Care*.

122 Dimmitt, R.A., Moss, R.L., Rhine, W.D. *et al.* (2001) Venoarterial versus venovenous extracorporeal membrane oxygenation in congenital diaphragmatic hernia: the Extracorporeal Life Support Organization Registry, 1990–1999. *Journal of Pediatric Surgery* **36**, 1199–1204.

123 Dinner, M., Tjeuw, M., Artusio, J.F. (1987) Bacteremia as a complication of nasotracheal intubation. *Anesthesia and Analgesia* **66**, 460–462.

124 Dobyns, E.L., Griebel, J., Kinsella, J.P. *et al.* (1999) Infant lung function after inhaled nitric oxide therapy for persistent pulmonary hypertension of the newborn. *Pediatric Pulmonology* **28**, 24–30.

125 Donn, S. (1982) Cost-effectiveness of home management of bronchopulmonary dysplasia. *Pediatrics* **70**, 330–331.

126 Donn, S.M., Greenough, A., Sinha, S.K. (2000) Patient triggered ventilation. *Archives of Disease in Childhood* **83**, F225–F226.

127 Dorkin, H.L., Frantz, I.D. (1981) Frequency-dependent impedance of the respiratory system in paralyzed intubated infants. *Pediatric Research* **15**, 717 abstract.

128 Durand, D.J., Goodman, A., Ray, P. *et al.* (1987) Theophylline treatment in the extubation of infants weighing less than 1250 grams: a controlled trial. *Pediatrics* **80**, 684–688.

129 Durand, M., McCann, E., Brady, J.P. (1983) Effect of continuous positive airway pressure on the ventilatory response to CO_2 in preterm infants. *Pediatrics* **71**, 634–638.

130 Easa, D., Mundie, T.G., Finn, K.C. *et al.* (1994) Continuous negative extrathoracic pressure versus positive end-expiratory pressure in piglets after saline lung lavage. *Pediatric Pulmonology* **17**, 161–168.

131 Elias-Jones, A.C., Dhillon, S., Greenough, A. (1985) The efficacy of oral theophylline in ventilated premature infants. *Early Human Development* **12**, 9–14.

132 Engle, W.A., Yoder, M.C., Andreoli, S.P. *et al.* (1997) Controlled prospective randomized comparison of high frequency jet ventilation and conventional ventilation in neonates with respiratory failure and persistent pulmonary hypertension. *Journal of Perinatology* **17**, 3–9.

133 Epstein, R.A. (1971) The sensitivities and response times of ventilatory assists. *Anesthesiology* **34**, 321–326.

134 Extracorporeal Life Support Organization (ELSO) Registry. (1990) University of Michigan. Ann Arbor.

135 Farstad, T., Bratlid, D. (1991) Effects of endotracheal tube size and ventilator settings on the mechanics of a test system during intermittent flow ventilation. *Pediatric Pulmonology* **11**, 15–21.

136 Ferrara, B., Johnson, D.E., Chang, P.-N., Thompson, T.R. (1984) Efficacy and neurologic outcome of profound hypocapneic alkalosis for the treatment of persistent pulmonary hypertension in infancy. *Journal of Pediatrics* **105**, 457–461.

137 Fiastro, J.F., Habib, M.P., Quan, S.F. (1988) Pressure support compensation for inspiratory work due to endotracheal tubes and demand continuous positive airway pressure. *Chest* **92**, 499–505.

138 Field, D., Milner, A.D., Hopkin, I.E. (1985) Calculation of mean airway pressure during neonatal intermittent positive pressure ventilation and high frequency positive pressure ventilation. *Pediatric Pulmonology* **1**, 141–144.

139 Field, D., Milner, A.D., Hopkin, I.E. (1985) Inspiratory time and tidal volume during intermittent positive pressure ventilation. *Archives of Disease in Childhood* **60**, 259–261.

140 Field, D., Milner, A.D., Hopkin, I.E. (1985) Manipulation of ventilator settings to reduce expiration against positive pressure inflation. *Archives of Disease in Childhood* **60**, 1036–1040.

141 Field, D., Milner, A.D., Hopkin, I.E. (1989) Inspiratory-to-expiratory ratio during ventilation for idiopathic respiratory distress syndrome. *Pediatric Pulmonology* **7**, 2–7.

142 Finer, N.N., Barrington, K.J. (1999) Nitric oxide for respiratory failure in infants born at or near term (Cochrane review). In *The Cochrane Library*, Issue 4. Oxford: Update Software,

143 Finer, N.N., Moriartey, R.R., Boyd, J. *et al.* (1979) Post extubation atelectasis: a retrospective review and a prospective controlled study. *Journal of Pediatrics* **94**, 110–113.

144 Fok, T.F., Ng, P.C., Wong, W. *et al.* (1997) High frequency oscillatory ventilation in infants with increased intra-abdominal pressure. *Archives of Disease in Childhood* **76**, F123–F125.

145 Fox, W.W., Spiker, A.R., Musci, M. (1984) Tracheal secretion impaction during hyperventilation for persistent pulmonary hypertension of the neonate. *Pediatric Research* **18**, 323A.

146 Frampton, M.W., Morrow, P.E., Cox, C. *et al.* (1991) Effects of nitrogen dioxide exposure on pulmonary function and airway reactivity in normal humans. *American Review of Respiratory Disease* **143**, 522–527.

147 Frantz, I.D., Werhammer, J., Stark, A.R. (1983) High frequency ventilation in premature infants with lung disease: adequate gas exchange at low tracheal pressures. *Pediatrics* **71**, 438–488.

148 Frantz, I.D., Werthammer, J., Stark, A.R. (1983) Improvements in pulmonary interstitial emphysema with high frequency ventilation. *Pediatric Research* **15**, 719 (abstract).

149 Freeland, A.P. (1988) The laryngologist in the neonatal unit. In *Recent Advances in Otolaryngology*. Edinburgh: Churchill Livingstone, 495–502.

150 Friedlich, P., Lecart, C., Posen, R. *et al.* (1999) A randomized trial of nasopharyngeal synchronized intermittent mandatory ventilation versus nasopharyngeal continuous positive airway pressure in very low birth weight infants after extubation. *Journal of Perinatology* **19**, 413–418.

151 Froese, A.B., Bryan, A.C. (1987) High frequency ventilation. *American Review of Respiratory Disease* **135**, 1363–1374.

152 Frostell, C. (1994) Nitric oxide inhalation – future drug or an invitation to disaster? *Paediatric Anaesthesia* **4**, 147–150.

153 Gappa, M., Costeloe, K., Southall, D.P. *et al.* (1994) Effect of continuous negative extrathoracic pressure on respiratory

mechanics and timing in infants recovering from neonatal respiratory distress syndrome. *Pediatric Research* **36**, 364–372.

154 Garg, M., Kurzner, S.I., Bautista, D.B., Keens, T.G. (1988) Clinically unsuspected hypoxia during sleep and feeding in infants with bronchopulmonary dysplasia. *Pediatrics* **81**, 635–642.

155 Garland, J.S., Nelson, D.B., Rice, T., Neu, J. (1985) Increased risk of gastrointestinal perforations in neonates mechanically ventilated with either face mask or nasal prongs. *Pediatrics* **76**, 406–410.

156 Garland, J.S., Buck, R.K., Allred, E.N., Leviton, A. (1995) Hypocarbia before surfactant therapy appears to increase bronchopulmonary dysplasia risk in infants with respiratory distress syndrome. *Archives of Pediatrics and Adolescent Medicine* **149**, 617–622.

157 Gau, G.S., Ryder, T.A., Mobberley, M.A. (1987) Iatrogenic epithelial change caused by endotracheal intubation in neonates. *Early Human Development* **15**, 221–229.

158 Gauger, P.G., Hirschl, R.B., Delosh, T.N. *et al.* (1995) A matched pairs analysis of venoarterial and venovenous extracorporeal life support in neonatal respiratory failure. *ASAIO Journal* **41**, M573–579.

159 Gauger, P.G., Pranikoff, T., Schreiner, R.J. *et al.* (1996) Initial experience with partial liquid ventilation in pediatric patients with the acute respiratory distress syndrome. *Critical Care Medicine* **24**, 16–22.

160 George, T.N., Johnson, K.J., Bates, J.N., Segar, J.L. (1998) The effect of inhaled nitric oxide therapy on bleeding time and platelet aggregation in neonates. *Journal of Pediatrics* **132**, 731–734.

161 Gerhardt, T., Reifenberg, L., Goldberg, R.N., Bancalari, E. (1989) Pulmonary function in preterm infants whose lungs were ventilated conventionally or by high frequency oscillation. *Journal of Pediatrics* **115**, 121–126.

162 Gerstmann, D.R., deLemos, R.A., Clark, R.H. (1991) High frequency ventilation: issues of strategy. *Clinics in Perinatology* **18**, 563–580.

163 Gerstmann, D.R., Minton, S.D., Stoddard, R.A. *et al.* (1996) The Provo multicenter early high frequency oscillatory ventilation trial: improved pulmonary and clinical outcome in respiratory distress syndrome. *Pediatrics* **98**, 1044–1057.

164 Gerstmann, D.R., Wood, K., Miller, A. *et al.* (2001) Childhoood outcome after early high-frequency oscillatory ventilation for neonatal respiratory distress syndrome. *Pediatrics* **108**, 617–623.

165 Gill, B.S., Neville, H.L., Khan, A.M. *et al.* (2002) Delayed institution of extracorporeal membrane oxygenation is associated with increased mortality rate and prolonged hospital stay. *Journal of Pediatric Surgery* **37**, 7–10.

166 Gittermann, M.K., Fusch, C., Gittermann, A.R. *et al.* (1997) Early nasal continuous positive airway pressure treatment reduces the need for intubation in very low birth weight infants. *European Journal of Pediatrics* **156**, 384–388.

167 Glass, P., Wagner, A.E., Papero, P.H. *et al.* (1995) Neurodevelopmental status at age five years of neonates treated with extracorporeal membrane oxygenation. *Journal of Pediatrics* **127**, 447–457.

168 Goldberg, L.A., Marmon, L.M., Keszler, M. (1992) High-frequency jet ventilation decreases air flow through a tracheoesophageal fistula. *Critical Care Medicine* **20**, 547–549.

169 Goldman, A.P., Tasker, R.C., Haworth, S.G. *et al.* (1996) Four patterns of response to inhaled nitric oxide for persistent pulmonary hypertension of the newborn. *Pediatrics* **98**, 706–713.

170 Goldman, S.L., Brady, J.-P., Dumpit, R.M. (1979) Increased work of breathing associated with nasal prongs. *Pediatrics* **64**, 160–164.

171 Goldman, S.L., McCann, E.M., Lloyd, B.W., Yup, G. (1991) Inspiratory time and pulmonary function in mechanically ventilated babies with chronic lung disease. *Pediatric Pulmonology* **11**, 198–201.

172 Gonzalez, F., Harris, T., Black, P., Richardson, P. (1987) Decreased gas flow through pneumothoraces in neonates receiving high frequency jet versus conventional ventilation. *Pediatrics* **110**, 464–466.

173 Gotteiner, N.L., Harper, W.R., Gidding, S.S. *et al.* (1997) Echocardiographic prediction of neonatal ECMO outcome. *Pediatric Cardiology* **18**, 270–275.

174 Govindaswami, B., Heldt, G.P., Bernstein, G., Bejar, R. (1993) Reduction in cerebral blood flow velocity (CBFV) variability in infants <1500 g during synchronized ventilation (SIMV). *Pediatric Research* **33**, 213A.

175 Grammatikopoulos, T., Devane, S.P., Hannam, S., Greenough, A. (2003) Method of endotracheal tube fixation and iatrogenic ear deformities. *European Journal of Pediatrics* **162**: 41–43.

176 Greenough, A. (1988) The premature infant's respiratory response to mechanical ventilation. *Early Human Development* **17**, 1–5.

177 Greenough, A., Greenall, F. (1987) Performance of respirators at fast rates commonly used in the neonatal intensive care unit. *Pediatric Pulmonology* **3**, 357–361.

178 Greenough, A., Greenall, F. (1988) Observation of spontaneous respiratory interaction with artificial ventilation. *Archives of Disease in Childhood* **63**, 168–171.

179 Greenough, A., Milner, A.D. (1987) High frequency ventilation in the neonatal period. *European Journal of Pediatrics* **146**, 446–449.

180 Greenough, A., Morley, C.J. (1982) Oesophageal pressure measurements in ventilated preterm babies. *Archives of Disease in Childhood* **57**, 851–855.

181 Greenough, A., Pool, J. (1988) Neonatal patient triggered ventilation. *Archives of Disease in Childhood* **63**, 394–397.

182 Greenough, A., Morley, C.J., Davis, J.A. (1983) Respiratory reflexes in ventilated premature babies. *Early Human Development* **8**, 65–75.

183 Greenough, A., Dixon, A., Roberton, N.R.C. (1984) Pulmonary interstitial emphysema. *Archives of Disease in Childhood* **59**, 1046–1051.

184 Greenough, A., Wood, S., Morley, C.J., Davis, J.A. (1984) Pancuronium prevents pneumothoraces in ventilated premature babies who actively expire against positive pressure inflation. *Lancet* **1**, 1–3.

185 Greenough, A., Elias-Jones, A., Pool, J., Morley, C.J. (1985) The therapeutic actions of theophylline in preterm ventilated infants. *Early Human Development* **12**, 15–22.

186 Greenough, A., Greenall, F., Gamsu, H. (1987) Synchronous respiration: which ventilator rate is best? *Acta Paediatrica Scandinavica* **76**, 713–718.

187 Greenough, A., Greenall, F., Gamsu, H.R. (1987) Inspiratory times when weaning from mechanical ventilation. *Archives of Disease in Childhood* **62**, 1269–1270.

188 Greenough, A., Pool, J., Greenall, F. *et al.* (1987) Comparison of different rates of artificial ventilation in preterm neonates with the respiratory distress syndrome. *Acta Paediatrica Scandinavica* **76**, 706–712.

189 Greenough, A., Gamsu, H.R., Greenall, F. (1989) Investigation of the effects of paralysis by pancuronium on heart rate variability, blood pressure and fluid balance. *Acta Paediatrica Scandinavica* **78**, 829–834.

190 Greenough, A., Pool, J., Gamsu, H.R. (1989) A randomised controlled trial of two methods of weaning from high

frequency positive pressure ventilation. *Archives of Disease in Childhood* **64**, 834–838.

191 Greenough, A., Hird, M.F., Gamsu, H.R. (1991) Home oxgyen therapy following neonatal intensive care. *Early Human Development* **26**, 29–35.

192 Greenough, A., Chan, V., Hird, M.F. (1992) Positive end expiratory pressure in acute and chronic neonatal respiratory distress. *Archives of Disease in Childhood* **67**, 320–323.

193 Greenough, A., Milner, A., Dimitriou, G. (1998) Volume controlled and time cycled pressure limited ventilation. *Archives of Disease in Childhood Fetal and Neonatal Edition* **79**, F79–F80.

194 Greenough, A., Alexander, J., Burgess, S. *et al.* (2001) Home oxygen status on rehospitalisation and primary care requirements of chronic lung disease infants. *Archives of Disease in Childhood* **85**, 463–468.

195 Greenough, A., Milner, A.D., Dimitriou, G. (2001) Synchronized ventilation (Cochrane review). In *The Cochrane Library*, Issue 1. Update Software, Oxford.

196 Greenspan, J.S., Wolfson, M.R., Rubenstein, D., Shaffer, T.H. (1990) Liquid ventilation of human preterm neonates. *Journal of Pediatrics* **117**, 106–111.

197 Greenspan, J.S., Fox, W.W., Rubenstein, S.D. *et al.* (1997) Partial liquid ventilation in critically ill infants receiving extracorporeal life support. *Pediatrics* **99**, e2.

198 Gregory, G.A. (1986) Devices for applying continuous positive airway pressure. In Thibeault, D.W., Gregory, G.A. (eds), *Neonatal Pulmonary Care.* Norwalk CT: Appleton Century Crofts, 307–320.

199 Gregory, G.A., Kitterman, J.A., Phibbs, R.H. *et al.* (1971) Treatment of idiopathic respiratory distress syndrome with continuous positive pressure. *New England Journal of Medicine* **284**, 1333–1340.

200 Groothuis, J.R., Rosenberg, A.A. (1987) Home oxygen promotes weight gain in infants with bronchopulmonary dysplasia. *American Journal of Diseases in Children* **141**, 992–995.

201 Gullberg, N., Winberg, P., Sellden, H. (1996) Pressure support ventilation increases cardiac output in neonates and infants. *Paediatric Anaesthesia* **6**, 311–315.

202 Hamilton, P.P., Onayemi, A., Smyth, J.A. *et al.* (1983) Comparison of conventional and high frequency ventilation: oxygenation and lung pathology. *Journal of Applied Physiology* **55**, 131–138.

203 Han, V.K.M., Beverly, D.W., Clarson, C. *et al.* (1987) Randomized controlled trial of very early continuous distending pressure in the management of preterm infants. *Early Human Development* **15**, 21–23.

204 Harris, H., Wilson, S., Brans, Y. *et al.* (1976) Nasal continuous positive airway pressure. *Biology of the Neonate* **29**, 231–237.

205 Harris, M.C., Baumgart, S., Rooklin, A.R., Fox, W.W. (1983) Successful extubation of infants with respiratory distress syndrome using aminophylline. *Journal of Pediatrics* **103**, 303–306.

206 Hatcher, D., Watanabe, H., Ashbury, T. *et al.* (1998) Mechanical performance of clinically available, neonatal, high frequency, oscillatory-type ventilators. *Critical Care Medicine* **26**, 1081–1088.

207 Heaf, D.P., Helms, P., Dinwiddie, R., Matthew, D.J. (1982) Nasopharyngeal airways in Pierre–Robin syndrome. *Journal of Pediatrics* **100**, 698–703.

208 Heicher, D.A., Kasting, D.S., Harrod, J.R. (1981) Prospective clinical comparison of two methods for mechanical ventilation of neonates: rapid rate and short inspiratory time versus slow rate and long inspiratory time. *Journal of Pediatrics* **98**, 957–961.

209 Henderson-Smart, D.J., Bhuta, T., Cools, F., Offringa, M. (2001) Elective high frequency oscillatory ventilation versus conventional ventilation for acute pulmonary dysfunction in preterm infants. (Cochrane review). In *The Cochrane Library*, Issue 3. Update Software, Oxford.

210 Hendricks-Munoz, K.D., Walton, J.P. (1988) Hearing loss in infants with persistent fetal circulation. *Pediatrics* **81**, 650–656.

211 Herman, S., Reynolds, E.O.R. (1973) Methods for improving oxygenation in infants mechanically ventilated for severe hyaline membrane disease. *Archives of Disease in Childhood* **48**, 612–617.

212 Herrera, C.M., Gerhardt, T., Everett, R. *et al.* (1994) Randomized, crossover study of volume guarantee (VG) versus synchronized intermittent mandatory ventilation (SIMV) in very low birth weight (VLBW) infants recovering from respiratory failure. *Pediatric Research* **45**, 304A.

213 Hibbs, A., Evans, J.R., Gerdes, M. *et al.* (2001) Outcome of infants with bronchopulmonary dysplasia who receive extracorporeal membrane oxygenation therapy. *Journal of Pediatric Surgery* **36**, 1479–1484.

214 HIFO Study Group. (1993) Randomized study of high-frequency oscillatory ventilation in infants with severe respiratory distress. *Journal of Pediatrics* **122**, 609–619.

215 Hintz, S.R., Suttner, D.M., Sheehan, A.M. *et al.* (2000) Decreased use of neonatal extracorporeal membrane oxygenation (ECMO): how new treatment modalities have affected ECMO utilization. *Pediatrics* **106**, 1339–1343.

216 Hirani, W.M., Shanon, D.C., Kacmarek, R. *et al.* (1996) Inhaled nitric oxide in infants and children with bronchopulmonary dysplasia. *American Journal of Respiratory and Critical Care Medicine* **153**, A499.

217 Hird, M., Greenough, A., Gamsu, H. (1990) Gas trapping during high frequency positive pressure ventilation using conventional ventilators. *Early Human Development* **22**, 51–56.

218 Hird, M.F., Greenough, A. (1990) Gestational age: an important influence on the success of patient triggered ventilation. *Clinical Physics and Physiological Measurement* **11**, 307–312.

219 Hird, M.F., Greenough, A. (1991) Comparison of triggering systems for neonatal patient triggered ventilation. *Archives of Disease in Childhood* **66**, 426–428.

220 Hird, M.F., Greenough, A. (1991) Patient triggered ventilation using a flow triggered system. *Archives of Disease in Childhood* **66**, 1140–1142.

221 Hird, M.F., Greenough, A. (1991) Spontaneous respiratory effort during mechanical ventilation in infants with and without acute respiratory distress. *Early Human Development* **25**, 69–73.

222 Hirschl, R.B., Pranikoff, T., Gauger, P. *et al.* (1995) Liquid ventilation in adults, children and full term neonates. *Lancet* **346**, 1201–1202.

223 Hoehn, T., Krause, M.F. (2000) Effective elimination of carbon dioxide by nasopharyngeal high-frequency ventilation. *Respiratory Medicine* **94**, 1132–1134.

224 Hoehn, T., Krause, M.F., Buhrer, C. (2000) Inhaled nitric oxide in premature infants – a meta-analysis. *Journal of Perinatal Medicine* **28**, 7–13.

225 Hofkosh, D., Thompson, A.E., Nozza, R.J. *et al.* (1991) Ten years of extracorporeal membrane oxygenation: neurodevelopmental outcome. *Pediatrics* **87**, 549–555.

226 Hogman, M., Frostell, C., Arnberg, H., Hedenstierna, G. (1993) Bleeding time prolongation and NO inhalation. *Lancet* **341**, 1664–1665.

227 Hoskyns, E.N., Milner, A.D., Hopkin, I.E. (1991) Combined conventional ventilation with high frequency oscillation in neonates. *European Journal of Pediatrics* **150**, 357–361.

228 Howell, J., Clozel, M., Aranda, J.V. (1981) Adverse effects of caffeine and theophylline in the newborn infant. *Seminars in Perinatology* **5**, 359–369.

229 Hummler, H., Gerhardt, T., Gonzalez, A. *et al.* (1996) Influence of different methods of synchronized mechanical ventilation on ventilation, gas exchange, patient effort and blood pressure fluctuations in premature neonates. *Pediatric Pulmonology* **22**, 305–313.

230 Hummler, H.D., Gerhardt, T., Gonzalez, A. *et al.* (1996) Patient triggered ventilation in neonates: comparison of a flow and an impedance triggered system. *American Journal of Respiratory and Critical Care Medicine* **154**, 1049–1054.

231 Hummler, H., Schulze, A., Pohlandt, F., Thome, U. (2000) Dynamics of breathing during partial liquid ventilation in spontaneously breathing rabbits supported by elastic and resistive unloading. *Pediatric Research* **47**, 392–397.

232 Hummler, H., Thome, U., Schulze, A. *et al.* (2001) Spontaneous breathing during partial liquid ventilation in animals with meconium aspiration. *Pediatric Research* **49**, 572–580.

233 Isomura, K., Chikahira, M., Teranishi, K., Hamada, K. (1984) Induction of mutations and chromosome aberrations in lung cells following *in vivo* exposure of rats to nitrogen oxides. *Mutation Research* **136**, 119–125.

234 Jackson, J.C., Truog, W.E., Standaert, T.A. *et al.* (1991) Effect of high-frequency ventilation on the development of alveolar edema in premature monkeys at risk for hyaline membrane disease. *American Review of Respiratory Disease* **143**, 865–871.

235 Jacobsen, T., Gronvall, J., Petersen, S., Andersen, G.E. (1993) 'Minitouch' treatment of very low birth weight infants. *Acta Paediatrica* **82**, 934–938.

236 Jaillard, S., Peierrat, V., Truffert, P. *et al.* (2000) Two years' follow-up of newborn infants after extracorporeal membrane oxygenation (ECMO). *European Journal of Cardiothoracic Surgery* **18**, 328–333.

237 Jardine, E., O'Toole, M., Paton, J.Y., Wallis, C. (1999) Current status of long term ventilation of children in the United Kingdom: questionnaire survey. *British Medical Journal* **318**, 295–299.

238 Jirapaet, K.S., Kiatchuskul, P., Kolatat, T., Srisuparb, P. (2001) Comparison of high-frequency flow interruption ventilation and hyperventilation in persistent pulmonary hypertension of the newborn. *Respiratory Care* **46**, 586–594.

239 Jouvet, P., Hubert, P., Jarreau, P.H. *et al.* (1995) Assessment of neonatal ventilator performances. *Intensive Care Medicine* **21**, 753–758.

240 Kalenga, M., Battisti, O., Francois, A. *et al.* (1998) High frequency oscillatory ventilation in neonatal RDS: initial volume optimization and respiratory mechanics. *Journal of Applied Physiology* **84**, 1174–1177.

241 Kamitsuka, M.D., Boynton, B.R., Villanueva, D. *et al.* (1990) Frequency, tidal volume and mean airway pressure combinations that provide adequate gas exchange and low alveolar pressure during high frequency oscillatory ventilation in rabbits. *Pediatric Research* **27**, 64–69.

242 Kamper, J., Ringsted, C. (1990) Early treatment of idiopathic respiratory distress syndrome using binasal continuous positive airway pressure. *Acta Paediatrica Scandinavica* **79**, 581–586.

243 Kamper, J., Wulff, K., Larsen, C., Lindequist, S. (1993) Early treatment with nasal continuous positive airway pressure in very low-birth-weight infants. *Acta Paediatrica* **82**, 193–197.

244 Kavvadia, V., Greenough, A., Lilley, J. *et al.* (1999) Plasma arginine levels and the response to inhaled nitric oxide in neonates. *Biology of the Neonate* **76**, 340–347.

245 Kavvadia, V., Greenough, A., Dimitriou, G. (2000) Effect on lung function of continuous positive airway pressure administered by either infant flow driver or single nasal prong. *European Journal of Pediatrics* **159**, 289–292.

246 Kavvadia, V., Greenough, A., Dimitriou, G. (2000) Prediction of extubation failure in preterm neonates. *European Journal of Pediatrics* **159**, 227–231.

247 Kavvadia, V., Greenough, A., Boylan, G. *et al.* (2001) Effect of a high volume strategy high frequency oscillation on cerebral haemodynamics. *European Journal of Pediatrics* **160**, 140–141.

248 Kelly, M.A., Finer, N.N. (1984) Nasotracheal intubation in the neonate: physiologic responses and effects of atropine and pancuronium. *Journal of Pediatrics* **26**, 1016–1022.

249 Keszler, M., Durand, D.J. (2001) Neonatal high-frequency ventilation. Past, present, and future. *Clinics in Perinatology* **28**, 579–607.

250 Keszler, M., Donn, S.M., Bucciarelli, R.L. *et al.* (1991) Multicenter controlled trial comparing high-frequency jet ventilation and conventional mechanical ventilation in newborn infants with pulmonary interstitial emphysema. *Journal of Pediatrics* **119**, 85–93.

251 Keszler, M., Ryckman, F.C., McDonald, J.V. *et al.* (1992) A prospective, multicenter, randomized study of high versus low positive end expiratory pressure during extracorporeal membrane oxygenation. *Journal of Pediatrics* **120**, 107–113.

252 Keszler, M., Modanlou, H.D., Brudno, S. *et al.* (1997) Multicenter controlled clinical trial of high frequency jet ventilation in preterm infants with uncomplicated respiratory distress syndrome. *Pediatrics* **100**, 593–599.

253 Kiciman, N.M., Andreasson, B., Bernstein, G. *et al.* (1998) Thoracabdominal motion in newborns during ventilation delivered by endotracheal tube or nasal prongs. *Pediatric Pulmonology* **25**, 175–181.

254 Kinsella, J.P., Gerstmann, D.R., Clark, R.H. *et al.* (1991) High frequency oscillatory ventilation versus intermittent mandatory ventilation: early hemodynamic effects in the premature baboon with hyaline membrane disease. *Pediatric Research* **29**, 160–166.

255 Kinsella, J.P., Nash, S.R., Shaffer, E., Abman, S.H. (1992) Low dose inhalational nitric oxide in persistent pulmonary hypertension of the newborn. *Lancet* **340**, 819–820.

256 Kinsella, J.P., Truog, W.E., Walsh, W.F. *et al.* (1997) Randomized, multicenter trial of inhaled nitric oxide and high-frequency oscillatory ventilation in severe, persistent pulmonary hypertension of the newborn. *Journal of Pediatrics* **131**, 55–62.

257 Kinsella, J.P., Walsh, W.F., Bose, C.L. *et al.* (1999) Inhaled nitric oxide in premature neonates with severe hypoxaemic respiratory failure: a randomised controlled trial. *Lancet* **354**, 1061–1065.

258 Kraybill, E.N., Runyan, D.K., Bose, C.L., Khan, J.H. (1989) Risk factors for chronic lung disease in infants with birth weights of 751 to 1000 grams. *Journal of Pediatrics* **115**, 115–120.

259 Krouskop, R.W., Brown, E.H., Sweet, A.Y. (1975) The early use of continuous positive airway pressure and the treatment of idiopathic respiratory distress syndrome. *Journal of Pediatrics* **87**, 263–267.

260 Krummel, T.M., Greenfield, L.J., Kirkpatrick, B.O. (1984) Alveolar arterial oxygen gradient versus the neonatal pulmonary insufficiency index for prediction of mortality in ECMO candidates. *Journal of Pediatric Surgery* **19**, 380–384.

261 Lagneaux, D., Mossay, C., Geubelle, F., Christiaens, G. (1988) Alveolar data in healthy awake neonates during

spontaneous ventilation, a preliminary investigation. *Pediatric Pulmonology* **5**, 225–231.

262 Laing, I.A., Cowan, D.L., Hume, R. (1988) Prevention of subglottic stenosis. *Journal of Laryngology and Otology Supplement* **17**, 11–14.

263 Langham, M.R., Krummel, T.M., Bartlett, R.H. *et al.* (1987) Mortality with extracorporeal membrane oxygenation following repair of congenital diaphragmatic hernia in 93 infants. *Journal of Pediatric Surgery* **22**, 1150–1154.

264 Laubscher, B., Greenough, A., Costeloe, K. (1996) Performance of four neonatal high frequency oscillators. *British Journal of Intensive Care* **6**, 148–152.

265 Laubscher, B., Greenough, A., Kavvadia, V., Devane, S.P. (1997) Response to nitric oxide in term and preterm infants. *European Journal of Pediatrics* **156**, 639–642.

266 Leach, C.L., Greenspan, J.S., Rubenstein, S.D. *et al.* (1996) Partial liquid ventilation with Perflubron in premature infants with severe respiratory distress syndrome. *New England Journal of Medicine* **335**, 761–767.

267 Lee, K.-S., Dunn, M.S., Fenwick, M., Shennan, A.T. (1998) A comparison of underwater bubble continuous positive airway pressure with ventilator-derived continuous positive airway pressure in premature neonates ready for extubation. *Biology of the Neonate* **73**, 69–75.

268 Lee, S., Milner, A.D. (2000) Resonant frequency in respiratory distress syndrome. *Archives of Disease in Childhood* **83**, F203–F206.

269 Lehtinen, A.-M., Hovorka, J., Widholm, O. (1984) Modification of aspects of the endocrine response to tracheal intubation by lignocaine, halothane and thiopentone. *British Journal of Anaesthesia* **56**, 239–246.

270 Lemyre, B., Davis, P.G., De Paoli, A.G. (2001) Nasal intermittent positive pressure ventilation (NIPPV) versus nasal continuous positive airway pressure (NCPAP) for apnea of prematurity (Cochrane review). In *The Cochrane Library*, Issue 2. Update Software, Oxford.

271 Lin, C.H., Wang, S.T., Lin, Y.J., Yeh, T.F. (1998) Efficacy of nasal intermittent positive pressure ventilation in treating apnea of prematurity. *Pediatric Pulmonology* **26**, 349–353.

272 Linden, V., Palmer, K., Reinhard, J. *et al.* (2001) Inter-hospital transportation of patients with severe acute respiratory failure on extracorporeal membrane oxygenation – national and international experience. *Intensive Care Medicine* **27**, 1643–1648.

273 Linsao, L.S., Levison, H., Sawyer, P.R. (1970) Negative pressure artificial respiration: use in treatment of respiratory distress syndrome of the newborn. *Canadian Medical Assocation Journal* **102**, 602–606.

274 Locke, R., Greenspan, J.S., Shaffer, T.H. *et al.* (1991) Effect of nasal CPAP on thoracoabdominal motion in neonates with respiratory insufficiency. *Pediatric Pulmonology* **11**, 259–264.

275 Locke, R.G., Wolfson, M.R., Shaffer, T.H. *et al.* (1993) Inadvertent administration of positive end distending pressure during nasal cannula flow. *Pediatrics* **91**, 135–138.

276 Loe, E.A., Graves, E.D., Ochsner, J.L. *et al.* (1985) ECMO for newborn respiratory failure. *Journal of Pediatric Surgery* **20**, 684–688.

277 Lonnqvist, P.A., Winberg, P., Lundell, B. *et al.* (1994) Inhaled nitric oxide in neonates and children with pulmonary hypertension. *Acta Paediatrica* **83**, 1132–1136.

278 Lundstrom, K.E., Greisen, G. (1993) Early treatment with nasal-CPAP. *Acta Paediatrica* **82**, 856.

279 MacDonald, M.G., Chou, M.M. (1986) Preventing complications from lines and tubes. *Seminars in Perinatology* **10**, 224–233.

280 Madar, J., Richmond, S. (1996) Role of extracorporeal membrane oxygenation. *Lancet* **348**, 823.

281 Mammel, M.C., Boros, S.J. (1987) Airway damage and mechanical ventilation. *Pediatric Pulmonology* **3**, 443–447.

282 Manczur, T., Greenough, A., Nicholson, G.P., Rafferty, G.F. (1999) Resistance of pediatric and neonatal endotracheal tubes – influence of flow rate, size and shape. *Critical Care Medicine* **28**, 1595–1598.

283 Marchak, B.E., Thompson, W.K., Duffty, P. *et al.* (1981) Treatment of respiratory distress syndrome by high frequency oscillatory ventilation: A preliminary report. *Journal of Pediatrics* **99**, 287–292.

284 McCulloch, P.R., Fokert, P.G., Froese, A.B. (1988) Lung volume maintenance prevents lung injury during high frequency oscillatory ventilation in surfactant deficient rabbits. *American Review of Respiratory Disease* **137**, 1185–1192.

285 McGuire, G., Crossley, D., Richards J., Wong, D. (1997) Effects of varying levels of positive end-expiratory pressure on intracranial pressure and cerebral perfusion pressure. *Critical Care Medicine* **25**, 1059–1062.

286 Mehta, A., Callan, K., Wright, B.M., Stacey, T.E. (1986) Patient triggered ventilation in the newborn. *Lancet* **2**, 17–19.

287 Mercier, J.C., Zupan, V., Delian, M. *et al.* (1993) Device to monitor concentration of inhaled nitric oxide. *Lancet* **342**, 431–432.

288 Meredith, K.S., DeLemos, R.A., Coalson, J.J. *et al.* (1989) Role of lung injury in the pathogenesis of hyaline membrane disease in premature baboons. *Journal of Applied Physiology* **66**, 2150–2158.

289 Merritt, T.A., Stuard, I.D., Puccia, J. *et al.* (1981) Newborn tracheal aspirate cytology: classification during respiratory distress syndrome and bronchopulmonary dysplasia. *Journal of Pediatrics* **98**, 949–956.

290 Miller, M.J., Carlo, W.A., Martin, R.J. (1985) Continuous positive airway pressure selectively reduces obstructive apnea in preterm infants. *Journal of Pediatrics* **106**, 91–94.

291 Millet, V., Lacroze, V., Bartoli, J.M. *et al.* (1997) [Early continuous positive pressure in the labor room]. *Archives de Pediatrie* **4**, 15–20.

292 Milner, A.D., Saunders, R.A., Hopkin, I.E. (1977) Effects of continuous distending pressure on lung volumes and lung mechanics in the immediate neonatal period. *Biology of the Neonate* **31**, 111–115.

293 Mitchell, A., Greenough, A., Hird, M. (1989) Limitations of patient triggered ventilation in neonates. *Archives of Disease in Childhood* **64**, 924–929.

294 Moa, G., Nilsson, K. (1993) Nasal continuous positive airway pressure: experiences with a new technical approach. *Acta Paediatrica* **82**, 210–211.

295 Moa, G., Nilsson, K., Zetterstrom, H., Jonsson, L.O. (1988) A new device for administration of nasal continuous positive airway pressure in the newborn: an experimental study. *Critical Care Medicine* **16**, 1238–1242.

296 Moncada, S., Palmer, R.M.J., Higgs, E.A. (1991) Nitric oxide: physiology, pathophysiology and pharmacology. *Pharmacology Reviews* **43**, 109–142.

297 Moretti, C., Marzetti, G., Agostino, R. *et al.* (1981) Prolonged intermittent positive pressure ventilation by nasal prongs in intractable apnea of prematurity. *Acta Paediatrica Scandinavica* **70**, 211–216.

298 Moretti, C., Gizzi, C., Papoff, P. *et al.* (1999) Comparing the effects of nasal synchronized intermittent positive pressure ventilation (nSIPPV) and nasal continuous positive airway pressure (nCPAP) after extubation in very low birth weight infants. *Early Human Development* **56**, 167–177.

299 Moriette, G., Paris-Llado, J., Walti, H. *et al.* (2001) Prospective randomized multicenter comparison of

high-frequency oscillatory ventilation and conventional ventilation in preterm infants of less than 30 weeks with respiratory distress syndrome. *Pediatrics* **107**, 363–372.

300 Mrozek, J.D., Bendel-Stenzel, E.M., Meyers, P.A. *et al.* (2000) Randomized controlled trial of volume-targeted synchronized ventilation and conventional intermittent mandatory ventilation following initial exogenous surfactant therapy. *Pediatric Pulmonology* **29**, 11–18.

301 Musante, G., Schulze, A., Gerhardt, T. *et al.* (2001) Respiratory mechanical unloading decreases thoraco-abdominal asynchrony and chest wall distortion in preterm infants. *Pediatric Research* **49**, 175–180.

302 Nagaya, M., Kato, J., Niimi, N., Tanaka, S. (2001) Extracorporeal membrane oxygenation for newborns with gastric rupture. *Pediatric Surgery International* **17**, 35–38.

303 Nelle, M., Zilow, E.P., Linderkamp, O. (1997) Effects of high-frequency oscillatory ventilation on circulation in neonates with pulmonary interstitial emphysema or RDS. *Intensive Care Medicine* **23**, 671–676.

304 Nicklaus, P.J. (1995) Airway complications of jet ventilation in neonates. *Annals of Otology, Rhinology & Laryngology* **104**, 24–30.

305 Nugent, J., Matthews, B., Goldsmith, J. (1988) Pulmonary care. In Carlon, W.A., Chatburn, R.L. (eds), *Assisted Ventilation of the Neonate*. Chicago: Yearbook Publishers Inc., 107–129.

306 Ogawa, Y., Miyasaka, K., Kawano, T. *et al.* (1993) Multicentre randomized trial of high frequency oscillatory ventilation as compared with conventional ventilation in preterm infants with respiratory failure. *Early Human Development* **32**, 1–10.

307 O'Rourke, P.P., Cronke, R.K., Vacanti, J.P. *et al.* (1989) Extracorporeal membrane oxygenation and conventional medical therapy in neonates with persistent pulmonary hypertension of the newborn: a prospective randomised study. *Pediatrics* **84**, 957–963.

308 Outerbridge, E.W., Roloff, D.W., Stern, L. (1972) Continuous negative pressure in the management of severe respiratory distress syndrome. *Journal of Pediatrics* **81**, 384–391.

309 Palmisano, J.M., Moler, F.W., Custer, J.R. *et al.* (1992) Unsuspected congenital heart disease in neonates receiving extracorporeal life support: a review of ninety-five cases from the Extracorporeal Life Support Organization Registry. *Journal of Pediatrics* **121**, 115–117.

310 Pandit, P.B., Courtney, S.E., Pyon, K.H. *et al.* (2001) Work of breathing during constant- and variable-flow nasal continuous positive airway pressure in preterm neonates. *Pediatrics* **108**, 682–685.

311 Pape, K.E., Armstrong, D.L., Fitzhardinge, P.M. (1976) Cerebral nervous system pathology associated with mask ventilation in the very low birthweight infant. A new aetiology for intracerebellar haemorrhages. *Pediatrics* **58**, 473–483.

312 Pardou, A., Vermeylen, D., Muller, M.F., Detemmerman, D. (1993) High frequency ventilation and conventional mechanical ventilation in newborn babies with respiratory distress syndrome: a prospective randomized trial. *Intensive Care Medicine* **19**, 406–410.

313 Parker, T.A., Kinsella, J.P., Abman, S.H. (1998) Response to inhaled nitric oxide in persistent pulmonary hypertension of the newborn: relationship to baseline oxygenation. *Journal of Perinatology* **18**, 221–225.

314 Pearl, J.M., Nelson, D.P., Raake, J.L. *et al.* (2002) Inhaled nitric oxide increases endothelin-1 levels: a potential cause of rebound pulmonary hypertension. *Critical Care Medicine* **30**, 89–93.

315 Pedersen, J.E., Neilsen, K. (1994) Oropharyngeal and esophageal pressures during mono- and binasal CPAP in neonates. *Acta Paediatrica* **83**, 143–149.

316 Pelioski, A., Finer, N.N. (1990) A blinded, randomized, placebo-controlled trial to compare theophylline and doxapram for the treatment of apnea of prematurity. *Journal of Pediatrics* **116**, 648–653.

317 Peliowski, A., Finer, N.N., Etches, P.C. *et al.* (1995) Inhaled nitric oxide for premature infants after prolonged rupture of the membranes. *Journal of Pediatrics* **126**, 450–453.

318 Pepe, P.E., Marini, J.J. (1982) Occult positive end-expiratory pressure in mechanically ventilated patients with airflow obstruction. *American Review of Respiratory Disease* **126**, 166–170.

319 Pianosi, P.T., Fisk, M. (2000) High frequency ventilation trial. Nine year follow up of lung function. *Early Human Development* **57**, 225–234.

320 Pillow, J.J., Neil, H., Wilkinson, M.H., Ramsden, C.A. (1999) Effect of I/E ratio on mean alveolar pressure during high-frequency oscillatory ventilation. *Journal of Applied Physiology* **87**, 407–414.

321 Pinney, M.A., Cotton, E.K. (1976) Home management of bronchopulmonary dysplasia. *Pediatrics* **58**, 856–859.

322 Piotrowski, A., Sobala, W., Kawczynski, P. (1997) Patient-initiated, pressure-regulated, volume-controlled ventilation compared with intermittent mandatory ventilation in neonates: a prospective, randomised study. *Intensive Care Medicine* **23**, 975–981.

323 Poets, C.F. (1998) When do infants need additional inspired oxygen? A review of the current literature. *Pediatric Pulmonology* **26**, 424–428.

324 Poets, C.F., Sens, B. (1996) Changes in intubation rates and outcome of very low birth weight infants: a population-based study. *Pediatrics* **98**, 24–27.

325 Pohlandt, F., Saule, H., Schröder, H. *et al.* (1992) Decreased incidence of extra-alveolar air leakage or death prior to air leakage in high versus low rate positive pressure ventilation: results of a randomised seven-centre trial in preterm infants. *European Journal of Pediatrics* **151**, 904–909.

326 Poon, C.S., Ward, S.A. (1986) A device to provide respiratory-mechanical unloading. *IEEE Transactions on Biomedical Engineering BME* **33**, 361–364.

327 Poon, C.S., Lebowitz, H.H., Sidney, D.A., Li, S.X. (1997) Negative-impedance ventilation and pressure support ventilation: a comparative study. *Respiration Physiology* **108**, 117–127.

328 Pranikoff, T., Gauger, P.G., Hirschl, R.B. (1996) Partial liquid ventilation in newborn patients with congenital diaphragmatic hernia. *Journal of Pediatric Surgery* **31**, 613–618.

329 Quiney, R.E., Spencer, M.G., Bailey, C.M. *et al.* (1986) Management of subglottic stenosis, experience from two centres. *Archives of Disease in Children* **61**, 686–690.

330 Quinn, M.W., de Boer, R.C., Ansari, N., Baumer, J.H. (1998) Stress response and mode of ventilation in preterm infants. *Archives of Disease in Childhood Fetal and Neonatal Edition* **78**, F195–F198.

331 Raine, J., Redington, A.N., Benatar, A. *et al.* (1993) Continuous negative extrathoracic pressure and cardiac output – a pilot study. *European Journal of Pediatrics* **152**, 595–598.

332 Rais-Bahrami, K., Wagner, A.E., Coffman, C. *et al.* (2000) Neurodevelopmental outcome in ECMO vs near-miss ECMO patients at 5 years of age. *Clinical Pediatrics (Philadelphia)* **39**, 145–152.

333 Raju, T.N.K., Vidyasagar, D., Torres, C. *et al.* (1980) Intracranial pressure during intubation and anaesthesia in infants. *Journal of Pediatrics* **96**, 860–862.

334 Raval, N.C., Leef, K.H., Antunes, M.J., Stefano, J.L. (1994) Effect of aerosolised furosemide on pulmonary function in infants with BPD: a randomized, blinded placebo controlled trial. *Pediatric Research* **35**, 350A.

335 Rettwitz-Volk, W., Veldman, A., Roth, B. *et al.* (1998) A prospective, randomized, multicenter trial of high frequency oscillatory ventilation compared with conventional ventilation in preterm infants with respiratory distress syndrome receiving surfactant. *Journal of Pediatrics* **132**, 249–254.

336 Revenis, M.E., Glass, P., Short, B.L. (1992) Mortality and morbidity rates among lower birthweight infants (2000 to 2500 grams) treated with extracorporeal membrane oxygenation. *Journal of Pediatrics* **121**, 452–458.

337 Reynolds, E.O.R. (1970) Indications for mechanical ventilation in infants with hyaline membrane disease. *Pediatrics* **46**, 193–202.

338 Reynolds, E.O.R. (1971) Effect of alterations in mechanical ventilator settings on pulmonary gas exchange in hyaline membrane disease. *Archives of Disease in Childhood* **46**, 152–159.

339 Rhodes, P.G., Graves, G.R., Patel, D.M. *et al.* (1983) Minimizing pneumothorax and BPD in ventilated infants with hyaline membrane disease. *Journal of Pediatrics* **103**, 634–637.

340 Rimensberger, P.C., Beghetti, M., Hanquinet, S., Berner, M. (2000) First intention high-frequency oscillation with early lung volume optimization improves pulmonary outcome in very low birth weight infants with respiratory distress syndrome. *Pediatrics* **105**, 1202–1208.

341 Roberton, N.R.C. (1993) *Manual of Neonatal Intensive Care.* London: Edward Arnold.

342 Roberts, J.D., Fineman, J.R., Morin, F.C. *et al.* (1997) Inhaled nitric oxide and persistent pulmonary hypertension of the newborn. *New England Journal of Medicine* **336**, 605–610.

343 Roberts, J.D.J., Polaner, D.M., Lang, P., Zapol, W.M. (1992) Inhaled nitric oxide in persistent pulmonary hypertension of the newborn. *Lancet* **340**, 818–819.

344 Roberts, T.E. (1998) Economic evaluation and randomised controlled trial of extracorporeal membrane oxygenation: UK collaborative trial. *British Medical Journal* **317**, 911–916.

345 Robertson, N.J., McCarthy, L.S., Hamilton, P.A., Moss, A.L.H. (1996) Nasal deformities resulting from flow driver continuous positive airway pressure. *Archives of Disease in Childhood* **75**, F209–F288.

346 Rooklin, A.R., Moomjian, A.S., Shutack, J.G. *et al.* (1979) Theophylline therapy in bronchopulmonary dysplasia. *Journal of Pediatrics* **95**, 882–885.

347 Rost, J.R., Frush, D.P., Auten, R.L. (1999) Effect of neck position on endotracheal tube location in low birth weight infants. *Pediatric Pulmonology* **27**, 199–202.

348 Roy, B.J., Rycus, P., Conrad, S.A., Clark, R.H. (2000) The changing demographics of neonatal extracorporeal membrane oxygenation patients reported to the Extracorporeal Life Support Organization (ELSO) Registry. *Pediatrics* **106**, 1334–1338.

349 Roze, J.C., Liet, J.M., Gournay, V. *et al.* (1997) Oxygen cost of breathing and weaning process in newborn infants. *European Respiratory Journal* **10**, 2583–2585.

350 Ryan, C.A., Finer, N.N., Peters, K.L. (1989) Nasal intermittent positive pressure ventilation offers no advantages over nasal continuous positive airway pressure in apnoea of prematurity. *American Journal of Diseases in Children* **143**, 1196–1198.

351 Saari, A.F., Rossing, T.H., Solway, J., Drazen, J.M. (1984) Lung inflation during high frequency oscillation. *American Review of Respiratory Disease* **129**, 333–336.

352 Sakakihara, Y., Yamanaka, T., Kajii, M., Kamoshita, S. (1996) Long-term ventilator-assisted children in Japan: a national survey. *Acta Paediatrica Japonica* **38**, 137–142.

353 Samuels, M.P., Southall, D.P. (1989) Negative extrathoracic pressure in treatment of respiratory failure in infants and young children. *British Medical Journal* **299**, 1253–1257.

354 Samuels, M.P., Raine, J., Wright, T. *et al.* (1996) Continuous negative extrathoracic pressure in neonatal respiratory failure. *Pediatrics* **98**, 1154–1160.

355 Sauve, R.S., McMillan, D.D., Mitchell, I. *et al.* (1989) Home oxygen therapy. Outcome of infants discharged from NICU on continuous treatment. *Clinical Pediatrics (Philadelphia)* **28**, 113–118.

356 Schaller, P., Schulze, A. (1991) A ventilator generating a positive or negative internal compliance. *Uppsala Journal of Medical Sciences* **96**, 219–234.

357 Schindler, M., Seear, M. (1991) The effect of lung mechanics on gas transport during high frequency oscillation. *Pediatric Pulmonology* **11**, 335–339.

358 Schreiner, M.S., Donar, M.E., Kettrick, R.G. (1987) Pediatric home mechanical ventilation. *Pediatric Clinics of North America* **34**, 47–60.

359 Schulze, A. (2000) Enhancement of mechanical ventilation of neonates by computer technology. *Seminars in Perinatology* **24**, 429–444.

360 Schulze, A., Bancalari, E. (2001) Proportional assist ventilation in infants. *Clinics in Perinatology* **28**, 561–578.

361 Schulze, A., Schaller, P. (1997) Assisted mechanical ventilation using resistive and elastic unloading. *Seminars in Neonatology* **2**, 105–114.

362 Schulze, A., Schaller, P., Gerhardt, B. *et al.* (1990) An infant ventilator technique for resistive unloading during spontaneous breathing. Results in a rabbit model of airway obstruction. *Pediatric Research* **28**, 79–82.

363 Schulze, A., Schaller, P., Jonzon, A., Sedin, G. (1993) Assisted mechanical ventilation using elastic unloading: a study in cats with normal and injured lungs. *Pediatric Research* **34**, 600–605.

364 Schulze, A., Schaller, P., Toepfer, A., Kirpalani, H. (1993) Resistive and elastic unloading to assist spontaneous breathing does not change functional residual capacity. *Pediatric Pulmonology* **16**, 170–176.

365 Schulze, A., Jonzon, A., Schaller, P., Sedin, G. (1996) Effects of ventilator resistance and compliance on phrenic nerve activity in spontaneously breathing cats. *American Journal of Respiratory and Critical Care Medicine* **153**, 671–676.

366 Schulze, A., Rich, W., Schellenberg, L. *et al.* (1998) Effects of different gain settings during assisted mechanical ventilation using respiratory unloading in rabbits. *Pediatric Research* **44**, 132–138.

367 Schulze, A., Suguihara, C., Gerhardt, T. *et al.* (1998) Effects of respiratory mechanical unloading on thoracoabdominal motion in meconium-injured piglets and rabbits. *Pediatric Research* **43**, 191–197.

368 Schulze, A., Gerhardt, T., Musante, G. *et al.* (1999) Proportional assist ventilation in low birth weight infants with acute respiratory disease. A comparison to assist/control and conventional mechanical ventilation. *Journal of Pediatrics* **135**, 339–344.

369 Schulze, A., Jonzon, A., Sindelar, R. *et al.* (1999) Assisted mechanical ventilation using combined elastic and resistive unloading in cats with severe respiratory failure: effects on gas exchange and phrenic nerve activity. *Acta Paediatrica* **88**, 636–641.

370 Schulze, A., Suguihara, C., Gerhardt, T. *et al.* (2001) Inductance plethysmography: an alternative signal to servocontrol the airway pressure during proportional assist ventilation. *Pediatric Research* **49**, 169–174.

371 Schumacher, R.E., Baumgart, S. (2001) Extracorporeal membrane oxygenation 2001. The odyssey continues. *Clinics in Perinatology* **28**, 629–653.

372 Schumacher, R.E., Barks, J.D.E., Johnston, M.V. *et al.* (1988) Right-sided brain lesions in infants following extracorporeal membrane oxygenation. *Pediatrics* **82**, 155–161.

373 Schumacher, R.E., Palmer, T.W., Roloff, D.W. *et al.* (1991) Follow-up of infants treated with extracorporeal membrane oxygenation for newborn respiratory failure. *Pediatrics* **87**, 451–457.

374 Scott, E.M., Hoskinds, D.D. (1958) Hereditary methaemoglobinaemia in Alaskans, Eskimos and Indians. *Blood* **13**, 795–802.

375 Shaffer, T.H., Wolfson, M.R. (1994) Liquid ventilation. In Boynton, B.R., Carlo, W.A., Jobe, A. (eds), *New Therapies for Neonatal Respiratory Failure: a Physiologic Approach.* Cambridge: Cambridge University Press, 279–301.

376 Shaffer, T.H., Wolfson, M.R. (1996) Liquid ventilation: an alternative ventilation strategy for management of neonatal respiratory distress. *European Journal of Pediatrics* **155**, 530–534.

377 Shaffer, T.H., Wolfson, M.R. (1998) Liquid ventilation. In Polin, R.A., Fox, W.W. (eds), *Fetal and Neonatal Physiology.* Philadelphia: W.B. Saunders, 1219–1242.

378 Shaffer, T.H., Wolfson, M.R. (1998) Liquid ventilation. In Polin, R.A., Fox, W.W. (eds), *Fetal and Neonatal Physiology.* Philadelphia: W.B. Saunders, 1237.

379 Shaffer, T.H., Koen, P.A., Moskowitz, G.D. *et al.* (1978) Positive end expiratory pressure: effects on lung mechanics of premature lambs. *Biology of the Neonate* **34**, 1–10.

380 Shaffer, T.H., Wolfson, M.R., Clark, L.C.J. (1992) State of art review: liquid ventilation. *Pediatric Pulmonology* **14**, 102–109.

381 Shah, N., Jacob, T., Exler, R. *et al.* (1994) Inhaled nitric oxide in congenital diaphragmatic hernia. *Journal of Pediatric Surgery* **29**, 1010–1015.

382 Shribhan, A.J., Smith, G., Achola, K.J. (1987) Cardiovascular and catecholamine responses to laryngoscopy with and without intubation. *British Journal of Anaesthesia* **59**, 295–299.

383 Sills, J.H., Cvetnic, W.G., Pietz, J. (1989) Continuous negative pressure in the treatment of infants with pulmonary hypertension and respiratory failure. *Journal of Perinatology* **9**, 43–48.

384 Silva, D.T., Hagan, R., Sly, P.D. (1995) Home oxygen management of neonatal chronic lung disease in Western Australia. *Journal of Paediatrics and Child Health* **31**, 185–188.

385 Silverman, W.A., Sinclair, J.C., Gandy, G.M., *et al.* (1967) A controlled trial of management of respiratory distress syndrome in a body-enclosing respirator. *Pediatrics* **39**, 740–748.

386 Simbruner, G. (1986) Inadvertent positive end expiratory pressure in mechanically ventilated newborn infants: detection and effect on lung mechanics and gas exchange. *Journal of Pediatrics* **108**, 589–595.

387 Simma, B., Skladal, D., Falk, M. (2000) Predicting survival infants ventilated with high-frequency oscillation. *Weiner Klinische Wochenschrift* **112**, 804–810.

388 Sims, M.E., Rangasamy, R., Lee, S. *et al.* (1989) Comparative evaluation of caffeine and theophylline for weaning premature infants from the ventilator. *American Journal of Perinatology* **6**, 72–75.

389 Sinha, S.K., Donn, S.M., Gavey, J., McCarty, M. (1997) Randomised trial of volume controlled versus time cycled, pressure limited ventilation in preterm infants with respiratory distress syndrome. *Archives of Disease in Childhood* **77**, F202–F205.

390 Skimming, J.W., Bender, K.A., Hutchison, A.A., Drummond, W.H. (1997) Nitric oxide inhalation in infants with respiratory distress syndrome. *Journal of Pediatrics* **130**, 225–230.

391 Sokol, G.M., Fineberg, N.S., Wright, L.L., Ehrenkranz, R.A. (2001) Changes in arterial oxygen tension when weaning neonates from inhaled nitric oxide. *Pediatric Pulmonology* **32**, 14–19.

392 Solis, A., Harrison, G., Shaw, B.N.J. (2002) Assessing oxygen requirement after discharge in chronic lung disease. *European Journal of Pediatrics* **161**, 428–430.

393 South, M., Morley, C.J. (1986) Spontaneous respiratory tracing in intubated neonates with RDS. *Early Human Development* **14**, 147–148 (abstract).

394 Southgate, W.M., Annibale, D.J., Hulsey, T.C., Purohit, D.M. (2001) International experience with trisomy 21 infants placed on extracorporeal membrane oxygenation. *Pediatrics* **107**, 549–552.

395 Stahlman, M.T., Malan, A.F., Shepard, F.M., *et al.* (1970) Negative pressure assisted ventilation in infants with hyaline membrane disease. *Journal of Pediatrics* **76**, 174–182.

396 Steinhorn, R.H., Cox, P.N., Fineman, J.R. *et al.* (1997) Inhaled nitric oxide enhances oxygenation but not survival in infants with alveolar capillary dysplasia. *Journal of Pediatrics* **130**, 417–422.

397 Stern, L. (1970) Description and utilization of the negative pressure apparatus. *Biology of the Neonate* **16**, 24–29.

398 Stolar, C., Dillon, P., Reyes, C. (1988) Selective use of extracorporeal membrane oxygenation in the management of congenital diaphragmatic hernia. *Journal of Pediatric Surgery* **23**, 207–211.

399 Subhedar, N.V., Ryan, S.W., Shaw, N.J. (1997) Open randomized controlled trial of inhaled nitric oxide and early dexamethasone in high risk preterm infants. *Archives of Disease in Childhood* **77**, F185–F190.

400 Sun, S.C., Tein, H.C. (1999) Randomized controlled trial of two methods of nasal CPAP (nCPAP): flow driver versus conventional nCPAP. *Pediatric Research* **45**, 322A.

401 Tanswell, A.K., Clubb, R.A., Smith, B.T., Boston, R.W. (1980) Individualised continuous distending pressure applied within 6 hours of delivery in infants with respiratory distress syndrome. *Archives of Disease in Childhood* **55**, 33–39.

402 Tarnow-Mordi, W.O., Reid, E., Griffiths, P., Wilkinson, A.R. (1985) Lack of association of barotrauma and air leak in hyaline membrane disease. *Archives of Disease in Childhood* **60**, 555–559.

403 Tarnow-Mordi, W.O., Fletcher, M., Suton, P., Wilkinson, A.R. (1986) Evidence of inadequate humification of inspired gas during artificial ventilation of newborn infants in the British Isles. *Lancet* **2**, 909–910.

404 Tarnow-Mordi, W.O., Reid, E., Griffiths, P., Wilkinson, A.R. (1989) Low inspired gas temperature and respiratory complications in very low birth weight infants. *Journal of Pediatrics* **114**, 438–442.

405 Tellez, D.W., Galvis, A.G., Storgion, S.A. *et al.* (1991) Dexamethasone in the prevention of postextubation stridor in children. *Journal of Pediatrics* **118**, 289–294.

406 The Franco-Belgium Collaborative NO Trial Group. (1999) Early compared with delayed inhaled nitric oxide in moderately hypoxaemic neonates with respiratory failure: a randomised controlled trial. *Lancet* **354**, 1066–1071.

407 The Neonatal Inhaled Nitric Oxide Study Group. (1997) Inhaled nitric oxide in full-term and nearly full-term infants with hypoxic respiratory failure. *New England Journal of Medicine* **336**, 597–604.

408 The Neonatal Inhaled Nitric Oxide Study Group (NINOS). (1997) Inhaled nitric oxide and hypoxic respiratory failure in infants with congenital diaphragmatic hernia. *Pediatrics* **99**, 838–845.

409 The Neonatal Inhaled Nitric Oxide Study Group (NINOS). (2000) Inhaled nitric oxide in term and near-term infants: neurodevelopmental follow-up of The Neonatal Inhaled Nitric Oxide Study Group (NINOS). *Journal of Pediatrics* **136**, 611–617.

410 Thome, U., Toepfer, A., Schaller, P., Pohlandt, F. (1998) Effect of mean airway pressure on lung volume during high-frequency oscillatory ventilation of preterm infants. *American Journal of Respiratory and Critical Care Medicine* **157**, 1213–1218.

411 Thome, U., Kossel, H., Lipowsky, G. *et al.* (1999) Randomized comparison of high-frequency ventilation with high-rate intermittent positive pressure ventilation in preterm infants with respiratory failure. *Journal of Pediatrics* **135**, 39–46.

412 Thome, U., Schulze, A., Schnabel, R. *et al.* (2001) Partial liquid ventilation in severely surfactant-depleted spontaneously breathing rabbits supported by proportional assist ventilation. *Critical Care Medicine* **29**, 1175–1180.

413 Thompson, M.W., Bates, J.N., Klein, J.M. (1995) Treatment of respiratory failure in an infant with bronchopulmonary dysplasia infected with respiratory syncytial virus using inhaled nitric oxide and high frequency ventilation. *Acta Paediatrica* **84**, 100–102.

414 Thompson, W.K., Marchak, B.E., Bryan, A.C., Froese, A.B. (1981) Vagotomy reverses apnoea induced by high frequency oscillatory ventilation. *Journal of Applied Physiology* **51**, 1484–1487.

415 Thomson, M.A., on behalf of the IFDAS Study Group. (2002) Early nasal continuous positive airways pressure (nCPAP) with prophylactic surfactant for neonates at risk for RDS. The IFDAS multi-centre randomised trial. *Archives of Disease in Childhood* **86** (Suppl), A7.

416 Tobias, J.D., Grueber, R.E. (1999) High-frequency jet ventilation using a helium-oxygen mixture. *Paediatric Anaesthesia* **9**, 451–455.

417 Toomasian, J.M., Snedecor, S.M., Cornell, R.G. *et al.* (1983) National experience with ECMO for newborn respiratory failure: data from 715 cases. *Transactions of the American Society for Artificial Internal Organs* **34**, 140–147.

418 Torielli, F., Fashaw, L.M., Knudson, O. *et al.* (2001) Echocardiographic outcome of infants treated as newborns with inhaled nitric oxide for severe hypoxemic respiratory failure. *Journal of Pediatrics* **138**, 349–354.

419 Toro-Figueroa, L.O., Meliones, J.N., Curtis, S.E., *et al.* (1996) Perflubron partial liquid ventilation (PLV) in children with ARDS: a safety and efficacy pilot study. *Critical Care Medicine* **24**, 150A.

420 Trittenwein, G., Golej, J., Burda, G. *et al.* (2001) Neonatal and pediatric extracorporeal membrane oxygenation using nonocclusive blood pumps: the Vienna experience. *Artificial Organs* **25**, 994–999.

421 UK Collaborative ECMO Trial Group. (1996) UK collaborative randomized trial of neonatal extracorporeal membrane oxygenation. *Lancet* **348**, 75–82.

422 Upton, C.J., Milner, A.D., Stokes, G.M. (1990) The effect of changes in inspiratory time on neonatal triggered ventilation. *European Journal of Pediatrics* **149**, 648–650.

423 van der Hoeven, M., Brouwer, E., Blanco, C.E. (1998) Nasal high frequency ventilation in neonates with moderate respiratory insufficiency. *Archives of Disease in Childhood Fetal and Neonatal Edition* **79**, F61–F63.

424 van Meurs, K.P., Rhine, W.D., Asselin, J.M. *et al.* (1997) Response of premature infants with severe respiratory failure to inhaled nitric oxide. *Pediatric Pulmonology* **24**, 319–323.

425 Vazquez de Anda, G.F., Gommers, D., Verbrugge, S.J. *et al.* (2000) Mechanical ventilation with high positive end-expiratory pressure and small driving pressure amplitude is as effective as high-frequency oscillatory ventilation to preserve the function of exogenous surfactant in lung-lavaged rats. *Critical Care Medicine* **28**, 2921–2925.

426 Veness-Meehan, K.A., Richter, S., Davis, J.M. (1990) Pulmonary function testing prior to extubation in infants with respiratory distress syndrome. *Pediatric Pulmonology* **9**, 2–6.

427 Verder, H., Robertson, B., Greisen, G. *et al.* (1994) Surfactant therapy and nasal continuous positive airway pressure for newborns with respiratory distress syndrome. *New England Journal of Medicine* **331**, 1051–1055.

428 Verder, H., Albertsen, P., Ebbesen, F. *et al.* (1999) Nasal continuous positive airway pressure and early surfactant therapy for respiratory distress syndrome in newborns of less than 30 weeks' gestation. *Pediatrics* **103**, E24.

429 Vidyasagar, D., Chernick, V. (1971) Continuous positive transpulmonary pressure in hyaline membrane disease – a simple device. *Pediatrics* **48**, 296–299.

430 Viscardi, R.M., Faix, R.G., Nicks, J.J., Grasela, T.H. (1985) Efficacy of theophylline for prevention of post-extubation respiratory failure in very low birth weight infants. *Journal of Pediatrics* **107**, 469–472.

431 Visveshwara, N., Freeman, B., Peck, M. *et al.* (1991) Patient triggered synchronized assisted ventilation of newborns (SAVI): report of a preliminary study and three years' experience. *Journal of Perinatology* **11**, 347–354.

432 Volsko, T.A., Chatburn, R.L. (1997) Comparison of two methods for securing the endotracheal tube in neonates. *Neonatal Intensive Care* **10**, 52–58.

433 Vosatka, R.J., Kashyap, S., Trifiletti, R.R. (1994) Arginine deficiency accompanies persistent pulmonary hypertension of the newborn. *Biology of the Neonate* **66**, 65–70.

434 Walsh-Sukys, M.C., Bauer, R.E., Cornell, D.J. *et al.* (1994) Severe respiratory failure in neonates: mortality and morbidity rates and neurodevelopmental outcomes. *Journal of Pediatrics* **125**, 104–110.

435 Walther, F.J., Erickson, R.N., Sims, M.E. (1990) Cardiovascular effects of caffeine therapy in preterm infants. *American Journal of Diseases of Children* **144**, 1164–1166.

436 Weber, K., Courtney, S.E., Pyon, K.H. *et al.* (2000) Detecting lung overdistention in newborns treated with high-frequency oscillatory ventilation. *Journal of Applied Physiology* **89**, 364–372.

437 Wertheim, H.F., Albers, M.J., Piena-Spoel, M., Tibboel, D. (2001) The incidence of septic complications in newborns on extracorporeal membrane oxygenation is not affected by feeding route. *Journal of Pediatric Surgery* **36**, 1485–1489.

438 Wessel, D.L., Adatia, I., van Marter, L.J. *et al.* (1997) Improved oxygenation in a randomized trial of inhaled nitric oxide for persistent pulmonary hypertension of the newborn. *Pediatrics* **100**, e7.

439 Wilson, B.J., Becker, M.A., Linton, M.E., Donn, S.M. (1998) Spontaneous minute ventilation predicts readiness for extubation in mechanically ventilated preterm infants. *Journal of Perinatology* **18**, 436–439.

440 Wiswell, T.E., Graziani, L.J., Kornhauser, M.S. *et al.* (1996) High-frequency jet ventilation in the early management of

respiratory distress syndrome is associated with a greater risk for adverse outcomes. *Pediatrics* **98**, 1035–1043.

441 Wiswell, T.E., Graziani, L.J., Kornhauser, M.S. *et al.* (1996) Effects of hypocarbia on the development of cystic periventricular leukomalacia in premature infants treated with high frequency jet ventilation. *Pediatrics* **98**, 918–924.

442 Wolfson, M.R., Shaffer, T.H. (1999) Liquid assisted ventilation update. *European Respiratory Journal* **158**, S27–S31.

443 Wolfson, M.R., Greenspan, J.S., Shaffer, T.H. (1998) Liquid-assisted ventilation: an alternative respiratory modality. *Pediatric Pulmonology* **26**, 42–63.

444 Wong, W., Fok, T.F., Ng, P.C. *et al.* (1997) Vascular air embolism: a rare complication of nasal CPAP. *Journal of Paediatrics and Child Health* **33**, 444–445.

445 Wood, K.S., McCaffrey, M.J., Donovan, J.C. *et al.* (1999) Effect of initial nitric oxide concentration on outcome in infants with persistent pulmonary hypertension of the newborn. *Biology of the Neonate* **75**, 215–224.

446 Wung, J.T., James, L.S., Kilchevsky, E., James, E.P. (1985) Management of infants with severe respiratory failure and persistence of the fetal circulation, without hyperventilation. *Pediatrics* **76**, 488–494.

447 Wyman, M.L., Kuhns, L.R. (1977) Lobar opacification of the lungs after tracheal extubation in neonates. *Journal of Pediatrics* **91**, 109–112.

448 Wyszogrodski, I., Kyei-Aboagye, K., Taeusch, H.W.J. (1975) Surfactant inactivation by hyperventilation: conservation by end expiratory pressure. *Journal of Applied Physiology* **38**, 461–466.

449 Younes, M. (1992) Proportional assist ventilation, a new approach to ventilatory support theory. *American Review of Respiratory Diseases* **145**, 114–120.

450 Younes, M., Puddy, A., Roberts, D. *et al.* (1992) Proportional assist ventilation: results of an initial clinical trial. *American Review of Respiratory Disease* **145**, 121–129.

451 Yu, V.Y.H., Rolfe, P. (1977) Effect of continuous positive airway pressure breathing on cardiorespiratory function in infants with respiratory distress syndrome. *Acta Paediatrica Scandinavica* **66**, 59–64.

Intensive care

NEENA MODI

Intensive care requirements for the infant with respiratory failure encompass the full range of organ support techniques and require close collaboration between nursing, medical and other support staff. When conducting an evaluation of such an infant, a systematic approach is recommended. This chapter addresses the principal areas that should be addressed during the course of such an evaluation with the exception of issues specific to respiratory support, intensive care monitoring, physiotherapy and nutrition, which are discussed elsewhere (Chapters 15, 16B, 17, 18).

FLUID THERAPY

Fluid therapy during neonatal intensive care is dictated by need to maintain normal hydration as well as to deliver an adequate nutritional intake within the limits of metabolic tolerance. These demands may not always be compatible, but it is important to appreciate them as distinct goals.

Assessing renal function and fluid balance

Fluid balance should be monitoring meticulously in infants receiving intensive care and is the responsibility of both medical and nursing staff. Clinical assessment of hydration should be accompanied by consideration of weight change and biochemical indices.

CHANGES IN BODY WEIGHT

Newborn infants lose extracellular fluid in the first days after birth. This is a normal physiological process and is marked clinically by early postnatal weight loss.[54] The loss of extracellular fluid may be delayed if an excessive early sodium intake is administered.[31] Consideration of daily weight change is an important part of the assessment of renal function and fluid balance. Failure to lose weight after birth is associated with increased risk of adverse outcome, principally from chronic lung disease, symptomatic patent ductus arteriosus and necrotizing enterocolitis.[31] Once the period of postnatal weight loss is complete, failure to gain weight at a rate of around 14–16 g/kg/day suggests that nutritional support is inadequate.

SERUM SODIUM AND POTASSIUM

The assessment of serum sodium and potassium is usually carried out at least daily in infants receiving intensive care. These should be maintained within the normal range but minor fluctuations within the normal range should be disregarded. The serum sodium is a guide to both water and sodium balance. A low serum sodium when accompanied by weight gain or failure to lose weight after birth suggests water overload. Hyponatremia accompanied by weight loss or poor weight gain despite an adequate nutritional intake suggests sodium depletion (Table 16.1). Hypernatremia is usually seen as a consequence of dehydration from excessive transepidermal water loss.

Table 16.1 *Hyponatremia and hypernatremia*

- A normal serum sodium does not necessarily mean that fluid balance is satisfactory.
- Inappropriate weight gain or failure to lose weight after birth, in the presence of a normal serum sodium, suggests isotonic expansion of the extracellular compartment. This common problem will be missed if babies are not weighed regularly during intensive care.
- Hyponatremia accompanied by weight gain implies water overload; hyponatremia and weight loss, or poor weight gain, implies sodium depletion.
- Hypernatramia and weight loss occurs with water depletion; total body sodium is usually normal or reduced.
- Hypernatremia and weight gain imply an excess of both sodium and water.
- A diagnosis of the syndrome of inappropriate secretion of antidiuretic hormone (SIADH) should only be made when circulating ADH is raised in the absence of both osmotic and baroreceptor-mediated stimuli.

Hypokalemia may result from inadequate intake, renal loss as in diuretic therapy or excessive base administration, during the recovery phase after acute renal failure or rarely in Bartter's syndrome, hyperaldosteronism or Cushing's syndrome. Excessive gastrointestinal loss of potassium may result from failure to replace gastric aspirate, vomiting and in ileostomy fluid.

SERUM CREATININE

The serum creatinine is a useful guide to renal function. Serum urea is less helpful as it is subject to non-renal influences such as sequestered blood, an excessive protein intake and steroid therapy. The serum creatinine at birth is influenced by maternal concentration. Thereafter, the serum creatinine falls at a rate dependent on creatinine production, dependent on muscle mass, and the clearance rate, dependent on glomerular filtration.[33] The serum creatinine may rise transiently after birth, as the extracellular compartment contracts, but thereafter should exhibit a decline. The normal range for serum creatinine is wide and a more helpful pointer to renal insufficiency is failure to observe a postnatal decline.

SERUM OSMOLALITY

Most well preterm infants are able to achieve a minimum urine osmolality of around 100 mosm/kg and a maximum of 600–800 mosm/kg. A urine osmolality of between 200 and 400 mosm/kg suggests that water intake is neither too little nor excessive. Occasionally, extremely immature infants (born before 26 weeks of gestation) have much more limited concentrating ability and may become dehydrated while continuing to pass urine of low osmolality.

URINE FLOW RATE

It is generally held that a urine flow rate of less than 1 ml/kg/h is indicative of impaired renal function. This is because a fully fed infant needs to excrete a renal solute load of about 15 mosm/kg/day. Given a maximum urinary concentration of 600–800 mosm/kg water, solute retention would occur if the urine flow rate were less than 19–25 ml/kg/24 h, that is approximately 1 ml/kg/h. Urine flow rate should be assessed continuously during intensive care. Oliguria is usually the first sign of renal impairment. Early detection is essential if the situation is to be reversed by restoration of renal perfusion. Similarly, in established renal failure, the continued infusion of large fluid volumes will further compromise the infant.

WATER BALANCE

The maintenance of normal hydration requires that an infant is given sufficient water to replace losses and excrete the renal solute load without the need to pass either very concentrated or very dilute urine. In the neonate, especially if born extremely prematurely and less than a first few days old, the major source of water loss is insensible water loss through the skin and the respiratory tract. The latter may be minimized by adequate humidification of inspired gases. The former may be extremely high, with measured rates of transepidermal water loss exceeding 125 ml/kg/day in infants below 28 weeks of gestation when nursed in an ambient humidity of 50 percent (Figure 16.1).

Transepidermal water loss should be minimized by maintaining a high humidity microenvironment around the infant, careful attention to skin care and avoidance of draughts. Failure to minimize transepidermal water loss will predispose to hypernatremic dehydration and the infant will show excessive weight loss and a raised serum sodium concentration. Transepidermal water loss falls exponentially over the first days after birth as skin maturation is accelerated by birth and exposure to a gaseous environment.

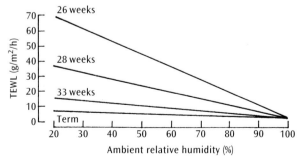

Figure 16.1 *The effect of ambient humidity and gestational age on transepidermal water loss (TEWL) (based on the data of Hammerlund and Sedin[19]). Reproduced with permission from Rutter.[43]*

A starting fluid prescription may be arrived at by estimating transepidemal water loss, taking into account the humidity in which the infant will be cared for and adding 60 ml/kg/day to cover urinary requirements. If ambient humidity is about 50 percent, this equates to a starting intake of around 90 ml/kg/day for neonates of around 28 weeks of gestation. If ambient humidity is higher, the starting prescription may be correspondingly reduced.

If an infant is being given 90 ml/kg of 10 percent glucose on day 1 and has normal hydration, is there any need to increase to 120 ml/kg of 10 percent glucose on day 2, a common practice in neonatal intensive care units? In terms of hydration, the answer is 'no'. The water requirement for urine production would be unchanged, and transepidermal water loss would be decreasing, not increasing. In terms of nutrition the answer is 'very little'. An increase of 30 ml/kg of 10 percent glucose would provide only an extra 3 g of carbohydrate or 12 kcal. If, however, the infant were receiving parenteral nutrition, with a balanced energy density of 0.66 kcal/ml, an increase of 30 ml/kg/day would mean an increase in nutrition delivered of 20 kcal/kg/day. Is there any reason to restrict the daily increase to 30 ml/kg rather than a larger increase in order to provide a better nutritional intake? The answer here is 'no'. In an elegant experiment Coulthard and Hey showed that if sodium intake is held constant, preterm infants are well able to cope with abrupt increases in the volume of intravenous intake from 100 to 200 ml/kg/day.[13] There therefore seems little justification to advocate small stepwise daily increases in fluid intake rather than a more rapid increase that would allow the delivery of a more favorable nutritional intake. The only caveat is that renal function should be normal. This should be assessed by demonstrating that the infant is showing normal postnatal weight loss, with a falling serum creatinine, normal serum sodium and potassium and a normal urine flow rate. Evidence to suggest that fluid restriction, in the perinatal period, may improve outcome from randomized studies demonstrated a higher survival without CLD[53] and less need for postnatal dexamethasone[25] are probably a consequence of sodium, not water restriction.

SODIUM BALANCE

In contrast to the relatively well developed ability to handle a water load, the preterm neonate has a limited ability to regulate sodium excretion and retention.[30] In a randomized, single-blind, controlled trial involving neonates below 32 weeks of gestation, the administration of a routine sodium intake of 4 mmol/kg/day from the second day after birth was compared with a sodium intake commencing when the infant had lost 6 percent of birth weight. The results of the study demonstrated that infants receiving routine early supplementation had a delayed loss of extracellular fluid[20] and an increased risk of prolonged oxygen dependency.[21] The loss of extracellular fluid after birth is a normal physiological response. It is triggered by atrial natriuretic peptide-driven natriuresis,[35] as sodium is the principal electrolyte in extracellular fluid. The causal pathway for these observations is that an unnecessary sodium supplement prior to the onset of the postnatal natriuresis will promote persistent expansion of the extracellular compartment, including lung interstitial fluid. The persistence of lung interstitial fluid will predispose to prolonged oxygen dependency. After the period of postnatal extracellular fluid loss, preterm infants below 32 weeks of gestation require a sodium intake of the order of 4 mmol/kg/day to support growth.

Syndrome of inappropriate antidiuretic hormone secretion (SIADH)

Antidiuretic hormone (ADH) secretion is triggered by alterations in the tonicity of the extracellular fluid and by baroreceptors located in the heart and great vessels. An increase in tonicity will stimulate the release of ADH and reduce urinary water loss. In addition to increasing permeability by the insertion of water channels in the apical membranes of the cells of the renal collecting ducts, ADH causes arteriolar vasoconstriction and a rise in blood pressure. The maintenance of central blood pressure overrides the defence of tonicity. If intravascular volume depletion goes unrecognized and only salt-poor fluid is administered, baroreceptor-driven ADH release will lead to water retention and hyponatremia. In this situation, ADH secretion is appropriate. It is likely that this clinical picture often goes unrecognized in neonates, as hypovolemia may be difficult to recognize. The correct management is to maintain central blood pressure and to use salt-containing fluid if intravascular volume support is required. True inappropriate ADH secretion is probably very rare in infants receiving intensive care.[31]

ACUTE RENAL FAILURE (ARF)

ARF is defined as a sudden and severe reduction in glomerular filtration rate. This will result in a rise in serum creatinine and subsequently in further metabolic disturbance. There are many causes of ARF, but in neonatal intensive care it is most commonly seen in the context of perinatal asphyxia, septic shock and necrotizing enterocolitis. ARF is often reversible in the early stages, emphasizing the importance of early detection through clinical vigilance. The most helpful early sign is the acute onset of oliguria or anuria. When this is recognized, the bladder should be palpated and an urgent ultrasound scan performed to detect an obstructed renal tract. If post-renal failure is excluded, the adequacy of the circulation should be assessed (p. 71). Renal perfusion should be optimized. A fluid challenge should be administered, consisting of 15–20 ml/kg normal saline over 1 hour followed by a single intravenous dose of furosemide of 4 mg/kg. The half-life

Table 16.2 *Management of hyperkalemia*

Serum potassium >6.5 mmol/l:

- Check serum potassium again, ensuring sample is not hemolysed.
- Monitor ECG.
- Calcium resonium, 150 mg/kg/dose rectally every 6 hours; remove rectal plug by irrigation with 2 ml normal saline.

Serum potassium >8.0 mmol/l or ECG evidence of toxicity (peaked T wave, widened QRS complexes):

- Calcium gluconate 10 percent, 0.5 ml/kg IV, diluted 10-fold with glucose 5 percent, at a maximum rate of 0.1 ml/min.
- Sodium bicarbonate 4.2%, 4 ml/kg (2 mmol/kg), IV over 5 minutes; check base deficit.
- Glucose and insulin; add 25 units neutral insulin to 500 ml 10 percent glucose; infuse at 1–2 ml/kg/h (0.05–0.1 units/kg/h); monitor blood glucose closely.
- Salbutamol, 4 μg/kg/dose IV over 20 minutes.
- Prepare for peritoneal dialysis.

of furosemide is long (approximately 24 hours in healthy preterm infants) and repeated doses are both unnecessary, as well as potentially harmful as they can increase the risks of interstitial nephritis, ototoxicity and ductal patency. If there is an increase in urine flow rate in response to the fluid challenge, the problem is one of pre-renal failure, and therapy should be directed to optimizing hydration and renal perfusion. If there is no increase in urine flow rate, the management is that of established renal failure. The mainstay of management of established renal failure is meticulous supportive care. Central vascular access should be established to allow the infusion of glucose solution, in high concentration if necessary. Fluid intake should be limited to insensible losses plus urine output and gastro-intestinal losses. These should be calculated for 6- to 8-hourly intervals. Intravenous fluid should consist of a glucose solution with calcium if necessary, without added sodium or potassium. Blood pressure and perfusion should be carefully supported. Hyponatremia in the anuric infant is indicative of water overload and the need to reduce infused volumes. The serum potassium needs careful monitoring and appropriate action taken (Table 16.2) if the level becomes too high.

Meticulous medical management, avoiding fluid overload, will usually allow even an anuric baby to remain in stable water and electrolyte balance for several days. The role of low-dose dopamine (2 μg/kg/min) in renal failure or incipient renal failure is unclear. In a large multicenter, randomized, placebo-controlled trial, the administration of low-dose dopamine by continuous intravenous infusion to critically ill adults at risk of renal failure did not confer clinically significant protection from renal dysfunction.[9] There is no direct evidence in infant populations that low-dose dopamine is a useful prophylactic therapy

when the risk of ARF is high, nor that it improves renal perfusion in established renal failure.

THERMOREGULATION

Infants lose heat by evaporation, convection, radiation and to a small extent, conduction. At delivery the infant should be rapidly dried, wrapped in warm blankets and have a hat put on. Hypothermia is associated with increased oxygen consumption, increased energy expenditure, impaired surfactant function and increased risk of infection. Cold stress is associated with increased mortality. Overheating is not as common, but is also associated with a range of problems including increased transepidermal water loss, hypernatremic dehydration and apnea.

The desired environmental temperature lies within the thermoneutral range, the range in which an infant's heat production is at a minimum and body temperature is normal. The ambient temperature appropriate for neonates when nursed fully clothed ranges from 25°C for infants of birthweight greater than 2 kg to 32°C for infants of less than 1.5 kg in weight. If it is necessary to nurse a baby naked, an incubator or radiant warmer is essential. Radiant warmers have the disadvantage of causing a large evaporative water and heat loss, but this can be minimized through the concurrent use of a humidified body box or plastic bubble 'blanket'. Radiant heaters are best reserved for use in infants above 34 weeks of gestation or for a short period during initial stabilization before transferring into a high-humidity incubator. Condensation is reduced by using double-walled incubators and maintaining a high environmental temperature in the intensive care unit.

SEDATION AND PAIN RELIEF (p. 316)

Adequate pain relief for acutely painful procedures is an essential component of good neonatal intensive care. Significant physiological perturbations occur with frequently performed procedures, such as venepuncture and tracheal suctioning. Evidence is mounting that exposure to pain during the neonatal period has adverse long-term effects.[4]

Many neonatal units now have clear policies incorporating the use of analgesia for invasive procedures such as non-emergency intubation and for blood sampling. There is good evidence to guide practice for obtaining blood samples from neonates.[39] Venepuncture is the preferred method for blood sampling as it appears less painful than heel lancing. If heel lancing is used, an automated device (e.g. Autolet, Tenderfoot) should be used rather than a standard lance. Sucrose and glucose decrease the pain response associated with heel lancing, but it is unclear if they are similarly effective during venepuncture. Paracetamol and heel warming do not reduce the pain response

Table 16.3 *Pharmacological agents for sedation or procedural analgesia*

Oral agents

Sucrose 12 percent, 0.5–2 ml 2 minutes before procedure
Paracetamol 20 mg/kg every 6 hours (may be
  administered rectally)
Morphine, 80 µg/kg every 4 hours
Chloral hydrate 25–50 mg/kg every 4–8 hours (may be
  administered rectally)

Topical/skin infiltration

Lidocaine (lignocaine) skin infiltration, maximum dose
  0.5 ml/kg, 1 percent solution
EMLA cream
Amethocaine gel

Intravenous agents

Morphine, IV bolus, 50–100 µg/kg over 30 minutes
Fentanyl, IV bolus 2–10 µg/kg over 30 minutes
Midazolam, IV bolus, 50–200 µg/kg over 30 minutes

of heel lancing. There is evidence that both EMLA cream and amethocaine gel reduce the pain of venipuncture,[24] but not heel lancing. The safety of repeated applications of EMLA or amethocaine, however, has yet to be determined.

Analgesia should always be provided for painful conditions, such as necrotizing enterocolitis and cryotherapy for retinopathy of prematurity (Table 16.3). The possible need for respiratory support as a result of opiate-induced respiratory depression should not be viewed as a contraindication to adequate pain relief. We use morphine by intravenous infusion and electively intubate and ventilate prior to cryotherapy. There is considerable evidence now that 'awake' intubation is unacceptable except in an emergency situation. For non-emergency intubation we use atropine for vagal blockade, followed by fentanyl for analgesia and suxamethonium (succinylcholine) for short-action muscle relaxation.[6]

In contrast to procedural pain relief, it is less clear whether routine sedation/analgesia is necessary during ventilation. The rationale for this approach is to reduce discomfort and pain, to enhance physiological stability and to reduce asynchrony with the ventilator (p. 316). There may be long-term benefits. Anand *et al.*[5] randomized 67 ventilated infants, born between 24 and 33 weeks of gestation, to infusions of morphine, midazolam or placebo. They showed that, though both morphine and midazolam reduced pain responses and stabilized vital signs, morphine was associated with a reduction in death and ultrasound evidence of major brain injury. Assessment of long-term outcomes of the infants entered into the study is awaited. A regimen of morphine 50–100 µg/kg over 30 minutes followed by 10–20 µg/kg/hour appears widely used in ventilated infants. Many ventilated infants, however, appear comfortable without regular analgesia. In these, the use of intermittent boluses of analgesics or sedatives may be appropriate. A drawback of long-term

opioid use is the development of tolerance, necessitating dose escalation, and resulting in signs of withdrawal following cessation of therapy. The latter may be managed by gradual weaning. Opioids are widely used to relieve suffering during terminal care. Intravenous morphine may be used to relieve dyspnea associated with respiratory failure when ventilator support is withdrawn. Oral morphine preparations are available when intravenous access is not present or when a baby is being cared for at home.

The use of the benzodiazepine, midazolam, for sedation is increasing in neonatal intensive care as it is reported to have a much shorter half-life than diazepam (6.5 hours versus 20–50 hours[23]). In our experience, continuous infusions of midazolam are inadvisable in extremely preterm neonates as sedation following cessation may be prolonged. In addition, concerns have been raised about the safety of midazolam, including description of a midazolam withdrawal syndrome.[37]

CARDIOVASCULAR SUPPORT

Adequacy of perfusion and consideration of the need for circulatory support are an integral part of intensive care. This requires assessment of adequacy of intravascular volume as well as cardiac output. Cardiac output is the product of ventricular stroke volume and heart rate (the Fick equation). Stroke volume is influenced by preload (venous filling pressure), myocardial contractility and afterload (vascular resistance). Each of these components requires individual consideration if therapy is to be tailored to cause.

Circulatory failure in the neonatal intensive care unit commonly results from either hypovolemia or poor myocardial contractility. It also occurs in septic shock, with peripheral vasodilatation and capillary leak syndrome and as a result of large left-to-right ductal shunting. Other recognized, but less common causes are cardiac tamponade secondary to pericardial effusion and the cardiomyopathies. A common easily remedied cause of impaired venous filling is inadvertent pulmonary overdistention during high frequency oscillatory ventilation. This leads to impaired cardiac output, reduced pulmonary perfusion and a paradoxical worsening in oxygenation at a time when the infant would be expected to be improving. It can be confirmed by demonstrating overdistention on a chest radiograph and responds to a reduction in mean airway pressure.

Detection of hypovolemia

Tachycardia is insufficiently sensitive at detecting hypovolemia. Regular blood pressure measurements are essential, but it should be borne in mind that in the newborn, the normal range for blood pressure is wide. In addition, blood pressure may well be maintained within the normal range until significant compromise has occurred. Blood pressure correlates poorly with blood volume[7,8] and a blood pressure within the normal range does not necessarily exclude hypovolemia. Neonates are at risk of intravascular volume depletion for several reasons. Immediate cord clamping can result in a 50 percent lower blood volume than delayed clamping. Unwell infants are subjected to frequent blood sampling that will further reduce circulating volume.

The recognition of an inadequate intravascular volume is difficult. Gerigk et al.[17] found that only a third of infants and children with intravascular volume depletion had concomitant clinical signs. Evaluation of capillary refill time and core-peripheral temperature gap are useful and simple to perform. Though capillary refill times correlate poorly with hypovolemia in adults, normal ranges have been established in neonates in different thermal environments.[50] The mid-sternum or forehead are the preferred sites for assessment. The capillary refill time should not exceed 3 seconds.[50]

Lyon et al.[28] studied central–peripheral temperature differences in infants with birthweights below 1000 g and concluded that in the first few days after birth, central and peripheral temperatures are similar because thermoregulation is immature. Central–peripheral temperature gaps of greater than 2°C became more frequent after 3 days from birth, when babies were more competent at mounting a vasoconstrictive response, but even then was more likely to represent thermal stress than hypovolemia. Despite these caveats, the central–peripheral temperature gap does correlate with circulating arginine vasopressin (AVP) levels[26] and, in the absence of thermal stress, should be regarded as an index of hypovolemia.

Central venous pressure (CVP) measurements, though infrequently used, may be helpful and are easy to measure from an umbilical venous catheter tip in the right atrium. Skinner et al.[46] published normative data from 13 infants with respiratory disease, eight of whom were born prematurely. These authors concluded that CVP monitoring was useful for detecting trends. In ventilated neonates a CVP of 0 mmHg suggested hypovolemia, but in spontaneously breathing infants, negative values did not necessarily represent hypovolemia. The benefits of this approach need to be weighed against the potential risks of invasive monitoring.

Echocardiography (p. 102)

In hypovolemia the chambers of the underfilled heart appear small and the inferior vena cava periodically collapses. In severe hypovolemia the ventricles appear hypertrophic since the muscle collapses down on the small ventricular cavities. The skilled operator may undertake serial evaluation of aortic and pulmonary stroke distances and ejection times.[58] The failing heart appears large and 'baggy'. Doppler assessment may show a low output and atrioventricular valve regurgitation. Again, serial assessment of aortic and pulmonary stroke distances and fractional shortening may be helpful in assessing the response to therapy.

Management

Unfocused approaches, such as blindly pursuing a 'normal' blood pressure without heed to other signs, cannot be condoned. Evidence of hypovolemia demands volume support whereas poor myocardial contractility requires inotropic support with, if necessary, a reduction of afterload. Inotropes are contraindicated in hypertrophic cardiomyopathy.

WHICH FLUID?

The choice of fluid for volume support is controversial. In many instances, whole blood would be the preferred product but concerns over excessive use of blood products has meant that in many parts of the world only component therapy is available. It is now widely accepted that fresh frozen plasma should be reserved for use only when specifically indicated by coagulation disturbance.

In a meta-analysis of randomized controlled trials, Alderson et al. assessed the effect on mortality of colloids compared to crystalloids for fluid resuscitation in critically ill patients.[2] The risk of death in the albumin-treated group was 6 percent higher than in the crystalloid-treated group. Unfortunately, neonates were excluded from this meta-analysis but the authors concluded:

> there is no evidence from randomized controlled trials that resuscitation with colloids reduces the risk of death compared to crystalloids in patients with trauma, burns and following surgery. As colloids are not associated with an improvement in survival, and as they are more expensive than crystalloids, it is hard to see how their continued use in these patient types can be justified outside the context of randomized controlled trials.

Osborn and Evans carried out a meta-analysis evaluating the need for volume expansion and the choice of fluid.[40] They concluded that there is insufficient evidence to determine what type of volume expansion should be used in preterm infants or for the use of early red cell transfusions. This meta-analysis included the only trial to compare colloid and crystalloid in preterm neonates.[47] This compared infants randomized to albumin 5 percent or normal saline 10 ml/kg over 30 minutes, with a maximum of three doses given if hypotension persisted. The authors found no benefit in using albumin. There was no significant difference in mortality (RR 1.36, 95 % CI 0.48, 3.82), but the albumin group showed significantly greater weight gain at 24 and 48 hours of life. As discussed above, a number of studies have shown that failure to lose weight after birth is associated with increased risk of adverse outcome. Others have shown that colloid administration is associated with prolonged oxygen dependency[25] and adverse neurological developmental outcome.[18] Those results are from non-randomized trials and albumin was usually given to treat hypotension. Nevertheless, the results would argue against giving albumin to treat hypotension when saline is equally effective.[47] The same group has also shown that both isotonic saline and 5 percent albumin are effective when used as replacement fluid in partial exchange transfusion for the treatment of neonatal polycythemia.[57] As isotonic saline is cheaper and does not carry the infective risks of blood products, the balance of evidence to date then favors the use of crystalloid in the form of normal saline, over colloid, for volume replacement.

WHICH AGENT?

Dopamine is widely held to be an effective agent for increasing blood pressure. It may, however, peripherally vasoconstrict without increasing ventricular output[42] and may exacerbate pulmonary vasoconstriction (Table 16.4).[42] Dobutamine is a less effective pressor,[42] but it appears to be an effective inotrope. Dobutamine has minimal chronotropic effect. Subhedar and Shaw included four trials enrolling a total of 143 infants into their meta-analysis comparing dopamine and dobutamine.[51] Only one of the four included studies assessed changes in left ventricular output[42] and this did not show a statistically significant effect when dopamine was compared with dobutamine (weighted mean difference −83 ml/kg/min, 95 percent CI −174 to 8 ml/kg/min). This review did not assess potential adverse consequences of dopamine-induced peripheral vasoconstriction such as worsening of respiratory disease, impaired renal perfusion and necrotizing enterocolitis. They found that if short-term treatment of systemic hypotension is considered to be the goal of cardiovascular support, dopamine should be used

in preference to dobutamine. The authors also point out that it is possible that higher doses of dobutamine than were used in these studies may be required to elicit the desired response. They conclude that in the absence of data confirming the long-term benefit and safety of dopamine compared to dobutamine, no firm recommendations can be made between these two agents. Low-dose dopamine (3–5 μg/kg/min) may improve urine output in very immature infants (median gestational age 27 weeks).[15] Epinephrine has both inotropic and chronotropic effects, but may cause renal and myocardial ischemia. As both epinephine and norepinephrine cause vasoconstriction, they are best reserved for use only when the first-line agents, dobutamine and dopamine, are insufficient. Left ventricular afterload reduction is commonly employed after open heart surgery as these infants invariably have some degree of myocardial impairment. This may be achieved with the use of a vasodilator such as sodium nitroprusside or with a phosphodiesterase inhibitor such as milrinone. These agents provide inotropic support combined with afterload reduction. The role of glucocorticoids remains controversial, as they have not been subjected to adequate evaluation. Hydrocortisone has been used in doses ranging from 2 to 6 mg/kg/day in hypotension resistant to standard pressor agents[45] and dexamethasone in a single dose of 0.25 mg/kg.[16]

TRANSFUSION THERAPY

Although believed to be small, blood products do carry a finite infection risk. It is, therefore, recommended that every effort should be made to reduce exposure to blood products. Fresh frozen plasma should no longer be used for volume support but its use should be limited to the management of coagulation disorders. Nevertheless, infants below 1500 g birthweight remain a frequently transfused patient group. Our own audit demonstrated that they receive a median of four red cell transfusions (range 0–12) during their initial hospital stay. Deciding when to transfuse a neonate in intensive care has always been a difficult and controversial issue.[34] We maintain the hemoglobin level above 12 g/dl when infants are acutely unwell, but would not transfuse well preterm infants on the basis of a low hemoglobin level alone, but only if accompanied by symptoms of anemia (poor weight gain, lethargy, slowing in suck ability, increase in apneic/bradycardic episodes). The routine use of furosemide during red cell transfusions is illogical and may expose infants to the risks of furosemide toxicity and transient polycythemia.[10] Infants should be protected from multiple donor exposure and as red cells may be safely used up to 35 days from collection, the allocation of a dedicated 'octopus pack' (donor unit divided into eight satellite packs) to each infant admitted to the neonatal intensive

Table 16.4 *Inotropic agents*

Dobutamine	10–20 μg/kg/min IV; may increase to 40 μg/kg/min
Dopamine	5–10 μg/kg/min IV; may increase to 20 μg/kg/min
Epinephrine	0.05–1.0 μg/kg/min IV
Norepinephrine	0.05–1.0 μg/kg/min IV
Milrinone	0.75 μg/kg/min over 2 hours; then 0.25–0.75 μg/kg/min; reduce dose in renal failure

care unit greatly assists in this. We do not irradiate red cells for neonatal use as they are leukodepleted. The role of erythropoietin (EPO) has still to be fully evaluated. Although benefit from EPO is detected across high-quality studies using conservative transfusion criteria, there is variation in the findings of available trials.[56] We administer erythropoietin, 250 units/kg subcutaneously three times per week, from day 8 after birth for 6 weeks, also ensuring a protein intake greater than 3 g/kg/day and an intake of elemental iron greater than 2 mg/kg/day, to all babies of less than 28 weeks of gestation and to babies of between 28 and 32 weeks of gestation if also less than the third centile for birthweight. It may be, however, that EPO reduces red cell requirements only in relatively well preterm babies but not in those who have severe, prolonged illness in whom the causes of anemia are many and varied.

NEUROLOGICAL ASSESSMENT

Infants receiving intensive care are at increased risk of neurological injury and neurological status must be routinely evaluated. Detailed neurological evaluation may not be possible in an infant requiring respiratory support. Nevertheless, once stable, a formal clinical neurological assessment is recommended. In babies born preterm, a normal neurological assessment on reaching full term, in conjunction with lack of evidence of major abnormality on cranial ultrasound scan, has good positive predictive value for a favorable long-term outcome.[49] At the very least, weekly measurement of head circumference as an index of brain growth should be considered mandatory.[29] Regular cranial ultrasound scans are useful, but due care must be taken to ensure high quality scans. Appropriate senior advice must be sought before conveying prognostic information to parents on the basis of ultrasound imaging.[41] A cranial ultrasound scan should be obtained on admission to the neonatal intensive care unit and at regular intervals thereafter.

The electroencephalogram (EEG) is widely used in full-term infants with acute neonatal encephalopathy, and its prognostic value has now been confirmed by several studies. The amplitude-integrated EEG (cerebral function monitoring) is a technique that is likely to increase in use.[36] It is easy to use at the cotside and allows continuous monitoring over prolonged periods. Its utility has been demonstrated in full-term infants with neonatal encephalopathy[1] and familiarity with preterm patterns is increasing.[11]

PREVENTION OF NOSOCOMIAL INFECTION

Neonates are particularly vulnerable to infection, especially bacteremia. This affects less than 7 percent of full-term babies, but as many as 50 percent of extremely premature babies. Bacteremia substantially increases the risks of death and long-term impairment. Infections diagnosed after the first 72 hours after birth are arbitrarily considered to be acquired nosocomially (hospital-acquired). This terminology may unfortunately detract from the importance of recognizing the immunological compromise of the preterm neonate as a major factor underlying these high infection rates. Immature immune responses include reduced phagocytosis, opsonization and intracellular killing,[12] decreased immunoglobulin concentrations, as well as poor skin[44] and gut barrier function.[22] The risk of sepsis is further increased by the use of invasive devices and parenteral nutrition.

Coagulase-negative staphylococci (CoNS) are now the most common cause of bacteremia in neonatal intensive care units in the developed world.[55] There are difficulties in the diagnosis of CoNS septicemia, as the organism is a ubiquitous skin commensal, which often results in contamination of blood cultures. A positive diagnosis should include both the presence of clinical signs of sepsis and a positive blood culture.

Several adjunctive therapeutic approaches have and are being explored for both prophylaxis against sepsis and its treatment. Until these trials report good general hygiene, the disciplined use of infection control protocols and obsessional hand hygiene, remain the mainstay of practice. The anti-infective properties of raw maternal breast milk are well known and the use of expressed maternal breast milk should be promoted in intensive care units. Another simple measure of benefit is keeping the cord clean which appears to be as effective and safe as using antibiotics or antiseptics.[59]

Prophylactic vancomycin in low doses reduces the incidence of total nosocomial sepsis and coagulase-negative staphylococcal sepsis in neonates. Meta-analysis of controlled trials, however, did not find mortality or length of stay to be significantly altered.[14] No increase in vancomycin toxicity was detected, but there was insufficient evidence to ascertain the risks of development of vancomycin-resistant organisms in the nurseries involved. As few clinically important benefits were demonstrated, routine prophylaxis with vancomycin cannot be recommended at present.

In two small studies, prophylactic application of emollient ointment decreased transepidermal water loss, decreased the severity of dermatitis, and decreased the risk of suspected and proven sepsis.[48] Further studies are required to test the efficacy of this simple intervention.

Intravenous immunoglobulin (IVIG) has been widely studied. Approximately 5000 preterm and/or low birthweight infants have been recruited into 19 randomized controlled trials of IVIG as prophylaxis against infection.[38] IVIG administration resulted in a 3 percent reduction in sepsis and a 4 percent reduction in one or more episodes of any serious infection, but was not associated with reductions in other important clinical outcomes or in length of hospital stay. IVIG administration did not have any effect on mortality from any cause or from infections. Though prophylactic use of IVIG is not associated with any short-term serious side-effects, from a clinical perspective a 3–4 percent reduction in nosocomial infections without a reduction in mortality or other important clinical outcomes is of marginal importance. By contrast, IVIG as an adjunctive therapy during sepsis does appear to merit further evaluation. A review by Ohlsson and Lacy found that treatment with IVIG in neonates with suspected infection resulted in a reduction in mortality of borderline statistical significance.[38] Treatment with IVIG in cases of subsequently proved infection did result in a statistically significant reduction in mortality [typical RR 0.55; 95 percent CI 0.31, 0.98; number necessary to treat 11 (95 percent CI; 5.6, 100)]. If confirmed, this would be an important advance in clinical management.

Other modalities that are currently being explored in planned or current randomized controlled trials in neonates are the use of the hemopoietic colony-stimulating factors (CSFs), granulocyte and granulocyte-macrophage CSF (G-CSF and GM-CSF),[32] probiotics and the phosphodiesterase inhibitor, pentoxifylline.[27] It is also relevant to emphasize the need to avoid instituting measures that have not been shown to be of benefit, such as routine gowning, gloving and masking, or that are detrimental, such as limiting the mother's contact with her baby.

DEVELOPMENTAL CARE

Developmental care includes vestibular, auditory, visual and tactile stimuli, clustering of nursery care activities, and positioning of the infant. Individual strategies have also been combined to form programs, such as the 'Neonatal Individualized Developmental Care and Assessment Program' (NIDCAP).[3] Whether developmental care interventions are of benefit is as yet uncertain. A Cochrane review detected 31 eligible randomized controlled trials involving developmental care interventions.[52] The review showed that, although analysis demonstrated developmental care interventions were of benefit to preterm infants with respect to decreased respiratory support, decreased length and cost of hospital stay and improved neurodevelopmental outcomes to 2 years corrected age, those analyses were not of more than two trials for any one outcome and there were a large number of outcomes for which no effect or conflicting effects were demonstrated. Before recommending the adoption of developmental care practices, consistent evidence of long-term benefit for infants and/or mothers would seem desirable. The cost of the interventions and personnel was not considered in any of the studies. Although no major harmful effects were reported, the economic implications of implementing

and supporting developmental care interventions also require consideration.

OTHER ROUTINE MEASURES

The focus on acute management issues during neonatal intensive care should not be allowed to detract from due attention to sometimes less acute, but just as important concerns. These include ensuring that screening for inborn errors of metabolism, hemoglobinopathies, retinopathy of prematurity and hearing are carried out at the appropriate times. Vitamin K prophylaxis against hemorrhagic disease of the newborn is recommended for all infants and should be given as soon as possible after birth. Contraindications to routine immunizations are rare and these should usually be offered to all infants.

FAMILY AND STAFF SUPPORT

Support for the infant's family should be regarded an essential component of good intensive care. This will include careful, repeated and patient explanation of what are often difficult clinical issues, encouragement to visit and undertake appropriate care and comfort-related tasks and explanation of research issues and the uncertainties that underlie many practices.

Sadly, death is a not infrequent occurrence in neonatal intensive care units and paradoxically may be more difficult to manage when it does not occur acutely or when it occurs after a long and difficult clinical course. In these circumstances, counselling and support for staff are as essential as for the family. Junior staff may not appreciate the classic course of bereavement, with initial disbelief and denial, followed by guilt, despair and anger until finally a stage of resolution is reached. They often need support in dealing with their own grief as well as in coping with parental anger that may appear to be directed towards them.

Administrative procedures in the event of an infant death should be both efficient and considerate. Parents should be offered an appointment with, ideally, a senior member of both nursing and medical staff to afford the opportunity to discuss issues and have questions answered, regardless of whether or not a postmortem examination has been carried out. Though difficult to evaluate, it is believed that counselling reduces the risk of psychiatric and pyschosomatic morbidity following bereavement. Many organizations have drawn up guidelines for bereavement support. These recommendations include the need to emphasize the reality of the event by encouraging parents to see, hold and name their baby and be involved in funeral arrangements and stress the importance of expert counselling and sympathetic listening by well informed and well trained professionals.

REFERENCES

1 Al Naqeeb, N., Edwards, A.D., Cowan, F.M., Azzopardi, D. (1999) Assessment of neonatal encephalopathy by amplitude-integrated electroencephalography. *Pediatrics* **103**, 1263–1271.

2 Alderson, P., Schierhout, G., Roberts, I., Bunn, F. (2001) Colloids versus crystalloids for fluid resuscitation in critically ill patients (Cochrane Review). In *The Cochrane Library*, Issue 2. Update Software, Oxford.

3 Als, H., Lawhon, G., Duffy, F. *et al.* (1994) Individualized developmental care for the very low-birth-weight preterm infant: medical and neurofunctional effects. *Journal of the American Medical Association* **272**, 853–858.

4 Anand, K.J.S. (2000) Pain, plasticity and premature birth: a prescription for permanent suffering. *Nature Medicine* **6**, 971–973.

5 Anand, K.J.S., McIntosh, N., Lagercrantz, H. *et al.* (1999) Analgesia and sedation in preterm neonates who require ventilatory support. *Archives of Pediatrics and Adolescent Medicine* **153**, 331–338.

6 Azzopardi, D., Edwards, D., Harvey, D. *et al.* (2000) *Neonatal Formulary*. London: Hammersmith Hospitals NHS Trust.

7 Barr, P.A., Bailey, P.E., Sumners, J., Cassady, G. (1977) Relation between arterial blood pressure and blood volume and effect of infused albumin in sick premature infants. *Pediatrics* **60**, 282–289.

8 Bauer, K., Linderkamp, O., Versmold, H.T. (1993) Systolic blood pressure and blood volume in preterm infants. *Archives of Disease in Childhood* **69**, 521–522.

9 Bellomo, R., Chapman, M., Finfer, S. *et al.* (2000) Low-dose dopamine in patients with early renal dysfunction: a placebo-controlled randomised trial. Australian and New Zealand Intensive Care Society (ANZICS) Clinical Trials Group. *Lancet* **356**, 2139–2143.

10 Betremieux, P., Hartnoll, G., Modi, N. (1997) Should frusemide be prescribed after packed red cell transfusion in the newborn? *European Journal of Pediatrics* **156**, 88–89.

11 Biagioni, E., Frisone, M.F., Laroche, S. *et al.* (2000) Occipital sawtooth: a physiological EEG pattern in very premature infants. *Clinical Neurophysiology* **111**, 2145–2149.

12 Carr, R. (2000) Neutrophil production and function in newborn infants. *British Journal of Haematology* **110**, 18–28.

13 Coulthard, M.G., Hey, E.N. (1985) Effect of varying water intake on renal function in healthy preterm babies. *Archives of Disease in Childhood* **60**, 614–620.

14 Craft, A.P., Finer, N.N., Barrington, K.J. (2001) Vancomycin for prophylaxis against sepsis in preterm neonates (Cochrane Review). In *The Cochrane Library*, Issue 2. Update Software, Oxford.

15 Emery, E.F., Greenough, A. (1993) Efficacy of low dose dopamine infusion. *Acta Paediatrica* **82**, 430–432.

16 Gaissmaier, R.E., Pohlandt, F. (1999) Single-dose dexamethasone treatment of hypotension in preterm infants. *Journal of Pediatrics* **134**, 701–705.

17 Gerigk, M., Gnehm, H.E., Rascher, W. (1996) Arginine vasopressin and renin in acutely ill children: implication for fluid therapy. *Acta Paediatrica* **85**, 550–553.

18 Greenough, A., Cheeseman, P., Kavvadia, V. *et al.* (2002) Colloid infusion in the perinatal period and abnormal neurodevelopmental outcome in very low birthweight infants. *European Journal of Pediatrics* **161**, 319–323.

19 Hammerlund, K., Sedin, G. (1979) Transepidermal water loss in newborn infants. *Acta Paediatrica Scandinavica* **68**, 795–801.

20 Hartnoll, G., Betremieux, P., Modi, N. (2000) Randomized controlled trial of postnatal sodium supplementation on body composition in 25 to 30 week gestational age infants. *Archives of Disease in Childhood Fetal and Neonatal Edition* **82**, F24–F28.

21 Hartnoll, G., Betremieux, P., Modi, N. (2000) Randomized controlled trial of postnatal sodium supplementation on oxygen dependency and body weight in 25–30 week gestational age infants. *Archives of Disease in Childhood Fetal and Neonatal Edition* **82**, F19–F23.

22 Insoft, R.M., Sanderson, I.R., Walker, W.A. (1996) Development of immune function in the intestine and its role in neonatal diseases. *Pediatric Clinics of North America* **43**, 551–571.

23 Jacqz-Aigrain, E., Wood, C., Robieux, I. (1990) Phamacokinetics of midazolam in critically ill neonates. *European Journal of Clinical Pharmacology* **39**, 191–192.

24 Jain, A., Rutter, N. (2000) Does topical amethocaine gel reduce the pain of venepuncture in newborn infants? A randomized double blind controlled trial. *Archives of Disease in Childhood Fetal and Neonatal Edition* **83**, F207–F210.

25 Kavvadia, V., Greenough, A., Dimitriou, G., Hooper, R. (2000) Randomized trial of fluid restriction in ventilated very low birthweight infants. *Archives of Disease in Childhood* **83**, F91–F96.

26 Lambert, J.H., Baylis, P.H., McAulay, J.A., Coulthard, M.G. (1998) Does positive pressure ventilation increase arginine vasopressin in preterm neonates? *Archives of Disease in Childhood* **78**, F38–F42.

27 Lauterbach, R., Pawlik, D., Tomaszczyk, B., Cholewa, B. (1994) Pentoxifylline treatment of sepsis of premature infants: preliminary clinical observations. *European Journal of Pediatrics* **153**, 672–674.

28 Lyon, A.J., Akaar, M.E., Badger, P., McIntosh, N. (1997) Temperature control in very low birthweight infants during the first five days of life. *Archives of Disease in Childhood Fetal and Neonatal Edition* **76**, F47–F50.

29 Mercuri, E., Ricci, D., Cowan, F.M. *et al.* (2000) Head growth in infants with hypoxic-ischemic encephalopathy: correlation with neonatal magnetic resonance imaging. *Pediatrics* **106**, 235–243.

30 Modi, N. (1993) Sodium intake and preterm babies. *Archives of Disease in Childhood* **69**, 87–91.

31 Modi, N. (1998) Hyponatremia in the newborn. *Archives of Disease in Childhood* **78**, F81–F84.

32 Modi, N., Carr, R. (2000) Promising stratagems for reducing the burden of neonatal sepsis. *Archives of Disease in Childhood Fetal and Neonatal Edition* **83**, F150–F153.

33 Modi, N., Hutton, J. (1990) Urinary creatinine excretion and estimation of muscle mass in infants of 25–34 weeks gestation. *Acta Paediatrica Scandinavica* **79**, 1156–1162.

34 Modi, N., Murray, N. (in press) Neonatal red cell infusions. *Vox Sanguinis*.

35 Modi, N., Bétrémieux, P., Midgley, J., Hartnoll, G. (2000) Postnatal weight loss and contraction of the extracellular compartment is triggered by atrial natriuretic peptide. *Early Human Development* **59**, 201–208.

36 Murdoch-Eaton, D., Darowski, M., Livingston, J. (2001) Cerebral function monitoring in paediatric intensive care: useful features for predicting outcome. *Developmental Medicine and Child Neurology* **43**, 91–96.

37 Ng, E., Taddio, A., Ohlsson, A. (2001) Intravenous midazolam infusion for sedation of infants in the neonatal intensive care unit. (Cochrane Review). In *The Cochrane Library*, Issue 1. Update Software, Oxford.

38 Ohlsson, A., Lacy, J.B. (2000) Intravenous imunoglobulin for suspected or subsequently proven infection in neonates

(Cochrane Review). In *The Cochrane Library*, Issue 1. Update Software, Oxford.

39 Ohlsson, A., Taddio, A., Jadad, A.R., Stevens, B. (2000) Evidence-based decision making, systematic reviews and the Cochrane collaboration: implications for neonatal analgesia. In McGrath, P.J. (ed:), *Pain in Neonates. Pain Research and Clinical Management*, Vol. 10. Amsterdam: Elsevier-Science, 251–268.

40 Osborn, D.A., Evans, N. (2001) Early volume expansion for prevention of morbidity and mortality in very preterm infants (Cochrane Review). In *The Cochrane Library*, Issue 2. Update Software, Oxford.

41 Reynolds, P.R., Dale, R.C., Cowan, F.M. (2001) Neonatal cranial ultrasound interpretation: a clinical audit. *Archives of Disease in Childhood Fetal and Neonatal Edition* **84**, F92–F95.

42 Roze, J.C., Tohier, C., Maingueneau, C. *et al.* (1993) Response to dobutamine and dopamine in the hypotensive very preterm infant. *Archives of Disease in Childhood* **69**, 59–63.

43 Rutter, N. (1999) Hazards of an immature skin. In Levitt, G., Harvey, D., Cooke, R. (eds), *Practical Perinatal Care: the Baby under 1000 g*. Oxford: Butterworth-Heinemann, 76.

44 Rutter, N. (2000) The newborn skin. *Seminars in Neonatology* **5**, 271.

45 Seri, I., Tan, R., Evans, J. (2001) Cardiovascular effects of hydrocortisone in preterm infants with pressor-resistant hypotension. *Pediatrics* **107**, 1070–1074.

46 Skinner, J.R., Milligan, D.W.A., Hunter, S., Hey, E.N. (1992) Central venous pressure in the ventilated neonate. *Archives of Disease in Childhood Fetal and Neonatal Edition* **67**, 374–377.

47 So, K.W., Fox, T.F., Ng, P.C. *et al.* (1997) Randomized controlled trial of colloid or crystalloid in hypotensive preterm infants. *Archives of Disease in Childhood* **76**, F43–F46.

48 Soll, R.F., Edwards, W.H. (2001) Emollient ointment for preventing infection in preterm infants (Cochrane Review). In *The Cochrane Library*, Issue 2. Update Software, Oxford.

49 Stewart, A., Hope, P.L., Hamilton, P. *et al.* (1988) Prediction in very preterm infants of satisfactory neurodevelopmental progress at 12 months. *Developmental Medicine and Child Neurology* **30**, 53–63.

50 Strozik, K.S., Pieper, C.H., Roller, J. (1997) Capillary refilling time in newborn babies: normal values. *Archives of Disease in Childhood Fetal and Neonatal Edition* **76**, F193–F196.

51 Subhedar, N.V., Shaw, N.J. (2001) Dopamine versus dobutamine for hypotensive preterm infants (Cochrane Review). In *The Cochrane Library*, Issue 2. Update Software, Oxford.

52 Symington, A., Pinelli, J. (2001) Developmental care for promoting development and preventing morbidity in preterm infants (Cochrane Review). In *The Cochrane Library*, Issue 2. Update Software, Oxford.

53 Tammela, O.K.T., Kovisto, M.E. (1992) Fluid restriction for preventing bronchopulmonary dysplasia? Reduced fluid intake during the first weeks of life improves the outcome of low birthweight infants. *Acta Paediatrica* **81**, 207–212.

54 Tang, W., Ridout, D., Modi, N. (1997) The influence of respiratory distress syndrome on body composition during the first week after birth. *Archives of Disease in Childhood Fetal and Neonatal Edition* **77**, F28–F31.

55 Thompson, P.J., Greenough, A., Hird, M.F. *et al.* (1992) Nosocomial bacterial infections in very low birthweight infants. *European Journal of Pediatrics* **151**, 451–454.

56 Vamvakas, E.C., Strauss, R.G. (2001) Meta-analysis of controlled clinical trials studying the efficacy of rHuEPO in reducing blood transfusions in the anemia of prematurity. *Transfusion* **41**, 406–415.

57 Wong, W., Fok, T.F., Lee, C.H. *et al.* (1997) Randomized controlled trial: comparison of colloid or crystalloid for partial exchange transfusion or treatment of neonatal polycythemia. *Archives of Disease in Childhood* **77**, F115–F118.

58 Wyllie, J.P., Skinner, J. (2000) The infant with heart failure, hypotension or shock: evaluating the infant with non-structural heart disease. In Skinner, J., Alverson, D., Hunter, S. (eds), *Echocardiography for the Neonatologist*. London: Churchill-Livingstone, Harcourt Publishers Limited, 219–223.

59 Zupan, J., Garner, P. (2001) Topical umbilical cord care at birth (Cochrane Review). In *The Cochrane Library*, Issue 2. Update Software, Oxford.

16B

Feeding

SEAN P DEVANE

Nutritional support for preterm infants attempts to reproduce *in utero* growth rates. This requires additional amounts to compensate for factors such as thermogenesis and infection. Allowance for the metabolic cost of growth must be made, being between 20 and 30 percent of the energy value of the incorporated tissues.[65,73] Aggressive attention to nutrition has been shown to improve growth rates and biochemical parameters of well-being.[99] Attention to nutritional support has also been shown to influence developmental indices.[7,31,37,59] It may also interact with many of the factors thought to predispose to lung damage.[29] While it is logical to pay attention to nutritional support, it has not been shown *per se* to reduce respiratory morbidity or to improve survival chances. Undernutrition in newborn pups exposed to oxygen, however, doubles mortality,[29] and lung weight decreases during starvation.[81] In addition, malnutrition has been shown to weaken diaphragmatic function in adults.[3]

GUT MATURATION

Antenatal aspects

Swallowing activity has been observed from 16 weeks in the human fetus, with an appreciable amount of amniotic fluid being swallowed at that gestation.[77] Observation of contrast medium *in utero* has suggested that there is little intestinal activity before 30 weeks of gestation; motor activity reaching the colon is present by 34 weeks.[63]

Postnatal aspects

SUCKING

In premature infants, effective sucking develops at 34 weeks of gestation, although sucking activity is present earlier. An increase in both the number of sucks per burst of sucking and the frequency of sucks and improved coordination of sucking with swallows occurs with increasing maturity.[19,20]

ESOPHAGEAL FUNCTION

Immature contractions of the esophagus have been shown in premature infants, with poor propagation and abnormalities of the peristaltic waves.[33] Immaturity of the coordination of esophageal motor function, not inadequate lower esophageal sphincter pressure, is the cause of poor esophageal function in preterm infants.[70] Above 33 weeks postmenstrual age, the motor mechanisms regulating the upper esophageal sphincter are developed.[69] Parameters of normal esophageal acid reflux are different from those seen in adults and in older children.[12] In infants, the upper limits of normality are higher.[97] Considerably more reflux occurs in the supine position.[96]

GASTRIC EMPTYING

Gastric motor activity is similar in children and adults. The pressure generated by contractions of the gastric antrum increases with increasing gestational age.[9] Gastric emptying of glucose solutions in infants was slower with higher concentrations of glucose, although the total amount of glucose entering the duodenum per unit time was increased.[40] Starch is emptied more quickly than glucose,[41] which is the reverse of what is found in adults. Breast milk empties more rapidly than formula milk,[16] without any demonstrable difference in motor activity patterns,[92] suggesting that the faster emptying is not mediated by a simple increase in motor activity.

In preterm infants, gastric emptying follows a biphasic time course for human milk and a linear time course for formula milk, being faster for the former.[15] The emptying rate increases with weight, but not with gestational age. Osmolality does not influence the gastric emptying rate in preterm infants, but increasing caloric content slows emptying. Medium chain triglycerides are emptied more rapidly than long chain triglycerides, and glucose polymers are emptied more rapidly than glucose monomers.[84–86] The feedback mechanism that slows gastric emptying with increased caloric density may be more sensitive in preterm than term infants.[8] Non-nutritive sucking leads to an increase in gastric emptying[98] and may improve growth.[6]

INTESTINAL ACTIVITY

In the preterm infant, small intestinal motor activity shows developmental maturation.[9,10,45,67] Association of antral and duodenal activity increases significantly with increasing gestational age. Feeding influences activity patterns in a manner that correlates better with both bolus feed volume and length of time during which the infant has been exposed to milk, rather than with gestational age.[10] Feeding leads to disruption of the fasting pattern of activity in premature infants greater than 35 weeks of gestation. Exposure to feeding enhances the maturation of gastrointestinal hormonal concentrations[58] and of intestinal enzyme concentrations.[39] The duration of the disrupted pattern of activity is shorter in those fed human rather than formula milk.[92] Postprandial rises in hormonal concentrations have been shown in term infants with blunted rises in prematurely born infants.[58] Those results suggest early introduction of enteral feeds should lead to earlier tolerance of feeding. A number of clinical studies have supported that hypothesis.[64] Premature infants older than 30 weeks of postmenstrual age have normal anorectal pressures and a normal anal reflex.[5]

Illness causes ileus. This may be due to excessive inhibitory enteric nervous system activity. In adult studies, administration of sympathetic blockers had no effect, however. The effect of chronic lung disease on the gut of preterm infants has been studied. These infants have less reflux of gastric acid to the upper esophagus than control infants.[88] What reflux occurs is due to transient lower esophageal sphincter relaxations, and esophageal clearance mechanisms are fully functional.[68] Morphine is known to have an inhibitory effect on gut motor action (p. 209). Hypokalemia, if severe, may also inhibit motor function.

ENERGY REQUIREMENT AND METABOLISM

Very low birthweight (VLBW) infants have low energy reserves.[27] Infants, particularly those born prematurely, require proportionately greater intakes of energy, fluid, protein and micronutrients. In malnutrition, lean body mass and the mass of essential organs is greater. Basal energy expenditure may appear to be high if body weight is used as the denominator. Conversely, severe starvation may result in reduced basal energy expenditure. The preterm infant has a lower resting metabolic rate than the term infant when expressed per unit surface area and lacks the ability to increase metabolic rate in response to cold stress. Hormonal adaptation to stress in preterm infants is suboptimal.[57] Nitrogen balance in preterm infants in the first days after birth is frequently negative using current feeding regimens.[66] It is also negative for up to 96 hours after surgery.[78] In term infants, respiratory quotient (RQ) studies show an increase in the use of fat by 30 hours of age.[101] The energy expenditure of ventilated infants is less than that of spontaneous breathing infants.[26] Energy expenditure was shown to be increased in five infants with CLD.[21]

INFLUENCE OF NUTRITION ON SHORT- AND LONG-TERM OUTCOME

Major nutrients

A two to one ratio of carbohydrate and lipid is usually considered optimal for growth in well children. Ill infants may be unable to metabolize lipids. One influential source has recommended restricting lipid intake to that required to support essential fatty acid needs (0.5–1 g/day) (p. 403) in infants requiring supplementary oxygen, because of concern over increasing the pulmonary artery pressure.[44] Respiratory quotients are 0.71 for fatty acids, 0.81 (on average) for proteins and 1.0 for carbohydrate. The work required of the lungs to eliminate carbon dioxide should then be lower if the lipid content of the diet is increased. When a high fat formula was tried in ten infants with CLD,[72] a decrease in CO_2 production was seen with no difference in tolerance, but there was no change in pulmonary function and growth was slower. In addition, use of a higher density feed in a study of 60 infants failed to identify any improvement in pulmonary status or growth, despite a higher energy intake.[24] Lipid intake may have detrimental effects on lung function. Adult studies have shown that lipid infusion lowers PaO_2. This may be due to an effect of the lipids on eicosanoid production, leading to ventilation–perfusion mismatch.[34] Suggestions that preterm infants given generous quantities of lipids were more likely to develop CLD have not been confirmed.[1] Histological studies, however, have shown deposition of lipid in perivascular lung tissue.[82] There has been concern that intravenous intralipid emulsions might induce thrombocytopenia; reduced platelet numbers, however, were not found in preterm infants who received a range of lipid intakes for up to 4 weeks.[90] Similarly, studies have demonstrated normal immune function in infants receiving intravenous lipid emulsions.

Essential fatty acid deficiency has detrimental effects on respiratory function, perhaps by reducing surfactant production.[30] Illness affects essential fatty acid metabolism. Plasma arachidonic and decosahexaenoic acid levels decrease during acute illness in infants, suggesting preferential oxidation.[42] A recommended essential fatty acid composition of 3 percent fat intake may be insufficient to obtain normal profiles in sick infants.[61] Adequate simultaneous energy intake is required to prevent oxidation of lipid.

Other nutrients

Glutamine administration has been shown to have beneficial effects on gut barrier function in adults and in neonatal pigs.[14] Meta-analysis of the results of three trials of supplementation in preterm infants, however, did not show a clinical benefit,[94] but a reduced length of time of administration of parenteral nutrition was noted in supplemented infants in another study.[55] Inositol supplementation may produce significant improvements in short-term outcomes[35,38] and nucleotide supplementation in a growth retarded group of infants can improve catch-up growth.[18] Hypophosphatemia may lead to impaired oxygen transport, due to its effect on red cell membranes and to weakened respiratory muscle function.[4]

Antioxidants

Oxygen is toxic to lungs (p. 403) as it produces reactive intermediates such as hydrogen peroxide and hydroxyl radicals. Prevention of free radical damage is achieved by many intracellular and extracellular substances including acute phase proteins and intracellular catalase and superoxide dismutase. Nutritional substances including vitamins C and E, taurine, selenium and the drug N-acetylcysteine have been given in an attempt to protect against the effects of excess free radicals during severe illness. In very preterm infants, however, total antioxidant activity has not yet been correlated with outcome.[22] Polyunsaturated fatty acids have been shown to protect against free radical lung injury in rat models[89] and saturated fatty acid supplementation improves survival of newborn piglets challenged with high oxygen saturations. Results from VLBW infants categorized by their fatty acid status have suggested that essential fatty acid deficiency increases measures of red cell susceptibility to oxidative stress.[93]

Method of administration

The relationship between morbidity and the method of administration of nutrition is complex. It includes aspiration associated with enteral feeding, infection associated with indwelling lines, delay in gut maturation associated with excessive early reliance on total parenteral nutrition and direct interference with immunological (e.g. complement) function and lung physiology by intravenous nutrition (p. 411). Infection causes respiratory morbidity, and a major source of pathogenic organisms in the gastrointestinal (GI) tract. In a study of surgical neonates, 15 of 24 episodes of sepsis were due to translocation of enteral organisms. The organisms which caused septicemia were always present in the GI tract, often at high concentration.[74] Maintaining the transepithelial barrier in the gut reduces the theoretical risk of infection. Enteral nutrition is important for maintaining mucosal integrity.[2]

MODE OF ENTERAL FEEDING

Clinicians are appropriately concerned about the effect of enteral feeding on pulmonary function, particularly in infants with respiratory illness. In a study examining feeding methods, tidal volume, minute volume and dynamic compliance were lower in VLBW infants with respiratory distress given bolus feeds.[11] Continuous feeding may, therefore, be preferable in patients with respiratory instability. Small decreases in cerebral blood flow velocity (about 10 percent) were seen 5–11 minutes after bolus feeding.[50] Comparison of continuous and bolus feeds (over 5 minutes every 2–3 hours) in preterm infants demonstrated that peak energy expenditure was 15 percent higher and mean energy expenditure was 4 percent higher in the bolus-fed group.[32] There are, however, animal data suggesting that bolus feeding stimulates small intestinal growth[82] and bolus feeding may be associated with more physiological endocrine function and promotion of more normal biliary kinetics. These results illustrate the difficulties of balancing longer-term gastrointestinal advantages against possibly detrimental immediate respiratory disadvantages.

ADMINISTRATION OF NUTRITION

The specific questions of whether the addition of carbohydrate, fat and protein to the feeds of preterm infants are beneficial have been addressed.[51–53]

Enteral feeding

TYPE OF FEED

There is considerable evidence for the beneficial effects of human milk feeding.[60] Growth may be less than that noted on preterm formula, but better developmental indices in later infancy and a reduced risk of necrotizing enterocolitis are associated with human milk feeding.[56] Adapted preterm formula, with its increased content of protein, energy and sodium, produces better growth. Fortification of breast milk with multicomponent additives, however, can improve growth while offering the benefits of human milk.[54,79] It is the author's practice to preferentially use human milk; if mother's milk is unavailable then banked donor milk is used, adding a human milk fortifier at half strength for 24 hours then at full strength once full enteral feeding (at least 150 ml/kg/day) is established. If human milk is not available or not desired, term formula is used until full enteral feeding is established, and then intake is converted to a preterm formula over 24 hours.

WHEN TO FEED

Clinical researchers have attempted to show the benefits of aggressive feeding policies.[99]

Early or late

Feeds may be introduced early or late, and may then be progressive or trophic (also called minimal enteral nutrition). In a review updated in 1999, Kennedy et al. found only two eligible studies comparing early progressive feeding with late progressive feeding.[48] Early feeding was defined as introduction by 4 days of age and late feeding as introduction after 4 days of age. While some benefits of early feeding were suggested, the data were not enough to convince the authors of the superiority of either policy. It is the author's practice to start feeds (in infants born less than 1800 g) within the first three days if appropriate for gestational age (greater than the tenth percentile), and without obstetric evidence of antenatal reversed end-diastolic blood flow velocities in the umbilical arteries, at a rate of less than 15 ml/kg/day. For infants with documented antenatal reversed end-diastolic flow, feeding should be delayed for at least seven days.

Trophic feeding

Tyson and Kennedy[95] identified eight eligible studies comparing minimal enteral feeding with delayed feeding. Minimal enteral feeding ranged from 12 ml/kg/day to 24 ml/kg/day and was introduced as early as the first day to as late as the eighth day. The data suggested that minimal enteral feeding had a significant advantage in terms of days to achieving full enteral nutrition and total hospital days. There was no increased risk of necrotizing enterocolitis. Since that review, further evidence for the benefit of trophic feeding has been produced. In a study including 100 infants with birthweights of less than 1750 g who required ventilatory support, mean reduced times to full enteral feeding, requirement for supplementary oxygen and hospital stay were found.[62] In that study, trophic feeding was defined as enteral feeding from day 3 to the end of ventilatory support at a rate of 0.5–1.0 ml/h (probably

equivalent to a maximum of approximately 20 ml/kg/day). In another study of 171 infants born between 26 and 30 weeks of gestation, improved biochemical indices were found in infants who experienced trophic feeding.[80] In that study, trophic feeding meant 20 ml/kg/day for 10 days.

RATE OF INCREASING FEEDS

Kennedy et al.[49] reported on three studies comparing slow versus rapid increase in feeds. A slow increase meant 10, 15 and 20 ml/kg/day and a fast increase meant 20, 30 and 35 ml/kg/day. No effect on the rate of necrotizing enterocolitis was demonstrated, but the confidence intervals were large. It is the author's policy to increase feeds at a rate not exceeding 35 ml/kg/day for well infants, and not exceeding 20 ml/kg/day for infants with particular risk factors for necrotizing enterocolitis.

MODE OF ADMINISTRATION

Milk may be given by continuous or by bolus administration. In a well-designed stratified study including 171 infants born between 26 and 30 weeks of gestation, infants given bolus feeds had a greater rate of weight gain and significantly less feeding intolerance.[80] In this study, bolus feeding consisted of administration of the feed over 20-minute periods every 3 hours. In another smaller study, however, no differences in retention of nitrogen, fat, total carbohydrate and lactose, or in days to regain birthweight, to full enteral feedings or to discharge, or in complications were found between the two methods.[87] Infants who received continuous rather than intermittent tube feeding, however, did take longer to reach full enteral feeds (weighted mean difference 3.0 days, 95 percent CI 0.7, 5.2).[76]

In keeping with the development of coordinated effective swallowing, breast or teat feeds become possible at 34 weeks of gestation. Delivery of oxygen by nasal cannulae facilitates these types of feeding and should be introduced at this stage of development, in oxygen-dependent infants.

It is the author's practice to use hourly bolus enteral feeds, progressing to 2- and then 3-hourly bolus feeds; introducing teat feeds at 33–34 weeks of gestation. It is important to be aware that undernutrition, in relation to planned nutrition, may arise in bolus feeding if residual milk aspirated prior to following feeds is not returned.

Nasojejunal tubes and gastrostomies

Nasojejunal feeding can be useful in infants who are at risk of recurrent aspiration of enteral feeds due to severe gastroesophageal reflux. In infants who require prolonged tube feeding and/or have delayed gastric emptying and/or gastroesophageal reflux, then siting of a gastrostomy is useful. Overnight gastric or gastrojejunal feeding can be given to nutritionally support infants whose oral feeding is inadequate. Provision of a multidisciplinary team including dietitians and nutritional support nurses allows such infants to be cared for in the community rather than have a protracted hospital admission.[71]

Intravenous nutrition

PROTEIN

In general, 1.5 g/kg/day of protein is sufficient to avoid catabolism in all neonatal populations and perhaps can be achieved by as low as 1–1.5 g/kg/day of parenteral protein in extremely low birthweight (ELBW) infants.[91] This latter intake has been suggested to be the lower limit at which to start intravenous protein delivery.[91] In critically ill malnourished infants, protein intakes in excess of 2 g/kg/day, however, were required to increase nutritional markers above baseline.[43] In ELBW infants protein intakes need to be advanced to 3.7–4 g/kg/day to achieve *in utero* protein deposition rates.[91] Infants who receive only dextrose infusions lose 1 percent of their protein stores each day.[47] A number of studies have demonstrated that infusion of amino acids with glucose as early as the first day after birth reduces protein catabolism.[23,100] Monitoring of blood urea nitrogen and ammonia concentrations and assessment of pH and base excess levels has suggested that early and aggressive intravenous protein administration is safe.[91]

GLUCOSE

The minimal glucose requirement to provide for basic metabolic needs is approximately 6 mg/kg/min. Glucose administration is also needed to support protein deposition and this means an additional glucose intake of 2–3 mg/kg/min per gram of protein intake.[91] Glucose administration is frequently limited by the development of hyperglycemia. Administration of insulin is the preferred strategy to deal with hyperglycemia, as reduction in the glucose intake will prevent adequate nutrition. Insulin administration has been shown to successfully lower the glucose concentration and increase weight gain without undue risk of hypoglycemia.[17] In normoglycemic ELBW infants, administration of insulin resulted in a significant elevation of plasma lactate and the development of a metabolic acidosis.[75] The upper limit of glucose administration is that which exceeds the maximal glucose oxidative capacity and excess glucose is converted into fat.[91] The upper limit in neonates is probably about 12–13 mg/kg/min,[46] but unexplained carbon dioxide production may indicate a lower limit is needed in certain individuals.

LIPID

In ELBW infants, essential fatty acid (EFA) deficiency can develop within 72 hours if exogenous fat is not given.[25] This can be prevented by administering as little as 0.5–1.0 g/kg/day of intravenous lipid.[91] Current recommendations suggest that lipid intake should not exceed 3 g/kg/day. An increased alveolar arteriolar gradient of oxygen occurred when 4 g/kg/day of lipid was administered over 24 hours as compared to over 16 hours.[13] Lipid emulsions of 20 percent rather than 10 percent are recommended, because the 10 percent emulsions have a higher phospholipid content which impedes plasma triglyceride clearance.[36]

FUTURE DEVELOPMENTS

Animal studies, supported by some human evidence, have shown a relationship with measures of lung function and development. Further developments in this field will undoubtedly relate to how nutritional status affects the lungs' ability to resist hyperoxic damage, effect repair, and resist infection, and how it influences the development of chronic lung damage such as that found in bronchopulmonary dysplasia in surviving preterm infants.[29]

REFERENCES

1 Alwaidh, M.H., Bowden, L., Shaw, B., Ryan, S.W. (1996) Randomized trial of effect of delayed intravenous lipid administration on chronic lung disease in preterm neonates. *Journal of Pediatric Gastroenterology and Nutrition* **22**, 303–306.

2 Aranow, J.S., Fink, M.P. (1996) Determinants of intestinal barrier failure in critical illness. *British Journal of Anaesthesia* **77**, 71–81.

3 Arora, N.S., Rochester, D.F. (1982) Effects of body weight and muscularity on human diaphragm mass, thickness and area. *Journal of Applied Physiology* **52**, 64.

4 Aubier, M., Murciano, D., Lecocguic, Y. *et al.* (1985) Effect of hypophosphatemia on diaphragmatic contractility in patients with acute respiratory failure. *New England Journal of Medicine* **313**, 420–424.

5 Benninga, M.A., Omari, T.I., Haslam, R.R., Barnett, C.P., Dent, J., Davidson, G.P. (2001) Characterization of anorectal pressure and the anorectal inhibitory reflex in healthy preterm and term infants. *Journal of Pediatrics* **139**, 233–237.

6 Bernbaum, J.C., Gilberto, R.P., Warkins, J.B., Peckham, G.J. (1983) Non-nutritive sucking during gavage feeding enhances growth and maturation in premature infants. *Pediatrics* **71**, 41–45.

7 Birch, E.E., Garfield, S., Hoffman, D.R., Uauy, R., Birch, D.G. (2000) A randomized controlled trial of early dietary supply of long-chain polyunsaturated fatty acids and mental development in term infants. *Developmental Medicine and Child Neurology* **42**, 174–181.

8 Bisset, W.M. (1991) Development of intestinal motility. *Archives of Disease in Childhood* **66**, 3–5.

9 Bisset, W.M., Watt, J.B., Rivers, R.P.A., Milla, P.J. (1988) Ontogeny of fasting small intestinal motor activity in the human infant. *Gut* **29**, 483–488.

10 Bisset, W.M., Watt, J., Rivers, R.P.A., Milla, P.J. (1989) The postprandial motor response of the small intestine to enteral feeds in the preterm human infant. *Archives of Disease in Childhood* **64**, 1356–1361.

11 Blondheim, O., Abbasi, S., Fox, W.W., Bhutani, V.K. (1993) Effect of enteral gavage feeding rate on pulmonary functions

of very low birth weight infants. *Journal of Pediatrics* **122**, 751–755.

12 Boix-Ochoa, J., Lafuente, J.M., Gil-Vernet, J.M. (1980) 24 hr esophageal monitoring in gastro-oesophageal reflux. *Journal of Pediatric Surgery* **15**, 74–78.

13 Brans, Y.W., Dutton, E.B., Andrew, D.S., Menchaca, E.M., West, D.L. (1986) Fat emulsion tolerance in very low birth weight neonates: effect on diffusion of oxygen in the lungs and on blood pH. *Pediatrics* **78**, 79–84.

14 Burrin, D.G., Shulman, R.J., Langston, C., Storm, M.C. (1994) Supplemental alanylglutamine, organ growth, and nitrogen metabolism in neonatal pigs fed by total parenteral nutrition, *Journal of Parenteral and Enteral Nutrition* **18**, 313–319.

15 Cavell, B. (1979) Gastric emptying in preterm infants. *Acta Paediatrica Scandinavica* **68**, 725–730.

16 Cavell, B. (1981) Gastric emptying in infants fed human milk and infant formula. *Acta Paediatrica Scandinavica* **70**, 639.

17 Collins, J.W., Jr, Hoppe, M., Brown, K., Edidin, D.V., Padbury, J., Ogata, E.S. (1991) A controlled trial of insulin infusion and parenteral nutrition in extremely low birth weight infants with glucose intolerance. *Journal of Pediatrics* **118**, 921–927.

18 Cosgrove, M., Davies, D.P., Jenkins, H.R. (1996) Nucleotide supplementation and the growth of term small for gestational age infants. *Archives of Disease in Childhood* **74**, F122–F125.

19 Crump, E.P., Gore, P.M., Horton, C. (1958) The sucking behavior of preterm infants. *Human Biology* **30**, 128–141.

20 Daniels, H., Devlieger, H., Casaer, P., Callens, M., Eggermont, E. (1986) Nutritive and non-nutritive sucking in preterm infants. *Journal of Developmental Physiology* **8**, 117–121.

21 de Gamarra, E. (1992) Energy expenditure in premature newborns with bronchopulmonary dysplasia. *Biology of the Neonate* **61**, 337–344.

22 Drury, J.A., Nycyk, J.A., Baines, M., Cooke, R.W. (1998) Does total antioxidant status relate to outcome in very preterm infants? *Clinical Science* **94**, 197–201.

23 Duffy, B., Gunn, J., Collinge, J. *et al.* (1981) The effect of varying protein quality and energy intake on the nitrogen metabolism of parenterally fed very low birthweight (<1600 g) infants. *Pediatric Research* **15**, 1040–1044.

24 Fewtrell, M.S., Adams, C., Wilson, D.C., Cairns, P., McClure, G., Lucas, A. (1997) Randomized trial of high nutrient density formula versus standard formula in chronic lung disease. *Acta Paediatrica* **86**, 577–582.

25 Foote, K.D., MacKinnon, M.J., Innis, S.M. (1991) Effect of early introduction of formula vs fat-free parenteral nutrition on essential fatty acid status of preterm infants. *American Journal of Clinical Nutrition* **54**, 93–97.

26 Forsyth, J.S., Crighton, A. (1992) An indirect calorimetry system for ventilator dependent very low birthweight infants. *Archives of Disease in Childhood* **67**, 315–319.

27 Frank, L. (1999) Development of lung defences against free radical injury. In Ziegler, E.E., Lucas, A., Moro, G.E. (eds), *Nutrition of the Very Low Birthweight Infant.* Philadelphia: Lippincott Williams & Wilkins.

28 Frank, L., Groseclose, E. (1982) Oxygen toxicity in newborn rats: the adverse effects of undernutrition. *Journal of Applied Physiology: Respiratory, Environmental and Exercise Physiology* **53**, 1248–1255.

29 Frank, L., Sosenko, I.R. (1988) Undernutrition as a major contributing factor in the pathogenesis of bronchopulmonary dysplasia. *American Review of Respiratory Diseases* **138**, 725–729.

30 Friedman, Z., Rosenberg, A. (1979) Abnormal lung surfactant related to essential fatty acid deficiency in a neonate. *Pediatrics* **76**, 447–452.

31 Georgieff, M.K., Hoffman, J.S., Pereira, G.R., Bernbaum, J., Hoffman Williamson, M. (1985) Effect of neonatal caloric deprivation on head growth and 1-year developmental status in preterm infants. *Journal of Pediatrics* **107**, 581–587.

32 Grant, J., Denne, S.C. (1991) Effect of intermittent versus continuous enteral feeding on energy expenditure in premature infants. *Journal of Pediatrics* **118**, 928–932.

33 Gryboski, J.D. (1965) The swallowing mechanism of the neonate. 1. Esophageal and gastric motility. *Pediatrics* **35**, 445–452.

34 Hageman, J.R., McCullogh, K., Gora, P. *et al.* (1983) Intralipid alterations in pulmonary prostaglandin metabolism and gas exchange. *Critical Care Medicine* **11**, 794.

35 Hallman, M., Bry, K., Hoppu, K., Lappi, M., Pohjavuori, M. (1992) Inositol supplementation in premature infants with respiratory distress syndrome. *New England Journal of Medicine* **326**, 1233–1239.

36 Haumont, D., Deckelbaum, R.J., Richelle, M. *et al.* (1989) Plasma lipid and plasma lipoprotein concentrations in low birth weight infants given parenteral nutrition with twenty or ten percent lipid emulsion. *Journal of Pediatrics* **115**, 787–793.

37 Hoffman, D.R., Birch, E.E., Birch, D.G. *et al.* (2000) Impact of early dietary intake and blood lipid composition of long-chain polyunsaturated fatty acids on later visual development. *Journal of Pediatric Gastroenterology and Nutrition* **31**, 540–553.

38 Howlett, A., Ohlsson, A. (1997) Inositol in preterm infants with RDS (Cochrane Review). *The Cochrane Library 2001.* Oxford, Update Software.

39 Hughes, C.A., Dowling, R.H. (1980) Speed of onset of adaptive mucosal hypoplasia and hypofunction in the intestine of parenterally fed rats. *Clinical Science* **59**, 317–327.

40 Husband, J., Husband, P. (1969) Gastric emptying of water and glucose solutions in the newborn. *Lancet* 409–411.

41 Husband, J., Husband, P., Mallinson, C.N. (1970) Gastric emptying of starch meals in the newborn. *Lancet* 290–292.

42 Innis, S.M. (1992) n-3 fatty acid requirements of the newborn. *Lipids* **27**, 879–885.

43 Innis, S.M. (1992) Plasma and red blood cell fatty acid values as indexes of essential fatty acids in the developing organs of infants fed with milk or formulas. *Journal of Pediatrics* **120**, S78–S86.

44 Innis, S.M. (1993) Fat. In Tsang, R.S. *et al.* (eds), *Nutritional Needs of the Preterm Infant.* Baltimore: Williams & Wilkins, 65–86.

45 Ittmann, P.I., Amarnath, R., Berseth, C.L. (1992) Maturation of antroduodenal motor activity in preterm and term infants. *Digestive Diseases and Sciences* **37**, 14–19.

46 Jones, M.O., Pierro, A., Hammond, P., Nunn, A., Lloyd, D.A. (1993) Glucose utilization in the surgical newborn infant receiving total parenteral nutrition. *Journal of Pediatric Surgery* **28**, 1121–1125.

47 Kashyap, S., Heird, W.C. (1993) Protein requirements of low birthweight, very low birthweight and small for gestational age infants. In Raiha, N.C.R. (ed.), *Protein Metabolism During Infancy.* New York: Raven Press, 133.

48 Kennedy, K.A., Tyson, J.E., Chamnanvanikij, S. (2001) Early versus delayed initiation of progressive enteral feedings for parenterally fed low birth weight or preterm infants (Cochrane Review). *The Cochrane Library.* Update Software, Oxford.

49 Kennedy, K.A., Tyson, J.E., Chamnanvanikij, S. (2001) Rapid versus slow rate of advancement of feedings for promoting growth and preventing necrotizing enterocolitis in

parenterally fed low-birth-weight infants (Cochrane Review). *The Cochrane Library*. Update Software, Oxford.

50 Kraeft, K., Roos, R., Mrozik, E. (1986) Influence of feeding tubes and gastrostomy on the colonization of the stomach in neonates. *Annali dell' Istituto Superiore di Sanita* **22**, 899–903.

51 Kuschel, C.A., Harding, J.E. (2000) Carbohydrate supplementation of human milk to promote growth in preterm infants. (Cochrane Review). *The Cochrane Library*. Update Software, Oxford.

52 Kuschel, C.A., Harding, J.E. (2000) Fat supplementation of human milk for promoting growth in preterm infants. (Cochrane Review). *The Cochrane Library*. Update Software, Oxford.

53 Kuschel, C.A., Harding, J.E. (2000) Protein supplementation of human milk for promoting growth in preterm infants. (Cochrane Review). *The Cochrane Library*. Update Software, Oxford.

54 Kuschel, C.A., Harding, J.E. (2001) Multicomponent fortified human milk for promoting growth in preterm infants (Cochrane Review). *The Cochrane Library*. Update Software, Oxford.

55 Lacey, J.M., Crouch, J.B., Benfell, K. *et al.* (1996) The effects of glutamine-supplemented parenteral nutrition in premature infants. *Journal of Parenteral and Enteral Nutrition* **20**, 74–80.

56 Lucas, A., Cole, T.J. (1990) Breast milk and neonatal necrotising enterocolitis. *Lancet* **336**, 1519–1523.

57 Lucas, A., Bloom, S.R., Green, A.A. (1985) Gastrointestinal peptides and the adaptation to extrauterine nutrition. *Canadian Journal of Physiology and Pharmacology* **63**, 527–537.

58 Lucas, A., Bloom, S.R., Aynsley-Green, A. (1986) Gut hormones and 'minimal enteral feeding'. *Acta Paediatrica Scandinavica* **75**, 719–723.

59 Lucas, A., Morley, R., Cole, T.J. *et al.* (1990) Early diet in preterm babies and developmental status at 18 months. *Lancet* **335**, 1477–1481.

60 Lucas, A., Morley, R., Cole, T.J., Lister, G., Leeson-Payne, C. (1992) Breast milk and subsequent intelligence quotient in children born preterm. *Lancet* **339**, 261–264.

61 McClead, R.E., Jr., Meng, H.C., Gregory, S.A., Budde, C., Sloan, H.R. (1985) Comparison of the clinical and biochemical effect of increased alpha-linolenic acid in a safflower oil intravenous fat emulsion. *Journal of Pediatric Gastroenterology and Nutrition* **4**, 234–239.

62 McClure, R.J., Newell, S.J. (2000) Randomized controlled study of clinical outcome following trophic feeding. *Archives of Disease in Childhood: Fetal and Neonatal Edition* **82**, F29–F33.

63 McLain, C.R., Jr. (1963) Amniographic studies of the gastrointestinal motility of the human fetus. *American Journal of Obstetrics and Gynecology* **86**, 1079–1087.

64 Meetze, W.H., Valentine, C., McGuigan, J.E., Conlon, M., Sacks, N., Neu, J. (1992) Gastrointestinal priming prior to full enteral nutrition in very low birth weight infants. *Journal of Pediatric Gastroenterology and Nutrition* **15**, 163–170.

65 Micheli, J.L., Schutz, Y. (1987) Protein metabolism and postnatal growth in very low birthweight infants. *Biology of the Neonate* **52**(Suppl 1), 25–40.

66 Mitton, S.G., Calder, A.G., Garlick, P.J. (1991) Protein turnover rates in sick, premature neonates during the first few days of life. *Pediatric Research* **30**, 418–422.

67 Morriss, F.H., Jr., Moore, M., Weisbradt, N.W., West, M.S. (1986) Ontogenic development of gastrointestinal motility. IV. Duodenal contractions in preterm infants. *Pediatrics* **78**, 1106–1113.

68 Omari, T., Barnett, C., Snel, A. *et al.* (1999) Mechanism of gastroesophageal reflux in premature infants with chronic lung disease. *Journal of Pediatric Surgery* **34**, 1795–1798.

69 Omari, T., Snel, A., Barnett, C., Davidson, G., Haslam, R., Dent, J. (1999) Measurement of upper esophageal sphincter tone and relaxation during swallowing in premature infants. *American Journal of Physiology* **277**, G862–G866.

70 Omari, T.I., Barnett, C., Snel, A. *et al.* (1998) Mechanisms of gastroesophageal reflux in healthy premature infants. *Journal of Pediatrics* **133**, 650–654.

71 Pencharz, P., Chaiit, P., Savoie, S., Mullan, C. (1994) Enteral support in the hospitalised infant. In Ghraf, R., Aggett, P., Lifschitz, C., Walker Smith, J., Moran, J. (eds), *Infant Nutrition in Special Situations*. Madrid, Spain: Ediciones Ergon SA, 239–251.

72 Pereira, G.R., Baumgart, S., Bennett, M.J. *et al.* (1994) Use of high-fat formula for premature infants with bronchopulmonary dysplasia: metabolic, pulmonary, and nutritional studies. *Journal of Pediatrics* **124**, 605–611.

73 Pierro, A., Carnielli, V., Filler, R.M., Kicak, L., Smith, J., Heim, T.F. (1991) Partition of energy metabolism in the surgical newborn. *Journal of Pediatric Surgery* **26**, 581–586.

74 Pierro, A., van Saene, H.K., Donnell, S.C. *et al.* (1996) Microbial translocation in neonates and infants receiving long-term parenteral nutrition. *Archives of Surgery* **131**, 176–179.

75 Poindexter, B.B., Karn, C.A., Denne, S.C. (1998) Exogenous insulin reduces proteolysis and protein synthesis in extremely low birth weight infants. *Journal of Pediatrics* **132**, 948–953.

76 Premji, S., Chessell, L. (2001) Continuous nasogastric milk feeding versus intermittent bolus milk feeding for premature infants less than 1500 grams (Cochrane review). In *The Cochrane Library*, Issue 1. Update Software, Oxford.

77 Pritchard, J.A. (1966) Fetal swallowing and amniotic fluid volume. *Obstetrics and Gynecology* **28**, 606–610.

78 Rickham, P.P. (1957) *The Metabolic Response to Neonatal Surgery*. Cambridge, MA: Harvard University Press.

79 Schanler, R.J. (1998) The role of human milk fortification for premature infants. *Clinics in Perinatology* **25**, 645–657.

80 Schanler, R.J., Shulman, R.J., Lau, C., Smith, E.O., Heitkemper, M.M. (1999) Feeding strategies for premature infants: randomized trial of gastrointestinal priming and tube-feeding method. *Pediatrics* **103**, 434–439.

81 Shabeljami, H., Vassallo, C.L. (1979) Lung mechanics and ultrastructure in prolonged starvation. *American Review of Respiratory Disease* **117**, 77.

82 Shulman, R.J., Langston, C., Schanler, R.J. (1987) Pulmonary vascular lipid deposition after administration of intravenous fat to infants. *Pediatrics* **79**, 99–102.

83 Shulman, R.J., Redel, C.A., Stathos, T. (1994) Bolus versus continuous feedings stimulate small-intestinal growth and development in the newborn piglet. *Journal of Pediatric Gastroenterology and Nutrition* **18**, 350–354.

84 Siegel, M., Lebenthal, E., Topper, W. (1982) Gastric emptying in prematures of isocaloric feedings with differing osmolalities. *Pediatric Research* **16**, 141–147.

85 Siegel, M., Lebenthal, E., Krantz, B. (1984) Effect of caloric density on gastric emptying in premature infants. *Journal of Pediatrics* **104**, 118–122.

86 Siegel, M., Krantz, B., Lebenthal, E. (1985) Effect of fat and carbohydrate composition on the gastric emptying of isocaloric feeding in premature infants. *Gastroenterology* **89**, 785–790.

87 Silvestre, M.A., Morbach, C.A., Brans, Y.W., Shankaran, S. (1996) A prospective randomized trial comparing continuous

versus intermittent feeding methods in very low birth weight neonates. *Journal of Pediatrics* **128**, 748–752.

88 Sindel, B.D., Maisels, J., Thomas, V., Ballantine, N. (1989) Gastroesophageal reflux to the proximal esophagus in infants with bronchopulmonary dysplasia. *American Journal of Diseases of Children* **143**, 1103–1106.

89 Sosenko, I.R., Innis, S.M., Frank, L. (1988) Polyunsaturated fatty acids and protection of newborn rats from oxygen toxicity. *Journal of Pediatrics* **112**, 630–635.

90 Spear, M.L., Spear, M., Cohen, A.R., Pereira, G.R. (1990) Effect of fat infusions on platelet concentration in premature infants. *Journal of Parenteral and Enteral Nutrition* **14**, 165–168.

91 Thureen, P.J., Hay, W.W. (2000) Intravenous nutrition and postnatal growth of the micropreme. *Clinics in Perinatology* **27**, 197–219.

92 Tomomasa, T., Hyman, P.E., Itoh, K. (1987) Gastroduodenal motility in neonates response to human milk compared with cow's milk formula. *Pediatrics* **80**, 434–438.

93 Tomsits, E., Rischak, K., Szollar, L. (2000) Effects of early nutrition on free radical formation in VLBW infants with respiratory distress. *Journal of the American College of Nutrition* **19**, 237–241.

94 Tubman, T.R., Thompson, S.W. (2000) Glutamine supplementation for preventing morbidity in preterm infants. (Cochrane Review). *The Cochrane Library*. Update Software, Oxford.

95 Tyson, J.E., Kennedy, K.A. (2001) Minimal enteral nutrition for promoting feeding tolerance and preventing morbidity in parenterally fed infants (Cochrane Review). *The Cochrane Library*. Update Software, Oxford.

96 Vandenplas, Y., Sacre-Smits, L. (1985) Seventeen-hour continuous esophageal pH monitoring in the newborn. *Journal of Pediatric Gastroenterology and Nutrition* **4**, 356–361.

97 Vandenplas, Y., Sacre-Smits, L. (1987) Continuous 24 hour esophageal pH monitoring in 285 asymptomatic infants (from 0 to 15 months old). *Journal of Pediatric Gastroenterology and Nutrition* **6**, 220–224.

98 Widstrom, A.M., Marchini, G., Matthiesen, A.S. (1988) Nonnutritive sucking in tube-fed preterm infants effects on gastric motility and gastric contents of somatostatin. *Journal of Pediatric Gastroenterology and Nutrition* **7**, 517–523.

99 Wilson, D.C., Cairns, P., Halliday, H.L., Reid, M., McClure, G., Dodge, J.A. (1997) Randomized controlled trial of an aggressive nutritional regimen in sick very low birthweight infants. *Archives of Disease in Childhood Fetal and Neonatal Edition* **77**, F4–F11.

100 Zlotkin, S.H., Bryan, M.H., Anderson, G.H. (1981) Intravenous nitrogen and energy intakes required to duplicate in utero nitrogen accretion in prematurely born human infants. *Journal of Pediatrics* **99**, 115–120.

101 Zoppi, G., Luciano, A., Cinquetti, M., Graziani, S., Bolognani, M. (1998) Respiratory quotient changes in full term newborn infants within 30 hours from birth before start of milk feeding. *European Journal of Clinical Nutrition* **52**, 360–362.

Monitoring

ANDREW LYON AND BEN STENSON

Developments in the care of neonatal respiratory disorders have relied on close monitoring of the physiological state of the infant. Measurements of heart rate, respiratory rate and temperature form the basis of the monitoring of any sick child, while measurement of blood gases and acid–base state are particularly important in respiratory disease. In ventilated infants, it is also possible to monitor the interaction of the infant with the ventilator (p. 157). The clinical interpretation of data provided by monitoring requires a knowledge of the underlying physiology and an understanding of the limitations of the measuring devices.

BLOOD GASES

Measurement of blood gases and acid–base balance provides important information about ventilation, perfusion, gas exchange and control of breathing.

Oxygen

The monitoring of oxygenation is fundamental to the assessment of infants with respiratory problems. The gold standard is the partial pressure of oxygen in arterial blood (PaO_2). This can be measured intermittently by arterial puncture or sampling from an indwelling catheter, or continuously by an intravascular electrode.

ARTERIAL PUNCTURE

Arterial punctures are painful. If the infant is crying or struggling, the PaO_2 can change significantly from the true value.[27] Blood is usually obtained from the radial artery. The femoral artery should be avoided in the newborn as there is an increased risk of nerve and vascular damage as well as a risk of serious infection if the hip joint is entered. If the ductus arteriosus is patent, right to left shunt may result in a higher PaO_2 in the right arm and head/neck compared with other areas of the body. A survey of UK and Ireland neonatal units highlighted that only 39 percent of units used arterial stabs, preferring continuous monitoring.[79]

CAPILLARY SAMPLES

Arterialized capillary blood samples are used commonly to estimate blood gas values. Results can be misleading if the infant is poorly perfused or the sample is not free flowing. Exposure of the blood to air will significantly change both PO_2 and PCO_2. In general, capillary samples significantly underestimate PaO_2 and are of little use in assessing oxygenation.[50]

INDWELLING ARTERIAL LINES

The use of indwelling arterial lines allows repeated blood sampling without disturbing the infant and permits continuous blood pressure monitoring.

Umbilical artery catheter (UAC)

These are commonly used in newborn infants. The catheter tip is positioned in the descending aorta to avoid the renal arteries. It is usually placed either above the diaphragm (high) or just above the aortic bifurcation (low). High catheters are associated with fewer complications and can remain *in situ* for longer.[14,39] Concern has been raised about the effect of high catheters on splanchnic blood flow. During the first week after birth no difference was seen in mesenteric arterial blood between high and low catheters. After 7 days, however, reduced flow was seen in infants with high catheters,[44] although this did not translate into any difference in incidence of necrotizing enterocolitis.[45]

UACs have been associated with a number of complications including thrombus formation, although clinically significant events are rare. There is no evidence that the material used alters the risk of thrombus,[12] but side-hole catheters carry a higher risk of thrombus formation than end-hole catheters.[11] Low-dose heparin added to the infusion fluid has no apparent adverse effect and reduces the risk of the catheter becoming blocked.[13] Sampling from the umbilical catheter has been shown to affect cerebral blood flow,[68] but the clinical importance of this is unknown. Most studies report only short-term follow-up, but long-term thrombotic complications have also been documented.[1]

To facilitate appropriate positioning of the catheter, many reference charts have been produced,[72,74] but an x-ray is needed to confirm the site of the tip.

Peripheral artery catheters

Cannulation of a peripheral artery allows rapid access to the arterial circulation. The radial or posterior tibial arteries are most commonly used but the dorsalis pedis artery is a suitable alternative. In preterm infants, the brachial and femoral arteries should be avoided. Transillumination of the limb, using cold light, can delineate the arteries in premature infants.

Complications are rare but vasospasm and thrombus formation can cause major problems in the distal limb. Low-dose heparin must be added to the infusion and the limb observed closely. Glyceryl trinitrate patches can be helpful.

Continuous intravascular blood gas monitoring

A drawback of intermittent sampling is that major fluctuations in condition may be difficult to follow in unstable infants. Increasing the frequency of sampling introduces significant blood loss in small infants. Continuous intravascular PaO_2 monitoring using a Clarke electrode has been possible for many years.[34] Although reliable, the accuracy of the electrode deteriorates due to fibrin deposition. More recently, an intravascular catheter which measures PO_2, PCO_2, pH and temperature continuously has been developed (Neotrend – Diametrics Medical Ltd, High Wycombe, UK). There can be difficulties with insertion of these catheters but once *in situ* they have been shown to work well, giving continuous blood gas data.[52]

NON-INVASIVE MONITORING

Non-invasive methods of oxygen monitoring are now in widespread use because of the limitations of intra-arterial lines and repeated blood sampling.

Transcutaneous oxygen monitoring

Electrodes capable of measuring transcutaneous PO_2 (TcO_2) were introduced in the early 1970s. A heater arterializes the blood in the skin and oxygen diffuses through a membrane into the electrode where it is reduced, setting up an electric current, the size of which is related to the partial pressure. Calibration takes several minutes and is required before, and at intervals during, use. Once sited, the electrode takes around 15 minutes to equilibrate and start giving meaningful readings. The heat from the electrode will burn the skin if it is not moved to a new site regularly. In term infants, using a temperature of 43°C, resiting may only be needed 8-hourly.[61] In some preterm infants, if a temperature of 44°C is used, resiting every 2 hours may be required.[35] The combination of resiting and recalibration can mean that the sensor is not recording on the baby for substantial periods of time.

Falsely low readings are obtained if the sensor is placed over thick or poorly perfused skin, for example a bony surface,[86] if the infant lies on the electrode or if there is poor peripheral circulation.[61] Falsely high readings occur if poor contact between the sensor and the skin allows air to get under the electrode.

The time taken for diffusion causes a delay before changes in PaO_2 are registered by the monitor. In 16 infants with recurrent acute life-threatening events, the median delay between the oxygen saturation falling to 60 percent and the transcutaneous monitoring registering 2.5 kPa (20 mmHg) was 16 seconds with the longest delay being 30 seconds.[61] Transcutaneous oxygen values depend on the temperature of the electrode.[70] For every 1°C reduction in temperature below the optimal 44°C, the measured oxygen tension falls by approximately 2 kPa (15 mmHg).[47] There is a larger difference between TcO_2 and PaO_2 in older infants with thicker skin.[92] Within infants, however, the ratio between TcO_2 and PaO_2 remains constant so that, although absolute values may not be accurate, the trend of changes in TcO_2 can still be reliable. Difficulties in the use of transcutaneous oxygen monitoring have been reported in infants with chronic lung disease, possibly due to changes in skin perfusion.[69]

The sensitivity and specificity of transcutaneous monitors at detecting hypoxia [defined as a PaO_2 less than 6.6 kPa (50 mmHg)] have been estimated at 85 percent and 97 percent, respectively. For hyperoxia [defined as a PaO_2 greater than 13.3 kPa (100 mmHg)], the sensitivity is 87 percent and specificity 89 percent. This means that the monitors will miss approximately 15 percent of both hypoxic and hyperoxic events, defined by these limits.[59] Target values for TcO_2 depend on maturity, severity of illness and underlying diagnosis. It is common practice in preterm infants to aim for TcO_2 between 6 and 10 kPa. Marked variability in TcO_2 in the first week of life has been associated with significant retinopathy of prematurity.[22]

Saturation monitoring

Pulse oximetry is now the predominant method of oxygen monitoring. It is based on the principle that oxygenated hemoglobin absorbs light in the infrared region of the spectrum (85–1000 nm) whereas deoxygenated hemoglobin absorbs light in the visible red band (600–750 nm). The probe transmits light at 660 and 940 nm through the tissue which is then measured by a photodetector. The ratio of the light absorbed at the two wavelengths correlates with the proportions of oxygenated and deoxygenated hemoglobin in the tissues. The pulsation of the blood vessels changes the path length of the light and this alters the amount of light transmitted during each pulse. The oximeter uses this property to measure only light absorbed by pulsating parts of tissue, that is, the hemoglobin in the blood vessels.

The probes are easily attached and require no calibration, so they provide immediate information. There are, however, several problems which can result in incorrect readings. An optical shunt occurs when light is received by the photodetector that has not passed through tissue; this may result from misalignment of the sensor or from exposure to ambient light. With ambient light the saturation trends to 85 percent – the value at which the ratio of red to infrared light equals one. In most probes there are two transmitting diodes, for the two wavelengths, placed 2–3 mm apart, and the effect of any optical shunt depends on which wavelength is bypassing the tissue. Poor perfusion can affect function. Most pulse oximeters need a pulse pressure of greater than 20 mmHg,[29,53] or a systolic blood pressure greater than 30 mmHg.[77] With lower pulse pressures, there is an increase in missing and incorrect values.[53,77] The use of tight, non-compliant tape can affect the signal by impairing the arterial pulsation.

An important source of artifact is movement of the patient. Interpretation of the saturation readings is impossible without some means of assessing whether there is movement artifact. Most oximeters show the light plethysmography waveform, which gives good information on signal quality.[59] Another validation method is to compare the pulse rate measured by the oximeter with that from an ECG monitor.[60] Saturation readings are reliable when the heart rates are similar (Figure 17.1). Oximeters differ in the way they deal with poor quality signals and possible artifact. Some show no value, but others continue to display a reading but with an alarm. The precision of the measurements is not affected by fetal hemoglobin[64] or bilirubin.[6] To reduce artifact, pulse oximeters often average their values over periods between 2 and 15 seconds. Longer averaging time slows the reaction to rapidly changing values, reducing the rate of false alarms. This, however, also slows the response to true changes in oxygenation so that brief desaturations will be missed. It may also be more difficult to interpret the temporal relationship between changes in oxygenation and cardiorespiratory events, such as apnea or bradycardia. Newer oximeters are addressing the problem of movement artifact. One instrument (Masimo Signal extraction technology) reduces false alarms by mathematically manipulating the red and infrared light absorbance to identify and subtract the noise components associated with these signals.[28] In preterm infants this monitor identified true desaturations and bradycardias at least as reliably as a conventional oximeter,[17] but with 93 percent fewer false alarms.[16]

On the same infant, two oximeters may display different saturation readings[36] and data from one make of monitor cannot be transferred to another.[59] Oximeters determine saturation values from 'look up' tables based on data from healthy adults and may not have been validated for infants and young children. Some instruments display 'functional' saturation and others 'fractional' saturation. The latter allows for levels of carboxyhemoglobin and

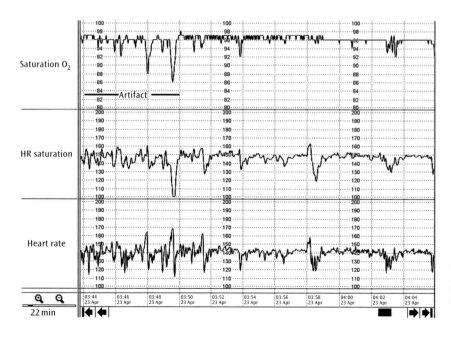

Figure 17.1 *Artifact on the saturation recording as evidenced by the lack of agreement by the heart rate (HR) traces.*

methemoglobin and is in general 2 percent lower. As pulse oximeters use data from healthy adults to determine saturation values, low saturations will not be included in the reference data and these have been derived by extrapolation from higher values. This may lead to an underestimate of the true degree of hypoxemia and this imprecision will be exacerbated by the effects of movement artifact. Sensitivity and specificity for the detection of hypoxemia have been estimated at 92 percent and 97 percent, respectively.[59] These data, however, were derived from studies where conditions were optimal and the values may well be lower in 'real life'. Because of the shape of the hemoglobin dissociation curve, pulse oximeters are not suitable for detecting hyperoxia.

Baseline oxygen saturation during quiet sleep, and at times free from apneic pauses, varies between 95 and 100 percent in preterm and 97 and 100 percent in older infants.[62,63,66] Episodic desaturations are common and their frequency varies with age. In preterm infants at the time of discharge from hospital, episodes of desaturation to below 80 percent for more than 4 seconds were found in most patients but this became relatively rare by 6 weeks later.[63] Such episodes were rare in full-term infants at 6 weeks of age but shorter episodes were still common.[80] These studies were done using an oximeter in beat-to-beat mode. A recent report looked at saturation levels in healthy infants over the first 6 months after birth using an oximeter with a short averaging time (3 seconds). The median baseline oxygen saturation was 98 percent with the tenth percentile at 95.2 percent, and this did not change with age. Acute decreases in saturation of at least 10 percent of baseline were normal phenomena, occurring in almost two-thirds of the infants.[40] Several studies now confirm that the normal range for oxygen saturation in infants is relatively narrow and a functional saturation below 95 percent, obtained repeatedly while the infant is breathing regularly, should be regarded as abnormal, irrespective of age. Occasional falls in saturation by at least 10 percent of baseline or to below 80 percent can be regarded as normal during the first 6 months after birth.[58] There are, however, no data that tell us at what baseline saturation level intervention should be considered or how often, or for how long, and to what nadir, saturation may be allowed to fall. In other words we know a lot about saturation monitoring in normal infants, but remain uncertain about how to apply this technology to infants with respiratory disease.

It is, therefore, difficult to recommend limits for oxygen saturation in infants with lung disease. Applying data from normal infants may increase their exposure to supplementary oxygen. This may itself be damaging, particularly in preterm infants where oxygen free radicals contribute to much of the morbidity seen in these infants.[75] Low saturations in infants with chronic lung disease have been associated with acute life-threatening events.[41] Maintaining saturations above 95 percent, however, may increase the incidence of chronic lung disease and retinopathy of prematurity.[9,88] Many recommend that oxygen therapy be considered in infants whose baseline saturation is less than 93 percent.[57] The safe upper limit is uncertain, but recent outcome data point to this being around 95 percent. In clinical practice it is impossible to set such tight limits without there being an unacceptable number of false alarms and infants in hospital may be allowed lower saturations than 93 percent. If being discharged home in oxygen, however, infants should be nursed with a saturation above 93 percent.[57]

Artifact makes the interpretation of single values from a pulse oximeter pointless. Continuous display of the saturation with heart rate from the monitor and an ECG allows visual exclusion of artifact and shows trends (Figure 17.1). The use of oxygen saturation profiles have also been shown to be a helpful way of guiding supplemental oxygen treatment.[55]

Carbon dioxide

Monitoring the partial pressure of carbon dioxide (PCO_2) is important in determining the adequacy of alveolar ventilation and interpreting the acid–base balance. PCO_2 is affected by crying, which commonly occurs during arterial puncture or capillary sampling. Capillary samples are useful for monitoring stable infants with chronic respiratory problems, but care must be exercised in their interpretation.[20] The new generation of multiparameter intravascular sensors (Neotrend) include continuous PCO_2 monitoring.

TRANSCUTANEOUS CARBON DIOXIDE MONITORING

Transcutaneous CO_2 (TcCO_2) is commonly combined with oxygen monitoring in the same probe. Most TcCO_2 electrodes work by measuring the change in pH of an electrolyte solution, separated from the skin by a hydrophobic membrane, which is permeable to carbon dioxide but not to hydrogen ions. As carbon dioxide diffuses more readily than oxygen, the electrodes can operate at lower temperatures, although there is better correlation with arterial blood gas tension at higher temperatures.[38] The electrodes are affected by poor perfusion. TcCO_2 is in general 27 percent higher than the corresponding arterial measurement, due partly to local tissue production of carbon dioxide (approximately 0.5 kPa) and partly to the heating coefficient of blood. This difference is greater in the hypercapnic range. The electrodes need calibration against a known concentration of carbon dioxide every 4 hours. This can take 10 minutes, adding to the time that the probe is not in use monitoring the infant. Over a 4-hour period there is an upward drift in the TcCO_2 but, in general, there remains a good correlation between transcutaneous and arterial CO_2. The electrodes give a good

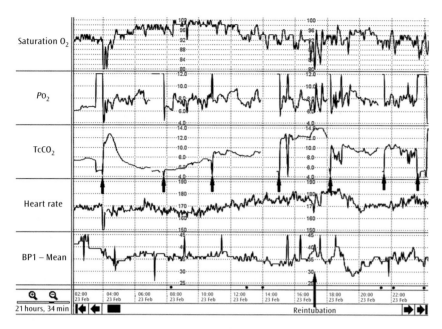

Figure 17.2 *Trend graphs of transcutaneous CO₂ (TcCO₂). This demonstrates the high Pco₂ associated with a blocked endotracheal tube, necessitating an emergency reintubation. Although the clinical deterioration was sudden, it can be seen that the Pco₂ had been rising slowly for several hours. Earlier assessment may well have avoided the subsequent collapse. (Black arrows show times when the probes were off the infant for recalibration.)*

indication of trends in the baby's $PaCO_2$. Repeated blood gas estimations are still required but changes in $TcCO_2$ can give early warning of developing problems (Figure 17.2). Even at lower temperatures (40°C), $TcCO_2$ probes have been shown to give useful information on CO_2 trends[15] and, used in this way, can be safely left on the skin for several hours. Transcutaneous CO_2 monitoring has proven useful in long distance transport, resulting in babies arriving in the referral unit with lower ventilator pressures and better blood gases.[56]

There are no data on normal values for $TcCO_2$. Our experience with these monitors has shown that each baby has its own individual relationship between arterial and $TcCO_2$ and these probes are more useful as a means of following trends than as a measurement of true arterial PCO_2. In the first days after birth, hypocapnia has been associated with a higher incidence of chronic lung disease (low CO_2 being a measure of aggressive overventilation),[32] and with an increased risk of periventricular leukomalacia,[31] probably as a consequence of reduced cerebral blood flow. In the same period, hypercapnia has been associated with an increased risk of intraventricular hemorrhage.[85] During the management of acute lung disease, $TcCO_2$ is helpful in ensuring that carbon dioxide levels are kept within an acceptable range. Once an infant can compensate metabolically, many clinicians allow the PCO_2 to rise in the hope that gentler ventilation will reduce the risks of long-term lung damage.

END TIDAL CO₂ MONITORING

Capnography measures the concentration of CO_2 in exhaled gas and has been used extensively in children and adults under general anesthesia as well as in adult intensive care. Small tidal volumes, rapid respiratory rates and inhomogeneous alveolar ventilation–perfusion in neonates

with lung disease had limited the value of capnography in the newborn, particularly the preterm infant.[37] The problem of inhomogeneous lung disease, however, has been reduced in infants with RDS by surfactant administration and studies using newer mainstream monitors, with low dead space and low resistance, have shown capnography to have some place in the monitoring of trends in carbon dioxide.[73] It may be useful in recognizing esophageal intubation.[67] In infants with respiratory disease, $TcCO_2$ monitoring provides a more accurate estimation of $PaCO_2$ than capnography.[89]

Acid–base balance

The pH, bicarbonate and base excess are important in the assessment of the respiratory status of the infant and help to determine the need for intervention. The multiparameter umbilical arterial catheter (Neotrend) records pH continuously and can also derive bicarbonate and base excess. Newborn infants with respiratory disease often have mixed respiratory and metabolic acidosis. What constitutes an optimal pH in these infants is unknown. Many clinicians attach different importance to metabolic and respiratory acidosis, accepting pH values around 7.20, rather than risking further lung injury by using aggressive ventilation to reduce respiratory acidosis. Lactate measurements can help to refine decision-making.

BLOOD PRESSURE

Blood pressure can be monitored directly with transducers attached to arterial lines. It is important to ensure that these are calibrated to zero. Changes in position of the transducer relative to the height of the heart may alter the reading. Damping of the arterial trace affects systolic and diastolic blood pressure. Mean pressure remains more reliable but even this can be affected by damping of the trace.[21] Non-invasive oscillometric methods are frequently used to measure blood pressure. These machines significantly overestimate blood pressure at the lower end of the range and are therefore poor at detecting and measuring hypotension. They therefore are not likely to be reliable in verifying low-pressure readings from arterial lines.

CENTRAL–PERIPHERAL TEMPERATURE DIFFERENCE

Continuous measurement of a central (abdominal) and a peripheral (foot) temperature is useful in detecting cold stress but also can give an early indication of poor tissue perfusion. A widening central–peripheral temperature gap with an increasing heart rate can indicate poor perfusion, due to hypovolemia or decreased venous return, even before the blood pressure starts to fall.[46] Recordings from over 400 healthy neonates of different gestational ages demonstrated that the upper limit of normal for capillary refill time was 3 seconds.[84] CRT (capillary refill time) values of the midpoints of the sternum and the forehead were found to be the most consistent. Routine nursing procedures can cause widening of the central peripheral temperature gap.[51]

CONTINUOUS TREND MONITORING

Readings from monitors and blood gas machines give information on the condition of the baby at a single moment. Display of the physiological parameters as continuous graphs allows developing trends to be detected and may facilitate earlier intervention (Figure 17.2). Trend monitoring of $TcCO_2$ may also facilitate earlier diagnosis of pulmonary air leak.[49] Although in retrospect diagnostic trends appear obvious, these patterns are difficult to recognize in evolution, even by experienced staff.[2] A randomized controlled trial of computerized trend monitoring in neonatal intensive care failed to show that it improved outcome.[23] Computerized pattern recognition and decision support may need to be developed to realize the full potential of this information.[3]

CONTINUOUS ON-LINE RESPIRATORY FUNCTION MONITORING

This is a standard feature on some infant ventilators and is obtainable as an add-on for most others. The data are presented as numerical values, time-based waveforms of flow, volume and airway pressures, and flow–volume and pressure–volume loops. To date, there is little evidence that this information improves clinical outcome. In a retrospective study of two cohorts of infants cared for before and after the introduction of continuous monitoring, Rosen et al. found a reduction in the incidence of pneumothorax and intraventricular hemorrhage, but no change in survival rates, duration of ventilation or incidence of bronchopulmonary dysplasia.[71] In a prospective randomized controlled trial of respiratory system compliance measurements, Stenson et al. showed no change in incidence of death or chronic lung disease.[82] On post hoc analysis there was a 40 percent reduction in the duration of ventilation of surviving infants in the group with regular lung function testing.[82] Randomized trials in adults, however, have shown that the use of graphical and numerical data from on-line respiratory monitors to guide ventilator management is associated with a significant reduction in the mortality and morbidity of ARDS.[5,10,65] Continuous on-line monitoring, therefore, is likely to become established as part of the routine management of ventilated infants in the coming years. Further critical evaluation is required as not all the information used in the adult trials can be obtained reliably in newborn infants.

Flow monitoring

Continuous monitoring requires a flow sensor to be connected directly to the endotracheal tube. Attempts to measure flow elsewhere in the ventilator circuit are inaccurate in small patients because the compliance of the circuit and variations in set-up cannot be corrected for with confidence.[18] Present devices add around 1 ml to the infant's respiratory dead space. In the smallest infants this could necessitate increased minute ventilation to maintain CO_2 elimination,[33,83] but this has not been fully evaluated. The most commonly used on-line monitoring device is a hot-wire anemometer which measures gas flow by its cooling effect on a pair of heated wires. Alternatively, a differential pressure transducer, which measures the change in pressure generated by a gas flow across a fixed resistance mounted within a pneumotachograph, can be used. Ultrasonic flow meters, which utilize Doppler effects, are also under evaluation.[76] Flow can be integrated with time to give volume.

Changes in gas composition affect the measurements. Pure oxygen is 12 percent more viscous than room air, so reducing the inspired oxygen concentration can be associated with an apparent increase in tidal volume, unless the monitor corrects for gas composition.[95] Errors may be particularly large during partial liquid ventilation where the exhaled gas contains perfluorocarbon vapour, but the inspired gas does not. This can result in overestimates of exhaled tidal volume of 35–41 percent when a hot-wire anemometer is used.[24] Data from different devices may not be comparable as some earlier devices overestimate or underestimate flow and volume measurements significantly.[19,90] Some manufacturers give little detail about the performance characteristics of their device and the methods used to calculate derived data. Devices are becoming increasingly accurate,[91] but optimal performance cannot be assumed.[25,26]

TIDAL VOLUME

A healthy, spontaneously breathing term infant with no lung disease has a tidal volume of around 7–9 ml/kg body weight.[8] The optimum tidal volume in a ventilated infant is uncertain. If there is lung disease, then the number of fully functional airspaces is likely to be less than normal and there may be regional inhomogeneity of pressure volume characteristics within the lungs. 'Normal' tidal volumes may therefore expose parts of the lungs to excess end inspiratory volume. Because of this, target tidal volumes are generally set around the 4–6 ml/kg range in ventilated infants, although if CO_2 elimination is adequate, lower tidal volumes are entirely acceptable. In a randomized trial in adults with ARDS, tidal volumes of 6 ml/kg were associated with less morbidity than tidal volumes of 12 ml/kg.[10] In immature newborn animals there was a dose-dependent relationship between tidal volume and degree of lung injury when tidal volumes of 5 ml/kg, 10 ml/kg and 20 ml/kg were compared.[93] In another study, high rate, low tidal volume ventilation was associated with less histological chronic lung disease than low rate, high tidal volume ventilation.[4] Some devices display tidal volume breath by breath, others display a rolling average. Spontaneous breaths are generally smaller than ventilator breaths, so if averaging is used it will not give a true impression of the ventilator tidal volumes if there is significant spontaneous breathing. Displayed values are not corrected for bodyweight.

MINUTE VENTILATION

A rolling average of expired minute ventilation can be calculated and subdivided into the relative proportions attributable to ventilator breaths and spontaneous breaths. Some have suggested that it may help in assessing weaning and readiness for extubation,[94] but whether this is any more useful than looking at tidal volumes is unclear. There is no evidence that measuring minute ventilation is any more useful than monitoring transcutaneous PCO_2.

Compliance and resistance

There are a variety of methods for deriving these data from continuous dynamic pressure–volume traces. The values obtained are affected by the lung volume at the time of the measurement. They are also unreliable if inappropriately short inspiratory or expiratory times are used and are made inaccurate by leaks around the endotracheal tube. The variable nature of infant–ventilator interactions (p. 159) also complicate their interpretation in real time. As a consequence, continuous on-line monitoring of compliance and resistance is unlikely to be useful in everyday clinical practice. The C_{20}:C ratio is a derived index of lung overdistension which compares the inflation compliance during the last 20 percent of inflation with that of the whole breath.[30] This index is unreliable in newborn infants because it requires a ventilator which generates a slow rise in inflation pressure, or a constant flow of gas into the lungs during inflation, and little or no air leak to compute it meaningfully.[54] These conditions are seldom met in neonatal ventilation.

Functional residual capacity

Ideally, to avoid high end inspiratory lung volumes and low end expiratory lung volumes, both the tidal volume and the functional residual capacity (FRC) must be known. FRC varies considerably over the course of an illness and can change rapidly with treatments such as surfactant[43] or high frequency oscillation. There is currently no readily applicable method to make repeated FRC measurements that is suitable for routine clinical use. FRC, however, can be inferred from the inspired oxygen concentration required to achieve adequate oxygenation and the chest radiograph appearance. The relationship between the radiographic and the measured lung volume has been reported to be inconsistent,[87] but can be improved by using computer-assisted analysis.[25]

LEAKS

There is generally some leak around the uncuffed endotracheal tubes used in newborn infants, although this can be minimal if shouldered endotracheal tubes are used (p. 154). The leak is only clinically apparent when it is large, but it makes derived data, such as compliance and resistance, unreliable. Leaks also complicate the interpretation of loops and waveforms. Airway pressure is higher in inspiration; therefore, most of the leak occurs in this phase of ventilation. As a consequence, usually the expired tidal volume is displayed by monitors. Leak is calculated as inspired volume minus expired volume and expressed as a percentage of the inspired volume.

Waveforms

Simultaneous time-based traces of flow, volume and pressure are the most commonly used graphical representation of respiratory function and provide the most readily interpretable information. The scaling of the graphs is important. If set to autoscale, then changes in the size of

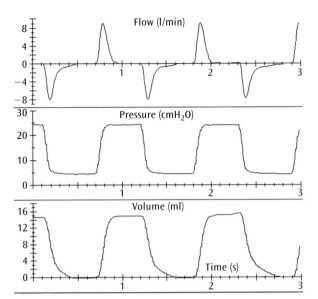

Figure 17.3 *Simultaneous time-based traces of flow, volume and pressure from a ventilated infant. With the onset of inflation, pressure rapidly rises to a peak and is maintained at this level for the duration of inspiration. As the pressure has risen, gas flows into the baby's lungs until the pressure in the lungs has equilibrated with that in the ventilator circuit. Inspiratory flow (shown above the line) is seen to rise rapidly to a peak and then fall back to zero. No further volume passes into the lungs for the remainder of the set inspiratory time. The volume trace rises rapidly to a peak and then stays at a plateau, with the inspired tidal volume held in the lungs until the onset of expiration.*

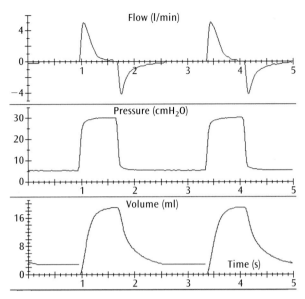

Figure 17.4 *Time-based waveforms from an infant with a modest leak around the endotracheal tube. If there is an air leak around the endotracheal tube, the volume plateau is not horizontal but slopes upward from left to right. The gradient of the slope reflects the size of the leak. Under these circumstances the flow trace does not return all the way to zero but continues at a low level after the initial rapid rise and fall. In the case of a very large leak, or when the endotracheal tube has slipped out of the trachea, the volume trace continues to rise steeply until it goes off the screen and the flow remains high throughout inspiration. Under these circumstances, little or no expiratory flow is seen at the onset of expiration.*

the waveforms due to variation in respiratory function, which would be obvious at a glance, may be obscured by the system re-drawing the waveforms on a new scale. Autoscaling should therefore only be used with caution. The time-based waveforms are helpful for determining whether inspiratory and expiratory times are appropriate (Figures 17.3 and 17.4). In human infants with RDS, fast rate, short inspiratory time ventilation is associated with fewer complications compared with slow rate, long inspiratory time ventilation.[7] In surfactant-depleted animals, shortening the inspiratory time to the point that inspiratory flow has returned to zero, thereby eliminating the inspiratory volume plateau, achieves equivalent gas exchange at lower mean airway pressure.[48] Some ventilators automate this and the term used to describe the process is termination sensitivity. In order for the automation to work in the presence of leak around the endotracheal tube, termination sensitivity switches to expiration when inspiratory flow has fallen to a low level rather than to zero (p. 167). This could result in uneven distribution of ventilation and has not yet been proven to be beneficial.

The expiratory waveforms can be analysed in a similar way. At the onset of expiration the pressure in the ventilator circuit rapidly falls to the set PEEP level. Gas now flows out

of the infant's lungs until the intrapulmonary pressure has equilibrated with the circuit pressure. The expiratory flow (conventionally displayed below the baseline) accelerates to a peak and then falls to zero (Figure 17.3). The volume trace rapidly falls from the inspiratory volume peak back to zero. If there is an air leak around the endotracheal tube, the volume trace does not return to zero because the gas that leaked around the endotracheal tube in inspiration cannot be exhaled (Figure 17.4). Monitoring devices are usually set to re-zero the volume baseline at the onset of the next inspiratory flow. If the next inflation begins before the expiratory flow has returned to zero, gas is trapped in the lungs. This means that the pressure in the lungs remains higher than the set PEEP at all times. This phenomenon is called occult PEEP or inadvertent PEEP.[78] It is common in ventilated infants and can result in impaired gas exchange. In some cases it may be life-threatening.[81] Inspection of the expired flow waveform allows the clinician to ensure that expiratory flow has returned to zero (Figure 17.3) or not (Figure 17.5) before the onset of the next inflation. If the endotracheal tube is becoming obstructed with secretions, the height of the peak flow on the inspiratory and expiratory flow

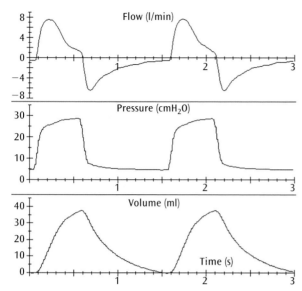

Figure 17.5 *Simultaneous waveforms from an infant with a long expiratory phase. After 1 second in expiration, expiratory flow has not reached zero before the onset of the next inflation.*

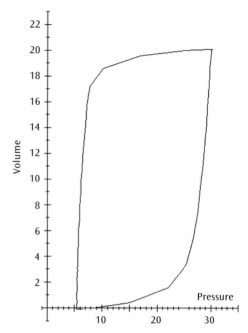

Figure 17.6 *Pressure–volume loop from an infant on pressure-limited ventilation.*

waveforms lessens, and the width of the expiratory flow pattern broadens because the increase in airway resistance makes gas movements take longer.

Excessive rain-out of humidity in the ventilator tubing can partially obstruct the bias flow in the circuit as the continuous gas flow bubbles through a column of water. This causes small fluctuations in airway pressure that result in small flow oscillations at the airway. These can be sufficient to cause autocycling of the ventilator. The fluctuations are usually visible as an oscillation of the flow baseline at times when there would otherwise usually be no flow. The presence of an oscillating flow baseline should prompt an inspection of the circuit for the site of the trapped water.

Loops

The commonest loops displayed are pressure–volume and flow–volume. Their use is difficult because many are distorted by infant–ventilator interactions, making them uninterpretable. If the screen is watched in real time, breaths that are relatively free from interaction can be identified when the infant is settled. It is suggested that pressure–volume loops can be inspected to determine the critical opening pressure of the airspaces and the upper inflection point where the slope of the pressure–volume relationship begins to flatten because of overdistention. This has been used in adults to facilitate less damaging ventilation strategies.[65] In order to plot the progressive change in lung volume that occurs for a given change in pressure, however, the pressure has to rise slowly enough to allow changes in volume to keep pace. Pressure-limited

neonatal ventilators typically generate relatively square pressure waves with a very rapid rise to peak inspiratory pressure and an equally rapid fall to the PEEP level in expiration. This means that the changes in lung volume during inspiration are mostly plotted against the peak inspiratory pressure and during expiration against the end pressure. This gives the loops a rectangular appearance that bears little or no relationship to the underlying pressure–volume characteristics of the lung (Figure 17.6). Unless the ventilator generates a slow-rise pressure waveform, pressure–volume loops should not be used. Significant leaks around the endotracheal tube make interpretation more difficult. Inspection of flow–volume loops can give information about airway resistance. If resistance is increased, flow is slower. This can readily be observed from the time-based waveforms without the need to look at flow–volume loops. If there is an excess of secretions in the endotracheal tube, the expiratory limb of the loop can show a sawtooth pattern, indicating the need for endotracheal suction.[42]

REFERENCES

1   Adelman, R.D., Morrell, R.E. (2000) Coarctation of the abdominal aorta and renal artery stenosis related to an umbilical artery catheter placement in a neonate. *Pediatrics* **106**, E36.

2   Alberdi, E., Becher, J.C., Gilhooly, K. *et al.* (1998) Decision support in the neonatal intensive care unit: expertise differences in the interpretation of monitored physiological data. In *Anonymous Proceedings of the 2nd International*

Conference on Engineering Psychology and Cognitive Ergonomics, Oxford.

3 Alberdi, E., Gilhooly, K., Hunter, J. *et al.* (2000) Computerization and decision making in neonatal intensive care: a cognitive engineering investigation. *Journal of Clinical Monitoring* **16**, 85–94.

4 Albertine, K.H., Jones, G.P., Starcher, B.C. *et al.* (1999) Chronic lung injury in preterm lambs. Disordered respiratory tract development. *American Journal of Respiratory and Critical Care Medicine* **159**, 945–958.

5 Amato, M.B., Barbas, C.S., Medeiros, D.M. *et al.* (1998) Effect of a protective-ventilation strategy on mortality in the acute respiratory distress syndrome. *New England Journal of Medicine* **338**, 347–354.

6 Anderson, J.V. (1987) The accuracy of pulse oximetry in neonates: effects of fetal hemoglobin and bilirubin. *Journal of Perinatology* **7**, 323.

7 Anonymous (1991) Multicentre randomised controlled trial of high against low frequency positive pressure ventilation. Oxford Region Controlled Trial of Artificial Ventilation OCTAVE Study Group. *Archives of Disease in Childhood* **66**, 770–775.

8 Anonymous (1993) Respiratory mechanics in infants: physiologic evaluation in health and disease. American Thoracic Society/European Respiratory Society. *American Review of Respiratory Disease* **147**, 474–496.

9 Anonymous (2000) Supplemental Therapeutic Oxygen for Prethreshold Retinopathy Of Prematurity (STOP-ROP), a randomized, controlled trial. I: Primary outcomes. *Pediatrics* **105**, 295–310.

10 Anonymous (2000) Ventilation with lower tidal volumes as compared with traditional tidal volumes for acute lung injury and the acute respiratory distress syndrome. The Acute Respiratory Distress Syndrome Network. *New England Journal of Medicine* **342**, 1301–1308.

11 Barrington, K.J. (2000) Umbilical artery catheters in the newborn: effects of catheter design (end vs side hole). Cochrane Database Systematic Review CD000508.

12 Barrington, K.J. (2000) Umbilical artery catheters in the newborn: effects of catheter materials. Cochrane Database Systematic Review CD000949.

13 Barrington, K.J. (2000) Umbilical artery catheters in the newborn: effects of heparin. Cochrane Database Systematic Review CD000507.

14 Barrington, K.J. (2000) Umbilical artery catheters in the newborn: effects of position of the catheter tip. Cochrane Database Systematic Review CD000505.

15 Binder, N., Atherton, H., Thorkelsson, T., Hoath, S.B. (1994) Measurement of transcutaneous carbon dioxide in low birthweight infants during the first two weeks of life. *American Journal of Perinatology* **11**, 237–241.

16 Bohnhorst, B., Poets, C.F. (1998) Major reduction in alarm frequency with a new pulse oximeter. *Intensive Care Medicine* **24**, 277–278.

17 Bohnhorst, B., Peter, C.S., Poets, C.F. (2000) Pulse oximeters' reliability in detecting hypoxemia and bradycardia: comparison between a conventional and two new generation oximeters. *Critical Care Medicine* **28**, 1565–1568.

18 Cannon, M.L., Cornell, J., Tripp-Hamel, D.S. *et al.* (2000) Tidal volumes for ventilated infants should be determined with a pneumotachometer placed at the endotracheal tube. *American Journal of Respiratory and Critical Care Medicine* **162**, 2109–2112.

19 Chow, L., Vanderhal, A., Raber, J., Sola, A. (1999) Tidal volume measurements in neonatal pressure control ventilation: are they meaningful? *Pediatric Research* **45**, 297A (Abstract).

20 Courtney, S.E., Weber, K.R., Breakie, L.A. *et al.* (1990) Capillary blood gases in the neonate. A reassessment and review of the literature. *American Journal of Disease of Children* **144**, 168–172.

21 Cunningham, S., Symon, A.G., McIntosh, N. (1994) Changes in mean blood pressure caused by damping of the arterial pressure waveform. *Early Human Development* **36**, 27–30.

22 Cunningham, S., Fleck, B.W., Elton, R.A., McIntosh, N. (1995) Transcutaneous oxygen levels in retinopathy of prematurity. *Lancet* **346**, 1464–1465.

23 Cunningham, S., Deere, S., Symon, A., Elton, R.A., McIntosh, N. (1998) A randomized, controlled trial of computerized physiologic trend monitoring in an intensive care unit. *Critical Care Medicine* **26**, 2053–2060.

24 Davies, M.W., Dunster, K.R. (2000) The effect of perfluorocarbon vapour on the measurement of respiratory tidal volume during partial liquid ventilation. *Physiological Measurement* **21**, N23–N30.

25 Dimitriou, G., Greenough, A., Alvares, B.R., Shute, M., Karani, J., Peacock, J. (2002) Chest radiograph lung area and oxygenation optimisation on transfer to HFO. *British Journal of Intensive Care* **11**, 78–82.

26 Dimitriou, G., Greenough, A., Sumi, K. (2002) Performance of a commercially available neonatal respiration monitor. *British Journal of Intensive Care* **11**, 42–46.

27 Dinwiddie, R., Patel, B.D., Kumar, S.P., Fox, W.W. (1979) The effects of crying on arterial oxygen tension in infants recovering from respiratory distress. *Critical Care Medicine* **7**, 50–53.

28 Dumas, C., Wahr, J.A., Tremper, K.K. (1996) Clinical evaluation of a prototype motion artifact resistant pulse oximeter in the recovery room. *Anesthesia and Analgesia* **83**, 269–272.

29 Falconer, R.J., Robinson, B.J. (1990) Comparison of pulse oximeters: accuracy at low arterial pressure in volunteers. *British Journal of Anaesthetics* **65**, 552–557.

30 Fisher, J.B., Mammel, M.C., Coleman, J.M., Bing, D.R., Boros, S.J. (1988) Identifying lung overdistension during mechanical ventilation by using volume–pressure loops. *Pediatric Pulmonology* **5**, 10–14.

31 Fujimoto, S., Togari, H., Yamaguchi, N., Mizutani, F., Suzuki, S., Sobajima, H. (1994) Hypocarbia and cystic periventricular leukomalacia in premature infants. *Archives of Disease in Childhood* **71**, F107–F110.

32 Garland, J.S., Buck, R.K., Allred, E.N., Leviton, A. (1995) Hypocarbia before surfactant therapy appears to increase bronchopulmonary dysplasia risk in infants with respiratory distress syndrome. *Archives of Pediatrics and Adolescent Medicine* **149**, 617–622.

33 Giuffre, M., Stenson, B. (1998) Evaluation of on-line respiratory function monitoring. *Pediatric Research* **44**, 456 (Abstract).

34 Goddard, P., Keith, I., Marcovitch, H., Roberton, N.R., Rolfe, P., Scopes, J.W. (1974) Use of a continuously recording intravascular oxygen electrode in the newborn. *Archives of Disease in Childhood* **49**, 853–860.

35 Golden, S.M. (1981) Skin craters – a complication of transcutaneous oxygen monitoring. *Pediatrics* **67**, 514–516.

36 Grieve, S.H., McIntosh, N., Laing, I.A. (1997) Comparison of two different pulse oximeters in monitoring preterm infants. *Critical Care Medicine* **25**, 2051–2054.

37 Hand, I.L., Shepard, E.K., Krauss, A.N., Auld, P.A. (1989) Discrepancies between transcutaneous and end-tidal carbon dioxide monitoring in the critically ill neonate with respiratory distress syndrome. *Critical Care Medicine* **17**, 556–559.

38 Herrell, N., Martin, R.J., Pultusker, M., Lough, M., Fanaroff, A. (1980) Optimal temperature for the measurement of

transcutaneous carbon dioxide tension in the neonate. *Journal of Pediatrics* **97**, 114–117.

39 Horbar, J.D., Wright, L.L., Soll, R.F. *et al.* (1993) A multicenter randomized trial comparing two surfactants for the treatment of neonatal respiratory distress syndrome. National Institute of Child Health and Human Development Neonatal Research Network. *Journal of Pediatrics* **123**, 757–766.

40 Hunt, C.E., Corwin, M.J., Lister, G. *et al.* (1999) Longitudinal assessment of hemoglobin oxygen saturation in healthy infants during the first 6 months of age. Collaborative Home Infant Monitoring Evaluation (CHIME) Study Group. *Journal of Pediatrics* **135**, 580–586.

41 Iles, R., Edmunds, A.T. (1996) Prediction of early outcome in resolving chronic lung disease of prematurity after discharge from hospital. *Archives of Disease in Childhood* **74**, 304–308.

42 Jubran, A., Tobin, M.J. (1994) Use of flow-volume curves in detecting secretions in ventilator-dependent patients. *American Journal of Respiratory and Critical Care Medicine* **150**, 766–769.

43 Kavvadia, V., Greenough, A., Dimitriou, G., Forsling, M. (1998) Comparison of respiratory function and fluid balance in very low birthweight infants given artificial or natural surfactant or no surfactant treatment. *Journal of Perinatal Medicine* **26**, 469–474.

44 Kempley, S.T., Gamsu, H.R. (1992) Randomized trial of umbilical arterial catheter position: Doppler ultrasound findings. *Archives of Disease in Childhood* **67**, 855–859.

45 Kempley, S.T., Bennett, S., Loftus, B.G., Cooper, D., Gamsu, H.R. (1993) Randomized trial of umbilical arterial catheter position: clinical outcome. *Acta Paediatrica* **82**, 173–176.

46 Lambert, H.J., Baylis, P.H., Coulthard, M.G. (1998) Central–peripheral temperature difference, blood pressure, and arginine vasopressin in preterm neonates undergoing volume expansion. *Archives of Disease in Childhood* **78**, F43–F45.

47 Lofgren, O., Jacobson, L. (1979) The influence of different electrode temperatures on the recorded transcutaneous Po_2 level. *Pediatrics* **64**, 892–897.

48 Mammel, M.C., Boros, S.J., Bing, D.R., Holloman, K.K., Connet, J.R. (1989) Determining optimum inspiratory time during intermittent positive pressure ventilation in surfactant depleted cats. *Pediatric Pulmonology* **7**, 223–229.

49 McIntosh, N., Becher, J.C., Cunningham, S. *et al.* (2000) Clinical diagnosis of pneumothorax is late: use of trend data and decision support might allow preclinical detection. *Pediatric Research* **48**, 408–415.

50 McLain, B.I., Evans, J., Dear, P.R. (1988) Comparison of capillary and arterial blood gas measurements in neonates. *Archives of Disease in Childhood* **63**, 743–747.

51 Mok, Q., Bass, C.A., Ducker, D.A., McIntosh, N. (1991) Temperature instability during nursing procedures in preterm neonates. *Archives of Disease in Childhood* **66**, 783–786.

52 Morgan, C., Newell, S.J., Ducker, D.A. *et al.* (1999) Continuous neonatal blood gas monitoring using a multiparameter intra-arterial sensor. *Archives of Disease in Childhood* **80**, F93–F98.

53 Morris, R.W., Nairn, M., Torda, T.A. (1989) A comparison of fifteen pulse oximeters. Part I: A clinical comparison; Part II: A test of performance under conditions of poor perfusion. *Anaesthesia and Intensive Care* **17**, 62–73.

54 Neve, V., de la Roque, E.D., Leclerc, F. *et al.* (2000) Ventilator-induced overdistension in children: dynamic versus low-flow inflation volume–pressure curves.

American Journal of Respiratory and Critical Care Medicine **162**, 139–147.

55 Ng, A., Subhedar, N., Primhak, R.A., Shaw, N.J. (1998) Arterial oxygen saturation profiles in healthy preterm infants. *Archives of Disease in Childhood* **79**, F64–F66.

56 O'Connor, T.A., Grueber, R. (1998) Transcutaneous measurement of carbon dioxide tension during long-distance transport of neonates receiving mechanical ventilation. *Journal of Perinatology* **18**, 189–192.

57 Poets, C.F. (1998) When do infants need additional inspired oxygen? A review of the current literature. *Pediatric Pulmonology* **26**, 424–428.

58 Poets, C.F. (1999) Assessing oxygenation in healthy infants. *Journal of Pediatrics* **135**, 541–543.

59 Poets, C.F., Southall, D.P. (1994) Noninvasive monitoring of oxygenation in infants and children: practical considerations and areas of concern. *Pediatrics* **93**, 737–746.

60 Poets, C.F., Stebbens, V.A. (1997) Detection of movement artifact in recorded pulse oximeter saturation. *European Journal of Pediatrics* **156**, 808–811.

61 Poets, C.F., Samuels, M.P., Noyes, J.P., Jones, K.A., Southall, D.P. (1991) Home monitoring of transcutaneous oxygen tension in the early detection of hypoxemia in infants and young children. *Archives of Disease in Childhood* **66**, 676–682.

62 Poets, C.F., Stebbens, V.A., Alexander, J.R., Arrowsmith, W.A., Salfield, S.A., Southall, D.P. (1991) Oxygen saturation and breathing patterns in infancy. 2: Preterm infants at discharge from special care. *Archives of Disease in Childhood* **66**, 574–578.

63 Poets, C.F., Stebbens, V.A., Alexander, J.R., Arrowsmith, W.A., Salfield, S.A., Southall, D.P. (1992) Arterial oxygen saturation in preterm infants at discharge from the hospital and six weeks later. *Journal of Pediatrics* **120**, 447–454.

64 Rajadurai, V.S., Walker, A.M., Yu, V.Y., Oates, A. (1992) Effect of fetal haemoglobin on the accuracy of pulse oximetry in preterm infants. *Journal of Paediatrics and Child Health* **28**, 43–46.

65 Ranieri, V.M., Suter, P.M., Tortorella, C. *et al.* (1999) Effect of mechanical ventilation on inflammatory mediators in patients with acute respiratory distress syndrome: a randomized controlled trial. *Journal of the American Medical Association* **282**, 54–61.

66 Richard, D., Poets, C.F., Neale, S., Stebbens, V.A., Alexander, J.R., Southall, D.P. (1993) Arterial oxygen saturation in preterm neonates without respiratory failure. *Journal of Pediatrics* **123**, 963–968.

67 Roberts, W.A., Maniscalco, W.M., Cohen, A.R., Litman, R.S., Chhibber, A. (1995) The use of capnography for recognition of esophageal intubation in the neonatal intensive care unit. *Pediatric Pulmonology* **19**, 262–268.

68 Roll, C., Huning, B., Kaunicke, M., Krug, J., Horsch, S. (2000) Umbilical artery catheter blood sampling decreases cerebral blood volume and oxygenation in very low birthweight infants. *Acta Paediatrica* **89**, 862–866.

69 Rome, E.S., Stork, E.K., Carlo, W.A., Martin, R.J. (1984) Limitations of transcutaneous PO_2 and PCO_2 monitoring in infants with bronchopulmonary dysplasia. *Pediatrics* **74**, 217–220.

70 Rooth, G., Huch, A., Huch, R. (1987) Transcutaneous oxygen monitors are reliable indicators of arterial oxygen tension (if used correctly). *Pediatrics* **79**, 283–286.

71 Rosen, W.C., Mammel, M.C., Fisher, J.B. *et al.* (1993) The effects of bedside pulmonary mechanics testing during infant mechanical ventilation: a retrospective analysis. *Pediatric Pulmonology* **16**, 147–152.

72 Rosenfeld, W., Biagtan, J., Schaeffer, H. *et al.* (1980) A new graph for insertion of umbilical artery catheters. *Journal of Pediatrics* **96**, 735–737.

73 Rozycki, H.J., Sysyn, G.D., Marshall, M.K., Malloy, R., Wiswell, T.E. (1998) Mainstream end-tidal carbon dioxide monitoring in the neonatal intensive care unit. *Pediatrics* **101**, 648–653.

74 Rubin, B.K., McRobert, E., O'Neill, M.B. (1986) An alternate technique to determine umbilical arterial catheter length. *Clinical Pediatrics* **25**, 407–408.

75 Saugstad, O.D. (2001) Update on oxygen radical disease in neonatology. *Current Opinion in Obstetrics and Gynecology* **13**, 147–153.

76 Scalfaro, P., Cotting, J., Sly, P.D. (2000) *In vitro* assessment of an ultrasonic flowmeter for use in ventilated infants. *European Respiratory Journal* **15**, 566–569.

77 Severinghaus, J.W., Spellman, M.J.J. (1990) Pulse oximeter failure thresholds in hypotension and vasoconstriction. *Anesthesiology* **73**, 532–537.

78 Simbruner, G. (1986) Inadvertent positive end-expiratory pressure in mechanically ventilated newborn infants: detection and effect on lung mechanics and gas exchange. *Journal of Pediatrics* **108**, 589–595.

79 Spencer, S.A., Dimmock, P.W., Brookfield, D.S.K. (2000) Survey in current neonatal practice in relation to preterm monitoring. *Journal of Clinical Excellence* **2**, 15–27.

80 Stebbens, V.A., Poets, C.F., Alexander, J.R., Arrowsmith, W.A., Southall, D.P. (1991) Oxygen saturation and breathing patterns in infancy. 1: Full term infants in the second month of life. *Archives of Disease in Childhood* **66**, 569–573.

81 Stenson, B.J., Glover, R.M., Wilkie, R.A., Laing, I.A., Tarnow-Mordi, W.O. (1995) Life-threatening inadvertent positive end-expiratory pressure. *American Journal of Perinatology* **12**, 336–338.

82 Stenson, B.J., Glover, R.M., Wilkie, R.A., Laing, I.A., Tarnow-Mordi, W.O. (1998) Randomised controlled trial of respiratory system compliance measurements in mechanically ventilated neonates. *Archives of Disease in Childhood* **78**, F15–F19.

83 Stokes, G.M., Milner, A.D., Wilson, A.J., Morgan, D.B., Carman, P.G., Oliver, M.R. (1986) Ventilatory response to increased dead spaces in the first week of life. *Pediatric Pulmonology* **2**, 89–93.

84 Strozik, K.S., Pieper, C.H., Roller, J. (1997) Capillary refilling time in newborn infants: normal values. *Archives of Disease in Childhood* **76**, F193–F196.

85 Szymonowicz, W., Yu, V.Y., Wilson, F.E. (1984) Antecedents of periventricular hemorrhage in infants weighing 1250 g or less at birth. *Archives of Disease in Childhood* **59**, 13–17.

86 Takiwaki, H., Nakanishi, H., Shono, Y., Arase, S. (1991) The influence of cutaneous factors on the transcutaneous pO_2 and pCO_2 at various body sites. *British Journal of Dermatology* **125**, 243–247.

87 Thome, U., Topfer, A., Schaller, P., Pohlandt, F. (1998) Comparison of lung volume measurements by antero-posterior chest X-ray and the SF6 washout technique in mechanically ventilated infants. *Pediatric Pulmonology* **26**, 265–272.

88 Tin, W., Milligan, D.W., Pennefather, P., Hey, E. (2001) Pulse oximetry, severe retinopathy, and outcome at one year in babies of less than 28 weeks gestation. *Archives of Disease in Childhood* **84**, F106–F110.

89 Tobias, J.D., Meyer, D.J. (1997) Noninvasive monitoring of carbon dioxide during respiratory failure in toddlers and infants: end-tidal versus transcutaneous carbon dioxide. *Anesthesia and Analgesia* **85**, 55–58.

90 Vanderhal, A., Chow, L., Raber, J., Sola, A. (1999) Tidal volume measurements in neonates: are they reliable? *Pediatric Research* **45**, 324A (Abstract).

91 Vanderhal, A., Chow, L.C., Raber, J., Sola, A. (2001) Accuracy of tidal volume measurement in neonatal ventilators (using a disposable heated wire neonatal ventilator circuit). *Pediatric Research* **49**, 416A (Abstract).

92 Vyas, H., Helms, P., Cheriyan, G. (1988) Transcutaneous oxygen monitoring beyond the neonatal period. *Critical Care Medicine* **16**, 844–847.

93 Wada, K., Jobe, A.H., Ikegami, M. (1997) Tidal volume effects on surfactant treatment responses with the initiation of ventilation in preterm lambs. *Journal of Applied Physiology* **83**, 1054–1061.

94 Wilson, B.J.J., Becker, M.A., Linton, M.E., Donn, S.M. (1998) Spontaneous minute ventilation predicts readiness for extubation in mechanically ventilated preterm infants. *Journal of Perinatology* **18**, 436–439.

95 Yeh, M.P., Adams, T.D., Gardner, R.M., Yanowitz, F.G. (1984) Effect of O_2, N_2, and CO_2 composition on nonlinearity of Fleisch pneumotachograph characteristics. *Journal of Applied Physiology* **56**, 1423–1425.

18

Physiotherapy

ANNETTE PARKER AND ANNE GREENOUGH

Physiotherapy is frequently used in neonatal units as part of respiratory management.[54] Careful assessment by staff qualified and experienced in the use of physiotherapy techniques is essential prior to any intervention. The techniques have possible detrimental effects and, as a consequence, should not be used routinely. The physiotherapy techniques used in the treatment of neonates are similar to those used in adults, but it may not be appropriate to extrapolate the results of studies involving adults to the newborn. Respiratory physiotherapy has rarely been investigated in the neonate. In those studies which have been performed, a full description of the physiotherapy techniques used is frequently lacking and the infants have often been of greater gestational age and weight than the majority of infants nursed in neonatal units today.[18]

HUMIDIFICATION

Inadequate humidification of the inspired gases of an intubated infant can cause tracheobronchial secretions to become more viscous and reduces mucociliary clearance.[74] This may lead to mucus plugging of small airways and blockage of the endotracheal tube. Lomholt et al., using a thermocouple in the inspiratory tube, found that endotracheal tube blockage was ten times less likely to occur and frequent suction unnecessary when humidity was consistently kept above 70 percent of body humidity.[49] Over-humidification, however, may result in pyrexia and fluid overload.[75] Most neonatal ventilators are used in conjunction with heated humidifiers in the ventilator circuit. The amount of humidity received by the infant is dependent upon the temperature of the humidifier, the ambient room and incubator temperature, the gas flow rate, the level of water in the humidifier chamber, the length of ventilator tubing and the position of the temperature probe in the ventilator circuit.[76] It has been claimed that the incidence of pneumothorax and chronic lung disease in infants weighing less than 1500 g may be reduced when a humidifier temperature greater than 36.5°C is used.[76]

SUCTIONING

Suctioning of intubated patients is required to maintain a clear airway, but it is a potentially hazardous technique.[84] Hypoxia, trauma, atelectasis, pneumothorax and raised blood and intracranial pressure are all recognized side-effects of suctioning.[61,84] Elevation of blood and intracranial pressure may be secondary to hypoxia and hypercapnia,[84] directly related to tracheal stimulation or the associated increase in intrathoracic pressure.[22] These effects are less common in paralyzed and sedated infants.[24]

Hypoxia following suctioning has been well documented[45,59,69,72] and incriminated in the causation of cardiac arrhythmias[71] and bradycardia,[72] although the latter may also be due to vagal stimulation.[44] The adverse effect of suctioning on heart rate and oxygenation do not depend on the ventilation mode.[47] Cerebral hemodynamics, as assessed by non-invasive near-infrared spectroscopy, were also similarly affected by suctioning (as evidenced by a decrease in the cerebral concentration of oxygenated hemoglobin and an increase in deoxygenated hemoglobin) during high-frequency oscillation (HFO) and conventional mechanical ventilation (CMV).[47] The etiology of the hypoxia may be multifactorial, including removal from the oxygen source, suction-induced atelectasis and reflex bronchoconstriction.[53] The length of time the patient is disconnected from the ventilator affects the degree of hypoxia, thus the suctioning time should be kept to a minimum. The maximum suctioning time for a term neonate should be 15 seconds and 7–10 seconds for a preterm infant. In many neonatal nurseries, adaptors are used which allow suctioning while the infant remains connected to the ventilator. This modification has been demonstrated to reduce the hypoxia associated with suctioning.[38] In a crossover study involving 12 premature infants,[8] closed compared to open suctioning was associated with a smaller deterioration in their oxygen saturation levels and a trend towards a faster recovery of heart rate and saturation levels.

Some method of preoxygenation may be necessary to prevent suctioning-induced hypoxia.[68] In the preterm infant, however, preoxygenation should be used cautiously, as it is imperative to avoid hyperoxia and the attendant risk of retinopathy of prematurity.[33] Inspired oxygen levels should be carefully increased prior to suctioning in those infants who are already hypoxic to bring their arterial oxygen levels to a satisfactory level. Preterm infants who are well oxygenated should only have their inspired oxygen concentration (FiO_2) increased by 10 percent, for example 30 percent to 40 percent immediately prior to passing the suction catheter. Following suctioning, the FiO_2 can again be increased if the infant continues to be hypoxic. Once recovery begins, the inspired oxygen should be reduced to the pretreatment level to avoid a swing into hyperoxia.

Tracheobronchial trauma has long been recognized as a hazard of suctioning.[60] Prolonged tracheobronchial trauma leads to destruction and ulceration of the ciliated epithelium. This is repaired by formation of granulation and fibrous tissue, which may cause bronchial obstruction leading to segmental or lobar collapse.[52] Pneumothorax secondary to perforation of a segmental bronchus has been reported in several studies.[3,4,80] The infants at greatest risk are those with severe lung disease, although poor suction technique is also implicated. The risk of perforation and mucosal trauma can be reduced by passing catheters to only 1 cm past the end of the endotracheal tube.[5,46] Suction catheters with graduations which correspond to markings on endotracheal tubes are available. The amount of trauma depends on the frequency of suction, the size and type of catheter used, the vigor of insertion and the magnitude of applied negative pressure employed.[84] Trauma to the mucosa, however, has been described after just one pass of the catheter[84] and insertion and passing of the catheter should always be gentle

and without application of negative pressure. If a resistance is met, the catheter should be withdrawn 0.5–1 cm before negative pressure is applied to avoid invagination of mucosa.

There are many different types of catheter available. The optimum catheter should have a smooth end and be neither too rigid nor so soft that it becomes easily misshapen and difficult to pass. There should be small side holes to act as pressure relief outlets when the end hole becomes totally occluded.[84] The combined diameter of the side holes, however, must be less than the diameter of the end hole or the suction pressure will be applied through the side holes rather than the end holes and this will reduce the effectiveness of suctioning and increase trauma from invagination of the mucosa into the side holes. Large catheters can increase tracheobronchial trauma due to greater mucosal contact. A large catheter wedged into a small bronchus may, in addition, cause airway collapse and atelectasis when suction is applied.[84] Ideally, the diameter of the catheter should be less than 70 percent of the internal diameter of the narrowest part of the endotracheal tube.[73] Practically, the smallest, but effective catheter is size 6FG.

Neonates should only be suctioned with catheters that have control valves or are used with a 'Y' connector. Catheters without these modifications have to be pinched or bent over during insertion to prevent application of negative pressure; this results in a build-up of negative pressure, which is suddenly transmitted to the airway when the catheter is released.[84] The amount of applied negative pressure is also relevant to tracheobronchial trauma; the higher the negative pressure the greater the tissue damage[70] and atelectasis.[73] The negative pressure, however, needs to be high enough to aspirate secretions up narrow-bore catheters. It has been suggested that the maximum pressure that should be used is between 100 and 150 mmHg, but in clinical practice this may need to be increased to 200 mmHg if the secretions are very viscid.[84] An intermittent suction technique has been advocated when using higher negative pressures to avoid prolonged pressure build-up but, if this is done too rapidly, it is ineffective in removing secretions and sudden release of pressure can cause mucosal trauma.[42] A careful controlled reduction of pressure by partially removing the thumb from the control port is a more effective technique.[42]

Upper airway secretions should be cleared by nasopharyngeal suction in non-ventilated infants as these may cause apneic spells.[58] Vigorous nasopharyngeal suction immediately after delivery, however, may result in apnea and bradycardia.[11] Care must also be taken when suctioning an infant who has recently been extubated as irritation of the larynx may exacerbate laryngeal edema. Suctioning reduces respiratory resistance, if there are retained secretions.[62] It is also necessary in intubated infants to clear secretions and thus reduce the risk of tube blockage and apneic spells.[58] The reported hazardous side-effects are such (see above) that it should never be performed on a routine basis.

LAVAGE

In many neonatal units, suctioning of the endotracheal tube is commonly preceded by instillation of a diluent or mucolytic. The solutions are instilled directly into the endotracheal tube or via a suction catheter.[17] The solution is likely to reach only the trachea and major bronchi.[39] In unparalyzed infants, instillation of the diluent often stimulates a cough which may encourage movement of secretions up the bronchial tree. This practice is thought to facilitate removal of secretions and therefore avoid blockage of the endotracheal tube, but the literature supporting this is relatively limited. The results of a trial, in which 86 infants intubated and ventilated for respiratory distress syndrome (RDS) were randomized to receive or not to receive saline prior to suctioning, demonstrated that routine instillation of saline was necessary only when the endotracheal tube size was 2.5 mm or less.[20] Routine instillation of a diluent or mucolytic is less important when infants are systemically well hydrated and there is efficient humidification of the inspired gases.[1]

Normal saline (0.9 percent sodium chloride solution) is the most commonly used diluent, but some units use N-acetylcysteine solution as a mucolytic. The mucolytic effect of N-acetylcysteine is thought to be due to its action of breakage of the disulfide links in mucus. There is, however, no clinical evidence for its effectiveness when used as a solution for instillation down endotracheal tubes and important side-effects have been described. The 5 percent aerosol solution completely inactivates penicillin and cephalosporins *in vitro* and the 10 percent aerosol solution has been shown to cause bronchoconstriction when inhaled by asthmatics.[57] The intravenous solution used to treat acetaminophen (paracetamol) overdose can cause hypersensitivity reactions.[57] In view of these side-effects, routine use of N-acetylcysteine should be avoided.

POSITIONING

Body position affects ventilation–perfusion matching and arterial oxygen levels. The prone position improves arterial oxygen levels in the newborn; the supine position is the least beneficial.[14] Unlike adults, neonates and young children preferentially ventilate the uppermost areas of their lung.[13] The head-up tilt position is associated with an increase in the transcutaneous arterial oxygen tension in spontaneously breathing infants.[77] If, however, the infant is left in one position for long periods of time, pooling of secretions and atelectasis tend to occur in dependent lung areas. In infants, the area of lung most commonly affected by retention of secretions and lobar collapse is the right upper lobe, particularly following extubation.[73] Regular position changes ensure that the uppermost areas of lung are periodically drained and preferentially ventilated.

Gravity-assisted positioning (postural drainage) involves placing infants in specific positions, thereby allowing gravity to aid drainage of secretions from different areas of the lung (Figure 18.1). It is often not practical to drain the apical segments of the upper lobes in infants who are intubated. The middle and lower lung zones are drained by placing the infant in the head-down position. This position is often poorly tolerated by spontaneously breathing infants, particularly those born prematurely who show a fall in transcutaneous PaO_2.[77] This effect is less marked when infants are fully mechanically ventilated. The head-down position also impairs venous return, which causes intracranial pressure to rise, thereby increasing the risk of intraventricular hemorrhage. In addition, it is ill-tolerated by infants with abdominal distention and may increase the risk of reflux.

Gravity-assisted positioning of the right lung consists of turning the infant on to the left side and vice versa. Specific gravity-assisted positioning may not be appropriate in sick neonates, particularly the very preterm. Infants

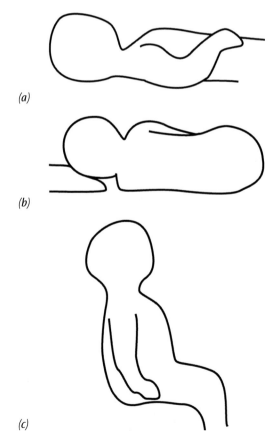

(a)

(b)

(c)

Figure 18.1 *Positioning for right upper lobe drainage: (a) anterior segment; (b) posterior segment – shoulder should be turned forwards into prone; (c) apical segment.*

who have unilateral lung disease may not tolerate the affected lung being uppermost for drainage of secretions. Treatment may need to be carried out in the prone position and the infant nursed with the unaffected lung uppermost in order to optimize gas exchange.[13] There should be regular changes of position from prone to alternate side lying for infants who can tolerate those positions. Care should be taken to position infants with a view to preventing future postural deformities.[19] Conventional postural therapy is associated with 12–24 changes per day. There is some evidence to suggest that more frequent postural changes might further improve pulmonary function.[51,66]

CHEST PERCUSSION

Chest percussion (clapping) is used to move secretions from peripheral to central airways so that they can be removed by coughing or suction. Percussion can be as effective as bronchoscopy in clearing lobar collapse when this is due to mucus plugging.[31,50] It is, however, only effective in patients who produce copious amounts of sputum.[32] In patients with minimal amounts of sputum, chest percussion can cause a fall in arterial oxygen tension.[10] Indeed, percussion is frequently associated with an increase in heart rate and desaturations.[2,21,29,41]

In full-term infants, percussion can be carried out using the cupped hand. The middle three fingers in a tenting position should be used for preterm infants. Various padded, cup-shaped objects, for example a face mask (Figure 18.2), have been used for percussion in preterm infants. Contact-heel percussion using the thenar and hypothenar eminences is used, but it is not widely taught or used in the United Kingdom. Contact-heel percussion combined with postural drainage, however, may be more effective than postural drainage alone.[25] Contact-heel percussion, face mask percussion and vibrations with the electric toothbrush were compared in 15 infants (median gestational age of 31 weeks and

median birthweight of 1537 g).[78] Arterial oxygen tension increased following contact-heel and face mask percussion. The greatest effect was with face mask percussion. The electric toothbrush vibration technique did not improve oxygenation.

VIBRATION

The vibratory technique is applied with the fingertips during expiration and moves secretions up the bronchial tree. Vibrations to the left side of the chest can provide external cardiac massage. This technique is particularly effective in moving secretions in neonates, because of the compliant chest wall, but it may not be tolerated by the very preterm infant. It is less useful in infants who are breathing or being ventilated at very fast rates, because of the short expiratory time. Vibrations increase intrathoracic pressure, which reduces venous return to the heart thereby lowering cardiac output[48] and raising intracranial pressure.[34]

Precautions to be taken when performing chest percussion or vibration

Percussion with the hand or fingertips should always be performed over clothing or a sheet to reduce the risk of skin damage. Face masks should have a soft plastic cuff and other cup-shaped objects should be well padded. Percussion and vibrations should not be applied over surgical incisions and their use should be avoided in infants with osteoporosis and those born very preterm whose skin is fragile and liable to bruise easily. Percussion and vibrations have been implicated as a cause of rib fractures (p. 513)[35] and associated with the formation of periosteal new bone formation.[83] Percussion is probably better tolerated and more useful than vibrations in preterm infants, but should only be used if the infant has large amounts of secretions or lobar collapse due to mucus plugging.

MANUAL HYPERINFLATION

Manual hyperinflation, when used as a physiotherapy technique, consists of a large volume, slow inspiration followed by rapid release of pressure to propel secretions up the bronchial tree on expiration. It is frequently performed in conjunction with vibration. This technique is used to inflate areas of collapse, loosen secretions and fully expand areas of lung in ventilated patients who are only receiving tidal volume breaths. It is, however, less useful in infants, than in older children or adults, as the collateral ventilation which allows diffusion of air between bronchioles and alveoli is not well developed in the newborn.[44] Gas under

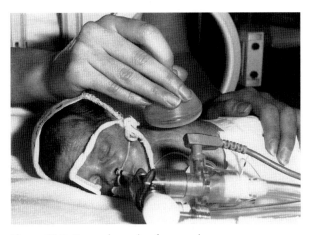

Figure 18.2 *Percussion using face mask.*

positive pressure takes the line of least resistance, so collapsed areas of lung will tend to remain collapsed, while being surrounded by areas of hyperinflation. Manual hyperinflation increases the risk of barotrauma, leading to pulmonary interstitial emphysema (PIE) or pneumothorax. It also can increase intrathoracic pressure, reducing venous return; this causes a rise in intracranial pressure and a drop in cardiac output which may impair oxygenation.[36]

Manual hyperinflation should not be used in preterm infants and only with great caution in full-term babies. It may result in a more rapid return in oxygenation to pre-physiotherapy levels.[30] If hyperinflation is used, the peak inspiratory pressures (PIPs) should be limited to no more than 20 percent above the PIP of the preceding mechanical ventilation. Pressure should be monitored throughout by a manometer in the bagging circuit.[43] Detrimental effects can be reduced by giving one large hyperinflation interspersed with three to four tidal volume breaths.[44]

ROUTINE VERSUS INDIVIDUALIZED PHYSIOTHERAPY

Comparison of 2-hourly chest physiotherapy and suction with suction alone for the clearance of secretions in infants in whom the clinician deemed there was a 'secretion problem requiring physiotherapy' highlighted that significantly more secretions were aspirated when physiotherapy was performed prior to suction.[23] The study, however, included only six infants. A subsequent study suggested routine physiotherapy was not well tolerated by certain individuals. Fifteen infants with a median birthweight of 1831 g and gestational age 32 weeks tolerated physiotherapy better at 5 than at 3 days of age.[27] Post-physiotherapy oxygenation improved progressively from day 3 to day 5. A third study, which included children who had undergone cardiac surgery,[67] indicated that routine chest physiotherapy was associated with more atelectasis on chest radiograph than breathing exercises, coughing or suction alone.

COMPLICATIONS OF PHYSIOTHERAPY

Chest physiotherapy has been associated with a number of important complications. These include intraventricular hemorrhage,[64] multiple rib fractures,[63] and a generalized periosteal reaction.[83] Physiotherapy may also increase the risk of encephaloclastic porencephaly. In a New Zealand nursery, physiotherapy using a soft latex face mask was suspected to have caused the death of five babies and brain damage in another eight infants.[9] Subsequently, a retrospective study was undertaken of 454 VLBW infants; 13 were identified who had developed encephaloclastic porencephaly. Comparison with 26 infants matched for birthweight and gestational age demonstrated that the

infants with porencephaly had received two to three times more (median 79 versus 19) treatments of chest physiotherapy in the second, third and fourth weeks than the controls. The infants with porencephaly were also more likely to have had a breech presentation and suffer hypotension. Once chest physiotherapy was no longer routinely given to VLBW infants during the first month after birth, no further cases of encephaloclastic porencephaly were identified, although the incidence of hypotension and breech presentation had not changed.[40] It was suggested that head movements during physiotherapy might be responsible for the lesions.[9] The pathological findings were consistent with those seen in older infants with shaking injuries. In addition, once the infant's head was held steady during chest physiotherapy, fewer cases of porencephaly were experienced.[9] Others have reported they could find no evidence that chest physiotherapy was associated with abnormal neurological outcome in extremely preterm infants.[6] In that unit, however, only 45 percent of the infants received physiotherapy and the chest physiotherapy was provided by trained physiotherapists. In addition, chest physiotherapy was reserved for infants with secretions causing obstruction to the airway or for babies with evidence of collapse and/or consolidation.

Thus, individualized care is most appropriate and only after careful and thorough assessment. Physiotherapy should never be undertaken routinely, but only when there are clear indications and the infant is in a fit state to tolerate physiotherapy.[9] Suction should only be performed if secretions are present and other physiotherapy techniques added only if suction is ineffective or there is lobar collapse.

CLINICAL INDICATIONS FOR PHYSIOTHERAPY

Lobar or lung collapse

Lobar or lung collapse, caused by mucus plugging, is a strong indication for physiotherapy (Figure 18.3). Positioning and percussion are the techniques of choice providing they are tolerated by the infant. Lobar collapse due to other etiologies, for example severe PIE in adjacent lung tissue or bronchomalacia, will not respond to physiotherapy.

Meconium aspiration

If initial attempts to remove meconium at delivery have been unsuccessful, then physiotherapy is essential.[12,55] Positioning and vigorous percussion should be given as soon as possible, preferably within 1 hour of aspiration.[56] Physiotherapy is usually well tolerated in these infants who are mature. Arterial oxygenation frequently improves during treatment as plugs of meconium are removed.

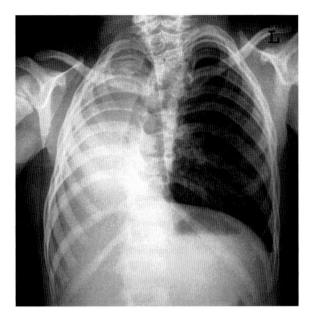

Figure 18.3 *Mucus plugging of right main bronchus resulting in collapse of the right lung; this was cleared by appropriate positioning and physiotherapy.*

If early treatment is not given, plugs of meconium cause partial obstruction of the small airways, leading to air trapping, increasing the risk of air leak. Later, a chemical pneumonitis develops which, being an inflammatory reaction, is unresponsive to physiotherapy. At that time, infants are often acutely unwell and tolerate handling badly; physiotherapy is therefore then not indicated and suction should only be given as required. Resolution of the pneumonitis may result in an increase of secretions, at which stage percussion and vibrations help removal of secretions if suction alone is unsuccessful.

Aspiration of feed/vomit

Infants who have aspirated feed or vomit should be suctioned immediately to clear the airway. If it is thought that aspiration into the small airways has occurred, then appropriate positioning and percussion should be commenced as soon as possible. Following aspiration, chemical pneumonitis will occur unless the aspirate is removed swiftly. Further physiotherapy treatment is as for meconium aspiration.

Physiotherapy may be unsatisfactory in patients with recurrent aspiration due to gastroesophageal reflux. Techniques of positioning, percussion and vibrations used to clear secretions may exacerbate existing gastroesophageal reflux. To avoid this, treatment should not be given in the horizontal or head-down positions and nasal, rather than oropharyngeal, suction should be used.[15] Physiotherapy should always be prior to feeds and never immediately afterwards. At least 1 hour should elapse after the end of a feed prior to any treatment. In some cases, the benefit

of physiotherapy is outweighed by increased reflux and aspiration.

Pneumonia

Physiotherapy is frequently requested for the infant with pneumonia. If, however, the pneumonia is in the inflammatory, consolidated phase, it is non-productive and physiotherapy is of no benefit.[7,37,79] As consolidation resolves, the infant may have secretions and appropriate positioning and percussion may be helpful if tolerated.

Postoperatively

Reduction of functional residual capacity, decreased mucociliary clearance due to immobility and the effects of anesthesia predispose the postoperative infant to atelectasis and retention of secretions.[44] Regular position changes are important, although this may not be possible in those patients who are cardiovascularly unstable or in infants with omphalocele where primary repair of the defect has not been possible. If secretion retention has been identified as a problem, then percussion may assist in removal if suction alone is ineffective. Specific positioning will be required if there is lobar collapse.

Meconium ileus

A large proportion of infants with meconium ileus suffer from cystic fibrosis.[16] If surgical intervention is necessary, the infant will require intensive physiotherapy postoperatively as copious amounts of viscid secretions are often present. Treatment will need to be given to all areas of lung so positioning, percussion and suction are required. Following resolution of the postoperative problems, positioning and percussion should continue unless the infant does not have cystic fibrosis.[56] If the diagnosis of cystic fibrosis is confirmed, then physiotherapy should be continued at least once a day, even if the chest is clear. Infants who continue to produce excess secretions should have physiotherapy two to three times daily. Parents and other relatives should be taught appropriate techniques, preferably by a physiotherapist experienced in the management of cystic fibrosis patients.

Chronic lung disease

Infants with chronic lung disease may have persistent problems with increased secretions and so positioning with percussion may be helpful in assisting removal. Wheeze and airway collapse, however, are also frequent problems in chronic lung disease and these are aggravated by physiotherapy techniques which increase intrathoracic pressure. Thus, careful assessment of the effects of physiotherapy in an individual patient is necessary to indicate if and when physiotherapy is beneficial.

Peri-extubation

It has been suggested that post-extubation physiotherapy prevented atelectasis.[26,81] The results of more recent studies, however, have questioned whether peri-extubation physiotherapy has a useful role. No benefit was demonstrated in a randomized trial.[2] Meta-analysis[28] of three randomized trials[2,25,26,81] confirmed that active chest physiotherapy was not associated with a reduction in post-extubation lobar collapse (relative risk 0.69, 95 percent CI 0.33–1.45), but a reduction in the need for reintubation (relative risk 0.24, 95 percent CI 0.08–0.78). Insufficient data were available to assess other short- and long-term outcomes, including adverse effects. Following extubation, infants are often at their most fragile and, particularly those born prematurely, are unlikely to tolerate frequent handling. Individual assessment is necessary to determine whether physiotherapy should be instigated rather than relying on rigid regimes.

CONTRAINDICATIONS TO PHYSIOTHERAPY

Respiratory distress syndrome

There is no place for physiotherapy in early, uncomplicated RDS as the main problem is lack of surfactant, with secretions being scant. Infrequent suctioning, that is 12-hourly, is sufficient to maintain a clear airway in early RDS.[82] Routine chest physiotherapy in the first 24 hours after birth has been associated with an increased incidence of grade III to IV intraventricular hemorrhage, when compared to suction alone.[65]

Pulmonary hemorrhage (Chapter 25)

Percussion and vibration are likely to prevent clotting and exacerbate bleeding, so are contraindicated in acute pulmonary hemorrhage. Instead, careful position changes and gentle suctioning to maintain a clear airway should be given, but as infrequently as possible. When fresh blood is no longer being aspirated and the secretions produced are brown and tenacious, then percussion and vibrations may be helpful to assist clearance. If, however, fresh blood is again aspirated, treatment should be discontinued.

Tracheo- and bronchomalacia

The floppy airways of infants with tracheo- and bronchomalacia will easily collapse if intrathoracic pressure increases, for example, during percussion and vibration or if a high negative pressure is used on suctioning. Careful positioning in affected infants may aid drainage if secretions retention is a problem.

REFERENCES

1 Ackerman, M.H. (1985) The use of bolus normal saline installations in artificial airways: is it useful or necessary? *Heart and Lung* **14**, 505–506.

2 Al-Alaiyan, S., Dyer, D., Khan, B. (1996) Chest physiotherapy and post-extubation atelectasis in infants. *Pediatric Pulmonology* **21**, 227–230.

3 Alpan, G., Glick, B., Peleg, O. *et al.* (1984) Pneumothorax due to endotracheal tube suction. *American Journal of Perinatology* **1**, 345–348.

4 Anderson, K., Chandra, K. (1976) Pneumothorax secondary to perforation of sequential bronchi by suction catheters. *Journal of Pediatric Surgery* **11**, 687–693.

5 Bailey, C., Kattwinkel, J., Teja, K., Buckley, T. (1988) Shallow versus deep endotracheal suctioning in young rabbits; pathologic effects on the tracheobronchial wall. *Pediatrics* **82**, 746–751.

6 Beeby, P.J., Henderson-Smart, D.J., Lacey, J.L., Rieger, I. (1998) Short- and long-term neurological outcomes following neonatal chest physiotherapy. *Journal of Paediatrics and Child Health* **34**, 60–62.

7 Britton, S., Bejsted, M., Vedin, L. (1985) Chest physiotherapy in primary pneumonia. *British Medical Journal* **290**, 1703–1704.

8 Castling, D., Giffin, F., Greenough, A. (1995) Neonatal endotracheal suction. Comparison of open and closed suction techniques. *British Journal of Intensive Care* **5**, 218–221.

9 Coney, S. (1995) Physiotherapy technique banned in Auckland. *Lancet* **345**, 510.

10 Connors, A.F., Hammon, W.E., Martin, R.J., Rogers, R.M. (1980) Chest physical therapy. The immediate effect on oxygenation in acutely ill patients. *Chest* **78**, 559–564.

11 Cordero, L., Hon, E. (1971) Neonatal bradycardia following nasopharyngeal stimulation. *Journal of Pediatrics* **78**, 441–447.

12 Crane, L. (1981) Physical therapy for neonates with respiratory dysfunction. *Physical Therapy* **61**, 1764–1773.

13 Davies, H., Kitchman, R., Gordon, I., Helms, P. (1985) Regional ventilation in infancy. *New England Journal of Medicine* **313**, 1626–1628.

14 Dean, E. (1985) Effect of body position on pulmonary function. *Physical Therapy* **65**, 613–618.

15 Demont, B., Escorrou, P., Vincon, C. *et al.* (1991) Effects of respiratory physical therapy and nasopharyngeal suction on gastroesophageal reflux in infants less than a year of age with or without abnormal reflux. *Archives Francaises de Pediatrie* **48**, 621–625.

16 Dinwiddie, R. (1990) Cystic fibrosis. In Dinwiddie, R. (ed.), *The Diagnosis and Management of Paediatric Respiratory Disease*. Edinburgh: Churchill Livingstone, 177–222.

17 Downs, J. (1989) Endotracheal suction: a method of tracheal washout. *Physiotherapy* **75**, 54.

18 Downs, J., Parker, A. (1991) Chest physiotherapy for preterm infants. *Paediatric Nursing* **3**, 14–17.

19 Downs, J., Edwards, A.D., McCormick, D.C. *et al.* (1991) Effect of intervention on development of hip posture in very

preterm babies. *Archives of Disease in Childhood* **66**, 797–801.

20 Drew, J.H., Padoms, K., Clabburn, S.L. (1986) Endotracheal management in newborn infants with hyaline membrane disease. *Australian Journal of Physiotherapy* **36**, 3–5.

21 Duara, S., Bessard, K., Keszler, L. et al. (1983) Evaluation of different percussion time intervals of chest physiotherapy on neonatal pulmonary function parameters. *Pediatric Research* **17**, 310A.

22 Durand, M., Sangha, B., Cabal, L.A. et al. (1989) Cardiopulmonary and intracranial pressure changes related to endotracheal suctioning in preterm infants. *Critical Care Medicine* **17**, 506–510.

23 Etches, P., Scott, B. (1978) Chest physiotherapy in the newborn: effects on secretions removed. *Pediatrics* **62**, 713–715.

24 Fanconi, S., Duc, G. (1987) Intratracheal suctioning in sick preterm infants: prevention of intracranial hypertension and cerebral hypoperfusion by muscle paralysis. *Pediatrics* **79**, 538–543.

25 Finer, N.N., Boyd, J. (1978) Chest physiotherapy in the neonate: a controlled study. *Pediatrics* **61**, 282–285.

26 Finer, N.N., Moriartey, R.R., Boyd, J. et al. (1979) Post extubation atelectasis: a retrospective review and a prospective controlled study. *Journal of Pediatrics* **94**, 110–113.

27 Fitzpatrick, M., Bullock, M., Tudehope, D. (1988) Chest physiotherapy for intubated infants with hyaline membrane disease. *New Zealand Journal of Physiotherapy* **16**, 15–18.

28 Flenady, V.J., Gray, P.H. (2001) Chest physiotherapy in babies being extubated from mechanical ventilation. Update Software, Oxford.

29 Fox, W., Schwartz, J., Shaffer, T. (1978) Pulmonary physiotherapy in neonates: physiological changes and respiratory management. *Journal of Pediatrics* **92**, 977–981.

30 Fox, W.W., Schwartz, J.G., Shaffer, T.H. (1977) Alterations in neonatal respiratory function following chest physiotherapy. *Pediatric Research* **11**, 570.

31 Gallon, A. (1987) A case history. *Association of Chartered Physiotherapists in Respiratory Care Newsletter* **10**, 32–33.

32 Gallon, A. (1992) The use of percussion. *Physiotherapy* **78**, 85–89.

33 Gandy, G., Roberton, N.R.C. (1987) *Lecture Notes on Neonatology*. Oxford: Blackwell Scientific.

34 Garrard, J., Bullock, M. (1986) The effect of respiratory therapy on intracranial pressure in ventilated neurosurgical patients. *Australian Journal of Physiotherapy* **32**, 107–111.

35 Geggel, R.L., Pereira, G.R., Spackman, T.J. (1978) Fractured ribs: unusual presentation of rickets in premature infants. *Journal of Pediatrics* **93**, 680–682.

36 Gormezano, J., Branthwaite, M. (1972) Effects of physiotherapy during intermittent positive pressure ventilation. Changes in arterial blood gas tensions. *Anaesthesia* **27**, 258–264.

37 Graham, W.G.B., Bradley, D.A. (1978) Efficacy of chest physiotherapy and intermittent positive pressure breathing in the resolution of pneumonia. *New England Journal of Medicine* **299**, 624–627.

38 Gunderson, L., McPhee, A., Donovan, E. (1986) Partially ventilated endotracheal suction. Use in newborns with respiratory distress syndrome. *American Journal of Diseases of Children* **140**, 462–465.

39 Hanley, M.V., Rudd, T., Butler, J. (1978) What happens to intratracheal saline instillations? *American Review of Respiratory Disease* **117**, 124.

40 Harding, J.E., Miles, F.K.I., Becroft, D.M.O. et al. (1998) Chest physiotherapy may be associated with brain damage in extremely premature infants. *Journal of Pediatrics* **132**, 440–444.

41 Holloway, R., Adams, E., Desai, S., Thambiran, A. (1969) Effect of chest physiotherapy on blood gases of neonates treated by intermittent positive pressure respiration. *Thorax* **24**, 421–426.

42 Hough, A. (1991) Methods to clear secretions. In Hough, A. (ed.), *Physiotherapy in Respiratory Care*. London: Chapman and Hall, 86–95.

43 Howard-Glenn, L., Koniak-Griffin, D. (1990) Evaluation of manometer use in manual ventilation of infants in neonatal intensive care units. *Heart and Lung* **19**, 620–627.

44 Hussey, J. (1992) Effects of chest physiotherapy for children in intensive care after surgery. *Physiotherapy* **78**, 109–113.

45 Kerem, E., Yatsiv, I., Gotein, K. (1990) Effect of endotracheal suctioning on arterial blood gases in children. *Intensive Care Medicine* **16**, 95–99.

46 Kleiber, C., Krutzfield, N., Rose, E. (1988) Acute histologic changes in the tracheobronchial tree associated with different suction catheter insertion techniques. *Heart and Lung* **17**, 10–14.

47 Kohlhauser, C., Bernert, G., Hermon, M. et al. (2000) Effects of endotracheal suctioning in high-frequency oscillatory and conventionally ventilated low birth weight neonates on cerebral hemodynamics observed by near infrared spectroscopy (NIRS). *Pediatric Pulmonology* **29**, 270–275.

48 Laws, A., Macintyre, R. (1969) Chest physiotherapy. The physiological assessment during intermittent position pressure ventilation in respiratory failure. *Canadian Anaesthetic Society Journal* **16**, 487–493.

49 Lomholt, N., Cooke, R., Lundin, M. (1968) A method of humidification in ventilator treatment of neonates. *British Journal of Anaesthesia* **40**, 335–339.

50 Marini, J., Pierson, D., Hudson, L. (1979) Acute lobar atelectasis – a prospective comparison of fibreoptic bronchoscopy and respiratory therapy. *American Review of Respiratory Disease* **122**, 133–146.

51 Murai, D.T., Whatley Grant, J. (1994) Continuous oscillation therapy improves the pulmonary outcome of intubated newborns: results of a prospective, randomized, controlled trial. *Critical Care Medicine* **22**, 1147–1154.

52 Nagaraj, H.S., Shott, R., Fellows, R., Yacoub, U. (1980) Recurrent lobar atelectasis due to acquired bronchial stenosis in neonates. *Journal of Pediatric Surgery* **15**, 411–415.

53 Naigow, D., Pavaser, M. (1977) The effect of different endotracheal suction procedures on arterial blood gases in a controlled experimental model. *Heart and Lung* **6**, 808–816.

54 Parker, A., Downs, J. (1991) Chest physiotherapy in neonatal ITU. *Paediatric Nursing* **3**, 319–321.

55 Parker, A.E. (1985) Chest physiotherapy in the neonatal intensive care unit. *Physiotherapy* **71**, 63–65.

56 Parker, A.E. (1993) Paediatrics. In Webber, B., Pryor, J. (eds), *Physiotherapy for Respiratory and Cardiac Problems*. Edinburgh: Churchill Livingstone.

57 Paterson, J.W. (1988) Antiallergic drugs and antitussives. In Dukes, M. (ed.), *Meyler's Side Effects of Drugs*. Amsterdam: Elsevier, 322–332.

58 Pickens, D., Schefft, G., Thach, B. (1988) Prolonged apnea associated with upper airway protective reflexes in apnea of prematurity. *American Review of Respiratory Disease* **137**, 113–118.

59 Pierce, J., Piazza, D. (1987) Differences in post suctioning arterial blood oxygen concentration values using two post oxygenation methods. *Heart and Lung* **16**, 34–38.

60 Plum, F., Dunning, M. (1956) Techniques for minimizing trauma to the tracheobronchial tree after tracheostomy. *New England Journal of Medicine* **254**, 193–200.

61 Prasad, A., Tasker, R. (1990) Guidelines for the physiotherapy management of critically ill children with acutely raised intracranial pressure. *Physiotherapy* **76**, 248–250.

62 Prendiville, A., Thomson, A., Silverman, M. (1986) Effect of tracheobronchial suction on respiratory resistance in intubated preterm babies. *Archives of Disease in Childhood* **16**, 1178–1183.

63 Purohit, D.M., Caldwell, C., Levkoff, A.H. (1975) Multiple rib fractures due to physiotherapy in a neonate with hyaline membrane disease. *American Journal of Diseases of Children* **129**, 1103–1104.

64 Raval, D., Yeh, T.F., Mora, A. *et al.* (1987) Chest physiotherapy in preterm infants with respiratory distress syndrome in the first 24 hours of life. *Journal of Perinatology* **7**, 301–304.

65 Ravel, D., Cuevas, A., Mora, A. *et al.* (1985) The efficacy of chest physiotherapy (CPT) on the first postnatal day in infants with RDS. *Pediatric Research* **19**(Suppl), 359A.

66 Ray, J.F., Yost, L., Moallem, S. (1974) Immobility hypoxaemia and pulmonary arteriovenous shunting. *Archives of Surgery* **109**, 537–541.

67 Reines, H., Sade, R., Bradford, B., Marshall, J. (1982) Chest physiotherapy fails to prevent post-operative atelectasis in children after cardiac surgery. *Annals of Surgery* **195**, 451–455.

68 Riegal, B., Forshee, T. (1985) A review and critique of the literature on pre-oxygenation for endotracheal suctioning. *Heart and Lung* **14**, 11–17.

69 Rux, M., Pavaser, M. (1979) Effect of apnea and three levels of negative pressure on the fall in arterial oxygen tension produced by endotracheal suctioning in dogs. *American Review of Respiratory Disease* **119**, 193.

70 Sackner, M., Landa, J., Greeneltch, N., Robinson, J. (1973) Pathogenesis and prevention of tracheobronchial damage with suction procedures. *Chest* **64**, 284–290.

71 Shim, C., Fine, N., Fernandez, R., Williams, M.H.J. (1969) Cardiac arrhythmias resulting from tracheal suctioning. *Annals of Internal Medicine* **71**, 1149–1153.

72 Simbruner, G., Coradello, H., Fodor, M. *et al.* (1981) Effect of tracheal suction on oxygenation, circulation and lung mechanics in newborn infants. *Archives of Disease in Childhood* **56**, 326–330.

73 Sumner, E. (1990) Artificial ventilation of children. In Dinwiddie, R. (ed.), *The Diagnosis and Management of Paediatric Respiratory Disease*. Edinburgh: Churchill Livingstone, 267–287.

74 Tarnow-Mordi, W. (1991) Is routine endotracheal suction justified? *Archives of Disease in Childhood* **66**, 374–375.

75 Tarnow-Mordi, W.O., Fletcher, M., Suton, P., Wilkinson, A.R. (1986) Evidence of inadequate humification of inspired gas during artificial ventilation of newborn infants in the British Isles. *Lancet* **ii**, 909–910.

76 Tarnow-Mordi, W.O., Reid, E., Griffiths, P., Wilkinson, A.R. (1989) Low inspired gas temperature and respiratory complications in very low birth weight infants. *Journal of Pediatrics* **114**, 438–442.

77 Thoresen, M., Cowan, F., Whitelaw, A. (1988) Effect of tilting oxygenation in newborn infants. *Archives of Disease in Childhood* **63**, 315–317.

78 Tudehope, D., Bagley, C. (1980) Techniques of physiotherapy in intubated babies with the respiratory distress syndrome. *Australian Paediatric Journal* **16**, 226–228.

79 Tydeman, D. (1989) An investigation into the effectiveness of physiotherapy in the treatment of patients with community acquired pneumonia. *Physiotherapy Practice* **5**, 75–81.

80 Vaughan, R., Menke, J., Giacoia, G. (1978) Pneumothorax: a complication of endotracheal tube suctioning. *Journal of Pediatrics* **92**, 633–634.

81 Vivian-Beresford, A., King, C., Macauley, H. (1987) Neonatal post-extubation complications: the preventive role of physiotherapy. *Physiotherapy Canada* **39**, 184–190.

82 Wilson, G., Hughes, G., Rennie, J., Morley, C. (1991) Evaluation of two endotracheal suction regimes in babies ventilated for respiratory distress syndrome. *Early Human Development* **25**, 87–90.

83 Wood, B.P. (1987) Infants ribs: generalized periosteal reaction resulting from vibrator chest physiotherapy. *Radiology* **162**, 811–812.

84 Young, C. (1984) A review of the adverse effects of airway suction and recommended guidelines for suction. *Physiotherapy* **70**, 104–108.

PART 4

Neonatal respiratory problems

19

Respiratory distress syndrome

HENRY L HALLIDAY

Respiratory distress syndrome (RDS) is an acute illness, usually of preterm infants, developing within 4–6 hours of birth, characterized by a rapid respiratory rate (>60 breaths/min), respiratory distress (intercostal, subcostal and sternal retraction or indrawing), expiratory grunting and cyanosis. In very prematurely born infants (less than 26 weeks of gestation) it may present as apnea at birth, in which case the characteristic clinical features described above will be absent. On the chest radiograph, there is a typical appearance of reticulogranular mottling with air bronchograms, but in severe cases the lungs may be completely white due to fluid retention in the airspaces and widespread atelectasis (the so-called 'white-out' picture). The basic etiology of RDS is surfactant deficiency.

INCIDENCE

Approximately 2–3 percent of infants develop respiratory distress soon after birth: 2.9 percent in Sweden,[100] 2.1 percent in Nottingham, UK,[55] and 2.8 percent in Italy.[178] Most of these infants have transient respiratory distress not fulfilling the criteria for RDS outlined above. In the Swedish study, only 0.33 percent had RDS, although this figure was probably an underestimate. In the UK series from Nottingham, 1.12 percent had RDS and from Italy the rate was 1.24 percent. Using a risk of 1 percent, approximately 7000 babies in the UK and 20 000 in the USA should develop RDS every year. Recent trends have shown a decrease in mortality from RDS with surfactant replacement therapy having a major effect.[122]

The risk of RDS is inversely proportional to gestational age (Figure 19.1). The proportion of preterm births in a given population will determine the incidence of RDS. The introduction of treatments such as prenatal corticosteroids and prophylactic surfactant has reduced the rates

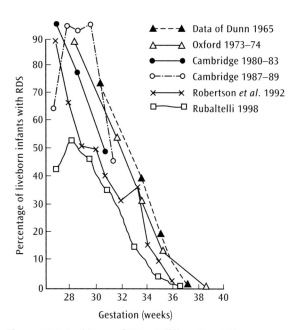

Figure 19.1 *Incidence of RDS at different gestations. (Adapted from Greenough, A., Morley, C.J., Roberton, N.R.C. (1992) Acute respiratory disease in the newborn. In Roberton, N.R.C. (ed.), Textbook of Neonatology, 2nd edn. Edinburgh: Churchill Livingstone, 385–504.)*

of RDS at each gestational age. Data from a study from Italy suggest a risk of RDS of about 50 percent up to 30 weeks of gestation, decreasing to 37 percent from 31 to 32 weeks, 12 percent from 33 to 34 weeks and 2 percent from 35 to 36 weeks.[178] Other factors predisposing to or protecting against RDS are discussed later (p. 249).

PATHOLOGY

On macroscopic examination, the lungs appear deflated, have the consistency of liver and do not float in water. Microscopically there are characteristic hyaline membranes, which gave rise to the earlier name of hyaline membrane disease (HMD). The presence of hyaline membranes, however, is not unique to RDS and they merely indicate damage to epithelial–endothelial integrity which may be found in cases of acute lung injury from any cause such as congenital infection.

Within 2 hours of birth, necrosis of bronchiolar epithelium is seen.[65,235] Prior to this there is edema of both the interstitial tissues and the basement membranes. Epithelial cells and capillary endothelial cells show fine vacuoles, indicating injury to both cell types. Capillaries become congested and lymphatics are dilated because of the delayed clearance of fetal lung liquid. After 2 hours, the pink amorphous material overlying the denuded portions of epithelium takes on a basophilic, amphophilic or eosinophilic appearance. By 10 hours hyaline membranes are usually well developed and they line the overdistended terminal and respiratory bronchioles.[188] The alveolar ducts appear overdistended with air and adjacent saccules are collapsed in most postmortem studies. The most distal component of the respiratory unit, the terminal sacs, although collapsed, are not lined by hyaline membranes. Their pink color in hematoxylin and eosin stains indicates the presence of a protein-rich substance which also contains fibrin and nuclear debris. In infants with severe hyperbilirubinemia, the membranes may become yellow, reflecting the presence of unconjugated bilirubin.[222]

In RDS, surfactant deficiency causes collapse of terminal air sacs at end expiration. Attempts to expand these sacs, either by spontaneous efforts to breathe or by positive pressure ventilation, will generate uneven transpulmonary pressure.[173] The shear forces so generated will damage the lining epithelium, giving rise to bronchiolar necrotic lesions,[154] which may be markers of subsequent chronic lung disease or bronchopulmonary dysplasia. Ischemia and increased pulmonary intravascular coagulation may contribute to this lung injury.[183]

After 24 hours, the repair phase begins and a few inflammatory cells appear within the airway lumen. Macrophages are usually the most prominent cell type, although some polymorphs may also be present.[142] After 5–7 days, the membranes start to disappear and the remnants are phagocytosed by macrophages. Macrophages are also present beneath the membrane within the interstitium. Regeneration of epithelia is detectable after 48 hours, usually beneath the separating membranes. Cuboidial cells from the unaffected transitional ducts become large and mitotic before flattening out to spread beneath the hyaline membranes. In the course of resolution, dilated airspaces alternate with lobular areas or atelectasis.[65] Interstitial edema is mobilized and a diuresis occurs after 72–96 hours. Congested capillaries in the acinus sometimes disrupt to give frank intrasaccular or intraductal hemorrhage, which may become confluent and extensive.[188]

By 7 days of age in uncomplicated RDS, the hyaline membranes will have disappeared. In babies treated with positive pressure ventilation, however, the healing process may be markedly altered and delayed. There is a hyperplastic healing process with massive shedding of bronchiolar epithelial cells and type II pneumocytes. Hyaline membranes may remain prominent and the terminal airways may be plugged with secretions. There is progressive scarring and fibrosis of the alveoli and airways, leading to the picture of CLD (p. 402).

Treatment with surfactant may also modify the pathologic features of RDS. Globular deposits of hyaline material in parenchymal airspaces, absence of hyaline membranes, and increased interstitial cellularity and edema without associated fibrosis have been described.[165] Reduction of epithelial necrosis and interstitial emphysema in the lungs of infants treated with surfactant was also reported. In another study, there was an increased incidence of intra-alveolar hemorrhage with an associated decreased incidence of pulmonary interstitial hemorrhage in surfactant-treated lungs.[158] Our own experience is that whilst surfactant treatment has reduced neonatal mortality, it has not significantly altered the histologic findings in the lungs of those infants who die.[217]

PATHOPHYSIOLOGY

Deficiency of surfactant leads to alveolar collapse, especially at end expiration, reduced lung volume and decreased lung compliance. Pressure–volume loops of lungs excised at postmortem examination from infants who have died with RDS have a characteristic pattern. During inflation, the volume change for a given increase in pressure is very small and the hysteresis loop is flatter than seen in the healthy newborn. Furthermore, as the pressure drops to zero, very little or no air is retained within the surfactant-less alveoli, corresponding to the very low FRC measured *in vivo* (see below). Infants with severe RDS will typically have a compliance of 0.3 mL/cmH$_2$O/kg,[46] which leads to an increased work of breathing.[138] The work of breathing in RDS is approximately twice that seen in healthy newborns.[138] Inspiratory resistance is usually normal in RDS, but expiratory resistance may be increased due to closure of the airways associated with the expiratory grunt. The endotracheal tube also affects the resistance. Functional residual capacity (p. 121) may be as low as 3–5 mL/kg.[43] Once recovery from the disease takes place, then FRCs of 25–30 mL/kg are reported.[46] There is also right-to-left shunting of blood, both intrapulmonary through collapsed lung and extrapulmonary across the ductus arteriosus and foramen ovale, if pulmonary vascular resistance remains high.[89,190] Persistent hypoxemia [PaO_2 less than 4 kPa (30 mmHg)] leads to metabolic acidosis, reduced cardiac output, hypotension and peripheral edema due to poor renal function. Hypercapnia occurs as a result of hypoventilation, decreased tidal volume and increased dead space. The blood gas and pH findings in severe RDS thus reflect a mixed metabolic and respiratory acidosis. Acidosis will further reduce surfactant production and may also increase pulmonary vascular resistance.

The normal surfactant pool size at birth is about 100 mg phospholipid/kg.[112] In preterm babies the pool size is greatly reduced (less than 25 mg/kg and, if severe RDS is present, less than 5 mg/kg).[93] Some infants appear to have sufficient surfactant at birth to sustain normal respiration,[172] but after a few hours the surfactant is used up and if surfactant replacement therapy is not given there is continued deterioration in respiratory function. Surfactant may also be inactivated by leakage of inhibitory proteins from the plasma[106,175] and this can be a feature of infants born to mothers with severe pregnancy-induced hypertension (pre-eclampsia). Endogenous surfactant production begins from 2–3 days of age[115] and heralds clinical recovery from the illness. Treatment with exogenous surfactant does not delay recovery of endogenous surfactant production and it might even enhance it.[28] Studies with stable isotopes have confirmed these findings and they show promise in further elucidating the interaction between endogenous and exogenous surfactant in preterm infants.[219]

ETIOLOGY

When hyaline membranes were first described in RDS they were thought to have resulted from the aspiration of vernix in the amniotic fluid.[52,101] Later, in the 1950s, it was known that prematurity, delivery by cesarean section and birth asphyxia were major predisposing factors. In 1959, Avery and Mead first demonstrated that extracts from the lungs of infants dying from HMD were missing a surface tension lowering agent.[7] They were the first to demonstrate that surfactant deficiency was the underlying cause of RDS. In the 1960s, the biochemical composition of surfactant was determined and the first trials of exogenous surfactant administraton began.[88] Successful exogenous surfactant administration was not reported until 1980.[63]

Factors predisposing to RDS (Table 19.1)

PREMATURITY

Premature birth is the greatest risk factor for the development of RDS. About half of all infants born prior to 30 weeks of gestation will develop RDS (Figure 19.1). Boys are also more likely to develop RDS than girls (male to female ratio about 1.7:1) and are more likely to die from the disease.[54] The delay in producing mature surfactant found in male fetuses may be due to an androgen effect on type II pneumocytes.[218]

CESAREAN SECTION

Cesarean section increases the risk of neonatal respiratory distress twofold for elective procedures and tenfold for emergency procedures.[178] The combination of elective cesarean section and delivery before term increases the risk of respiratory distress in a progressive manner. At 37 weeks of gestation, 7.4 percent of infants develop respiratory distress after an elective cesarean section compared to 4.2 percent at 38 weeks, and 1.8 percent at 38 weeks.[148] Not all of these infants have RDS; some have transient tachypnea of the newborn but a few develop severe respiratory failure and need extracorporeal membrane oxygenation.[119] Indeed, the need for mechanical ventilation after elective delivery at 37–38 weeks of gestation is 120 times greater than after delivery at 39–41 weeks,[134] and some infants die despite having intensive care.[86] The reasons for this increased risk of respiratory morbidity near term following cesarean section are probably a combination of delayed removal of lung fluid[228] and exaggerated pulmonary hypertension.[109] In very preterm infants the effect of cesarean section on the risk of RDS is less clear.

Table 19.1 *Factors predisposing to RDS*

Maternal factors
Diabetes
Hypertension
Multiple pregnancy
Malnutrition
Familial disposition

Perinatal factors
Premature delivery
Cesarean section
Male gender
Birth depression
Timing of cord clamping
Hypothermia
Hemolytic disease of the newborn

The risks are reduced if cesarean section is carried out after the onset of labor compared to elective delivery.[25]

ASPHYXIA

Asphyxia also increases the risk of developing RDS.[214] During asphyxia, lung perfusion falls to very low levels, causing ischemic damage to pulmonary capillaries. On recovery there is overperfusion of the lungs, which may allow protein-rich fluid to leak from damaged capillaries[110] into the alveoli where surfactant will be inactivated. Asphyxia is also associated with hypoxemia and acidemia, which will reduce surfactant production[141] and in addition cause pulmonary hypertension. Respiratory distress following asphyxia may therefore be more like acute respiratory distress syndrome (ARDS) (p. 396), where there is surfactant inactivation, than RDS where there is a primary surfactant deficiency.

MATERNAL DIABETES

Infants of diabetic mothers (IDM) are also more likely to develop RDS than other infants at equivalent gestational ages.[175] These babies have an abnormal pattern of surfactant synthesis with delayed appearance of phosphatidylglycerol,[35] although this is not a consistent finding.[92] Insulin has been shown to delay the maturation of type II pneumocytes and decrease the proportion of saturated phosphatidylcholine in surfactant.[76] Delivery at term rather than at 36–37 weeks has reduced the risks of severe RDS in IDM. Strict management of diabetic pregnancy in a regional center has probably contributed to successful outcomes with reduced risk of RDS.[220]

MATERNAL HYPERTENSION

Maternal hypertension increases the risk of RDS,[13] probably as a result of preterm delivery by elective cesarean section before the onset of labor.[221] Some of these babies may have ARDS rather than typical RDS.

FAMILIAL DISPOSITION

Cases of familial RDS in term babies have been reported and it is now believed that some of these are due to congenital deficiency of SP-B.[95] In cases where SP-B is totally absent, death is inevitable despite intensive care and surfactant treatment unless lung transplantation can be performed.[96] Gene therapy may prove to be successful in the future. Partial deficiency of SP-B has also been reported[26] and this may be compatible with survival. For preterm infants the risk of recurrent RDS is quite high,[151] suggesting an important genetic effect. Certain SP-A and SP-B alleles appear to associated with increased or decreased risk for RDS.[58] There is an interaction between genetic factors, prematurity, gender, response to antenatal steroids and ethnic background which determines the presence and severity of RDS in any given individual.

MULTIPLE PREGNANCY

In twin pregnancies, the second twin is usually at greater risk of developing RDS.[79] The excess risk of RDS in the second twin increases with gestation and is significant above 29 weeks of gestation.[79] It is not clear whether this increased risk is due to delayed maturation of the lungs[231] or an increased risk of asphyxia[6] in the second twin.

HYPOTHERMIA

Hypothermia worsens the outlook for preterm babies[202] and this may be for a number of reasons. Coagulation disturbances and defective surfactant function,[68] which is worsened by hypoxemia and acidemia,[141] are clearly detrimental to the preterm infant. Conversely, in the term infant who has suffered from asphyxia, hypothermia may be beneficial as a means of neuroprotection.[9] In the preterm infant both hypothermia and hyperthermia should be avoided.

NUTRITION

Nutrition is important to ensure normal surfactant synthesis. In animal studies, maternal malnutrition affects surfactant synthesis and lung growth.[127] Anecdotally, women with anorexia nervosa who manage to conceive, have a high risk of giving birth to infants who develop RDS. Deficiency of inositol might be important in these cases and supplementation of preterm infants has been shown to promote maturation of surfactant phospholipids.[94] A systematic review has shown that inositol supplementation reduces the risk of death or CLD, and severe retinopathy of prematurity (ROP) in treated infants.[104]

HEMOLYTIC DISEASE OF THE NEWBORN (HDN)

HDN has been associated with delayed fetal lung maturation,[234] but this is not universally accepted.[168] A possible mechanism is via elevation of insulin levels, due to B-islet cell hypertrophy as occurs in IDM. In the presence of severe erythroblastosis with anemia, heart failure and hydrops fetalis, surfactant inactivation can occur and pulmonary hypoplasia is also a possible complication increasing the risk of respiratory problems after birth.[162]

CORD CLAMPING

The timing of cord clamping is a controversial issue. In term infants, very delayed cord clamping at 3–5 minutes has been associated with increased respiratory morbidity.[240] In preterm infants, however, delayed cord clamping may improve lung function and reduce the incidence of RDS and the need for surfactant therapy.[121] This observation needs to be confirmed in a larger randomized controlled trial.

Table 19.2 *Factors protecting against RDS*

Antenatal corticosteroid treatment
Intrauterine growth restriction
Prolonged rupture of the membranes
Maternal drugs and smoking
Female gender
Non-Caucasian ethnic group

Factors protecting against RDS (Table 19.2)

INTRAUTERINE STRESS

It has been suggested that a stressful intrauterine environment might increase the production of glucocorticoids and catecholamines in fetal plasma, leading to earlier maturation of the fetal lungs and a reduced risk of RDS.[232] Clinical studies, however, have shown conflicting results; Procianoy et al.[167] found that small for gestational age (SGA) infants had a lower incidence of RDS and periventricular hemorrhage than gestation-matched controls but Thompson et al.[215] found the opposite. Tubman et al.[221] found that infants born after pregnancies complicated by pre-eclampsia had a higher risk of RDS. The crucial effect of gestational age and the presence of pre-eclampsia was confirmed in a study from Sweden.[125] These authors found that at a gestational age of 25–28 weeks, SGA infants had double the risk of RDS compared to appropriate for gestational age (AGA) infants. At a gestational age of 29–32 weeks, however, SGA infants had half the risk of RDS of the AGA infants. After adjustment for confounding variables, infants born at a gestational age of 25–28 weeks from mothers with pre-eclampsia appeared to be a high-risk group for RDS, whereas at 29–32 weeks of gestation being SGA protected against RDS. Furthermore, antenatal corticosteroid treatment appeared to have less beneficial effects on mortality, RDS and cerebral hemorrhage in infants born SGA compared to those who were AGA.[125]

PROLONGED RUPTURE OF THE MEMBRANES (PROM)

PROM was first suggested to reduce the incidence of RDS in 1973.[239] A large review, however, did not confirm the benefits of PROM.[140] One of the difficulties might be that PROM over a short period of time might help mature the fetal lungs as a result of 'stress hormones' but in the longer term the risk of congenital pneumonia is increased and this may be difficult to distinguish from RDS. More recent studies suggest that there is a positive benefit from PROM[21,221] and this may in part be mediated through increased use of antenatal steroids.[216]

MATERNAL DRUGS AND SMOKING

Maternal narcotic addiction,[67] cocaine use,[242] smoking[233] and alcohol intake[108] all reduce the incidence of RDS

in preterm babies. The mechanism is probably due to stimulation of surfactant synthesis, but the other more serious adverse effects of these drugs prohibits their use in pregnancy.

GENDER

Girls have less RDS at each gestational age compared with boys. Male fetuses have a delayed appearance of a mature lecithin:sphingomyelin (L:S) ratio and phosphatidyl-glycerol. This is probably due to androgen-induced delayed maturation of surfactant synthesis found in males.[218]

ETHNICITY

There are ethnic differences in the incidence of RDS.[117] Black infants have a lower incidence of RDS than white infants, probably due to enhanced lung maturation. The effect, however, may be restricted to infants with gestational ages above 32 weeks.[105] In a series of preterm infants of 23–32 weeks of gestation, those of African origin had a risk of RDS of 40 percent, Caucasians 75 percent and those of Caribbean origin 54 percent.[117] Infants from the Indian subcontinent also appear to have a reduced risk of RDS compared to white infants.

ANTENATAL CORTICOSTEROIDS

Antenatal corticosteroid treatment reduces the risk of RDS.[126] Meta-analysis of all randomized controlled trials suggests an approximate halving of the risk of RDS and a 40 percent reduction of neonatal mortality (p. 256).[32,33]

CLINICAL SIGNS

The classical diagnostic criteria for RDS were developed by Rudolph and Smith in 1960:[180]

- Tachypnea: respiratory rate above 60/min
- Grunting expiration
- Indrawing of sternum, intercostal spaces and lower ribs during inspiration
- Cyanosis without oxygen supplementation.

It has been stated that these signs must develop before the infant is 4 hours old and must persist beyond 24 hours of age. These classical signs of RDS, however, are outdated because very immature infants may present with apnea at birth and intubation at birth for assisted ventilation and surfactant treatment modifies the course of RDS. Walther and Taeusch have updated the clinical and radiological criteria for the diagnosis of RDS:[229]

- Evidence of prematurity
- Lung immaturity

- Abnormal signs, such as intercostal and sternal retraction, nasal flaring, tachypnea, expiratory grunt and cyanosis evident within hours of birth
- Evidence of reduced lung compliance, reduced functional residual capacity (FRC) and increased work of breathing
- Evidence of abnormal gas exchange (hypoxemia, hypercapnia, cyanosis) of sufficient severity to require oxygen and/or continuous or intermittent positive pressure ventilatory support for more than 24 hours
- An abnormal chest radiograph with diffuse, parenchymal reticulogranular densities and air bronchograms (atelectasis) and underinflation during a good inspiratory effort at 6–24 hours of age.

Natural history

The widespread introduction of surfactant therapy has meant that the natural history of RDS is unfamiliar to most residents in neonatal units. By definition, the disease presents within the first 4 hours after birth. Over the next 24–36 hours in untreated cases the lungs become progressively stiffer as protein leaks into the alveoli and inactivates any surfactant that is present. The infant has increased work of breathing and eventually tires with the development of worsening dyspnea and edema. Some infants progressively continue to deteriorate and without assisted ventilation would die of intractable respiratory failure. In most infants, however, the disease begins to abate after 48–72 hours when surfactant is again synthesized by the recovering type II pneumocytes. A spontaneous diuresis occurs around the time of improvement in lung function, but the precise temporal relationship remains controversial.[116] With continued recovery the infant is usually asymptomatic and in room air by 7–10 days of age.

Respiratory signs

The normal respiratory rate of a newborn is 40/min and tachypnea is usually defined as a rate in excess of 60/min. Reduced lung compliance and low lung volumes lead to the increased respiratory rate. Tachypnea is a good prognostic sign compared to apnea,[201] which may be a sign of respiratory decompensation.[42] Other features of dyspnea are intercostal and sternal recession and flaring of the alae nasi. The respiratory effort is primarily diaphragmatic and the compliant rib cage allows marked retractions to occur. The magnitude of retractions has been used to score the severity of the disease.[186]

Grunting is very common in infants with RDS. It is produced by expiration through a partially closed glottis. The infant attempts to sustain functional residual capacity (FRC) by delaying the escape of air from the lungs during expiration.[42] Harrison et al.[98] demonstrated the physiologic basis of grunting and showed that when it was eliminated by endotracheal intubation arterial oxygen tension decreased.

Cyanosis is common if oxygen supplementation is not provided. Clinical cyanosis becomes apparent when arterial oxygen tension falls below 40 mmHg (5.3 kPa).

Cardiorespiratory findings

Heart rate in mild to moderate RDS is usually in the normal range of 140–160/min with normal variability. In severe RDS, however, there may be tachycardia (heart rate greater than 160/min) and reduced variability.[111] Neonates with RDS are often hypotensive.[152,181] Some of these infants have a low blood volume and hypovolemia is associated with hypotension, low central venous pressure and a low hematocrit. Affected infants need volume expansion and correction of associated acidosis but rapid correction with sodium bicarbonate is associated with an increase in intracranial hemorrhage.[187,208] Early hypotension is a risk factor for periventricular leukomalacia (PVL),[61,143] so it should be corrected but not too rapidly.

Heart failure is not a feature of RDS and if there are suggestive signs, an alternative or additional diagnosis must be sought. After a few days, a persistent ductus arteriosus (PDA) may become apparent and lead to worsening of the cardiopulmonary condition. Following surfactant treatment, the signs of a PDA may appear earlier, sometimes within 12 hours of birth. The unmasking of a PDA following surfactant treatment has been associated with the development of pulmonary hemorrhage.[169] In these circumstances there may be hypotension with a low diastolic blood pressure before the appearance of the characteristic continuous murmur and bounding pulses. Early use of intravenous indomethacin or ibuprofen has been advocated to prevent PDA[40] and also to reduce the risk of intraventricular hemorrhage (IVH).[59]

Central nervous system findings

The preterm baby with severe RDS is prone to develop IVH and/or PVL as a result of loss of cerebral autoregulation. Autoregulation is a mechanism whereby a constant cerebral blood flow is maintained over a wide range of perfusion pressures and also in response to various biochemical stimuli. Cerebral autoregulation varies with gestational age and is frequently abolished in the presence of hypoxia, acidosis and hypercapnia.[131] In hypoxic preterm neonates who have no cerebral autoregulation, a sudden increase in blood pressure can increase cerebral perfusion pressure and lead to disruption of capillaries in the germinal matrix, causing IVH. When this occurs there may be neurological signs such as apnea, cycling or seizures or catastrophic deterioration with reduced levels of consciousness and overt convulsions.

Renal functional changes

Hypoxia, hypercapnia, acidosis and hypotension affect renal function. There will be reduced glomerular filtration rate, oliguria (<1 mL/kg/h), poor sodium excretion leading to hypernatremia, raised blood urea and hyperkalemia with generalized edema. Improvement in the infant's condition is often associated with a spontaneous diuresis,[49,73] which can lead to dehydration and hyponatremia if extra fluid and sodium are not provided.

Gastrointestinal signs

Most babies with severe RDS, as with any neonatal illness, have an ileus.[45] Their bowel sounds are absent, they do not pass meconium and gastric emptying is delayed.[241] Improvement in their general condition is often heralded by the reappearance of bowel sounds and the passage of meconium.

DIFFERENTIAL DIAGNOSIS

A number of conditions cause respiratory distress in the first 4 hours after birth (Table 19.3). Good history taking is most important in distinguishing the various causes of early respiratory distress. Gestational age and the presence of perinatal risk factors such as chorioamnionitis, meconium staining and asphyxia are important in determining the cause of early respiratory distress. Prenatal diagnosis of congenital pulmonary or cardiac anomalies will also guide towards the correct diagnosis. A careful physical examination and a chest radiograph are also helpful in making a definitive diagnosis. It is important to be aware that two or more respiratory disorders may coexist in the one infant: for example, RDS and congenital pneumonia in preterm infants after prolonged rupture of

Table 19.3 *Differential diagnosis of early respiratory distress*

Respiratory distress syndrome (RDS)
Transient tachypnea of the newborn (TTN)
Congenital pneumonia
Meconium aspiration syndrome (MAS)
Other aspiration syndromes
Pneumothorax
Congenital pulmonary malformations
Pulmonary hypoplasia
Congenital heart disease
Persistent pulmonary hypertension
Inborn errors of metabolism
Neurologic disorders
Upper airway obstruction
Anemia
Polycythemia

the membranes or in the presence of chorioamnionitis, and meconium aspiration and congenital sepsis in term infants with respiratory distress.

INVESTIGATIONS

These are aimed at confirming the diagnosis of RDS and excluding other diagnoses (Table 19.3). The chest radiograph is the best method of making a definitive diagnosis of RDS, but congenital pneumonia can coexist and have radiological findings similar to those of RDS (p. 281).

Chest radiograph

Classically, the chest radiograph shows diffuse reticulogranular opacification or mottling in both lung fields with air bronchograms, where the air-filled bronchi stand out against the atelectatic alveoli. The appearance varies from a slight granularity (Figure 19.2) to completely opaque lung fields where the cardiac shadow is obliterated – the so-called 'white-out' picture (Figure 19.3). The radiological severity of RDS may be graded in four categories (Table 19.4).[66,238] Grade 1 consists of a fine granularity with superimposed air bronchograms confined within the borders of the cardiothymic silhouette. The cardiac margins are clearly seen (Figure 19.2). In grade 2, the typical generalized reticulogranular pattern is seen and the lungs show a slight overall reduction in radiolucency. The air bronchograms are projected beyond the cardiothymic borders. The lungs of infants with grade 3 show more confluent densities produced by the summation of numerous

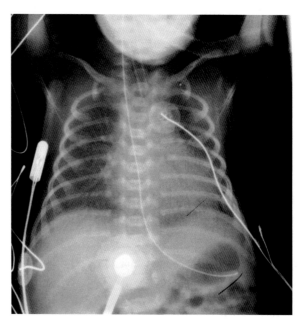

Figure 19.2 *Chest radiograph showing changes of mild RDS (grade 1).*

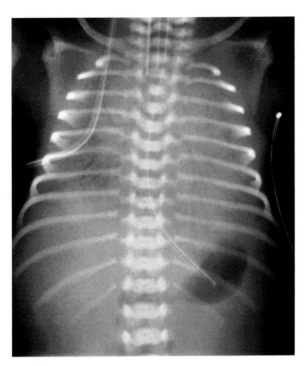

Figure 19.3 *Chest radiograph showing changes of severe RDS equivalent to 'white-out' (grade 4).*

Table 19.4 *Radiological grading of severity of RDS*

Grade	Characteristics
Grade 1	Very fine granularity
	Air bronchograms within heart borders
Grade 2	Generalized reticulogranular mottling
	Air bronchograms projected beyond heart borders
Grade 3	More confluent densities
	More extensive air bronchograms
	Extending to second and third bronchial divisions
	Heart borders still visible
Grade 4	Complete opacification of lung fields
	Absence of air bronchograms
	Heart borders no longer visible
	'White-out' appearance

reticulogranular densities. Air bronchograms are more extensive, extending into the second and third bronchial divisions. Grade 4 is characterized by complete opacification of the lungs with absence of air bronchograms and the heart borders are no longer visible (Figure 19.3).[57] Before assisted ventilation became available, the appearance of grade 4 RDS usually indicated impending death. Assisted ventilation, including positive end expiratory pressure (PEEP) or CPAP, however, can produce rapid improvement in the radiological severity of the lung disease.[66] Cases have been reported where a striking change from grade 3 or 4 to grade 1 or 2 has occurred after the application of PEEP. Early intervention with high-frequency oscillatory ventilation (HFOV) or surfactant prophylaxis, especially with rapidly acting protein-containing surfactants, can also dramatically improve the radiological appearances of RDS.[17]

Changes on the chest radiograph are usually apparent within 5 hours of birth;[238] they coincide with the onset of clinical signs. The appearances, however, may occasionally be delayed for as long as 24 hours, which might be the radiologic correlate of surfactant becoming used up.[172] In untreated cases, the radiologic picture progressively deteriorates as the reticulogranularity becomes more prominent during the first 12–24 hours (Table 19.4). In infants treated with positive pressure and/or surfactant, the improved radiologic findings reduce the prognostic significance of the chest radiograph.[43] There are, however, other reasons for performing chest radiography in infants with signs of respiratory distress: first, to exclude other diagnoses or coexistent disorders such as congenital pneumonia, pneumothorax, pulmonary interstitial emphysema, congenital pulmonary anomalies or abnormalities of the ribs; second, to check for position of the endotracheal tube and/or umbilical arterial catheter.

The radiologic findings in RDS may sometimes be atypical.[57] There may occasionally be a fine bubbly pattern due to maximal distention of terminal airways.[207] This pattern can precede the development of pulmonary interstitial emphysema. Perhaps the most common variation in the usual pattern is an increase in density of the posterior basal portion of the lung.[170] This is due to atelectasis and fluid accumulation in the more dependent alveoli of the supine neonate. MRI scanning has recently been used to confirm these findings.[3] Asymmetric changes are surprisingly common occurring in about 30 percent of chest radiographs.[213] In these cases the RDS pattern is almost always more pronounced on the right and most infants have mild disease with a good outcome. Less commonly, RDS may be confined to the lower lobes or clear more rapidly from the upper lobes. In animal studies, the upper lobes show earlier physiologic maturation than the lower lobes.[1] When the chest radiograph shows uneven distribution of reticulogranularity, the presence of underlying or superimposed pneumonia should be considered.[179] Another cause of asymmetric parenchymal involvement is surfactant treatment,[199] due to uneven distribution of the drug.

Recently, ultrasound has been used to diagnose RDS, the appearance of retrohepatic hyperechogenicity being described as pathognomonic.[8] The technique, however, is difficult to apply and involves more handling of preterm infants than the standard anterior-posterior chest radiograph. Ultrasound has also been proposed as a method for determining the position of an endotracheal tube,[191] but this requires expertise and does have a significant failure rate of about 14 percent, which means that it is not widely used.

Biochemical

Blood gas and pH measurements are probably the most useful biochemical investigations. Hypoxemia, hypercapnia and a combined metabolic and respiratory acidosis are characteristic findings in RDS. From arterial oxygen tension (PaO_2) measurements, the size of the right-to-left shunt can be calculated. The P_{50} is the point on the oxyhemoglobin dissociation curve at which the hemoglobin is 50 percent saturated and in preterm infants is usually between 2.9 and 3.1 kPa (22–23 mmHg) on the first day. By term the P_{50} has increased to 3.3–3.5 kPa (25–26 mmHg) and shows the expected variation with pH.[136] Some degree of hypercapnia is present in nearly all cases of RDS prior to treatment and its absence should suggest an alternative diagnosis such as transient tachypnea of the newborn (Table 19.3).

The objectives of treatment of RDS are to prevent hypoxemia, severe hypercapnia and acidosis, which lead to hypotension and poor perfusion of organs such as the brain and kidneys. Arterial blood gases and pH need to be assessed regularly in infants with moderate to severe RDS and this will usually necessitate insertion of an indwelling arterial catheter. The right radial artery or an umbilical artery may be used for this purpose. Neonatal units should have their own blood gas analyzer on site to allow frequent arterial blood analysis, every 2–4 hours if necessary. Continuous blood gas and pH monitoring is now possible using specially developed sensing catheters,[144] but these are expensive and sometimes not easy to insert and, therefore, have not gained widespread popularity to date. Pulse oximetry provides a continuous display of oxygen saturation and is now used widely in neonatal units as a surrogate measure for PaO_2.[74] Its main drawback, however, is that hyperoxia cannot be completely excluded and in infants at risk of retinopathy of prematurity (ROP), other forms of monitoring which measure PaO_2 must be used in addition.[166]

Hypernatremia and hyperkalemia occur in RDS.[159,223] The risk of hypernatremia can be reduced by avoiding the use of overhead radiant warmers after the initial period of resuscitation and stabilization, the provision of adequate fluids, use of high humidity in incubators and avoidance of sodium supplements including bicarbonate in the early neonatal period. Serum sodium will usually increase a little despite these measures, but levels above 150 mmol/L should be avoided. Occasionally hyponatremia is found soon after birth, but this usually means that there has been excessive fluid and oxytocin administration to the mother during labor.[211] On recovery from RDS, impaired renal tubular reabsorption results in excessive sodium losses in the urine, leading to hyponatremia unless adequate replacement is given during this phase. Hyperkalemia can occur in VLBW infants, despite apparently normal renal function.[20,77] This is probably due to a shift of potassium ions from blood cells and is not usually dangerous until levels above 7.0 mmol/L have been reached.[185] In the presence of reduced renal function, hyperkalemia will be exaggerated.[19,78] The kidneys of infants with RDS are also poor at excreting hydrogen ions[5] and this contributes to their metabolic acidosis. The reduction in renal function can be exacerbated by excessive fluid restriction, which will lead to increased plasma urea and creatinine.[78]

Serum albumin is often low in infants with RDS and this is due to a combination of leak into the subcutaneous tissues,[107] poor protein intake and impaired hepatic synthesis. Low albumin levels are associated with low colloid osmotic pressure, which is close to the level at which tissue and pulmonary edema develop.[16]

Immediately after birth, preterm infants with RDS may develop hypoglycemia as a result of inadequate glucose intake and reduced glycogen stores,[29] but later they may develop hyperglycemia,[163] which is due to a combination of stress hormones, excessive intake from intravenous supplementation and relative tissue resistance to insulin.[71,164]

Hematologic

There are no specific hematologic features of RDS, although infants with this condition can develop anemia from blood losses (sampling for investigations or intracranial hemorrhage). The white blood cell count is usually normal for gestation.[135] If it is raised ($>35\,000/mm^3$) or lowered ($<6000/mm^3$) then congenital sepsis should be suspected.[91] Thrombocytopenia is not normally a feature of RDS, unless there is sepsis or disseminated intravascular coagulation (DIC). Thrombocytopenia has, however, been reported as a complication of mechanical ventilation in the newborn.[11] Other measurements of coagulation (prothrombin time and partial thromboplastin time) are prolonged in preterm infants compared to adults and illness such as RDS may aggravate these findings. Overt DIC, however, is rare in infants with RDS unless there has been coexistent birth asphyxia, hypothermia or sepsis.[22,137]

Microbiological

Since sepsis is one of the most important differential diagnoses of RDS, cultures of blood and gastric aspirates should be taken on admission to the neonatal unit (p. 281). A history of chorioamnionitis or a positive maternal high vaginal swab for group B β-hemolytic streptococci (GBS) makes these investigations even more important. The place of lumbar puncture in the investigation of RDS is somewhat controversial. In most cases it is not necessary[82,230] as blood cultures are sufficient to isolate any infecting organism. In the presence of neurological signs, however, a lumbar puncture is recommended as soon as the infant is likely to tolerate the extra manipulation involved. After cultures have been taken, treatment with antibiotics should be started in all infants with respiratory signs to eradicate GBS infection which may be present (p. 283).[91]

Echocardiography

Echocardiography can be helpful to exclude unrecognized congenital heart disease and to look for pulmonary hypertension and/or depressed myocardial function.[114] Later echocardiography can be used to diagnose PDA and assess whether treatment with indomethacin or ibuprofen is required.

Measurement of surfactant

Gastric or tracheal aspirate or amniotic fluid may be examined for surfactant activity. L:S ratio was formerly used to determine the presence of sufficient amounts of surface-active phospholipids but it is now rarely used. Assessment of surfactant protein levels, SP-A or SP-B, may be used to determine pulmonary maturity, but the assays are relatively expensive and take time to perform. Rapid tests for diagnosis of RDS soon after birth include the 'shake test'[24] and the 'click test'.[189] The 'shake test' relies upon the fact that surfactant generates stable foam when shaken with ethanol. The 'click test' is said to be quick, simple, inexpensive, reproducible, unaffected by contamination with blood and capable of being used to permit early and optimal treatment with surfactant. Despite this, it has not found favor as a routine investigation in most perinatal centers.

PREVENTION

Prevention of prematurity

As most infants with RDS are born prematurely, the avoidance of prematurity would largely prevent this respiratory disorder.[161] Premature birth is associated with poverty and its covariates (drug use, alcohol abuse, smoking, stress and poor diet).[209] Availability and access to prenatal care may reduce risks of premature birth,[157,237] but the results of these studies may not be generalizable. In countries with comparatively low rates of premature birth, interventions in the antenatal period probably have limited effects even in the high-risk groups.[56,227] The pathophysiology of preterm birth, like that of normal birth, remains uncertain[69] and until more is known it is unlikely that prevention of prematurity will become a reality for many years.

Some obstetric interventions, such as *in vitro* fertilization, increase the risk of preterm birth at least partly because of the increase in higher multiple births.[123] Other interventions such as cervical cerclage,[150] control of hypertension and tocolytic therapy have had limited effects on preventing premature birth. As an example, if cervical cerclage is used in women with a previous mid-trimester loss, it will prevent one preterm labor for every 25–30 cerclages performed.[87,150] Beta-mimetic drugs, such as ritodrine, have been shown to be effective in prolonging pregnancy for up to 48 hours but not longer.[118] This intervention, however, might be beneficial to allow time for drugs which mature the fetal lungs to be given and to organize transfer to a tertiary perinatal center for delivery.[51]

Antenatal drugs

CORTICOSTEROIDS

Prenatal treatment with a total of 24 mg betamethasone reduces the risk of RDS by about 60 percent and neonatal mortality by about 40 percent (Table 19.5) and VLBW infants seem to derive the same benefit as more mature infants.[44,156] The reduction in the risk of RDS is accompanied by decreases in periventricular hemorrhage and necrotizing enterocolitis,[83] but not chronic lung disease (Table 19.5).

Guidelines for antenatal corticosteroids

There are very few contraindications to antenatal corticosteroid treatment when preterm labor is likely. Diabetic control may be more difficult, hypertension may need additional treatment and infectious indicators in the mother and newborn may be obscured, but these are not contraindications to therapy.[209] In 1994, a Consensus Conference organized by the National Institutes for Health in the USA suggested the following recommendations for use of corticosteroids to prevent RDS:[153]

- All fetuses between 24 and 34 weeks of gestation at risk of preterm birth should be considered candidates for antenatal treatment with corticosteroids.
- The decision to use antenatal corticosteroids should not be altered by fetal race or gender or by the availability of surfactant replacement therapy.
- Patients eligible for therapy with tocolytics should also be eligible for treatment with corticosteroids.
- Treatment consists of two doses of 12 mg betamethasone given intramuscularly 24 hours apart or four doses of dexamethasone given intramuscularly 12 hours apart. Optimal benefit begins 24 hours after initiation of therapy and lasts for 7 days.
- Treatment with corticosteroids for less than 24 hours is associated with significant reductions in neonatal mortality, RDS and intraventricular hemorrhage (IVH), thus antenatal corticosteroids should be given unless immediate delivery is anticipated.
- In preterm premature rupture of the membranes at less than 30–32 weeks of gestation, in the absence of

Table 19.5 *Meta-analysis of outcome of antenatal corticosteroid treatment*

Outcome	Number Trials	Number Babies	Odds ratio	95% CI
RDS (all babies)	18	3735	0.53	0.44–0.63
RDS (<28 wk)	4	48	0.64	0.16–2.50
RDS (<30 wk)	8	349	0.48	0.30–0.77
RDS (<32 wk)	7	393	0.33	0.21–0.50
RDS (<34 wk)	7	1048	0.36	0.27–0.48
RDS (>34 wk)	8	744	0.65	0.33–1.29
RDS (<24 h after 1st dose)	6	349	0.70	0.43–1.16
RDS (<48 h after 1st dose)	1	42	0.34	0.08–1.16
RDS (24 h–7 d after 1st dose)	4	728	0.38	0.25–0.57
RDS (>7 d after 1st dose)	3	265	0.41	0.18–0.98
RDS (dexamethasone)	5	1400	0.56	0.43–0.73
RDS (betamethasone)	11	2176	0.49	0.39–0.63
RDS (hydrocortisone)	2	172	0.69	0.32–1.47
RDS (males)	3	627	0.43	0.29–0.64
RDS (females)	3	555	0.36	0.23–0.57
RDS (twins/triplets)	2	140	0.72	0.31–1.68
NND (all)	14	3517	0.60	0.48–0.75
NND (<1980)	8	2133	0.51	0.38–0.68
NND (>1980)	6	1384	0.78	0.54–1.12
IVH (autopsy)	4	863	0.29	0.14–0.61
IVH (US)	5	596	0.48	0.32–0.72
NEC	4	1154	0.59	0.32–1.09
CLD	3	411	1.57	0.87–2.84
Surfactant use	1	121	0.41	0.18–0.89
Stillbirth (all)	12	3306	0.83	0.57–1.22
Stillbirth (hypertension)	4	239	3.75	1.24–11.30
Infection (fetal & neonatal)	15	2675	0.82	0.57–1.19
Infection (PROM > 24 h)	2	163	2.31	0.77–6.99
Infection (PROM at trial entry)	4	329	1.11	0.50–2.43
Maternal infection (PROM > 24 h)	11	2109	1.31	0.99–1.73
Maternal infection (PROM > 24 h)	1	42	6.04	1.47–24.7
Maternal infection (PROM at trial entry)	3	320	1.26	0.69–2.28
Long-term neurological abnormality	3	778	0.62	0.36–1.08

Adapted from Crowley.[32]

clinical chorioamnionitis, antenatal corticosteroid use is recommended because of the high risk of IVH at these early gestational ages.

- In complicated pregnancies where delivery prior to 34 weeks' gestation is likely, antenatal corticosteroid use is recommended unless there is evidence that corticosteroids will have an adverse effect on the mother or delivery is imminent.

The Royal College of Obstetricians and Gynaecologists (RCOG) published similar guidelines for use of antenatal corticosteroids, but extended the upper gestational age limit to 36 weeks.[176]

Betamethasone is preferable to dexamethasone as the latter was associated with a greater risk of periventricular leukomalacia in an observational study from France.[14] There is no evidence that a single course of antenatal corticosteroids causes any harmful long-term effects,[133,192]

but there is some doubt about the safety of multiple courses.[60] Until the results of ongoing randomized trials comparing a single course with multiple courses of antenatal corticosteroids are available, multiple courses cannot be recommended as routine treatment.[70]

There is now accumulating evidence that the combination of antenatal corticosteroids and postnatal surfactant leads to improved outcomes compared to either treatment alone.[53,113] Indeed, the combination of antenatal corticosteroids and prophylactic surfactant is the most cost-effective intervention for RDS in infants of less than 30 weeks of gestation.[47]

THYROTROPIN-RELEASING HORMONE (TRH)

TRH has been used with corticosteroids in three studies; a reduction in the risk of CLD was found in one.[10] Subsequent studies, however, have shown that TRH and corticosteroids increase the risk of RDS and the need for assisted ventilation[2] and at follow-up there was an increased risk of motor delay and sensory impairment in surviving infants.[34] Administration of TRH to women at risk of preterm delivery can no longer be recommended.

AMBROXOL

Ambroxol, a metabolite of bromhexine, has been used in some centers in Europe to promote fetal lung maturation.[205] The few studies showing benefit, however, were poorly designed and either too small or failed to analyze outcomes in all of the treated infants.[132] One further study showed no benefit from antenatal ambroxol[39] and this, together with the need for 5 days of intravenous treatment, make this intervention of limited use.

Prevention of intrapartum asphyxia

Asphyxia increases the risk and severity of RDS. If asphyxia is absent and the preterm fetus is presenting by the vertex, there seems to be no need to proceed to cesarean section on a routine basis,[4] but if fetal distress develops, delivery by cesarean section should be considered at gestations of 24 weeks and above. For preterm fetuses who are presenting by the breech, it is likely that cesarean section leads to improved outcomes with less asphyxia and a reduced risk of intracranial hemorrhage.[120] There have been no successful randomized trials of method of delivery in preterm pregnancies, but the risk of entrapment of the aftercoming head is likely to be reduced by cesarean delivery.[18] A recent randomized trial of method of delivery in term breech presentations demonstrated significant benefits for mother and baby when delivery was by cesarean section.[97] Asphyxia and the associated hypoxemia and acidosis affect surfactant synthesis. Hypothermia has a similar effect and both should be avoided following preterm birth to reduce the risk and severity of RDS.

MANAGEMENT

Treatment of RDS comprises a number of interventions which should begin immediately after birth. The initial care of preterm infants at risk of developing RDS may be critical in reducing the severity of the condition and preventing deterioration and its associated complications. Delivery room management, surfactant treatment, ventilatory support and general supportive care are the important components of treatment of RDS.

Delivery room management

Appropriate resuscitation of preterm infants at risk of developing RDS is vitally important. These deliveries must always be attended by the most experienced pediatric staff. Transfer to a tertiary perinatal center before birth has been shown to improve outcome. Resuscitation might require endotracheal intubation,[129] which will allow the prophylactic administration of surfactant.[112] Prevention of asphyxia and early or prophylactic administration of surfactant are both beneficial interventions but unnecessary intubation and overtreatment with surfactant might be harmful and wasteful of resources. An alternative strategy is the early use of CPAP, which has been associated with a reduced risk of chronic lung disease in non-randomized trials (p. 151).[146] Furthermore, studies from Scandinavia have shown that intubation for surfactant administration followed by extubation to nasal CPAP can reduce the need for positive pressure ventilation.[225,226] This leaves the clinician attending the birth of a preterm infant with a dilemma about the best way to undertake initial resuscitation and management.[129] Guidelines for early management of RDS have been proposed (Figure 19.4).[84,177] In general, these guidelines are based upon the perceived risk of an infant developing RDS and they take into account gestational age, use of antenatal corticosteroids, method of delivery, complications of pregnancy such as

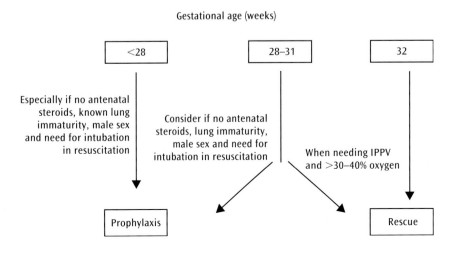

Gestational age (weeks)

<28   28–31   32

Especially if no antenatal steroids, known lung immaturity, male sex and need for intubation in resuscitation

Consider if no antenatal steroids, lung immaturity, male sex and need for intubation in resuscitation

When needing IPPV and >30–40% oxygen

Prophylaxis   Rescue

Figure 19.4 *Flow chart to guide timing of surfactant treatment. (Reproduced with permission from Halliday.[84])*

hypertension or antepartum hemorrhage and the infant's condition at birth (need for endotracheal intubation for resuscitation).

Surfactant therapy

A number of surfactant preparations are used in clinical practice (Table 19.6). Natural surfactants (derived from animal lungs) have some clear advantages over synthetic, protein-free preparations (Table 19.7). There have been many randomized controlled trials of surfactant replacement therapy.[36,112,174] These have used synthetic or natural surfactants, in doses ranging from 50 to 200 mg/kg given at various times after birth (prophylaxis and early and late treatment). The results of these trials have been synthesized as a number of meta-analyses published in the Cochrane Library.[193–198] Both natural and synthetic surfactants, given as either prophylaxis (Tables 19.8 and 19.9) or treatment (Table 19.10), reduce mortality rates and the incidence of pulmonary air leaks compared with control infants receiving only mechanical ventilation. Prophylactic surfactant has advantages over selective use of surfactant (Table 19.11). Multiple doses of surfactant give better outcomes than a single dose in those infants who relapse (Table 19.12).

PROPHYLACTIC SURFACTANT

A meta-analysis has shown that prophylactic surfactant, that is, given within 10–15 minutes of birth, leads to reduced mortality for infants of 31 weeks of gestation or less,[48] but the benefit is likely to be relatively greater at lower gestational ages. The cost of surfactant also needs

Table 19.6 *Some surfactant preparations in clinical use*

Generic name	Trade name	Composition	Concentration (mg/mL)	Dose (mg/kg)	No. doses	Dose volume (mL/kg)
Natural[a]						
Surfactant TA	Surfacten® (Tokyo Tanabe)	Bovine mince plus DPPC, tripalmitin and palmitic acid	30	120	3	4
Beractant	Survanta® (Ross)	Bovine mince plus DPPC, tripalmitin and palmitic acid	25	100	4	4
Bovactant	Alveofact® (Thomae)	Bovine lavage	41.7	50	4	1.2
Poractant alfa	Curosurf® (Chiesi)	Porcine mince (polar lipids)	80	100–200	3	1.25–2.5
Calfactant	Infasurf® (Forest)	Calf lung lavage	33.3	100	3	3
Synthetic						
Colfosceril palmitate	Exosurf® (Glaxo-Wellcome)	DPPC 13.5 mg, hexadeconal 1.5 mg, tyloxapol 1.0 mg	13.5	67.5	3	5

[a]All these drugs contain SP-B and SP-C in concentrations of 1–2 percent.
*In the US the dose is 200 mg/kg.

Table 19.7 *Meta-analysis comparing outcome of natural versus synthetic surfactants*

Outcome	Number		RR	95% CI	NNT	95% CI
	Trials	Babies				
Pneumothorax	9	4550	0.63	0.53–0.75	23	17–37
PDA	7	3283	0.98	0.91–1.06	–	–
Sepsis	8	4413	1.00	0.90–1.12	–	–
IVH	7	4220	1.09	1.00–1.19	36	18–∞
Severe IVH	8	4202	1.08	0.92–1.28	–	–
ROP	4	2396	0.95	0.88–1.01	–	–
BPD	8	3515	1.02	0.93–1.11	–	–
CLD	5	3179	1.01	0.90–1.12	–	–
Mortality	10	4588	0.86	0.76–0.98	40	22–334

BPD, bronchopulmonary dysplasia; CLD, chronic lung disease; IVH, intraventricular hemorrhage; PDA, patent ductus arteriosus; ROP, retinopathy of prematurity.
Adapted from Soll and Blanco.[197]

Table 19.8 *Meta-analysis of outcome of prophylactic natural surfactant*

Outcome	Number Trials	Number Babies	RR	95% CI	NNT	95% CI
Pneumothorax	8	988	0.35	0.26–0.49	7	5–9
PDA	8	988	1.08	0.94–1.24	–	–
IVH	8	986	0.98	0.84–1.15	–	–
Severe IVH	7	961	1.22	0.90–1.66	–	–
BPD	7	932	0.93	0.80–1.07	–	–
Neonatal mortality	7	932	0.60	0.44–0.83	14	9–35
Mortality before discharge	6	402	0.70	0.47–1.06	–	–
ROP	2	92	1.37	0.63–2.98	–	–
Severe ROP	3	250	0.58	0.27–1.24	–	–
PIE	5	749	0.46	0.35–0.60	6	4–8

BPD, bronchopulmonary dysplasia; IVH, intraventricular hemorrhage; PDA, patent ductus arteriosus; PIE, pulmonary interstitial emphysema; ROP, retinopathy of prematurity. Adapted from Soll.[194]

Table 19.9 *Meta-analysis of outcome of prophylactic synthetic surfactant*

Outcome	Number Trials	Number Babies	RR	95% CI	NNT	95% CI
Pneumothorax	6	1252	0.67	0.50–0.90	20	12–67
IVH	4	1146	0.96	0.81–1.14	–	–
BPD	4	1086	1.06	0.83–1.36	–	–
Neonatal mortality	7	1500	0.70	0.58–0.85	15	10–31
Mortality before discharge	5	729	0.86	0.71–1.04	–	–
PDA	7	1560	1.11	1.00–1.22	21	11–500
PIE	2	831	0.68	0.50–0.93	16	9–77
Necrotizing enterocolitis	7	1543	1.11	0.78–1.59	–	–
Severe IVH	4	1117	1.01	0.75–1.38	–	–
Pulmonary hemorrhage	4	1120	3.28	1.50–7.16	32	19–84
Cerebral palsy (1–2 years)	4	670	0.93	0.64–1.33	–	–
ROP	3	645	0.96	0.86–1.07	–	–
Severe ROP	3	645	0.89	0.58–1.36	–	–
Mortality (1 year)	3	1046	0.83	0.70–0.98	18	10–200

BPD, bronchopulmonary dysplasia; IVH, intraventricular hemorrhage; PDA, patent ductus arteriosus; PIE, pulmonary interstitial emphysema; ROP, retinopathy of prematurity. Adapted from Soll.[195]

to be taken into account, as overtreatment of infants who are less likely to develop RDS represents a waste of limited resources. For these reasons prophylactic surfactant has been recommended only for infants of less than 27–28 weeks of gestation unless the mother has not received antenatal corticosteroids.

EARLY RESCUE SURFACTANT

For infants of 32 weeks of gestation and greater, early rescue treatment when endotracheal intubation becomes necessary to treat RDS is recommended. At gestational ages in between, that is from 28 to 31 weeks, early CPAP is recommended with surfactant given as soon as endotracheal

intubation is needed. If intubation at birth is needed for resuscitation, surfactant should be given at that time. This in effect will mean that those resuscitating preterm babies need to have surfactant available in the delivery room from 23 or 24 weeks of gestation to 31 weeks of gestation, aiming to give surfactant to those under 27–28 weeks of gestation and to have it in reserve for others who might need intubation for resuscitation.

RESCUE SURFACTANT

For infants not given prophylactic surfactant, the decision to give surfactant treatment must be based upon factors such as gestational age and severity of RDS assessed by

Table 19.10 *Meta-analysis of outcome of synthetic surfactant for RDS*

Outcome	Number Trials	Babies	RR	95% CI	NNT	95% CI
Pneumothorax	5	2328	0.64	0.55–0.76	12	9–18
PIE	4	2224	0.62	0.54–0.71	8	6–12
Pulmonary hemorrhage	5	2328	1.44	0.68–3.05	–	–
PDA	5	2328	0.90	0.84–0.97	18	11–59
Necrotizing enterocolitis	5	2328	1.32	0.76–2.29	–	–
Apnea	4	2224	1.20	1.09–1.31	13	9–26
IVH	4	2224	0.88	0.77–0.99	27	14–500
Severe IVH	5	2328	0.84	0.63–1.12	–	–
BPD		2248	0.75	0.61–0.92	27	16–91
Neonatal mortality	6	2352	0.73	0.61–0.88	22	14–53
ROP	3	605	0.93	0.80–1.09	–	–
Severe ROP	3	605	0.73	0.46–1.17	–	–
Mortality before discharge	6	2352	0.79	0.68–0.92	23	14–63
Mortality at 1 year	4	2224	0.80	0.69–0.94	25	14–91
Cerebral palsy	5	1557	0.76	0.55–1.05	–	–

BPD, bronchopulmonary dysplasia; IVH, intraventricular hemorrhage; PDA, patent ductus arteriosus; PIE, pulmonary interstitial emphysema; ROP, retinopathy of prematurity. Adapted from Soll.[196]

Table 19.11 *Meta-analysis of outcome of prophylactic versus selective use of surfactant*

Outcome	Number Trials	Babies	RR	95% CI	NNT	95% CI
Pneumothorax	6	2515	0.62	0.42–0.89	48	27–200
PIE	5	2037	0.54	0.36–0.82	39	24–112
Necrotizing enterocolitis	5	2368	1.01	0.73–1.40	–	–
PDA	6	2515	0.96	0.85–1.09	–	–
IVH	7	2508	0.92	0.82–1.03	–	–
Severe IVH	7	2508	0.84	0.66–1.06	–	–
BPD	8	2816	0.96	0.82–1.12	–	–
Neonatal mortality	7	2613	0.61	0.48–0.77	22	15–42
Mortality before discharge	5	1207	0.75	0.59–0.96	20	11–125
ROP	4	1919	1.09	0.72–1.66	–	–
Severe ROP	2	388	0.97	0.45–2.10	–	–
Neonatal mortality < 30 weeks	7	1822	0.62	0.49–0.78	16	11–30

BPD, bronchopulmonary dysplasia; IVH, intraventricular hemorrhage; PDA, patent ductus arteriosus; PIE, pulmonary interstitial emphysema; ROP, retinopathy of prematurity. Adapted from Soll and Morley.[198]

Table 19.12 *Meta-analysis of multiple versus single dose of natural surfactant*

Outcome	Number Trials	Babies	RR	95% CI	NNT	95% CI
Pneumothorax	2	394	0.51	0.30–0.88	12	7–50
IVH	2	394	0.98	0.77–1.25	–	–
PDA	2	394	1.12	0.93–1.36	–	–
BPD	1	343	1.10	0.63–1.93	–	–
Sepsis	1	343	0.66	0.41–1.08	–	–
Mortality	2	394	0.63	0.39–1.02	15	8–∞

BPD, bronchopulmonary dysplasia; IVH, intraventricular hemorrhage; PDA, patent ductus arteriosus. Adapted from Soll.[193]

Table 19.13 *Recommendations for surfactant treatment*

	Recommendations
Type of surfactant	Natural preferred
	Synthetic may still be used for mild disease
Timing	Early rather than late (e.g. $FiO_2 > 0.40$)
Initial dose	100–200 mg phospholipids/kg
Re-treatment	Flexible (6–12-hourly) when $FiO_2 > 0.30$ and still on ventilator
Action after treatment	*For natural surfactants*:
	Lower FiO_2 immediately
	Reduce inspiratory time
	Lower PIP according to chest wall movement and blood gases
	For synthetic surfactant:
	Lower FiO_2 cautiously and maintain PEEP
Some causes of a poor response	*Wrong diagnosis*: lung hypoplasia, pneumonia, ARDS, congenital heart disease
	Wrong dose: inadequate to overcome surfactant inactivation
	Wrong place: given into one lung or into esophagus
	Wrong condition: correct hypothermia, acidosis and hypotension before treatment
Causes of early relapse and its management	*Inadequate dose*: re-treat
	PDA (Doppler, low diastolic BP): early use of indomethacin or ibruprofen
	Pneumonia (Gram stain and culture of tracheal aspirate): early treatment with antibiotics
	Pulmonary hemorrhage: increase pressures, close the PDA, give diuretics, consider re-treatment.

Adapted from Halliday and Speer.[90]

clinical signs, blood gas results and chest radiographic appearances (Table 19.13). Clearly, giving surfactant earlier rather than later improves the outcome (Table 19.11) and if the infant is able to tolerate extubation to CPAP then this has added advantages.[226] Natural surfactant preparations, containing SP-B and SP-C, are now preferred to the slower acting synthetic preparations. For infants who relapse, second and occasionally third doses of surfactant are usually indicated and lead to improved outcomes compared with a single dose (Table 19.13).

Transportation to the neonatal intensive care unit (NICU)

After resuscitation and stabilization, it is important that the preterm infant is transferred to the NICU without any deterioration. This means keeping the infant warm in a transport incubator and avoiding hypoxemia by giving oxygen, CPAP or intermittent positive pressure ventilation as needed. The adequacy of oxygenation can be assessed using a pulse oximeter, remembering that hyperoxia will not be detected.[74] If a longer transport is needed, for example, to a regional center, then this should be carried out by a dedicated neonatal transport team. Assisted ventilation in preference to CPAP, and adequate cardiorespiratory monitoring with chest leads and transcutaneous blood gas sensors[23] are prerequisites of efficient and safe neonatal transportation. In general, surfactant should be

given before transportation if this is indicated,[30] but it should be remembered that after surfactant the infant may need to be stabilized at the referral hospital before transfer.

Stabilization on the NICU

On arrival at the neonatal unit the infant must have a further period of assessment and stabilization and this may be best performed under a radiant warmer. To prevent excessive water losses, infants should not stay under a radiant warmer for longer than 1–2 hours. This time is needed to place further lines for intravenous fluids, arterial blood gas monitoring and to carry out chest and abdominal radiography to confirm line positions. Rescue surfactant may also need to be given at this time (p. 260). After further stabilization, the infant should be transferred to a warm, humidified incubator for further care.

FLUID MANAGEMENT

This will depend upon a number of factors, for example, gestational age, which correlates with insensible water losses, presence of asphyxia or hydrops, and severity of the respiratory distress. Generally, insensible water losses are high in the first 3 days after birth, especially in the most immature infants. Radiant warmers and phototherapy further increase insensible water losses. The presence of a PDA may be an indication for fluid restriction. Fluid restriction in the acute stage of RDS has been recommended with the aim of improving respiratory function. The results of a randomized trial, however, demonstrated that when sodium supplementation was controlled, restriction of maintenance fluids did not result in improvements in perinatal lung function.[116] Use of diuretics is not recommended even though oliguria and peripheral edema may be present. Diuretic-promoting agents such as furosemide or albumin do not improve respiratory function in infants with RDS.

MEDICATION

Infants requiring mechanical ventilation may need sedation with morphine or fentanyl[182] and in the presence of hypotension inotropic agents may occasionally be required (p. 211).

Ventilatory support

CPAP and positive pressure ventilation are both effective interventions and they reduce mortality in neonates with RDS.[85] Widespread use of antenatal corticosteroids and prophylactic surfactant means that these interventions may not be needed. CPAP should be used for babies with vigorous spontaneous respiration (usually more than 25–26 weeks of gestation). Initial pressures of 5–6 cmH$_2$O are used, but sometimes higher pressures of 7–8 cmH$_2$O may be needed (p. 151).[160] Intermittent positive pressure ventilation, if needed, should start at high rates (60–80/min) and peak pressures sufficient to achieve chest wall expansion, but preferably 20 cmH$_2$O or less. Inspiratory times should be 0.3–0.4 seconds. Inspiratory times and ventilator rates should be manipulated to achieve synchrony (p. 159). PEEP levels of at least 3 cmH$_2$O initially should be employed, but increased if the RDS is severe. After surfactant has been administered, ventilator settings can usually be adjusted downwards. To reduce the risks of chronic lung disease, the lowest ventilator settings possible should be used. HFOV cannot yet be recommended as a starting treatment for infants with RDS.[99,145] For infants receiving mechanical ventilation, it is important that there is adequate humidification of the inspired gases.[212] Endotracheal tube suction is rarely needed early in the course of RDS (p. 236).[210,236]

COMPLICATIONS

Complications of RDS may arise because of prematurity, as sequelae of RDS, and/or as a result of treatment. Examples of acute pulmonary complications are pneumothorax (p. 311), pulmonary interstitial emphysema and pulmonary hemorrhage (p. 365). Acute extrapulmonary complications include intraventricular hemorrhage and persistent ductus arteriosus. Chronic complications include retinopathy of prematurity, neurodevelopmental sequelae, chronic lung disease and adverse effects of treatment such as subglottic stenosis.

Air leaks

The incidence of pneumothorax depends upon the severity of RDS, the need for assisted ventilation and whether or not surfactant treatment has been given (p. 312). In the surfactant trials infants, in the control groups had rates of pneumothorax varying between 11 and 80 percent with lower rates in the prophylaxis trials. Surfactant treatment reduces the risk of pneumothorax by more than 60 percent if natural surfactants are given prophylactically. This means that most neonatal units experience a rate of pneumothorax of less than 5–10 percent, so that resident doctors are often inexperienced in the placement of chest drains. The incidence of pulmonary interstitial emphysema (PIE) in control infants in the surfactant trials ranged from 22 to 73 percent, being greater in the treatment trials. Treatment with natural surfactant reduces the risk of PIE by about 70 percent. PIE is associated with raised elastase levels in tracheal aspirates,[62] suggesting that intrauterine infection may be a predisposing factor. Severe bilateral or even unilateral PIE (more common on the right side) is often difficult to manage (p. 319).

Pulmonary hemorrhage

Pulmonary hemorrhage (p. 365) is a rare, but serious complication of RDS which may be increased after surfactant therapy, especially with synthetic surfactants.[169,203] There is also an association with persistent ductus arteriosus,[203] which is consistent with the view that it is really hemorrhagic pulmonary edema secondary to left ventricular failure and damage to the pulmonary capillaries.[27] The onset is frequently between the second and fourth day,[80] when there may be sudden deterioration with pink or red frothy fluid aspirated from the lungs or endotracheal tube. The chest radiograph may show massive consolidation. Treatment should include increased ventilator pressures to produce tamponade and reduce pulmonary capillary bleeding, diuretics to treat pulmonary edema and indomethacin or ibuprofen to close the ductus arteriosus if it appears to be patent.[80] Re-treatment with surfactant may be beneficial.[155] With timely treatment this formerly fatal condition can be controlled, but the associated sudden deterioration can lead to periventricular hemorrhage or leukomalacia.

Periventricular hemorrhage (PVH)

This is a relatively common association of severe RDS; the incidence ranges from 14 to 72 percent in infants who had been enrolled in trials of surfactant replacement.[87] The effect of surfactant treatment on the risk of periventricular hemorrhage (PVH) has been variable, with some trials showing a reduction,[50,64,139,147] but one an increase.[103] Systematic reviews, however, suggest that the overall effect is a non-significant reduction in PVH following surfactant treatment.[124,200] Pneumothorax is commonly associated with PVH[130] and as surfactant treatment reduces the risk of pulmonary air leak this may be one mechanism whereby surfactant exerts a positive effect. The development of a PVH is often associated with clinical deterioration characterized by increasing ventilatory needs and neurologic signs, which may be subtle. Small PVH and periventricular leukomalacia (PVL) are generally asymptomatic. Maintenance of normal blood pressure can prevent or reduce these neurologic complications. Recently, it has become apparent that PVL can be caused by an inflammatory process, which may have its origin in utero[37,38] and in these cases prevention requires a prenatal intervention.

Persistent ductus arteriosus (PDA)

The ductus arteriosus is likely to remain open in babies with severe RDS for a number of reasons: prematurity is associated with poorly developed circular musculature in the ductus, there are reduced arterial oxygen tensions and inadequate metabolism of vasodilatory prostaglandins in the lungs.[81] Fluid overload may also be an important factor in the etiology of PDA.[15] The incidence of PDA in the surfactant trials ranged from 14 to 83 percent and there is a suggestion from the meta-analyses of an increased risk after surfactant treatment.[195,200] The greatest risk would appear to be in very immature male babies treated with prophylactic synthetic surfactant.[203] An association has been made between PDA and pulmonary hemorrhage in these infants.[224] For this reason early use of either intravenous indomethacin or ibuprofen has been recommended.[40] Late signs of PDA include a continuous murmur, active precordium and bounding pulses often associated with a deterioration in pulmonary status. Early signs include hypotension with diastolic blood pressure particularly being reduced, and echocardiography is also helpful at this stage to confirm the diagnosis.

Chronic lung disease (CLD)

Most infants developing chronic lung disease (CLD) weigh less than 1100 g and about half of them have mild or no initial respiratory disease.[12] CLD, sometimes referred to as the 'new bronchopulmonary dysplasia (BPD)', is probably due to abnormal repair following acute lung injury. There is evidence of a chronic inflammatory process in the airways,[75] which may have its origins in utero associated with chorioamnionitis. CLD can be defined as an

oxygen requirement beyond 28 days (mild disease) or beyond 36 weeks corrected age (severe disease).[206] Using these definitions the incidence varies between 40 and 70 percent.[102] Prevention of CLD is difficult (p. 409) and the effects of both antenatal corticosteroids and surfactant treatment appear minimal.[184,206]

Retinopathy of prematurity (ROP)

Retinopathy of prematurity (ROP) remains an important cause of blindness. With the introduction of surfactant treatment there were concerns that the risk of ROP would increase, but this has not been confirmed and, indeed, it would appear that the incidence has decreased.[171] Gestational age, severe systemic illness and hyperoxia are all important factors in the pathogenesis of ROP and the size and quality of hospital providing neonatal care also determine the risks of mortality and severe ROP.[41]

Subglottic stenosis (p. 443)

This is an uncommon complication of endotracheal intubation.[149] It has been associated with the use of cuffed or shouldered endotracheal tubes, insertion of tubes that were too wide, inadequate humidification, too frequent or vigorous tracheal suction and repeated intubations.

Neurodevelopmental outcome and prognosis

During the past 25 years, survival of very preterm infants with RDS has greatly increased,[122] but the population of disabled survivors has generally remained constant. Infants of gestational ages 22–25 weeks have a particularly poor long-term prognosis.[31,239] In addition to immaturity, factors such as intrauterine growth retardation, neonatal signs of cerebral depression and low social class are significant predictors of neurodevelopmental problems at 9 years of age.[128] Cerebral ultrasound scans can also be used to predict outcome[204] and absence of large PVH or PVL is usually a good prognostic sign.[72]

REFERENCES

1 Ablow, R.C., Orzalesi, M.M. (1971) Localized roentgenographic pattern of hyaline membrane disease. *American Journal of Radiology* 112, 23–27.

2 Actobat Study Group. (1995) Australian collaborative trial of antenatal thyrotropin releasing hormome (ACTOBAT) for prevention of neonatal respiratory disease. *Lancet* 345, 877–882.

3 Adams, E.W., Counsell, S.J., Hajnal, J.V. et al. (2000) Investigation of lung disease in preterm infants using magnetic resonance imaging. *Biology of the Neonate* 77(Suppl 1), 17–20.

4   Ahn, M.O., Cha, K.Y., Phelan, J.P. (1992) The low birthweight infant: is there a preferred route of delivery? *Clinics in Perinatology* **19**, 411–423.

5   Allen, A.C., Usher, R.H. (1971) Renal acid excretion in infants with respiratory distress syndrome. *Pediatric Research* **5**, 345–355.

6   Arnold, C., McLean, F.H., Dramer, M.S., Usher, R.H. (1987) Respiratory distress syndrome in second-born versus first-born twins. *New England Journal of Medicine* **317**, 1121–1124.

7   Avery, M.E., Mead, J. (1959) Surface properties in relation to atelectasis and hyaline membrane disease. *American Journal of Diseases in Childhood* **97**, 517–523.

8   Avni, E.F., Braude, P., Pardou, A., Matos, C. (1990) Hyaline membrane disease in the newborn: diagnosis by ultrasound. *Pediatric Radiology* **20**, 143–146.

9   Azzopardi, D., Robertson, N.J., Cowan, F.M. *et al.* (2000) Pilot study of treatment with whole body hypothermia for neonatal encephalopathy. *Pediatrics* **106**, 684–694.

10 Ballard, R.A., Ballard, P.L., Creasy, R.K. *et al.* (1992) Respiratory disease in very low birthweight infants after prenatal thyrotropin-releasing hormone and glucocorticoids. *Lancet* **339**, 510–515.

11 Ballin, A., Koren, G., Kohelet, D. *et al.* (1987) Reduction of platelet counts induced by mechanical ventilation in newborn infants. *Journal of Pediatrics* **111**, 445–449.

12 Bancalari, E., del Moral, T. (2001) Bronchopulmonary dysplasia and surfactant. *Biology of the Neonate* **80**(Suppl 1), 7–13.

13 Banias, B.B., Devoe, L.T., Nolan, T.E. (1983) Severe pre-eclampsia in preterm pregnancy between 26 and 32 weeks' gestation. *American Journal of Perinatology* **9**, 357–360.

14 Baud, O., Foix-L'Helias, L., Kaminski, M. *et al.* (1999) Antenatal glucocorticoid treatment and cystic periventricular leukomalacia in very premature infants. *New England Journal of Medicine* **341**, 1190–1196.

15 Bell, E.F., Warburton, D., Stonestreet, B., Oh, W. (1980) Effect of fluid administration on the development of symptomatic patent ductus arteriosus and congestive heart failure in premature infants. *New England Journal of Medicine* **302**, 598–604.

16 Bhat, R., Malacis, L., Shurla, A., Vidyasagar, D. (1983) Colloid osmotic pressure in infants with hyaline membrane disease. *Chest* **83**, 776–779.

17 Bick, U., Muller-Leisse, C., Troger, J. *et al.* (1992) Therapeutic use of surfactant in neonatal respiratory distress syndrome. *Pediatric Radiology* **22**, 169–173.

18 Bodmer, B., Benjamin, A., McLean, F., Usher, R.H. (1986) Has the use of cesarean section reduced the risks of delivery in the preterm breech presentation? *American Journal of Obstetrics and Gynecology* **154**, 244–250.

19 Brem, A.S. (1992) Electrolyte disorders associated with respiratory distress syndrome and bronchopulmonary dysplasia. *Clinics in Perinatology* **19**, 223–231.

20 Brion, L.P., Schwartz, G.J., Campbell, D., Fleischman, A.R. (1989) Early hyperkalaemia in very low birthweight infants in the absence of oliguria. *Archives of Disease in Childhood* **64**, 270–272.

21 Bryan, H., Hawrylyshyn, P., Hogg-Johnson, S. *et al.* (1990) Perinatal factors associated with the respiratory distress syndrome. *American Journal of Obstetrics and Gynecology* **162**, 476–481.

22 Chessels, J.M., Wigglesworth, J.S. (1972) Coagulation studies in preterm infants with respiratory distress and intracranial haemorrhage. *Archives of Disease in Childhood* **47**, 564–570.

23 Clarke, T.A., Zmora, E., Chen, J.H. *et al.* (1980) Transcutaneous oxygen monitoring during neonatal transport. *Pediatrics* **65**, 884–886.

24 Clements, J.A., Platzker, A.C.G., Rierney, D.F. *et al.* (1972) Assessment of the risk of respiratory distress syndrome by a rapid test for surfactant in amniotic fluid. *New England Journal of Medicine* **286**, 1077–1081.

25 Cohen, M., Carson, B.S. (1985) Respiratory morbidity benefit of awaiting onset of labor after elective cesarean section. *Obstetrics and Gynecology* **65**, 818–824.

26 Cole, F.S., Hamvas, A., Rubenstein, P. *et al.* (2000) Population-based estimates of surfactant protein B deficiency. *Pediatrics* **105**, 538–541.

27 Cole, V.A., Normand, I.C.S., Reynolds, E.O.R., Rivers, R.P.A. (1973) Pathogenesis of hemorrhagic pulmonary edema and massive pulmonary hemorrhage in the newborn. *Pediatrics* **51**, 175–187.

28 Corcoran, J.D., Sheehan, O., O'Hare, M.M.T., Halliday, H.L. (1995) Tracheal aspirate surfactant protein A following treatment with Curosurf. *Applied Cardiopulmonary Pathophysiology* **5**, 245–248.

29 Cornblath, M., Schwartz, R. (1976) *Disorders of Carbohydrate Metabolism in Infancy*. Philadelphia: WB Saunders.

30 Costakos, D., Allen, D., Kraus, A. *et al.* (1996) Surfactant therapy prior to the interhospital transport of preterm infants. *American Journal of Perinatology* **13**, 309–316.

31 Costeloe, K., Hennessy, E., Gibson, A.T. *et al.* (2000) The EPICure study: outcomes to discharge from hospital for infants born at the threshold of viability. *Pediatrics* **106**, 659–671.

32 Crowley, P. (2003) Prophylactic corticosteroids for preterm birth (Cochrane Review). In *The Cochrane Library*, Issue 1. Update Software, Oxford.

33 Crowley, P., Chalmers, I., Keirse, M. (1990) The effects of corticosteroid administration before preterm delivery: an overview of the evidence from controlled trials. *British Journal of Obstetrics and Gynaecology* **97**, 11–25.

34 Crowther, C.A., Hiller, J.E., Haslam, R.R. *et al.* (1997) Australian collaborative trial of antenatal thyrotropin-releasing hormone: adverse effects at 12-month follow-up. *Pediatrics* **99**, 311–317.

35 Cunningham, M.D., Desai, N.F., Thompson, S.A., Greene, J.M. (1978) Amniotic fluid phosphatidylglycerol in diabetic pregnancies. *American Journal of Obstetrics and Gynecology* **131**, 719–724.

36 Curley, A.E., Halliday, H.L. (2001) The present status of exogenous surfactant for the newborn. *Early Human Development* **61**, 67–83.

37 Dammann, O., Leviton, A. (1997) Maternal intrauterine infection, cytokines and brain damage in the preterm neonate. *Pediatric Research* **42**, 1–8.

38 Dammann, O., Leviton, A. (2000) Role of the fetus in perinatal infection and neonatal brain damage. *Current Opinion in Pediatrics* **12**, 99–104.

39 Dani, C., Crella, P.V., Lazzarin, L. *et al.* (1997) Antenatal ambroxal treatment does not prevent the respiratory distress syndrome in premature infants. *European Journal of Pediatrics* **156**, 392–393.

40 Dani, C., Bertini, G., Reali, M.F. *et al.* (2000) Prophylaxis of patent ductus arteriosus with ibuprofen in preterm infants. *Acta Paediatrica* **89**, 1369–1374.

41 Darlow, B.A., Harwood, L.J., Clemett, R.S. (1992) Retinopathy of prematurity: risk factors in a prospective population-based study. *Paediatric and Perinatal Epidemiology* **6**, 62–80.

42 Davis, G.M., Bureau, M.A. (1987) Pulmonary and chest wall mechanics in the control of respiratory distress in the newborn. *Clinics in Perinatology* **14**, 551–579.

43 Dimitriou, G., Greenough, A. (1995) Measurement of lung volume and optimal oxygenation during high frequency

oscillation. *Archives of Disease in Childhood Fetal and Neonatal Edition* **72**, F180–F183.

44 Doyle, L.W., Kitchen, W.H., Ford, G.W. *et al.* (1986) Effects of antenatal steroid therapy on mortality and morbidity in very low birthweight infants. *Journal of Pediatrics* **108**, 287–292.

45 Dunn, P.M. (1963) Intestinal obstruction in the newborn with special reference to transient functional ileus associated with respiratory distress syndrome. *Archives of Disease in Childhood* **38**, 459–467.

46 Edberg, K.E., Sandberg, K., Silberberg, A. *et al.* (1991) Lung volume, gas mixing and mechanics of breathing in mechanically ventilated very low birthweight infants with idiopathic respiratory distress syndrome. *Pediatric Research* **30**, 496–500.

47 Egberts, J. (1995) Theoretical changes in neonatal hospitalisation costs after the introduction of porcine-derived lung surfactant ('Curosurf'). *Pharmaco Economics* **8**, 324–342.

48 Egberts, J., Brand, R., Walti, H. *et al.* (1997) Mortality, severe respiratory distress syndrome and chronic lung disease of the newborn are reduced more after prophylactic than after therapeutic administration of the surfactant Curosurf. *Pediatrics* **100**, e4.

49 Engle, W.D., Araut, B.S., Wiriyathian, S., Rosenfeld, C.R. (1983) Diuresis and respiratory distress syndrome: physiologic mechanisms and therapeutic implications. *Journal of Pediatrics* **102**, 912–917.

50 Enhorning, G., Shennan, A., Possmayer, F. *et al.* (1985) Prevention of neonatal respiratory distress syndrome by tracheal instillation of surfactant: a randomized clinical trial. *Pediatrics* **76**, 145–153.

51 Fanaroff, A.A., Merkatz, I.R. (1993) Antenatal and intrapartum care of the high-risk infant. In Klaus, M.H., Fanaroff, A.A. (eds), *Care of the High-risk Neonate.* Philadelphia: W.B. Saunders, 1–37.

52 Farber, S., Sweet, L.K. (1931) Amniotic sac contents in the lungs of infants. *American Journal of Diseases of Children* **42**, 1372–1383.

53 Farrell, E.E., Silver, R.K., Kimberlin, L.V. *et al.* (1989) Impact of antenatal dexamethasone administration in respiratory distress in surfactant treated infants. *American Journal of Obstetrics and Gynecology* **161**, 628–633.

54 Farrell, P.M., Avery, M.E. (1975) Hyaline membrane disease. *American Review of Respiratory Disease* **111**, 657–688.

55 Field, D.J., Milner, A.D., Hopkin, I.E., Madeley, R.J. (1987) Changing patterns in neonatal respiratory diseases. *Pediatric Pulmonology* **3**, 231–235.

56 Fink, A., Yano, E.M., Goya, D. (1992) Prenatal programs. What the literature reveals. *Obstetrics and Gynecology* **80**, 867–872.

57 Fletcher, B.D. (1984) The radiology of respiratory distress syndrome and its sequelae. In Stern, L. (ed.), *Hyaline Membrane Disease: Pathogenesis and Pathophysiology.* Orlando: Grune and Stratton, 119–143.

58 Floros, J., Fan, R. (2001) Surfactant protein A and B genetic variants and respiratory distress syndrome: allele interactions. *Biology of the Neonate* **80**(Suppl 1), 22–25.

59 Fowlie, P.W. (1996) Prophylactic indomethacin: systematic review and meta-analysis. *Archives of Disease in Childhood* **74**, F81–F87.

60 French, N.P., Hagan, R., Evans, S.F. *et al.* (1999) Repeated antenatal corticosteroids: size at birth and subsequent development. *American Journal of Obstetrics and Gynecology* **180**, 114–121.

61 Fujimara, M., Salisbury, D.M., Robinson, R.O. (1979) Clinical events relating to intraventricular hemorrhage in the newborn. *Archives of Disease in Childhood* **54**, 409–414.

62 Fujimura, M., Kitajima, H., Nakayama, M. (1993) Increased leucocyte elastase of the tracheal aspirate at birth and neonatal pulmonary emphysema. *Pediatrics* **92**, 564–569.

63 Fujiwara, T., Chida, S., Watabe, Y. *et al.* (1980) Artificial surfactant therapy in hyaline membrane disease. *Lancet* **1**, 55–59.

64 Fujiwara, T., Konishi, M., Chida, S. *et al.* (1990) Surfactant replacement therapy with a single post-ventilatory dose of a reconstituted bovine surfactant in preterm neonates with respiratory distress syndrome: final analysis of a multicenter, double-blind, randomized trial and comparison with similar trials. *Pediatrics* **86**, 753–764.

65 Gandy, G.M., Jacobson, W., Gairdner, D. (1970) Hyaline membrane disease. I. Cellular changes. *Archives of Disease in Childhood* **45**, 289–295.

66 Giedion, A., Haefliger, H., Dangel, P. (1973) Acute pulmonary X-ray changes in hyaline membrane disease treated with artificial ventilation and positive end-expiratory pressure (PEP). *Pediatric Radiology* **1**, 145–152.

67 Glass, J., Rajecowda, B.K., Evans, H.E. (1971) Absence of respiratory distress syndrome in premature infants of heroin-addicted mothers. *Lancet* **ii**, 685–686.

68 Gluck, L., Kulovich, M.V., Eidelman, A.I. *et al.* (1972) Biochemical development of surface activity in mammalian lung. IV. Pulmonary lecithin synthesis in the human fetus and newborn and etiology of the respiratory distress syndrome. *Pediatric Research* **6**, 81–99.

69 Goldenberg, R.L., Rouse, D.J. (1998) Prevention of premature birth. *New England Journal of Medicine* **339**, 313–320.

70 Goldenberg, R.L., Wright, R.L. (2001) Repeated courses of antenatal corticosteroids. *Obstetrics and Gynecology* **97**, 316–317.

71 Goldman, S.L., Hirata, T. (1980) Attenuated response to insulin in very low birthweight infants. *Pediatrics Research* **14**, 50–53.

72 Graham, M., Levene, M., Trounce, J.Q., Rutter, N. (1987) Reduction of cerebral palsy in very low birthweight infants: prospective ultrasound study. *Lancet* **1**, 593–596.

73 Green, T.P., Thompson, T.R., Johnson, D.E., Lock, J.E. (1983) Diuresis and pulmonary function in premature infants with respiratory distress syndrome. *Journal of Pediatrics* **103**, 618–623.

74 Greenough, A. (1994) Pulse oximetry. *Current Paediatrics* **4**, 196–199.

75 Groneck, P., Götze-Speer, B., Oppermann, M. *et al.* (1994) Association of pulmonary inflammation and increased microvascular permeability during the development of bronchopulmonary dysplasia: a sequential analysis of inflammatory mediators in respiratory fluids of high risk preterm neonates. *Pediatrics* **93**, 712–718.

76 Gross, I., Smith, G.J., Wilson, C.M. *et al.* (1980) The influence of hormones on the biochemical development of fetal rat lung in organ culture. II: Insulin. *Pediatric Research* **14**, 834–838.

77 Gruskay, J., Costarino, A.T., Polin, R.A., Baumgart, S. (1988) Nonoliguric hyperkalemia in the premature infant weighing less than 1000 grams. *Journal of Pediatrics* **113**, 381–386.

78 Guignard, J.P., Tarado, A., Mazouni, S.M., Gautier, E. (1976) Renal function in respiratory distress syndrome. *Journal of Pediatrics* **88**, 845.

79 Hacking, D., Watkins, A., Fraser, S. *et al.* (2001) Respiratory distress syndrome and birth order in premature twins. *Archives of Disease in Childhood Fetal and Neonatal Edition* **84**, F117–F121.

80 Halahakoon, C.N., Halliday, H.L. (1995) Other acute lung disorders. In Yu, V.Y.H. (ed.), *Pulmonary Problems in the Neonatal Period and Their Sequelae.* London: Baillière Tindall, 87–114.

81 Halliday, H.L. (1988) Neonatal patent ductus arteriosus. *Pediatric Reviews and Communications* **3**, 1–17.

82 Halliday, H.L. (1989) When to do a lumbar puncture in a neonate. *Archives of Disease in Childhood* **64**, 313–316.

83 Halliday, H.L. (1993) Current views on the use of surfactant. *Contemporary Reviews of Obstetrics and Gynaecology* **5**, 65–70.

84 Halliday, H.L. (1997) Prophylactic surfactant for preterm infants. In Cockburn, F. (ed.), *Advances in Perinatal Medicine.* New York: The Parthenon Publishing Group, 360–370.

85 Halliday, H.L. (1998) Which interventions for neonatal respiratory failure are effective? *Croatian Medical Journal* **39**, 165–170.

86 Halliday, H.L. (1999) Elective delivery at 'term': implications for the newborn. *Acta Paediatrica* **88**, 1180–1181.

87 Halliday, H.L. (1999) Prevention and management of respiratory distress syndrome. In Levitt, G., Harvey, D., Cooke, R. (eds), *Practical Perinatal Care: the Baby under 1000 g.* Oxford: Butterworth-Heinemann, 33–51.

88 Halliday, H.L. (2000) The Bengt Robertson Lecture. Surfactant replacement: from the laboratory to routine clinical practice. *Prenatal Neonatal Medicine* **5**, 204–208.

89 Halliday, H.L., Hirschfeld, S.S., Riggs, T. *et al.* (1977) Respiratory distress syndrome: echocardiographic assessment of cardiovascular function and pulmonary vascular resistance. *Pediatrics* **60**, 444–449.

90 Halliday, H.L., Speer, C.P. (1995) Strategies for surfactant therapy in established neonatal respiratory distress syndrome. In Robertson, B., Taeusch, H.W. (eds), *Surfactant Therapy for Lung Disease.* New York: Marcel Dekker, 443–459.

91 Halliday, H.L., McClure, G., Reid, M.McC. (1998) *Handbook of Neonatal Intensive Care* 4th edition. London: W.B. Saunders.

92 Hallman, M., Teramo, K., Kankaanpaa, K. *et al.* (1980) Prevention of respiratory distress syndrome: current view of lung maturity studies. *Annals of Clinical Research* **12**, 36–44.

93 Hallman, M., Merritt, T.A., Pohjavuori, M., Gluck, L. (1986) Effect of surfactant substitution on lung effluent phospholipids in respiratory distress syndrome: evaluation of surfactant phospholipid turnover, pool size, and the relationship to severity of respiratory failure. *Pediatric Research* **20**, 1228–1235.

94 Hallman, M., Arjomaa, P., Hoppu, K. (1987) Inositol supplementation in respiratory distress syndrome: relationship between serum concentration, renal excretion and lung effluent phospholipids. *Journal of Pediatrics* **110**, 604–610.

95 Hamvas, A., Cole, S., de Mello, D.E. *et al.* (1994) Surfactant protein B deficiency: antenatal diagnosis and prospective treatment with surfactant replacement. *Journal of Pediatrics* **125**, 356–361.

96 Hamvas, A., Nogee, L.M., deMello, D.E., Cole, F.S. (1995) Pathophysiology and treatment of surfactant protein-B deficiency. *Biology of the Neonate* **67**(Suppl 1), 18–31.

97 Hannah, M.E., Hannah, W.J., Hewson, S.A. *et al.* (2000) Planned caesarean section versus planned vaginal birth for breech presentation at term: a randomised multicentre trial. Term Breech Trial Collaborative Group. *Lancet* **356**, 1375–1383.

98 Harrison, V.C., Heese, H.D., Klein, M. (1968) The significance of grunting in hyaline membrane disease. *Pediatrics* **41**, 549–559.

99 Henderson-Smart, D.J., Bhuta, T., Cools, F., Offringa, M. (2003) Elective high frequency oscillatory ventilation versus conventional ventilation for acute pulmonary dysfunction in preterm infants. (Cochrane review). In *The Cochrane Library,* Issue 1. Update Software, Oxford.

100 Hjalmarson, O. (1981) Epidemiology and classification of acute neonatal respiratory disorders. A prospective study. *Acta Paediatrica Scandinavica* **70**, 773–783.

101 Hochheim, K. (1903) Ueber einige befunde in den lungen von neugeborenen und die beziehung derselben zuraspiration von fruchtwasser. *Zentralbl Pathologie* **14**, 537–542.

102 Horbar, J.D., McAuliffe, T.L., Adler, S.M. *et al.* (1988) Variability in 28-day outcomes for very low birth weight infants: an analysis of 11 neonatal intensive care units. *Pediatrics* **82**, 554–559.

103 Horbar, J.D., Soll, R.F., Schachinger, M. *et al.* (1990) A European multicentre randomized controlled trial of single dose surfactant therapy for idiopathic respiratory distress syndrome. *European Journal of Pediatrics* **149**, 416–423.

104 Howlett, A., Ohlsson, A. (2003) Inositol for respiratory distress syndrome in preterm infants (Cochrane Review). In *The Cochrane Library,* Issue 2. Update Software, Oxford.

105 Hulsey, T.C., Alexander, G.R., Robillard, P.Y. *et al.* (1993) Hyaline membrane disease: the role of ethnicity and maternal risk characteristics. *American Journal of Obstetrics and Gynecology* **168**, 572–576.

106 Ikegami, M., Jacobs, H., Jobe, A. (1983) Surfactant function in respiratory distress syndrome. *Journal of Pediatrics* **102**, 443–447.

107 Ingomar, C.J., Klebe, J.C. (1974) The transcapillary escape rate of T1824 in newborn infants of diabetic mothers and newborn infants with respiratory distress or birth asphyxia. *Acta Paediatrica Scandinavica* **63**, 565–570.

108 Ioffe, S., Chernick, V. (1987) Maternal alcohol ingestion and the incidence of respiratory distress syndrome. *American Journal of Obstetrics and Gynecology* **156**, 1231–1235.

109 Jacobsen, M.D., Hirschfeld, S.S., Finn, C. *et al.* (1982) Neonatal circulatory changes following elective cesarean section: an echocardiographic study. *Pediatrics* **69**, 374–376.

110 Jeffries, A.L., Coates, G., O'Brodovich, H. (1984) Pulmonary epithelial permeability in hyaline membrane disease. *New England Journal of Medicine* **311**, 1075–1080.

111 Jenkins, J.G., Reid, M.McC., McClure, B.G. (1989) Study of heart rate variability in sick newborn infants. *Acta Paediatrica Scandinavica* **69**, 393–396.

112 Jobe, A.H. (1993) Pulmonary surfactant therapy. *New England Journal of Medicine* **328**, 861–868.

113 Jobe, A.H., Michell, B.R., Gunkel, J.H. (1993) Beneficial effects of the combined use of prenatal corticosteroids and postnatal surfactant on preterm infants. *American Journal of Obstetrics and Gynecology* **168**, 508–513.

114 Johnson, G.L., Cunningham, M.D., Desai, N.S. *et al.* (1980) Echocardiography in hypoxemic neonatal pulmonary disease. *Journal of Pediatrics* **96**, 716–720.

115 Kanto, W.P., Borer, R.C., Barr, M., Roloff, D.W. (1976) Tracheal aspirate lecithin:sphingomyelin ratios as predictors of recovery from respiratory distress syndrome. *Journal of Pediatrics* **89**, 612–616.

116 Kavvadia, V., Greenough, A., Dimitriou, G., Forsling, M. (1998) Comparison of respiratory function and fluid balance in very low birthweight infants given artificial or natural surfactant or no surfactant treatment. *Journal of Perinatal Medicine* **26**, 469–474.

117 Kavvadia, V., Greenough, A., Dimitriou, G., Hooper, R. (1998) Influence of ethnic origin on respiratory distress in very premature infants. *Archives of Disease in Childhood* **78**, F25–F28.

118 Keirse, M.J.N.C. (1995) Betamimetic tocolytics in preterm labour. In Enkin, MN, Keirse, M.J.N.C., Renfrew, M.J., Neilson, J.P., Crowther, C. (eds), *Pregnancy and Childbirth Module of the Cochrane Collaboration,* Issue 2. Update Software, Oxford.

119 Keszler, M., Carbone, M.T., Cox, C., Schumacher, R.E. (1992) Severe respiratory failure after elective repeat cesarean delivery: a potentially preventable condition leading to

extracorporeal membrane oxygenation. *Pediatrics* **89**, 670–672.

120 Kiely, J.L. (1991) Mode of delivery and neonatal death in 17,587 infants presenting by the breech. *British Journal of Obstetrics and Gynaecology* **98**, 989–904.

121 Kinmond, S., Aitchison, T.C., Holland, B.M. *et al.* (1993) Umbilical cord clamping and preterm infants: a randomised trial. *British Medical Journal* **306**, 172–175.

122 Lee, K.-S., Khoshnood, B., Wall, S.N. *et al.* (1999) Trend in mortality from respiratory distress syndrome in the United States, 1970–1995. *Journal of Pediatrics* **134**, 434–440.

123 Levene, M.I. (1991) Assisted reproduction and its implications for paediatrics. *Archives of Disease of Childhood* **66**, 1–3.

124 Leviton, A., Van Marter, L., Kuban, K.C.K. (1989) Respiratory distress syndrome and intracranial hemorrhage: cause or association. Inferences from surfactant clinical trials. *Pediatrics* **84**, 915–922.

125 Ley, D., Wide-Swensson, D., Lindroth, M. *et al.* (1997) Respiratory distress syndrome in infants with impaired intrauterine growth. *Acta Paediatrica* **86**, 1090–1096.

126 Liggins, G.C., Howie, R.N. (1972) A controlled trial of antepartum glucocorticoid treatment for prevention of the respiratory distress syndrome in premature infants. *Pediatrics* **50**, 515–520.

127 Lin, Y., Lechner, A.J. (1991) Surfactant content and type II cell development in fetal guinea pig lungs during prenatal starvation. *Pediatric Research* **29**, 288–291.

128 Lindahl, E., Michelsson, K., Helenns, M., Parre, M. (1988) Neonatal risk factors and later neurodevelopmental disturbances. *Developmental Medicine and Child Neurology* **30**, 571–589.

129 Lindner, W., Vossbeck, S., Hummler, H., Pohlandt, F. (1999) Delivery room management of extremely low birthweight infants: spontaneous breathing or intubation? *Pediatrics* **103**, 961–967.

130 Lipscombe, A.P., Reynolds, E.O.R., Blackwell, R.J. *et al.* (1981) Pneumothorax and cerebral haemorrhage in preterm infants. *Lancet* **1**, 414–417.

131 Lou, H.C., Lassen, N.A., Hansen Friis, B. (1992) Impaired autoregulation of cerebral blood flow in the distressed newborn infant. *Journal of Pediatrics* **94**, 118–121.

132 Luerti, M., Lazzarin, A., Corbella, E. *et al.* (1987) An alternative to steroids for prevention of respiratory distress syndrome (RDS): multicentre controlled study to compare ambroxal and betamethasone. *Journal of Perinatal Medicine* **15**, 227–238.

133 MacArthur, B.A., Howie, R.N., Dezoete, J.A., Elkins, J. (1982) School progress and cognitive development of 6-year-old children whose mothers were treated antenatally with betamethasone. *Pediatrics* **70**, 99–105.

134 Madar, J., Richmond, S., Hey, E. (1999) Surfactant-deficient respiratory distress after elective delivery at 'term'. *Acta Paediatrica* **88**, 1244–1248.

135 Manroe, B.L., Weinberg, A.G., Rosenfield, C.R., Browne, R. (1979) The neonatal blood count in health and disease. I. Reference values for neutrophil cells. *Journal of Pediatrics* **95**, 89–98.

136 Manzke, H. (1972) Relationship between extracellular and intracellular hydrogen ion concentrations and hemoglobin oxygen affinity in the blood of premature infants with respiratory distress syndrome. *Biology of the Neonate* **20**, 321–333.

137 Margolis, C.Z., Orzalesi, M.M., Schwartz, A.D. (1973) Disseminated intravascular coagulation in the respiratory distress syndrome. *American Journal of Diseases in Children* **125**, 324–326.

138 McCann, E.M., Goldman, S.L., Brady, J.P. (1987) Pulmonary function in the sick newborn infant. *Pediatric Research* **21**, 313–324.

139 McCord, F.B., Curstedt, T., Halliday, H.L. *et al.* (1988) Surfactant treatment and incidence of intraventricular haemorrhage in severe respiratory distress syndrome. *Archives of Disease in Childhood* **63**, 10–16.

140 Mead, P.B. (1980) Management of the patient with premature rupture of the membranes. *Clinics in Perinatology* **7**, 243–255.

141 Merritt, T.A., Farrell, P.M. (1976) Diminished pulmonary lecithin synthesis in acidosis. Experimental findings as related to the respiratory distress syndrome. *Pediatrics* **57**, 32–40.

142 Merritt, T.A., Stuard, I.D., Puccia, J. *et al.* (1981) Newborn tracheal aspirate cytology: classification during respiratory distress syndrome and bronchopulmonary dysplasia. *Journal of Pediatrics* **98**, 949–956.

143 Miall-Allen, V.M., de Vries, L.S., Dubowitz, L.M.S. (1989) Blood pressure fluctuation and intraventricular hemorrhage in the preterm infant less than 31 weeks of gestation. *Pediatrics* **83**, 657–661.

144 Morgan, C., Newell, S.J., Ducker, D.A. *et al.* (1999) Continuous neonatal blood gas monitoring using a multiparameter intra-arterial sensor. *Archives of Disease in Childhood Fetal and Neonatal Edition* **80**, F93–F98.

145 Moriette, G., Paris-Llado, J., Walti, H. *et al.* (2001) Prospective randomized multicenter comparison of high-frequency oscillatory ventilation and conventional ventilation in preterm infants of less than 30 weeks with respiratory distress syndrome. *Pediatrics* **107**, 363–372.

146 Morley, C.J. (1999) Continuous distending pressure. *Archives of Disease in Childhood Fetal and Neonatal Edition* **81**, F152–F156.

147 Morley, C.J., Greenough, A., Miller, N.G. *et al.* (1988) Randomised trial of artificial surfactant (ALEC) given at birth to babies from 23–34 weeks gestation. *Early Human Development* **17**, 41–54.

148 Morrison, J.J., Rennie, J.M., Milton, P.J. (1995) Neonatal respiratory morbidity and mode of delivery at term: influence of timing of elective caesarean section. *British Journal of Obstetrics and Gynaecology* **102**, 101–106.

149 Morrissey, M.S.C., Bailey, C.M. (1990) Diagnosis and management of subglottic stenosis after neonatal ventilation. *Archives of Disease in Childhood* **65**, 1103–1108.

150 MRC/RCOG Working Party on Cervical Cerclage (1998) Interim report of the Medical Research Council / Royal College of Obstetrics and Gynaecologist's multicentre randomized trial of cervical cerclage. *British Journal of Obstetrics and Gynaecology* **95**, 437–445.

151 Nagourney, B.A., Kramer, M.S., Klebanoff, M.A., Usher, R.H. (1996) Recurrent respiratory distress syndrome in successive preterm pregnancies. *Journal of Pediatrics* **129**, 591–596.

152 Neligan, G.A., Smith, C.A. (1960) The blood pressure of newborn infants in asphyxial states and hyaline membrane disease. *Pediatrics* **26**, 735–744.

153 NIH Consensus Development Panel. (1995) Effect of corticosteroids of fetal maturation on perinatal outcomes. *Journal of the American Medical Association* **273**, 413–418.

154 Nilsson, R., Grossmann, G., Robertson, B. (1978) Lung surfactant and the pathogenesis of neonatal bronchiolar lesions induced by artificial ventilation. *Pediatric Research* **12**, 249–255.

155 Pandit, P.B., Dunn, M.S., Colucci, E.A. (1995) Surfactant therapy in neonates with respiratory deterioration due to pulmonary hemorrhage. *Pediatrics* **95**, 32–36.

156 Papageorgiou, A.N., Doray, J.-L., Ardila, R., Kunos, I. (1989) Reduction of mortality, morbidity and respiratory distress

syndrome in infants weighing less than 1000 grams by treatment with betamethasone and ritodrine. *Pediatrics* **83**, 493–497.

157 Papiernik, E., Bruyer, J., Dreyfus, J. *et al.* (1985) Prevention of preterm births: a perinatal study in Haguenau, France. *Pediatrics* **76**, 154–158.

158 Pappin, A., Shenker, N., Hack, M., Redline, R.W. (1994) Extensive intraalveolar pulmonary hemorrhage in infants dying after surfactant therapy. *Journal of Pediatrics* **124**, 621–626.

159 Payne, W.W., Acharya, P.T. (1965) The effect of abnormal birth on blood biochemistry during the first 48 hours of life. *Archives of Disease in Childhood* **40**, 436–441.

160 Pedersen, J.E., Neilsen, K. (1994) Oropharyngeal and oesophageal pressures during mono- and binasal CPAP in neonates. *Acta Paediatrica* **83**, 143–149.

161 Phelan, J.P. (1992) Prevention of prematurity. *Clinics in Perinatology* **19**, 275–281.

162 Phibbs, R.H., Johnson, P., Kitterman, J.A. *et al.* (1972) Cardiorespiratory status of erythroblastotic infants: I. Relationship of gestational age, severity of hemolytic disease, and birth asphyxia to idiopathic respiratory distress syndrome and survival. *Pediatrics* **49**, 5–14.

163 Pildes, R.S. (1986) Neonatal hyperglycemia. *Journal of Pediatrics* **109**, 905–907.

164 Pildes, R.S., Pyati, S.P. (1986) Hypoglycemia and hyperglycemia in tiny infants. *Clinics in Perinatology* **13**, 351–376.

165 Pinar, H., Makarova, N., Rubin, L., Singer, D.B. (1994) Pathology of the lung in surfactant treated neonates. *Pediatric Pathology* **14**, 627–636.

166 Poets, C.F. (1998) When do infants need additional inspired oxygen? A review of the current literature. *Pediatric Pulmonology* **26**, 424–428.

167 Procianoy, R.S., Garcia-Prats, J.A., Adams, J.M. *et al.* (1980) Hyaline membrane disease and intraventricular haemorrhage in small for gestational age infants. *Archives of Disease in Childhood* **55**, 502–505.

168 Quinlan, R.W., Buhi, W.C., Cruz, A.C. (1984) Fetal pulmonary maturity in isoimmunized pregnancies. *American Journal of Obstetrics and Gynecology* **148**, 787–789.

169 Raju, T.N.K., Langerberg, P. (1993) Pulmonary hemorrhage and exogenous surfactant therapy: a meta-analysis. *Journal of Pediatrics* **123**, 603–610.

170 Reilly, B.J. (1975) Regional distribution of atelectasis and fluid in the neonate with respiratory distress. *Radiological Clinics of North America* **13**, 225–250.

171 Repka, M.X., Hudak, M.L., Parsa, C.F., Tielsch, J.M. (1992) Calf lung surfactant extract prophylaxis and retinopathy of prematurity. *Ophthalmology* **99**, 531–536.

172 Reynolds, E.O.R., Roberton, N.R.C., Wigglesworth, J.S. (1968) Hyaline membrane disease, respiratory distress syndrome and surfactant deficiency. *Pediatrics* **42**, 758–765.

173 Robertson, B. (1991) The origin of neonatal lung injury (editorial). *Pediatric Pathology* **11**, iii–vi.

174 Robertson, B., Halliday, H.L. (1998) Principles of surfactant replacement. *Biochimica et Biophysica Acta* **1408**, 346–361.

175 Robertson, B., Berry, D., Curstedt, T. *et al.* (1985) Leakage of protein in the immature rabbit lung: effect of surfactant replacement. *Respiratory Physiology* **61**, 265–276.

176 Royal College of Obstetricians and Gynaecologists. (1996) Antenatal corticosteroids to prevent respiratory distress syndrome. www.rcog.org.uk/guidelines/corticosteroids

177 Royal College of Paediatrics and Child Health. (2000) Guidelines for Good Practice – management of neonatal respiratory distress syndrome. www.rcpch.ac.uk/library

178 Rubaltelli, F.F., Bonafe, L., Tangucci, M. *et al.* (1998) Epidemiology of neonatal acute respiratory disorders. *Biology of the Neonate* **74**, 7–15.

179 Rudhe, U., Margolin, F.R., Robertson, B. (1970) Atypical roentgen appearances of the lung in hyaline membrane disease of the newborn. *Acta Radiologica* **10**, 57–68.

180 Rudolph, A.J., Smith, C.A. (1960) Idiopathic respiratory distress syndrome of the newborn. *Journal of Pediatrics* **57**, 905–921.

181 Rudolph, A.M., Drorbaugh, J.E., Auld, P.A.M. *et al.* (1961) Studies on the circulation in the neonatal period: the circulation in respiratory distress syndrome. *Pediatrics* **27**, 551–556.

182 Saarenmaa, E., Huttunen, P., Leppaluoto, J. *et al.* (1999) Advantages of fentanyl over morphine in analgesia for ventilated newborn infants after birth: a randomized trial. *Journal of Pediatrics* **134**, 144–150.

183 Schmidt, B., Vegh, P., Weitz, H. *et al.* (1992) Thrombin/antithrombin III complex formation in the neonatal respiratory distress syndrome. *American Review of Respiratory Disease* **145**, 767–770.

184 Shaw, B. (1999) Chronic lung disease of prematurity. In Levitt, G., Harvey, D., Cooke, R. (eds), *Practical Perinatal Care: the Baby under 1000 g.* Oxford: Butterworth-Heinemann, 64–72.

185 Shortland, D., Trounce, J.Q., Levene, M.I. (1987) Hyperkalaemia, cardiac arrhythmias and cerebral lesions in high risk neonates. *Archives of Disease in Childhood* **62**, 1139–1143.

186 Silverman, W.A., Anderson, A.H. (1956) A controlled clinical trial of effects of water mist in obstructive respiratory signs, death rate and necropsy findings in premature infants. *Pediatrics* **17**, 1–9.

187 Simmons, M.A., Adcock, E.W.I., Bard, H., Battaglia, F.C. (1974) Hypernatremia and intracranial hemorrhage in neonates. *New England Journal of Medicine* **291**, 6–10.

188 Singer, D.B. (1984) Morphology of hyaline membrane disease and its pulmonary sequelae. In Stern, L. (ed.), *Hyaline Membrane Disease. Pathogenesis and Pathophysiology.* Orlando: Grune and Stratton, 63–96.

189 Skelton, R., Jeffery, H. (1994) 'Click test': rapid diagnosis of the respiratory distress syndrome. *Pediatric Pulmonology* **17**, 383–389.

190 Skinner, J.R., Boys, R.J., Hunter, S., Hey, E.N. (1992) Pulmonary and systemic arterial pressure in hyaline membrane disease. *Archives of Disease in Childhood* **67**, 366–373.

191 Slovis, T.L., Poland, R.L. (1986) Endotracheal tubes in neonates: sonographic positioning. *Radiology* **160**, 262–263.

192 Smolders-de Haas, H., Neuvel, J., Schmand, B. *et al.* (1990) Physical development and medical history of children who were treated antenatally with corticosteroids to prevent respiratory distress syndrome: a 10- to 12-year follow-up. *Pediatrics* **86**, 65–70.

193 Soll, R.F. (2003) Multiple versus single dose natural surfactant extract for severe neonatal respiratory distress syndrome (Cochrane review). In *The Cochrane Library*, Issue 1. Update Software, Oxford.

194 Soll, R.F. (2003) Prophylactic natural surfactant extract for preventing mortality and morbidity in preterm infants (Cochrane Review). In *The Cochrane Library*, Issue 1. Update Software, Oxford.

195 Soll, R.F. (2003) Prophylactic synthetic surfactant for preventing morbidity and mortality in preterm infants (Cochrane Review). In *The Cochrane Library*, Issue 4. Update Software, Oxford.

196 Soll, R.F. (2001) Synthetic surfactant for respiratory distress syndrome in preterm infants (Cochrane Review). In *The Cochrane Library*, Issue 1. Update Software, Oxford.

197 Soll, R.F., Blanco, F. (2003) Natural surfactant extract versus synthetic surfactant for neonatal respiratory distress

syndrome (Cochrane Review). In *The Cochrane Library*, Issue 1. Update Software, Oxford.

198 Soll, R.F., Morley, C.J. (2003) Prophylactic versus selective use of surfactant for preventing morbidity and mortality in preterm infants (Cochrane Review). In *The Cochrane Library*, Issue 1. Update Software, Oxford.

199 Soll, R.F., Horbar, J.F., Grissom, N.T. *et al.* (1991) Radiographic findings associated with surfactant treatment. *American Journal of Perinatology* **8**, 114–118.

200 Speer, C.P., Halliday, H.L. (1994) Surfactant therapy in the newborn. *Current Paediatrics* **4**, 5–9.

201 Stahlman, M.T., Battersby, E.J., Shepard, F.M. *et al.* (1967) Prognosis in hyaline membrane disease: use of a linear discriminant. *New England Journal of Medicine* **276**, 303–306.

202 Stanley, F.J., Alberman, E.D. (1978) Infants of very low birthweight. I: Perinatal factors affecting survival. *Developmental Medicine and Child Neurology* **20**, 300–312.

203 Stevenson, D., Walther, F., Long, W. *et al.* (1992) Controlled trial of a single dose of synthetic surfactant at birth in premature infants weighing 500–699 grams. *Journal of Pediatrics* **120**, S3–S12.

204 Stewart, A.L., Reynolds, E.O.R., Hope, P.L. *et al.* (1987) Probability of neurodevelopmental disorders estimated from ultrasound appearance of brain in very preterm infants. *Developmental Medicine and Child Neurology* **29**, 3–11.

205 Sweet, D.G., Halliday, H.L. (1999) Current perspectives on the drug treatment of neonatal respiratory distress syndrome. *Paediatric Drugs* **1**, 19–30.

206 Sweet, D.G., Halliday, H.L. (2000) A risk–benefit assessment of drugs used for neonatal chronic lung disease. *Drug Safety* **22**, 389–404.

207 Swischuk, L.E. (1977) Bubbles in hyaline membrane disease. Differentiation of three types. *Radiology* **122**, 417–426.

208 Synnes, A.R., Chien, L.-Y., Peliowski, A. *et al.* (2001) Variations in intraventricular hemorrhage incidence rates among Canadian neonatal intensive care units. *Journal of Pediatrics* **138**, 525–531.

209 Taeusch, H.W., Boncuk-Dayaniku, P. (1995) Respiratory distress syndrome. In Yu, V.Y.H. (ed.), *Pulmonary Problems in the Perinatal Period and their Sequelae.* London: Baillière Tindall, 71–85.

210 Tarnow-Mordi, W. (1991) Is routine endotracheal suction justified? *Archives of Disease in Childhood* **66**, 374–375.

211 Tarnow-Mordi, W.O., Shaw, J.C., Liu, D. *et al.* (1981) Iatrogenic hyponatraemia of the newborn due to maternal fluid overload – a prospective study. *British Medical Journal* **283**, 639–642.

212 Tarnow-Mordi, W.O., Sutton, P., Wilkinson, A.R. (1986) Inadequate humidification of respiratory gases during mechanical ventilation of the newborn. *Archives of Disease in Childhood* **61**, 698–700.

213 Tchou, C.-S., Fletcher, B.D., Franke, P. *et al.* (1972) Asymmetric distribution of the roentgen pattern in hyaline membrane disease. *Journal of the Canadian Association of Radiologists* **23**, 85–90.

214 Thibeault, D.W., Hall, F.K., Sheehan, M.D., Hall, R.J. (1984) Post-asphyxial lung disease in newborn infants with severe perinatal acidosis. *American Journal of Obstetrics and Gynecology* **150**, 393–399.

215 Thompson, P.J., Greenough, A., Gamsu, H.R., Nicolaides, K.H. (1992) Ventilatory requirements for respiratory distress syndrome in small for gestational age infants. *European Journal of Pediatrics* **151**, 528–531.

216 Thompson, P.J., Greenough, A., Nicolaides, K.H. (1993) Steroid usage in pregnancies complicated by premature rupture of the membranes. *Journal of Perinatal Medicine* **21**, 219–224.

217 Thornton, C.M., Halliday, H.L., O'Hara, M.D. (1994) Surfactant replacement therapy in preterm neonates: a comparison of postmortem pulmonary histology in treated and untreated infants. *Pediatric Pathology* **14**, 945–953.

218 Torday, J. (1992) Cellular timing of fetal lung development. *Seminars in Perinatology* **16**, 130–139.

219 Torresin, M., Zimmermann, L.J.I., Cogo, P.E. *et al.* (2000) Exogenous surfactant kinetics in infant respiratory distress syndrome: a novel method with stable isotopes. *American Journal of Respiratory and Critical Care Medicine* **161**, 1584–1589.

220 Traub, A.I., Harley, J.M., Cooper, T.K. *et al.* (1987) Is centralised hospital care necessary for all insulin-dependent pregnant diabetics? *British Journal of Obstetrics and Gynaecology* **94**, 957–962.

221 Tubman, T.R.J., Rollins, M.D., Patterson, C.C., Halliday, H.L. (1990) Increased incidence of respiratory distress syndrome in babies of hyptertensive mothers. *Archives of Disease in Childhood* **66**, 52–54.

222 Turkel, S.P., Mapp, J.R. (1983) A ten year retrospective study of pink and yellow neonatal hyaline membrane disease. *Pediatrics* **72**, 170–175.

223 Usher, R.H. (1959) The respiratory distress syndrome of prematurity. I. Changes in potassium in the serum and ECG and effects of therapy. *Pediatrics* **24**, 562–576.

224 van Houten, J., Long, W., Mullett, M. *et al.* (1992) Pulmonary hemorrhage in premature infants after treatment with synthetic surfactant. An autopsy evaluation. The American Exosurf Neonatal Study Group I and the Canadian Exosurf Neonatal Study Group. *Journal of Pediatrics* **120**, S40–S44.

225 Verder, H., Robertson, B., Greisen, G. *et al.* (1994) Surfactant therapy and nasal continuous positive airway pressure for newborns with respiratory distress syndrome. *New England Journal of Medicine* **331**, 1051–1055.

226 Verder, H., Albertsen, P., Ebbesen, F. *et al.* (1999) Nasal continuous positive airway pressure and early surfactant therapy for respiratory distress syndrome in newborns of less than 30 weeks' gestation. *Pediatrics* **103**, E24.

227 Villar, J., Farnot, U., Barros, F. (1992) A randomized trial of psychosocial support during high risk pregnancy. *New England Journal of Medicine* **327**, 1266–1271.

228 Walters, D.V., Olver, R.E. (1978) The role of catecholamines in lung liquid absorption at birth. *Pediatric Research* **12**, 239–242.

229 Walther, F., Taeusch, H.W. (1991) New approaches to surfactant therapy. *Neonatal Respiratory Disease* **1**, 1–12.

230 Weiss, M.G., Ionides, S.P., Anderson, S.L. (1991) Meningitis in premature infants with respiratory distress. Role of admission lumbar puncture. *Journal of Pediatrics* **119**, 973–975.

231 Weller, P.H., Jenkins, P.A., Gupta, J., Baum, J.D. (1976) Pharyngeal lecithin:sphingomyelin ratio in newborn infants. *Lancet* **i**, 12–15.

232 White, E., Shy, K.K., Benedetti, R.J. (1986) Chronic fetal stress and the risk of infant respiratory distress syndrome. *Obstetrics and Gynecology* **67**, 57–62.

233 White, E., Shy, K.K., Daling, J.R., Guthrie, R.D. (1986) Maternal smokers and infants' respiratory distress syndrome. *Obstetrics and Gynecology* **67**, 365–370.

234 Whitfield, C.R., Chan, W.H., Sproule, W.B., Stewart, A.D. (1972) Amniotic fluid lecithin:sphingomyelin ratio and fetal lung development. *British Medical Journal* **2**, 85–86.

235 Wigglesworth, J.S. (1977) Pathology of neonatal respiratory distress. *Proceedings of the Royal Society of Medicine* **70**, 861–863.

236 Wilson, G., Hughes, G., Rennie, J., Morley, C. (1991) Evaluation of two endotracheal suction regimes in babies

ventilated for respiratory distress syndrome. *Early Human Development* **25**, 87–90.

237 Wise, P.H. (1990) Poverty, technology and recent trends in the United States infant mortality rate. *Paediatric and Perinatal Epidemiology* **4**, 390–401.

238 Wolfson, S.L., Frech, R., Hewitt, C. *et al.* (1969) Radiographic diagnosis of hyaline membrane disease. *Radiology* **93**, 339–343.

239 Wood, N.S., Marlow, N., Costeloe, K. *et al.* (2000) Neurologic and developmental disability after extremely preterm birth. *New England Journal of Medicine* **343**, 378–384.

240 Yao, A.C., Lind, J. (1974) Placental transfusion. *American Journal of Diseases of Children* **127**, 128–141.

241 Yu, V.Y.H. (1975) Effect of body position on gastric emptying in the neonate. *Archives of Disease in Childhood* **50**, 500–504.

242 Zuckerman, B., Maynard, E.C., Cabral, H. (1991) A preliminary report of prenatal cocaine exposure and respiratory distress syndrome in premature infants. *American Journal of Diseases of Children* **145**, 696–698.

20

Transient tachypnea of the newborn (TTN)

ANNE GREENOUGH

Transient tachypnea of the newborn (TTN) was first described by Avery and colleagues.[2] It has also been called wet lung,[49] benign unexplained respiratory distress in the newborn,[44] neonatal tachypnea[26] and type two respiratory distress syndrome (RDS).[32]

INCIDENCE

In two epidemiological surveys of neonatal respiratory disease, the incidence of pulmonary maladaption, which corresponds very largely to TTN, was 9.3/1000,[19] and 3.6–4.5/1000.[12] In another series,[28] amongst infants delivered between 37 and 42 weeks of gestation, the incidence of TTN was 5.7/1000. Others have suggested rates of 0.8/1000[46] and 4/1000[35] in infants born at term. In prematurely born infants, a higher rate of 10/1000 has been observed.[9] It has been suggested that TTN is the commonest cause of neonatal respiratory distress, accounting for 41 percent of cases in one series[45] and 32 percent in another.[19] Others[4] have commented that this condition is underdiagnosed and as many as 77 percent of cases of RDS are in fact TTN.

PATHOPHYSIOLOGY

Infants with TTN appear to have abnormal epithelial ion transport.[14] At birth the mature lung switches from lung fluid secretion to absorption in response to circulating catecholamines, steroids and vasopressin (p. 27). Changes in oxygen tension are thought to augment the sodium ion (Na^+) transporting capacity of the epithelium and increase gene expression for the epithelial Na^+ channel (p. 29).[29] In 85 term neonates, measurements of the change in ion transport function were made during the first 72 hours after birth by assessing the basal transepithelial potential difference across the ciliated epithelium of the nose. The measurements revealed that basal potential differences in the first 24 hours were higher in neonates delivered by cesarean section without labor and in those with TTN than in neonates born during normal spontaneous vaginal delivery (SVD) or cesarean section with prior labor.[14]

It has been suggested that surfactant deficiency may be important in the pathogenesis of TTN.[6] Seven infants with TTN who had a low lecithin:sphingomyelin (L:S) ratio (<2) were reported by Hallman and Teramo.[18] Infants with TTN compared to controls were found to have less desaturated phosphatidylcholine (lecithin) and phosphatidylinositol and much less phosphatidylglycerol in their gastric aspirates.[20]

ETIOLOGY

In a population based study of 63 537 newborns enrolled in a 12-month survey in Italy,[9] risk factors for TTN were gestational age, maternal diseases, twinning, birthweight, operative vaginal delivery, elective and emergency cesarean section and male sex. The relationship of TTN to prematurity has been noted previously.[5] Results from a retrospective study[48] suggest that above 28 weeks of gestation, the heavier compared to the lighter twin is at increased risk of short-term, mild respiratory problems following delivery, but this was not as strong a risk factor as birth order or male gender.

Asphyxia

TTN was originally attributed to delay in fetal lung fluid clearance.[2] Newborn lambs with retained fetal fluid have similar clinical signs and radiological features to infants with TTN.[13] Alveolar fluid normally has a very low protein content and thus can be absorbed into the circulation. Avery[2] postulated that the protein content could be increased during an episode of asphyxia, either by alteration of the permeability of the lung capillaries or inhalation of amniotic fluid. The resultant fluid would have more difficulty passing into the pulmonary circulation.[1] Rawlings and Smith noted an association between TTN and prolonged labor and fetal macrosomia, both factors likely to be associated with fetal asphyxia.[34]

Cesarean section

TTN is increased in infants born by cesarean section with[33] or without labor; in such infants the incidence of TTN may be as high as 23 percent.[31] RDS occurs in the setting of elective[28] or repeat[30] cesarean section. TTN and RDS were found to be more common in twins delivered by cesarean section if this was performed before labor and prior to 38 weeks of gestation.[7] This may be due to the lower epinephrine (adrenaline) levels associated with such elective deliveries[24] as, in animals, epinephrine surges result in lung fluid clearance.[47] Comparison of non-asphyxiated (cord pH >7.25 and/or Apgar score >7 at 5 minutes) prematurely born infants with infants who did or did not develop TTN, revealed that eight of 10 infants with TTN were delivered by cesarean section compared to only two of 13 controls ($P < 0.01$). In addition, norepinephrine (noradrenaline) levels were significantly lower in the infants with TTN (median 3.1 nmol/l compared to 6.4 nmol/l; $P < 0.01$).[15] An alternative explanation is that since during cesarean section birth, the infant's thorax is not subjected to the same pressure as when delivered by the vaginal route, fetal lung liquid is not squeezed out of the lung. Certainly lung function is relatively impaired following cesarean section compared with vaginal delivery. The crying vital capacity has been noted to be lower[8,39] and the mean thoracic gas volume (TGV) 6 hours after birth was 19.7 ml/kg after cesarean section compared to 32.7 ml/kg after a vaginal delivery.[27] As the chest circumferences were the same in both groups, the difference in volumes may be explained by high residual volumes of interstitial and alveolar fluid in infants delivered by cesarean section.[27] The timing of delivery by cesarean section is important with regard to the development of respiratory distress. The relative risk for respiratory distress after delivery by cesarean

section before the onset of labor, during the week 37^{+0} to 37^{+6} compared with the week 38^{+0} to 38^{+6} was 1.74 (95 percent CI 1.1–2.8, $P < 0.02$) and during the week 38^{+0} to 38^{+6} compared to 39^{+0} to 39^{+6} was 2.4 (95 percent CI 1.2–4.8, $P < 0.02$).[28] If an infant born at term develops respiratory distress following an elective cesarean, it should not be assumed they have TTN.[25] An area-based retrospective study of all 179 701 babies of 34 or more weeks of gestation born alive in a defined area of the north of England in 1988–92 identified 149 babies with features of respiratory distress typical of surfactant deficiency severe enough to be managed with ventilatory support and with no evidence of aspiration or intrapartum infection. Thirty-six of the infants were born at or after 37 weeks of gestation.[25] Those born between 37 and 38 weeks were 20 times more likely to receive ventilatory support for surfactant deficiency than those born between 39 and 41 weeks.

Maternal asthma

Two hundred and ninety-four asthmatic patients registering between 1978 and 1984 for prenatal care were matched with non-asthmatic controls according to age and smoking status. TTN occurred in 3.7 percent of the infants of asthmatic subjects compared to only 0.8 percent of controls ($P = 0.003$).[38] Multiparity was commoner in the asthmatic subjects but, even when this was allowed for, the difference in the incidence of TTN between the groups remained significant. The occurrence of TTN, however, did not significantly relate to the asthma severity or medication variables. The finding[37] of an increased incidence of TTN in maternal asthma is supported by the data of Shohat et al.[40] who reported a trend towards a higher occurrence of a family history of atopy in babies who developed TTN. Comparison of mothers with asthma and their infants to a fourfold larger randomly selected control sample demonstrated that, after controlling for the confounding effects of important variables, infants of asthmatic mothers were more likely (OR 1.79, 95 percent CI 1.35–2.37) than infants of control mothers to exhibit TTN (Demissie et al. 1998). The proposed mechanism for the association between TTN and maternal asthma is that the mothers and infants of asthmatic mothers have a genetic predisposition to β-adrenergic hyporesponsiveness.[3,38] In support of that hypothesis are the findings that 58 children aged 4–5 years who were diagnosed as having had TTN, were more likely to have recurrent episodes of wheezy breathlessness and symptoms consistent with asthma and signs of atopy.[40]

CLINICAL SIGNS

TTN is more frequently diagnosed in term than preterm infants, but in the latter group coexisting respiratory problems mask the presentation. Affected infants are tachypneic with respiratory rates up to 100–120 breaths/min. Grunting and retractions are uncommon. The chest is barrel shaped due to hyperinflation and the liver and spleen are palpable because of downward displacement of the diaphragm. Peripheral edema with puffiness of the hands, feet and face may be present. On auscultation there may be added moist sounds, similar to those heard in heart failure. There is frequently an associated tachycardia, but the blood pressure is usually within the normal range, unless the infant develops severe respiratory failure.

Sundell et al. described type II respiratory distress as a variation of TTN in preterm infants.[43] This followed mild depression at birth. Infants with type II respiratory distress could be distinguished from those with RDS as they all had a prompt response to oxygen administration and the course of their illness was always benign.

TTN usually settles within 24 hours but may persist for up to 8 days.[41] In one study,[45] the signs had abated by 48 hours in 74 percent of babies. In some infants the course is more prolonged, in 19 percent of cases in one series[4] and in 26 percent of cases in another.[45] In this latter series the disorder lasted for a mean of 5.7 days in nine infants who were male, marginally premature, born by cesarean section and mildly asphyxiated at birth, but did not differ with regard to their chest radiograph appearance on the day of delivery to those of infants with transient symptoms. Halliday et al. reported six infants they described as suffering from severe TTN as they required more than 60 percent oxygen in order to maintain normal arterial oxygen tensions and six of the nine babies required intubation and mechanical ventilation.[17] The infants, however, had evidence of perinatal asphyxia with both low Apgar scores and arterial pHs immediately after birth, and thus may have been suffering from post-asphyxial lung edema,[42] rather than TTN.

Pulmonary hypertension has been reported in infants with TTN with right-to-left shunting of blood across the ductus arteriosus.[17] The pulmonary hypertension following elective section may be so severe that extracorporeal membrane oxygenation (ECMO) is required.[22] The increase in pulmonary vascular resistance may be due to the lung hyperinflation associated with retained fetal lung fluid.[5] Alternatively, the increase in pulmonary vascular resistance may be the result of perinatal asphyxia and acidosis. Pulmonary air leaks have been reported in infants with TTN.[16]

Lung function

In the only large study of lung mechanics in infants with established TTN, Sandberg et al. found a reduced tidal volume, but as the respiratory rate was increased, the minute volume was higher than that measured after recovery.[36] There was some gas trapping, an increased total lung resistance and reduction in dynamic lung compliance. The changes were attributed to lung liquid retained within the lung causing narrowing of the small airways.

DIFFERENTIAL DIAGNOSIS

The diagnosis of TTN is inevitably a retrospective one when the transience of the illness has been documented and other potentially more serious conditions have been excluded. At the mild end of its spectrum, TTN merges into minimal respiratory disease (p. 247) and, at the severe end, where there are abnormalities of pulmonary vascular tone and cardiac function, it merges into persistent pulmonary hypertension (p. 373). It can usually be differentiated from post-asphyxial tachypnea (p. 396) on the basis of the clinical features (p. 396), blood gases and chest radiograph appearance. In post-asphyxia tachypnea there may be cardiac enlargement, which is unusual in TTN. In addition, there will usually be a low pH, with a base deficit $>10 \, mmol/l$ and a low or normal $PaCO_2$, whereas in TTN usually a base deficit is absent and the pH will be normal or elevated. TTN is differentiated from RDS by the chest radiograph appearance. The most important and difficult differential is from early-onset sepsis, particularly due to group B streptococcus (GBS). As this diagnosis can only be excluded once the blood culture results are known to be negative, antibiotics must be administered to all infants with respiratory distress, including those with TTN.

DIAGNOSIS

Criteria for the diagnosis of TTN have been suggested to include any supplementary oxygen requirement during the first 6 hours which does not increase during the subsequent 18 hours; improvement in the clinical condition within 3–6 hours and a chest radiograph appearance, which is either normal or shows reduced translucency, infiltrates or hyperinsufflation of the lungs.[9]

Chest radiograph

The chest radiograph demonstrates hyperinflation with prominent perihilar vascular markings, edema of the interlobar septa and fluid present in the fissures (Figure 20.1).[23] The prominent perihilar streaking (Figure 20.2) is probably engorgement of the periarterial lymphatics that appear to participate in the clearance of alveolar fluid. Fluid may be present in the costophrenic angles with intercostal bulging of the pleura. Clearing of fluid from the lungs on the chest radiograph is usually apparent by the next day, although complete clearing may take up to 3–7 days.

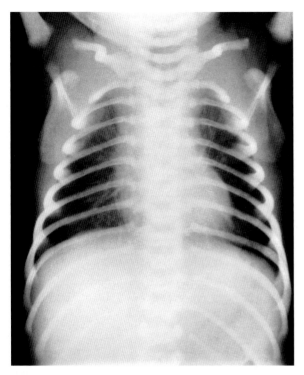

Figure 20.1 *Characteristic features of retained pulmonary fluid with airspace filling and fluid in the horizontal fissure.*

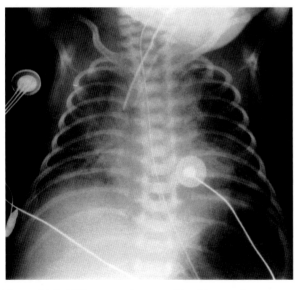

Figure 20.2 *TTN: severe changes with widespread consolidation indistinguishable radiologically from infection at this stage. Rapid clearance of the abnormalities within 24 hours confirmed the diagnosis.*

Echocardiography

Infants with mild or classic TTN have only mild left ventricular failure with disordered left ventricular contractility in the first 24 hours after birth, but no right

ventricular dysfunction or increased pulmonary vascular resistance.[17] Severe TTN may be associated with generalized myocardial failure, pulmonary hypertension, right-to-left shunting and abnormalities of systolic time intervals of both ventricles lasting up to 72 hours. The left ventricular pre-ejection period to ejection time (LPEP/LVET) ratio has been found to correlate with the duration of treatment with oxygen; this ratio increased for the first 3 days after birth in those infants with severe TTN.[17]

Inflammatory markers

Interleukin-6 (IL-6) levels at the onset of symptoms in newborns evaluated for sepsis in the perinatal period differed in infants with TTN to those with proven and/or clinical sepsis. Initial CRP results, however, had no value in distinguishing infants with TTN.[21]

MONITORING

Oxygen requirements should initially be monitored by intermittent arterial sampling, pulse oximetry or transcutaneous oxygen monitoring. An umbilical arterial catheter should be sited if the infant continues to require an FiO_2 of greater than 0.4 for 6 hours and/or mechanical ventilation.

PROPHYLAXIS

In a randomized placebo-controlled trial, a continuous infusion of terbutaline given to mothers prior to elective cesarean section was associated with higher lung compliance and lower airway resistance. None of the infants whose mothers had received terbutaline, but two controls, developed TTN. No adverse effects were seen in the neonates, but the mothers who received terbutaline had significantly higher levels of bleeding.[11]

MANAGEMENT

Respiratory support

The majority of infants require no form of respiratory support. If oxygen is required, it is usually at a concentration of less than 40 percent oxygen delivered into a headbox for up to 2–3 days. Some infants, however, require up to 100 percent inspired oxygen concentration[5] and a few infants positive pressure ventilation.[45] Continuous positive airways pressure is not recommended for infants with TTN because of the theoretical increased risk of pneumothorax in the presence of an already hyperinflated chest.

Fluid management

Nasogastric feeds should be withheld until the infant's respiratory rate settles. Infants with TTN lose weight less rapidly than infants without TTN (J.S. Rawlings and F.R. Smith presented to the Californian Perinatal Association 1985). Fluid restriction to 40 ml/kg/day should be instituted until a diuresis occurs, usually by 48 hours of age. Diuretics, however, do not influence outcome. In a controlled randomized prospective study, Wiswell et al.[50] demonstrated that treatment with frusemide at a dose of 2 mg/kg given orally at the time of diagnosis and 1 mg/kg 12 hours later, made no significant difference to the duration of tachypnea or the duration of hospitalization.

Antibiotics

Early-onset sepsis may mimic TTN; as a consequence antibiotics should be given to all infants with respiratory distress. In most cases it is adequate to just give penicillin until the cultures are known to be negative. If, however, there are suspicious features in the history (prolonged membrane rupture, maternal pyrexia, gestational age less than 37 weeks), worrying clinical features (apnea, hypotension) or abnormalities of the blood count or a raised CRP level (p. 74), then both penicillin and gentamicin should be given. If by 48 hours of age the baby is clinically improving and the cultures are negative the antibiotics can be stopped.

PROGNOSIS

Mortality

A mortality of 1.3 percent in infants with TTN was found in a 12-month survey which included 63 537 newborns.[9] The 594 infants who developed TTN, however, included 350 born prior to 36 weeks of gestational age and if only those born at term are considered the mortality rate was 0.8 percent.[9] In low birthweight infants, an early study reported a mortality rate of 7.8 percent in TTN.[34]

Morbidity

RESPIRATORY

The condition is self-limiting and usually improves within 2–4 days. Some infants with TTN have a longer course resulting in prolonged hospital admission.[33] Bronchopulmonary dysplasia is not seen in TTN survivors. At follow-up it has been suggested that young children who had TTN may have an increased incidence of wheeze.[40] Comparison at 4–5 years of age of 59 children who had suffered from TTN with 58 controls of similar birthweight and gestational age, revealed that the 'TTN group' had a significantly higher incidence of recurrent (more than two) episodes of wheezy breathlessness ($P < 0.02$). There was a trend towards a higher incidence of a family history of atopy and symptoms consistent with childhood asthma and other atopic conditions were significantly more common in the TTN group. In contrast, others[38] have reported none of their TTN infants manifested wheezing by the age of 15 months. A prospective follow-up study is required to accurately determine the occurrence and extent of chronic respiratory morbidity following TTN.

NEUROLOGICAL

Long-term neurological sequelae have not been described in infants who had TTN and would not be anticipated in a group of term babies who were not seriously hypoxic nor hypotensive and not susceptible to intracranial hemorrhage.

REFERENCES

1 Aherne, W., Dawkins, M.J.R. (1964) The resorption of fluid from pulmonary airways in the rabbit and the effect of this on prematurity and prenatal hypoxia. Biology of the Neonate 7, 214–218.

2 Avery, M.E., Gatewood, O.B., Brumley, G. (1966) Transient tachypnea of the newborn. American Journal of Diseases of Children 111, 380–385.

3 Barnes, P.J. (1986) Endogenous catecholamine and asthma. Journal of Allergy and Clinical Immunology 77, 791–795.

4 Brice, J.E., Walker, C.H. (1977) Changing pattern of respiratory distress in the newborn. Lancet 2, 752–754.

5 Bucciarelli, R.L., Egan, E.R., Gessner, I.H., Eitzman, D.V. (1976) Persistence of fetal cardiopulmonary circulation: one manifestation of transient tachypnea of the newborn. Pediatrics 58, 192–197.

6 Callen, P., Goldsworthy, S., Graves, I. et al. (1979) Mode of delivery and the lecithin/sphingomyelin ratio. British Journal of Obstetrics and Gynaecology 86, 965–968.

7 Chasen, S.T., Madden, A., Chervenak, F.A. (1999) Cesarean delivery of twins and neonatal respiratory disorders. American Journal of Obstetrics and Gynecology 181, 1052–1056.

8 Chiswick, M.L., Milner, R.D.G. (1976) Crying vital capacity measurement of neonatal lung function. Archives of Disease in Childhood 51, 22–27.

9 Dani, C., Reali, M.F., Bertini, G. et al. (1999) Risk factors for the development of respiratory distress syndrome and transient tachypnoea in newborn infants. European Respiratory Journal 14, 155–159.

10 Demissie, K., Marcella, S.W., Breckenridge, M.B., Rhoads, G.G. (1998) Maternal asthma and transient tachypnea of the newborn. Pediatrics 102, 84–90.

11 Eisler, G., Hjertberg, R., Lagercrantz, H. (1999) Randomized controlled trial of effect of terbutaline before elective cesarean section on postnatal respiration and glucose homeostasis. Archives of Disease in Childhood Fetal and Neonatal Edition 80, F88–F92.

12 Field, D.J., Milner, A.D., Hopkin, I.E., Madeley, R.J. (1987) Changing patterns in neonatal respiratory diseases. *Pediatric Pulmonology* **3**, 231–235.

13 Fletcher, B.D., Sachs, B.F., Kotas, R.V. (1970) Radiological demonstration of post-natal liquid in the lungs of newborn lambs. *Pediatrics* **46**, 252–257.

14 Gowen, C.W., Lawson, E.E., Gingras, J. et al. (1988) Electrical potential differences and ion transport across nasal epithelium of term neonates. Correlation with mode of delivery, transient tachypnea of the newborn and respiratory rate. *Journal of Pediatrics* **113**, 121–127.

15 Greenough, A., Lagercrantz, H. (1992) Catecholamine abnormalities in transient tachypnoea of the premature newborn. *Journal of Perinatal Medicine* **20**, 223–226.

16 Gross, T.L., Sokol, R.J., Kwong, M.S. et al. (1983) Transient tachypnea of the newborn: the relationship to preterm delivery and significant neonatal morbidity. *American Journal of Obstetrics and Gynecology* **146**, 236–241.

17 Halliday, H.L., McClure, G., Reid, M.M. (1981) Transient tachypnea of the newborn: two distinct clinical entities? *Archives of Disease in Childhood* **56**, 322–325.

18 Hallman, M., Teramo, K. (1981) Measurement of the lecithin/sphingomyelin ratio and phosphatidylglycerol in amniotic fluid: an accurate method for the assessment of fetal lung maturity. *British Journal of Obstetrics and Gynaecology* **88**, 860–813.

19 Hjalmarson, O. (1981) Epidemiology and classification of acute neonatal respiratory disorders. A prospective study. *Acta Paediatrica Scandinavica* **70**, 773–783.

20 James, D.K., Chiswick, M.L., Harkes, A. et al. (1984) Non-specificity of surfactant deficiency in neonatal respiratory distress. *British Medical Journal* **288**, 1635–1638.

21 Kallman, J., Ekholm, L., Eriksson, M. et al. (1999) Contribution of interleukin-6 in distinguishing between mild respiratory disease and neonatal sepsis in the newborn infant. *Acta Paediatrica* **88**, 880–884.

22 Keszler, M., Carbone, M.T., Cox, C., Schumacher, R.E. (1992) Severe respiratory failure after elective repeat cesarean delivery: a potentially preventable condition leading to extracorporeal membrane oxygenation. *Pediatrics* **89**, 670–672.

23 Kuhn, M.P., Fletcher, B.D., deLemos, R.A. (1969) Roentgen findings in transient tachypnoea of the newborn. *Radiology* **92**, 751–757.

24 Lagercrantz, H., Bistoletti, P., Nylund, L. (1981) Sympathoadrenal activity in the fetus during delivery and at birth. In Stern, L. et al. (eds), *Intensive Care of the Newborn*. New York: Mason Press, 1–12.

25 Madar, J., Richmond, S., Hey, E. (1999) Surfactant-deficient respiratory distress after elective delivery at 'term'. *Acta Paediatrica* **88**, 1244–1248.

26 Malan, A.F. (1966) Neonatal tachypnoea. *Australian Paediatric Journal* **3**, 159–163.

27 Milner, A.D., Saunders, R.A., Hopkin, I.E. (1978) Effects of delivery by cesarian section on lung mechanics and lung volume in human neonates. *Archives of Disease in Childhood* **53**, 545–548.

28 Morrison, J.J., Rennie, J.M., Milton, P.J. (1995) Neonatal respiratory morbidity and mode of delivery at term: influence of timing of elective caesarean section. *British Journal of Obstetrics and Gynaecology* **102**, 101–106.

29 O'Brodovich, H.M. (1996) Immature epithelial Na$^+$ channel expression is one of the pathogenetic mechanisms leading to human neonatal respiratory distress syndrome. *Proceedings of the Asssociation of American Physicians* **108**, 345–355.

30 Parilla, B.V., Dooley, S.L., Jansen, R.D., Socol, M.L. (1993) Iatrogenic respiratory distress syndrome following elective repeat cesarean delivery. *Obstetrics and Gynecology* **81**, 392–395.

31 Patel, D.M., Donovan, E.F., Keenan, W.J. (1983) Transient respiratory difficulty following cesarian delivery. *Biology of the Neonate* **43**, 146–151.

32 Prod'hom, L.S., Leveson, H., Cherry, R.B., Smith, C.A. (1965) Adjustment of ventilation, intrapulmonary gas exchange and acid balance in the first day of life. *Pediatrics* **35**, 662–676.

33 Rawlings, J.S., Scott, J.S. (1996) Postconceptional age of surviving preterm low birthweight infants at hospital discharge. *Archives of Pediatrics and Adolescent Medicine* **150**, 260–262.

34 Rawlings, J.S., Smith, F.R. (1984) Transient tachypnea of the newborn: an analysis of neonatal and obstetric risk factors. *American Journal of Diseases of Children* **138**, 869–871.

35 Rubaltelli, F.F., Dani, C., Reali, M.F. et al. (1998) Acute neonatal respiratory distress in Italy: a one-year prospective study. *Acta Paediatrica* **87**, 1261–1268.

36 Sandberg, K., Sjoqvist, B.A., Hjalmarson, O. Olsson, T. (1987) Lung function in newborn infants with tachypnea of unknown cause. *Pediatric Research* **22**, 581–586.

37 Schatz, M. (1999) Asthma and pregnancy. *Lancet* **353**, 1202–1204.

38 Schatz, M., Zeiger, R.S., Hoffman, C.P. et al. (1991) Increased transient tachypnea of the newborn in infants of asthmatic mothers. *American Journal of Diseases of Children* **145**, 156–158.

39 Segal, S., Chu, J. (1963) *Neonatal Respiratory Adaptation*. US Department of Health, Education and Welfare, National Institutes of Health.

40 Shohat, M., Levy, G., Levy, I. et al. (1989) Transient tachypnea of the newborn and asthma. *Archives of Disease in Childhood* **64**, 277–279.

41 Stahlman, M.T. (1977) Respiratory disorders in the newborn: type II respiratory distress. In Kendig, E.L. (ed.), *Disorders of the Respiratory Tract in Children*. Philadelphia: W.B. Saunders, 290–292.

42 Strang, L.B. (1965) The lungs at birth. *Archives of Disease in Childhood* **40**, 575–582.

43 Sundell, H., Garrott, J., Blankenship, W.J. et al. (1971) Studies on infants with type II respiratory distress syndrome. *Journal of Pediatrics* **78**, 754–758.

44 Taylor, P.M., Allen, A.C., Stinson, D.A. (1971) Benign unexplained respiratory distress of the newborn. *Pediatric Clinics of North America* **18**, 975–1004.

45 Tudehope, D.I., Smyth, M.H. (1979) Is transient tachypnoea of the newborn always a benign condition? *Australian Paediatric Journal* **15**, 160–165.

46 van Rijswijk, P., Ingle, R.F. (1996) Causes of early neonatal respiratory distress in the former Venda – a community-based study. *South African Medical Journal* **86**, 1413–1416.

47 Walters, D.V., Olver, R.E. (1978) The role of catecholamines in lung liquid absorption at birth. *Pediatric Research* **12**, 239–242.

48 Webb, R.D., Shaw, N.J. (2001) Respiratory distress in heavier versus lighter twins. *Journal of Perinatal Medicine* **29**, 60–63.

49 Wesenberg, R.L., Graven, S.N., McCabe, E.B. (1971) Radiological findings in wet lung disease. *Radiology* **98**, 69–74.

50 Wiswell, M.T., Rawlings, J.S., Smith, F.R., Goo, E.D. (1985) Effect of furosemide on the clinical couse of transient tachypnea of the newborn. *Pediatrics* **75**, 908–910.

21

Pneumonia

PETER RF DEAR, with contributions from AMANDA FIFE

Invasion of lung tissue by pathogenic microorganisms is relatively common during the newborn period because of the immaturity and naiveté of the immune system, including specific pulmonary defenses, and the fragility of the mechanical barriers provided by skin and mucous membranes. Premature birth increases the susceptibility but, as with all infections, host factors are but one part of the story. Other important concerns are the characteristics and dose of the microorganisms encountered, the balance struck between colonization and invasion and the existence of abnormal portals of entry such as endotracheal tubes. Pneumonia is an exceptionally serious condition for the newborn and is responsible for the deaths of some two million infants per year worldwide.[256] In the developing world, pneumonia occurring during the neonatal period carries a ten times greater mortality than when it occurs at any other time in infancy.[33] Pneumonia is particularly dangerous when respiratory reserve is already limited by conditions such as RDS (p. 245), CLD (p. 399) or congenital anomalies. Neonatal pneumonia may be an isolated focal infection but is commonly part of a more widespread infective illness.[221] Definition and ascertainment of cause is generally more difficult with pneumonia than with other focal infections. This is partly because non-infective pulmonary pathology is so common in babies, and often impossible to distinguish radiologically, and partly because the isolation of microorganisms from respiratory secretions is not synonymous with pneumonia in the same way that microorganisms in the CSF are synonymous with meningitis. Indeed, bacteria can be found in the lungs at postmortem examination in a large proportion of babies who show no histological evidence of pneumonia.[35,37,38,329] The facts that neonatal pneumonia is relatively common, potentially life-threatening and difficult to diagnose makes it a challenging condition for the neonatologist.

INCIDENCE

Reliable incidence figures for neonatal pneumonia are hard to find, mainly on account of case definition problems. The most commonly quoted figures are 1 percent for term infants and 10 percent for preterm infants, but a reliable source for these data is difficult to locate. Using a rigorous approach to diagnosis, in a prospective study, the incidence of neonatal pneumonia in an Oxford hospital was reported to be 3.7 per 1000 live births.[444] This was among a population of almost 20 000 babies born in a tertiary referral center and included all cases of pneumonia occurring before discharge. This probably represents the best available estimate of the current incidence of neonatal pneumonia among hospitalized newborn infants in the UK. There are, of course, additional cases occurring in infants under the age of 1 month in the community, but these data are not available. Among preterm infants the incidence is much higher. In the Oxford study 92 percent of infants with late-onset pneumonia were preterm and 87 percent were ventilated at the time of onset.[444] The mean postnatal age at onset was 35 days. The reported incidence of pneumonia in intubated babies varies from 10 to 35 percent.

Halliday et al.[191] reported an incidence of pneumonia of 35 percent among intubated babies with RDS. Using more stringent immunological criteria Giacoia et al.[159] diagnosed pneumonia in 24 percent of intubated babies, but in the Oxford study, using strict radiological and laboratory criteria, only 10 percent of intubated babies had late-onset pneumonia. Pneumonia is an important cause of perinatal mortality, contributing 36 percent of cases in the British Perinatal Mortality Survey,[22] and 20 percent of neonatal deaths in the US Collaborative Perinatal Project.[302]

PATHOGENESIS

The fetus normally encounters no microorganisms during development and the newborn infant becomes harmlessly colonized by bacteria acquired from the birth canal and the environment. This happy state of affairs is evidence of the integrity of the barrier to infection provided by the placenta and membranes, the low pathogenicity of most colonizing organisms, and the relative competence of the infant's defense mechanisms. It is usually when one or other of these factors is altered that fetal or neonatal infection occurs.

Pulmonary defense mechanisms

The lining of the airways and alveoli is essentially an external surface which is readily accessible through breathing to microorganisms present in the atmosphere, colonized upper airways, ventilator circuits and endotracheal tubes. Mechanisms to deal with this constant invasion of potential pathogens are fundamental to health and must operate with minimal adverse effect on gas exchange.

AIRWAYS

In the upper airway, the main line of defense is mucociliary clearance. Inhaled microorganisms adhere to the mucus secreted by glandular cells in the columnar epithelium of the airway and are subsequently expelled by ciliary action and coughing. Respiratory mucus also exhibits bactericidal properties effected by secretory IgA, lysozyme, lactoferrin and peroxidases.[124,226] Several respiratory pathogens, though, such as Haemophilus influenzae, Pseudomonas aeruginosa and Streptococcus pneumoniae, have a high affinity for mucus, although they do not adhere well to respiratory epithelium.[36,136,416] Many of these organisms produce factors which slow down and disorganize ciliary action.[454,456] A relatively static, thick film of mucus allows many bacteria to thrive and in this biofilm they are relatively safe from opsonophagocytic killing by neutrophils.[229]

In the newborn, mucociliary clearance is relatively poor but in the preterm infant with CLD, intubation, excessive mucus production and the virtual absence of coordinated ciliary function are strong predisposing factors to persistent pulmonary infection.[28,245,253,274,349,434] In the upper airway, pulmonary epithelial cells create an effective mechanical barrier by the maintenance of tight junctions just below the luminal surface,[335] although some bacteria, such as P. aeruginosa, produce toxins which can disrupt these tight junctions.[170] The epithelial cells produce and respond to a variety of eicosanoids, cytokines and growth factors. These have important roles such as the chemoattraction of neutrophils and lymphocytes to the lung, upregulating the expression of adhesion molecules such as ICAM-1 and expression of both class I and II major histocompatibility complexes (MHC) involved in antigen presentation to lymphocytes.[360] Respiratory epithelium also contains dendritic cells, which are the most efficient antigen-presenting cells, expressing both class I and II MHC molecules.[310] There is relatively little information on the relative competence of the respiratory epithelial defense mechanisms of the newborn and there are some conflicting data.[213,398]

ALVEOLI

The defenses against microorganisms at alveolar level are both cellular and humoral. The main defense cell of the lung is the alveolar macrophage whose phagocytic and microbicidal capacity exceeds that of macrophages from other tissues. The developing lung contains few macrophages until term,[11] but there is a rapid increase following birth. In a monkey model, RDS attenuates this postnatal increase in alveolar macrophages, leading to the suggestion that surfactant may have a role in attracting circulating macrophages to the lung.[225] An important function of the alveolar macrophage is to ingest foreign antigens and transport them to the cell surface, where they bind to MHC molecules. This allows the antigen to be recognized by T cells, which then proliferate, develop functional effector capabilities (such as immunoglobulin synthesis, cytotoxic activity) and communicate with other cells through the liberation of cytokines and leukotrienes. Other cell types, such as polymorphonuclear leukocytes, are attracted to the lower respiratory tract[389] and leukotrienes are probably especially important in this respect.[330] An important mechanism in this is binding of circulating immune cells to adhesion molecules expressed on pulmonary endothelium.[270,320] As the population of immunocompetent memory cells in the inflamed lung increases so does the possibility of antigen recognition and a more efficient killing response. In the newborn, antigen presentation on the cell surface appears to be an efficient process but the T-cell effector response is reduced in comparison to adults (p. 50).[125,260] Leukotriene synthesis by alveolar macrophages is also reduced by adult standards[266] and there is some evidence of reduced expression of the nitric oxide synthetase enzyme.[9]

The humoral response to inhaled antigens is brisk as antigen-specific B cells initiate the synthesis of secretory IgA in the upper airway and IgG in lung parenchyma, which is then released onto the alveolar surface. One of the functions of the IgG is to act as a bacterium-specific opsonin to facilitate phagocytosis by alveolar macrophages,[353] which are otherwise not good at ingesting viable bacteria.[388] Specific IgG is essential for the killing of Gram-negative organisms such as *P. aeruginosa*. In the newborn, the B-cell repertoire increases throughout gestation, but even at term IgG responses to both protein and polysaccharide antigens is relatively poor compared with adults. This limits resistance to lung invasion by microorganisms to which the mother has little or no IgG antibody.

Both surfactant and its associated proteins may have direct effects on bacteria and also interact with lung defense mechanisms in a variety of ways.[386] For example, it has been shown that Curosurf enhances the phagocytosis of *Cryptococcus deformans* by alveolar macrophages *in vitro*, whether or not the yeast was opsonized by IgG.[182] In another study, a modified Curosurf preparation was shown to inhibit the multiplication of Group B streptococci in the lungs of rabbit fetuses.[201]

CONGENITAL OR INTRAUTERINE PNEUMONIA

Pneumonia which is established at the time of birth has occurred either as a result of transplacental hematogenous spread or else as a result of ascending infection from the birth canal. Infection usually occurs via the ascending route in the setting of prolonged rupture of the membranes, but may rarely be introduced by procedures such as amniocentesis or fetal blood transfusion.[380,421] The microorganisms responsible for transplacentally acquired pneumonia include rubella virus, cytomegalovirus (CMV), herpes simplex virus (HSV), adenovirus,[309] varicella zoster virus,[325] enterovirus,[296] mumps virus,[351] influenza A virus,[282] *Toxoplasma gondii*, *Listeria monocytogenes*, *Mycobacterium tuberculosis*[401] and *Treponema pallidum*. In most of these cases pneumonia is but one feature of a serious generalized infection.

Established pneumonia at birth as a result of ascending infection is rare and when pneumonia is acquired in this way it is much more usual for the initial signs to develop during the first few days after birth. There is no doubt, though, that many of the histological features of pneumonia can be found in some infants who are stillborn or else die shortly after birth. There are usually diffuse inflammatory changes, with increased numbers of polymorphs and alveolar macrophages and an infiltration of round cells in the interstitial tissue of small airways and interalveolar septa.[8,16,382]

Some of the histological changes usually associated with pneumonia are absent in congenital cases, particularly evidence of a pleural reaction and of infiltration and destruction of bronchopulmonary tissue.[98] Evidence of aspiration of amniotic fluid, in the form of vernix and squamous cells in the alveoli, is common. Bacteria are uncommon and cultures are often negative.[99] These features have led to the suggestion that many cases of so-called congenital pneumonia are predominantly, or even exclusively, cases of asphyxia. This view is supported by evidence of widespread asphyxial injury in infants dying of congenital pneumonia[54] and that asphyxia and infection may produce similar inflammatory changes in the lung.[37] An appealing way of linking the concurrence of asphyxia and congenital pneumonia is to say that pneumonia does not develop while there is a continuous outflow of lung liquid, but when asphyxia leads the fetus to gasp deeply, infected liquor is aspirated into the depths of the lung.

The microorganisms associated with congenital pneumonia are the same as those causing early-onset infection. The mortality rate for congenital pneumonia is very high. Amongst extremely low birthweight infants, congenital pneumonia has been reported to be the main cause of death, although the difficulty in distinguishing between asphyxia combined with infection and infection alone remains problematic.[39]

EARLY-ONSET PNEUMONIA

Pneumonia secondary to contact with microorganisms from the mother's vagina during, or just prior to, birth is much commoner than congenital pneumonia and typically presents with symptoms during the first 48 hours after birth. There is often systemic sepsis in addition to pulmonary involvement. The reported incidence of such early-onset pneumonia is 1.79 per 1000 live births.[444]

Microbiology

Numerous microorganisms can cause early-onset pneumonia, but in the developed world *Streptococcus agalactiae* (group B streptococcus, GBS) accounts for some 60–70 percent of cases.[444] Other important bacteria causing early-onset pneumonia include *H. influenzae*,[242,262,365] *S. pneumoniae*,[51,154,186,223,236,339,458] *L. monocytogenes*,[206] pseudomonads,[418] and the Gram-negative enteric bacilli such as *Escherichia coli*, *Klebsiella pneumoniae* and *Proteus mirabilis*. Rarely, anaerobic bacteria such as *Bacteroides fragilis* are implicated.[67,68,460] Some unusual organisms may also cause early-onset pneumonia (Table 21.1).

Table 21.1 *Unusual causes of neonatal pneumonia*

Organism	Reference
Serratia marcescens	Duggan et al.[110]
Bacteroides fragilis	Yohannan et al.[460]
	Brook et al.[68]
Pasteurella multicoda	Andersson et al.[17]
Bacillus cereus	Jevon et al.[230]
Stenotrophomonas maltophilia	Ozkan et al.[321]
Nocardia asteroides	Johnston et al.[231]
Flavobacterium meningosepticum	Tam et al.[408]
Coccidioides immitis	Fukuda[145]
Branhamella catarrhalis	Dyson et al.[115]
	Ohlsson and Bailey[315]
Citrobacter diversus	Shamir et al.[384]
Morganella morganii	Rowen and Lopez[361]
Trichomonas vaginalis	Hiemstra et al.[205]
Lactobacillus leichmannii	Lorenz et al.[265]
HSV 6	Cone[89]
Influenza A virus	Kao et al.[235]
Mumps virus	Jones et al.[233]
Measles virus	Drut and Drut[109]
	Radoycich et al.[345]
Varicella zoster virus	Isaacs[215]
CMV	Hocker et al.[207]

Non-bacterial pathogens causing pneumonia include yeasts, especially *Candida albicans*[157,307,452] and numerous viruses, including adenovirus,[3,79,299,334,406] CMV,[379] HSV[34] and echovirus.[61,413] *Chlamydia trachomatis* is reported to cause early-onset disease,[12,24,88,273,312] as are mycoplasmas.[75,342,422]

Pathogenesis

Most cases of early-onset pneumonia are the result of inhalation of infected amniotic fluid or secretions from the birth canal, but pneumonia may occasionally occur as a result of the blood-borne spread of infection to the lung. Apart from the presence of pathogenic organisms in the birth canal, the most important predisposing factors to early-onset pneumonia are prolonged rupture of the membranes,[10,107,180,246,258,275,354] prematurity and maternal urinary tract infection.[374] Bronchoalveolar lavage fluid from ventilated infants, born following prolonged rupture of the membranes, contains increased numbers of white blood cells and a high concentration of interleukin-6.[180]

The histology of early-onset neonatal pneumonia is little different from that seen in other age groups. There is usually a diffuse infiltration of leukocytes, vascular congestion, hemorrhage and patchy necrosis. Fibrin deposition is common in later presenting cases but unusual in very early ones. Bacteria are commonly seen. Hyaline membranes, similar to those seen in surfactant-deficient RDS, are often observed in babies dying of pneumonia caused by GBS, *H. influenzae* and Gram-negative enteric bacteria. In the case of infants dying very soon after birth, the hyaline membranes are full of bacteria.[225] Abscess, empyema or pneumatocele formation is very unusual in early-onset pneumonia, because it is rarely caused by organisms such as *Staphylococcus aureus* or *K. pneumoniae* with which these phenomena are strongly associated. Occasionally, though, abscesses or pneumatoceles have been reported in early-onset cases caused by *Streptococcus pneumoniae*,[339] *Escherichia coli*[185,249] and *H. influenzae*.[81]

Clinical features

The clinical features of early-onset pneumonia vary to some extent according to the causative agent. Typically, though, signs of progressive respiratory distress accompanied by signs of systemic sepsis develop within a few hours of birth and progress rapidly. Less often, the illness has a more insidious onset with signs of sepsis predominating over respiratory signs. Pneumonia must be on the list of differential diagnoses for all cases of suspected sepsis and all cases of respiratory distress.

Investigation

CULTURE

Blood culture is usually positive and culture of nasopharyngeal aspirates grows the same organism as the blood culture in a high proportion of cases.[444] If intubation is necessary, tracheal secretions should be obtained for microscopy and culture. Positive cultures from respiratory secretions do not prove pneumonia, but there is a much better correlation between bacteria in tracheal aspirates and invasive lung infection in early-onset infection[385] than in late-onset infection.[294] Cultures are also valuable in rationalizing the choice of antibiotics so as to cover all organisms isolated. Cultures from other sites are less helpful, although almost all infants with GBS pneumonia will have positive Gram stains and cultures from gastric aspirate, throat and ear swabs.[257]

RADIOLOGY

The radiological features vary according to the causative agent, the duration of infection and the coexistence of other lung pathology (Figures 21.1 and 21.2). They comprise infiltrative patterns, changes in lung volume, pleural effusions and, rarely, abscess or pneumatocele formation. Infiltrative patterns can be categorized as lobar or segmental consolidation, patchy alveolar infiltrates, hilar and peribronchial infiltrates, reticular or reticulogranular infiltrates, nodular infiltrates and diffuse haziness or opacification. Whilst these, and other, descriptive terms are needed in order to communicate

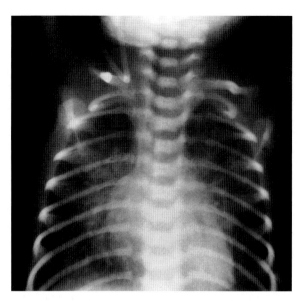

Figure 21.1 *Bacterial pneumonia due to* E. coli. *Diffuse consolidation associated with hyperinflation indicating large and small airway disease.*

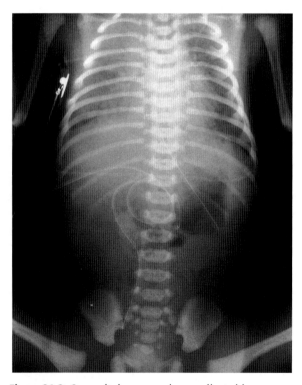

Figure 21.2 *Congenital pneumonia complicated by meconium aspiration syndrome.*

radiological descriptions, none of them is specific to a given pathogen and several different patterns may be seen during the evolution of a pulmonary infection. Changes in lung volume occur in pneumonia as a result of partial or complete airway obstruction by inflammatory

swelling or secretions. Partial obstruction leads to hyperaeration and complete obstruction to absorption atelectasis. Pleural effusions occur when fluid from the inflammatory process overflows into the pleural space. Effusions are commoner in bacterial and fungal infection than in viral or mycoplasma infection.

NON-SPECIFIC TESTS

In addition to clinical, microbiological and radiological evidence, the diagnosis of pneumonia is usually supported by evidence of an inflammatory process, such as a rise in the C-reactive protein (CRP) (or other inflammatory marker) or an abnormal white blood cell count. Infants with pneumonia have higher concentrations of interleukin-1 and TNF-α in tracheal aspirates than infants with uncomplicated RDS.[69]

DIFFERENTIAL DIAGNOSIS

The principal differential diagnosis in the preterm infant is RDS and, since pneumonia can damage surfactant production and function, the two conditions may coexist.[252] Bacterial pneumonia should always be suspected in preterm infants with respiratory distress, but especially when there are risk factors for sepsis such as premature rupture of the membranes (PROM) or maternal pyrexia and when there are features such as early onset of apnea, hypotension, poor tissue perfusion and metabolic acidosis. In terms of investigations, those with the highest positive predictive value for bacterial pneumonia, as opposed to RDS, are a positive Gram stain from surface sites, a low total neutrophil count ($<4 \times 10^9$/l) and an increased ratio of immature neutrophils to total neutrophil number (>0.4).[257] Since it is impossible, however, to exclude a diagnosis of bacterial pneumonia in preterm infants with apparent RDS, the only safe approach is to prescribe antibiotics for 48 hours, until cultures are known to be negative and the CRP level, or other indicator of infection, has been seen not to rise. If a previously well infant becomes dyspneic after 6 hours of age, pneumonia is the most likely diagnosis. Pulmonary edema in infants with heart disease, and the very rare infant who presents late with a pneumothorax or an intrathoracic malformation can usually be differentiated easily by a clinical examination, chest radiograph and, if necessary, an echocardiograph. Care must be taken to exclude other causes of tachypnea, in particular that secondary to metabolic acidemia.

Treatment

All infants showing signs of respiratory distress which does not have a clear non-infective cause must be treated with antibiotics pending the results of further observation,

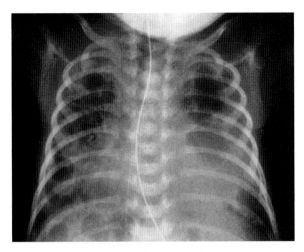

Figure 21.3 *Pneumatoceles in a case of pneumonia caused by* Staphylococcus aureus.

cultures and CRP levels. If the cultures are negative, the inflammatory markers do not rise and the baby makes a rapid recovery (as is often the case), treatment can be stopped. The safest 'blind' choice of antibiotic for presumed neonatal pneumonia is a combination of ampicillin or benzylpenicillin and an aminoglycoside. A third generation cephalosporin is an alternative, if there is little likelihood of the pneumonia being due to *L. monocytogenes* or enterococci and it does offer the benefit of reliable cover against *H. influenzae* as increasing numbers are resistant to ampicillin. Antibiotic therapy for proven pneumonia should continue for 10 days, unless the pathogen is *Staphylococcus aureus*, in which case at least 3 weeks of therapy should be administered.

In infants with staphylococcal or coliform pneumonia, pneumatoceles may develop[249] as, rarely, may lung abscesses and empyema (Figure 21.3).[185] Abscesses and pneumatoceles should be treated conservatively in the first place, using long-term intravenous antibiotics if there is an abscess. If the infant has an empyema, a thoracentesis tube for closed-chest drainage should be inserted and intravenous antibiotics administered for several weeks.

Outcome

Mortality rates for early-onset pneumonia are influenced by the identity of the pathogen and whether the infection is confined to the lung or disseminated. In the late 1970s, early-onset sepsis and pneumonia with GBS had a mortality rate of approximately 50 percent,[29] rising to 100 percent for VLBW infants.[340] Results have improved since then. The overall mortality rate for early-onset disease is now 15 percent or less.[218,459] For mature babies, the mortality should now be less than 10 percent,[63,218,459] but low birthweight babies do less well, with reported mortality rates of 27 percent[447] to 50 percent.[444]

GBS pneumonia

There are seven identifiable subtypes of GBS based on capsular polysaccharide antigens – Ia, Ib, II, III, IV, V, VI – and one non-typable group. All are implicated in early-onset pneumonia but most neonatal infections are caused by types I, II and III. Simultaneous infection with more than one serotype has been reported.[136] In addition to the polysaccharide antigens, there are surface-exposed protein antigens which may also contribute to the pathogenicity of particular strains,[83] although tissue invasiveness seems unrelated to known surface antigens.[426] The incidence of early-onset GBS sepsis is 1.8 per 1000 live births in the USA,[62] 1.75 per 1000 in Canada,[85] 1.3 per 1000 in Australia,[218] 1.2 per 1000 in Spain,[202] and 0.76 per 1000 in Finland.[234] In the UK, reported incidences ranged from 0.3 to 1 per 1000.[228,279,350] More recently, reported incidences show regional variation, from 1.15 culture-proven cases of early-onset GBS sepsis per 1000 live births in Bedfordshire[43] to 0.5 per 1000 in Oxford.[301] From time to time, major outbreaks are reported during which the incidence may be as high as 14 per 1000 live births.[5]

The two major factors influencing the prevalence of GBS sepsis are vaginal carriage rates among pregnant women and the effectiveness of strategies to prevent contamination of the infant at birth. During the last 5 years, vaginal and rectal carriage rates have been variously reported as 18.5 percent,[160] 12 percent,[227] 16.3 percent,[341] 23 percent[19] and 7.1 percent.[202] The lowest rates are reported from European centers and this is mirrored in the lower reported incidence of early-onset GBS sepsis in Europe compared with the USA.

CLINICAL PICTURE

Most cases of GBS pneumonia develop within the first 4–6 hours and almost 90 percent of cases present within 24 hours of birth.[149,459] Pneumonia may complicate bacteremia, but can occur without bacteremia in about 30 percent of cases.[120] GBS sepsis may masquerade as severe birth asphyxia,[268,328] or present immediately after resuscitation with respiratory failure, cyanosis and shock. More often, the infant presents with the early signs of sepsis. Without prompt recognition and treatment, the infant's condition rapidly worsens and they require intubation and ventilation for apnea and severe hypoxemia, often demonstrating the cardiorespiratory features of persistent pulmonary hypertension of the newborn. Hypotension, metabolic acidemia, tachycardia and poor peripheral perfusion develop in severe cases and then the prognosis is poor.[70]

PATHOPHYSIOLOGY

The hypotension, hypoxemia and lung injury which characterize early-onset GBS sepsis in the newborn are very reminiscent of the septic shock syndrome caused by the endotoxin of Gram-negative organisms. Gram-negative endotoxin exerts its effects mainly by stimulating the release of cytokines, such as TNF-α, interleukin-1,[427] and interleukin-6 from antigen-presenting cells, including macrophages and monocytes. TNF-α causes progressive hypotension, decreased cardiac output, hypoxemia and lung injury when infused directly into animals. TNF-α can be detected in the serum and urine of infants with GBS sepsis (but not from healthy controls) and in the laboratory, heat-killed, washed GBS can induce the production of TNF-α from monocytes and macrophages.[453] Interestingly, mixed mononuclear cells from neonates produced significantly more TNF-α in response to GBS than cells from adults.[453] The cellular component of GBS responsible for TNF-α release is not yet identified, but seems not to be the polysaccharide surface antigen. These observations could shed fresh light on the pathophysiology of GBS sepsis and may lead to novel immunological therapies, such as antibodies directed against TNF-α.

Pulmonary hypertension with hypoxemia secondary to right-to-left shunting is a relatively common feature. In the case of GBS, pulmonary hypertension has been shown to relate to an ability to invade pulmonary endothelial cells,[127] especially the cells of the microvasculature, and lead to the release of the eicosanoids, such as prostacyclin and PGE$_2$,[161,313] and leukotrienes.[376] In animals, injection of heat-killed GBS causes dose-dependent increases in pulmonary arterial pressure and pulmonary and systemic vascular resistance, and decreases in cardiac output and heart rate. The quantitative response of the pulmonary vascular resistance is strain-dependent, with serotype Ib having a greater effect than serotype III.[94] Infection with different strains might go some way towards explaining different severities of illness.

Host defenses against GBS include polymorphonuclear leukocytes, complement and type-specific antibodies directed against the polysaccharide and protein antigens. An infant is most susceptible to GBS when his mother, although having GBS in her vagina, has little or no circulating anti-GBS IgG.[30,435] This is particularly likely if the infant is born prematurely.[15] A concentration of IgG specific antibody of greater than 2 μg/ml in the serum of newborns seems protective.[164] Neonatal white blood cells find it difficult to kill the organism[405] and, if antibody is present, GBS antigen causes neutrophil aggregation in the lung with the consequent release of a multiplicity of cytokines which further contribute to tissue injury.[281]

HISTOLOGY

There are no specific features though many infants have alveolar hyaline membranes, as well as pneumonia.[1,337] In the preterm infant, surfactant-deficient RDS may coexist,[222] but in term infants the hyaline membranes are a non-specific change caused by GBS toxicity.[359] The presence of hyaline membranes may in the past, in the absence of adequate bacteriological investigation, have resulted in many deaths due to GBS or other similar infections being attributed to surfactant-deficient RDS.

INVESTIGATION

The treatment of suspected early-onset pneumonia should not be delayed pending the results of investigations. The objective of performing investigations is to provide retrospective confirmation of the diagnosis and to identify the responsible organism.

Microbiological

The blood culture will almost invariably be positive, if the mother has not been treated with antibiotics. GBS is easy to culture and will usually grow from most surface swabs and from the gastric aspirate (which often contains numerous Gram-positive cocci). GBS antigen can be identified by latex particle agglutination tests on the infant's serum and concentrated urine.[144,344] In a multi-center study evaluating the latex particle agglutination test on urine samples from infants with culture-proven GBS, only 53.5 percent of infected infants had a positive test.[46] The organism is invariably present in the mother's high vaginal swab, and new techniques may enable rapid detection of the organism in this site when the mother is admitted in labor.[403] The specificity of these tests appears to be good, but their sensitivity is relatively poor.[173]

Hematological

Neutropenia and the presence of primitive cells in the peripheral blood are common[64,272] and neutropenia $<1.5 \times 10^9$/l is an ominous sign.[327] The sensitivity, specificity and predictive values of hematological variables, however, in the diagnosis of early-onset sepsis is poor.[174,187] Anemia and thrombocytopenia may develop in survivors. Acute-phase reactants such as the C-reactive protein are generally highly elevated in GBS sepsis, but there may be a delay of 12 hours or so between the onset of signs and the rise in CRP.[331]

Radiological

The chest radiograph may be virtually normal or show widespread homogeneous opacity in those with coexisting RDS[436] and is rarely helpful in differential diagnosis (Figures 21.4–21.6). Pleural effusions may occur.[87,327]

TREATMENT

Intravenous antibiotics, at the high end of the recommended dose range, must be started immediately the diagnosis is suspected. A combination of ampicillin or benzylpenicillin and gentamicin is a good choice for blind treatment of early-onset pneumonia in the newborn, because of synergism between these antibiotics against GBS,[261,428] and because it is necessary to cover other organisms responsible for the syndrome. A cephalosporin alone is unsatisfactory initial therapy for early-onset sepsis

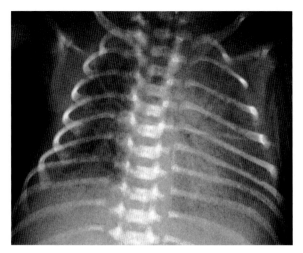

Figure 21.4 *GBS pneumonia indistinguishable from RDS.*

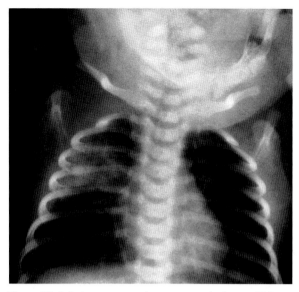

Figure 21.6 *Lobar pneumonia uncommonly due to GBS.*

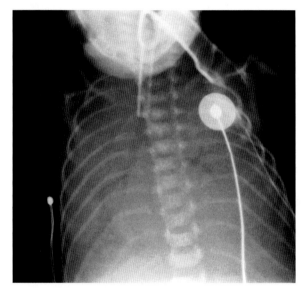

Figure 21.5 *GBS pneumonia. A widespread consolidation pattern without specific diagnostic features.*

as it will not treat *L. monocytogenes* or enterococci. Intravenous antibiotics should be given for 10 days. GBS is very sensitive to penicillin with most isolates having a minimal inhibitory concentration of less than 0.06 μg/ml.

Exchange transfusions using blood from a donor with anti-GBS antibodies have been considered helpful.[211,356,431] Infusions of immunoglobulins have been advocated and are used by some clinicians as supplementary therapy. The published evidence relating to the benefits of immunoglobulin infusions in the treatment of early-onset neonatal sepsis is fairly persuasive but is based mainly on small studies which are not amenable to meta-analysis, because of significant differences in study design and evaluation criteria.[86,448] The immunological activity of standard immunoglobulin preparations is highly variable.[164] Specially prepared GBS-hyperimmune globulin will produce higher antibody titers and such a

product has been effective in the experimental animal.[449] Immunoglobulin infusions, however, may increase the risk of white cells aggregating in the lungs and they should be used cautiously.[446]

Studies of GBS disease in experimental animals have shown a halving of mortality rate with the use of recombinant human granulocyte-macrophage colony-stimulating factor as adjunctive therapy.[165] There is some evidence of surfactant deficiency or dysfunction in animal models of infective pneumonia and there may be a role for surfactant therapy. There are few studies examining the efficacy of surfactant in neonatal pneumonia,[178] but benefit has been reported.[26]

PREVENTING GBS PNEUMONIA

Maternal prophylaxis

Approximately 1 percent of infants born vaginally to mothers who carry GBS at the time of birth become infected. Important predisposing factors are: evidence of chorioamnionitis such as maternal pyrexia, prolonged labor, prolonged rupture of the membranes, frequent pelvic examinations in labor and low birthweight.[5,84,149,160,285] One or more of these predisposing factors is present in 82 percent of cases of early-onset neonatal GBS sepsis and pneumonia.[149]

The main approach to preventing vertical transmission is intrapartum antibiotic prophylaxis, given to women who have been shown to carry GBS on screening during pregnancy and/or have obstetric risk factors.[52,333] Many individual studies have reported significant benefits of this policy with regard to reducing neonatal colonization and infection,[150,227,341,417] although this finding has not been universal.[21] A meta-analysis of all published, randomized controlled trials up to 1994 concluded that, although there was convincing evidence of a reduction in neonatal colonization with GBS, there was no demonstrated significant reduction in the incidence of serious maternal or neonatal outcome.[316] The observation that the use of antibiotics to prevent neonatal GBS infection can be associated with serious neonatal infection with resistant Enterobacteriaceae is of concern.[280] On the balance of the existing evidence, it seems advisable to use maternal antibiotic prophylaxis in an attempt to prevent neonatal infection and the American Academy of Pediatrics has recommended two possible approaches.[13] One approach is to screen all pregnant women for GBS at 35–37 weeks of gestation and to give intrapartum penicillin or ampicillin to all who screen positive regardless of other risk factors. The second approach is not to screen, but to give intrapartum antibiotics to all women with a risk factor. Risk factors include a previous infant with GBS disease, GBS bacteriuria during pregnancy, preterm labor, ruptured membranes for more than 18 hours prior to delivery and intrapartum fever. Cost-benefit analyses have suggested that a risk-factor approach should be implemented at an incidence of greater than 0.6 per 1000 and a screening program at an incidence of greater than 0.2 per 1000.[214]

Management of premature rupture of the membranes[169,291]

Once the amnion ruptures, the amniotic cavity and the fetus become accessible to microorganisms present in the vagina. The likelihood of such ascending infection increases with time. When the membranes rupture prior to the onset of labor (PROM), the interval between membrane rupture and the birth of the infant may be prolonged. When the membranes rupture at less than 37 weeks of gestation (preterm, premature rupture of the membranes, PPROM), an even greater interval between membrane rupture and birth often occurs. The evidence concerning the risk of neonatal sepsis following premature rupture of the membranes at term is conflicting. Some studies suggest relatively little increased risk,[263] while others show a high risk and a high mortality.[10] Meconium staining of the liquor increases the risk of intra-amniotic infection.[451] A randomized controlled trial of the management of PROM at term has recently been concluded and shows no benefit in terms of neonatal sepsis of induction of labor over expectant management for up to 4 days.[194] The overall rate of neonatal sepsis in this study was approximately 2–3 percent.

PPROM carries a significant risk of sepsis and pneumonia,[27,60,204,258,263,429] although when membrane rupture occurs before 28 weeks of gestation pulmonary hypoplasia is probably the greater threat to survival (p. 450).[284] The risk of neonatal sepsis following PPROM has been reported to be about 3.5 times the risk without PPROM.[258] The risk can be reduced by prompt delivery following membrane rupture but this has to be balanced against the risk of premature birth. There have been no satisfactory randomized trials comparing different delivery strategies following PPROM.

There have been numerous studies examining the value of prophylactic antibiotics in preterm labor, with or without ruptured membranes, but the results have often been inconclusive because of small sample sizes.[121,122,128,283,290] The largest study to date of the effect of maternal antibiotics for preterm, prelabor rupture of the membranes is the ORACLE I trial.[239] ORACLE did not look specifically at pneumonia as an outcome measure, but infants whose mothers were treated with erythromycin had a lower rate of positive blood cultures, less need for surfactant and a lower rate of oxygen dependency at 28 days of age than those whose mothers received placebo. There was also evidence of prolongation of pregnancy, confirming a previous finding.[169] In the ORACLE trial, there was no increased rate of neonatal sepsis and pneumonia with resistant organisms, such as E. coli, as has been reported elsewhere.[280]

Neonatal prophylaxis

Administration of prophylactic antibiotics to asymptomatic infants considered to be at risk of GBS sepsis is a controversial issue. Some studies have shown that giving prophylactic penicillin to all infants[317,456] or just those of birthweight less than 2 kg[255] will cause a significant reduction in the incidence of GBS sepsis, but others have failed to demonstrate this benefit.[340] Administration of prophylactic penicillin to all infants is not justified, but giving penicillin to asymptomatic infants of women who have grown GBS from vaginal swabs, but have not themselves received appropriate antibiotics, is a common and appropriate practice.

Escherichia coli

Escherichia coli (E. coli) is the second commonest cause of early neonatal sepsis. Pneumonia arises as a result of hematogenous spread. Approximately 40 percent of E. coli strains causing early-onset sepsis and meningitis possess the capsule type K1.[371] The K1 polysaccharide capsule is an important virulence factor which confers antiphagocytic properties and resistance of complement mediated killing. Pregnancy is associated with increased carriage of K1 strains, which are then vertically transmitted.[371] Ampicillin resistance in community-acquired E. coli infections is seen in approximately 40 percent of isolates. Third-generation cephalosporins, cefotaxamine and ceftriaxone, are used for E. coli sepsis.

Streptococcus pneumoniae

The pneumococcus accounts for about 5 percent of early-onset neonatal pneumonia.[300] It is the commonest cause of childhood pneumonia outside of the neonatal period.[105] Unlike GBS, the pneumococcus cannot be regarded as part of the normal vaginal flora and prolonged rupture of the membranes is a less common feature of early-onset pneumococcal pneumonia than it is with other causes of early-onset disease.[186] There is also a higher mortality rate when the membranes have been ruptured for less than 24 hours, than there is with more prolonged membrane rupture–delivery intervals. These observations suggest that the pathogenesis of early-onset pneumococcal pneumonia may differ from that of other bacteria. The majority of cases present as a fulminant systemic illness within a few hours of birth. Typically, both lungs are diffusely involved, with radiological features indistinguishable from RDS. The lobar distribution typical of pneumococcal infections in older children and adults is not described. The mortality rate has been reported to be high,[154,186] but there are no recent data.

Haemophilus influenzae

PATHOGENESIS

Haemophilus influenzae, especially the non-capsulate, non-serotypable strains, has an affinity for the female genital tract and is responsible for almost 10 percent of early-onset pneumonia.[289] This organism is the third most common cause of early-onset pneumonia, after GBS and *E. coli*.[365] The incidence of neonatal *H. influenzae* infection was reported to be 4.6 per 100 000 births in the Oxford region.[133] The same obstetric risk factors operate as for GBS and a recent study of early-onset *H. influenzae* sepsis reported preterm labor in 92 percent of cases, PROM for longer than 12 hours in 63 percent, maternal fever in 64 percent, chorioamnionitis in 43 percent and vaginal discharge in 44 percent.[242] In comparison with GBS, the rate of vaginal carriage of *H. influenzae* is low, but the risk of invasive disease in colonized infants is much greater, at around 50 percent.[74]

CLINICAL SIGNS

Most infants present immediately after birth, with respiratory distress due to pneumonia, which is clinically and radiologically indistinguishable from RDS or pneumonia caused by other bacteria. Meningitis and conjunctivitis are relatively common. The reported mortality rate is approximately 50 percent.[457] Most *H. influenzae* causing early-onset pneumonia in newborn infants in the UK are currently sensitive to ampicillin. Ampicillin resistance, however, is emerging and cefotaxime should be added when there is reason to suspect *H. influenzae* sepsis.

Listeria monocytogenes

INCIDENCE

Early-onset neonatal sepsis with *L. monocytogenes* occurred in 25.3 cases per 100 000 livebirths in Denmark in 1986.[141]

Laboratory proven cases of pregnancy associated listeriosis in England and Wales increased markedly in the late 1980s. Following a national campaign to increase awareness amongst pregnant women and food producers, the number of cases has fallen from 86 per year during 1985–1989 to 18 per year during 1995–1999.[338]

PATHOGENESIS

L. monocytogenes is a short Gram-positive rod which can be found both inside and outside cells. The most important reservoir for transmission to humans is probably food, especially dairy products, contaminated by infected farm animals.[137,156] Almost half of all documented infections occur in pregnant women.[232] Women infected with HIV are considerably more susceptible to *L. monocytogenes* than the general population.[130] Newborn infants are particularly susceptible to infection by *L. monocytogenes* for a variety of immunological reasons, including defects in macrophage response[220] and low opsonic activity.[59,141] At least two-thirds of infants who acquire listeria infection intrapartum are preterm and almost all become ill within 24 hours of birth.[129,269]

CLINICAL SIGNS

L. monocytogenes causes a non-specific influenzal or gastroenteritic illness in pregnant women, during which the organism may infect the fetus, either by hematogenous spread across the placenta or via infection of the amniotic fluid. First- or second-trimester infection can cause fetal death or miscarriage. Recurrent abortion due to listeria has been recorded in humans.[172] Later in pregnancy, infection can precipitate preterm labor,[156] with fetal distress and meconium staining of the liquor.[254] Since meconium staining of the liquor is rare at gestations below 34 weeks, its presence should raise the suspicion of bacterial infection. Congenitally infected babies are often extremely ill at birth. They have a severe pneumonia and hepatomegaly; meningitis may already be present. Blood and stool cultures are invariably positive. Characteristically, small (2–3 mm) pinkish-grey cutaneous granulomas are present and, at autopsy, similar small granulomatous lesions are widespread in lung, liver, CNS and many other organs. The mortality rate recently reported from a UK center is about 15 percent.[232]

INVESTIGATIONS

The vast majority of babies with early-onset infection caused by *L. monocytogenes* have pneumonia as a prominent feature. The radiological features may mimic RDS, but in some cases a much coarser pattern of infiltration is seen, reminiscent of meconium aspiration pneumonia. Diarrhea and an erythematous skin rash may occur. The routine investigations of early-onset sepsis and meningitis reveal the diagnosis. The organism can be isolated from the first meconium passed. Listeria, however, can pose problems for the microbiologist since its take-up of the Gram stain can be variable and it may be slow growing.

MANAGEMENT

The most effective antibiotic therapy is ampicillin plus gentamicin and in units where listeria is a common pathogen this combination should be considered as the routine treatment for early-onset sepsis. Listeria is resistant to all third-generation cephalosporins. Extracorporeal membrane oxygenation (ECMO) has been used successfully in the treatment of severe, early-onset pneumonia caused by *L. monocytogenes*.[206]

LATE-ONSET PNEUMONIA

Most neonatal pulmonary infections which begin more than 48 hours after birth are caused by organisms acquired from the postnatal environment rather than transplacentally or from the birth canal. The vast majority of cases of late-onset pneumonia on a neonatal intensive care unit occur in preterm infants, especially those who are on ventilatory support.[444] Late-onset pneumonia is rare in infants born at term.

Among hospitalized infants, the commonest bacteria causing late-onset pneumonia are Gram-negative bacilli (such as *Klebsiella* spp., *E. coli*, *Serratia marcescens*, *Pseudomonas* spp. and *Proteus* spp.), coagulase-negative staphylococci and *Staphylococcus aureus*.[77] Unusual bacterial causes of nosocomial neonatal pneumonia include *Legionella pneumophila*.[73,176,208,267] Several viral agents have also been implicated, including RSV,[189,293] influenza virus,[41,286] parainfluenza virus,[287] rhinovirus,[78,425] enterovirus,[53] coronavirus,[394] CMV and varicella zoster virus.[184] Among very immature infants, nosocomial fungal infections are a significant problem.[288]

In the community, neonatal bacterial pneumonia is fairly unusual, although pertussis[304] and late-presenting, perinatally acquired chlamydial infections[112,400] can occur. Viral infections acquired from household members are relatively common and may progress to pneumonia.[2] Important causes are influenza A,[97,322] RSV,[463] parainfluenza,[463] enterovirus,[117] adenovirus and rhinovirus.

Epidemiology of nosocomial infection

The important reservoirs of microorganisms involved in late-onset pneumonia are people, including the infant's own skin and gastrointestinal tract, other infants, hospital staff and visitors. Colonization of the skin and aerodigestive tract in the normal neonate begins within 24 hours of birth with organisms derived from the genital tract, skin and oropharynx of the mother. Skin colonization with coagulase-negative staphylococci

(particularly *Staphylococcus epidermidis*) begins round the umbilicus and nose. The oropharynx is colonized by α-hemolytic streptococci, *Escherichia coli*, enterococci, lactobacilli and *Bifidobacterium* species colonize the gastrointestinal tract. Colonization of the nose, throat, umbilicus and gut of neonates admitted to neonatal intensive care units is delayed, even beyond 3 days after birth, and the colonization is abnormal.[168] Stool colonization with nosocomial Gram-negative bacilli, particularly species of *Klebsiella*, *Enterobacter* and *Citrobacter*, has been reported to occur in more than 50 percent of infants. Increased rates of throat and surface colonization with these organisms were also noted. Antibiotic therapy for more than 3 days was significantly associated with acquisition of carriage. An inverse relationship between the number of days of antibiotic therapy and number of microbial species present in the stool of infants with a birthweight of less than 1000 g and a significant positive effect of breast milk on the diversity of gut flora have been observed.[158] The inhibitory effect of the presence of α-hemolytic streptococci on oral colonization on methicillin-resistant *Staphylococcus aureus* (MRSA) has been described in a unit with endemic MRSA.[419] Failure to establish a diverse microflora renders neonates requiring intensive care vunerable to colonization and thus infection from organisms derived from the hospital environment via the hands of healthcare workers or contaminated equipment. Infected family members of healthcare staff may transmit viruses by aerosols or fomites. *Bordetella pertussis* infection has been transmitted to neonates of non-immune mothers from non-immunized siblings. Rarely, the source is the physical environment. Occasionally, a specific contaminated source is discovered, for example mineral oil containing *Listeria* sp.[377] or parenteral nutrition solutions containing *Acinetobacter* sp.[306]

Modern methods of identifying specific strains of bacteria are proving useful in understanding the ecology of nosocomial pathogens, a step which is essential if the increasing rates of nosocomial infection and antibiotic resistance on the NICU are to be controlled.[134,183,237,326] There is a strong relationship between prematurity and low birthweight and the risk of late-onset pneumonia.[45,171,218,219,240,375,404] In two studies of infants on NICUs, rates of nosocomial infection amongst those weighing less than 1000 g have been reported to be 44.4 and 22.6 percent and amongst those weighing more than 2000 g to be 10.1 and 0.6 percent, respectively.[108,219] These figures reflect the inherent susceptibility of such infants to infection,[71] but also are strongly influenced by factors in the NICU environment, such as the adverse microbiological ecology and the use of medical devices. Many studies have demonstrated a strong positive correlation between the rate of nosocomial infection and use, and duration of use, of ventilators, lines for central vascular access, intravenous fat emulsions and implanted shunts for hydrocephalus.[47,72,142,148,152,155,336,357] The importance of exposure to these risk factors has been illustrated by the finding of a positive association between the rate of nosocomial infection and the overall average duration of stay on the NICU,[153] as well as the individual duration of stay on the NICU.[171] These findings show the importance of correcting for average duration of admission when making inter-hospital comparisons of nosocomial infection rates. Pneumonia developing more than 48 hours after birth is commonest among preterm infants who are being ventilated. Pneumonia in ventilated infants can occur secondary to septicemia or secondary to colonization of the endotracheal tube. In contrast to early-onset cases, blood cultures are negative in most instances of late-onset pneumonia.

Microbiology

COAGULASE-NEGATIVE STAPHYLOCOCCI

Coagulase-negative staphylocooci, particularly *Staphylococcus epidermidis*, have emerged as the commonest cause of nosocomial bloodstream infection in neonates, causing more than 50 percent of episodes in many series.[153,332,409] Intravascular catheters are well recognized risk factors for nosocomial infection with these organisms[438] and pneumonia may arise from hematogenous dissemination. Coagulase-negative staphylococci were the commonest cause of late-onset bacteremic pneumonia in one series, causing 57 percent of cases.[444] Nosocomial strains are often resistant to multiple antibiotics, including methicillin. Molecular typing of strains isolated from ventilated neonates has demonstrated that clonal dissemination does occur, suggesting that adherence to infection control procedures may be helpful.[433]

STAPHYLOCOCCUS AUREUS

Staphylococcus aureus colonization is acquired at birth or via the hands of personnel and family. It was reported to be the cause of 44 percent of nosocomial pneumonia cases, but only infants with positive respiratory cultures were considered.[200] Phage typing demonstrated multiple strains.[200] MRSA, which causes the same spectrum of infection as sensitive *Staphylococcus aureus*, has become endemic in some units, although most will see sporadic cases.

ENTEROBACTERIACEAE

Neonatal gut colonization with members of the Enterobacteriaceae is the major source of nosocomial infection with these organisms. Outbreaks of invasive infection caused by strains of *Klebsiella pneumoniae* harboring plasmids encoding for extended spectrum-based lactamases (conferring resistance to third-generation cephalosporins) have been frequently reported.[143,363]

Resistance to gentamicin is common in these strains. *Escherichia coli* and *Enterobacter* species are also common isolates.[153] *Enterobacter* species possess a chromosomal β-lactamase which is not usually expressed (as do *Citrobacter* and *Serratia* species). Selective pressure from use of third-generation cephalosporins can lead to the emergence of stably depressed mutants (resistant to all β-lactams with the exception of the carbapenems) in hospital settings.[100,139]

PSEUDOMONAS AERUGINOSA

Pseudomonas aeruginosa thrives in moist environments and colonization of ventilated infants has been widely documented.[91,151,217] It is an uncommon cause of nosocomial infection, but outbreaks have been linked to environmental sources and hand colonization.[138,151] Infection is associated with significant morbidity and mortality. In one series, the mortality of bacteremic pneumonia was 87 percent.[91]

CANDIDA SPECIES

Invasive infections with *Candida albicans* and other species, particularly *Candida parapsilosis*, are described increasingly in neonates requiring intensive care. An incidence of 12.3 per 1000 admissions has been reported, with marked variation between units.[347] Intravascular lines and lipid-rich parenteral nutrition are risk factors, but more important is exposure to prolonged antibiotics, particularly third-generation cephalosporins.[50,445] Pneumonia arises as a result of blood-borne spread in disseminated infection.

VIRUSES

Nosocomial infection with RSV, rhinoviruses, adenoviruses, influenza and parainfluenza viruses and enteroviruses reflect high levels of infection in the community, although sporadic cases are reported.[461] Neonatal adenovirus infection is often disseminated and fatal.[3]

Clinical features

In an infant with primary lung disease already on a ventilator, pneumonia presents with deteriorating lung function and non-specific signs of infection. An increase in endotracheal tube aspirate suggests infection, but can be confused with the bronchorrhea seen in BPD (p. 405). Localized and generalized crepitations may be heard. Initial symptoms may be those of an unspecified respiratory tract infection (URTI) accompanied by a low-grade pyrexia.[95,247,287,425] More severe viral pneumonia, however, can also occur at any time in the neonatal period and adenoviruses and coronaviruses are often responsible.[277,334,394]

Investigation

A possible routine surveillance strategy is to perform routine, twice-weekly, CRP estimations on all ventilated infants and to undertake a chest radiograph, blood cultures and culture of respiratory secretions in any infant whose ventilatory requirement increases significantly or who develops a raised CRP. Interpretation of the results of tracheal secretion cultures, however, poses difficulties (p. 73). Microorganisms recovered from the upper airway may be those causing lower respiratory tract infection. This has been shown in the case of coagulase-negative staphylococci, using ribotyping techniques,[56] and with *Candida* spp.[362] The results of cultures of respiratory secretions should, therefore, be used to inform the choice of antimicrobial agents for suspected pulmonary infection. It is, however, naïve to base the diagnosis of pulmonary infection solely on the results of culture of respiratory secretions, as illustrated by a recent study comparing tracheal aspirate cultures from infants showing signs of respiratory deterioration with cultures from babies who were stable. No significant difference was found in the rate of positive cultures for bacteria, viruses, chlamydia or ureaplasmas. Cultures were positive in about one-third of the infants in each group.[411] Other studies, however, have reported that culturing respiratory secretions has clinical value[196,251,385] and it has been suggested that using a bronchial brush technique may give better results.[355] In older infants, viral cultures and immunofluorescence studies for mycoplasma, chlamydia and respiratory viruses are indicated.

Management

The choice of initial antibiotic therapy for late-onset neonatal pneumonia is difficult, because the list of potential pathogens is long. It is important to cover coagulase-negative staphylococci. Unless local knowledge suggests otherwise, a third-generation cephalosporin plus vancomycin is a good choice. Therapy should subsequently be modified to cover organisms grown from the blood or tracheal secretions.

If the infant is already on antibiotics when the deterioration from the presumed pneumonia occurs, it is usually advisable to change the drugs and to broaden the spectrum of cover, often to include an antibiotic effective against *Pseudomonas* spp. In infants who have been ventilated for several weeks, in whom *Chlamydia* spp., *Mycoplasma* spp., *Bordetella pertussis* or even *Pneumocystis carinii* are possible pathogens, antibiotics such as erythromycin and septrin should be considered.

LUNG ABSCESS

This is a rare occurrence in the newborn, presenting usually with dyspnea and an area of opacification on chest rediograph. CT scanning is a useful diagnostic aid.[278] A lung abscess usually follows previous pneumonia and is usually caused by Gram-negative organisms, but can be caused by *Staphylococcus aureus* and occasionally *Serratia marcescens*[241] It should be treated initially with broad-spectrum antibiotics. If the lesion does not resolve, bronchoscopy or surgery may be indicated.[384,390]

PNEUMONIA IN THE INFANT WITH CLD

In infants with long-term respiratory disease, pneumonia should always be at the top of the list of differential diagnoses if their respiratory status deteriorates. Some of these infants are several months old and, in addition to the usual pathogens, the respiratory viral infections characteristic of that age group are common.[334] Respiratory tract colonization with Gram-negative organisms may be associated with more severe CLD.[90] Infants with CLD who develop added pulmonary infection often become extremely ill, and frequently require ventilatory support.[337] There is often a marked deterioration in the radiological appearances (Figure 21.7). *Staphylococcus epidermidis* may be

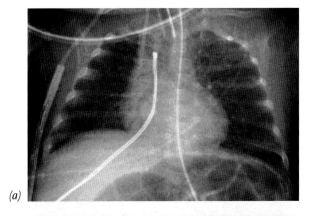

(a)

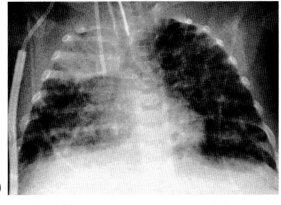

(b)

Figure 21.7 *(a) Deterioration in an infant with CLD complicated by pneumonia caused by* P. aeruginosa. *(b) Chest radiograph appearance 3 days later demonstrating right upper lobe collapse.*

the infective agent (Figure 21.8). Antibiotics should always be given. Strategies to prevent pneumonia in ventilated patients have been reviewed.[244] Underlying viral, or indeed non-viral, infection may play a significant role in the pathogenesis of CLD.[442] In one study, adenovirus DNA was detected in tracheal aspirate samples, obtained at 1 week of age, in 27 percent of infants who went on to develop CLD, but only 3 percent of otherwise comparable infants who did not develop CLD.[93] Viral respiratory infections in infants with CLD led to a worsening of chronic respiratory morbidity with signs of increased airway resistance compared to those who did not develop viral infection.[462] In a randomized trial in a cohort of CLD infants with acute deterioration (but without a diagnosis of RSV infection), infants treated with the antiviral agent ribavirin had both short- and medium-term benefit in clinical signs and lung function.[162]

BACTERIAL LUNG INFECTIONS

Bordetella pertussis

Infants may acquire the infection from their non-immunized mother who developed the disease perinatally.[48,82]

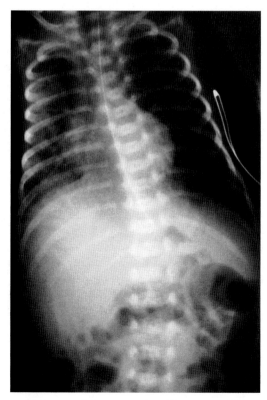

Figure 21.8 *Bacterial pneumonia with asymmetrical consolidation.* Staphylococcus epidermidis *was isolated from the infant.*

CLINICAL SIGNS

Severe pertussis can occur in the neonatal period, presenting with paroxysmal cough, vomiting, apnea and choking spells. Whooping is rare. Prolonged ventilatory support is often required.[195]

INVESTIGATIONS

A marked leukocytosis and lymphocytosis is typical. The chest radiograph shows bilateral coarse infiltrates. Diagnosis is by culture of nasopharyngeal swabs or, in the case of infants who have started antibiotic therapy, by PCR.[119]

MANAGEMENT

Erythromycin and sedation should be given; ventilatory support may be required.[163]

Chlamydia (Figure 21.9)

Chlamydia trachomatis is probably the commonest sexually transmitted pathogen in the western world. Birth by cesarean section with intact membranes does not preclude the possibility of vertical transmission[49] and the organism can cross the intact membranes, causing fetal pneumonic stillbirth.[410] The chlamydial species responsible for causing neonatal pneumonia is *C. trachomatis* and it is usually vertically transmitted. Between 10 and 20 percent of infants born to infected mothers will develop pneumonia[373] and about a half of these will have conjunctivitis.[412]

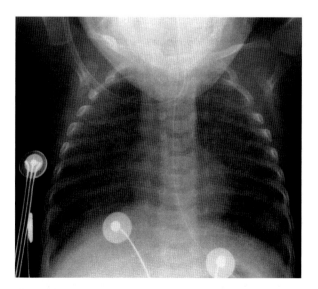

Figure 21.9 *Chlamydia pneumonia with features of an interstitial pneumonitis and characteristic widespread interstitial changes.*

CLINICAL SIGNS

Chlamydial pneumonia in term infants characteristically occurs beyond the neonatal period,[197] but it can occur in the first weeks after birth.[179,312,318,367] Chlamydial pneumonia is characterized by tachypnea, paroxysmal cough and apneic episodes.[66,197] There are usually also signs of infection in the upper respiratory tract and often the conjunctivae. Eosinophilia is a common feature. The chest radiograph characteristically shows hyperexpansion and diffuse bilateral infiltrates. A distinctive form of early-onset chlamydial pneumonia has been described in preterm infants. The presentation is very similar to early-onset pneumonia caused by organisms such as GBS or *H. influenzae* and the same difficulty of distinguishing the condition from RDS applies.[12,24,88,273,397] The eosinophilia and hyperinflation of the lung characteristic of later infection in term infants is replaced by a neutrophilia and either atelectasis or diffuse infiltrations. Some reports have described a biphasic pattern of illness with an initial picture similar to RDS followed by improvement and then deterioration.[24,397] It may be that surfactant deficiency was the main cause of the first phase and chlamydial pneumonia the cause of the second phase. Like other neonatal lung diseases, chlamydial pneumonia can cause long-term pulmonary damage.[450]

DIAGNOSIS

This has traditionally been made by culturing chlamydia from respiratory secretions and by the detection of specific IgM in blood. There are also direct immunofluorescence tests.[358] Increasingly, tests based on the detection of DNA are being employed.[57,318] These provide a rapid result and have diagnostic sensitivity and specificity equal or superior to culture.[192]

MANAGEMENT

The treatment of chlamydial pneumonia is a 2-week course of erythromycin, given intravenously in severe and early-onset cases. Chlamydial infection during pregnancy should be treated with either ampicillin or erythromycin in order to prevent perinatal transmission.[369] An alternative strategy, where a lack of compliance is anticipated, is a single dose of azithromycin.[4]

Tuberculosis

Congenital transmission is very rare, but has been reported in the infants of mothers who acquire primary infection during pregnancy. It usually presents in the first month after birth with evidence of disseminated infection including respiratory distress.[401] The global increase in the prevalence of tuberculosis, in part fuelled by the HIV pandemic, may result in an increased incidence of perinatally acquired tuberculosis.[6] Neonatal tuberculosis is acquired vertically either transplacentally or through inhalation of tubercle bacilli during or soon after birth or nosocomially through intimate contact with an adult with active pulmonary tuberculosis.

CLINICAL SIGNS

A large proportion of newborn infants with tuberculosis suffer from a progressive pneumonia,[6] usually with radiological evidence of widespread pulmonary infection involving both lungs and mediastinal and hilar lymph nodes. There is usually no hepatic involvement in this clinical syndrome, the source of infection probably being the amniotic fluid or maternal genital tract.[167]

DIAGNOSIS

In most cases there are no clinical features which point directly to the diagnosis, therefore, detection relies mainly on good maternal history taking and a high index of suspicion.[40,248] Examination of the gastric aspirate for acid-fast bacilli is the best diagnostic test. The infected neonate is not sensitive to tuberculin.

MANAGEMENT

Treatment of proven infection is with isoniazid 20 mg/kg daily plus rifampicin (10–20 mg/kg/day) together with a third drug such as streptomycin or ethambutol for short-term use. Rifampicin should not be given continuously for more than 3 months because of its effects on liver function, while streptomycin should be withdrawn after 8 weeks, as it is ototoxic. Steroids have no place in treatment, because of the lack of a host reaction. The infant with congenital tuberculosis should be vaccinated with isoniazid-resistant BCG to encourage active immunity. Breast feeding should be encouraged and, if the mother is infected, she must also be treated with antituberculous drugs.

Legionella

Legionella pneumophilia is a fastidious Gram-negative organism well known as a cause of pneumonia in adults. Since 1989, several reports of cases in the newborn have appeared.[25,176,208,209,259,267] Most affected infants were either born prematurely or in some way unusually susceptible to infection. The age at diagnosis in reported neonatal cases has varied from 4 to 28 days. Most have developed a severe bilateral pneumonia requiring ventilatory support and mortality is high. The source of infection has commonly been hot water systems or incubators.

DIAGNOSIS

This is mainly by culture although the organism will not grow on ordinary culture media. A rapid diagnostic test using real-time PCR has recently been reported.[199]

MANAGEMENT

Treatment is with intravenous erythromycin for 14–21 days.

Syphilis

Syphilis is most likely to be transmitted to the infants of untreated or inadequately treated mothers who are in the early stages of infection during pregnancy.[415] In the most severe cases, late fetal loss and stillbirth occur. In liveborn infants, who are severely affected, neonatal death from generalized infection including pneumonia occurs. Many infants with congenitally acquired syphilis, however, do not have obvious signs of infection at birth.

Mycoplasmas

Ureaplasmas are members of the family of Mycoplasmataceae of the class Mollicutes. They are commensals of the genitourinary and respiratory tracts of humans and animals. If present in the mother's birth canal, these organisms may colonize as many as 50 percent of infants,[103,370] but their importance in causing infectious disease remains incompletely understood. *Ureaplasma urealyticum* has been implicated in some cases of chorioamnionitis and premature delivery,[114,370] along with *Mycoplasma hominis*.[424] There is growing evidence that these organisms may cause acute neonatal pneumonia[319,323] and have a role in the pathogenesis of CLD.[76,114,147] There are case reports of fatal early-onset pneumonia, in which ureaplasmas were grown in pure culture from inflamed lung tissue obtained at autopsy.[342,440] Clinically, radiologically and in terms of the white blood cell response, there was nothing to distinguish these cases from early-onset pneumonia caused by common bacteria such as GBS or *H. influenzae*. Interestingly, some of the cases were associated with persistent pulmonary hypertension[440] and there may be a similar mechanism at work as occurs with GBS infection, as ureaplasmas have been shown to produce phospholipases capable of inducing thromboxane formation.[101] Cases of early-onset neonatal pneumonia with negative cultures for the usual bacterial pathogens should be investigated for mycoplasma infection as well as for viruses such as herpes. The evidence that *M. hominis* can cause neonatal pneumonia is based on serology and culture from blood and the upper respiratory tract,[364,381,422,423] but there are few reports of recovery of the organism from the lung itself.[104] The role of *M. pneumoniae* and other mycoplasma species in causing neonatal pneumonia is currently uncertain, although congenital pneumonia probably caused by *M. pneumoniae* has been reported.[423]

DIAGNOSIS

Unfortunately, mycoplasmas are not visible with Gram's stain using standard cytological methods. *M. hominis* may be grown and presumptively identified on blood agar but *U. urealyticum* needs a special culture medium and may take several weeks to grow. Recently, a detection method for ureaplasma antibody has been described which should be useful in both clinical and research contexts.[343] Other improved methods of detecting these organisms, such as PCR, should help to define their role further.[58,195]

MANAGEMENT

Mycoplasmas have no cell wall and so antimicrobial agents such as penicillin and cephalosporins are ineffective against them. Erythromycin is the antibiotic of choice for ureaplasma infections in the newborn[441] and is also effective against most strains of *M. pneumoniae*. *M. hominis* is more difficult to treat as it is erythromycin resistant, although some of the newer macrolides, such as clarithromycin, and quinolones, such as sparfloxacin, are reported to show promise.[44,116,238,352,439]

Pneumocystis carinii

Cases of *P. carinii* pneumonia were common, mainly in premature infants in post-war Europe.[146] Infected infants usually presented just outside the neonatal period with progressive dyspnea and increasing oxygen requirements, and with symptomatic treatment the mortality rate was approximately 50 percent. *P. carinii* infection in the developed world now occurs predominantly among infants with an underlying immunodeficiency state,[210] often in combination with CMV infection, but may also affect apparently immunocompetent preterm infants.[324] Vertically transmitted HIV infection has been reported to cause *P. carinii* infection in the neonate.[42] The presentation is usually insidious, with progressive respiratory distress and a diffusely hazy chest radiograph.

INVESTIGATIONS

The diagnosis requires a high level of clinical suspicion and acumen and may be confirmed by direct microscopy of bronchial lavage material, although lung biopsy is much more likely to be successful. A PCR-based test is available.[393]

MANAGEMENT

Treatment is with high-dose co-trimoxazole or, if that does not prove successful, with pentamidine.

FUNGI

Congenital infection with *Candida* spp.

Vaginal candidiasis is common in pregnancy and ascending fetal infection occasionally occurs, especially if an intrauterine contraceptive device is left *in situ* or a cervical suture is inserted.[452] It is associated with preterm labor.[430] The infection spreads over the external and internal body surface rather than invading the bloodstream and congenitally infected infants characteristically have skin and mucosal involvement as well as pneumonia.[212,307,452]

INVESTIGATION

Candida spp. can be cultured from gastric aspirates, superficial lesions and the lung, but rarely from the blood or CSF.

MANAGEMENT

Treatment is with amphotericin and flucytosine (see below) but, as with postnatally acquired systemic candidiasis, the mortality is high. *C. albicans* amnionitis has been successfully treated by amnioinfusion with amphotericin.[383]

Acquired systemic candidiasis

This affects 2–3 percent of VLBW survivors of neonatal intensive care.[288] The majority have been colonized by *C. albicans* from birth,[32] although around 15 percent acquire the organism nosocomially. Risk factors include the presence of central lines,[368] ventriculo-peritoneal shunts,[80] endotracheal tubes[362] and extensive antibiotic use.[31,132]

CLINICAL SIGNS

Disseminated candidiasis presents like bacterial sepsis.[31,396] As well as pneumonia, infected infants may have septicemia with or without endocarditis, septic arthritis, osteomyelitis, endophthalmitis, intraperitoneal infection, liver abscesses, meningitis and renal tract infection. Preceding mucocutaneous candidiasis is common[132] and skin lesions are almost universal. Neonatal sepsis caused by other *Candida* species such as *C. parapsilosis*[123,396] and *C. lusitaniae* presents a clinical picture indistinguishable from that caused by *C. albicans*.[131]

INVESTIGATION

It is harder to diagnose fungal infection than bacterial infection because positive blood cultures are less common. Even when the organisms are in the blood it takes several days longer for cultures to become positive than is the case with most bacteria.[396] In one study, the average time between the onset of symptoms and the initiation of antifungal therapy was 11 days.[31] When there is no typical mucocutaneous rash or some other clue to suggest fungal infection, the diagnosis is usually made during the routine investigation of an infant with suspected sepsis. In addition to culturing blood, urine and CSF where indicated, endotracheal tube aspirate and tubes removed from the infant, including chest drains and intravascular cannulae, can be examined microscopically for budding yeasts or fungal hyphae. A useful additional test is to examine a buffy coat smear for the characteristic intracellular inclusions. Thrombocytopenia is common[113] and should raise the level of suspicion. Acute-phase proteins are usually very elevated in systemic candida infection.

MANAGEMENT

Immediately the diagnosis has been made, or even when there is a high level of suspicion in a sick infant, treatment with intravenous amphotericin B should be started. It is preferable to use the liposomal form of the amphotericin, ambisome, when infants are at risk of toxicity from the non-liposomal form.[96,250] Ambisome should be started at a dose of 1.0 mg/kg/day, given as a single infusion over 1 hour, and increased to 2 mg/kg/day after 3 or 4 days.[166] Flucytosine acts synergistically with amphotericin and their combined use is advocated in the initial treatment of systemic fungal infection in the newborn. The dose of flucytosine is 100 mg/kg/day, given as a single infusion. Flucytosine may depress the marrow and damage the liver; plasma levels should be monitored and weekly blood counts checked. Miconazole has been used successfully, but there are limited data on the newer agents, such as ketoconazole, fluconazole or itraconazole. Central vascular catheters should be removed if systemic candidiasis is diagnosed or strongly suspected.[366,368]

VIRUSES

Respiratory syncytial virus (RSV)
(Figures 21.10 and 21.11)

RSV infections are comparatively rare on the neonatal unit, but small epidemics occur from time to time and the effects on individual infants can be devastating, especially among those with severe chronic lung disease.[181,189,287,303,420,425] Such infants may develop almost complete airway obstruction and become impossible to ventilate. Recurrent bradycardia is a common presenting feature[140] and the clinical course is occasionally

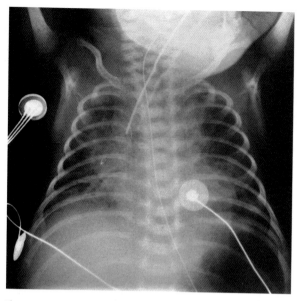

Figure 21.10 *RSV infection with atelectasis and perihilar consolidation.*

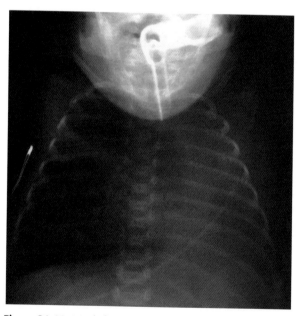

Figure 21.11 *RSV infection resulting in left lung collapse and right lung hyperinflation.*

complicated by atrial tachycardia.[20,106] RSV infection must always be considered when an infant with CLD experiences a deterioration in lung function, even if the typical physical signs of a bronchiolitis are absent.[181] RSV is easily diagnosed by immunofluorescence on respiratory secretions. Stringent measures to limit cross-infection are required if a case of RSV infection occurs on a NICU.[271] Babies with CLD remain very vulnerable to RSV infection for many months after discharge from the NICU.[391]

PROPHYLAXIS

Prevention of RSV infection in preterm infants and those with BPD using the monoclonal anti-RSV antibody preparation palivizumab has been shown to be effective (p. 413). In a multicenter, randomized, double-blind, placebo-controlled trial, the rate of hospitalization was reduced by 55 percent.[18] A subsequent non-randomized study, following the fairly widespread introduction of palivizumab prophylaxis in the USA, showed a hospitalization rate for RSV-infected babies with CLD of only 4 percent and for preterm infants without chronic lung disease of 2.3 percent.[399] These rates are far lower than the 12.8 and 8.1 percent, respectively, found in the control arm of the original study. Debate continues concerning whether prophylaxis is cost-effective.[23,102,111,198,308] Another approach to prevention is immunization of pregnant women, on the grounds that the infants of mothers with high levels of neutralizing RSV antibody seem protected.[126]

MANAGEMENT

Apart from mechanical ventilation and supportive measures, the antiviral agent ribavirin has been used. Published data on efficacy are, however, conflicting[118,298,346,432] and there is no sound evidential basis for recommending the treatment at the present time. Natural surfactant has been used in the treatment of severe RSV pneumonia and anecdotal reports suggest benefit, with an increase in lung compliance and a reduction in inspired oxygen requirement,[437] but there are no randomized, controlled trials. ECMO should be considered in deteriorating cases.

Parainfluenza virus

Parainfluenza type 3 is the most frequent cause of bronchiolitis and pneumonia after RSV. In common with RSV, parainfluenza virus has caused outbreaks of pneumonia in neonatal nurseries[287,392] with some babies requiring ventilatory support. Associated upper respiratory signs and wheezing are frequently seen.

Herpes simplex virus (HSV) (Figure 21.12)

Neonatal herpes in the UK is rare, around only one case per 50 000 births,[190,414] but it is potentially devastating.[92] The mother may have either a primary or secondary infection, the former carrying a greater risk to the infant. Transplacental or immediate postnatal acquisition of herpes infection is rare. Pneumonia may occur in isolation,[14,34,175,264,276,348] but more often is part of a disseminated systemic infection involving many organs and tissues, especially the liver and the brain.[292] Twenty percent have no cutaneous manifestations, making diagnosis difficult.[443] Approximately 70 percent of infections are

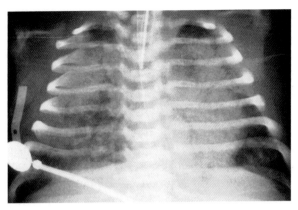

Figure 21.12 *Pneumonia caused by HSV virus.*

caused by HSV-2. Women acquiring primary infection late in pregnancy are at highest risk of transmitting infection and cesarean section for women with active lesions can prevent disease. Seventy percent of neonatal HSV cases are born to mothers without symptoms at delivery.

CLINICAL SIGNS

Infection usually presents clinically around 9–11 days, as a non-specific illness. Approximately 50 percent of infections become disseminated and 20 percent of neonates die despite antiviral treatment. Infants with disseminated disease present like any critically ill septic infant. They have respiratory distress as a result of pneumonia and usually require ventilatory support. They are often hypotensive, peripherally vasoconstricted, and have renal failure. Severe hepatitis[177] may occur and disseminated intravascular coagulation (DIC), causing petechiae and generalized bleeding, is common.[216] Hypotonia, seizures and coma are common whether or not meningoencephalitis is present. Primary neonatal herpes simplex virus pneumonia presents with fever and progressive respiratory insufficiency. Marked hyperammonemia has been described in association with primary HSV pneumonia.[378] The mortality is high (57 percent)[224] and morbidity in survivors is common.

DIAGNOSIS

Radiologically there are patchy or reticular infiltrates, often progressing to complete opacification of the lung fields. Cutaneous vesicles, ocular or oral lesions strongly suggest herpes. The most rapid and useful diagnostic test that is widely available is immunofluorescence performed on vesicle fluid. Cultures may show cytopathic changes within a few days. The virus may also grow from blood. CSF samples from the neonate and genital swabs from the mother should be obtained. Serology is much less useful because of the difficulty in distinguishing between passively acquired maternal antibody and endogenously produced antibody. DNA amplification

tests are also available.[311] In the absence of a maternal history of genital disease or of suspicious skin, eye or mouth lesions, HSV infection will only be diagnosed if viral cultures are a routine part of the investigation of all babies with early-onset pneumonia from whom no bacterial pathogen is grown after 24–48 hours. The transaminase level is markedly increased in HSV infection.

MANAGEMENT

If there is even a suspicion that the pneumonia is due to herpes, treatment should be started pending a definite diagnosis. Treatment is with aciclovir. Aciclovir-resistant neonatal HSV infection has been reported.[314] In the experimental animal, a combination of anti-HSV antibody and aciclovir is far superior to aciclovir alone in reducing mortality,[65] but there is no such study in newborn infants. Aciclovir is given intravenously, 8-hourly, in a total daily dose of 30 mg/kg for no fewer than 14 days. Topical aciclovir should be applied to eye and skin lesions. ECMO has been used successfully to treat HSV pneumonia.[402]

Adenovirus (Figure 21.13)

Although adenoviruses are a common cause of upper and lower respiratory tract infection in children more than 3 months old, neonatal adenovirus pneumonia is relatively rare. This probably relates to the fact that more than 90 percent of adults have detectable antibody. Neonatal adenovirus pneumonia is probably vertically transmitted and about half of the mothers are unwell with fever and upper respiratory symptoms in the perinatal period. The onset of neonatal pneumonia is within 10 days of birth and apnea is a prominent feature. Fever and hepatomegaly commonly occur.

The mortality rate is extremely high and deterioration is accompanied by DIC and neurological signs.[3,387,406] Successful treatment with ECMO has been reported.[243] Adverse long-term respiratory sequelae are common after neonatal adenovirus infection.[395]

DIAGNOSIS

The chest radiograph typically shows coarse bilateral infiltrates and sometimes pleural effusions but more confluent areas of consolidation may also be seen. Adenovirus isolated from nasopharyngeal aspirates can be visualized by electron microscopy or produce a cytopathic effect in cell culture.

Echovirus

The echoviruses are enteroviruses and rare, but potent causes of neonatal pneumonia.[55,61,188,295,413] Several

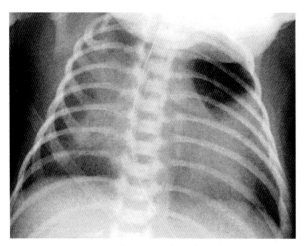

Figure 21.13 *Pneumonia caused by adenovirus.*

serotypes are implicated but echovirus 11 is the most notorious. Echovirus infection may be vertically transmitted but nosocomial spread is responsible for epidemics.

DIAGNOSIS

Severe early-onset echovirus pneumonia is similar to that caused by GBS and persistent pulmonary hypertension is well described.[413] The chest radiograph of infected infants usually shows diffuse infiltration with perihilar streaking. Diagnosis is by viral culture, but this can take up to 4 days, or the detection of viral DNA, for example by PCR.[407] Swabs should be sent in viral transport medium. The large number of serotypes renders immunological tests less useful.

Coxsackie (Figure 21.14)

Neonatal respiratory illnesses, including pneumonia, have been reported with coxsackie A and B infections. Fatal pneumonia has been described.[297] Infection occurs via vertical transmission, aspiration or ingestion of infected secretions or blood from the mother at birth or, rarely, transplacentally.

Cytomegalovirus (CMV)

CMV is a DNA virus of the herpes group. Diffuse interstitial pneumonitis occurs in less than 1 percent of congenitally infected infants. CMV-associated pneumonitis is more likely to occur in infants with perinatally acquired CMV. Prematurely born and ill full-term infants are at greater risk. Most serious congenital infections are acquired following maternal primary disease early in gestation, although 90 percent of neonates so infected are asymptomatic at birth. Clinical disease following maternal reinfection or reactivation of latent virus during pregnancy is usually less severe, but may be an important

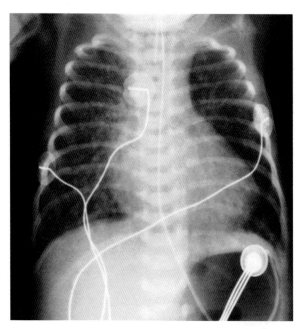

Figure 21.14 *Coxsackie pneumonia with widespread consolidation and hyperinflation.*

mode of infection in terms of number of infants.[216] Perinatally acquired CMV is likely to be acquired primarily from the mother, either in the birth canal or sometimes via breast milk and is usually asymptomatic, although severe infection with pneumonia has been reported in association with blood transfusion of VLBW infants.[7]

DIAGNOSIS

CMV infected infants have elevated levels of one or more immunoglobulin classes, leukocytosis and an absolute eosinophilia. Diagnosis is by viral culture or CMV DNA detection by PCR in the urine or saliva. Infected fetuses usually produce specific IgM antibodies, which can be detected in cord or neonatal blood. IgG is transmitted from mother to fetus (p. 55). A negative antibody titer in cord and maternal sera excludes the diagnosis of congenital CMV infection. In uninfected fetuses of seropositive mothers, IgG antibodies will decrease and finally disappear between 4 and 9 months of age. IgG will persist in infants infected congenitally or perinatally.

MANAGEMENT

A humanized monoclonal antibody is available and has been used in infants with perinatally acquired infections.

Varicella zoster virus (VSV)

Pneumonia has been reported in vertically acquired neonatal VSV infections.[325] VSV can cause severe infection in the fetus during the first trimester, with fetal damage due to scarring and interference with normal development in 2–5 percent of cases. The subsequent high-risk period is around the time of birth, particularly in those infants whose mothers developed the rash in the period 5 days before to 2 days after delivery. Affected infants may develop a severe pneumonic illness with a mortality rate as high as 30 percent.

DIAGNOSIS

VSV can be isolated from tissue culture of the vesicular fluid, but this can take up to 6–14 days. Electron microscopy does not permit distinguishing between varicella and herpes viruses. IgG and IgM rise 2–5 days after the rash appears and, although the IgG response in the infant is poor, it can be detected by ELISAs or immunofluorescence.

MANAGEMENT

To prevent neonatal chicken pox, passive immunization is indicated. Zoster immunoglobulin (ZIG) should be given to an infant whose mother develops chickenpox up to 7 days before delivery or up to 28 days after delivery.[203] If varicella occurs, aciclovir treatment should be promptly administered.[372]

REFERENCES

1 Ablow, R.C., Driscoll, S.G., Effmann, E.L. *et al.* (1976) A comparison of early-onset group B steptococcal neonatal infection and the respiratory-distress syndrome of the newborn. *New England Journal of Medicine* **294**, 65–70.

2 Abzug, M.J., Beam, A.C., Gyorkos, E.A., Levin, M.J. (1990) Viral pneumonia in the first month of life. *Pediatric Infectious Disease Journal* **9**, 881–885.

3 Abzug, M.J., Levin, M.J. (1991) Neonatal adenovirus infection: four patients and review of the literature. *Pediatrics* **87**, 890–896.

4 Adair, C.D., Gunter, M., Stovall, T.G., McElroy, G., Veille, J.C., Ernest, J.M. (1998) Chlamydia in pregnancy: a randomized trial of azithromycin and erythromycin. *Obstetrics and Gynecology* **91**, 165–168.

5 Adams, W.G., Kinney, J.S., Schuchat, A. *et al.* (1993) Outbreak of early onset group B streptococcal sepsis. *Pediatric Infectious Disease Journal* **12**, 565–570.

6 Adhikari, M., Pillay, T., Pillay, D.G. (1997) Tuberculosis in the newborn: an emerging disease. *Pediatric Infectious Disease Journal* **16**, 1108–1112.

7 Adler, S.P., Chandrika, T., Lawrence, L., Baggett, J. (1983) Cytomegalovirus infection in neonates acquired by blood transfusions. *Pediatric Infectious Disease Journal* **2**, 114–118.

8 Ahvenainen, E. K. (1951) On congenital pneumonia. *Acta Paediatrica* **40**, 1–21.

9 Aikio, O., Vuopala, K., Pokela, M.L., Hallman, M. (2000) Diminished inducible nitric oxide synthase expression in fulminant early-onset neonatal pneumonia. *Pediatrics* **105**, 1013–1019.

10 Airede, A.I. (1992) Prolonged rupture of membranes and neonatal outcome in a developing country. *Annals of Tropical Paediatrics* **12**, 283–288.

11 Alenghat, E., Esterly, J.R. (1984) Alveolar macrophages in perinatal infants. *Pediatrics* **74**, 221–223.

12 Amato, M., Inaebnit, D. (1988) Perinatal *Chlamydia trachomatis* infection in a low birth weight infant. *Journal of Perinatal Medicine* **16**, 487–489.

13 American Academy of Pediatrics Committee on Infectious Diseases and Committee on Fetus and Newborn (1997) Revised guidelines for prevention of early-onset group B streptococcal (GBS) infection. *Pediatrics* **99**, 489–496.

14 Andersen, R.D. (1987) Herpes simplex virus infection of the neonatal respiratory tract. *American Journal of Diseases of Children* **141**, 274–276.

15 Anderson, D.C., Hughes, B.J., Edwards, M.S., Buffone, G.J., Baker, C.J. (1983) Impaired chemotaxigenesis by type III group B streptococci in neonatal sera: relationship to diminished concentration of specific anticapsular antibody and abnormalities of serum complement. *Pediatric Research* **17**, 496–502.

16 Anderson, G.S., Green, C.A., Neligan, G.A. (1962) Congenital bacterial pneumonia. *Lancet* **2**, 585.

17 Andersson, S., Larinkari, U., Vartia, T. *et al.* (1994) Fatal congenital pneumonia caused by cat-derived *Pasteurella multocida*. *Pediatric Infectious Disease Journal* **13**, 74–75.

18 Anonymous (1998) Palivizumab, a humanized respiratory syncytial virus monoclonal antibody, reduces hospitalization from respiratory syncytial virus infection in high-risk infants. The Impact-RSV Study Group. *Pediatrics* **102**, 531–537.

19 Armer, T., Clark, P., Duff, P., Saravanos, K. (1993) Rapid intrapartum detection of group B streptococcal colonization with an enzyme immunoassay. *American Journal of Obstetrics and Gynecology* **168**, 39–43.

20 Armstrong, D.S., Menahem, S. (1993) Cardiac arrhythmias as a manifestation of acquired heart disease in association with paediatric respiratory syncytial virus infection. *Journal of Paediatrics and Child Health* **29**, 309–311.

21 Ascher, D.P., Becker, J.A., Yoder, B.A. *et al.* (1993) Failure of intrapartum antibiotics to prevent culture-proved neonatal group B streptococcal sepsis. *Journal of Perinatology* **13**, 212–216.

22 Askin, F. (1991) Respiratory tract disorders in the fetus and neonate. In Wigglesworth, J.S., Singer, D.B. (eds), *Textbook of Fetal and Perinatal Pathology*. Boston: Blackwell Scientific Publications, 643–688.

23 Atkins, J.T., Karimi, P., Morris, B.H., McDavid, G., Shim, S. (2000) Prophylaxis for respiratory syncytial virus with respiratory syncytial virus–immunoglobulin intravenous among preterm infants of thirty-two weeks gestation and less: reduction in incidence, severity of illness and cost. *Pediatric Infectious Disease Journal* **19**, 138–143.

24 Attenburrow, A.A., Barker, C.M. (1985) Chlamydial pneumonia in the low birthweight neonate. *Archives of Disease in Childhood* **60**, 1169–1172.

25 Aubert, G., Bornstein, N., Rayet, I., Pozzetto, B., Lenormand, P.H. (1990) Nosocomial infection with *Legionella pneumophila* serogroup 1 and 8 in a neonate. *Scandinavian Journal of Infectious Diseases* **22**, 367–370.

26 Auten, R.L., Notter, R.H., Kendig, J.W., Davis, J.M., Shapiro, D.L. (1991) Surfactant treatment of full-term newborns with respiratory failure. *Pediatrics* **87**, 101–107.

27 Averbuch, B., Mazor, M., Shoham Vardi, I. *et al.* (1995) Intrauterine infection in women with preterm premature rupture of membranes: maternal and neonatal characteristics. *European Journal of Obstetrics & Gynecology and Reproductive Biology* **62**, 25–29.

28 Awasthi, S., Coalson, J.J., Crouch, E., Yang, F., King, R.J. (1999) Surfactant proteins A and D in premature baboons with chronic lung injury (bronchopulmonary dysplasia). Evidence for an inhibition of secretion. *American Journal of Respiratory and Critical Care Medicine* **160**, 942–949.

29 Baker, C.J., Edwards, M.S. (1983) Group B streptococcal infections. In Remington, J.S., Klein, J.O. (eds), *Infectious Diseases of the Fetus and Newborn Infant*. Philadelphia: W.B. Saunders, 820–881.

30 Baker, C.J. Kasper, D.L. (1976) Correlation of maternal antibody deficiency with susceptibility to neonatal group B streptococcal infection. *New England Journal of Medicine* **294**, 753–756.

31 Baley, J.E., Kliegman, R.M., Fanaroff, A.A. (1984) Disseminated fungal infections in very low birthweight infants: clinical manifestations and epidemiology. *Pediatrics* **73**, 144–152.

32 Baley, J.E., Kliegman, R.M., Boxerbaum, B., Fanaroff, A. (1986) Fungal colonization in the very low birthweight infant. *Pediatrics* **78**, 225–232.

33 Bang, A.T., Bang, R.A., Morankar, V.P., Sontakke, P.G., Solanki, J.M. (1993) Pneumonia in neonates: can it be managed in the community? *Archives of Disease in Childhood* **68**, 550–556.

34 Barker, J.A., McLean, S.D., Jordan, G.D., Krober, M.S., Rawlings, J.S. (1990) Primary neonatal herpes simplex virus pneumonia. *Pediatric Infectious Disease Journal* **9**, 285–289.

35 Barson, A.F. (1990) A postmortem study of infection in the newborn from 1976 to 1988. In de Luvois, J., Harvey, D (eds), *Infection in the Newborn*. New York: John Wiley, 13–34.

36 Barsum, W., Wilson, R., Read, R.C. (1995) Interaction of fimbriated and non-fimbriated strains of unencapsulated *Haemophilus influenzae* with human respiratory tract mucus in vitro. *European Respiratory Journal* **8**, 709–714.

37 Barter, R.A. (1962) Congenital pneumonia. *Lancet* **1**, 165–167.

38 Barter, R.A. (1974) Bacteriological findings in perinatal pneumonia. *Pathology* **6**, 226.

39 Barton, L., Hodgman, J.E., Pavlova, Z. (1999) Causes of death in the extremely low birth weight infant. *Pediatrics* **103**, 446–451.

40 Bate, T.W., Sinclair, R.E., Robinson, M.J. (1986) Neonatal tuberculosis. *Archives of Disease in Childhood* **61**, 512–514.

41 Bauer, C.R., Elie, K., Spence, L., Stern, L. (1973) Hong Kong influenza in a neonatal unit. *Journal of the American Medical Association* **223**, 1233–1235.

42 Beach, R.S., Garcia, E.R., Sosa, R., Good, R.A. (1991) *Pneumocystis carinii* pneumonia in a human immunodeficiency virus 1-infected neonate with meconium aspiration. *Pediatric Infectious Disease Journal* **10**, 953–955.

43 Beardsall, K., Thompson, M.H., Mulla, R.J. (2000) Neonatal group B streptococcal infection in South Bedfordshire, 1993–1998. *Archives of Disease in Childhood Fetal and Neonatal Edition* **82**, F205–F207.

44 Bebear, C.M., Renaudin, H., Schaeverbeke, T., Leblanc, F., Bebear, C. (1999) In-vitro activity of grepafloxacin, a new fluoroquinolone, against mycoplasmas. *Journal of Antimicrobial Chemotherapy* **43**, 711–714.

45 Beck Sague, C.M., Azimi, P., Fonseca, S.N. *et al.* (1994) Bloodstream infections in neonatal intensive care unit patients: results of a multicenter study. *Pediatric Infectious Disease Journal* **13**, 1110–1116.

46 Becker, J.A., Ascher, D.P., Mendiola, J. *et al.* (1993) False-negative urine latex particle agglutination testing in neonates with group B streptococcal bacteremia. A function of improper test implementation? *Clinical Pediatrics (Philadelphia)* **32**, 467–471.

47 Beganovic, N., Verloove-Vanhorick, S.P., Brand, R., Ruys, J.H. (1988) Total parenteral nutrition and sepsis. *Archives of Disease in Childhood* **63**, 66–67.

48 Beiter, A., Lewis, K., Pineda, E.F., Cherry, J.D. (1993) Unrecognized maternal peripartum pertussis with subsequent fatal neonatal pertussis. *Obstetrics and Gynecology* **82**, 691–693.

49 Bell, T.A., Stamm, W.E., Kuo, C.C., Wang, S.P., Holmes, K.K., Grayston, J.T. (1994) Risk of perinatal transmission of *Chlamydia trachomatis* by mode of delivery. *Journal of Infection* **29**, 165–169.

50 Benjamin, D.K., Ross, K., McKinney, R.E. *et al.* (2000) When to suspect fungal infection in neonates: a clinical comparison of *Candida albicans* and *Candida parapsilosis* fungaemia with coagulase-negative staphylococcal bacteraemia. *Pediatrics* **106**, 712–718.

51 Bergqvist, G., Trovik, M. (1985) Neonatal infections with *Streptococcus pneumoniae*. *Scandinavian Journal of Infectious Diseases* **17**, 33–35.

52 Beri, R., Lourwood, D.L. (1997) Chemoprophylaxis for group B streptococcus transmission in neonates. *Annals of Pharmacotherapy* **31**, 110–112.

53 Berkovich, S., Pangan, J. (1968) Recoveries of virus from premature infants during outbreaks of respiratory disease: the relation of ECHO virus type 22 to disease of the upper and lower respiratory tract in the premature infant. *Bulletin of the New York Academy of Medicine* **44**, 377–387.

54 Bernstein, J., Wang, J. (1961) The pathology of neonatal pneumonia. *American Journal of Diseases of Children* **101**, 350–355.

55 Berry, P.J., Nagington, J. (1982) Fatal infection with echovirus 11. *Archives of Disease in Childhood* **57**, 22–29.

56 Betremieux, P., Donnio, P.Y., Pladys, P. (1995) Use of ribotyping to investigate tracheal colonization by *Staphylococcus epidermidis* as a source of bacteremia in ventilated newborns. *European Journal of Clinical Microbiology and Infectious Diseases* **14**, 342–346.

57 Black, C.M. (1997) Current methods of laboratory diagnosis of *Chlamydia trachomatis* infections. *Clinical Microbiology Reviews* **10**, 160–184.

58 Blanchard, A., Hentschel, J., Duffy, L., Baldus, K., Cassell, G.H. (1993) Detection of *Ureaplasma urealyticum* by polymerase chain reaction in the urogenital tract of adults, in amniotic fluid, and in the respiratory tract of newborns. *Clinical Infectious Diseases* **17**(Suppl 1), S148–S153.

59 Bortolussi, R., Issekutz, T.B., Faulkner, A. (1986) Opsonization of *Listeria monocytogenes* type 4b by human adult and newborn sera. *Infection and Immunity* **52**, 493–495.

60 Botet, F., Cararach, V., Sentis, J. (1994) Premature rupture of membranes in early pregnancy. Neonatal prognosis. *Journal of Perinatal Medicine* **22**, 45–52.

61 Boyd, M.T., Jordan, S.W., Davis, L.E. (1987) Fatal pneumonitis from congenital echovirus type 6 infection. *Pediatric Infectious Disease Journal* **6**, 1138–1139.

62 Boyer, K.M. (1995) Neonatal group B streptococcal infections. *Current Opinion in Pediatrics* **7**, 13–18.

63 Boyer, K.M., Gotoff, S.P. (1986) Prevention of early-onset neonatal group B streptococcal disease with selective intrapartum chemoprophylaxis. *New England Journal of Medicine* **314**, 1665–1669.

64 Boyle, R.J., Chandler, B.D., Stonestreet, B.S., Oh, W. (1978) Early identification of sepsis in infants with respiratory distress. *Pediatrics* **62**, 744–750.

65 Bravo, F.J., Bourne, N., Harrison, C.J. *et al.* (1996) Effect of antibody alone and combined with acyclovir on neonatal

herpes simplex virus infection in guinea pigs. *Journal of Infectious Diseases* **173**, 1–6.

66 Brayden, R.M., Paisley, J.W., Lauer, B.A. (1987) Apnea in infants with *Chlamydia trachomatis* pneumonia. *Pediatric Infectious Disease Journal* **6**, 423–425.

67 Brook, I. (1994) Anaerobic infections in the neonate. *Advances in Pediatrics* **41**, 369–383.

68 Brook, I., Martin, W.J., Finegold, S.M. (1980) Neonatal pneumonia caused by members of the *Bacteroides fragilis* group. *Clinical Pediatrics (Philadelphia)* **19**, 541–544.

69 Buck, C., Gallati, H., Pohlandt, F., Bartmann, P. (1994) Increased levels of tumor necrosis factor alpha (TNF-α) and interleukin 1 β (IL-1 β) in tracheal aspirates of newborns with pneumonia. *Infection* **22**, 238–241.

70 Cabal, L.A., Siassi, B., Cristofani, C., Cabal, C., Hodgman, J.E. (1990) Cardiovascular changes in infants with β-hemolytic streptococcus sepsis. *Critical Care Medicine* **18**, 715–718.

71 Cadnapaphornchai, M., Faix, R.G. (1992) Increased nosocomial infection in neutropenic low birth weight (2000 grams or less) infants of hypertensive mothers. *Journal of Pediatrics* **121**, 956–961.

72 Cairns, P.A., Wilson, D.C., McClure, B.G., Halliday, H.L., McReid, M. (1995) Percutaneous central venous catheter use in the very low birth weight neonate. *European Journal of Pediatrics* **154**, 145–147.

73 Campbell, J.R. (1996) Neonatal pneumonia. *Seminars in Respiratory Infection* **11**, 155–162.

74 Campognone, P., Singer, D.B. (1986) Neonatal sepsis due to nontypable *Haemophilus influenzae*. *American Journal of Diseases of Children* **140**, 117–121.

75 Cassell, G.H., Waites, K.B., Crouse, D.T. (1991) Perinatal mycoplasmal infections. *Clinics in Perinatology* **18**, 241–262.

76 Cassell, G.H., Waites, K.B., Watson, H.L., Crouse, D.T., Harasawa, R. (1993) *Ureaplasma urealyticum* intrauterine infection: role in prematurity and disease in newborns. *Clinical Microbiology Reviews* **6**, 69–87.

77 Chartrand, S.A., McCracken, G.H., Jr. (1982) Staphylococcal pneumonia in infants and children. *Pediatric Infectious Disease Journal* **1**, 19–23.

78 Chidekel, A.S., Rosen, C.L., Bazzy, A.R. (1997) Rhinovirus infection associated with serious lower respiratory illness in patients with bronchopulmonary dysplasia. *Pediatric Infectious Disease Journal* **16**, 43–47.

79 Chiou, C.C., Soong, W.J., Hwang, B., Wu, K.G., Lee, B.H., Wang, H.C. (1994) Congenital adenoviral infection. *Pediatric Infectious Disease Journal* **13**, 664–665.

80 Chiou, C.C., Wong, T.T., Lin, H.H. *et al.* (1994) Fungal infection of ventriculoperitoneal shunts in children. *Clinical Infectious Diseases* **19**, 1049–1053.

81 Chitayat, D., Diamant, S., Lazevnick, R., Spirer, Z. (1980) *Haemophilus influenzae* type B pneumonia with pneumatocele formation. *Clinical Pediatrics (Philadelphia)* **19**, 151–152.

82 Christie, C.D., Baltimore, R.S. (1989) Pertussis in neonates. *American Journal of Diseases of Children* **143**, 1199–1202.

83 Chun, C.S., Brady, L.J., Boyle, M.D., Dillon, H.C., Ayoub, E.M. (1991) Group B streptococcal C protein-associated antigens: association with neonatal sepsis. *Journal of Infectious Diseases* **163**, 786–791.

84 Churgay, C.A., Smith, M.A., Blok, B. (1994) Maternal fever during labor – what does it mean? *Journal of the American Board of Family Practitioners* **7**, 14–24.

85 Cimolai, N., Roscoe, D.L. (1995) Contemporary context for early-onset group B streptococcal sepsis of the newborn. *American Journal of Perinatology* **12**, 46–49.

86 Clark, H.W., Reid, K.B., Sim, R.B. (2000) Collectins and innate immunity in the lung. *Microbes and Infection* **2**, 273–278.

87 Cleveland, R.H. (1995) A radiologic update on medical diseases of the newborn chest. *Pediatric Radiology* **25**, 631–637.

88 Colarizi, P., Chiesa, C., Pacifico, L. *et al.* (1996) *Chlamydia trachomatis*-associated respiratory disease in the very early neonatal period. *Acta Paediatrica* **85**, 991–994.

89 Cone, R.W. (1995) Human herpesvirus 6 as a possible cause of pneumonia. *Seminars in Respiratory Infection* **10**, 254–258.

90 Cordero, L., Ayers, L.W., Davis, K. (1997) Neonatal airway colonization with gram-negative bacilli: association with severity of bronchopulmonary dysplasia. *Pediatric Infectious Disease Journal* **16**, 18–23.

91 Cordero, L., Sananes, M., Coley, B. *et al.* (2000) Ventilator-associated pneumonia in very low birthweight infants at the time of nosocomial bloodstream infection and during airway colonization with *Pseudomonas aeruginosa*. *American Journal of Infection Control* **28**, 333–339.

92 Corey, L. (2000) Herpes simplex virus. In Mandell, G.L., Bennett, J.E., Dolin, R. (eds), *Mandell, Douglas and Bennett's Principles and Practice of Infectious Diseases*, 5th edition. Philadelphia: Churchill Livingstone, 1564–1579.

93 Couroucli, X.I., Welty, S.E., Ramsay, P.L. *et al.* (2000) Detection of microorganisms in the tracheal aspirates of preterm infants by polymerase chain reaction: association of adenovirus infection with bronchopulmonary dysplasia. *Pediatric Research* **47**, 225–232.

94 Covert, R.F., Schreiber, M.D. (1993) Three different strains of heat-killed group B β-hemolytic streptococcus cause different pulmonary and systemic hemodynamic responses in conscious neonatal lambs. *Pediatric Research* **33**, 373–379.

95 Crain, E.F., Gershel, J.C. (1988) Which febrile infants younger than two weeks of age are likely to have sepsis? A pilot study. *Pediatric Infectious Disease Journal* **7**, 561–564.

96 da Silva, L.P., Amaral, J.M., Ferreiva, N.C. (1993) Which is the most appropriate dosage of liposomal amphotericin B for the treatment of fungal infections in infants of very low birthweight? *Pediatrics* **91**, 1217–1218.

97 Dagan, R., Hall, C.B. (1984) Influenza A virus infection imitating bacterial sepsis in early infancy. *Pediatric Infectious Disease* **3**, 218–221.

98 Davies, P.A. (1980) Pathogen or commensal? *Archives of Disease in Childhood* **55**, 169–170.

99 Davies, P.A., Aherne, W. (1962) Congenital pneumonia. *Archives of Disease in Childhood* **37**, 598–602.

100 De Man, P., Verhoeven, B.A., Verbrugh, H.A. *et al.* (2000) An antibiotic policy to prevent emergence of resistant Gram-negative bacilli. *Lancet* **355**, 973–978.

101 De Silva, N.S., Quinn, P.A. (1986) Endogenous activity of phospholipases A and C in *Ureaplasma urealyticum*. *Journal of Clinical Microbiology* **23**, 354–359.

102 Deshpande, S. (2000) RSV prevention. *Archives of Disease in Childhood* **82**, 88.

103 Dinsmoor, M.J., Ramamurthy, R.S., Gibbs, R.S. (1989) Transmission of genital mycoplasmas from mother to neonate in women with prolonged membrane rupture. *Pediatric Infectious Disease Journal* **8**, 483–487.

104 Dische, M.R., Quinn, P.A., Czegledy-Nagy, E., Sturgess, J.M. (1979) Genital mycoplasma infection. Intrauterine infection: pathologic study of the fetus and placenta. *American Journal of Clinical Pathology* **72**, 167–174.

105 Djuretic, T., Ryan, M.J., Miller, E., Fairley, C.K., Goldblatt, D. (1998) Hospital admissions in children due to pneumococcal pneumonia in England. *Journal of Infection* **37**, 54–58.

106 Donnerstein, R.L., Berg, R.A., Shehab, Z., Ovadia, M. (1994) Complex atrial tachycardias and respiratory syncytial virus infections in infants. *Journal of Pediatrics* **125**, 23–28.

107 Dowd, J., Permezel, M. (1992) Pregnancy outcome following preterm premature rupture of the membranes at less than 26 weeks' gestation. *Australian and New Zealand Journal of Obstetrics and Gynaecology* **32**, 120–124.

108 Drews, M.B., Ludwig, A.C., Leititis, J.U., Daschner, F.D. (1995) Low birth weight and nosocomial infection of neonates in a neonatal intensive care unit. *Journal of Hospital Infection* **30**, 65–72.

109 Drut, R., Drut, R.M. (1988) Measles pneumonia in a newborn. *Pediatric Pathology* **8**, 553–557.

110 Duggan, T.G., Leng, R.A., Hancock, B.M., Cursons, R.T. (1984) *Serratia marcescens* in a newborn unit – microbiological features. *Pathology* **16**, 189–191.

111 Duppenthaler, A., Gorgievski-Hrisoho, M., Aebi, C. (2001) Regional impact of prophylaxis with the monoclonal antibody palivizumab on hospitalisations for respiratory syncytial virus in infants. *Swiss Medical Weekly* **131**, 11–12, 146–151.

112 Dworsky, M.E., Stagno, S. (1982) Newer agents causing pneumonitis in early infancy. *Pediatric Infectious Disease* **1**, 188–195.

113 Dyke, M.P., Ott, K. (1993) Severe thrombocytopenia in extremely low birthweight infants with systemic candidiasis. *Journal of Paediatrics and Child Health* **29**, 298–301.

114 Dyke, M.P., Grauaug, A., Kohan, R., Ott, K., Andrews, R. (1993) *Ureaplasma urealyticum* in a neonatal intensive care population. *Journal of Paediatrics and Child Health* **29**, 295–297.

115 Dyson, C., Poonyth, H.D., Watkinson, M., Rose, S.J. (1990) Life threatening *Branhamella catarrhalis* pneumonia in young infants. *Journal of Infection* **21**, 305–307.

116 Echaniz, A.G., Conde, G.C., Juarez, F.L., Carnalla, B.N., Tamayo, L.E., Calderon, J.E. (1992) *In vitro* activity of several antimicrobial agents against genital mycoplasmas. *Clinical Therapeutics* **14**, 688–695.

117 Eckert, H.L., Portnoy, B., Salvatore, M.A., Ressler, R. (1967) Group B, Coxsackie virus infection in infants with acute lower respiratory disease. *Pediatrics* **39**, 526–531.

118 Edell, D., Bruce, E., Hale, K., Edell, D., Khoshoo, V. (1998) Reduced long-term respiratory morbidity after treatment of respiratory syncytial virus bronchiolitis with ribavirin in previously healthy infants: a preliminary report. *Pediatric Pulmonology* **25**, 154–158.

119 Edelman, K., Nikkari, S., Ruuskanen, O., He, Q., Viljanen, M., Mertsola, J. (1996) Detection of *Bordetella pertussis* by polymerase chain reaction and culture in the nasopharynx of erythromycin-treated infants with pertussis. *Pediatric Infectious Disease Journal* **15**, 54–57.

120 Edwards, M.S., Baker, C.J. (2000) *Streptococcus agalactiae* (group B streptococcus). In Mandell, G.L., Bennett, J.E., Dolin, R. (eds), *Mandell, Douglas and Bennett's Principles and Practice of Infectious Diseases*, 5th edition. Philadelphia: Churchill Livingstone, 2156–2167.

121 Egarter, C., Leitich, H., Husslein, P., Kaider, A., Schemper, M. (1996) Adjunctive antibiotic treatment in preterm labor and neonatal morbidity: a meta-analysis. *Obstetrics and Gynecology* **88**, 303–309.

122 Egarter, C., Leitich, H., Karas, H., Wieser, F., Husslein, P., Kaider, A., Schemper, M. (1996) Antibiotic treatment in preterm premature rupture of membranes and neonatal morbidity: a meta-analysis. *American Journal of Obstetrics and Gynecology* **174**, 589–597.

123 el Mohandes, A.E., Johnson Robbins, L., Keiser, J.F., Simmens, S.J., Aure, M.V. (1994) Incidence of *Candida parapsilosis* colonization in an intensive care nursery population and its association with invasive fungal disease. *Pediatric Infectious Disease Journal* **13**, 520–524.

124 Ellison, R.T., Giehl, T.J. (1991) Killing of gram-negative bacteria by lactoferrin and lysozyme. *Journal of Clinical Investigation* **88**, 1080–1091.

125 English, B.K., Hammond, W.P., Lewis, D.B. (1992) Decreased granulocyte-macrophage colony-stimulating factor production by human neonatal blood mononuclear cells and T-cells. *Pediatric Research* **31**, 211–216.

126 Englund, J.A. (1994) Passive protection against respiratory syncytial virus disease in infants: the role of maternal antibody. *Pediatric Infectious Disease Journal* **13**, 449–453.

127 Eriksen, N.L., Blanco, J.D. (1993) Group B streptococcal infection in pregnancy. *Seminars in Perinatology* **17**, 432–442.

128 Ernest, J.M., Givner, L.B. (1994) A prospective, randomized, placebo-controlled trial of penicillin in preterm premature rupture of membranes. *American Journal of Obstetrics and Gynecology* **170**, 516–521.

129 Evans, J.R., Allen, A.C., Stinson, D.A. (1985) Perinatal listeriosis; report of an outbreak. *Pediatric Infectious Disease Journal* **4**, 240.

130 Ewert, D.P., Lieb, L., Hayes, P.S., Reeves, M.W., Mascola, L. (1995) *Listeria monocytogenes* infection and serotype distribution among HIV-infected persons in Los Angeles County, 1985–1992. *Journal of Acquired Immune Deficiency Syndromes and Human Retrovirology* **8**, 461–465.

131 Faix, R.G. (1992) Invasive neonatal candidiasis: comparison of albicans and parapsilosis infection. *Pediatric Infectious Disease Journal* **11**, 88–93.

132 Faix, R.G., Kovarik, S.M., Shaw, T.R., Johnson, R.V. (1989) Mucocutaneous and invasive candidiasis among very low birth weight (less than 1500 grams) infants in intensive care nurseries: a prospective study. *Pediatrics* **83**, 101–107.

133 Falla, T.J., Dobson, S.R., Crook, D.W. *et al.* (1993) Population-based study of non-typable *Haemophilus influenzae* invasive disease in children and neonates. *Lancet* **341**, 851–854.

134 Fang, F.C., McClelland, M., Guiney, D.G. *et al.* (1993) Value of molecular epidemiologic analysis in a nosocomial methicillin-resistant *Staphylococcus aureus* outbreak. *Journal of the American Medical Association* **270**, 1323–1328.

135 Feldman, C., Read, R.C., Rutman, A. (1992) The interaction of *Streptococcus pneumoniae* with intact human respiratory mucosa *in vitro*. *European Respiratory Journal* **5**, 576–583.

136 Fernandez, M., Rench, M.A., Baker, C.J. (1999) Neonatal sepsis caused simultaneously by two serotypes of group B streptococcus. *Pediatric Infectious Disease Journal* **18**, 391–393.

137 Fleming, D.W., Cochi, S.L., MacDonald, K.L. (1985) Pasteurised milk as a vehicle of infection in an outbreak of listeriosis. *New England Journal of Medicine* **312**, 404–407.

138 Foca, M., Jakob, K., Whittier, S. *et al.* (2000) Endemic *Pseudomonas aeruginosa* infection in a neonatal intensive care unit. *New England Journal of Medicine* **343**, 695–700.

139 Fok, T.F., Lee, C.H., Wong, E.M.C. *et al.* (1998) Risk factors for *Enterobacter* septicaemia in a neonatal unit: a case control study. *Clinical Infectious Diseases* **27**, 1204–1209.

140 Forster, J., Schumacher, R.F. (1995) The clinical picture presented by premature neonates infected with the respiratory syncytial virus. *European Journal of Pediatrics* **154**, 901–905.

141 Frederiksen, B., Samuelsson, S. (1992) Feto-maternal listeriosis in Denmark 1981–1988. *Journal of Infection* **24**, 277–287.

142 Freeman, J., Goldmann, D.A., Smith, N.E., Sidebottom, D.G., Epstein, M.F., Platt, R. (1990) Association of intravenous lipid emulsion and coagulase-negative staphylococcal bacteremia in neonatal intensive care units. *New England Journal of Medicine* **323**, 301–308.

143 French, G.L., Shannon, K.P., Simmons, J. (1996) Hospital outbreak of *Klebsiella pneumoniae* resistant to broad spectrum cephalosporins and β-lactam–β-lactamase combinations by hyperproduction of SHV5 β-lactamase. *Journal of Clinical Microbiology* **34**, 358–365.

144 Friedman, C.A., Wender, D.F., Rawson, J.E. (1984) Rapid diagnosis of group B streptococcal infection utilizing a commercially available latex agglutination assay. *Pediatrics* **73**, 27–30.

145 Fukuda, Y. (1994) Fever and persistent pulmonary infiltrate in a one-month-old infant. *Pediatric Infectious Disease Journal* **13**, 241–245.

146 Gajdusek, D.C. (1957) *Pneumocystis carinii* – etiologic agent of interstitial plasma cell pneumonia of perinatal and young infants. *Pediatrics* **19**, 543–565.

147 Gannon, H. (1993) *Ureaplasma urealyticum* and its role in neonatal lung disease. *Neonatal Network* **12**, 13–18.

148 Garland, J.S., Dunne, W.M.J., Havens, P. *et al.* (1992) Peripheral intravenous catheter complications in critically ill children: a prospective study. *Pediatrics* **89**, 1145–1150.

149 Garland, S.M. (1991) Early onset neonatal group B streptococcus (GBS) infection: associated obstetric risk factors. *Australian and New Zealand Journal of Obstetrics and Gynaecology* **31**, 117–118.

150 Garland, S.M., Kelly, N. (1995) Early-onset neonatal group B streptococcal sepsis: economics of various prevention strategies. *Medical Journal of Australia* **162**, 413–417.

151 Garland, S.M., Mackay, S., Tabrizi, S., Jacobs, S. (1996) *Pseudomonas aeruginosa* outbreak associated with a contaminated blood-gas analyser in a neonatal intensive care unit. *Journal of Hospital Infection* **33**, 145–151.

152 Gaynes, R.P., Martone, W.J., Culver, D.H. *et al.* (1991) Comparison of rates of nosocomial infections in neonatal intensive care units in the United States. National Nosocomial Infections Surveillance System. *American Journal of Medicine* **91**, 192S–196S.

153 Gaynes, R.P., Edwards, J.R., Jarvis, W.R., Culver, D.H., Tolson, J.S., Martone, W.J. (1996) Nosocomial infections among neonates in high-risk nurseries in the United States. National Nosocomial Infections Surveillance System. *Pediatrics* **98**, 357–361.

154 Geelen, S.P., Gerards, L.J., Fleer, A. (1990) Pneumococcal septicemia in the newborn. A report on seven cases and a review of the literature. *Journal of Perinatal Medicine* **18**, 125–129.

155 Gellert, G.A., Ewert, D.P., Bendana, N. *et al.* (1993) A cluster of coagulase-negative staphylococcal bacteremias associated with peripheral vascular catheter colonization in a neonatal intensive care unit. *American Journal of Infection Control* **21**, 16–20.

156 Gellin, B.G., Broome, C.V. (1989) Listeriosis. *Journal of the American Medical Association* **261**, 1313–1320.

157 Gerberding, K.M., Eisenhut, C.C., Engle, W.A., Cohen, M.D. (1989) Congenital candida pneumonia and sepsis: a case report and review of the literature. *Journal of Perinatology* **9**, 159–161.

158 Gewolb, I.H., Schwalbe, R.S., Taciak, V.L., Harrison, T.S., Panigrahi, P. (1999) Stool flora in extremely low birthweight infants. *Archives of Disease in Childhood Fetal and Neonatal Edition* **80**, F167–F173.

159 Giacoia, G.P., Neter, E., Ogra, P. (1981) Respiratory infections in infants on mechanical ventilation: the immune response as a diagnostic aid. *Journal of Pediatrics* **98**, 691–695.

160 Gibbs, R.S., McDuffie, R.S.J., McNabb, F., Fryer, G.E., Miyoshi, T., Merenstein, G. (1994) Neonatal group B streptococcal sepsis during 2 years of a universal screening program. *Obstetrics and Gynecology* **84**, 496–500.

161 Gibson, R.L., Soderland, C., Henderson, W.R.J., Chi, E.Y., Rubens, C.E. (1995) Group B streptococci (GBS) injure lung endothelium *in vitro*: GBS invasion and GBS-induced eicosanoid production is greater with microvascular than with pulmonary artery cells. *Infection and Immunity* **63**, 271–279.

162 Giffin, F.J., Greenough, A., Yuksel, B. (1995) Antiviral therapy in neonatal chronic lung disease. *Early Human Development* **42**, 97–109.

163 Gillis, J., Grattan-Smith, T., Kilham, H. (1988) Artificial ventilation in severe pertussis. *Archives of Disease in Childhood* **63**, 364–367.

164 Givner, L.B. (1990) Human immunoglobulins for intravenous use: comparison of available preparations for group B streptococcal antibody levels, opsonic activity, and efficacy in animal models. *Pediatrics* **86**, 955–962.

165 Givner, L.B., Nagaraj, S.K. (1993) Hyperimmune human IgG or recombinant human granulocyte-macrophage colony-stimulating factor as adjunctive therapy for group B streptococcal sepsis in newborn rats. *Journal of Pediatrics* **122**, 774–779.

166 Glick, C., Graves, G.R., Feldman, S. (1993) Neonatal fungemia and amphotericin B. *Southern Medical Journal* **86**, 1368–1371.

167 Gogus, S., Umer, H., Akcoren, Z., Sanal, O., Osmanlioglu, G., Cimbis, M. (1993) Neonatal tuberculosis. *Pediatric Pathology* **13**, 299–304.

168 Goldman, D.A., Leclair, J., Macone, A. (1978) Bacterial colonization of neonates admitted to an intensive care unit. *Journal of Pediatrics* **93**, 288–293.

169 Gomez, R., Ghezzi, F., Romero, R., Munoz, H., Tolosa, J.E., Rojas, I. (1995) Premature labor and intra-amniotic infection. Clinical aspects and role of the cytokines in diagnosis and pathophysiology. *Clinics in Perinatology* **22**, 281–342.

170 Graham, A., Steel, D., Wilson, R. (1993) Effects of purified Pseudomonas rhamnolipids on bioelectrical properties of sheep tracheal epithelium. *Experimental Lung Research* **19**, 77–89.

171 Gray, J.E., Richardson, D.K., McCormick, M.C., Goldmann, D.A. (1995) Coagulase-negative staphylococcal bacteremia among very low birthweight infants: relation to admission illness severity, resource use, and outcome. *Pediatrics* **95**, 225–230.

172 Gray, M.L. (1960) Genital listeriosis as a cause of repeated abortion. *Lancet* **2**, 296–297.

173 Green, M., Dashefsky, B., Wald, E.R., Laifer, S., Harger, J., Guthrie, R. (1993) Comparison of two antigen assays for rapid intrapartum detection of vaginal group B streptococcal colonization. *Journal of Clinical Microbiology* **31**, 78–82.

174 Greenberg, D.N., Yoder, B.A. (1990) Changes in the differential white blood cell count in screening for group B streptococcal sepsis. *Pediatric Infectious Disease Journal* **9**, 886–889.

175 Greene, G.R., King, D., Romansky, S.G., Marble, R.D. (1983) Primary herpes simplex pneumonia in a neonate. *American Journal of Diseases of Childhood* **137**, 464–465.

176 Greene, K.A., Rhine, W.D., Starnes, V.A., Ariagno, R.L. (1990) Fatal postoperative *Legionella* pneumonia in a newborn. *Journal of Perinatology* **10**, 183–184.

177 Greenes, D.S., Rowitch, D., Thorne, G.M., Perez Atayde, A., Lee, F.S., Goldmann, D. (1995) Neonatal herpes simplex virus infection presenting as fulminant liver failure. *Pediatric Infectious Disease Journal* **14**, 242–244.

178 Greenough, A. (1996) Exogenous surfactant therapy in non-respiratory distress syndrome. *Turkish Journal of Pediatrics* **38**, 45–50.

179 Griffin, M., Pushpanathan, C., Andrews, W. (1990) *Chlamydia trachomatis* pneumonitis: a case study and literature review. *Pediatric Pathology* **10**, 843–852.

180 Grigg, J.M., Barber, A., Silverman, M. (1992) Increased levels of bronchoalveolar lavage fluid interleukin-6 in preterm ventilated infants after prolonged rupture of membranes. *American Review of Respiratory Disease* **145**, 782–786.

181 Groothuis, J.R., Gutierrez, K.M., Lauer, B.A. (1988) Respiratory syncytial virus infection in children with bronchopulmonary dysplasia. *Pediatrics* **82**, 199–203.

182 Gross, N.T., Camner, P., Chinchilla, M., Jarstrand, C. (1998) *In vitro* effect of lung surfactant on alveolar macrophage defence mechanisms against *Cryptococcus neoformans*. *Mycopathologia* **144**, 21–27.

183 Grundmann, H., Kropec, A., Hartung, D., Berner, R., Daschner, F. (1993) *Pseudomonas aeruginosa* in a neonatal intensive care unit: reservoirs and ecology of the nosocomial pathogen. *Journal of Infectious Diseases* **168**, 943–947.

184 Gustafson, T.L., Shehab, Z., Brunell, P.A. (1984) Outbreak of varicella in a newborn intensive care nursery. *American Journal of Diseases of Children* **138**, 548–550.

185 Gustavson, E.E. (1986) *Escherichia coli* empyema in the newborn. *American Journal of Diseases of Children* **140**, 408–411.

186 Guzzardo, M.B., Hacker, M.E., Walker, G. (1988) Neonatal pneumococcal pneumonia. Case report and literature review. *Journal of the Medical Association of Georgia* **77**, 313–315.

187 Hachey, W.E., Wiswell, T.E. (1992) Limitations in the usefulness of urine latex particle agglutination tests and hematologic measurements in diagnosing neonatal sepsis during the first week of life. *Journal of Perinatology* **12**, 240–245.

188 Haddad, J., Gut, J.P., Wendling, M.J. *et al.* (1993) Enterovirus infections in neonates. A retrospective study of 21 cases. *European Journal of Medicine* **2**, 209–214.

189 Hall, C.B., Kopelman, A.E., Douglas, R.G., Jr, Geiman, J.M., Meagher, M.P. (1979) Neonatal respiratory syncytial virus infection. *New England Journal of Medicine* **300**, 393–396.

190 Hall, S., Glickman, B. (1991) The British Paediatric Surveillance Unit. *New England Journal of Medicine* **363**, 344–346.

191 Halliday, H.L., McClure, G., Reid, M.M., Lappin, T.R., Meban, C., Thomas, P.S. (1984) Controlled trial of artificial surfactant to prevent respiratory distress syndrome. *Lancet* **1**, 476–478.

192 Hammerschlag, M.R., Roblin, P.M., Gelling, M., Tsumura, N., Jule, J.E., Kutlin, A. (1997) Use of polymerase chain reaction for the detection of *Chlamydia trachomatis* in ocular and nasopharyngeal specimens from infants with conjunctivitis. *Pediatric Infectious Disease Journal* **16**, 293–297.

193 Hampl, S.D., Olson, L.C. (1995) Pertussis in the young infant. *Seminars in Respiratory Infection* **10**, 58–62.

194 Hannah, M.E., Ohlsson, A., Farine, D. *et al.* (1996) Induction of labor compared with expectant management for prelabor

195 Hardegger, D., Nadal, D., Bossart, W., Altwegg, M., Dutly, F. (2000) Rapid detection of *Mycoplasma pneumoniae* in clinical samples by real-time PCR. *Journal of Microbiological Methods* **41**, 45–51.

rupture of the membranes at term. TERMPROM Study Group. *New England Journal of Medicine* **334**, 1005–1010.

196 Harris, H., Wirtschafter, D., Cassady, G. (1976) Endotracheal intubation and its relationship to bacterial colonization and systemic infection of newborn infants. *Pediatrics* **58**, 816–823.

197 Harrison, H.R., English, M.G., Lee, C.K., Alexander, E.R. (1978) *Chlamydia trachomatis* infant pneumonitis: comparison with matched controls and other infant pneumonitis. *New England Journal of Medicine* **298**, 702–708.

198 Hashmi, N.A., Cosgrove, J.F., MacMahon, P. (2000) Prophylaxis in RSV infection (Palivizumab) – is it worthwhile? *Irish Medical Journal* **93**, 284.

199 Hayden, R.T., Uhl, J.R., Qian, X. *et al.* (2001) Direct detection of legionella species from bronchoalveolar lavage and open lung biopsy specimens: comparison of lightcycler PCR, *in situ* hybridization, direct fluorescence antigen detection, and culture. *Journal of Clinical Microbiology* **39**, 2618–2626.

200 Hemming, V.G., Overall, J.C., Britt, M.R. (1976) Nosocomial infections in a newborn intensive care unit. *New England Journal of Medicine* **294**, 1310–1316.

201 Herting, E., Jarstrand, C., Rasool, O., Curstedt, T., Sun, B., Robertson, B. (1994) Experimental neonatal group B streptococcal pneumonia: effect of a modified porcine surfactant on bacterial proliferation in ventilated near-term rabbits. *Pediatric Research* **36**, 784–791.

202 Hervas, J.A., Gonzalez, L., Gil, J., Paoletti, L.C., Madoff, L.C., Benedi, V.J. (1993) Neonatal group B streptococcal infection in Mallorca, Spain. *Clinical Infectious Diseases* **16**, 714–718.

203 Heuchan, A.M., Isaacs, D. (2001) The management of varicella-zoster virus exposure and infection in pregnancy and the newborn period. Australasian Subgroup in Paediatric Infectious Diseases of the Australasian Society for Infectious Diseases. *Medical Journal of Australia* **174**, 288–292.

204 Hibbard, J.U., Hibbard, M.C., Ismail, M., Arendt, E. (1993) Pregnancy outcome after expectant management of premature rupture of the membranes in the second trimester. *Journal of Reproductive Medicine* **38**, 945–951.

205 Hiemstra, I., van Bel, F., Berger, H.M. (1984) Can *Trichomonas vaginalis* cause pneumonia in newborn babies? *British Medical Journal (Clinical Research Edition)* **289**, 355–356.

206 Hirschl, R.B., Butler, M., Coburn, C.E., Bartlett, R.H., Baumgart, S. (1994) *Listeria monocytogenes* and severe newborn respiratory failure supported with extracorporeal membrane oxygenation. *Archives of Pediatrics and Adolescent Medicine* **148**, 513–517.

207 Hocker, J.R., Cook, L.N., Adams, G., Rabalais, G.P. (1990) Ganciclovir therapy of congenital cytomegalovirus pneumonia. *Pediatric Infectious Disease Journal* **9**, 743–745.

208 Holmberg, R.E., Jr, Pavia, A.T., Montgomery, D., Clark, J.M., Eggert, L.D. (1993) Nosocomial *Legionella* pneumonia in the neonate. *Pediatrics* **92**, 450–453.

209 Horie, H., Kawakami, H., Minoshima, K. *et al.* (1992) Neonatal Legionnaires' disease. Histopathological findings in an autopsied neonate. *Acta Pathologica Japonica* **42**, 427–431.

210 Hostoffer, R.W., Litman, A., Smith, P.G., Jacobs, H.S., Tosi, M.F. (1993) *Pneumocystis carinii* pneumonia in a term newborn infant with a transiently depressed T lymphocyte

count, primarily of cells carrying the CD4 antigen. *Journal of Pediatrics* **122**, 792–794.

211 Hsieh, S., Goldstein, E., Lippert, W., Margulies, L. (1978) Effect of protein A on the antistaphylococcal defence mechanisms of the murine lung. *Journal of Infectious Diseases* **138**, 754–759.

212 Hung, F.C., Huang, C.B., Huang, S.C., Liu, S.T. (1994) Congenital cutaneous candidiasis – report of two cases. *Chang Keng I Hsueh* **17**, 63–67.

213 Hunt, D.W., Huppertz, H.I., Jiang, H.J. (1994) Studies of human cord blood dendritic cells: evidence for functional immaturity. *Blood* **84**, 4333–4343.

214 Isaacs, D. (1998) Prevention of early onset group B streptococcal infection: screen, treat, or observe? *Archives of Disease in Childhood Fetal and Neonatal Edition* **79**, F81–F82.

215 Isaacs, D. (2000) Neonatal chickenpox. *Journal of Paediatrics and Child Health* **36**, 76–77.

216 Isaacs, D., Moxon, E.R. (1991) *Neonatal Infections*. Oxford: Butterworth Heinemann, 149–166.

217 Isaacs, D., Wilkinson, A.R., Moxon, E.R. (1987) Surveillance of colonization and late-onset septicaemia in neonates. *Journal of Hospital Infection* **10**, 114–119.

218 Isaacs, D., Barfield, C.P., Grimwood, K., McPhee, A.J., Minutillo, C., Tudehope, D.I. (1995) Systemic bacterial and fungal infections in infants in Australian neonatal units. Australian Study Group for Neonatal Infections. *Medical Journal of Australia* **162**, 198–201.

219 Isaacs, D., Barfield, C., Clothier, T. *et al.* (1996) Late-onset infections of infants in neonatal units. *Journal of Paediatrics and Child Health* **32**, 158–161.

220 Issekutz, T.B., Evans, J., Bortolussi, R. (1984) The immune response of human neonates to *Listeria monocytogenes* infection. *Clinical and Investigative Medicine* **7**, 263–266.

221 Itoh, K., Aihara, H., Takada, S. *et al.* (1990) Clinicopathological differences between early-onset and late-onset sepsis and pneumonia in very low birthweight infants. *Pediatric Pathology* **10**, 757–768.

222 Jacob, J., Edwards, D., Gluck, L. (1980) Early-onset sepsis and pneumonia observed as respiratory distress syndrome: assessment of lung maturity. *American Journal of Diseases of Children* **134**, 766–768.

223 Jacobs, J., Garmyn, K., Verhaegen, J., Devlieger, H., Eggermont, E. (1990) Neonatal sepsis due to *Streptococcus pneumoniae*. *Scandinavian Journal of Infectious Diseases* **22**, 493–497.

224 Jacobs, R.F. (1998) Neonatal herpes simplex virus infections. *Seminars in Perinatology* **22**, 64–71.

225 Jacobs, R.F., Wilson, C.B., Smith, A.L. (1983) Age-dependent effects of aminobutyryl muramyl dipeptide on alveolar macrophage function in infant and adult Macaca monkeys. *American Review of Respiratory Disease* **128**, 862–867.

226 Jacquot, J., Puchelle, E., Zahm, J.M., Beck, G. (1987) Effect of human airway lysozyme on the *in vitro* growth of *Streptococcus pneumoniae*. *European Journal of Respiratory Diseases* **71**, 295–305.

227 Jeffery, H.E. McIntosh, E.D. (1994) Antepartum screening and non-selective intrapartum chemoprophylaxis for group B streptococcus. *Australian and New Zealand Journal of Obstetrics and Gynaecology* **34**, 14–19.

228 Jeffery, H.E., Mitchison, R., Wigglesworth, J.S., Davies, P.A. (1977) Early neonatal bacteraemia: comparison of group B streptococcal, other Gram-positive and Gram-negative infections. *Archives of Disease in Childhood* **52**, 683–686.

229 Jensen, E.T., Kharazmi, A., Lam, K., Costerton, J.W., Hoiby, N. (1990) Human polymorph leucocyte response to *Pseudomonas aeruginosa* grown in biofilms. *Infection and Immunity* **58**, 2383–2385.

230 Jevon, G.P., Dunne, W.M., Jr, Hicks, M.J., Langston, C. (1993) *Bacillus cereus* pneumonia in premature neonates: a report of two cases. *Pediatric Infectious Disease Journal* **12**, 251–253.

231 Johnston, H.C., Shigeoka, A.O., Hurley, D.C., Pysher, T.J. (1989) Nocardia pneumonia in a neonate with chronic granulomatous disease. *Pediatric Infectious Disease Journal* **8**, 526–528.

232 Jones, E.M., McCulloch, S.Y., Reeves, D.S., MacGowan, A.P. (1994) A 10 year survey of the epidemiology and clinical aspects of listeriosis in a provincial English city. *Journal of Infection* **29**, 91–103.

233 Jones, J.F., Ray, C.G., Fulginiti, V.A. (1980) Perinatal mumps infection. *Journal of Pediatrics* **96**, 912–914.

234 Kalliola, S., Vuopio-Varkila, J., Takala, A.K., Eskola, J. (1999) Neonatal group B streptococcal disease in Finland: a ten-year nationwide study. *Pediatric Infectious Disease Journal* **18**, 806–810.

235 Kao, H.T., Huang, Y.C., Lin, T.Y. (2000) Influenza A virus infection in infants. *Journal of Microbiology, Immunology and Infection* **33**, 105–108.

236 Kaplan, M., Rudensky, B., Beck, A. (1993) Perinatal infections with *Streptococcus pneumoniae*. *American Journal of Perinatology* **10**, 1–4.

237 Kazembe, P., Simor, A.E., Swarney, A.E. *et al.* (1993) A study of the epidemiology of an endemic strain of *Staphylococcus haemolyticus* (TOR-35) in a neonatal intensive care unit. *Scandinavian Journal of Infectious Diseases* **25**, 507–513.

238 Kenny, G.E., Cartwright, F.D. (1991) Susceptibilities of *Mycoplasma hominis* and *Ureaplasma urealyticum* to two new quinolones, sparfloxacin and WIN 57273. *Antimicrobial Agents and Chemotherapy* **35**, 1515–1516.

239 Kenyon, S.L., Taylor, D.J., Tarnow-Mordi, W. (2001) Broad-spectrum antibiotics for preterm, prelabour rupture of fetal membranes: the ORACLE I randomised trial. ORACLE Collaborative Group. *Lancet* **357**, 979–988.

240 Khadilkar, V., Tudehope, D., Fraser, S. (1995) A prospective study of nosocomial infection in a neonatal intensive care unit. *Journal of Paediatrics and Child Health* **31**, 387–391.

241 Khan, E.A., Wafelman, L.S., Garcia-Prats, J.A., Taber, L.H. (1997) *Serratia marcescens* pneumonia, empyema and pneumatocele in a preterm neonate. *Pediatric Infectious Disease Journal* **16**, 1003–1005.

242 Kinney, J.S., Johnson, K., Papasian, C., Hall, R.T., Kurth, C.G., Jackson, M.A. (1993) Early onset *Haemophilus influenzae* sepsis in the newborn infant. *Pediatric Infectious Disease Journal* **12**, 739–743.

243 Kinney, J.S., Hierholzer, J.C., Thibeault, D.W. (1994) Neonatal pulmonary insufficiency caused by adenovirus infection successfully treated with extracorporeal membrane oxygenation. *Journal of Pediatrics* **125**, 110–112.

244 Kollef, M.H. (1999) The prevention of ventilator-associated pneumonia. *New England Journal of Medicine* **340**, 627–634.

245 Konrad, F., Schiener, R., Marx, T., Georgieff, M. (1995) Ultrastructure and mucociliary transport of bronchial respiratory epithelium in intubated patients. *Intensive Care Medicine* **21**, 482–489.

246 Korbage de Araujo, M.C., Schultz, R., do Rosario Dias de Oliveira, Ramos, J.L., Vaz, F.A. (1999) A risk factor for early-onset infection in premature newborns: invasion of chorioamniotic tissues by leukocytes. *Early Human Development* **56**, 1–15.

247 Korones, S.B. (1988) Uncommon virus infections of the mother, fetus, and newborn: influenza, mumps and measles. *Clinics in Perinatology* **15**, 259–272.

248 Krishnan, L., Vernekar, A.V., Diwakar, K.K., Krishnanand, G., Gomes, R.G., Bhaskaranand, N. (1994) Neonatal tuberculosis: a case report. *Annals of Tropical Paediatrics* **14**, 333–335.

249 Kuhn, J.P., Lee, S.B. (1973) Pneumatoceles associated with *Escherichia coli* pneumonias in the newborn. *Pediatrics* **51**, 1008–1011.

250 Lackner, H., Schwinger, W., Urban, C. (1992) Liposomal amphotericin B for treatment of disseminated fungal infections in two infants of very low birthweight. *Pediatrics* **89**, 1259–1261.

251 Lau, Y.L., Hey, E. (1991) Sensitivity and specificity of daily tracheal aspirate cultures in predicting organisms causing bacteremia in ventilated neonates. *Pediatric Infectious Disease Journal* **10**, 290–294.

252 Lee, D.R., Moore, G.W., Hutchins, G.M. (1991) Lattice theory analysis of the relationship of hyaline membrane disease and fetal pneumonia in 96 perinatal autopsies. *Pediatric Pathology* **11**, 223–233.

253 Lee, R.M., Rossman, C.M., O'Brodovich, H., Forrest, J.B., Newhouse, M.T. (1984) Ciliary defects associated with the development of bronchopulmonary dysplasia. Ciliary motility and ultrastructure. *American Review of Respiratory Disease* **129**, 190–193.

254 Lennon, D., Lewis, B., Mantell, C. *et al.* (1984) Epidemic perinatal listeriosis. *Pediatric Infectious Disease* **3**, 30–34.

255 Lenz, A.G., Costabel, U., Maier, K.L. (1996) Oxidized BAL fluid proteins in patients with interstitial lung diseases. *European Respiratory Journal* **9**, 307–312.

256 Leowski, J. (1986) Mortality from acute respiratory infections in children under 5 years of age: global estimates. *World Health Statistics Quarterly* **39**, 138–144.

257 Leslie, G.I., Scurr, R.D., Barr, P.A. (1981) Early-onset bacterial pneumonia: a comparison with severe hyaline membrane disease. *Australian Paediatric Journal* **17**, 202–206.

258 Levine, C.D. (1991) Premature rupture of the membranes and sepsis in preterm neonates. *Nursing Research* **40**, 36–41.

259 Levy, I., Rubin, L.G. (1998) Legionella pneumonia in neonates: a literature review. *Journal of Perinatology* **18**, 287–290.

260 Lewis, D.B., Yu, C.C., Meyer, J. (1991) Cellular and molecular mechanisms for reduced interleukin 4 and interferon-gamma production by neonatal T-cells. *Journal of Clinical Investigation* **87**, 194–202.

261 Lidin-Janson, G., Hanson, L.A., Mattsby-Baltzer, I. (1980) Immunologic defence mechanisms. *European Journal of Respiratory Diseases Supplement* **108**, 12–15.

262 Lillien, L.D., Yeh, T.F., Novak, G.M. (1978) Early-onset haemophilus sepsis in newborn infants: clinical, roentgenographic and pathological features. *Pediatrics* **59**, 1006–1011.

263 Linder, N., Ohel, G., Gazit, G., Keidar, D., Tamir, I., Reichman, B. (1995) Neonatal sepsis after prolonged premature rupture of membranes. *Journal of Perinatology* **15**, 36–38.

264 Lissauer, T.J., Shaw, P.J., Underhill, G. (1984) Neonatal herpes simplex pneumonia. *Archives of Disease in Childhood* **59**, 668–670.

265 Lorenz, R.P., Appelbaum, P.C., Ward, R.M., Botti, J.J. (1982) Chorioamnionitis and possible neonatal infection associated with *Lactobacillus* species. *Journal of Clinical Microbiology* **16**, 558–561.

266 Lu, M.C., Peters-Golden, M., Hostetler, D., Robinson, N., Derksen, F. (1996) Age-related enhancement of 5-lipoxygenase metabolic capacity in cattle alveolar macrophages. *American Journal of Physiology* **271**, 547–554.

267 Luck, P.C., Dinger, E., Helbig, J.H. *et al.* (1994) Analysis of *Legionella pneumophila* strains associated with nosocomial pneumonia in a neonatal intensive care unit. *European Journal of Clinical Microbiology and Infectious Diseases* **13**, 565–571.

268 Maberry, M.C., Ramin, S.M., Gilstrap, L.C., III, Leveno, K.J., Dax, J.S. (1990) Intrapartum asphyxia in pregnancies complicated by intra-amniotic infection. *Obstetrics and Gynecology* **76**, 351–354.

269 MacGowan, A.P., Cartlidge, P.H., MacLeod, F., McLaughlin, J. (1991) Maternal listeriosis in pregnancy without fetal or neonatal infection. *Journal of Infection* **22**, 53–57.

270 Mackay, C.R. (1992) Migration pathways and immunologic memory among T-lymphocytes. *Seminars in Immunology* **4**, 51–58.

271 Madge, P., Paton, J.Y., McColl, J.H., Mackie, P.L. (1992) Prospective controlled study of four infection-control procedures to prevent nosocomial infection with respiratory syncytial virus. *Lancet* **340**, 1079–1083.

272 Manroe, B.L., Rosenfeld, C.R., Weinberg, A.G., Browne, R. (1977) The differential leukocyte count in the assessment and outcome of early-onset neonatal group B streptococcal disease. *Journal of Pediatrics* **91**, 632–637.

273 Mardh, P.A., Johansson, P.J., Svenningsen, N. (1984) Intrauterine lung infection with *Chlamydia trachomatis* in a premature infant. *Acta Paediatrica Scandinavica* **73**, 569–572.

274 Margraf, L.R., Tomashefski, J.F., Bruce, M.C., Dahms, B.B. (1991) Morphometric analysis of the lung in bronchopulmonary dysplasia. *American Review of Respiratory Disease* **143**, 391–400.

275 Martius, J.A., Roos, T., Gora, B. *et al.* (1999) Risk factors associated with early-onset sepsis in premature infants. *European Journal of Obstetrics & Gynecology and Reproductive Biology* **85**, 151–158.

276 Mascola, L., Cable, D.C., Walsh, P., Guinan, M.E. (1984) Neonatal herpes simplex virus death manifested as rapidly progressive pneumonia. *Clinical Pediatrics (Philadelphia)* **23**, 400–403.

277 Matsuoka, T., Naito, T., Kubota, Y. *et al.* (1990) Disseminated adenovirus (type 19) infection in a neonate. Rapid detection of the infection by immunofluorescence. *Acta Paediatrica Scandinavica* **79**, 568–571.

278 Mayer, T., Matlak, M.E., Condon, V., Shasha, I., Glasgow, L. (1982) Computed tomographic findings of neonatal lung abscess. *American Journal of Diseases of Children* **136**, 39–41.

279 Mayon White, D. (1982) The incidence of neonatal group B streptococcal disease in Britain. In Holm, S.E., Christensen, P. (eds), *Basic Concepts of Streptococci and Streptococcal Diseases*. Chertsey: Reedbooks Ltd, 305–306.

280 McDuffie, R.S.J., McGregor, J.A., Gibbs, R.S. (1993) Adverse perinatal outcome and resistant Enterobacteriaceae after antibiotic usage for premature rupture of the membranes and group B streptococcus carriage. *Obstetrics and Gynecology* **82**, 487–489.

281 McFall, T.L., Zimmerman, G.A., Augustine, N.H., Hill, H.R. (1987) Effect of group B streptococcal type-specific antigen on polymorphonuclear leukocyte function and polymorphonuclear leukocyte-endothelial cell interaction. *Pediatric Research* **21**, 517–523.

282 McGregor, J.A., Burns, J.C., Levin, M.J. (1984) Transplacental passage of influenza A/Bangkok mimicking amniotic fluid infection syndrome. *American Journal of Obstetrics and Gynecology* **149**, 856–859.

283 McGregor, J.A., French, J.I., Seo, K. (1991) Antimicrobial therapy in preterm premature rupture of membranes: results

of a prospective, double-blind, placebo-controlled trial of erythromycin. *American Journal of Obstetrics and Gynecology* **165**, 632–640.

284 McIntosh, N., Harrison, A. (1994) Prolonged premature rupture of membranes in the preterm infant: a 7 year study. *European Journal of Obstetrics & Gynecology and Reproductive Biology* **57**, 1–6.

285 McLaren, R.A., Chauhan, S.P., Gross, T.L. (1996) Intrapartum factors in early-onset group B streptococcal sepsis in term neonates: a case–control study. *American Journal of Obstetrics and Gynecology* **174**, 1934–1937.

286 Meibalane, R., Sedmak, G.V., Sasidharan, P., Garg, P., Grausz, J.P. (1977) Outbreak of influenza in a neonatal intensive care unit. *Journal of Pediatrics* **91**, 974–976.

287 Meissner, H.C., Murray, S.A., Kiernan, M.A., Snydman, D.R., McIntosh, K. (1984) A simultaneous outbreak of respiratory syncytial virus and parainfluenza virus type 3 in a newborn nursery. *Journal of Pediatrics* **104**, 680–684.

288 Melville, C., Kempley, S., Graham, J., Berry, C.L. (1996) Early onset systemic Candida infection in extremely preterm neonates. *European Journal of Pediatrics* **155**, 904–906.

289 Mendoza, J.C., Roberts, J.L. (1991) Early-onset *Haemophilus influenzae* sepsis in the neonate. *Journal of Perinatology* **11**, 126–129.

290 Mercer, B.M., Arheart, K.L. (1995) Antimicrobial therapy in expectant management of preterm premature rupture of the membranes. *Lancet* **346**, 1271–1279.

291 Merenstein, G.B., Weisman, L.E. (1996) Premature rupture of the membranes: neonatal consequences. *Seminars in Perinatology* **20**, 375–380.

292 Merritt, T.A., Anderson, V.M. (1983) Icterus, encephalopathy, and galloping neonatal pneumonia. *American Journal of Diseases of Children* **137**, 1001–1007.

293 Mintz, L., Ballard, R.A., Sniderman, S.H., Roth, R.S., Drew, W.L. (1979) Nosocomial respiratory syncytial virus infections in an intensive care nursery: rapid diagnosis by direct immunofluorescence. *Pediatrics* **64**, 149–153.

294 Miyamura, K., Malhotra, R., Hoppe, H.J. *et al.* (1994) Surfactant proteins A (SP-A) and D (SP-D): levels in human amniotic fluid and localization in the fetal membranes. *Biochimica Biophysica Acta* **1210**, 303–307.

295 Modlin, J.F. (1988) Perinatal echovirus and group B coxsackievirus infections. *Clinics in Perinatology* **15**, 233–246.

296 Modlin, J.F. (1994) Neonatal enterovirus infections. *Pediatric Infectious Disease* **5**, 70–77.

297 Modlin, J. (2000) Coxsackieviruses, echoviruses and newer enteroviruses. In Mandell, G.L., Bennett, J.E., Dolin, R. (eds), *Mandell, Douglas and Bennett's Principles and Practice of Infectious Diseases*, 5th edition. Philadelphia: Churchill Livingstone, 1904–1919.

298 Moler, F.W., Steinhart, C.M., Ohmit, S.E., Stidham, G.L. (1996) Effectiveness of ribavirin in otherwise well infants with respiratory syncytial virus-associated respiratory failure. Pediatric Critical Study Group. *Journal of Pediatrics* **128**, 422–428.

299 Montone, K.T., Furth, E.E., Pietra, G.G., Gupta, P.K. (1995) Neonatal adenovirus infection: a case report with *in situ* hybridization confirmation of ascending intrauterine infection. *Diagnostic Cytopathology* **12**, 341–344.

300 Moriartey, R.R., Finer, N.N. (1979) Pneumococcal sepsis and pneumonia in the neonate. *American Journal of Diseases of Children* **133**, 601–602.

301 Moses, L.M., Heath, P.T., Wilkinson, A.R., Jeffery, H.E., Isaacs, D. (1998) Early onset group B streptococcal neonatal infection in Oxford 1985–96. *Archives of Disease in Childhood Fetal and Neonatal Edition* **79**, F148–F149.

302 Naeye, R.L., Tafari, N. (1983) *Risk Factors in Pregnancy and Diseases of the Fetus and Newborn.* Baltimore: Williams & Wilkins.

303 Neligan, G.A., Steiner, H., Gardner, P.S., McQuillin, J. (1970) Respiratory syncytial virus infection of the newborn. *British Medical Journal* **3**, 146–147.

304 Nelson, J.D. (1978) The changing epidemiology of pertussis in young infants. The role of adults as reservoirs of infection. *American Journal of Diseases of Children* **132**, 371–373.

305 Ng, P.C. (1994) Systemic fungal infections in neonates. *Archives of Disease in Childhood* **71**, F130–F135.

306 Ng, P.C., Herrington, R.A., Beane, C.A., Ghonheim, A.T.M., Dear, P.R.F. (1989) An outbreak of *Acinetobacter* septicaemia in a neonatal intensive care unit. *Journal of Hospital Infection* **14**, 363–368.

307 Ng, P.C., Siu, Y.K., Lewindon, P.J., Wong, W., Cheung, K.L., Dawkins, R. (1994) Congenital *Candida* pneumonia in a preterm infant. *Journal of Paediatrics and Child Health* **30**, 552–554.

308 Nicoll, R.M. (2000) RSV prevention. *Archives of Disease in Childhood* **82**, 88.

309 Nicod, L.P. (1999) Pulmonary defence mechanisms. *Respiration* **66**, 2–11.

310 Nicod, L.P., El Habre, F. (1992) Adhesion molecules on human lung dendritic cells and their role for T-cell activation. *American Journal of Respiratory Cell and Molecular Biology* **7**, 207–213.

311 Nicoll, J.A., Love, S., Burton, P.A., Berry, P.J. (1994) Autopsy findings in two cases of neonatal herpes simplex virus infection: detection of virus by immunohistochemistry, *in situ* hybridization and the polymerase chain reaction. *Histopathology* **24**, 257–264.

312 Niida, Y., Numazaki, K., Ikehata, M., Umetsu, M., Motoya, H., Chiba, S. (1998) Two full-term infants with *Chlamydia trachomatis* pneumonia in the early neonatal period. *European Journal of Pediatrics* **157**, 950–951.

313 Nizet, V., Gibson, R.L., Rubens, C.E. (1997) The role of group B streptococci β-hemolysin expression in newborn lung injury. *Advances in Experimental Medicine and Biology* **418**, 627–630.

314 Nyquist, A.C., Rotbart, H.A., Cotton, M. *et al.* (1994) Acyclovir-resistant neonatal herpes simplex virus infection of the larynx. *Journal of Pediatrics* **124**, 967–971.

315 Ohlsson, A., Bailey, T. (1985) Neonatal pneumonia caused by *Branhamella catarrhalis*. *Scandinavian Journal of Infectious Diseases* **17**, 225–228.

316 Ohlsson, A., Myhr, T.L. (1994) Intrapartum chemoprophylaxis of perinatal group B streptococcal infections: a critical review of randomized controlled trials. *American Journal of Obstetrics and Gynecology* **170**, 910–917.

317 Ohlsson, A., Myhr, T.L. (1994) Intrapartum penicillin prophylaxis of early-onset streptococcal infection. *Canadian Medical Association Journal* **150**, 1197–1198, 1200.

318 Ohyama, M., Tanaka, Y., Sasaki, Y., Goto, A. (1990) Detection of *C. trachomatis* by *in situ* DNA hybridization: report of two cases with neonatal pneumonia. *Acta Paediatrica Japonica* **32**, 319–322.

319 Ollikainen, J., Hiekkaniemi, H., Korppi, M., Sarkkinen, H., Heinonen, K. (1993) *Ureaplasma urealyticum* infection associated with acute respiratory insufficiency and death in premature infants. *Journal of Pediatrics* **122**, 756–760.

320 Osborn, L. (1990) Leukocyte adhesion to endothelium in inflammation. *Cell* **62**, 3–6.

321 Ozkan, H., Pasaoglu, G., Olgac, N., Gunel, R., Yuce, A., Gulay, Z. (1999) *Stenotrophomonas maltophilia* pneumonia in a premature infant. *Turkish Journal of Pediatrics* **41**, 283–286.

322 Paisley, J.W., Bruhn, F.W., Lauer, B.A., McIntosh, K. (1978) Type A2 influenza viral infections in children. *American Journal of Diseases of Children* **132**, 34–36.

323 Panero, A., Pacifico, L., Rossi, N., Roggini, M., Chiesa, C. (1995) *Ureaplasma urealyticum* as a cause of pneumonia in preterm infants: analysis of the white cell response. *Archives of Disease in Childhood Fetal and Neonatal Edition* **73**, F37–F40.

324 Panero, A., Roggini, M., Papoff, P., Moretti, C., Contini, C., Bucci, G. (1995) *Pneumocystis carinii* pneumonia in preterm infants: report of two cases successfully diagnosed by non-bronchoscopic bronchoalveolar lavage. *Acta Paediatrica* **84**, 1309–1311.

325 Paryani, S.G., Arvin, A.M. (1986) Intrauterine infection with varicella-zoster virus after maternal varicella. *New England Journal of Medicine* **314**, 1542–1546.

326 Patrick, C.H., John, J.F., Levkoff, A.H., Atkins, L.M. (1992) Relatedness of strains of methicillin-resistant coagulase-negative *Staphylococcus* colonizing hospital personnel and producing bacteremias in a neonatal intensive care unit. *Pediatric Infectious Disease Journal* **11**, 935–940.

327 Payne, N.R., Burke, B.A., Day, D.L., Christenson, P.D., Thompson, T.R., Ferrieri, P. (1988) Correlation of clinical and pathologic findings in early onset neonatal group B streptococcal infection with disease severity and prediction of outcome. *Pediatric Infectious Disease Journal* **7**, 836–847.

328 Peevy, K.J., Chalhub, E.G. (1983) Occult group B streptococcal infection: an important cause of intrauterine asphyxia, *American Journal of Obstetrics and Gynecology* **146**, 989–990.

329 Penner, D.W., McInnis, A.C. (1955) Intrauterine and neonatal pneumonia. *American Journal of Obstetrics and Gynecology* **69**, 147–151.

330 Peters-Golden, M., Coffey, M. (1998) Role of leukotrienes in antimicrobial defense of the lung. *Journal of Laboratory and Clinical Medicine* **132**, 251–257.

331 Philip, A.G. (1985) Response of C-reactive protein in neonatal Group B streptococcal infection. *Pediatric Infectious Disease* **4**, 145–148.

332 Philip, A.G. (1994) The changing face of neonatal infection: experience at a regional medical center. *Pediatric Infectious Disease Journal* **13**, 1098–1102.

333 Philipson, E.H., Herson, V.C. (1996) Intrapartum chemoprophylaxis for group B streptococcus infection to prevent neonatal disease: who should be treated? *American Journal of Perinatology* **13**, 487–490.

334 Piedra, P.A., Kasel, J.A., Norton, H.J. *et al.* (1992) Description of an adenovirus type 8 outbreak in hospitalized neonates born prematurely. *Pediatric Infectious Disease Journal* **11**, 460–465.

335 Plopper, C.G., Mariassy, A.T., Wilson, D.W., Alley, J.L., Nishio, S.J., Nettesheim, P. (1983) Comparison of nonciliated tracheal epithelial cells in six mammalian species: ultrastructure and population densities. *Experimental Lung Research* **5**, 281–294.

336 Pople, I.K., Bayston, R., Hayward, R.D. (1992) Infection of cerebrospinal fluid shunts in infants: a study of etiological factors. *Journal of Neurosurgery* **77**, 29–36.

337 Pryce, C.J., Donn, S.M. (1991) Ventilatory casebook. Respiratory syncytial virus infection complicating bronchopulmonary dysplasia. *Journal of Perinatology* **11**, 390–393.

338 Public Health Laboratory Service (2001) Reports to Centre for Communicable Disease Control: PHLS Food Hygiene Laboratory.

339 Purdy, G.D., Cullen, M., Yedlin, S., Bedard, M.P. (1987) An unusual neonatal case presentation: *Streptococcus pneumoniae* pneumonia with abscess and pneumatocele formation. *Journal of Perinatology* **7**, 378–381.

340 Pyati, S.P., Pildes, R.S., Ramamurthy, R.S., Jacobs, N. (1981) Decreasing mortality in neonates with early-onset group B streptococcal infection: reality or artifact. *Journal of Pediatrics* **98**, 625–627.

341 Pylipow, M., Gaddis, M., Kinney, J.S. (1994) Selective intrapartum prophylaxis for group B streptococcus colonization: management and outcome of newborns. *Pediatrics* **93**, 631–635.

342 Quinn, P.A., Gillan, J.E., Markestad, T. *et al.* (1985) Intrauterine infection with *Ureaplasma urealyticum* as a cause of fatal neonatal pneumonia. *Pediatric Infectious Disease* **4**, 538–543.

343 Quinn, P.A., Li, H.C., Th'ng, C., Dunn, M., Butany, J. (1993) Serological response to *Ureaplasma urealyticum* in the neonate. *Clinical Infectious Diseases* **17**(Suppl 1), S136–S143.

344 Rabalais, G.P., Bronfin, D.R., Daum, R.S. (1987) Evaluation of a commercially available latex agglutination test for rapid diagnosis of group B streptococcal infection. *Pediatric Infectious Disease Journal* **6**, 177–181.

345 Radoycich, G.E., Zuppan, C.W., Weeks, D.A., Krous, H.F., Langston, C. (1992) Patterns of measles pneumonitis. *Pediatric Pathology* **12**, 773–786.

346 Randolph, A.G., Wang, E.E. (1996) Ribavirin for respiratory syncytial virus lower respiratory tract infection. A systematic overview. *Archives of Pediatrics and Adolescent Medicine* **150**, 942–947.

347 Rangel-Frausto, M.S., Wiblin, T., Blumberg, H.M. *et al.* (1999) Neonatal epidemiology of mycoses survey (NEMIS): variations in rates of bloodstream infections due to *Candida* species in seven surgical intensive care units and six neonatal intensive care units. *Clinical Infectious Diseases* **29**, 253–258.

348 Rawlings, J.S., Krober, M.S., Aamodt, L.W. (1989) Imaging case of the month: neonatal herpes simplex virus pneumonia. *American Journal of Perinatology* **6**, 304–306.

349 Reid, L. (1977) Influence of the pattern of structural growth of lung on susceptibility to specific infectious diseases in infants and children. *Pediatric Research* **11**, 210–215.

350 Reid, T.M.S. (1975) Emergence of Group B streptococci in obstetric and neonatal infections. *British Medical Journal* **2**, 533–536.

351 Reman, O., Freymuth, F., Laloum, D., Bonte, J.F. (1986) Neonatal respiratory distress due to mumps. *Archives of Disease in Childhood* **61**, 80–81.

352 Renaudin, H., Bebear, C. (1990) Comparative *in vitro* activity of azithromycin, clarithromycin, erythromycin and lomefloxacin against *Mycoplasma pneumoniae*, *Mycoplasma hominis* and *Ureaplasma urealyticum*. *European Journal of Clinical Microbiology and Infectious Diseases* **9**, 838–841.

353 Reynolds, H.Y. (1988) Immunoglobulin IgG and its function in the human respiratory tract. *Mayo Clinic Proceedings* **63**, 161–174.

354 Riegel, K., Sohne, B., Fischer, P., Ort, B., Wolke, D., Osterlund, K. (1999) Premature rupture of fetal membranes, risk of infection and infant prognosis – a comparison of 2 regions. *Zeitschrift fuer Geburtshilfe und Neonatologie* **203**, 152–160.

355 Rigal, E., Roze, J.C., Villers, D. *et al.* (1990) Prospective evaluation of the protected specimen brush for the

diagnosis of pulmonary infections in ventilated newborns. *Pediatric Pulmonology* **8**, 268–272.

356 Robertson, B. (1980) Basic morphology of the pulmonary defence system. *European Journal of Respiratory Diseases Supplement* **107**, 21–40.

357 Rocha, B.H., Christenson, J.C., Pavia, A., Evans, R.S., Gardner, R.M. (1994) Computerized detection of nosocomial infections in newborns. *Proceedings of the Annual Symposium on Computers in Applied Medical Care* 684–688.

358 Rodriguez, E.M., Hammerschlag, M.R. (1987) Diagnostic methods for *Chlamydia trachomatis* disease in neonates. *Journal of Perinatology* **7**, 232–234.

359 Rojas, J., Stahlman, M. (1984) The effects of group B streptococcus and other organisms on the pulmonary vasculature. *Clinics in Perinatology* **11**, 591–599.

360 Rossi, G.A., Sacco, O., Balbi, B. *et al.* (1990) Human ciliated bronchial epithelial cells; expression of HLA-DR alpha gene, modulation of the HLA-DR antigens by gamma interferon and antigen-presenting function in the mixed leucocyte reaction. *American Journal of Respiratory Cell and Molecular Biology* **3**, 431–439.

361 Rowen, J.L., Lopez, S.M. (1998) *Morganella morganii* early onset sepsis. *Pediatric Infectious Disease Journal* **17**, 1176–1177.

362 Rowen, J.L., Rench, M.A., Kozinetz, C.A., Adams, J.M.J., Baker, C.J. (1994) Endotracheal colonization with *Candida* enhances risk of systemic candidiasis in very low birthweight neonates. *Journal of Pediatrics* **124**, 789–794.

363 Royle, J., Halasz, S., Eagles, G. *et al.* (1999) Outbreak of extended spectrum β-lactamase producing *Klebsiella pneumoniae* in a neonatal unit. *Archives of Disease in Childhood Fetal and Neonatal Edition* **80**, F64–F68.

364 Rudd, P.T., Brown, M.B., Cassell, G.H. (1984) A prospective study of mycoplasma infection in the preterm infant. *Israel Journal of Medical Science* **20**, 899–901.

365 Rusin, P., Adam, R.D., Peterson, E.A., Ryan, K.J., Sinclair, N.A., Weinstein, L. (1991) *Haemophilus influenzae*: an important cause of maternal and neonatal infections. *Obstetrics and Gynecology* **77**, 92–96.

366 Sadiq, H.F., Devaskar, S., Keenan, W.J., Weber, T.R. (1987) Broviac catheterization in low birthweight infants: incidence and treatment of associated complications. *Critical Care Medicine* **15**, 47–50.

367 Sagy, M., Barzilay, Z., Yahav, J., Ginsberg, R., Sompolinsky, D. (1980) Severe neonatal chlamydial pneumonitis. *American Journal of Diseases of Children* **134**, 89–91.

368 Salzman, M.B., Rubin, L.G. (1995) Intravenous catheter-related infections. *Advances in Pediatric Infectious Diseases* **10**, 337–368.

369 Samson, L., MacDonald, N.E. (1995) Management of infants born to mothers who have *Chlamydia* infection. *Pediatric Infectious Disease Journal* **14**, 407–408.

370 Sanchez, P.J. (1993) Perinatal transmission of *Ureaplasma urealyticum*: current concepts based on review of the literature. *Clinical Infectious Diseases* **17**(Suppl 1), S107–S111.

371 Sarff, I.D., McCracken, G.H., Schiffer, M.S. *et al.* (1975) Epidemiology of *Escherichia coli* K1 in healthy and diseased newborns. *Lancet* **1**, 1099–1104.

372 Sauerbrei, A., Wutzler, P. (2001) Neonatal varicella. *Journal of Perinatology* **21**, 545–549.

373 Schacter, J., Ridgeway, G.L., Collier, L. (1998) Chlamydial diseases. In Collier, L., Balows, A., Sussman, M. (eds), *Topley and Wilson's Microbiology and Microbial Infections*, Volume 3, *Bacterial Infections*, 9th edition. London: Arnold, 977–995.

374 Schieve, L.A., Handler, A., Hershow, R., Persky, V., Davis, F. (1994) Urinary tract infection during pregnancy: its association with maternal morbidity and perinatal outcome. *American Journal of Public Health* **84**, 405–410.

375 Schiff, D.E., Stonestreet, B.S. (1993) Central venous catheters in low birth weight infants: incidence of related complications. *Journal of Perinatology* **13**, 153–158.

376 Schreiber, M.D., Covert, R.F., Torgerson, L.J. (1992) Hemodynamic effects of heat-killed group B beta-hemolytic streptococcus in newborn lambs: role of leukotriene D4. *Pediatric Research* **31**, 121–126.

377 Schuchat, A., Lizano, C., Broome, C.V., Swaminathan, B., Kim, C., Winn, K. (1991) Outbreak of neonatal listeriosis associated with mineral oil. *Pediatric Infectious Disease Journal* **10**, 183–189.

378 Schutze, G.E., Edwards, M.S., Adham, B.I., Belmont, J.W. (1990) Hyperammonemia and neonatal herpes simplex pneumonitis. *Pediatric Infectious Disease Journal* **9**, 749–750.

379 Schwebke, K., Henry, K., Balfour, H.H.J., Olson, D., Crane, R.T., Jordan, M.C. (1995) Congenital cytomegalovirus infection as a result of nonprimary cytomegalovirus disease in a mother with acquired immunodeficiency syndrome. *Journal of Pediatrics* **126**, 293–295.

380 Scott, J.M., Henderson, A. 1972 Acute villous inflammation in the placenta following intrauterine transfusion. *Journal of Clinical Pathology* **25**, 872–875.

381 Sethi, S., Sharma, M., Narang, A., Aggrawal, P.B. (1999) Isolation pattern and clinical outcome of genital mycoplasma in neonates from a tertiary care neonatal unit. *Journal of Tropical Pediatrics* **45**, 143–145.

382 Sgrignoli, A.R., Yen, D.R., Hutchins, G.M. (1994) Giant cell and lymphocytic interstitial pneumonia associated with fetal pneumonia. *Pediatric Pathology* **14**, 955–965.

383 Shalev, E., Battino, S., Romano, S., Blondhaim, O., Ben Ami, M. (1994) Intra-amniotic infection with *Candida albicans* successfully treated with transcervical amnioinfusion of amphotericin. *American Journal of Obstetrics and Gynecology* **170**, 1271–1272.

384 Shamir, R., Horev, G., Merlob, P., Nutman, J. (1990) *Citrobacter diversus* lung abscess in a preterm infant. *Pediatric Infectious Disease Journal* **9**, 221–222.

385 Sherman, M.P., Goetzman, B.W., Ahlfors, C.E., Wennberg, R.P. (1980) Tracheal asiration and its clinical correlates in the diagnosis of congenital pneumonia. *Pediatrics* **65**, 258–263.

386 Sherman, M.P., Campbell, L.A., Merritt, T.A. *et al.* (1994) Effect of different surfactants on pulmonary group B streptococcal infection in premature rabbits. *Journal of Pediatrics* **125**, 939–947.

387 Shikes, R.H., Ryder, J.W. (1989) Case 5. Adenovirus pneumonia in a newborn. *Pediatric Pathology* **9**, 199–202.

388 Sibille, Y., Reynolds, H.Y. (1990) Macrophages and polymorphonuclear neutrophils in lung defence and injury: state of the art. *American Review of Respiratory Disease* **141**, 471–501.

389 Sibille, Y., Naegel, G.P., Merrill, W., Young, K.R., Care, S.B., Reynolds, H.Y. (1987) Neutrophil chemotactic activity produced by normal and activated human bronchoalveolar lavage cells. *Journal of Laboratory and Clinical Medicine* **110**, 624–633.

390 Siegel, J.D., McCracken, G.H., Jr (1979) Neonatal lung abscess. A report of six cases. *American Journal of Diseases of Children* **133**, 947–949.

391 Simoes, E.A., King, S.J., Lehr, M.V., Groothuis, J.R. (1993) Preterm twins and triplets. A high-risk group for severe

respiratory syncytial virus infection. *American Journal of Diseases of Children* **147**, 303–306.

392 Singh-Naz, N., Willy, M., Riggs, N. (1990) Outbreak of parainfluenza virus type 3 in a neonatal nursery. *Pediatric Infectious Disease Journal* **9**, 31–33.

393 Sison, A.V. (1992) Maternal and fetal infections. *Current Opinion in Obstetrics and Gynecology* **4**, 48–54.

394 Sizun, J., Soupre, D., Legrand, M.C. *et al.* (1995) Neonatal nosocomial respiratory infection with coronavirus: a prospective study in a neonatal intensive care unit. *Acta Paediatrica* **84**, 617–620.

395 Sly, P.D., Soto-Quiros, M.E., Landau, L.I., Hudson, I., Newton-John, H. (1984) Factors predisposing to abnormal pulmonary function after adenovirus type 7 pneumonia. *Archives of Disease in Childhood* **59**, 935–939.

396 Smith, H., Congdon, P. (1985) Neonatal systemic candidiasis. *Archives of Disease in Childhood* **60**, 365–369.

397 Sollecito, D., Midulla, M., Bavastrelli, M. *et al.* (1992) *Chlamydia trachomatis* in neonatal respiratory distress of very preterm babies: biphasic clinical picture. *Acta Paediatrica* **81**, 788–791.

398 Sorg, S. (1998) Dendritic cell function in the neonate. *Vaccine* **100**, 1–10.

399 Sorrentino, M., Powers, T. (2000) Effectiveness of palivizumab: evaluation of outcomes from the 1998 to 1999 respiratory syncytial virus season. The Palivizumab Outcomes Study Group. *Pediatric Infectious Disease Journal* **19**, 1068–1071.

400 Stagno, S., Brasfield, D.M., Brown, M.B. *et al.* (1981) Infant pneumonitis associated with cytomegalovirus, *Chlamydia*, *Pneumocystis*, and *Ureaplasma*: a prospective study. *Pediatrics* **68**, 322–329.

401 Starke, J.R. (1994) Perinatal tuberculosis. *Seminars in Pediatric Infectious Diseases* **5**, 20–29.

402 Stewart, D.L., Cook, L.N., Rabalais, G.P. (1993) Successful use of extracorporeal membrane oxygenation in a newborn with herpes simplex virus pneumonia. *Pediatric Infectious Disease Journal* **12**, 161–162.

403 Stiller, R.J., Blair, E., Clark, P., Tinghitella, T. (1989) Rapid detection of vaginal colonization with group B streptococci by means of latex agglutination. *American Journal of Obstetrics and Gynecology* **160**, 566–568.

404 Stoll, B., Gordon, T., Korones, S.B. *et al.* (1996) Late-onset sepsis in very low birthweight neonates: a report from the National Institute of Child Health and Human Development Neonatal Research Network. *Journal of Pediatrics* **129**, 63–71.

405 Stroobant, J., Harris, M.C., Cody, C.S., Polin, R.A., Douglas, S.D. (1984) Diminished bactericidal capacity for group B Streptococcus in neutrophils from stressed and healthy neonates. *Pediatric Research* **18**, 634–637.

406 Sun, C.C., Duara, S. (1985) Fatal adenovirus pneumonia in two newborn infants, one case caused by adenovirus type 30. *Pediatric Pathology* **4**, 247–255.

407 Takami, T., Sonodat, S., Houjyo, H. *et al.* (2000) Diagnosis of horizontal enterovirus infections in neonates by nested PCR and direct sequence analysis. *Journal of Hospital Infection* **45**, 283–287.

408 Tam, A.Y., Yung, R.W., Fu, K.H. (1989) Fatal pneumonia caused by *Flavobacterium meningosepticum*. *Pediatric Infectious Disease Journal* **8**, 252–254.

409 Thompson, P.J., Greenough, A., Hird, M.F., Philpott-Howard, J., Gamsu, H.R. (1992) Nosocomial bacterial infections in very low birthweight infants. *European Journal of Pediatrics* **151**, 451–454.

410 Thorp, J.M., Jr, Katz, V.L., Fowler, L.J., Kurtzman, J.T., Bowes, W.A., Jr (1989) Fetal death from chlamydial infection across intact amniotic membranes. *American Journal of Obstetrics and Gynecology* **161**, 1245–1246.

411 Thureen, P.J., Moreland, S., Rodden, D.J., Merenstein, G.B., Levin, M., Rosenberg, A.A. (1993) Failure of tracheal aspirate cultures to define the cause of respiratory deteriorations in neonates. *Pediatric Infectious Disease Journal* **12**, 560–564.

412 Tipple, M.A., Beem, M.O., Saxon, E.M. (1979) Clinical characteristics of the afebrile pneumonia syndrome associated with *Chlamydia trachomatis* infection in infants less than six months. *Pediatrics* **63**, 192–197.

413 Toce, S.S., Keenan, W.J. (1988) Congenital echovirus 11 pneumonia in association with pulmonary hypertension. *Pediatric Infectious Disease Journal* **7**, 360–362.

414 Tookey, P., Peckham, C.S. (1996) Neonatal herpes simplex virus infection in the British Isles. *Paediatric and Perinatal Epidemiology* **10**, 432–442.

415 Tramont, E.C. (2000) *Treponema pallidum* (syphilis). In Mandell, G.L., Bennett, J.E., Dolin, R. (eds), *Mandell, Douglas and Bennett's Principles and Practice of Infectious Diseases*, 5th edition. Philadelphia: Churchill Livingstone, 2472–2490.

416 Tsang, K.W.T., Rutman, A., Kanthakumar, K. (1994) Interaction of *Pseudomonas aeruginosa* with human respiratory mucus *in vitro*. *European Respiratory Journal* **7**, 1746–1753.

417 Tuppurainen, N., Hallman, M. (1989) Prevention of neonatal group B streptococcal disease: intrapartum detection and chemoprophylaxis of heavily colonised parturients. *Obstetrics and Gynecology* **73**, 583–587.

418 Turkel, S.B., Pettross, C.W., Appleman, M.D., Salminen, C.A., Yonekura, M.L. (1986) Perinatal mortality associated with intrauterine infection due to pseudomonads. *Pediatric Pathology* **6**, 131–137.

419 Uehara, Y., Kikuchi, K., Nakamura, T. (2001) Inhibition of methicillin resistant *Staphylococcus aureus* colonization of oral cavities in newborns by viridans group streptococci. *Clinical Infectious Diseases* **32**, 1399–1407.

420 Unger, A., Tapia, L., Minnich, L.L., Ray, C.G. (1982) Atypical neonatal respiratory syncytial virus infection. *Journal of Pediatrics* **100**, 762–764.

421 United States National Institute of Child Health and Human Development Study Group (1976) Mid-trimester amniocentesis for prenatal diagnosis. Safety and efficacy. *Journal of the American Medical Association* **236**, 1471–1476.

422 Unsworth, P.F., Taylor-Robinson, D., Shoo, E.E., Furr, P.M. (1985) Neonatal mycoplasmaemia: *Mycoplasma hominis* as a significant cause of disease? *Journal of Infection* **10**, 163–168.

423 Ursi, D., Ursi, J.P., Ieven, M., Docx, M., Van Reempts, P., Pattyn, S.R. (1995) Congenital pneumonia due to *Mycoplasma pneumoniae*. *Archives of Disease in Childhood Fetal and Neonatal Edition* **72**, F118–F120.

424 Valencia, G.B., Banzon, F., Cummings, M., McCormack, W.M., Glass, L., Hammerschlag, M.R. (1993) *Mycoplasma hominis* and *Ureaplasma urealyticum* in neonates with suspected infection. *Pediatric Infectious Disease Journal* **12**, 571–573.

425 Valenti, W.M., Clarke, T.A., Hall, C.B., Menegus, M.A., Shapiro, D.L. (1982) Concurrent outbreaks of rhinovirus and respiratory syncytial virus in an intensive care nursery: epidemiology and associated risk factors. *Journal of Pediatrics* **100**, 722–726.

426 Valentin Weigand, P., Chhatwal, G.S. (1995) Correlation of epithelial cell invasiveness of group B streptococci with clinical source of isolation. *Microbial Pathogenesis* **19**, 83–91.

427 Vallette, J.D., Jr, Goldberg, R.N., Suguihara, C. et al. (1995) Effect of an interleukin-1 receptor antagonist on the hemodynamic manifestations of group B streptococcal sepsis. *Pediatric Research* **38**, 704–708.

428 van As, A. (1980) Pulmonary airway defence mechanisms: an appreciation of integrated mucociliary activity. *European Journal of Respiratory Diseases Supplement* **111**, 21–24.

429 Van Overmeire, B., Bleyart, S., Van Reempts, P., Van Assche, F.A. (1993) The use of intravenously administered immunoglobulins in the prevention of severe infections in very low birthweight neonates. *Biology of the Neonate* **64**, 110–115.

430 Van Winter, J.T., Ney, J.A., Ogburn, P.L.J., Johnson, R.V. (1994) Preterm labor and congenital candidiasis. A case report. *Journal of Reproductive Medicine* **39**, 987–990.

431 Vassallo, R., Thomas, C.F., Jr, Vuk-Pavlovic, Z., Limper, A.H. (2000) Mechanisms of defence in the lung: lessons from *Pneumocystis carinii* pneumonia. *Sarcoidosis and Vascular Diffuse Lung Disease* **17**, 130–139.

432 Ventura, F., Cheseaux, J.J., Cotting, J., Guignard, J.P. (1998) Is the use of ribavirin aerosols in respiratory syncytial virus infections justified? Clinical and economic evaluation. *Archives of Pediatrics* **5**, 123–131.

433 Villari, P., Sarnataro, C., Jacuzio, L. (2000) Molecular epidemiology of *Staphylococcus epidermidis* in a neonatal intensive care unit over a three-year period. *Journal of Clinical Microbiology* **38**, 1740–1746.

434 Villegas, C.H., Morales, J.M., Peralta, O.L., Najera, R.S., Flores, R.E. (1997) Ultrastructure of the tracheal epithelium in preterm neonates treated with mechanical ventilation. *Ginecologia y Obstetrica de Mexico* **65**, 194–201.

435 Vogel, L.C., Boyer, K.M., Gadzala, C.A., Gotoff, S.P. (1980) Prevalence of type-specific group B streptococcal antibody in pregnant women. *Journal of Pediatrics* **96**, 1047–1051.

436 Voisin, C., Carre, P., Piva, F., Wallaert, B. (1987) Alveolar macrophages and antibiotics. Review. *Pathologie Biologie (Paris)* **35**, 1412–1417.

437 Vos, G.D., Rijtema, M.N., Blanco, C.E. (1996) Treatment of respiratory failure due to respiratory syncytial virus pneumonia with natural surfactant. *Pediatric Pulmonology* **22**, 412–415.

438 Waggoner-Fountain, L.A., Donowitz, L.G. (1997) Infection in the newborn. In Wenzel, R.P. (ed.), *Prevention and Control of Nosocomial Infections*, 3rd edition. Baltimore: Williams & Wilkins, 1019–1038.

439 Waites, K.B., Cassell, G.H., Canupp, K.C., Fernandes, P.B. (1988) *In vitro* susceptibilities of mycoplasmas and ureaplasmas to new macrolides and aryl-fluoroquinolones. *Antimicrobial Agents and Chemotherapy* **32**, 1500–1502.

440 Waites, K.B., Crouse, D.T., Philips, J.B., III, Canupp, K.C., Cassell, G.H. (1989) Ureaplasmal pneumonia and sepsis associated with persistent pulmonary hypertension of the newborn. *Pediatrics* **83**, 79–85.

441 Waites, K.B., Crouse, D.T., Cassell, G.H. (1993) Therapeutic considerations for *Ureaplasma urealyticum* infections in neonates. *Clinical Infectious Diseases* **17**(Suppl 1), S208–S214.

442 Walti, H., Tordet, C., Gerbaut, L., Saugier, P., Moriette, G., Relier, J.P. (1989) Persistent elastase/proteinase inhibitor imbalance during prolonged ventilation of infants with bronchopulmonary dysplasia: evidence for the role of nosocomial infections. *Pediatric Research* **26**, 351–355.

443 Wareham, J., Harris, H., Whitman, I. (1995) Herpes simplex type II infection in monozygotic twins. *American Journal of Perinatology* **12**, 75–77.

444 Webber, S., Wilkinson, A.R., Lindsell, D., Hope, P.L., Dobson, S.R., Isaacs, D. (1990) Neonatal pneumonia. *Archives of Disease in Childhood* **65**, 207–211.

445 Weese-Mayer, D.E., Fondriest, D.W., Brouillette, R.T., Schulman, S.T. (1987) Risk factors associated with candidaemia in the neonatal intensive care unit. *Pediatric Infectious Disease Journal* **6**, 190–196.

446 Weisman, L.E., Lorenzetti, P.M. (1989) High intravenous doses of human immune globulin suppress neonatal group B streptococcal immunity in rats. *Journal of Pediatrics* **115**, 445–450.

447 Weisman, L.E., Stoll, B.J., Cruess, D.F. (1992) Early-onset group B streptococcal disease; a current assessment. *Journal of Pediatrics* **121**, 428–433.

448 Weisman, L.E., Stoll, B.J., Kueser, T.J. et al. (1992) Intravenous immune globulin therapy for early-onset sepsis in premature neonates. *Journal of Pediatrics* **121**, 434–443.

449 Weisman, L.E., Cruess, D.F., Fischer, G.W. (1993) Standard versus hyperimmune intravenous immunoglobulin in preventing or treating neonatal bacterial infections. *Clinics in Perinatology* **20**, 211–224.

450 Weiss, S.G., Newcomb, R.W., Beem, M.O. (1986) Pulmonary assessment of children after chlamydial pneumonia of infancy. *Journal of Pediatrics* **108**, 659–664.

451 Wen, T.S., Eriksen, N.L., Blanco, J.D., Graham, J.M., Oshiro, B.T., Prieto, J.A. (1993) Association of clinical intra-amniotic infection and meconium. *American Journal of Perinatology* **10**, 438–440.

452 Whyte, R.K., Hussain, Z., deSa, D. (1982) Antenatal infections with *Candida* species. *Archives of Disease in Childhood* **57**, 528–535.

453 Williams, P.A., Bohnsack, J.F., Augustine, N.H., Drummond, W.K., Rubens, C.E., Hill, H.R. (1993) Production of tumor necrosis factor by human cells *in vitro* and *in vivo*, induced by group B streptococci. *Journal of Pediatrics* **123**, 292–300.

454 Wilson, R. (1988) Secondary ciliary dysfunction. *Clinical Science* **75**, 113–120.

455 Wilson, R., Pitt, T., Taylor, G. et al. (1987) Pyocyanine and 1-hydroxyphenazine products by *Pseudomonas aeruginosa* inhibit the beating of human respiratory cilia *in vitro*. *Journal of Clinical Investigation* **79**, 221–229.

456 Wilson, R., Dowling, R.B., Jackson, A.D. (1996) The biology of bacterial colonization and invasion of the respiratory mucosa. *European Respiratory Journal* **9**, 1523–1530.

457 Wong, S.N., Ng, T.L. (1991) *Haemophilus influenzae* septicaemia in the neonate: report of two cases and review of the English literature. *Journal of Paediatrics and Child Health* **27**, 113–115.

458 Wright, E.D., Lortan, J.E., Perinpanayagam, R.M. (1990) Early-onset neonatal pneumococcal sepsis in siblings. *Journal of Infection* **20**, 59–63.

459 Yagupsky, P., Menegus, M.A., Powell, K.R. (1991) The changing spectrum of group B streptococcal disease in infants: an eleven-year experience in a tertiary care hospital. *Pediatric Infectious Disease Journal* **10**, 801–808.

460 Yohannan, M.D., Vijayakumaran, E., Remo, C., al Mofada, S. (1992) Congenital pneumonia and early neonatal septicemia due to *Bacteroides fragilis*. *European Journal of Clinical Microbiology and Infectious Diseases* **11**, 472–473.

461 Yuksel, B., Greenough, A. (1992) Acute deteriorations in neonatal chronic lung disease. *European Journal of Pediatrics* **151**, 697–700.

462 Yuksel, B., Greenough, A. (1994) Viral infections acquired during neonatal intensive care and lung function of preterm infants at follow-up. *Acta Paediatrica* **83**, 117–118.

463 Zollar, L.M., Krause, H.E., Mufson, M.A. (1973) Microbiologic studies on young infants with lower respiratory tract disease. *American Journal of Diseases of Children* **126**, 56–60.

Air leaks

ANNE GREENOUGH

Pulmonary air leaks are the result of alveolar overdistention with resultant tissue rupture at the alveolar bases. The alveolar overdistention occurs in conditions associated with high transpulmonary pressure swings, air trapping and uneven alveolar ventilation. The alveolar connecting channels, the pores of Kohn, are reduced in immature infants,[102] which exacerbates uneven ventilation. Once tissue rupture has occurred, gas tracks to the mediastinum along the sheaths of the pulmonary blood vessels, which are in apposition to the alveolar bases. The interstitial air may track to the mediastinum to form a pneumomediastinum or penetrate directly into the pleural cavity to cause a pneumothorax. A pneumothorax may also occur if a subpleural bleb ruptures.[135] Air from the pneumomediastinum can move to extrathoracic areas, resulting in subcutaneous emphysema or rupture into the pleural cavity to form a pneumothorax.[103] The type of pulmonary air leak produced is determined by the direction and ease with which the gas can then move. The movement of gas is impeded by the presence of connective tissue, which is more extensive in the immature infant than in the adult. High levels of interstitial water, also found in premature infants, particularly those with respiratory distress syndrome (RDS), impede gas flow along the perivascular spaces. In such patients, widespread interstitial emphysema is more likely to occur than a pneumothorax.[146]

PNEUMOTHORAX

Incidence

One percent of infants develop a spontaneous pneumothorax around the time of birth, although only 10 percent of these are symptomatic.[160] Fifteen to 20 percent are bilateral and two-thirds of unilateral pneumothoraces occur on the right. It might be predicted from the lung structure of the immature infant and findings in an animal model that greater pressures would be necessary to rupture lungs of preterm infants[2] and that the incidence of pneumothorax would correlate directly with postconceptional age. Clinical experience, however, does not corroborate that supposition; McIntosh[110] reported an inverse trend with gestational age and Greenough et al.[60] found no relationship between gestational age and pneumothorax occurrence. The incidence of air leaks amongst ventilated preterm infants during the 1980s and early 1990s decreased, but during the last few years the incidence appears relatively stable (Table 22.1).

Etiology

SPONTANEOUS

Spontaneous pneumothoraces occur in the immediate perinatal period.[25,160] These may result from high transpulmonary pressures sometimes generated during an infant's first breaths,[174] or as a result of congenital bullae. Familial spontaneous pneumothoraces have usually been reported in adolescents or adults with males predominating. The etiology in older children and adults includes pulmonary blebs, emphysematous changes in the lung, asthma, tuberculosis and Marfan's syndrome. Reports of familial spontaneous pneumothorax (FSP) in neonates are very rare.[42] The mode of inheritance of FSP has not been clearly defined. It may be autosomal dominant or an X-linked pattern, while others have suggested an HLA association.[1,134,153]

Table 22.1 *Incidence of air leaks data from Rosie Maternity Hospital Cambridge*

Year	Pneumothorax	PIE
1985	30	38
1986	33	28
1987	30	26
1988	25	22
1989	N/A	N/A
1990	25	18
1991	15	18
1992	20	22
1995	19	
1996	17	
1997	31	21
1998	16	18
1999	19	22

Data are expressed as the percentage of VLBW ventilated infants. N/A, not available. Reproduced with kind permission from J. Rennie and J. Ahluwahlia (all infants received artificial lung expanding compound).

COMPLICATIONS OF OTHER RESPIRATORY DISORDERS

Pneumothoraces are more likely to occur in infants with underlying lung pathology, particularly where there is non-uniform compliance and uneven alveolar ventilation. Infants with all types of aspiration syndrome are particularly at risk; the gas trapping which occurs can result in alveolar overdistension and hence a pneumothorax. The need for respiratory support is increased in infants with respiratory disease, further predisposing to air leak (see below).

RESPIRATORY SUPPORT

The incidence of air leak was reported to relate to the level of respiratory support used, being 4 percent in infants receiving oxygen only, 16 percent in infants on continuous positive airways pressure (CPAP) and 34 percent in those fully ventilated.[105] Studies performed in the 1970s and 1980s incriminated certain features of so-called 'conventional' ventilation as increasing the likelihood of air leak. In an uncontrolled study,[14] comparison to historical controls demonstrated that employment of PEEP during ventilatory support increased the pneumothorax rate from 21 to 34 percent. Long inflation times[140] and an inspiratory:expiratory (I:E) ratio $\geq$ 1:1[166] were also associated with an increased incidence of pneumothorax. A prolonged inspiratory time is more likely to provoke active expiration,[55] an interaction significantly associated with the development of pneumothorax (see below). High inflation pressures have been suggested to increase the pneumothorax rate,[60,129] but in a third study,[166] lowering peak pressures did not reduce the incidence of air leak. Nevertheless, a MAP greater than compared to less than 12 cmH$_2$O was associated with a 39 percent rather than a 17 percent pneumothorax rate.[165]

PATIENT–VENTILATOR INTERACTION

Infants who fight the ventilator, that is actively expire during positive pressure inflation, have an increased incidence of pneumothorax.[59] This interaction is a manifestation of the active expiratory component of the Hering–Breuer reflex.[77] Prolongation of inflation time or reducing ventilator rate while keeping the I:E ratio constant provokes active expiration,[44] particularly if the start of a square wave positive pressure inflation is delivered at the end of spontaneous inspiration.[55]

INSPIRED GAS TEMPERATURE

Amongst VLBW infants, maintaining the inspired gas temperature >36.5°C rather than at or below that temperature was associated with a reduction in the pneumothorax rate from 43 to 13 percent. As, at the lower gas temperature the inspired gas water content was only 28–36 mgH$_2$O/l, impaired mucociliary clearance precipitating airway obstruction might explain the higher pneumothorax rate.[167]

DIRECT INJURY

Suction catheters passed down the endotracheal tube rarely cause a pneumothorax (p. 236).[6] The most common site of injury is the right lower lobe bronchus.[173] Central venous catheter placement has also been associated with the development of a pneumothorax.[50]

Clinical signs

A large pneumothorax, particularly in an immature infant, is often heralded by a sudden deterioration, with a marked reduction in arterial blood pressure (this occurred in 77 percent of infants in one series[128]) and a fall in heart rate. Oxygenation deteriorates, but pH and PaCO$_2$ show no consistent change.[128] On examination, there is loss of air entry on the affected side. A tension pneumothorax results in shift of both the mediastinum and position of the cardiac impulse. Abdominal distention may occur due to downward displacement of the diaphragm by the tension pneumothorax. In a ventilated infant, reduced chest wall movement can indicate a tension pneumothorax, as the extra-alveolar air expands the chest wall to its elastic limit, reducing its compliance. Pneumothoraces are associated with raised arginine vasopressin levels.[161] This may lead to fluid retention, which may be further aggravated by administration of a neuromuscular blocking agent (p. 316).

'Paradoxical symmetry of the chest' has been described as a clinical sign of unilateral pneumothorax.[36] In health, rotation of the neck causes the hemithorax on the side to which the head is turned to be less prominent than on the other side. If the chest is symmetrical when the head is rotated, then the hemithorax on the side to which the head is turned is as prominent as the contralateral side, which is not the norm. Any space-occupying lesion, however, could be associated with this appearance. Thus, the differential diagnosis includes unilateral pneumothorax, lobar emphysema, hydrothorax, hemothorax, chylothorax and masses.

Retrospective evaluation of computerized trends in transcutaneous carbon dioxide ($TcCO_2$) and oxygen tensions demonstrated that the clinical diagnosis of pneumothorax occurs late when infants have decompensated.[112] Forty-two consecutive cases of pneumothorax were diagnosed at a median of 27 minutes (range 45–660 minutes) after the event. In at least 40 percent of cases the infants had been reintubated prior to the diagnosis being made. Trend analysis monitoring of $TcCO_2$ was suggested to allow earlier diagnosis. Reference centiles for the level of $TcCO_2$ and the slope of the trended $TcCO_2$ over various time intervals were constructed. The 5-minute $TcCO_2$ trend slopes were compared between those with pneumothorax and matched control infants. This revealed that the presence of five consecutive and overlapping 5-minute slopes greater than the ninetieth percentile showed good discrimination for a pneumothorax.

Differential diagnosis

The chest radiograph appearance may, rarely, be confused with lobar emphysema, cystic adenomatoid malformation of the lung or congenital diaphragmatic hernia.[95] A bronchogenic cyst may be mistaken for a medial pneumothorax.[152]

Diagnosis

Changes in the transthoracic electrical impedance signal[84] or intraesophageal pressure swings[124] have been suggested to indicate a pneumothorax. In addition, the electrocardiogram (ECG) may become of low amplitude. Transillumination[85] with an intense beam from a fiberoptic light can identify abnormal air collections by an increased transmission of light on the involved side. Unfortunately, a pneumothorax and pulmonary interstitial emphysema (PIE) give a similar appearance on transillumination.

Chest radiograph

The chest radiograph remains the gold standard in the diagnosis of pneumothorax. A small pneumothorax may

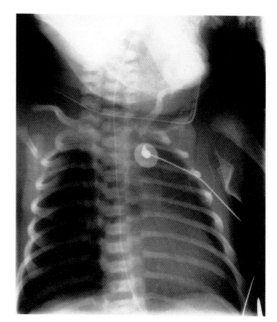

Figure 22.1 *Right-sided pneumothorax of the two lung fields with discrepant translucency.*

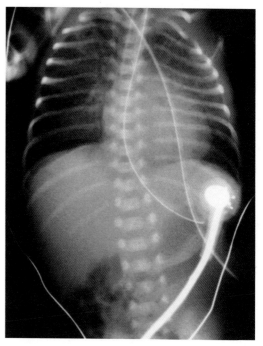

Figure 22.2 *Small right-sided anterior pneumothorax demonstrated by air just above the diaphragm and bulging of the intercostal spaces.*

only be recognized by the difference in radiolucency of the two lung fields (Figures 22.1 and 22.2).[164] The lack of lung markings and collapsed lung on the ipsilateral side will demonstrate a large pneumothorax, but if the lung is noncompliant it may not collapse and the visceral pleural line can be identified (Figures 22.3 and 22.4). In the presence of

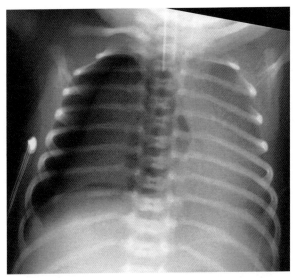

Figure 22.3 *Right-sided tension pneumothorax with mediastinal shift. Both lungs demonstrate opacification of alveolar collapse.*

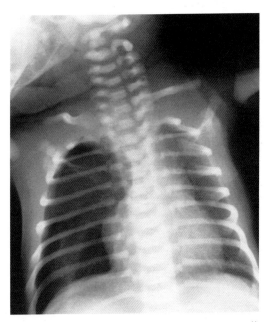

Figure 22.4 *Right-sided pneumothorax: the non-compliant lung has not collapsed completely and the visceral pleural line can be identified.*

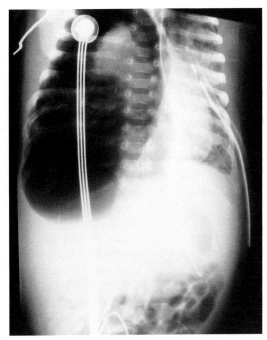

Figure 22.5 *Large right-sided pneumothorax under tension with herniation of air across the midline; there is compression of the underlying right lung.*

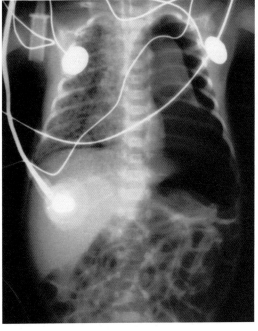

Figure 22.6 *Left-sided pneumothorax under tension. There is pulmonary interstitial emphysema in the right lung and a small basal right pneumothorax.*

a tension pneumothorax, the diaphragm may be everted, there is bulging of the intercostal spaces and mediastinal shift (Figures 22.5 and 22.6). The chest radiograph appearance may be confused by a coexistent pneumomediastinum (Figure 22.7). A film taken by a horizontal beam with the infant in the supine position is useful in demonstrating an anterior collection of air.[101] A lateral view will show whether there is any retrosternal air (Figures 22.7 and 22.8); this is a common position for extra-alveolar air, as air rises to the uppermost region and ill ventilated infants are usually nursed in the supine position.

Prophylaxis

RESPIRATORY SUPPORT MODES (p. 159)

The impact of ventilatory modes on pneumothorax rate has been investigated in a number of randomized trials;

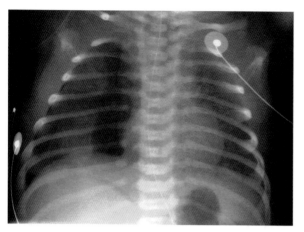

Figure 22.7 *Chest radiograph demonstrating a pneumothorax and a pneumomediastinum complicating RDS. Air is also noted outlying the posterior diaphragmatic recess of the pleura.*

they have yielded conflicting results. Thus, systematic reviews of the randomized trials will be considered.

High-frequency positive pressure ventilation (HFPPV)

In the 1980s, it was noted that increasing ventilator rates to 60 bpm or more using a 'conventional' ventilator reduced active expiration[44,62] and provoked synchronous respiration in the majority of patients.[57,62,63] Perhaps as a consequence, infants ventilated at rates in excess of 60 breaths/min rather than 30–40/min have been shown to have a lower incidence of air leaks in a number of studies.[71,131,136] Meta-analysis of the results of those randomized trials[66] demonstrated that fast versus slow rates on conventional ventilators are associated with a significantly lower rate of air leaks [relative risk (RR) 0.69, 95 percent CI 0.51, 0.93]. All of the trials, however, were performed prior to the routine use of antenatal steroids and postnatal surfactant and whether a similar advantageous effect would be seen in the present population of preterm infants is not known.

Patient-triggered ventilation (PTV)

Comparison with historical controls suggested that infants supported by PTV might have a lower pneumothorax rate.[29] That, however, has not been confirmed by meta-analysis of the results of six randomized trials; RR for air leak was 1.03 (95 percent CI 0.80,1.34).[66] In one trial,[13] amongst very immature infants, there was a tendency for a greater proportion of those supported on PTV rather than conventional mechanical ventilation (CMV) to develop air leaks. During PTV, if there is a long trigger delay, inflation will extend into expiration and thus could provoke active expiration and hence pneumothoraces (p. 163). In the multicenter trial,[13] the majority of the infants were supported by a ventilator which incorporates an airway pressure trigger. In very immature infants, that airway pressure trigger has a long trigger delay and high rate of

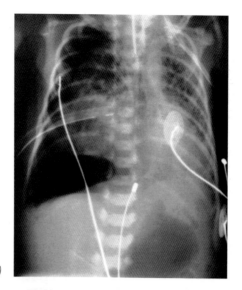

(a)

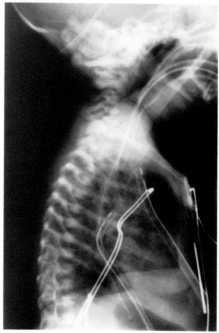

(b)

Figure 22.8 *(a) A loculated anterior pneumothorax with inadequate decompression by a posterior sited drain. (b) A lateral film of the same infant demonstrates the second drain has been directed into the anterior component and has drained the air.*

asynchrony.[38] Even in very immature infants, asynchrony can be dramatically reduced during PTV by employing a trigger device sensing not only the beginning but also the end of spontaneous inspiration and terminating each inflation accordingly.[39] Whether use of such devices will reduce the pneumothorax rate during PTV needs to be tested in a randomized trial.

High-frequency oscillation (HFO) (p. 172)

Meta-analysis of randomized trials comparing HFO and CMV commenced in the first 24 hours after birth has not

Table 22.2 *Non-depolarizing muscle blockers*

	Dose	Half-life (min)	Interactions
Pancuronium	0.06–0.1 mg/kg 0.05–0.2 mg/kg/h	30–40	No histamine release May be enhanced or prolonged
Vecuronium	2–10 µg/kg	20–30	by aminoglycosides or polymyxins Reduce dose in renal failure
Atracurium	0.3–0.6 mg/kg/h	15–35	Histamine release may occur

demonstrated that HFO reduces the pneumothorax rate. Indeed, if a high volume strategy was used, HFO was associated with a significant excess of air leaks (RR 1.40, 95 percent; CI 0.92, 2.15).[72] When HFO is used in infants with severe RDS, a more favorable result may be achieved. In the HIFO Study infants,[74] all receiving peak pressures >25 cmH$_2$O and less than 48 hours of age were randomized to receive CMV or HFO. The HFO group had a significantly lower incidence of new air leak (RR 0.73; 95 percent CI 0.55, 0.96). There were, however, no significant differences in the proportions suffering PIE, mortality and the rate of intraventricular hemorrhage (IVH) was increased in the infants supported by HFO (relative rate 1.77; 95 percent CI 1.06, 2.96).

Suppression of respiratory activity

As infants who fight the ventilator are at increased risk of pneumothorax, suppression of respiratory activity should then reduce that disadvantageous outcome. Initial studies, however, demonstrated that administration of neuromuscular blocking agents to all infants reduces mortality[73] and chronic lung disease[138] but not pneumothorax. The likely explanation for those results is that when treatment is given to all infants, this will include those whose respiratory efforts were synchronous with mechanical inflation. Paralysis of such infants will necessitate an increase in peak pressure to maintain adequate ventilation, thus exposing them to an increased risk of pneumothorax. Selective paralysis, that is paralyzing only infants thought to be fighting the ventilator, can prevent pneumothorax.[32,61] It is important to use a reliable method of detection of fighting the ventilator if selective paralysis is to be successful. In a study in which only a clinical diagnosis was used,[154] selective paralysis was no more efficacious in preventing pneumothoraces than universal paralysis. Fighting the ventilator can be diagnosed clinically, but this is not reliable unless infants are studied at two ventilator rates.[56] Fighting the ventilator is most accurately diagnosed by detailed physiological studies.[61,147] Others[94] have suggested increased fluctuation between the maximum and minimum systolic peaks and a high variability (a coefficient of variation exceeding 10 percent) on the arterial blood pressure recording may also be used as a diagnostic criterion for fighting the ventilator.

Agents used to suppress respiratory activity

In randomized trials, selective use of pancuronium has been found to reduce air leaks. Pancuronium is an

Table 22.3 *Major analgesics*

Analgesic	Dose	Infusion compatibilities
Morphine	10–40 µg/kg/h	5 percent dextrose
Pethidine	0.5–1.0 mg/kg/h	5 percent dextrose
Fentanyl	4–8 µg/mg/h 15 µg/kg	All
Diamorphine	15 µg/kg/h 50 µg/kg	10 percent dextrose

example of a non-depolarizing blocking agent (Table 22.2). Pancuronium and vecuronium are primarily renally excreted, although their duration of action may be prolonged in hepatic failure. The half-lives of the non-depolarizing blocking agents are prolonged in sick neonates. Accidental disconnection from the ventilator of a paralyzed infant leads to severe hypoxia. When a paralyzing agent is administered to an infant on a conventional ventilator, the inspiratory pressure should be increased by approximately 6 cmH$_2$O immediately prior to the first dose to ensure maintenance of oxygenation.[64] In addition, ventilator rate should be reduced to 60 breaths/min or less to avoid gas trapping.[76] Cardiovascular effects of pancuronium are uncommon;[111] this is not surprising as pancuronium has very little ganglion blockade action. Prolonged use of pancuronium has been associated with the development of contractures,[157] which can be avoided by regular passive physiotherapy.[54] This is particularly important for infants receiving medications with actions synergistic with pancuronium, for example gentamicin. Infants who receive neuromuscular blocking agents for a prolonged period become edematous. The likely mechanism is renal hypoperfusion and relative oliguria; paralyzed infants have been noted to have a high urine osmolality.[65] Chest wall edema can reduce respiratory compliance, necessitating use of higher inflating pressures to maintain adequate ventilation. Unfortunately, fluid restriction does not satisfactorily deal with this problem.[65]

In view of the side-effects of neuromuscular blocking agents, analgesics and sedatives (Table 22.3) have been used as alternatives, but have also been administered to minimize the discomfort infants might experience during respiratory support (p. 156). Morphine is metabolized in the liver to an inactive metabolite morphine-3-glucuronide (M3G) and a potent analgesic agent morphine-6-glucuronide (M6G), which is reported to have a greater respiratory depressant effect than morphine itself.[130] Morphine given at an infusion rate of 10 μg/kg/h during PTV had a variable effect on the triggered breath rate and this was not significantly different from placebo.[143] Infants, however, who produced M6G at 12 hours showed a significantly greater reduction in the triggered rate than those who did not.[143] Morphine, compared to placebo, significantly reduced epinephrine (adrenaline) concentrations in ventilated neonates, but did not lower the pneumothorax rate.[144] The rate of clearance of morphine and its metabolism to M6G are impaired in neonates. Morphine (bolus 100 μg/kg and 10 μg/kg/h) in 14 infants with RDS was not shown to have any significant effects on the triggered breath rates until the infusion had been *in situ* for 12 hours. Infants, however, who produced M6G had a greater reduction in the triggered breath rate than those who did not.[143] Diamorphine is more soluble than morphine, but may produce less respiratory depression than morphine in the neonate.[141] Use of diamorphine has been associated with a reduction in respiratory rate, which might indicate improved synchrony with the ventilator, but did cause a small, but significant reduction in blood pressure.[40] Diamorphine is hepatically metabolized by non-specific monamine oxidases. The half-lives of morphine and diamorphine vary with maturity, being 9–10 hours in premature infants,[11] 7 hours in term infants[100] and 2 hours in adults.[119] Fentanyl, a synthetic opioid which is renally excreted, has a half-life of around 2 hours in adults[97] and 4 hours in neonates.[5] An intravenous bolus, however, only has a 30-minute duration of action on pain because of rapid redistribution into fat and muscle. In a randomized trial,[88] premature infants ventilated for RDS who received a low-dose fentanyl infusion (mean 1.1 μg/kg/h) had lower behavioral stress scores and fewer oxygen desaturations than untreated controls. There were, however, no significant differences in ventilatory variables or short-term outcomes including air leak. Although fentanyl has a shorter duration of action and greater cardiovascular stability because of less histamine release than morphine, it does have disadvantages. Administration of fentanyl sometimes causes muscle rigidity requiring treatment with a muscle relaxant. Alfentanil might, on theoretical grounds, be a useful alternative because less tissue accumulation occurs, but muscle rigidity is even more commonly encountered. Withdrawal symptoms appear common in neonates; in one series,[126] more than 50 percent of babies treated with fentanyl developed withdrawal symptoms. Withdrawal symptoms include extreme irritability, tremor, myoclonus, ataxia and choreoathetosis; these can be avoided by reducing the drug dose gradually. Fentanyl can precipitate movement disorders.[16,89] Naloxone is an effective antidote to fentanyl. Acetaminophen (paracetamol) is also given to treat pain in neonates, although less commonly in critically ill prematurely born infants because of concerns of hepatoxicity and increased bilirubin concentrations. A recent study, however,[170] demonstrated a single 20 mg/kg

dose of acetaminophen can be safely given to preterm infants in whom sulfation is the major pathway of excretion. If the drug is administered rectally, higher doses will be required to achieve the therapeutic level quicker, as rectal absorption is prolonged. If multiple doses are required, then an interval of more than 8 hours should be used to prevent progressively increasing serum concentration.[170] The impact of acetaminophen administration on the outcome of ventilation has not been investigated, but acetaminophen administration should be considered in infants requiring moderate analgesia.

Benzodiazepines induce less respiratory depression than opiates. They are metabolized in the liver and excreted in the urine and have a very long half-life, which can result in extremely high plasma concentrations in patients who have received a continuous infusion. Midazolam and imidazo-benzodiazepine, have a shorter half-life of 1–12 hours, but their use in children has been associated with neurological abnormalities.[16] Midazolam is a sedative and anticonvulsant, but has no action on pain. In high doses it causes respiratory suppression, hypotension and reduced cerebral blood flow; paradoxical agitation may also occur. Long-term use may result in drug accumulation and a severe encephalopathic illness with drowsiness, dystonic posturing and choreoathetosis. This occurs 1–2 days after stopping treatment and can persist for a week or more. Midazolam can be reversed by 10 μg/kg of intravenous flumazenil. Comparative studies have suggested that midazolam is not as good a sedative as chloral.[125] Midazolam in a dose of 60 μg/kg/h has been used as a sedative for up to 4 days without apparent adverse effects in ventilated neonates. In infants born prior to 33 weeks of gestational age, however, the dose should be halved after 24 hours to prevent drug accumulation. Chloral can cause gastric irritation. It is metabolized to trichloroethanol, an active metabolite with a half-life of 8 hours. Trichloroacetic acid is hepatotoxic and has a half-life of several days. Toxic levels are frequently reported as absorption may vary considerably between patients. In adults administration of chloral with frusemide displaces thyroxine (T_4) from plasma proteins.[35] Unfortunately, there are no controlled trials demonstrating that use of either analgesics or sedatives reduce pneumothoraces.

Management

CONSERVATIVE

Asymptomatic pneumothoraces need no treatment other than careful observation of the infant. A small, symptomatic pneumothorax may respond to increasing the inspired oxygen content concentration to 100 percent, as resorption of the extra-alveolar air occurs via nitrogen washout. This strategy should not be used for preterm infants at risk of retinopathy of prematurity.

NEEDLE ASPIRATION

Drainage by aspiration using a syringe and butterfly is not recommended, other than as a diagnostic procedure when the infant is in extremis and there are no other diagnostic aids immediately available. Needle aspiration is undertaken using an 18 G butterfly attached to a three-way tap; the latter is held under water in a small sterile container. The needle is inserted through the skin and then the skin and needle moved sideways, before advancing the needle through the underlying muscle (Z-track); this reduces the likelihood of leaving an open needle track for entry of air once the needle has been removed. Care must be taken not to remove too much air, otherwise the lung may be punctured by the needle and when the drain is subsequently inserted, it is likely to be inserted directly into the lung parenchyma.

CHEST DRAIN PLACEMENT

A pneumothorax must always be drained in symptomatic preterm babies, in all babies who are receiving mechanical ventilation (unless the pneumothorax is very small and not associated with any deterioration in clinical condition) and in all those with tension pneumothoraces. A retrospective review of 149 cases of chest drain placement[4] revealed that effective drainage of extra-alveolar air was achieved in only 44 percent of posterior placements (Figures 22.8a and 22.8b), compared to 96 percent of anterior placements. The mid-axillary site, however, may be preferred for cosmetic reasons, as any resultant scarring is less obvious. The chest drain (FG 10–14) should be inserted, following local anesthetic, by blunt dissection through either the second intercostal space just lateral to the mid-clavicular line or the sixth space in the mid-axillary line. If the lower site is chosen, the infant should be turned so that the affected side is uppermost and the drain aimed anteriorly, otherwise achievement of a retrosternal position is unlikely.[85] The drain should be positioned with the trochar removed and the infant temporarily disconnected from the ventilator, as this reduces the likelihood of inserting the drain through the lung. The chest tube should then be connected to an underwater sealed drain and suction applied at a pressure of 5–10 cmH$_2$O. Heimlich valves are useful to attach to chest tubes during transport, but are not recommended for long-term use as they can block and without suction not all the extra-alveolar air will be removed. If the chest tube tip is placed anteriorly, the position should be confirmed by an appropriate chest radiograph. A second drain will occasionally be required to ensure complete drainage. The drain should then be left *in situ* for at least 48 hours, and certainly for 24 hours following effective drainage. The chest tube should be clamped and only removed if no pleural air then accumulates. In a ventilator-dependent infant, the unclamped drain should be left *in situ* for longer, but removed if blocked with serous fluid and a further drain inserted if

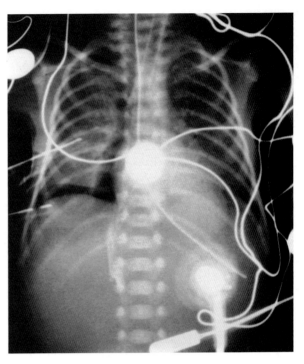

Figure 22.9 *Recurrent anterior basal pneumothorax following displacement of the lower chest drain.*

the extra-alveolar air accumulates and causes clinical compromise. Continuing leakage from a pneumothorax is usually detected by air bubbling in the bottle; the chest tube should be removed only once this has stopped. Continuous bubbling frequently indicates that the chest drain has been displaced which may result in recurrence of the pneumothorax (Figure 22.9). A vacuum pump allowing quantification of the volume of air through the chest tube has been used to indicate the appropriate timing of chest tube removal.[43] In adults, the time to successful chest drain removal was reduced from 8.1 to 4.8 days when the pump was employed. PVC tubes are usually employed to accomplish drainage, but alternatives have been described including a J chest tube (JCT).[81] The JCT has a pigtail configuration at the distal end, intended to simplify placement and minimize chest wall and lung trauma because of its reduced tube size and depth of insertion. A major cause for chest tube ineffectiveness is excessive depth of insertion.[4] In 35 of 38 infants, pneumothoraces were successfully drained using JCTs, although 12 pneumothoraces recurred after 24 hours and responded to irrigation or tube replacement. Pneumothorax drainage was also accomplished in 25 infants using a small-bore pigtail catheter.[178]

Complications of chest drain placement

Complications of chest drain placement include direct perforation of the lung by the drain. At autopsy, perforation was found in approximately 25 percent of cases.[117] This complication should be suspected if there is continuous drainage of air or the pneumothorax persists.

Perforation of the lung can be avoided by introducing the chest drain tube by blunt dissection, rather than using the sharp trochar. The chest tube, if inserted so as to enter the posterosuperior mediastinum, may traumatize the thoracic duct, resulting in a chylothorax.[87] Chest tubes may also enter the pericardium, resulting in a hemorrhagic pericardial effusion with cardiac tamponade.[142] Phrenic nerve injury secondary to insertion of a chest drain is uncommon; it may be unilateral[9,107] or bilateral.[8] Drainage tubes which are placed deep in the chest carry the greatest risk.[8,107,176] The phrenic nerve runs down the mediastinum over the pericardium and thus can be damaged by drains impinging on the mediastinum.[176]

Bronchopleural fistula If the chest drain is inserted into the lung, a bronchopleural fistula may result and, then, despite reduction of ventilator pressures, significant air leak will persist. In affected infants, single lung ventilation, surgical thoracotomy with oversewing of the fistula or lobectomy may be necessary as emergency measures.[15] High-frequency ventilation has allowed maintenance of ventilation and been claimed to assist in healing by decreasing the amount of air leak through the fistula.[53] In one neonate,[15] fibrin glue pleurodesis successfully sealed a pneumothorax which had persisted for more than 3 weeks despite high-frequency ventilation. In another infant,[86] recurrent pneumothorax was also successfully treated by fibrin glue, which was injected into the pleural cavity through the chest tube. Fibrin glue is a biological preparation composed of separate solutions of fibrinogen and thrombin and mimics the last phase of the normal clotting system. If not commercially available, it can be made with cryoprecipitate and topical bovine thrombin. The fibrin glue is believed to be cleaved by fibrinolytic enzymes and disappears within weeks, leaving no scars. An alternative, more conservative approach is to use selective bronchial occlusion. Occlusion of the right main bronchus with a Fogarty's catheter produced rapid improvement in a 26-week gestation infant who had developed severe right PIE of the right lung with a bronchopleural fistula, pneumothorax and mediastinal shift.[121]

Bronchocutaneous fistula This is a very rare complication and results in the development of subcutaneous gas in the chest wall. Resolution without drainage occurred in one case.[10]

Prognosis

MORTALITY

The occurrence of a pneumothorax in prematurely born infants with RDS increases mortality. On conventional ventilation and before the routine use of surfactant, the mortality of babies with a pneumothorax was inversely related to birthweight.[58] Infants may be more likely to die if they develop an air leak on day 1 or after day 4 than on day 2 or 3.[139]

MORBIDITY

Pneumothorax development is associated with hemorrhage into the germinal layer and ventricles of preterm infants.[96] When a pneumothorax occurs, there is a marked increase in cerebral blood flow velocity,[75] which correlates closely with systemic hemodynamic changes; the marked increase in flow is of importance in the genesis of intracranial hemorrhage (ICH). Acute hypotension resulting from pneumothorax is associated with severe ICH development.[114] Air leak development is associated with increased levels of antidiuretic hormone (ADH);[82] this can lead to further fluid retention in a paralyzed infant. If the pneumothorax is complicated by an air embolus, circulatory failure can result.

PULMONARY INTERSTITIAL EMPHYSEMA (PIE)

Incidence

PIE has an inverse relationship with birthweight.[68,180]

Pathology

PIE may be lobar in distribution, but more commonly affects both lungs diffusely. In acute PIE, small subpleural blebs are discernible macroscopically. At autopsy the blebs may be difficult to see, at least in part due to postmortem gas absorption. On the cut surface of the lung, there are variably sized cystic spaces, which are either round or oval if tracking in the interlobar septae. The 'spaces' occur in the pulmonary parenchyma or interlobular and subpleural loose connective tissue; they are also frequently present in the perivascular lymphatics and can simulate congenital lymphangiectasia. The cysts of chronic PIE microscopically have been found to have a fibrous wall lined by giant cells.

Etiology

Interstitial emphysema rarely occurs spontaneously in term infants and is almost entirely confined to preterm infants.[135,169] PIE occurs mainly in neonates with RDS.[23] In the surfactant-deficient lung, rupture of the small airways occurs distal to the termination of the fascial sheath; air then dissects into the interstitium, creating PIE (see above). PIE in the immature infant appears to be the result of volutrauma, as it is rare in infants who have not received positive pressure ventilation.[60,68] It is significantly related to the use of high peak inspiratory pressures,[60]

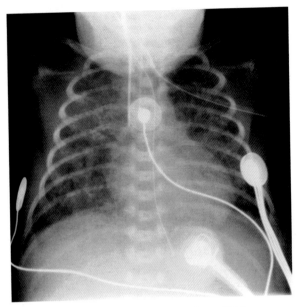

Figure 22.10 *Diffuse early pulmonary interstitial emphysema.*

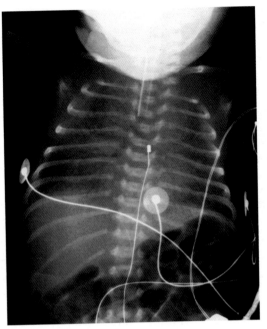

Figure 22.11 *Early pulmonary interstitial emphysema more marked in the right lung.*

although unusually low mean airway pressures (MAPs) during piston-type HFO may contribute to PIE in infants with non-compliant lungs.[149] PIE can also be a complication of resuscitation; a rare and extreme manifestation of this is the development of a large subpleural air cyst.[37] Asymmetrical PIE has been associated with a malpositioned endotracheal tube.[60]

Clinical signs

The trapped gas reduces pulmonary perfusion by compression of the blood vessels[150] and the emphysema splints the lung, impairing ventilation. As a consequence, infants suffer profound hypoxemia with carbon dioxide retention.

Differential diagnosis

The chest radiograph appearance may be confused with lobar emphysema or, if more localized, with cystic adenomatoid malformation of the lung.

Diagnosis

Transillumination of the chest of an infant with diffuse PIE yields the same appearance as a large pneumothorax.

CHEST RADIOGRAPH

There is a characteristic cystic appearance (Figure 22.10). Unusually, PIE may be unsuspected and found on the

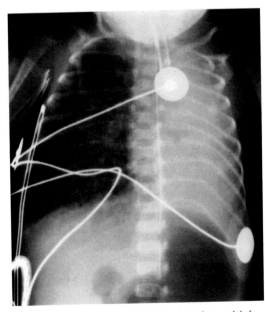

Figure 22.12 *Severe unilateral pulmonary interstitial emphysema with gross hyperinflation of the right hemithorax and consequent compression of the left lung.*

routine daily chest radiograph of a ventilated infant (Figure 22.11). At that stage the appearance may be of rounded non-confluent microradiolucencies; usually this progresses with further extravasation of air to the more typical picture (Figure 22.10). At a later stage, there may be large bullae and the affected areas will be hyperinflated (Figures 22.12 and 22.13).

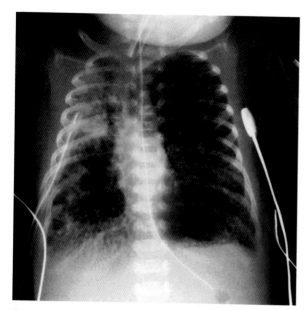

Figure 22.13 *Severe bilateral PIE affecting the right more than the left lung; there is gross cardiac compression. A chest drain is* in situ *in the right hemithorax.*

Management

GENERALIZED PIE

Ventilatory management is directed at reducing further trauma to the lung and this is accomplished by decreasing pressures to the minimum compatible with acceptable gases [PaO_2 6–7 kPa (45–53 mmHg), pH > 7.25, $PaCO_2$ < 8 kPa (60 mmHg)]. An infant who is obviously 'fighting' (p. 159), should be paralyzed to minimize the risk of extension of the air leak. Withdrawal of positive end expiratory pressure (PEEP) may result in disappearance of the PIE.[93,99] Using conventional ventilators at fast rates[60] can reduce the occurrence of pneumothorax in infants with PIE, but has the drawback that the PIE had no 'outlet' through which to decompress and potentially this can result in an increase in PIE severity. Transfer from conventional ventilators to high-frequency jet ventilation (HFJV),[18,83,137] high-frequency flow interruption[49] or oscillation[28] has improved oxygenation in infants with severe respiratory failure due to PIE. Maintenance of the same MAP during high-frequency oscillatory ventilation (HFOV) as on CMV in infants with PIE does not appear to impair cardiovascular function.[123] Results from a randomized trial,[83] however, suggested that HFJV has only short-term benefits in affected infants. Treatment with HFJV resulted in improved ventilation at lower peak and mean airway pressures with more rapid radiological improvement of the PIE, but survival, the incidences of chronic lung disease, IVH, patent ductus arteriosus, airway obstruction and new air leak did not differ significantly between infants supported on HFJV or CMV. A combination of continuous negative pressure and IMV

may also be useful to improve oxygenation in infants with respiratory failure due to PIE.[34]

If the above ventilatory strategies fail, decompression of the PIE can be accomplished by linear pleurotomies.[115] This procedure involves scarification of the surface of the lung at several sites; an uncapped 21 G needle can be used to puncture the lung and create an artificial pneumothorax. The outcome of infants so treated, however, is variable.[115] Performing a thoracotomy, at which all the blebs were lysed by multiple linear pleurotomies and the hilum skeletonized to release perihilar blebs, resulted in only 17 of 31 patients so treated surviving.[181] A poor prognosis was associated with very low birthweight, severe preoperative hypoxia, shock or a combination of these problems. Dexamethasone has been given to infants with PIE, apparently with good effect,[92,118] perhaps by reducing airway edema and inflammation and airway obstruction.[46] A 7–12 day course of dexamethasone led to decompression of acquired lobar emphysema complicating late-onset PIE in three infants.[118] Three days of treatment with 0.5 mg/kg/day resulted in lower oxygenation indices and MAP requirement and by day 7 the PIE had resolved in the majority. Only ten infants, however, were included in that retrospective series;[46] the efficacy of this treatment requires testing in a randomized trial.

LOCALIZED PIE

As with generalized PIE, a ventilatory mode should be employed which minimizes further trauma to the lung (see above). Short inflation times (0.10–0.15 seconds) have been used with a standard time-cycled, pressure-limited ventilator to direct the delivered volume preferentially towards units of the lung with relatively normal time constants while avoiding inflation of longer time-constant emphysematous areas.[113] Use of such short inflation times will adversely affect volume delivery[38] and hence are unlikely to be tolerated for prolonged periods. Additional strategies may be required if the PIE is causing respiratory embarrassment. Selective intubation of the contralateral lung can be associated with decompression of the PIE. Therapeutic intubation of the right rather than the left main bronchus is more commonly described,[20,22,104] as this is more easily achieved for anatomical reasons. Unfortunately, this also means that the right main bronchus is more commonly intubated unintentionally and the development of unilateral or more severe PIE is more common on the right than the left.[60] Intubation of the left main bronchus, however, can be accomplished[24] and is facilitated by positioning the bevel on the end of the endotracheal tube so that the long part of the tube is directed toward the main bronchus to be intubated. Turning the infant's head to the right moves the tip of the endotracheal tube to the contralateral side of the trachea and thus the left main bronchus is intubated. The outcome of selective intubation has been suggested to be further improved by cutting a side hole in the endotracheal tube as this reduces the problem of upper lobe collapse.[104] In one series, an elliptical hole 1 cm in length was cut through half the circumference 0.5 cm above the tip of the oblique distal end and the elliptical side hole was directed to the left lung.[175] It is, however, preferable for the manufacturers to make such modified endotracheal tubes, so that the 'hole' could be achieved without the risks of sharp edges or detachment of the distal part. Once selectively intubated, 'unilateral' ventilation can be carried out conventionally or by high-frequency jet[27] or oscillatory[145] ventilation. The 'bypassed' lung becomes atelectatic and the hyperinflation usually disappears within 48 hours of selective bronchial intubation.[20,24] It is controversial, however, how long selective intubation must be maintained, some reporting that PIE does not recur after only 48 hours of decompression,[24] while others[20] report that selective intubation should be maintained for 5 days to ensure non-recurrence of the PIE. In a single infant selective intubation was continued for 10 days.[127] Such a prolonged procedure, however, may be poorly tolerated and increases the risk of bronchial injury, subsequent scarring and stenosis. An alternative method to achieve decompression of PIE is to selectively obstruct a bronchus by insertion of a hand-made latex balloon under bronchoscopic control.[109] This procedure carries the risk of bronchial mucosal necrosis.

Placing the infant in the lateral decubitus position may promote atelectasis of affected segments.[31] Lateral decubitus positioning for 3 days was associated with radiological resolution of tension PIE in 19 of 21 infants whilst their respiratory status either improved or remained stable.[151] In such a position, the uppermost lung receives the greater proportion of the ventilation;[69] hence, by under-ventilation, decompression of the dependent lung is encouraged. A combination of placing the infant so that the hyperinflated lung is dependent at all times, minimal chest physiotherapy and suctioning and appropriate ventilation management (reduction of PEEP and decreasing the inspiratory time below 0.3 seconds) may be particularly useful.[163] A more complex approach involving hourly instillation of isotonic saline followed by endotracheal suction, vibration, percussion and changing the infant's position to favor drainage from the right main bronchus has been recommended,[93] but seems unlikely to be tolerated by VLBW infants (p. 238). A chest tube may be inserted directly into the blebs[148] and left there for 48 hours to drain them; such a procedure, however, carries the risk of causing a bronchopleural fistula. Percutaneous evacuation under computed tomographic guidance of larger focal interstitial air collections has been achieved using an 8 FG pigtail catheter.[48]

Although localized PIE may resolve spontaneously,[99] it can persist for many weeks. Sudden enlargement can result in deterioration of the infant's condition and progressive overdistention of the affected area may lead to compression of the adjacent normal lung parenchyma (Figures 22.12 and 22.13). Surgical resection of the affected area may be required to alleviate respiratory distress.[12,47] Resection of multiple lobes has been described. Resection of both the right upper and middle lobes of a VLBW infant with unilateral PIE allowed extubation within a few days of surgery.[3] Unfortunately, no information was given regarding the long-term lung function of the infant.

Prognosis

MORTALITY

Generalized PIE is associated with an increased mortality, which in the 1980s amongst infants supported by conventional ventilators varied from 24 percent[60] to 80 percent.[120] It is controversial whether PIE appearing on the first postnatal day is invariably fatal.[51,60,68] In one series, 94 percent mortality was experienced in infants with birthweight less than 1600 g, who required an oxygen level greater than 0.6 on the first day and had bilateral PIE in the first 48 hours.[120] Use of a peak pressure greater than 26 cmH$_2$O also discriminated between survivors and non-survivors.[120]

MORBIDITY

Chronic lung disease is greatly increased following diffuse PIE.[159,179] On the chest radiograph, the changes of PIE frequently merge imperceptibly with time into those of CLD and retrospectively it is often difficult to determine the exact time of the change. It has been suggested that PIE may persist and cause a form of chronic lung disease, persistent interstitial pulmonary emphysema.[162] Some infants develop localized cysts which may be up to 3 cm in diameter. These lesions usually resolve spontaneously, but if they result in progressive and persistent compression of normal areas of lung (Figure 22.14), they require decompression by direct puncture or surgical intervention has to be performed.

PNEUMOMEDIASTINUM

Incidence

Pneumomediastinum occurs in approximately 2.5 per 1000 live births. Postmature infants are at increased risk; this may relate to their higher rate of meconium aspiration syndrome (p. 334).

Etiology

Pneumomediastinum occurs when there is gas trapping associated with RDS, pneumonia and mechanical ventilation. Additional associations are birth trauma, positive pressure resuscitation at delivery, blood or meconium aspiration, trauma or mechanical obstruction as seen with a foreign body, or a tumor.

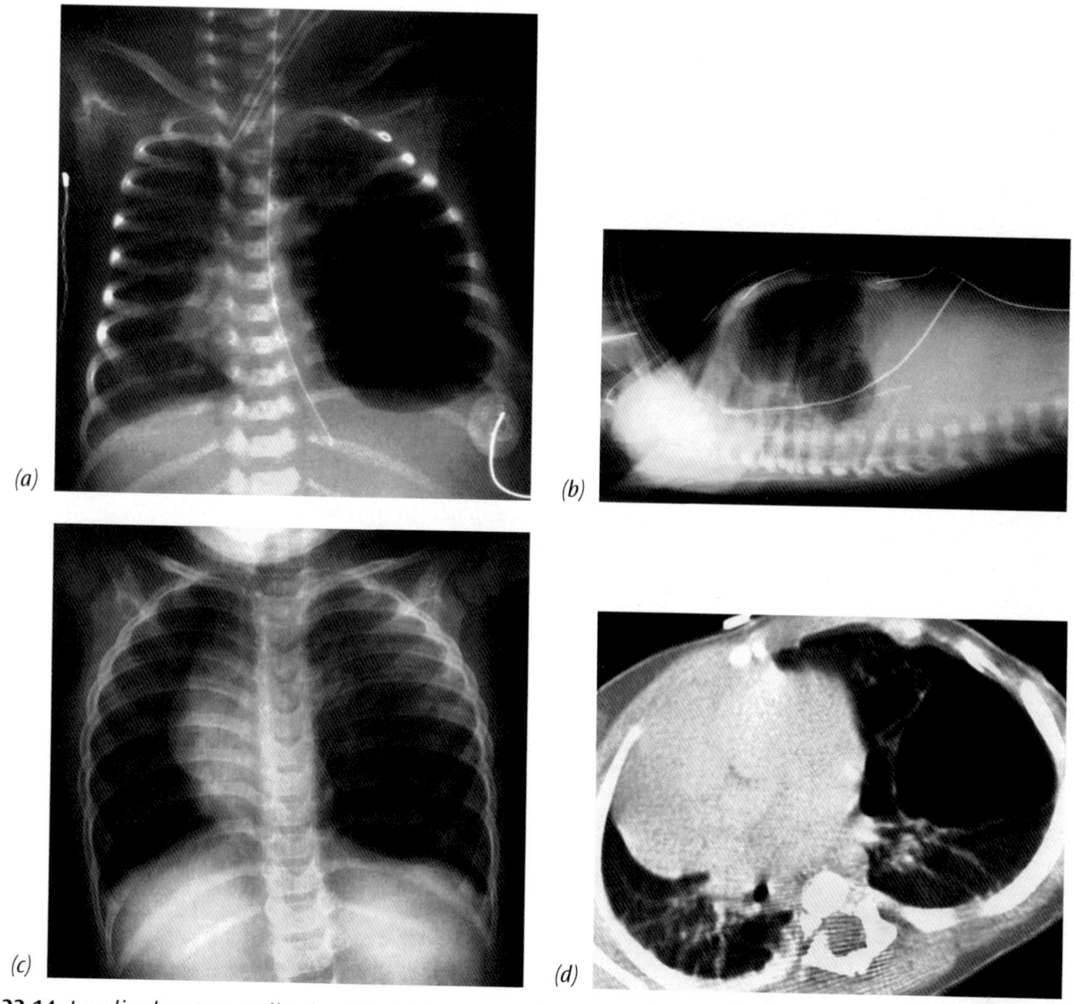

Figure 22.14 *Localized cysts complicating PIE. (a) Large cysts in the left lung causing mediastinal shift. (b) Lateral view. (c) A follow-up chest radiograph at 18 months demonstrates that the mediastinal shift is still present. (d) CT scan demonstrates large dominant cyst and multiple small cysts in the left lung causing mediastinal shift.*

Clinical signs

The infant may be asymptomatic or have mild respiratory distress; mediastinal shift rarely occurs. On examination the sternum may appear bowed and the heart sounds muffled. Rarely, air tracks up into the soft tissues of the neck. Pneumomediastinum is commonly associated with other forms of air leak, through which it decompresses. Under those circumstances the infant may have severe respiratory failure. Tension pneumomediastinum may cause compression of major bronchi or cardiovascular compromise by reducing venous return, but this is unusual.

Diagnosis

CHEST RADIOGRAPH

Pneumomediastinum appears as a halo of air adjacent to the borders of the heart (Figure 22.15). On a lateral

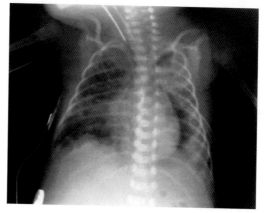

Figure 22.15 *Pneumomediastinum. Gas apparent adjacent to the left side of the heart. There is PIE present in the right lung.*

view it produces marked retrosternal hyperlucency. The mediastinal gas may elevate the thymus away from the pericardium, resulting in a crescenteric configuration resembling a spinnaker sail.[122]

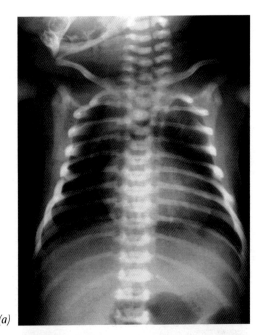

(a)

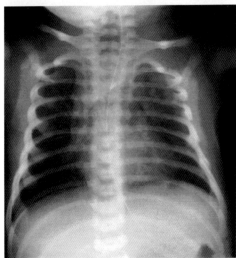

(b)

Figure 22.16 *(a) Pneumomediastinum with elevation of thymic shadows and hyperinflation of the underlying lungs. (b) 24 hours later the chest radiograph demonstrates almost complete resolution of the pneumomediastinum with only a small amount of air now present outlining the left heart border.*

Differential diagnosis

Bronchogenic cyst.[152]

Management

An isolated pneumomediastinum is often asymptomatic and requires no treatment (Figure 22.16). In term infants, use of a high inspired oxygen concentration can result in resorption of the extra-alveolar air, but this should not be attempted in preterm infants at risk from retinopathy of

prematurity. It may not be possible to drain an isolated pneumomediastinum as the gas is collected as multiple independent locules. Drainage is recommended for rare cases of tension pneumomediastinum causing cardiovascular compromise. Attempts, however, at draining mediastinal air are often unsuccessful despite needling or tube drainage and indeed may cause complications such as phrenic nerve damage.[168] If the infant requires ongoing ventilatory support, use of a lower airway mean airway pressure should be attempted. This may be achieved using HFO.[116]

PNEUMOPERICARDIUM

In a mixed population of term and preterm infants, the incidence of pneumopericardium was 1.3 percent.[21] It appears commoner in immature and ventilated infants, occurring in 2 percent of 2389 VLBW infants and 3.5 percent of 1349 ventilated infants.[78] Pneumopericardium frequently occurs with pneumomediastinum. It seems likely that gas enters the pericardium through a defect in the pericardial sac, probably at the pericardial reflection near the ostia of the pulmonary veins, which allows dissection of gas from the mediastinum or pleural space. It has been suggested that there is an anatomical predisposition to pneumopericardium.[171]

Etiology

This may rarely occur spontaneously.[80] The majority of cases are ventilated, prematurely born infants, but affected term infants have been described.[45] Pneumopericardium is usually secondary to barotrauma,[30,33,52,98,155] occurring during vigorous resuscitation or mechanical ventilation and/or the infants have significant lung pathology. In one series, pneumopericardia were commoner in infants supported with peak pressures greater than 32 cmH$_2$O, MAPs greater than 17 cmH$_2$O and inspiratory times greater than 0.7 seconds.[52] A tension pneumopericardium in an infant supported only by nasal CPAP has been described.[70]

A pneumopericardium can occur if a pneumothorax occurs in the absence of the pericardium;[133] the presence of a parietal pleural defect allows communication with the pericardial sac.[158] Congenital absence of the left pericardium results from maldevelopment of the left pleuropericardial membrane. Both partial and complete absence are quite rare and were seen in less than 0.01 percent of approximately 34 000 patients undergoing cardiovascular surgery.[132] Defects on the right are exceedingly rare. Several deaths have been reported when there was partial absence of the left pericardium; the deaths were due to herniation of the left ventricle through the defect. Complete absence is considered a benign condition, as it has a normal life expectancy. Patients with complete absence are usually asymptomatic, but some complain of vague chest pain, probably as a result of adhesions or abnormal traction on the great vessels.[133] Radiographic findings of complete absence of the left pericardium include an unusual cardiac silhouette with elongation of the left heart border, leftward shift and clockwise rotation of the heart, a radiolucent cleft between the ascending aorta and the main pulmonary artery and lucency separating the heart and the left hemidiaphragm. The first two findings related to the abnormal mobility of the heart, the later two result from interposition of lung that is normally restricted by the left pericardium. An unusual pattern of fluid collection may also suggest this condition. The ECG shows right axis deviation.

Clinical signs

Pneumopericardiums are rarely asymptomatic, usually causing cardiac tamponade with sudden hypotension, bradycardia and cyanosis. It has been suggested that early-onset cases often resolve spontaneously, whereas those of late onset are usually severe.[80] Symptoms occur when the pericardial pressure exceeds ventricular filling pressure, resulting in lowered stroke volume; this is particularly poorly tolerated in neonates because of their lower cardiac reserve.[98] The signs may be confused with those of a tension pneumothorax. The heart sounds are muffled, but a friction rub is occasionally audible. It is usually accompanied by other air leaks, such as widespread PIE or a tension pneumothorax, both with a pneumomediastinum.

Diagnosis

The ECG is of low voltage.

CHEST RADIOGRAPH

Gas can be seen completely surrounding the heart, outlining the base of the great vessels and contained within the pericardium (Figure 22.17). Gas does not rise above the upper border of the pericardium, whereas with a pneumomediastinum air is seen anterior to the heart with hyperlucency behind the sternum.[106] Gas occurs inferior to the diaphragmatic surface of the heart and this also differentiates this abnormality from a pneumomediastinum. Air behind the heart is virtually diagnostic of a pneumopericardium. Mediastinal gas is limited inferiorly by the attachment of the mediastinal pleura to the central tendon of the diaphragm. In a hemodynamically significant pneumopericardium, the transverse diameter of the heart is significantly reduced.

Management

A conservative approach can be adopted for the few asymptomatic lesions. Treatment with an oxygen hood

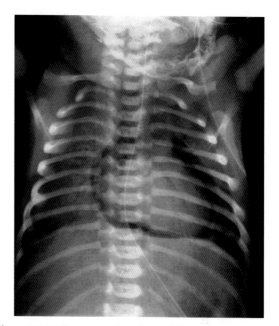

Figure 22.17 *Pneumopericardium with air completely surrounding the heart, demarcating the pericardial sac.*

(an inspired oxygen concentration of 100 percent) resulted within 12 hours in the complete resolution of a large isolated pneumopericardium that developed after delivery and resuscitation.[79] The infant, however, although cardiovascularly compromised, had only mild respiratory distress.[79] All symptomatic pneumopericardia should be drained immediately. Drainage is by direct pericardial tap via the subxiphoid route. The blood pressure should be monitored continuously and the tap repeated if bradycardia or hypotension recur. Catheter drainage has been recommended only if the pericardial air is not controlled by needle aspiration,[90] but some[41] dispute this. Emery *et al.* reported that recurrences occurred in 100 percent of neonates with severe respiratory illness in whom symptomatic pneumopericardia were treated by aspiration alone.[41] It is important to prevent further gas entry into the pericardium and attempts should be made to reduce ventilator pressures.

Prognosis

MORTALITY

This is between 70 and 90 percent,[45,78] although the pneumopericardium may not be the immediate cause of death.

MORBIDITY

Recurrent tension pneumopericardium has rarely been described. In our own practice, a term infant supported by HFO developed a pneumopericardium which was successfully drained prior to surgical repair of a CDH. Some days after the operation, the pneumopericardium recurred and required drainage; the infant survived. In one series,[78] neurodevelopmental delay was more likely in pneumopericardium survivors than other VLBW infants.

PNEUMOPERITONEUM

Etiology

This usually results from perforation of the gut (Figure 22.18), but can be caused by air under pressure dissecting from the chest via the diaphragmatic foramina into the intraperitoneal space.[7] Pneumoperitoneum usually occurs in infants who are ventilated and already have a pneumothorax and pneumomediastinum (Figures 22.19 and 22.20).

Differential diagnosis

Rupture of the gastrointestinal tract must be excluded. Bloody stools, bile-stained aspirate and the absence of respiratory disease will suggest bowel perforation. Differentiation of pneumoperitoneum resulting from air dissection transdiaphragmatically and gas leaking from perforated bowel can be made by aspiration of the intraperitoneal air.[172] Gas aspirated using a 20 G Quickcath inserted into the right lower quadrant is introduced into a blood gas analyzer. Surgical pneumoperitoneum will be

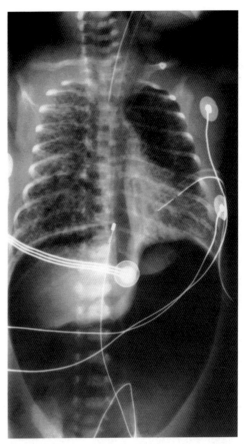

Figure 22.19 *Pneumoperitoneum developing secondary to barotrauma with associated pulmonary interstitial emphysema and pneumothoraces.*

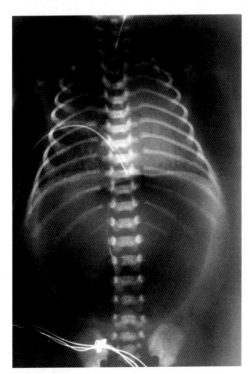

Figure 22.18 *Large pneumoperitoneum with air outlining the umbilical ligament. A chest drain noted in a suboptimal position.*

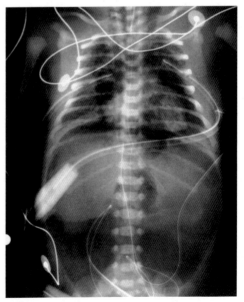

Figure 22.20 *Pneumoperitoneum may be seen in association with pneumomediastinum. There are pockets of loculated interstitial air in association with a left pneumothorax.*

indicated by a partial pressure of oxygen similar to room air. In ventilator-induced pneumoperitoneum the intraperitoneal oxygen tension reflects the partial pressure of oxygen in the alveolar gas deduced from the oxygen concentration delivered by the respirator.

Diagnosis

ABDOMINAL RADIOGRAPH

A horizontal beam lateral or right lateral radiograph will demonstrate the liver clearly defined from the anterior abdominal wall (Figure 22.21). The abdominal radiograph may also demonstrate the cause of the pneumoperitoneum, for example stomach perforation by a nasogastric tube (Figure 22.22).

Management

If the abdomen is not under sufficient tension to cause respiratory embarrassment, no further treatment is necessary. If the abdomen is under tension, however, it should be decompressed by temporary insertion of a large-bore needle.

PULMONARY GAS EMBOLISM

Intravascular gas is a rare complication of positive pressure ventilation.[91]

Pathophysiology

Pulmonary gas embolism results from direct communication between the airway, interstitium and small vascular channels and this has been demonstrated by barium studies at autopsy.[19] Such communications are more likely to

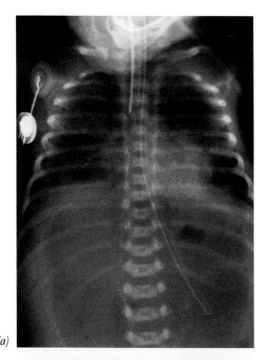
(a)

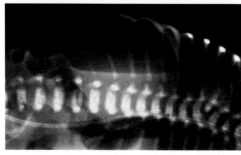
(b)

Figure 22.21 *Pneumoperitoneum resulting from a perforation in the rectosigmoid junction. (a) On the AP radiograph the 'football sign' can be seen. (b) Horizontal radiograph defining air within the peritoneum with a fluid interface. This technique allows small volumes of free air to be detected, which may not be recognized on a supine film.*

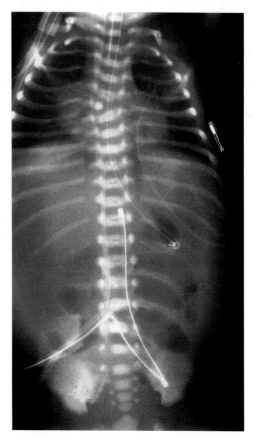

Figure 22.22 *A large pneumoperitoneum secondary to gastric perforation from a misplaced nasogastric tube. The stomach is demarcated by gas within the fundus. There are pulmonary changes of prematurity with multifocal airspace loss in the right upper lobe.*

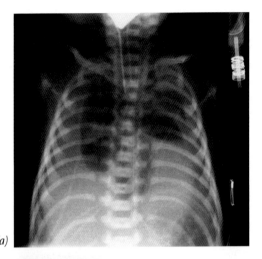

(a)

(b)

Figure 22.23 *Serial radiographs carried out at 24-hour intervals. (a) The initial chest radiograph demonstrates extensive air within the mediastinum, including the pericardium. Air is tracking into the supraclavicular fossa and the neck. The volume and the pressure effects of the non-anatomical air result in compression of the underlying lungs. (b) The second film demonstrates partial resolution of the mediastinal and superficial air, the lungs are now expanded and relatively normal.*

occur in air leak syndromes but also follow trauma to the lung. Laceration of lung tissue favors reversal of the intrabronchial pressure, pulmonary venous pressure gradient, thereby increasing the risk of pulmonary vascular air embolism.[26] Systemic embolus may result from the introduction of air into the pulmonary veins as a result of an alveolar-capillary fistula, but gas could also gain access to the systemic venous circulation via the lymphatics.[17]

Clinical signs

Affected infants are usually premature, have severe respiratory failure necessitating very high ventilatory pressures ($>40\,cmH_2O$), although this condition has also been reported on CPAP[177] and HFOV.[108] The majority (94 percent) have other air leak syndromes.[91] It causes a catastrophic deterioration in the patient's condition with sudden collapse, pallor or cyanosis, hypotension and bizarre electrocardiogram irregularities.

Diagnosis

In over half of the reported cases, gas can be withdrawn from the umbilical venous or arterial catheters.

CHEST RADIOGRAPH

On the chest radiograph, gas can be seen in the systemic and pulmonary arteries and veins.

Management

Early withdrawal of air from the umbilical artery catheter may be of benefit, particularly if the leak is small or has been introduced through an intravascular line. Placement of the infant in the Trendelenburg and left posterior-anterior position can be helpful.[156]

Prognosis

MORTALITY

This condition is usually fatal, only four of 53 infants reported survived.

SUBCUTANEOUS EMPHYSEMA

Subcutaneous emphysema, with air tracking up into the neck, is rare in the neonate and is usually associated with a pneumomediastinum (Figure 22.23). It requires no treatment.

REFERENCES

1 Abolnik, I.Z., Lossos, I.S., Zlotogora, J., Brauer, R. (1991) On the inheritance of primary spontaneous pneumothorax. *American Journal of Medical Genetics* **40**, 155–158.

2 Adler, S.M., Wyszogrodski, I. (1975) Pneumothorax as a function of gestational age: clinical and experimental studies. *Journal of Pediatrics* **87**, 771–776.

3 Ahluwalia, J.S., Rennie, J.M., Wells, F.C. (1996) Successful outcome of severe unilateral pulmonary interstitial emphysema after bi-lobectomy in a very low birthweight infant. *Journal of the Royal Society of Medicine* **89**, 167P–168P.

4 Allen, R.W., Jung, A.L., Lester, P.D. (1981) Effectiveness of chest tube evacuation of pneumothorax in neonates. *Journal of Pediatrics* **99**, 629–634.

5 Anand, K.J.S., Hickey, P.R. (1987) Pain and its effects in the human neonate and fetus. *New England Journal of Medicine* **317**, 1321–1329.

6 Anderson, K., Chandra, K. (1976) Pneumothorax secondary to perforation of sequential bronchi by suction catheters. *Journal of Pediatric Surgery* **11**, 687–693.

7 Aranda, J.V., Stern, L., Dunbar, J.S. (1972) Pneumothorax with pneumoperitoneum in a newborn infant. *American Journal of Diseases of Children* **123**, 163–166.

8 Arya, H., Williams, J., Ponsford, S.N., Bissenden, J.G. (1991) Neonatal diaphragmatic paralysis caused by chest drains. *Archives of Disease in Childhood* **66**, 441–442.

9 Ayalon, A., Anner, H., Moghilner, M., Schiller, M. (1979) Eventration of the diaphragm due to phrenic nerve injury caused by intercostals drainage. *Journal of Pediatric Surgery* **14**, 473–474.

10 Baildam, E.M., Dady, I.M., Chiswick, M.L. (1993) Surgical resection for pulmonary interstitial emphysema in the newborn infant. *Archives of Disease in Childhood* **69**, 525–526.

11 Barrett, D.A., Elias-Jones, A.C., Rutter, N. *et al.* (1991) Morphine kinetics after diamorphine infusion in premature neonates. *British Journal of Clinical Pharmacology* **32**, 31–37.

12 Bauer, B.R., Brennan, M.J., Doyle, C. (1978) Surgical resection for pulmonary interstitial emphysema in the newborn infant. *Journal of Pediatrics* **93**, 656–661.

13 Baumer, J.H. (2000) International randomized controlled trial of patient triggered ventilation in neonatal respiratory distress syndrome. *Archives of Disease in Childhood Fetal and Neonatal Edition* **82**, F5–F10.

14 Berg, T.J., Pagtakhan, T.D., Reed, M.H. *et al.* (1975) Bronchopulmonary dysplasia and lung rupture in hyaline membrane disease: influence of continuous distending pressure. *Pediatrics* **55**, 51–53.

15 Berger, J.T., Gilhooly, J. (1993) Fibrin glue treatment of persistent pneumothorax in a premature infant. *Journal of Pediatrics* **122**, 958–960.

16 Bergman, I., Steeves, M., Burckart, G., Thompson, A. (1991) Reversible neurologic abnormalities associated with prolonged intravenous midazolam and fentanyl administration. *Journal of Pediatrics* **119**, 644–648.

17 Booth, T.N., Allen, B.A., Royal, S.A. (1995) Lymphatic air embolism: a new hypothesis regarding the pathogenesis of neonatal sytemic air embolism. *Pediatric Radiology* **25**(Suppl 1), S220–S227.

18 Boros, S.J., Mammel, M.C., Coleman, J.M. *et al.* (1985) Neonatal high frequency jet ventilation: four years' experience. *Pediatrics* **75**, 657–663.

19 Bowen, F.W., Chandra, R., Avery, G.B. (1973) Pulmonary interstitial emphysema with gas embolism in hyaline membrane disease. *American Journal of Diseases of Children* **126**, 117–118.

20 Brooks, J.G., Bustamante, S.A., Koops, B.L. (1977) Selective bronchial intubation for the treatment of severe localized pulmonary interstitial emphysema in newborn infants. *Journal of Pediatrics* **91**, 648–652.

21 Burt, T.B., Lester, P.D. (1982) Neonatal pneumopericardium. *Pediatric Radiology* **142**, 81–84.

22 Campbell, N.A., Zarfin, Y., Perlman, M. (1984) Selective bronchial intubation for pulmonary emphysema. *Archives of Disease in Childhood* **59**, 890–892.

23 Campbell, R.E. (1970) Intrapulmonary interstitial emphysema. A complication of hyaline membrane disease. *American Journal of Radiology* **110**, 449–456.

24 Chan, V., Greenough, A. (1992) Severe localised pulmonary interstitial emphysema – decompression by selective bronchial intubation. *Journal of Perinatal Medicine* **20**, 313–316.

25 Chernick, V., Avery, M.E. (1963) Spontaneous alveolar rupture at birth. *Pediatrics* **32**, 816–824.

26 Chiu, C.J., Golding, M.R., Linder, J.B., Fries, C.C. (1967) Pulmonary venous air embolism: a hemodynamic reappraisal. *Surgery* **61**, 816–819.

27 Chua, R.N., Yoder, C. (1990) Management of unilateral pulmonary cystic emphysema with selective bronchial intubation and high frequency jet ventilation in two infants. *Pediatric Pulmonology* **9**, 121–124.

28 Clark, R.H., Gerstmann, D.R., Null, D.M. *et al.* (1986) Pulmonary interstitial emphysema treated by high frequency oscillatory ventilation. *Critical Care Medicine* **14**, 926–930.

29 Clifford, R.D., Whincup, G., Thomas, R. (1988) Patient triggered ventilation prevents pneumothoraces in premature babies. *Lancet* **1**, 529–530.

30 Cohen, D.J., Baumgart, S., Stephenson, L.W. (1983) Pneumopericardium in neonates – is it PEEP or is it PIP? *Annals of Thoracic Surgery* **35**, 179–183.

31 Cohen, R.S., Smith, D.W., Stevenson, D.K. *et al.* (1984) Lateral decubitus position as therapy for persistent focal pulmonary interstitial emphysema in neonates: A preliminary report. *Journal of Pediatrics* **104**, 441–443.

32 Cooke, R.W.I., Rennie, J.M. (1984) Pancuronium and pneumothorax. *Lancet* **i**, 286–287.

33 Cummings, R.G., Wesly, R.L.R., Adams, D.H., Lowe, J.R. (1984) Pneumopericardium resulting in cardiac tamponade. *Annals of Thoracic Surgery* **37**, 511–518.

34 Cvetnic, W.G., Waffarn, F., Martin, J.M. (1989) Continuous negative pressure and intermittent mandatory ventilation in the management of pulmonary interstitial emphysema. *Journal of Perinatology* **9**, 26–32.

35 Datasheet (1992) Association of the British Pharmaceutical Industry Data Sheet Compendium.

36 Delport, S.A. (1996) Paradoxical symmetry of the chest in neonates – a new clinical sign in the diagnosis of a unilateral pneumothorax. *South African Medical Journal* **86**, 1465–1466.

37 deRoux, S.J., Prendergast, N.C. (1998) Large sub-pleural air cysts: an extreme form of pulmonary interstitial emphysema. *Pediatric Radiology* **28**, 981–983.

38 Dimitriou, G., Greenough, A. (2000) Performance of neonatal ventilators. *British Journal of Intensive Care* **10**, 186–188.

39 Dimitriou, G., Greenough, A., Laubscher, B., Yamaguchi, N. (1998) Comparison of airway pressure triggered and airflow triggered ventilation in very immature infants. *Acta Paediatrica* **87**, 1256–1260.

40 Elias Jones, A.C., Barrett, D.A., Rutter, N. *et al.* (1991) Diamorphine infusion in the preterm neonate. *Archives of Disease in Childhood* **66**, 1155–1157.

41 Emery, R.W., Foker, J., Thompson, T.R. (1984) Neonatal pneumopericardium: a surgical emergency. *Annals of Thoracic Surgery* **37**, 128–132.

42 Engdahl, M.S., Gershan, W.M. (1998) Familial spontaneous pneumothorax in neonates. *Pediatric Pulmonology* **25**, 398–400.

43 Engdahl, O., Boe, J. (1990) Quantification of aspirated air volume reduces treatment time in pneumothorax. *European Respiratory Journal* **3**, 649–652.

44 Field, D., Milner, A.D., Hopkin, I.E. (1985) Manipulation of ventilator settings to reduce expiration against positive pressure inflation. *Archives of Disease in Childhood* **60**, 1036–1040.

45 Fiser, D.H., Walker, W.M. (1992) Tension pneumothorax in an infant. *Chest* **102**, 1888–1891.

46 Fitzgerald, D., Willis, D., Usher, R. *et al.* (1998) Dexamethasone for pulmonary interstitial emphysema in preterm infants. *Biology of the Neonate* **73**, 34–39.

47 Fletcher, D.B., Outerbridge, B.E., Youssef, S. (1974) Pulmonary interstitial emphysema in a newborn infant treated by lobectomy. *Pediatrics* **54**, 808–812.

48 Fox, R.B., Wright, A.M. (1998) Case 30–1997: pulmonary interstitial emphysema in infancy. *New England Journal of Medicine* **338**, 688–690.

49 Frantz, I.D., Werhammer, J., Stark, A.R. (1983) High frequency ventilation in premature infants with lung disease: adequate gas exchange at low tracheal pressures. *Pediatrics* **71**, 438–488.

50 Gabwell, C.E., Salzberg, A.M., Sonnino, R.E., Haynes, J.H. (2000) Potentially lethal complications of central venous catheter placement. *Journal of Pediatric Surgery* **35**, 709–713.

51 Gaylord, M.S., Thieme, R.E., Woodall, D.L., Quissell, B.J. (1985) Predicting mortality in low-birth-weight infants with pulmonary interstitial emphysema. *Pediatrics* **76**, 219–224.

52 Glenski, J.A., Hall, R.T. (1984) Neonatal pneumopericardium: analysis of ventilatory variables. *Critical Care Medicine* **12**, 439–442.

53 Gonzalez, F., Harris, T., Black, P., Richardson, P. (1987) Decreased gas flow through pneumothoraces in neonates receiving high frequency jet versus conventional ventilation. *Pediatrics* **110**, 464–466.

54 Greenough, A. (1984) Pancuronium bromide induced joint contractures in the newborn. *Archives of Disease in Childhood* **59**, 390–391.

55 Greenough, A. (1988) The premature infant's respiratory response to mechanical ventilation. *Early Human Development* **17**, 1–5.

56 Greenough, A., Greenall, F. (1988) Observation of spontaneous respiratory interaction with artificial ventilation. *Archives of Disease in Childhood* **63**, 168–171.

57 Greenough, A., Milner, A.D. (1987) High frequency ventilation in the neonatal period. *European Journal of Pediatrics* **146**, 446–449.

58 Greenough, A., Roberton, N.R.C. (1985) Morbidity and survival in neonates ventilated for the respiratory distress syndrome. *British Medical Journal* **290**, 597–600.

59 Greenough, A., Morley, C.J., Davis, J.A. (1983) The interaction of the infant's spontaneous respiration with ventilation. *Journal of Pediatrics* **103**, 769–773.

60 Greenough, A., Dixon, A., Roberton, N.R.C. (1984) Pulmonary interstitial emphysema. *Archives of Disease in Childhood* **59**, 1046–1051.

61 Greenough, A., Wood, S., Morley, C.J., Davis, J.A. (1984) Pancuronium prevents pneumothoraces in ventilated premature babies who actively expire against positive pressure inflation. *Lancet* **1**, 1–3.

62 Greenough, A., Morley, C.J., Pool, J. (1986) Fighting the ventilator – are fast rates an effective alternative to paralysis? *Early Human Development* **13**, 189–194.

63 Greenough, A., Greenall, F., Gamsu, H. (1987) Synchronous respiration: which ventilator rate is best? *Acta Paediatrica Scandinavica* **76**, 713–718.

64 Greenough, A., Pool, J.B., Lagercrantz, H. (1988) Catecholamine and blood pressure levels in paralyzed preterm ventilated infants. *Early Human Development* **16**, 219–224.

65 Greenough, A., Gamsu, H.R., Greenall, F. (1989) Investigation of the effects of paralysis by pancuronium on heart rate variability, blood pressure and fluid balance. *Acta Paediatrica Scandinavica* **78**, 829–834.

66 Greenough, A., Milner, A.D., Dimitriou, G. (2001) Update Software, Oxford.

67 Gregoire, R., Yulish, B., Martin, R. *et al.* (1979) Natural history of pulmonary interstitial emphysema in the preterm infant. *Pediatric Research* **13**, (1019).

68 Hart, S.M., McNair, M., Gamsu, H.R., Price, J.F. (1983) Pulmonary interstitial emphysema in very low birthweight infants. *Archives of Disease in Childhood* **58**, 612–615.

69 Heaf, D.P., Helms, P., Gordon, I., Turner, H.M. (1983) Postural effects on gas exchange in infants. *New England Journal of Medicine* **308**, 1505–1509.

70 Heckman, M., Lindner, W., Pohlandt, F. (1998) Tension pneumopericardium in a preterm infants without mechanical ventilation: a rare cause of cardiac arrest. *Acta Paediatrica* **87**, 346–348.

71 Heicher, D.A., Kasting, D.S., Harrod, J.R. (1981) Prospective clinical comparison of two methods for mechanical ventilation of neonates: rapid rate and short inspiratory time versus slow rate and long inspiratory time. *Journal of Pediatrics* **98**, 957–961.

72 Henderson-Smart, D.J., Bhuta, T., Cools, F., Offringa, M. (2001) Update Software, Oxford.

73 Henry, G.W., Stevens, D.C., Schreier, R.L. *et al.* (1979) Respiratory paralysis to improve oxygenation and mortality in large newborn infants with respiratory distress. *Journal of Pediatric Surgery* **14**, 761.

74 HIFO Study Group. (1993) Randomized study of high-frequency oscillatory ventilation in infants with severe respiratory distress. *Journal of Pediatrics* **122**, 609–619.

75 Hill, A., Periman, J.M., Volpe, J.J. (1982) Relationship of pneumothorax to occurrence of intraventricular haemorrhage in the premature newborn. *Pediatrics* **69**, 144–149.

76 Hird, M., Greenough, A., Gamsu, H. (1990) Gas trapping during high frequency positive pressure ventilation using conventional ventilators. *Early Human Development* **22**, 51–56.

77 Hird, M.F., Greenough, A. (1991) Spontaneous respiratory effort during mechanical ventilation in infants with and without acute respiratory distress. *Early Human Development* **25**, 69–73.

78 Hook, B., Hack, M., Morrison, S. *et al.* (1995) Pneumopericardium in very low birthweight infants. *Journal of Perinatology* **15**, 27–31.

79 Hummler, H.D., Badnstra, E.S., Abdenour, G.E. (1996) Neonatal fellowship. Neonatal pneumopericardium: successful treatment with nitrogen washout technique. *Journal of Perinatology* **16**, 490–493.

80 Itani, M.H., Mikati, M.A. (1998) Early onset neonatal spontaneous pneumopericardium. *J Med Lib* **46**, 165–167.

81 Jung, A.L., Nelson, J., Jenkins, M.B., Hodson, W.A. (1991) Clinical evaluation of a new chest tube used in neonates. *Clinical Pediatrics (Philadelphia)* **30**, 85–87.

82 Kavvadia, V., Greenough, A., Dimitriou, G., Forsling, M. (1998) Arginine vasopressin and prediction of neonatal chronic lung disease. *European Respiratory Journal* **12**, 925.

83 Keszler, M., Donn, S.M., Bucciarelli, R.L. *et al.* (1991) Multicenter controlled trial comparing high-frequency jet

ventilation and conventional mechanical ventilation in newborn infants with pulmonary interstitial emphysema. *Journal of Pediatrics* **119**, 85–93.

84 Korvenranta, H., Kero, P. (1983) Intraesophageal pressure monitoring in infants with respiratory disorders. *Critical Care Medicine* **11**, 276–279.

85 Kuhns, L.R., Bednarek, F.J., Wyman, M.L. *et al.* (1975) Diagnosis of pneumothorax or pneumomediastinum in the neonate by transillumination. *Pediatrics* **56**, 355–360.

86 Kuint, J., Lubin, D., Martinowitz, U., Linder, N. (1996) Fibrin glue treatment for recurrent pneumothorax in a premature infant. *American Journal of Perinatology* **13**, 245–247.

87 Kumar, S.P., Belik, J. (1984) Chylothorax – a complication of chest tube placement in a neonate. *Critical Care Medicine* **12**, 411–412.

88 Lago, P., Benini, F., Agosto, C., Zacchello, F. (1998) Randomised controlled trial of low dose fentanyl infusion in preterm infants with hyaline membrane disease. *Archives of Disease in Childhood: Fetal & Neonatal Edition* **79**, F194–F197.

89 Lane, J.C., Tennison, M.B., Lawless, S.T. *et al.* (1991) Movement disorder after withdrawal of fentanyl infusion. *Journal of Pediatrics* **119**, 649–651.

90 Lawson, E.E., Gould, T.B., Taeusch, W.J. (1980) Neonatal pneumopericardium: current management. *Journal of Pediatric Surgery* **15**, 181–185.

91 Lee, S.K., Tanswell, A.K. (1989) Pulmonary vascular air embolism in the newborn. *Archives of Disease in Childhood* **64**, 507–510.

92 Lefebvre, F. (1998) Case 30–1997: pulmonary interstitial emphysema in infancy. *New England Journal of Medicine* **338**, 688–689.

93 Leonidas, J.C., Hall, R.T., Rhodes, P.G. (1975) Conservative management of unilateral pulmonary interstitial emphysema under tension. *Journal of Pediatrics* **87**, 776–778.

94 Levene, M.I., Quinn, M.W. (1992) Use of sedatives and muscle relaxants in newborn babies receiving mechanical ventilation. *Archives of Disease in Childhood* **67**, 870–873.

95 Liang, J.S., Lu, F.L., Tang, J.R., Yau, K.I. (2000) Congenital diaphragmatic hernia misdiagnosed as pneumothorax in a newborn. *Tàiwan Erh kò i Hseh Hui Tsa Chih* **41**, 221–223.

96 Lipscombe, A.P., Reynolds, E.O.R., Blackwell, R.J. *et al.* (1981) Pneumothorax and cerebral haemorrhage in preterm infants. *Lancet* **1**, 414–417.

97 Lloyd-Thomas, A.R. (1990) Pain management in paediatric patients. *British Journal of Anaesthesia* **64**, 85–104.

98 Long, W.A. (1990) Pneumopericardium. In Long, W.A(Ed.), *Fetal and Neonatal Cardiology.* Philadelphia: W B Saunders, 377–388.

99 Lopez, J.B., Campbell, R.E., Bishop, H.C. (1977) Clinical note; non-operative resolution of prolonged localized intrapulmonary interstitial emphysema associated with hyaline membrane disease. *Journal of Pediatrics* **91**, 653–654.

100 Lynn, A.M., Slattery, J.T. (1987) Morphine pharmacokinetics in early infancy. *Anesthesiology* **66**, 136–139.

101 MacEwan, D.W., Dunbar, J.S., Smith, R.D., Brown, B.S.J. (1971) Pneumothorax in young infants – recognition and evaluation. *Journal of the Canadian Association of Radiologists* **22**, 264.

102 Macklin, C.C. (1936) Alveolar pores and their significance in the human lung. *Archives of Pathology* **21**, 202–210.

103 Macklin, C.C. (1939) Transport of air along sheaths of pulmonic blood vessels from alveoli to mediastinum, clinical implications. *Archives of Internal Medicine* **64**, 913–926.

104 MacMahon, P., Fleming, P.J., Thearle, M.J., Speidel, B.D. (1982) An improved selective bronchial intubation technique for managing severe localized interstitial emphysema. *Acta Paediatrica Scandinavica* **71**, 151–153.

105 Madansky, D.L., Lawson, E.E., Chernick, V., Taeusch, H.W. (1979) Pneumothorax and other forms of pulmonary air leak in newborns. *American Review of Respiratory Disease* **120**, 729–737.

106 Mansfield, P.B., Graham, C.B., Beckwith, J.B. *et al.* (1973) Pneumopericardium and pneumomediastinum in infants and children. *Journal of Pediatric Surgery* **8**, 691–699.

107 Marinelli, V., Ortiz, A., Alden, E. (1981) Acquired eventration of the diaphragm: a complication of chest tube placement in neonatal pneumothorax. *Pediatrics* **67**, 552–554.

108 Maruyama, K., Koizumi, T. (1996) Systemic air embolism in an extremely low birthweight infant treated with high-frequency oscillatory ventilation. *Acta Paediatrica Japonica* **38**, 681–683.

109 Matthew, O.P., Thach, B.T. (1980) Selective bronchial obstruction for treatment of bullous interstitial emphysema. *Journal of Pediatrics* **96**, 475–477.

110 McIntosh, N. (1983) Pulmonary air leaks in the newborn period. *British Journal of Hospital Medicine* **29**, 512–517.

111 McIntosh, N. (1985) Hypotension associated with pancuronium use in the newborn. *Lancet* **2**, 279.

112 McIntosh, N., Becher, J.-C., Cunningham, S. *et al.* (2000) Clinical diagnosis of pneumothorax is late: use of trend data and decision support might allow preclinical detection. *Pediatric Research* **48**, 408–415.

113 Meadow, W.L., Cheromcha, D. (1985) Successful therapy of unilateral pulmonary emphysema: mechanical ventilation with extremely short inspiratory time. *American Journal of Perinatology* **2**, 194–197.

114 Mehrabani, D., Gowen, C.W., Kopelman, A.E. (1991) Association of pneumothorax and hypotension with intraventricular haemorrhage. *Archives of Disease in Childhood* **66**, 48–51.

115 Milligan, D.W.A., Issler, H., Massam, M., Reynolds, E.O.R. (1984) Treatment of neonatal pulmonary interstitial emphysema by lung puncture. *Lancet* **1**, 1010–1011.

116 Miyahara, K., Ichihara, T., Watanabe, T. (1999) Successful use of high frequency oscillatory ventilation for pneumomediastinum. *Annals of Thoracic and Cardiovascular Surgery* **5**, 49–51.

117 Moessinger, A.C., Driscoll, J.M.J., Wigger, H.J. (1978) High incidence of lung perforation by chest tube in neonatal pneumothorax. *Journal of Pediatrics* **92**, 635–637.

118 Mohsini, K., Reid, D., Tanswell, K. (1987) Resolution of acquired lobar emphysema with dexamethasone therapy. *Journal of Pediatrics* **111**, 901–904.

119 Moore, R.A., Baldwin, D., Allen, M.C. *et al.* (1984) Sensitive and specific radioimmunoassay with iodine label: pharmacokinetics or morphine in man after intravenous administration. *Annals of Clinical Biochemistry* **21**, 318–325.

120 Morisot, C., Kacet, N., Bouchez, M.C. *et al.* (1990) Risk factors for fatal pulmonary interstitial emphysema in neonates. *European Journal of Pediatrics* **149**, 493–495.

121 Mosca, F., Lattanzio, M., Colnaghi, M.R., Pugliese, S. (1995) Bronchopleural fistula: successful selective bronchial occlusion with a Fogarty's catheter in a preterm infant. *Acta Paediatrica* **84**, 1079–1082.

122 Moseley, J.E. (1960) Loculated pneumomediastinum in the newborn. A thymic 'spinnaker' sign. *Radiology* **75**, 788–790.

123 Nelle, M., Zilow, E.P., Linderkamp, O. (1997) Effects of high-frequency oscillatory ventilation on circulation in neonates with pulmonary interstitial emphysema or RDS. *Intensive Care Medicine* **23**, 671–676.

124 Noack, G., Freyschuss, U. (1977) The early detection of pneumothorax with transthoracic impedance in newborn infants. *Acta Paediatrica Scandinavica* **66**, 677–680.

125 Northern Neonatal Network (2000) *Neonatal Formulary.* London: BMJ Books.

126 Norton, S. (1988) After effects of morphine and fentanyl analgesia: a retrospective study. *Neonatal Network* **7**, 25–28.

127 O'Donovan, D., Wearden, M., Adams, J. (1999) Unilateral pulmonary interstitial emphysema following pneumonia in a preterm infant successfully treated with prolonged selective bronchial intubation. *American Journal of Perinatology* **16**, 327–331.

128 Ogata, E.S., Gregory, G.A., Kitterman, J.A. *et al.* (1976) Pneumothorax in the respiratory distress syndrome: incidence and effect on vital signs, blood gases and pH. *Pediatrics* **58**, 177–183.

129 Oh, W., Stern, L. (1977) Diseases of the respiratory system. In Behrman, R.E. (ed.), *Neonatal and Perinatal Medicine: Diseases of the Fetus and Infant.* St Louis: CV Mosby, 558.

130 Osborne, R., Joel, S., Trew, D., Slevin, M. (1988) Analgesic activity of morphine-6-glucuronide. *Lancet* **1**, 828.

131 Oxford Region Controlled Trial of Artificial Ventilation (OCTAVE) Study Group. (1991) Multicentre randomised controlled trial of high against low frequency positive pressure ventilation. *Archives of Disease in Childhood* **66**, 770–775.

132 Perna, G. (1909) Sopra un arresto di sviluppo della sierosa pericardica nell'uomo. *Anatomische Anzelger* **35**, 323–338.

133 Pickhardt, P.J. (1998) Congenital absence of the pericardium confirmed by spontaneous pneumothorax. *Clinical Imaging* **22**, 404–407.

134 Pierce, J.A., Suarez, B., Reich, T. (1980) More on familial spontaneous pneumothorax. *Chest* **78**, 263.

135 Plenat, F., Vert, P., Didier, F., Andre, M. (1978) Pulmonary interstitial emphysema. *Clinics in Perinatology* **5**, 351–375.

136 Pohlandt, F., Bernsau, V., Feilen, K.D., *et al.* (1985) Reduction of barotrauma in ventilated neonates by increase in ventilation frequency. First results of a collaborative and randomized trial of two different ventilatory techniques. *Pediatric Research* **19**, 1077.

137 Pokora, T., Bing, D.R., Mammel, M.C., Boros, S. (1983) Neonatal high frequency jet ventilation. *Pediatrics* **72**, 27–32.

138 Pollitzer, M.J., Reynolds, E.O.R., Shaw, D.G., Thomas, R.M. (1981) Pancuronium during mechanical ventilation speeds recovery of lungs of infants with hyaline membrane disease. *Lancet* **1**, 346–348.

139 Powers, W.F., Clemens, J.D. (1993) Prognostic implications of age at detection of air leak in very low birth weight infants requiring ventilatory support. *Journal of Pediatrics* **123**, 611–617.

140 Primhak, R.A. (1983) Factors associated with pulmonary air leak in premature infants receiving mechanical ventilation. *Journal of Pediatrics* **102**, 764–769.

141 Purcell-Jones, G., Dormon, F., Sumner, E. (1987) The use of opioids in neonates. A retrospective study of 933 cases. *Anaesthesia* **42**, 1316–1320.

142 Quak, J.M.E., Szatmari, A., van den Anker, J.N. (1993) Cardiac tamponade in a preterm neonate secondary to a chest tube. *Acta Paediatrica* **82**, 490–491.

143 Quinn, M.W., Vokes, A. (2000) Effect of morphine on respiratory drive in triggered ventilated preterm infants. *Early Human Development* **59**, 27–35.

144 Quinn, M.W., Wild, J., Dean, H.G. *et al.* (1993) Randomised double blind controlled trial of effect of morphine on catecholamine concentrations in ventilated preterm infants. *Lancet* **342**, 324–327.

145 Randel, R., Mannino, F. (1989) One lung high frequency ventilation in the management of an acquired neonatal pulmonary cyst. *Journal of Perinatology* **98**, 66–68.

146 Reid, L., Rubino, M. (1958) The connective tissue septa in the foetal human lung. *Thorax* **14**, 3–13.

147 Rennie, J.M., Cooke, R.W.I., Morley, C.J. (1987) Failure of observation and impedance respirography to detect active expiration in ventilated preterm infants. *Early Human Development* **15**, 197–201.

148 Roberton, N.R.C. (1976) Treatment of cystic ventilator lung disease. *Proceedings of the Royal Society of Medicine* **69**, 344–345.

149 Sakai, T., Aiba, S., Takahashi, R. *et al.* (1996) Pulmonary interstitial emphysema during piston-type high-frequency oscillatory ventilation. *Tohoku Journal of Experimental Medicine* **180**, 327–335.

150 Salmon, G.W., Forbes, G.B., Davenport, H. (1947) Air block in the newborn infant. *Journal of Pediatrics* **30**, 260–265.

151 Schwartz, A.N., Graham, C.B. (1986) Neonatal tension pulmonary interstitial emphysema in bronchopulmonary dysplasia: treatment with lateral decubitus positioning. *Radiology* **161**, 351–354.

152 Shah, D.S., Lala, R., Rajegowda, B., Bhatia, J. (1999) Bronchogenic cyst and its progress in a premature infant. *Journal of Perinatology* **19**, 150–152.

153 Sharpe, I.K., Ahmad, M., Braun, W. (1980) Familial spontaneous pneumothorax and HLA antigens. *Chest* **78**, 264–268.

154 Shaw, N.J., Cooke, R.W.I., Gill, A.B. *et al.* (1993) Randomised trial of routine versus selective paralysis during ventilation for neonatal respiratory distress syndrome. *Archives of Disease in Childhood* **69**, 479–482.

155 Shennib, H.F., Barkun, A.N., Matouk, E., Blundell, P.E. (1988) Surgical decompression of a tension pneumomediastinum: a ventilatory complication of status asthmaticus. *Chest* **93**, 1301–1302.

156 Shook, D.R., Cram, K.B., Williams, H.J. (1975) Pulmonary venous air embolism in hyaline membrane disease. *American Journal of Radiology* **125**, 538–542.

157 Sinha, S.K., Levene, M.I. (1984) Pancuronium bromide induced joint contractures in the newborn. *Archives of Disease in Childhood* **59**, 73–75.

158 Southworth, H., Stevenson, C.S. (1938) Congenital defects of the pericardium. *Archives of Internal Medicine* **61**, 223–240.

159 Stahlman, M.T., Cheatham, W., Gray, M.E. (1979) The role of air dissection in bronchopulmonary dysplasia. *Journal of Pediatrics* **95**, 878–885.

160 Steele, R.W., Metz, J.R., Bass, J.W., DuBois, J.J. (1971) Pneumothorax and pneumomediastinum in the newborn. *Radiology* **98**, 629–632.

161 Stern, P., Larochelle, F.T., Little, G.A. (1981) Vasopressin and pneumothorax in the neonate. *Pediatrics* **68**, 499–503.

162 Stocker, T.J., Madewell, J.E. (1977) Persistent interstitial pulmonary emphysema: another complication of the respiratory distress syndrome. *Pediatrics* **59**, 847–857.

163 Swingle, H.M., Eggert, L.D., Bucciarelli, R.L. (1984) New approach to management of unilateral tension pulmonary interstitial emphysema in premature infants. *Pediatrics* **74**, 354–357.

164 Swischuk, L.E. (1976) Two lesser known but useful signs of neonatal pneumothorax. *American Journal of Roentgenology* **127**, 623–627.

165 Tarnow-Mordi, W.O., Wilkinson, A.R. (1985) Inspiratory:expiratory ratio and pulmonary interstitial emphysema. *Archives of Disease in Childhood* **60**, 496–497.

166 Tarnow-Mordi, W.O., Reid, E., Griffiths, P., Wilkinson, A.R. (1985) Lack of association of barotrauma and air leak in hyaline membrane disease. *Archives of Disease in Childhood* **60**, 555–559.

167 Tarnow-Mordi, W.O., Reid, E., Griffiths, P., Wilkinson, A.R. (1989) Low inspired gas temperature and respiratory complications in very low birth weight infants. *Journal of Pediatrics* **114**, 438–442.

168 Taylor, J., Dibbins, A., Sobel, D.B. (1993) Neonatal pneumomediastinum indications for and complications of treatment. *Critical Care Medicine* **21**, 296–298.

169 Thibeault, D.W., Lachman, R.S., Laul, V.R., Kwong, M.S. (1973) Pulmonary interstitial emphysema, pneumomediastinum and pneumothorax. Occurrence in the newborn infant. *American Journal of Diseases of Children* **126**, 611–614.

170 van Lingen, R.A., Deinum, J.T., Quak, J.M.E. *et al.* (1999) Pharmacokinetics and metabolism of rectally administered paracetamol in preterm neonates. *Archives of Disease in Childhood Fetal and Neonatal Edition* **80**, F59–F63.

171 van Norstrand, C., Beamish, W.E., Schiff, D. (1975) Neonatal pericardium. *Canadian Medical Association Journal* **112**, 186–192.

172 Vanhaesebrouck, P., Leroy, J.G., Depraeter, C. *et al.* (1989) Simple test to distinguish between surgical and non-surgical pneumoperitoneum in ventilated neonates. *Archives of Disease in Childhood* **64**, 48–49.

173 Vaughan, R., Menke, J., Giacoia, G. (1978) Pneumothorax: a complication of endotracheal tube suctioning. *Journal of Pediatrics* **92**, 633–634.

174 Vyas, H., Field, D., Hopkin, I.E., Milner, A.D. (1986) Determinants of the first inspiratory volume and functional residual capacity at birth. *Pediatric Pulmonology* **2**, 189–193.

175 Weintraub, Z., Oliven, A., Weissman, D., Sonis, Z. (1990) A new method for selective left main bronchus intubation in premature infants. *Journal of Pediatric Surgery* **25**, 604–606.

176 Williams, O., Greenough, A., Mustafa, N., Haughen, S., Rafferty, G.R. (2003) Extubation failure due to phrenic nerve injury. *Archives of Disease in Childhood* **88**, F72–F73.

177 Wong, W., Fok, T.F., Ng, P.C. *et al.* (1997) Vascular air embolism: a rare complication of nasal CPAP. *Journal of Paediatrics and Child Health* **33**, 444–445.

178 Wood, B., Dubik, M. (1995) A new device for pleural drainage in newborn infants. *Pediatrics* **96**, 955–956.

179 Yu, V.Y.H., Orgill, A.A., Lim, S.B. *et al.* (1983) Growth and development of very low birthweight infants recovering from bronchopulmonary dysplasia. *Archives of Disease in Childhood* **58**, 791–794.

180 Yu, V.Y.K., Wong, P.Y., Bajuk, B., Szymonowicz, W. (1986) Pulmonary air leak in extremely low birthweight infants. *Archives of Disease in Childhood* **71**, 239–241.

181 Zerella, J.T., Trump, D.S. (1987) Surgical management of neonatal interstitial emphysema. *Journal of Pediatric Surgery* **22**, 34–37.

23

Aspiration syndromes

THOMAS E WISWELL AND PINCHI SRINIVASAN, with contributions by NRC ROBERTON

Aspiration syndromes are one of the common causes of neonatal respiratory distress and include aspiration of meconium, amniotic fluid, gastric contents, and blood. Although the pathophysiology and epidemiological factors of meconium aspiration are relatively well studied, the same is not true for the other aspiration syndromes. The clinical symptoms in any aspiration syndrome most commonly result from airway obstruction (atelectasis, air trapping and air leaks), parenchymal injury (pneumonitis), right-to-left shunting, and ventilation–perfusion mismatch. The meconium aspiration syndrome (MAS) is the most commonly occurring and best described of the aspiration disorders. As such, we have focused on the pathophysiology and management of MAS as a basis to guide the clinician treating any of the aspiration syndromes.

MECONIUM ASPIRATION SYNDROME (MAS)

Incidence

MAS develops in approximately 5 percent of neonates born through meconium-stained amniotic fluid.[38,171] The incidence of MAS is reported to be 2 per 1000 live-born infants in the United Kingdom.[41] Higher incidence rates have been documented elsewhere.[38,168] Particularly high incidence rates are reported from Indian subcontinent[34,72,117] and Middle East.[185]

Pathology

A review of 123 autopsy cases with histological evidence of intrauterine exposure to meconium revealed the frequent presence of pulmonary and umbilical cord inflammation, as well as inflammation of the membranes and chorionic plate.[28] Focal necrotic injury of umbilical cord vessels and cord ulceration were also noted in many cases. Burgess and Hutchings[28] speculated meconium passage *in utero* occurred in response to fetal distress as, in more than 50 percent of cases, there was presence of definite or probable evidence of fetal distress; this suggested the inflammatory changes were due to *in utero* exposure to meconium. Sepulveda *et al.* described a dose-dependent vasoconstrictive effect by bile acids (such as cholic acid) on human placental chorionic vessels.[140] Umbilical cord vessel injury and vasoconstriction induced by meconium have been previously described.[6,7] These mechanisms are thought to play a role in the pathogenesis of ischemic injury to the fetus, either global or focal in nature. Wiswell *et al.* observed multiple ischemic changes in the umbilical cords and placenta of fetal rabbits exposed to *in utero* meconium in the absence of hypoxia.[174] MAS is the most common disorder in which pulmonary hemorrhage is described in full-term infants.[20] Such bleeding may be caused by direct toxicity of meconium or by hypoxic/ischemic damage. The effects of chronic intrauterine meconium aspiration were reported in three neonates by Kearney.[90] Pathological findings were manifested by fetal lung infarcts containing inspissated meconium with a granulomatous reaction, lung rupture and meconium embolism.

Petechial hemorrhages may be present on the lung surfaces of infants who died from MAS. These findings are likely to be due to acute hypoxemia, particularly if death has occurred rapidly after birth. The lungs are often grossly greenish-yellow in color. The cut surface can be normal or show congestion and hemorrhage. In some specimens, meconium is readily apparent within both large and small airways. The pathognomonic histological feature of MAS is the presence of amniotic squames and meconium in the terminal airways. Meconium itself appears as rather granular eosinophilic material. Vacuoles containing meconium are frequently found within the macrophages that are frequently present. Hyaline membranes are often noted in lungs of neonates with MAS. In this context, a direct hypoxemic-ischemic insult to pulmonary epithelium may play a greater role in the pathogenesis of these membranes than in RDS. Non-specific changes of an asphyxial insult to the lung may also be present, including interstitial edema and hemorrhage. In addition, as, since the 1980s, infants that die from MAS will frequently have been ventilated at high pressures and rates, there may be histological changes mimicking those of bronchopulmonary dysplasia.[133] Infants who die from MAS may have changes in their pulmonary vascular tree in which pulmonary vessels have hypertrophied medial musculature.[130] The increased muscularity of the pulmonary vessels may extend into normally non-muscularized arteries down to the level of alveolus.

Pathophysiology (Table 23.1)

MAS results from the aspiration of meconium-stained amniotic fluid into fetal or infant lungs. Meconium is fetal bowel content. The word meconium is derived from the Greek *mekonion*, meaning poppy juice or opium. Aristotle is credited with naming the substance, having drawn the analogy between the presence of meconium in the amniotic fluid and the 'sleepy' or depressed newborn. Meconium is a complex, sterile, viscous substance, composed of swallowed amniotic fluid, cholesterol, bile acids and salts, mucopolysaccharides, intestinal pancreatic enzymes, vernix caseosa, lanugo, squamous cells and other debris.

MECONIUM PASSAGE *IN UTERO* AND ASPIRATION

Meconium-stained amniotic fluid is noted in 10–15 percent of all term deliveries in North America.[38,70,119,171] The overall incidence of meconium-stained amniotic fluid in the United Kingdom is 11.5 percent.[31] There is an increased risk with advanced gestational age[53] and in African-American women.[4] Although meconium may be present in the gastrointestinal tract as early as 10–16 weeks of gestation, it is rarely passed before 37 weeks of gestation. As a consequence, MAS is generally a disease of term or post-term infants, being rare before 37 weeks and common after 42 weeks of gestation.[111] Between 22 and 44 percent of infants born beyond 42 weeks of gestation will pass meconium *in utero*.[81,96] Additionally, meconium staining has been reported in association with congenital listeriosis[74] and other *in utero* infections.[136]

Lack of passage of meconium in early gestation is related to the absence of strong intestinal peristaltic activity, presence of tonically contracted anal sphincter and a terminal cap of viscous meconium.[62] It is believed that *in utero* meconium passage is associated with maturation, fetal stress and/or high levels of intestinal hormones. The maturation factor is related to gestational age, as previously described. Stresses, such as cord compression or fetal hypoxia, are believed to relax the anal

Table 23.1 *The pathophysiological effects and the mediators of the MAS*

Pathophysiological changes	Mediators

Mechanical effects
  Airway obstruction
  Altered lung elastic forces
	Meconium, edema fluid, protein exudates, red blood cells and white blood cells

Inflammatory effects
  Alveolar and parenchymal inflammation
  Protein leak into the airways
	Chemotactants: neutrophils and macrophages
	Cytokines: TNF-α, IL-1β and IL-8
	Eicosanoids: thromboxane B_2, leukotrienes B_4 and D_4 and 6-ketoprostaglandin F1α

Vascular effects
  Altered pulmonary vasoreactivity
  Vasoconstriction of pulmonary arteries
  Pulmonary vascular remodeling
  Right-to-left shunting
	Vasoactive mediators: endothelin-1, PGE_2, thromboxane A_2
	Direct effects of meconium
	Hypoxia

Metabolic effects
  Surfactant dysfunction
  Surfactant inactivation
  Decreased levels of surfactant proteins (SP-A and SP-B)
	Meconium, proteins, inflammatory cells, blood and edema fluid

Toxic effects
  Tissue necrosis and umbilical cord ulceration
  Vasoconstriction of placental, umbilical and fetal blood vessels with decreased blood flow
	Direct effects of meconium and its constituents

sphincter and increase intestinal peristalsis. Investigators have described an association between low Apgar scores and fetal acidosis with the presence of meconium-stained amniotic fluid.[98,119,148,149] Increased passage of meconium with low umbilical venous oxygen (less than 30 percent) saturations has been reported.[163] Although aspiration of meconium-stained amniotic fluid is often associated with prenatal or perinatal asphyxia or acidosis,[89] no consistent relationship between meconium passage *in utero* and fetal distress has been established.[49,132] Motilin, a gut hormone that stimulates peristaltic activity, may play a role in meconium passage. Motilin levels have been noted to be increased fourfold in term infants with abnormal fetal heart rate patterns.[103] In addition, motilin concentrations were reported to be higher in term gestation infants that did rather than did not pass meconium *in utero*.[104] Concentrations of the hormone are higher in term-gestation infants compared to those born prematurely.

The presence of fetal asphyxia or fetal distress may lead to cessation of normal fetal respiratory movements, resulting in apnea (p. 39). With prolonged asphyxia, periods of deep gasps will occur between the periods of apnea.[32,107] Fetal gasping movements have been observed by ultrasound examination.[24] A gasping fetus is more apt to aspirate meconium. This phenomenon is more likely to occur in term and post-term infants than in those who are preterm.[62] *In utero* aspiration of meconium prior to delivery has been shown by presence of meconium in the lungs of stillborn babies as well as those that die within minutes of birth.[27,130]

Both the *in utero* gasping and the initial breaths after the delivery of the baby's head can result in aspiration of large amounts of amniotic fluid into the lungs. In surviving infants, there is no way known to date to accurately distinguish which particular mechanism occurred.[38] Autopsies of stillborn fetuses and of infants dying from MAS within hours of birth have revealed deeply inspissated meconium in the lungs. In these infants, aspiration has probably occurred prior to delivery. It is likely that the most severe MAS, that requiring high ventilatory support or extracorporeal membrane oxygenation, results from *in utero* aspiration.

Correlation of meconium consistency ('thick' versus 'thin' meconium) with fetal outcome is also a subject of controversy due to the subjective nature of assessing the consistency. Nevertheless, virtually all reports associate the likelihood of MAS to be substantially higher with the thickest consistency meconium-stained amniotic fluid compared to thin or moderately thick fluid. Thick meconium is often described as 'pea-soup', particulate, viscous, and opaque, in contrast with watery, transluscent, lightly stained thin meconium. Perhaps the most important value of meconium-stained amniotic fluid is to alert the obstetrician to look further for signs of fetal compromise.[43]

Meconium is normally sterile. However, meconium concentrations exceeding 1 percent enhance the ability of amniotic fluid to sustain bacterial growth.[57] The mechanism may involve inhibition of phagocytosis, neutrophil oxidative burst[35] and alterations in zinc concentration[82] that favor bacterial growth. In three studies, women with meconium-stained amniotic fluid who were in preterm labor[112,136] or term labor[165] were found to have higher rates of positive amniotic fluid cultures. In none of those studies, however, were the infants born through meconium-stained amniotic fluid more likely to have systemic infections.[38]

In a large, prospective trial assessing the delivery room management of apparently vigorous meconium stained infants,[175] the factors significantly associated with the subsequent development of MAS were delivery via cesarean section, fewer than five prenatal visits, lack of oropharyngeal suctioning before delivery, presence of meconium in the trachea of intubated infants, abnormal fetal heart rate tracings, presence of oligohydramnios, and male gender.

PULMONARY PARENCHYMAL, ALVEOLAR AND VASCULAR CHANGES

There are multiple mechanisms involved in the complex pathophysiology of MAS (Figure 23.1).[38] At any given time, one or more of these mechanisms may be contributing to the degree of respiratory distress manifested by the infant. Not infrequently, there is a vicious cycle of ventilation–perfusion mismatch, right-to-left shunting, hypoxemia, acidosis and increased pulmonary vascular resistance that may be difficult or impossible to treat successfully.

AIRWAY OBSTRUCTION

Although meconium is approximately 75 percent water,[168] more than 80 percent of the solid portion of meconium is composed of mucopolysaccharides. Hence, the material may very easily obstruct both large and small airways. Obstruction can be partial or complete. Partial obstruction, acting in a 'ball-valve' mechanism, may lead to air trapping and air leaks.[154,157] This mechanism is characterized by gas entering the airway with each inspiration from negative intrathoracic pressure. During exhalation the airway diameter normally decreases; as a result, exhaled gas may be trapped without expulsion in the distal airways. Complete airway obstruction results in atelectasis, ventilation–perfusion mismatch, right-to-left shunting, and hypoxemia.[154] Atelectasis may also result from decreased alveolar compliance due to surfactant dysfunction.[115,150]

PULMONARY PARENCHYMAL AND ALVEOLAR INFLAMMATION

In addition to causing mechanical obstruction to airways, meconium causes pulmonary parenchymal and alveolar injury by other mechanisms. Within hours of

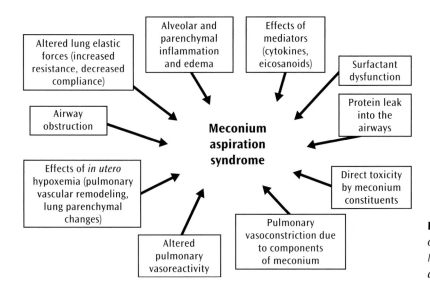

Figure 23.1 *The complex pathophysiology of the meconium aspiration syndrome. Multiple mechanisms may affect the lung and cause the infant's symptoms.*

meconium aspiration there is a profound inflammatory response within the pulmonary parenchyma and alveoli.[46,131,172,174] This is associated with the release of a variety of inflammatory cells and mediators (for example, cytokines and eicosanoids) that can directly injure the lung or influence vessel contractility.[2,46,86] The various inflammatory mediators released within the large airways, alveoli and lung parenchyma include interleukins such as IL-1β, IL-6 and IL-8, as well as tumor necrosis factor-α. Additionally, within 2 hours of aspiration, there is a marked influx of neutrophils and macrophages into the airways and lung parenchyma.

Meconium affects neutrophil function by inhibiting oxidative burst and phagocytosis.[35] The presence of IL-8 induces neutrophil chemotaxis.[47] The increased levels of inflammatory cytokines (TNF-α, IL-1β and IL-8) may directly injure lung parenchyma and lead to capillary leakage,[73] resulting in an injury pattern similar to acute respiratory distress syndrome (ARDS) (p. 396). The cytokines noted in animal models of MAS[184] cause airway and alveolar epithelial cell necrosis, as well as cell death from cellular apoptosis (non-inflammatory cell death). The enzyme phospholipase A$_2$ plays a key role in the pathogenesis of inflammatory lung diseases. High concentrations of phospholipase A$_2$ are found in meconium.[80] The substance has been shown to induce cellular injury and apoptosis in lung tissue.

EFFECTS ON SURFACTANT

The effect of meconium on endogenous surfactant has been extensively studied in the last two decades, both in animals and humans.[12,33,39,45,150] Both quantitative measures of surfactant components (for example, phospholipids and surfactant proteins) and biophysical measures of surfactant properties (for example, surface tension measurement or stable microbubble counts) are altered by meconium. Meconium displaces surfactant from the

Table 23.2 *Constituents of meconium that may contribute to surfactant dysfunction*

Proteolytic enzymes
Free fatty acids (especially oleic, steric, and palmitic acids)
Phospholipases
Bile salts
Blood
Lanugo
Squamous cells
Bilirubin
Multiple proteins
Steroid compounds
Cholesterol
Triglycerides

alveolar surface and inhibits its surface-lowering function.[69] Meconium can directly inhibit surfactant production and function.[38,62] There are many constituents of meconium that can contribute to the alteration of surfactant function (Table 23.2).[167] It inhibits surfactant in a concentration-dependent manner.[115,150] Decreased production of surfactant proteins A and B, as well as lower levels of large phospholipid aggregates, are associated with exudative lung injury occurring after meconium instillation in animal models.[8,39] Meconium diluted to as little as 1:6500 will adversely affect surface tension.[115] Surfactant inhibition has been demonstrated by both the water–methanol soluble phase of meconium (bilirubin and proteins), as well as the chloroform-soluble phase (free fatty acids, triglycerides and cholesterol) with highest specific inhibitory activity by the chloroform-soluble phase.[150]

Inhibition of surfactant function results from various lipophilic and hydrophilic substances (for example, glycolipids, free fatty acids, proteins and bilirubin) in meconium competing with surfactant molecules at the air–liquid interface.[71] Biochemical degradation of surfactant is caused by enzymes present in meconium, particularly phospholipase A$_2$.[138] The latter substance additionally causes asymmetry in the surfactant monolayer, as well as producing 'holes' in the type II pneumocyte.

Free fatty acids in meconium biophysically may disrupt the phospholipid layer at the air–liquid interface and inhibit the surface tension lowering activity of surfactant. Other phospholipases in meconium decrease surfactant activity in two ways, by directly hydrolyzing surfactant dipalmitoylphosphatidylcholine (DPPC) and, indirectly, the lysophosphatidylcholine (LPC) can also inhibit surfactant activity and secretion.[10,71] Bile salts in meconium induce intracellular calcium accumulation in type II pneumocytes,[123] which may alter how they function. Meconium can also alter surfactant morphological ultrastructure, thus decreasing the surface tension lowering ability.[12] The influx of neutrophils in the airways and alveoli produces proteases that degrade surfactant proteins. Hemorrhagic edema is a frequent histological finding in MAS.[45,172,174] Blood and edema fluid will adversely interfere with lowering of surface tension.

PULMONARY VASCULAR EFFECTS

Gersony and colleagues reported that hypoxia caused right-to-left shunting in fetal sheep due to pulmonary vascular obstruction and hypothesized a vicious cycle of hypoxia, pulmonary vasoconstriction, right-to-left shunting and hypoxia.[64] MAS is the most common respiratory disorder associated with persistent pulmonary hypertension of newborn (PPHN), making up at least 50 percent of the cases of PPHN. Pulmonary hypertension in association with perinatal aspiration syndromes was initially reported by Fox et al.[60] The increased pulmonary artery pressure is frequently greater than systemic arterial pressure. The pulmonary vascular resistance may be increased secondary to vasoconstriction of pulmonary vessels caused by vasoactive substances released with inflammatory response after meconium aspiration, platelet aggregation in pulmonary vessels in response to vasoactive substance and maldevelopment of pulmonary vessels secondary to chronic intrauterine hypoxia. In addition, prolonged in utero hypoxia may cause hypertrophy of muscular pulmonary artery walls and contribute to pulmonary hypertension.[85,116] There may be delayed adaptation of pulmonary hemodynamics in infants with mild and moderate MAS.[97] Elevated pulmonary artery pressure is seen in all infants as a response to hypoxemia and acidosis. The presence of hypoxemia and acidosis in infants at risk for delayed adaptation will have a significant additive effect contributing to PPHN, making it difficult to treat successfully. The inflammatory response to meconium leads to increased levels of various eicosanoids (thromboxane B$_2$, leukotrienes B$_4$ and D$_4$, and 6-ketoprostaglandin F1α) in the airways,[177,178] as well as increased blood levels of endothelin-1 (ET-1)[144]

and prostaglandin E$_2$.[141,142] These vasoactive mediators play a role in the pulmonary artery vasoconstriction of persistent pulmonary hypertension, which is frequently associated with MAS.[145–147]

Clinical signs

Approximately 20–30 percent of meconium-stained infants will be depressed at birth, typically manifesting decreased heart rate, poor color and abnormal respiratory effort. The occurrence of respiratory complications in an infant born through meconium-stained amniotic fluid may relate to in utero factors. Stresses such as hypoxia or oligohydramnios may lead to meconium passage. Subsequent gasping leads to aspiration of the material. Virtually all published reports confirm that the development of MAS is increased among infants who are depressed at birth, as well as those born through the thickest consistency meconium-stained amniotic fluid.[169] It must be recognized, however, that a significant proportion of infants with MAS are either born through thin-consistency meconium-stained amniotic fluid or are apparently vigorous at birth.[38,171,175] The incidence of MAS is about 1 percent with thin meconium-stained amniotic fluid and 7 percent in infants born through thick meconium-stained amniotic fluid. While it is likely that the most severe cases of MAS occur in infants that have aspirated in utero, postnatal aspiration of oropharyngeal meconium-stained fluid also plays a role. Incidence of many other respiratory disorders, including transient tachypnea of the newborn, pneumonia, pulmonary edema and pneumothorax, are significantly higher in infants born through meconium-stained amniotic fluid compared to those born through clear amniotic fluid.[175,182] The latter disorders are also more common in those born through thick, compared with thin, meconium-stained amniotic fluid.

Infants with MAS are often born after their due dates and manifest features of post-maturity, including long nails, a dysmature appearance, dry and scaling skin, and a dystrophic umbilical cord. The infant's skin, nails and umbilical cord are often stained by meconium and exhibit a range of different colors from green to brown to yellow. The latter manifestations generally take 3–12 hours of exposure to develop.

Approximately 50 percent of infants with MAS require mechanical ventilation, 15–33 percent develop pulmonary air leaks (most commonly pneumothoraces), and as many as 5–12 percent die.[38,171,175] As many as two-thirds of infants with persistent pulmonary hypertension have MAS as an associated disorder.[1,164] The proportion of babies admitted to newborn intensive care units is three- to tenfold higher among those born through meconium-stained amniotic fluid compared with those born through clear amniotic fluid.[9,105,119] In a report examining intrapartum and neonatal attributes associated with increased risk for severe MAS (that requiring assisted ventilation), the following factors were predictive in two-thirds of cases of severe MAS: fetal heart rate abnormalities during labor, low 5-minute Apgar scores, delivery by cesarean section and respiratory distress necessitating intubation following delivery.[77]

Over the past decade an association between intra-amniotic infection and meconium-stained amniotic fluid has been described.[38,136] It is difficult to ascertain whether the stress of intra-amniotic infection causes meconium passage or whether the presence of the substance enhances bacterial growth. The issue of increased risk for neonatal sepsis in infants born through meconium-stained amniotic fluid was studied by Wiswell and Henley.[170] No significant difference in culture-proven bacteremia in infants born through meconium-stained amniotic fluid (0.8 percent) was found compared with those born with clear amniotic fluid (0.7 percent). Krishman *et al.* have reported a similar lack of association between meconium-stained amniotic fluid and neonatal septicemia.[99] Although meconium-stained amniotic fluid has been described as a common feature of neonatal listeriosis,[25] the overwhelming majority of infants born through this fluid, as well as those who develop MAS, are not infected.

RESPIRATORY

Respiratory distress in the form of marked tachypnea, grunting, nasal flaring, intercostal and subcostal retractions and cyanosis is seen. Air trapping is recognized by an overdistended chest with a markedly increased anteroposterior diameter (a 'barrel-chest' appearance). Auscultation of the chest may reveal diffuse rales and rhonchi. Extensive consolidation of the lungs may be associated with diminished breath sounds. A more ominous feature is the presence of a pneumothorax, which is associated with diminished breath sounds on the involved side, as well as asymmetric chest expansion. Symptoms may persist for many days depending on the severity of the disease. Patients who are asphyxiated or born with neurological depression are frequently initially apneic. Nevertheless, when such patients are intubated and ventilated, they manifest physical signs in the respiratory tract that are identical to those in the spontaneously breathing neonate.[133]

CARDIOVASCULAR

In the absence of asphyxial damage or PPHN, there are no specific cardiovascular features associated with MAS. Due to delayed adaptation of normal pulmonary hemodynamics in infants with mild or moderate MAS, even in the absence of PPHN, careful cardiovascular monitoring is required for these infants during postnatal circulatory transition.[99] In the presence of PPHN there may exist cyanosis. On auscultation, a single S2 may be heard while the systolic heart murmur characteristic of tricuspid insufficiency is a common finding. Myocardial dysfunction may manifest in the form of hypotension and poor perfusion.

ABDOMINAL

The umbilical cord may be stained greenish-yellow if the meconium has been present in the liquor for 6–12 hours or longer. Not infrequently, the liver and spleen are palpable due to downward displacement of the diaphragm from air trapping.

CENTRAL NERVOUS SYSTEM

Approximately 20–30 percent of all infants born through meconium-stained amniotic fluid are depressed at birth, typically with 1-minute Apgar scores of less than 6.[38] Irritability and jitteriness may persist for the first 2–3 days, often aggravated by coexisting hypoxemia.[133] If there is a coexisting neurological insult, then the infant may have neurological features of birth asphyxia to a varying degree, including hypotonia, coma, and seizures.

Differential diagnosis

The major differential diagnoses in infants born through meconium-stained amniotic fluid include bacterial pneumonia, sepsis with pulmonary edema, ARDS, transient tachypnea of newborn (TTN), PPHN, aspiration of amniotic fluid or blood, and respiratory distress syndrome in a term-gestation infant. Additionally, congenital cyanotic heart disease needs to be ruled out in the presence of significant hypoxemia. Echocardiography is a useful tool to assess for structural cardiac lesions or for findings of PPHN. Based on clinical presentation and chest radiography, it may be difficult to initially differentiate MAS from sepsis or pneumonia. Infants with TTN usually require only oxygen therapy (p. 272). Moreover, those with TTN typically have their worst respiratory distress shortly after birth and improve steadily without any further deterioration. Aspiration of amniotic fluid or blood may have a presentation similar to MAS.

Investigations

Routine investigations such as complete and differential blood count, blood culture, serum electrolytes including calcium, serum glucose, arterial blood gases and chest radiography should be done in all babies born through meconium-stained amniotic fluid who are manifesting respiratory distress. If the patient is severely hypoxemic, other investigations such as echocardiography and electrocardiogram should be done. Investigations to evaluate suspected perinatal asphyxia are warranted as necessary,[62] including placental and umbilical cord histopathology, serial serum creatinine, blood urea nitrogen (BUN), serum glucose and calcium, urinalysis, complete blood count with differential and platelet count, prothrombin time (PT) and partial prothrombin time (PTT) (in the presence of disseminated intravascular coagulation), electroencephalogram and neuroimaging (if abnormal neurological findings are present).

HEMATOLOGY

Elevated nucleated red blood cell counts in infants with symptomatic meconium aspiration has been reported.[50] Leukocytosis is often present. The latter may be due to multiple factors, including the profound inflammatory response to meconium aspiration; stress from perinatal birth asphyxia; or concomitant infection.[108,113] Thrombocytopenia is often seen in MAS infants with PPHN,[139] those who are ventilated mechanically,[15] or who have had perinatal asphyxia.

BIOCHEMISTRY

Although no characteristic biochemical abnormalities are specific for MAS, metabolic abnormalities consistent with pre-existing asphyxia are often seen, including hypoglycemia, hypocalcemia, elevated BUN/creatinine, and hyponatremia.

ARTERIAL BLOOD GAS ANALYSIS

Due to ventilation–perfusion mismatch and right-to-left shunting in MAS, hypoxemia is common. In many cases ventilation may not be problem and $PaCO_2$ levels may even be low. Elevated $PaCO_2$ is found in patients with the most severe lung disease or when air leaks such as pneumothoraces occur. Persistent metabolic acidosis may indicate the presence of sepsis, hypotension, or renal failure.[133]

ECHOCARDIOGRAPHY AND ELECTROCARDIOGRAPHY

Echocardiography is often necessary to evaluate cardiac contractility and ventricular filling, as well as to look for the evidence of PPHN. Korhonen et al. prospectively evaluated serial Doppler echocardiograms during the first 72 hours after birth in infants with mild or moderately severe MAS.[97] They found evidence of delayed adaptation of pulmonary hemodynamics. The patients in the study group had bidirectional shunting significantly more common than the control (non-MAS) group in the first day, with a slower increase in the peak aortopulmonary pressure gradient. Following severe intrapartum asphyxia, the electrocardiogram may reveal ST segment changes suggestive of subendocardial ischemia. When concomitant PPHN is present, Doppler studies may reveal right-to-left shunting across the ductus arteriosus and/or the foramen ovale, as well as a 'jet' of tricuspid insufficiency that confirms elevated right ventricular pressures. Moreover, right ventricular and atrial hypertrophy may be present. The

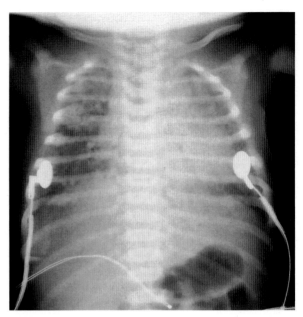

Figure 23.2 *Chest radiograph of an infant with MAS. There are diffuse, patchy infiltrates bilaterally.*

sickest infants often demonstrate poor ventricular functioning. Cyanotic congenital heart disease should be considered when persistent hypoxemia is encountered.

RADIOGRAPHY

The classic chest radiograph findings of MAS are generalized overaeration with diffuse, patchy infiltrates (Figures 23.2, 23.3). The differences in the quantity of meconium aspirated, the variations in the consistency of the meconium-stained amniotic fluid that is aspirated and the diverse mechanisms involved in the pathogenesis of the disorder, lead to a wide variety of radiographic findings. These include: consolidation (Figure 23.4), atelectasis, pleural effusions, air leaks (pneumomediastinum or pneumothorax), hyperaeration, 'wet-lung' picture, hypovascularity, or a relatively normal appearance.[38] Moreover, the radiographic appearance may also be influenced by other factors, such as pulmonary edema related to cerebral anoxia, ischemic myocardial dysfunction, or renal ischemia. In many patients recovering from MAS, radiographic clearing may be slow, over a period of days to weeks.[121] In others, the roentgenographic changes may revert to normal within days. Although Yeh et al. described a relationship between the severity of MAS and the degree of radiological abnormalities,[181] others have not confirmed this association.[83,162]

URINALYSIS

Spectrophotometric analysis of urine may reveal absorption at 405 nm, characteristic of bile pigments present in meconium. The urine may appear dark greenish brown in color due to meconium pigments excreted in urine

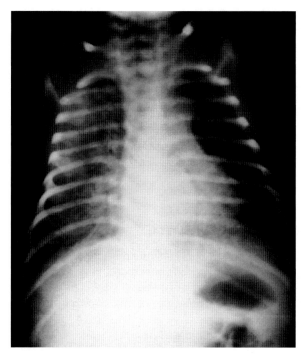

Figure 23.3 *In the chest radiograph of this infant with MAS who is not being mechanically ventilated, one notes the bilateral hyperexpansion of the lung fields. This is likely due to air trapping secondary to obstruction of airways by meconium.*

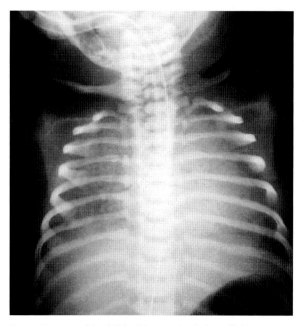

Figure 23.4 *In this child with MAS, both lung fields appear to be more globally affected as the lung fields progress to be consolidated.*

after absorption across the pulmonary epithelium into the plasma.[48] Decreased urine output (oliguria or anuria), proteinuria and hematuria may indicate renal injury due to acute tubular necrosis due to antenatal or intrapartum hypoxemia/ischemia. Concurrent elevations in serum BUN and creatinine can occur.

Monitoring

UMBILICAL ARTERIAL/VENOUS CATHETER PLACEMENT AND BLOOD GASES

Placement of umbilical arterial and venous catheters should be reserved for moderately or severely ill infants with MAS, such as those requiring mechanical ventilation or high levels of oxygen ($FiO_2 > 0.40$). Such access facilitates serial monitoring of arterial blood gases, acid–base status, and blood pressure, as well as providing central venous access for administration of drugs and nutrition. If it is not possible to place an umbilical arterial catheter, peripheral arterial lines are used; the PaO_2 should optimally be maintained in the range of 80–100 mmHg (10.6–13.3 kPa). Some clinicians try to achieve hyperoxemic levels, believing that this will prevent or mitigate concurrent PPHN; however, there is no evidence that this strategy improves outcome and it may increase the risk of oxygen toxicity to the lungs and other organs. Maintenance of $PaCO_2$ levels between 35 and

50 mmHg (5–6.6 kPa) is a reasonable approach. When arterial catheters are not available, capillary blood gases are often obtained to assess acid–base status and ventilation. It is important to be aware that a capillary sample represents a mixed-venous specimen in which the PCO_2 value is at best 6–7 mmHg (1 kPa) higher than the arterial $PaCO_2$.

PULSE OXIMETRY AND VITAL SIGN MONITORING

Vital signs of all infants with MAS need to be monitored continuously. This includes oxygen saturation (SaO_2) monitoring. During the early course of MAS, we recommend placement of preductal (right hand) and postductal (either lower extremity) SaO_2 probes. A greater than 10 percent difference in preductal and postductal oxygen saturation (SaO_2) is consistent with the diagnosis of PPHN. Transcutaneous $PaCO_2$ or end tidal CO_2 monitoring may be considered as non-invasive methods of assessing ventilation and CO_2 elimination.

LABORATORY MONITORING

In addition to serial monitoring of arterial blood gases, frequent monitoring of serum electrolytes, glucose, creatinine and calcium is essential in infants with severe MAS. Frequent chest radiographs are indicated in all infants with MAS who require mechanical ventilation or substantial oxygen supplementation, in order to facilitate early detection of complications such as air leaks or atelectasis.

Table 23.3 *Results of the international randomized, controlled trial assessing the effect of intrapartum oro- and nasopharyngeal suctioning in preventing meconium aspiration syndrome (MAS) and adverse outcomes of the disorder*

	Suction (n = 1245)	No suction (n = 1236)	Significance
Number with MAS (percent)	43 (3.5)	44 (3.6)	NS
Number needing mechanical ventilation (percent)	15 (1.2)	14 (1.1)	NS
Number of deaths (percent)	5 (0.4)	3 (0.2)	NS
Mean number of days on oxygen in patients with MAS ($\pm$SD)	5.0 ± 7.1	5.3 ± 7.3	NS
Mean number of days on mechanical ventilation in patients with MAS ($\pm$SD)	5.8 ± 5.5	4.2 ± 4.6	NS

*NS: not significant; SD: standard deviation.

Prevention

Several strategies to mitigate or lesson the effects of aspirated meconium-stained amniotic fluid have been proposed, but only a few have undergone sufficient study to be proven effective.

PRENATAL STRATEGIES

Several studies have evaluated amnioinfusion for preventing MAS. The amnioinfusion technique consists of infusing warmed fluid (typically saline or Ringer's lactate) into the uterus via an internal pressure catheter after the membranes have ruptured and thick-consistency meconium-stained amniotic fluid has been observed. Amnioinfusion is based on the principle that increasing the volume of amniotic fluid will dilute meconium and increase the amniotic fluid volume. Although it might be thought that diluting the meconium would make it easier for the fetus to aspirate the substance, respiratory complications are more likely in infants born through moderately thick and thick-consistency meconium-stained amniotic fluid. Additionally, meconium dilution may decrease its toxicity. Furthermore, if oligohydramnios is present, an increase in fluid volume might relieve cord compression and hence fetal hypoxia and acidosis, further meconium passage, gasping, and meconium aspiration. A meta-analysis concluded that the amnioinfusion technique would prevent MAS[52] and may be associated with improvements in perinatal outcome, particularly in settings where facilities for perinatal surveillence are limited.[79] Nevertheless, in several large retrospective studies,[94,135,160] investigators were unable to demonstrate any difference in neonatal outcomes between infants born to women who had received amnioinfusion for meconium-stained amniotic fluid compared to those born to women who did not. A higher incidence of fetal heart rate abnormalities, instrument-assisted deliveries and endometritis have been noted in women who received amnioinfusion. Currently a large international multicenter, randomized trial is under way to clarify the role of amnioinfusion in preventing MAS.[61]

INTRAPARTUM STRATEGIES

Routine oropharyngeal suctioning before delivery of the infant's shoulders has long been thought to play an important role in preventing or mitigating the course of MAS. This is largely based on the report of Carson et al.[30] Carson reported a comparison of the results of infants undergoing routine suction to those of historical controls. Although the decreased incidence of MAS following intrapartum suctioning was not significantly different from the control group, naso- and oropharyngeal suctioning is now routinely performed by obstetricians. Falciglia reported a similar analysis and did not find this technique to be of benefit.[55] Additionally, Falciglia and colleagues subsequently performed an observational study and again demonstrated no effect of intrapartum suctioning.[55] Vain and colleagues recognized the lack of adequate evidence supporting the technique and recently completed a large, randomized, controlled trial assessing its efficacy.[161] Almost 2500 infants were prospectively enrolled into their trial and randomized to either naso- and oropharyngeal suctioning prior to delivery of the shoulders or to no suctioning. There were no differences between the suction and no-suction groups in the incidence of MAS or in other major outcomes (Table 23.3). Additionally, in the subpopulations of infants at greater risk for developing MAS (those born through the thickest consistency meconium-stained amniotic fluid or those exhibiting fetal distress during labor), there were no differences due to intrapartum suctioning.

Some authors recommend cesarean sections for infants surrounded by meconium stained amniotic fluid. Coltart et al. proposed that cesarean sections be electively performed on woman who have meconium-stained amniotic fluid.[41] They speculated that preventing the stresses of vaginal delivery may decrease the risk of meconium aspiration. In most large reviews of meconium-stained amniotic fluid and MAS, however, babies born via cesarean section have higher rates of MAS than those delivered vaginally.[169] This is not surprising, as cesarean sections are usually performed on infants at greater risk for developing MAS, i.e. those with fetal distress. Meydanli et al. recently performed a randomized controlled trial in 70 consecutive women with singleton pregnancies complicated by thick-consistency meconium-stained amniotic fluid.[114] The women were randomized to either undergo elective abdominal delivery or spontaneous vaginal delivery. The incidence of MAS was significantly higher among the infants delivered by cesarean section (11/35, 31 percent) compared to those delivered vaginally (4/35, 11 percent) ($P = 0.041$).

One physician recommended the intrapartum administration of drugs such as morphine or paralytics to laboring mothers with meconium-stained amniotic fluid.[67,68] Theoretically, transplacental passage of these drugs could prevent gasping and aspiration of the meconium-stained amniotic fluid. Although the therapy was apparently successful in an animal model of meconium-stained amniotic fluid/MAS,[23] anecdotal data from human reports have not substantiated this approach.[29,51] No prospective, controlled trials have been performed to confirm the benefits of such a strategy. Indeed, the high chance of adverse effects on both the mother and the neonate (mainly respiratory depression) makes this therapy one that we would strongly advise against.

POSTNATAL STRATEGIES

In the infant born through meconium-stained amniotic fluid, several therapies performed immediately after birth are practiced or have been proposed as being beneficial. It has been suggested to perform them until the infant is intubated and suctioned: thoracic 'squeeze', manual epiglottal blockage and manual cricoid pressure. There are, however, no scientific data validating these therapies and none should be performed.

Postnatal tracheal suctioning has generated considerable controversy. The technique as described by Gregory et al.[70] is potentially risky to the infant's trachea, because of the uncontrolled degree of negative pressure generated by the mouth of the intubator.[14] Moreover, such suctioning is potentially hazardous and could result in transmission of infectious secretions from neonate to the intubator or vice versa.[13] Therefore, it is recommended that suction be provided only by mechanical devices attached to the proximal end of the endotracheal tube. In an in vitro trial to determine the optimal method comparing different mechanical devices available for this purpose, Bent and Wiswell found the meconium aspirator (Neotech Products, Inc., Chatsworth, CA) at a continuously applied negative pressure of 150 mmHg resulted in the greatest amount of meconium retrieval.[19] The airway histopathological findings in an in vivo model of newborn piglet models did not reveal substantial injury resulting from continuously applied negative pressure of 150 mmHg using the meconium aspirator.[19] A recent multicenter prospective randomized trial was unable to demonstrate any difference in the incidence of MAS or other respiratory complications in apparently vigorous infants who underwent intubation and tracheal suctioning compared with those who

received routine delivery room care. Only a few children (3.8 percent) experienced complications of intubation, and all the complications were transient.[175] The Neonatal Resuscitation Program of the American Academy of Pediatrics now recommends only intubating and suctioning newborn infants who are 'depressed' in the delivery room, depression being defined as having a heart rate less than 100/min, poor respiratory effort or poor tone.

Many believe that chest physiotherapy of meconium-stained infants will loosen adherent debris from the lungs and improve the retrieval of intra-airway meconium. There are, however, no data verifying the efficacy of chest physiotherapy either in preventing MAS or in treating the disorder. Similarly, although clinicians routinely perform gastric suctioning of meconium-stained infants with the belief it will lessen the risk of subsequent emesis or reflux and aspiration, this has yet to be evaluated in clinical trials. Routine gastric lavage prior to initiation of feeding in a group of infants born through meconium-stained amniotic fluid was not associated with a decrease in MAS in either the control or study group, regardless of thickness of meconium stained amniotic fluid.[118]

Many believe that the majority of infants with MAS have aspirated meconium-stained amniotic fluid before birth.[65,88] We believe that despite optimal management, infants born through meconium-stained amniotic fluid may still develop MAS and have morbid or even fatal outcomes.[153,168]

Treatment

It is easy to underestimate the severity of lung disease in mature term babies. It is, therefore, important to investigate infants appropriately in the first hour so that severe blood gas derangements, hypotension or radiological changes can be detected. Children with MAS often need prolonged hospitalization and make up the largest proportion (approximately 35 percent) of infants requiring extracorporeal membrane oxygenation (ECMO).[143] Treatment in MAS is largely supportive, yet crucial in avoiding morbidity and mortality. The general principles and goals of respiratory therapy in MAS include assuring adequate oxygen delivery to tissues, generally by maintaining PaO_2 or SaO_2 levels in acceptable ranges, improving the distribution of ventilation lowering pulmonary vascular resistance, avoiding hypo- or hypercapnia, avoiding metabolic or respiratory acidosis; and minimizing the oxygen demands. Preventing or ameliorating the vicious cycle of hypoxemia → acidosis → right-to-left shunting → hypoxemia, by directing the therapies at the underlying pathophysiology is essential.

GENERAL MANAGEMENT

First and foremost, sufficient supplementary oxygen should be provided to maintain oxygen saturation levels above 95 percent or PaO_2 levels between 80 and 100 mmHg (10.4–13 kPa). Other strategies that are often used include minimal stimulation, sedation, paralytic agents, routine chest physiotherapy and suctioning. None of these latter therapies has undergone the rigors of scientific scrutiny in the management of MAS. Maintaining infants in neutral thermal environment minimizes their oxygen consumption. Term babies with serious lung disease of all types become very agitated when disturbed and hypoxemia may result. Similarly, pulmonary vasoconstriction can be triggered as a response to noxious stimuli such as suctioning; therefore minimal stimulation and sedation are appropriate.

The systemic blood pressure should be kept greater than pulmonary pressure. Maintaining sufficient cardiac output may require volume replacement and/or use of inotropes. We advise maintaining hemoglobin concentrations of at least 13–15 g/dl by packed red cell transfusions. If there has been intrapartum asphyxia, fluid intake and output should be strictly monitored and the common metabolic problems such as oliguria, hypoglycemia and hypocalcemia anticipated and treated accordingly. Parenteral nutrition should be instituted in those patients with severe lung disease on ventilation who are not receiving enteral feedings by 3 days of age.

ANTIBIOTICS

Although there is little evidence to justify the routine use of prophylactic antibiotics for MAS, it is not easy to distinguish the early radiographic features of the disorder from those of neonatal pneumonia. We initially administer antibiotics to infants with apparent MAS. However, we discontinue this therapy once cultures have been negative for 48–72 hours.

STEROIDS

Systemic corticosteroid use has been suggested for the treatment of MAS because of the profound pulmonary inflammation that occurs soon after aspiration of meconium. Two small trials have demonstrated minimal benefits.[179,180] Major outcomes (mortality, chronic lung disease, and duration of hospitalization), however, were not improved by steroid use. In the aforementioned trials, the majority of study patients had mild MAS (only 20 percent and 40 percent, respectively, of the enrolled infants with MAS required mechanical ventilation). In a recently published pilot study, da Costa et al. treated 14 infants with MAS and PPHN who were on mechanical ventilation and severely ill.[44] Therapy was started on average more than 3 days after birth. Rapid improvement was reported in 13 of the 14 infants. There is a need for randomized, controlled trials in similar patients in order to verify this response.

RESPIRATORY THERAPY

Initially, most infants are treated with oxygen alone. Anecdotally, many physicians believe that oxygen alone up to an inspiratory fraction (FiO_2) of 1.00 should be used in order to avoid positive pressure ventilation, prevent air trapping and minimize air leaks.[180] Many babies with MAS can be managed by providing an adequate concentration of warmed humidified oxygen into a headbox (oxyhood) or via nasal cannula. We advise that sufficient oxygen should be provided to maintain oxygen saturation levels above 95 percent or PaO_2 levels between 80 and 100 mmHg (10.4–13 kPa).

Approximately 30–50 percent of infants diagnosed with MAS require mechanical ventilation. Assisted ventilation may be necessary for infants with MAS in order to treat hypoxemia, hypercapnia and acidosis. Clinicians vary in their desire to maintain certain arterial blood gas levels: some seek to achieve normal oxygen and carbon dioxide levels, whereas others wish to maintain oxygenation at higher than usual levels in an effort to prevent or mitigate PPHN. Hyperventilation is frequently employed to achieve alkalosis by hypocapnia in an attempt to attain pulmonary vasodilation and decreased pulmonary vascular resistances, while others have suggested that a more beneficial approach might be 'gentle ventilation', in which lower oxygen and pH levels, as well as higher carbon dioxide values, are accepted, in the belief this will decrease ventilator-induced trauma to the lungs. To date, there have been no trials comparing any of these strategies in infants with MAS.

Some consider application of low to moderate positive end expiratory pressures (PEEP) or continuous positive airway pressure (CPAP) at 4–7 cmH$_2$O to be of benefit.[59] It may improve oxygenation through resolution of atelectasis, stabilization of collapsing terminal airways[3] and diminished pulmonary shunting.[156] Others prefer using nasal CPAP at higher levels (J.-T. Wung, personal communication, 1999). We believe higher levels of PEEP or CPAP should be used with caution because of the potential for producing air trapping and pneumothoraces.

There are no strictly defined indications for mechanical ventilation in babies with MAS. Hypoxemia, hypercapnia and acidemia, however, are all undesirable in these babies who are frequently at risk for PPHN, as well as hypoxic-ischemic encephalopathy and cerebral edema. In these babies, it may be beneficial to maintain the $PaCO_2$ levels between 30 and 35 mmHg (4 and 4.5 kPa). Various conventional methods of ventilation including intermittent mandatory ventilation (IMV), patient-triggered ventilation (synchronized IMV or assist/control), pressure support ventilation, and volume-control ventilation have been used in infants with MAS. None of these methods has been compared to each other or to other therapies in clinical trials. We generally initiate mechanical ventilation using patient-triggered ventilation. We typically prefer a long expiratory time (0.35–0.45 seconds) and use low to moderate levels of PEEP (4–5 cmH$_2$O).

High-frequency ventilation

Infants with MAS may have unremittent respiratory failure while managed on conventional mechanical ventilation. This has led some to consider using high-frequency ventilation (HFV). The results of HFV trials in animal models of MAS have been conflicting.[91,106,155,169,173] The most commonly used high-frequency ventilators are high-frequency oscillators (HFOs) and high-frequency jet ventilators (HFJVs). To date, there have been no prospective, randomized, controlled trials performed comparing high-frequency ventilation with conventional ventilation or other therapies in infants with MAS only. Clark *et al.* performed a prospective RCT examining the use of high-frequency oscillatory ventilation (HFOV) in sick, term-gestation infants with respiratory failure, many of whom had MAS, comparing them with those treated conventionally.[36] No differences in the major outcomes were reported. Baumgart *et al.* retrospectively examined the outcomes of a group of near-term infants with respiratory failure, many of whom had MAS;[17] they found no advantages in those who had been supported by HFJV. Finally, HFOV appeared to be of benefit in infants with PPHN who concomitantly had MAS, especially in combination with inhaled nitric oxide (p. 381).[95] We believe that current evidence supports the role of HFV as rescue therapy in babies with MAS.

Surfactant

The surfactant dysfunction seen in MAS is from inhibited surfactant functions, alterations in surfactant composition, and disrupted production of endogenous surfactant. In the laboratory, the concentration-dependent inhibition by meconium is overcome by administering greater quantities of surfactant.[115] Conceivably, the course of MAS could be positively affected by the use of exogenous surfactant replacement therapy. The results in animal models of MAS, however, have been conflicting.[66,150,151,173] Two different methods of surfactant administration, intratracheal bolus or lung lavage, have been studied.

Several anecdotal reports of bolus surfactant therapy in human infants with MAS appeared in the 1990s.[11,22,74,93] Frequently, no substantial improvements were noted until second or third doses of surfactant were administered. In the sole randomized trial of 'bolus' therapy, Findlay *et al.* administered bovine surfactant at 1.5 times the standard 'RDS' dose and infused it over 20 minutes.[56] They found surfactant-treated infants to be significantly less likely to have pneumothoraces or require ECMO. The treated group also had fewer days of mechanical ventilation, oxygen therapy and hospitalization; improvements were only seen when multiple doses of surfactant had been given. Lotze *et al.* performed a randomized trial in which term-gestation infants with respiratory failure received four standard doses of bovine surfactant.[102] Approximately

half of the enrolled infants had MAS. A decreased need for ECMO was noted in treated infants, but there were no differences in mortality, air leaks or duration of mechanical ventilation, oxygen therapy, or hospitalization.

The lavage approach with dilute surfactant was initially described in an animal model of MAS.[127] Since surfactant is a detergent, it should have a cleansing action on the lungs. The theory behind the lavage approach is 'wash-out' of meconium, its constituents and the products of inflammation (cells, cytokines, etc.),[125] as well as dilution of the toxic effects of meconium. Multiple small volume dilute surfactant lavages have reportedly improved oxygenation in anecdotal reports.[100,124] A more vigorous lavage approach with a series of bronchoalveolar lavages using Surfaxin® (KL-4 surfactant, Discovery Laboratories, Inc., Doylestown, PA), both in animal models of MAS[40] and in a small randomized trial in infants,[176] has shown improvement in pulmonary function. Currently available evidence favors exogenous surfactant administration for MAS. Nevertheless, no surfactants have been approved by any regulatory agencies (for example the Food and Drug Administration) specifically for use in MAS. There have been no trials in human infants comparing the types of surfactants with each other. *In vitro* work has demonstrated that the protein-containing synthetic surfactant (KL-4 surfactant) and a surfactant containing recombinant surfactant protein C resist meconium inhibition better than commercially available natural surfactants, including Survanta, Alveofact and Curosurf.[78] Ongoing trials should further delineate the unanswered questions such as the timing of surfactant administration in the course of MAS, the optimal method (bolus versus lavage) of administration, the optimal dose (amount and concentration), the frequency of doses, and whether there are synergistic effects of addition of other substances or modes of therapy to surfactant administration in the management of MAS.

Inhaled nitric oxide (iNO)

Inhaled nitric oxide (iNO) as a pulmonary vascular relaxing agent in the treatment of PPHN in neonates has been assessed for the past decade. It is believed that iNO decreases extrapulmonary right-to-left shunting and ventilation–perfusion mismatch by dilating the blood vessels in well-aerated lung fields. Its efficacy depends on adequate delivery of the agent to the target resistance vessels within the lung. Some clinical trials have indicated that the response to iNO is disease-specific, with more consistent improvement in oxygenation in infants with extrapulmonary right-to-left shunting than in other infants. The use of iNO in term-gestation infants with respiratory failure (including MAS) has led to improvement in oxygenation and decreased need for ECMO compared to control infants (p. 179).[37,134,152] In these trials, however, there have been no significant differences in mortality, duration of mechanical ventilation or length of hospitalization. We believe iNO should be tried in the presence of significant unremitting hypoxemia when there is evidence of pulmonary hypertension.

Liquid ventilation

Liquid ventilation with perfluorocarbons appears promising, but remains an experimental therapy. Meconium-stained lambs with respiratory distress improve rapidly after treatment with partial or total liquid ventilation.[58] Increased survival, gas exchange and hemodynamic instability in a guinea pig model of MAS have been shown with perfluorochemical lavage compared with saline lavage.[109,110] Liquid ventilation with perfluorochemical compound may potentially alleviate MAS in several ways which include providing a cleaning action, improving ventilation–perfusion matching, recruiting alveoli, anti-inflammatory activity and reducing surface tension. It may be that the unique ability of perfluorocarbons to dissolve large quantities of oxygen and carbon dioxide at atmospheric pressure can be useful for ventilating neonates with MAS, providing much-needed time for the lungs to recuperate from the insult.[63]

Extracorporeal membrane oxygenation (p. 179)

A subgroup of patients with severe MAS progress to develop intractable pulmonary hypertension with profound hypoxemia, despite aggressive treatment measures. These infants have a variable degree of parenchymal lung injury. Extracorporeal membrane oxygenation (ECMO) is the treatment of last resort in such patients. Bartlett et al. first described the use of ECMO in the treatment of MAS.[16] The use of venoarterial ECMO during the 1980s was associated with encouraging results for neonates with severe MAS.[101]

The United Kingdom collaborative ECMO trial concluded that for every four infants receiving ECMO for MAS, there was one additional survivor.[159] ECMO support is typically required for 4–5 days in infants with MAS,[129] the shortest duration for any diagnosis. The worldwide survival rate for more than 5000 neonates with MAS managed with ECMO since the mid-1980s until 1999 is 94 percent, the highest survival rate for any condition supported by ECMO. The survivors of ECMO do not appear to have increased rate of disability or neurological damage compared to other severely hypoxic, conventionally treated neonates with MAS, despite a greater proportion surviving.[158,164]

Prognosis

MORTALITY

The mortality of MAS has fallen considerably from the 40 to 62 percent reported in the 1960s and 1970s. Nevertheless, during the past decade, reported mortality rates still ranged from 4 to 12 percent.[38] One must recognize that some babies will have suffered severe antenatal inhalation of meconium and may be unresuscitable in the delivery room or may die despite optimal intensive care. Other infants with MAS may die from the associated cardiac, pulmonary, neurological or renal sequelae of severe asphyxia.

MORBIDITY

Many infants with MAS have suffered in utero hypoxia-ischemia. These insults may result in myocardial dysfunction, PPHN, renal failure and brain or other organ injury.

Air leaks

The most common pulmonary complications of MAS are air leaks: pneumomediastinum, pneumothorax and pneumopericardium, with an incidence of 15–20 percent in non-ventilated babies and up to 50 per cent in those who require ventilation. Pulmonary interstial emphysema is rare in babies with MAS. Pneumothoraces may be bilateral and under tension and commonly cause acute deterioration in the infant's condition. Air leaks secondary to unwarranted aggressive traumatic intubation in delivery room are not uncommon.

Persistent pulmonary hypertension (PPHN)

The incidence of this complication varies. Approximately 50–66 percent of those with PPHN have MAS as an underlying respiratory disorder. One may expect 10–35 percent of infants with MAS to develop PPHN. A large proportion of mortality associated with MAS is attributable to PPHN.

Chronic lung disease Infants with MAS are at risk for chronic lung disease, particularly if they have required high ventilatory support or ECMO. As many as 5–10 percent of ventilated infants require oxygen beyond 28 days after birth. Moreover, many infants demonstrate reactive airway disease, decreased compliance and increased resistance at follow-up.[183] The abnormal lung function appears to be related to the degree of severity of MAS.

INFECTION

In non-ventilated babies with MAS, who are routinely treated with antibiotics, infection is not a clinical problem. During the acute stages of MAS, affected infants are at no higher risk for bacteremia than is the general population of neonates.[170] Infants with severe lung disease who are ventilated for longer periods are at increased risk for infections secondary to central line colonization, long-term intubation and other invasive procedures.

NEUROLOGICAL

Compared with those born through clear amniotic fluid, meconium-stained infants and those with MAS are at greater risk for having poor neurological outcomes, including cerebral palsy and seizures.[166] There are several speculated potential mechanisms of fetal injury and poor outcomes caused by meconium exposure.[5,18] These include direct injury of vascular smooth muscle or ulceration;[6,7] umbilical or placental vasoconstriction by meconium components such as eicosanoids or bile acid, the result of which is ischemia and hypoxemia; and diffusion of the latter substances into the fetal circulation where they could cause vasoconstriction of blood vessels in the fetal lungs, brain, or other organs. Severe neurological damage may be caused by antepartum hypoxia-ischemia and may occasionally follow extreme hypoxemia during the course of severe lung disease. Some neurological injury may be due to hypocapnia during hyperventilation in an effort to achieve alkalosis.

OTHER ASPIRATION SYNDROMES

These include aspiration of amniotic fluid, blood and gastric contents; their management is similar to that of MAS.

Aspiration of amniotic fluid

Aspiration of amniotic fluid reportedly occurs when a fetus experiences severe enough asphyxia to initiate deep gasping.[42] Other potential mechanisms are the inhalation of amniotic fluid during the cesarean section process or aspiration of cervical secretions during vaginal delivery. The support for amniotic fluid aspiration is from postmortem studies that have revealed amniotic squamous epithelial cells in both stillborn and liveborn infants. The importance of amniotic fluid aspiration as a clinical entity remains speculative. Amniotic fluid is substantially different from lung liquid and fetal lung fluid (p. 26) (Table 23.4).[21] These differences may contribute to the pathophysiology of the respiratory distress following amniotic fluid aspiration. Jose et al. instilled large volumes of amniotic fluid with squamous cells into the lungs of adult rabbits and found no adverse effects.[87] Infants with aspiration of amniotic fluid manifest with similar respiratory symptoms as in aspiration of

meconium-stained amniotic fluid. Animal comparison studies assessing amniotic fluid aspiration, however, have demonstrated the presence of normal resting volume, lung pressure volume curves, arterial PaO_2 and significantly less atelectasis than seen in meconium-stained amniotic fluid aspiration.[88] Maternal amniotic fluid may be contaminated with potentially infectious organisms. The mother may either be symptomatic (with signs of chorioamnionitis) or, more commonly, asymptomatic. Moreover, it may be difficult to distinguish the radiographic appearance from that of infectious pneumonia. Thus, clinicians should strongly consider starting antibiotic therapy in babies suspected of having amniotic fluid aspiration. Such therapy may be discontinued once blood cultures are negative for 48 hours and the child has no further signs of infection. In addition, vernix caseosa, the cheesy substance consisting of sebum and desquamated epithelial cells, covers the fetus during the latter part of pregnancy. The substance may be found floating in the amniotic fluid. Ohlsson et al. reported that aspiration of vernix caseosa caused clinical symptoms and radiographic findings similar to those of MAS.[126]

Aspiration of blood

Aspiration of blood has been described in neonates.[128] The process is believed to occur during birth through a bloody field, such as during a cesarean section or a vaginal birth in the presence of an abrupted placenta. Conceivably, a neonate who has had gastrointestinal bleeding could potentially have either reflux or vomit this material and aspirate it. The radiographic features of blood aspiration may vary from localized infiltrates to diffuse pulmonary consolidation. They are often similar to those of MAS (Figure 23.5). Saia and Gasparotto reported the finding of macroscopic hemoglobinuria in a neonate with massive blood aspiration.[137] The diagnosis of blood aspiration is typically made when there is a history of a bloody birth process in a child with respiratory distress and consistent radiographic features for which there is no other etiology.

Aspiration pneumonia

Aspiration of gastric contents is the disorder generally referred to by the term 'aspiration pneumonia'. Under various circumstances, the neonate may aspirate acidic gastric secretions, milk (breast milk or formula), or both. The clinical findings depend on host factors as well as the quantity and the type of the material aspirated. When the normal mechanisms that protect the larynx against inhalation of foreign material are overcome, milk, gastric contents or the mucus secretions of the upper airway can be inhaled.

Table 23.4 Composition of fetal lung fluid[22]

	Lung liquid	Interstitial fluid	Plasma	Amniotic fluid
Sodium (mEq/l)	150	147	150	113
Potassium (mEq/l)	6.3	4.8	4.8	7.6
Chloride (mEq/l)	157	107	107	87
Bicarbonate (mEq/l)	3	25	24	19
pH	6.27	7.31	7.34	7.02
Protein (g/dl)	0.03	3.27	4.09	0.10

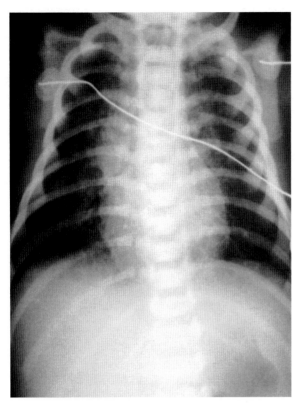

Figure 23.5 *Chest radiograph of an infant with blood aspiration. Note the diffuse coarse, stringy infiltrates and hyperexpansion of the lung fields. The appearance is very similar to that of MAS.*

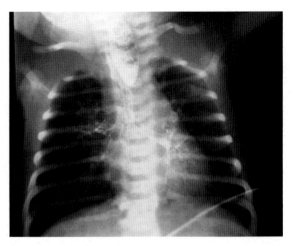

Figure 23.6 *Esophageal atresia. Barium swallow demonstrating a blind-ending esophagus and aspiration of contrast into the bronchial tree.*

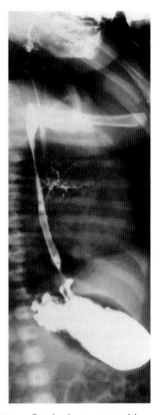

Figure 23.7 *H-type fistula demonstrated by an esophageal tube study. The fistula is at the level of the thoracic inlet.*

PATHOPHYSIOLOGY

Material aspirated into the airway may have different effects: physical obstruction of airways, acute chemical irritation (inflammation), and acute infectious injury or promotion of infection, and recurrent chemical injury. Aspiration of large particles can produce acute airway obstruction, smaller particles or liquid aspiration induce hypoxemia by different mechanisms such as reflex airway closure, hemorrhagic pneumonitis and destruction and dilution of surfactant with secondary atelectasis. The major problem is the irritant potential of the inhaled fluid. All fluids, including water, inhaled into the lung are damaging but gastric contents are the most devastating; this is related primarily to the pH. In the first few days after birth, the pH of a neonate's stomach contents can be 2.5 or less if he has not been fed. Gastric contents buffered with milk are probably less irritating. Inhaled curd is particulate and can obstruct airways and the areas of collapse consolidation, seen on the chest radiograph immediately after an episode of inhalation, are presumably due to obstruction behind inhaled secretions or a plug of inspissated, partially digested milk. The presence of organic material in the airway predisposes to infection.

ETIOLOGY

Aspiration occurs when there is sucking and swallowing incoordination, as can occur in an infant born prematurely or who has structural abnormalities in the upper airway (p. 437) or gastrointestinal tract (Figures 23.6 and 23.7) or neurological problems (p. 523). Gastroesophageal reflux is also a risk factor and there is a high incidence of this problem in prematurely born infants.[120]

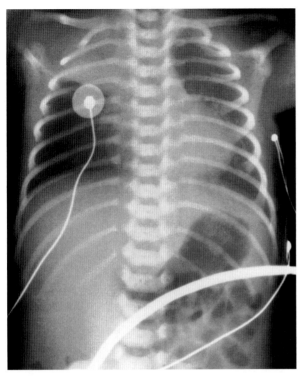

Figure 23.8 *Right upper lobe collapse from aspiration of gastric contents. Gastroesophageal reflux was diagnosed by pH monitoring.*

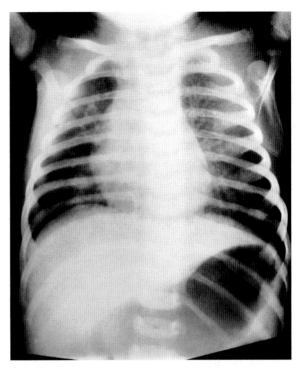

Figure 23.9 *Pulmonary inhalation pneumonia secondary to a tracheoesophageal fistula.*

INVESTIGATION

The diagnosis of gastroesophageal reflux should be suspected in an infant with apparently inexplicable and recurrent respiratory problems, particularly if there is recurrent apnea resistant to methylxanthines (p. 430),[120] a history suggesting reflux or recurrent vomiting or the right upper lobe collapse/consolidation on the chest radiograph. The diagnosis can be confirmed radiologically or using a pH probe.[92] Confirmation of milk aspiration may be made by finding of lipid-laden macrophages in tracheal aspirate samples.[122] Additionally, a colored dye can be added to the milk prior to feeding with recovery of dye in tracheal aspirate samples.[76] Aspiration of milk can be verified by examining immunohistochemical staining of lung secretions with antibodies against milk components.[84] If an underlying disorder is suspected, then the infant should be appropriately investigated (Figures 23.6 and 23.7).

Chest radiography

A new area of consolidation, particularly in the right upper lobe (Figure 23.8) is very suggestive of inhalation. More generalized, non-specific changes (Figure 23.9) can also occur.

PREVENTION

Infants with acute respiratory distress should not be fed enterally. Feeding should only be commenced when the infant has bowel sounds and passed meconium. Enteral feeds should not be started for 12–24 hours after extubation, the longer interval applying to infants who have had prolonged intubation. Progression from tube feeding should be done cautiously and only when the infant has spontaneous activity. It is clearly important to promptly diagnose any underlying disorder which would make the infant at increased risk of aspiration.

MANAGEMENT

During the acute episode, it is important to clear the airway and give appropriate resuscitation. The infant may require intubation and ventilation. If the infant has persisting respiratory distress, suction under direct vision within 15 minutes of the episode can be helpful and, if milk is obtained, the diagnosis is made. Appropriate positioning and percussion should be commenced if there is aspiration into the small airways (p. 238). Further physiotherapy is as for MAS. It is important to be aware that techniques of positioning, percussion and vibration may exacerbate existing gastroesophageal reflux. Broad-spectrum antibiotics should be given and continued for a week for infants with marked changes on their chest radiograph.

It is also important to treat any underlying cause. Infants with gastroesophageal reflux may become asymptomatic if changed to continuous or small, frequent feeds, particularly if nursed prone or with head-up tilt. Other infants require thickened feeds and, if there is evidence of esophagitis, antacids should be given. Cisapride is no longer prescribed for neonates with reflux, because of the reports of toxicity and lack of evidence of efficacy.[26] For infants who remain symptomatic despite thickened feeds and appropriate positioning, some clinicians prescribe another prokinetic agent, domperidone, but there is not robust evidence to support such a policy. Fundoplication is rarely required, but may be necessary in some older infants with BPD and infants post CDH repair (p. 497) who have severe, persistent reflux.

REFERENCES

1 Abu-Osba, Y.K. (1991) Treatment of persistent pulmonary hypertension of the newborn: update. *Archives of Disease in Childhood* **66**, 74–77.

2 Adeniyi-Jones, S., McCormick, M., Ramdial, H., *et al.* (1996) RT-PCR for cytokine MRNA expression by airway cells from term infants with acute respiratory failure. *Pediatric Research* **39**, 323A.

3 Ahumada, C.A., Goldsmith, J.P. (1996) Continuous distending pressure. In Goldsmith, J.P., Karotkin, E.H. (eds), *Assisted Ventilation of the Newborn*, 3rd edition. Philadelphia, PA: W.B. Saunders, 151–165.

4 Alexander, G.R., Hulsey, T.C., Robillard, P.-Y., *et al.* (1994) Determinants of meconium-stained amniotic fluid in term pregnancies. *Journal of Perinatology* **14**, 259–263.

5 Altshuler, G. (1995) Placental insights into neurodevelopmental and other childhood diseases. *Seminars in Pediatric Neurology* **2**, 90–103.

6 Altshuler, G., Hyde, S. (1989) Meconium induced vasocontraction: a potential cause of cerebral and other fetal hypoperfusion and poor pregnancy outcome. *Journal of Child Neurology* **4**, 137–141.

7 Altshuler, G., Arizawa, M., Molnar-Nadasdy, G. (1992) Meconium-induced umbilical cord vascular necrosis and ulceration: a potential link between the placenta and poor pregnancy outcome. *Obstetrics and Gynecology* **79**, 760–765.

8 Antunes, M.J., Friedman, M., Greenspan, J.S. *et al.* (1997) Meconium decreases surfactant protein B levels in rat fetal lung explants. *Pediatric Research* **41**, 137A.

9 Anyaegbunam, A., Fleischer, A., Whitty, J., Brustman, L., Randolph, G., Langer, O. (1991) Association between umbilical artery cord pH, five-minute Apgar scores and neonatal outcome. *Gynecology and Obstetrics Investigation* **32**, 220–223.

10 Arbibe, L., Koumanov, K., Vial, D. *et al.* (1998) Generation of lyso-phospholipids from surfactant in acute lung injury is mediated by type-II phospholipase A2 and inhibited by a direct surfactant protein A-phospholipase A2 protein interaction. *Journal of Clinical Investigation* **102**, 1152–1160.

11 Auten, R.L., Notter, R.H., Kendig, J. *et al.* (1991) Surfactant treatment of full-term newborns with respiratory failure. *Pediatrics* **87**, 101–105.

12 Bae, C.W., Takahashi, A., Chida, S., Sasaki, M. (1998) Morphology and function of pulmonary surfactant inhibited by meconium. *Pediatric Research* **44**, 187.

13 Ballard, J.L., Musial, M.J., Myers, M.G. (1986) Hazards of delivery room resuscitation using oral methods of endotracheal suctioning. *Pediatric Infectious Diseases* **5**, 198–200.

14 Ballard, J.L., Farley, A.J., Atherton, H. *et al.* (1988) Negative pressures used for delivery room neonatal resuscitation. *Journal of Pediatrics* **112**, 478–481.

15 Ballin, A., Koren, G., Kohelet, D. *et al.* (1987) Reduction of platelet counts induced by mechanical ventilation in newborn infants. *Journal of Pediatrics* **111**, 445–449.

16 Bartlett, R.H., Gazzinga, A.B., Huxtable, R.F. *et al.* (1977) Extracorporeal circulation (ECMO) in neonatal respiratory failure. *Journal of Thoracic and Cardiovascular Surgery* **74**, 826–833.

17 Baumgart, S., Hirschl, R.B., Butler, S.Z., Coburn, C.E., Spitzer, A.R. (1992) Diagnosis-related criteria in the consideration of extracorporeal membrane oxygenation in neonates previously treated with high-frequency jet ventilation. *Pediatrics* **89**, 491–494.

18 Beebe, L.A., Cowan, L.D., Altshuler, G. (1996) The epidemiology of placental features: associations with gestational age and neonatal outcome. *Obstetrics and Gynecology* **87**, 771–775.

19 Bent, R.C., Wiswell, T.E. (1992) Does intubation and suctioning for meconium cause airway damage? *Pediatric Research* **31**, 195A.

20 Berger, T.M., Allred, E.N., Van Marter, L.J. (2000) Antecedents of clinically significant pulmonary hemorrhage among newborn infants. *Journal of Perinatology* **20**, 295–300.

21 Bland, R.D. (1991) Formation of fetal lung liquid and its removal near birth. In Polin, R.A., Fox, W.W. (eds), *Fetal and Neonatal Physiology*. Philadelphia: W.B. Saunders, 504–505.

22 Blanke, J.G., Jorch, G. (1993) [Surfactant therapy in severe neonatal respiratory failure – multicenter study – II. Surfactant therapy in 10 newborn infants with meconium aspiration syndrome]. *Klinische Pädiatrie* **205**, 75–78.

23 Block, M.F., Kallenberger, D.A., Kern, J.D., Nepveux, R. (1981) In utero meconium aspiration by the baboon fetus. *Obstetrics and Gynecology* **57**, 37–40.

24 Boddy, K., Dawes, G.S. (1975) Fetal breathing. *British Medical Bulletin* **31**, 3–7.

25 Bortolussi, R., Seeliger, H.P.R. (1990) Listerosis. In Remington, J.S., Klein, J.O. (eds), *Infectious Diseases of the Fetus and Newborn Infant*, 3rd edition. Philadelphia: W.B. Saunders, 812–833.

26 Bourke, B., Drumm, B. (2002) Cochrane's epitaph for cisapride in childhood gastro-oesophageal reflux. *Archives of Disease in Childhood* **86**, 71–73.

27 Brown, B.L., Gleicher, N. (1981) Intrauterine meconium aspiration. *Obstetrics and Gynecology* **57**, 26–29.

28 Burgess, A.M., Hutchins, G.M. (1996) Inflammation of the lungs, umbilical cord, and placenta associated with meconium passage *in utero*: review of 123 autopsied cases. *Pathology, Research and Practice* **192**, 1121–1128.

29 Byrne, D.L., Gau, G. (1987) *In utero* meconium aspiration: an unpreventable cause of neonatal death. *British Journal of Obstetrics and Gynecology* **94**, 813–814.

30 Carson, B.S., Losey, R.W., Bowes, W.A. *et al.* (1976) Combined obstetric and pediatric approach to prevent meconium aspiration syndrome. *American Journal of Obstetrics and Gynecology* **126**, 712–716.

31 Chamberlain, R., Chamberlain, G., Howlett, B., Claireaux, A. (1975) *British Births 1970*. London: William Heinemann, 235–253.

32 Chapman, R.L., Dawes, G.S., Rurak, D.W., Wilds, P.L. (1978) Intermittent breathing before death in fetal lambs. *American Journal of Obstetrics and Gynecology* **131**, 894–898.

33 Chen, C.T., Toung, T.J.K., Rogers, M.C. (1985) Effect of intraalveolar meconium on pulmonary surface tension properties. *Critical Care Medicine* **13**, 233–236.

34 Chishty, A.L., Alvi, Y., Iftikhar, M. *et al.* (1996) Meconium aspiration in neonate: combined obstetric and paediatric intervention improves outcome. *Journal of the Pakistan Medical Association* **46**, 104–108.

35 Clark, P., Duff, P. (1995) Inhibition of neutrophil oxidative burst and phagocytosis by meconium. *American Journal of Obstetrics and Gynecology* **173**, 1301–1305.

36 Clark, R.H., Yoder, B.A., Sell, M.S. (1994) Prospective, randomized comparison of high-frequency oscillation and conventional ventilation in candidates for extracorporeal membrane oxygenation. *Journal of Pediatrics* **124**, 447–454.

37 Clark, R.H., Kueser, T.J., Walker, M.W. *et al.* (2000) Low-dose nitric oxide therapy for persistent pulmonary hypertension of the newborn. Clinical Inhaled Nitric Oxide Research Group. *New England Journal of Medicine* **342**, 469–474.

38 Cleary, G.M., Wiswell, T.E. (1998) Meconium-stained amniotic fluid and the meconium aspiration syndrome: an update. *Pediatrics Clinics of North America* **45**, 511–529.

39 Cleary, G.M., Antunes, M.J., Ciesielka, D.A. *et al.* (1997) Exudative lung injury is associated with decreased levels of surfactant proteins in a rat model of meconium aspiration. *Pediatrics* **100**, 998–1003.

40 Cochrane, C.G., Revak, S.D., Merritt, T.A. *et al.* (1998) Bronchoalveolar lavage with KL4-Surfactant in models of meconium aspiration syndrome. *Pediatric Research* **44**, 705–715.

41 Coltart, T.M., Byrne, D.L., Bates, S.A. (1989) Meconium aspiration syndrome: a six-year retrospective study. *British Journal of Obstetrics and Gynaecology* **96**, 411–414.

42 Cottancin, G., Bourgeois, J., Cordier, M.P. *et al.* (1980) Amniotic fluid aspiration: apropros of 225 cases. *Pediatrie*, **35**, 105–117.

43 Creasy, R., Resnik, R. (1999) *Maternal–Fetal Medicine*, 4th edition. Philadelphia: W.B. Saunders, 393–403.

44 da Costa, D.E., Nair, A.K., Pai, M.G., Al Khusaiby, S.M. (2001) Steroids in full term infants with respiratory failure and pulmonary hypertension due to meconium aspiration syndrome. *European Journal of Pediatrics* **160**, 150–153.

45 Dargaville, P.A., South, M., McDougall, P.N. (2001) Surfactant and surfactant inhibitors in meconium aspiration syndrome. *Journal of Pediatrics* **138**, 113–115.

46 Davey, A.M., Becker, J.D., Davis, J.M. (1993) Meconium aspiration syndrome: physiological and inflammatory changes in a newborn piglet model. *Pediatric Pulmonology* **16**, 101–108.

47 de Beaufort, A.I., Pelikan, D.M.V., Elferink, J.G.R., Berger, H.M. (1998) Effect of interleukin 8 in meconium on *in vitro* neutrophil chemotaxis. *Lancet* **352**, 102–105.

48 Dehan, M., Francoual, J., Londenbaum, A. (1978) Diagnosis of meconium aspiration by spectrophotometric analysis of urine. *Archives of Disease in Childhood* **53**, 74–76.

49 Dijxhoorn, M.J., Visser, G.H.A., Fidler, V.J. *et al.* (1986) Apgar scores, meconium and academia at birth in relation to neonatal neurological morbidity in term infants. *British Journal of Obstetrics and Gynaecology* **93**, 217–222.

50 Dollberg, S., Livny, S., Mordecheyev, N., Mimouni, F.B. (2001) Nucleated red blood cells in meconium aspiration syndrome. *Obstetrics and Gynecology* **97**, 593–596.

51 Dooley, S.L., Pesavento, D.J., Depp, R. *et al.* (1985) Meconium below the vocal cords at delivery: correlation with intrapartum events. *American Journal of Obstetrics and Gynecology* **153**, 767–770.

52 Dye, T., Aubry, R., Gross, S., Artal, R. (1994) Amnioinfusion and the intrauterine prevention of meconium aspiration. *American Journal of Obstetrics and Gynecology* **173**, 671–672.

53 Dysart, M., Graves, B.W., Sharp, E.S. *et al.* (1991) The incidence of meconium stained amniotic fluid from 1980 through 1986, by year and gestational age. *Journal of Perinatology* **11**, 245–248.

54 Falciglia, H.S. (1988) Failure to prevent meconium aspiration syndrome. *Obstetrics and Gynecology* **71**, 349–353.

55 Falciglia, H.S., Henderschott, C., Potter, P. *et al.* (1992) Does DeLee suction at the perineum prevent meconium aspiration syndrome? *American Journal of Obstetrics and Gynecology* **167**, 1243–1249.

56 Findlay, R.D., Taeusch, H.W., Walther, F.J. (1996) Surfactant replacement therapy for meconium aspiration syndrome. *Pediatrics* **97**, 48–52.

57 Florman, A.L., Tuebner, D. (1969) Enhancement of bacterial growth in amniotic fluid by meconium. *Journal of Pediatrics* **74**, 111–115.

58 Foust, R., Tran, N.N., Cox, C. *et al.* (1996) Liquid assisted ventilation: an alternative ventilatory strategy for acute meconium aspiration injury. *Pediatric Pulmonology* **21**, 316–322.

59 Fox, W.W., Berman, L.S., Downes, J.J. Jr, Peckham, G.J. (1975) The therapeutic application of end-expiratory pressure in the meconium aspiration syndrome. *Pediatrics* **56**, 214–217.

60 Fox, W.W., Gewitz, M.H., Dinwiddie, R., Drummond, W.H., Peckham, G.J. (1977) Pulmonary hypertension in the perinatal aspiration syndromes. *Pediatrics* **59**, 205–211.

61 Fraser, W., Marcoux, S., Prendiville, W. *et al.* (2000) Multicenter randomized trial of amnioinfusion. *Journal de Gynecologie, Obstetrique et Biologie de la Reproduction* **29**, 312–315.

62 Fuloria, M., Wiswell, T.E. (2000) Management of the meconium-stained infant. *Contemporary Pediatrics* **17**, 125–143.

63 Fuloria, M., Ying, W., Brandt, M.L. *et al.* (2002) Effect of meconium saline suspensions on the surface properties of perflubron. *Journal of Applied Physiology* (in press).

64 Gersony, W.M., Morishima, H.O., Daniel, S.S. *et al.* (1976) The hemodynamic effects of intrauterine hypoxia: an experimental model in newborn lambs. *Journal of Pediatrics* **89**, 631–635.

65 Ghidini, A., Spong, C.Y. (2001) Severe meconium aspiration syndrome is not caused by aspiration of meconium. *American Journal of Obstetrics and Gynecology* **185**, 931–938.

66 Giuseppetti, M.M., Wiswell, T.E. (1994) The use of saline lavage and surfactant therapy in the management of a piglet model of the meconium aspiration syndrome (MAS). *Pediatric Research* **35**, 333A.

67 Goodlin, R.C. (1970) Suppression of fetal breathing to prevent aspiration of meconium. *Obstetrics and Gynecology* **36**, 944–947.

68 Goodlin, R.C. (1988) *In utero* meconium aspiration: an unpreventable cause of neonatal death. *British Journal of Obstetrics and Gynaecology* **95**, 103.

69 Greenough, A. (1995) Surfactant replacement therapy for non-respiratory distress syndrome neonatal respiratory disease – research or clinical application? *European Journal of Pediatrics* **154**(Suppl 3), S2–S4.

70 Gregory, G.A., Gooding, C.A., Phibbs, R.H. *et al.* (1974) Meconium aspiration in infants: a prospective study. *Journal of Pediatrics* **85**, 848–852.

71 Grossman, G., Tashiro, K., Kobayashi, T. *et al.* (1999) Experimental neonatal respiratory failure induced by lysophosphatidylcholine: effect of surfactant treatment. *Journal of Applied Physiology* **86**, 633–640.

72 Gupta, V., Bhatia, B.D., Mishra, O.P. (1996) Meconium stained amniotic-fluid: antenatal, intrapartun, and neonatal attributes. *Indian Pediatrics* **33**, 293–297.

73 Hageman, J.R., Caplan, M.S. (1995) An introduction to the structure and function of inflammatory mediators for clinicians. *Clinics in Perinatology* **22**, 251–261.

74 Halliday, H.L., Hirata, T. (1979) Perinatal listeriosis – a review of twelve patients. *American Journal of Obstetrics and Gynecology* **133**, 405–410.

75 Halliday, H.L., Speer, C.P., Robertson, B. *et al.* (1996) Treatment of severe meconium aspiration syndrome with porcine surfactant. *European Journal of Pediatrics* **155**, 1047–1051.

76 Hansen, T., Corbet, A. (1998) Neonatal pneumonias. In Taeusch, H.W., Ballard, R.A. (eds), *Avery's Diseases of the Newborn*. Philadelphia: W.B. Saunders, 648–660.

77 Hernandez, C., Little, B.B., Dax, J.S. *et al.* (1993) Prediction of the severity of meconium aspiration syndrome. *American Journal of Obstetrics and Gynecology* **169**, 61–70.

78 Herting, E., Rauprich, P., Stichtenother, G. *et al.* (2001) Resistance of different surfactant preparations to inactivation by meconium. *Pediatric Research* **50**, 44–49.

79 Hofmeyr, G.J. (2002) Amnioinfusion for meconium-stained liquor in labour (Cochrane Review). *Cochrane Database of Systematic Reviews* **1**, CD000014.

80 Holopainen, R.L., Aho, H., Laine, J. *et al.* (1999) Human meconium has high phospholipase A2 activity and induces cellular injury and apoptosis in piglet lungs. *Pediatric Research* **46**, 626–632.

81 Holtzman, R.B., Banzhaf, W.C., Silver, R.K., Hageman, J.R. (1989) Perinatal management of meconium staining of the amniotic fluid. *Clinics in Perinatology* **16**, 825–838.

82 Hoskins, I.A., Hemming, V.G., Johnson, T.R., Winkel, C.A. (1987) Effects of alterations of zinc-to-phophorus ratios and meconium content on group B streptococcus growth in human amniotic fluid in vitro. *American Journal of Obstetrics and Gynecology* **157**, 770–773.

83 Houlihan, C.M., Knuppel, R.A. (1994) Meconium-stained amniotic fluid: current controversies. *Journal of Reproductive Medicine* **39**, 888–898.

84 Iwadate, K., Doy, M., Nishimaki, Y. *et al.* (2000) Immunohistochemical examination of the lungs in infant death cases using antibodies against milk components. *Forensic Science International* **110**, 19–28.

85 James, M.B., Rowe, R.D. (1957) The pattern of response of pulmonary and systemic arterial pressures in newborn and older infants to short periods of hypoxia. *Journal of Pediatrics* **51**, 5–10.

86 Jones, C.A., Cayabyah, R.G., Hamden, H. *et al.* (1994) Early production of proinflammatory cytokines in the pathogenesis of neonatal adult respiratory distress syndrome (ARDS) associated with meconium aspiration. *Pediatric Research* **35**, 339A.

87 Jose, J., Schreiner, R., Mirkin, L. *et al.* (1981) Non-association of cell content with respiratory distress in adult rabbits aspirating human amniotic fluid. *Pediatric Research* **15**, 1672–1675.

88 Jose, J.H., Schreiner, R.L., Lemons, J.A. *et al.* (1983) The effect of amniotic fluid aspiration on pulmonary function in the adult and newborn rabbit. *Pediatric Research* **17**, 976–981.

89 Katz, V.L., Bowes, W.A. (1992) Meconium aspiration syndrome: reflections on a murky subject. *American Journal of Obstetrics and Gynecology* **134**, 376–381.

90 Kearney, M.S. (1999) Chronic intrauterine meconium aspiration causes fetal lung infarcts, lung rupture, and meconium embolism. *Pediatric Developmental Pathology* **2**, 544–551.

91 Keszler, M., Molina, B., Butterfield, A.B., Subramanian, K.N.S. (1986) Combined high frequency jet ventilation in a meconium aspiration model. *Critical Care Medicine* **14**, 34–38.

92 Khalaf, M.N., Porat, R., Brodsky, N.L., Bhandari, V. (2001) Clinical correlations in infants in the neonatal intensive care unit with varying severity of gastroesophageal reflux. *Journal of Pediatric Gastroenterology and Nutrition* **32**, 45–49.

93 Khammash, H., Perlman, M., Wojtulewicz, J. *et al.* (1993) Surfactant therapy in full-term neonates with severe respiratory failure. *Pediatrics* **92**, 135–139.

94 Khosla, A.H., Sangwan, K., Ahuja, S.D. (1997) Prophylactic amnioinfusion during labour complicated by meconium. *Australian and New Zealand Journal of Obstetrics and Gynaecology* **37**, 294–296.

95 Kinsella, J.P., Truog, W.E., Walsh, W.F. *et al.* (1997) Randomized, multicenter trial of inhaled nitric oxide and high-frequency oscillatory ventilation in severe persistent pulmonary hypertension of the newborn. *Journal of Pediatrics* **131**, 55–62.

96 Knox, G.E., Huddleston, J.F., Flowers, C.E. (1979) Management of prolonged pregnancy: results of a prospective randomized trial. *American Journal of Obstetrics and Gynecology* **134**, 376–381.

97 Korhonen, K.O., Seppanen, M.P., Kero, P.O., Kääpä, P.O. (1999) Delayed adaptation of the pulmonary hemodynamics in infants with mild to moderate meconium aspiration syndrome. *Journal of Pediatrics* **134**, 355–357.

98 Krebs, H.B., Peters, R.E., Dunn, L.J. *et al.* (1980) Intrapartum fetal heart rate monitoring: III. Association of meconium with abnormal fetal heart rate patterns. *American Journal of Obstetrics and Gynecology* **137**, 936–942.

99 Krishnan, L., Nasruddin, U., Prabhakar, P. *et al.* (1995) Routine antibiotic cover for newborns intubated for aspirating meconium: is it necessary? *Indian Pediatrics* **32**, 529.

100 Lam, B.C., Yeung, C.Y. (1999) Surfactant lavage for meconium aspiration syndrome: a pilot study. *Pediatrics* **103**, 1014–1018.

101 Lillehei, C.W., O'Rourke, P.P., Vacanti, J.P., Crone, R.K. (1989) Role of extracorporeal membrane oxygenation in selected pediatric respiratory problems. *Journal of Thoracic and Cardiovascular Surgery* **98**, 968–970.

102 Lotze, A., Mitchell, B.R., Short, B.L. *et al.* (1998) Multicenter study of surfactant (Beractant) use in the treatment of term infants with severe respiratory failure. *Journal of Pediatrics* **132**, 40–47.

103 Lucas, A., Christofides, N.D., Adrian, T.E. *et al.* (1979) Fetal distress, meconium and motilin. *Lancet* **31**, 718.

104 Mahmoud, E.L., Benirschke, K., Vaucher, Y.E., Poitras, P. (1988) Motilin levels in term neonates who have passed meconium prior to birth. *Journal of Pediatric Gastroenterology* **7**, 95–99.

105 Mahomed, K., Nyoni, R., Masona, D. (1994) Meconium staining of the liquor in a low-risk population. *Paediatric and Perinatal Epidemiology* **8**, 292–300.

106 Mammel, M.C., Gordon, M.J., Connett, J.E., Barbs, S.J. (1983) Comparison of high frequency jet ventilation and conventional mechanical ventilation in a meconium aspiration model. *Journal of Pediatrics* **103**, 630–634.

107 Manning, F.A., Martin, C.B. Jr, Murata, Y. *et al.* (1979) Breathing movements before death in the primate fetus. *American Journal of Obstetrics and Gynecology* **135**, 71–76.

108 Manroe, B.L., Weinberg, A.G., Rosenfeld, C.R., Browne, R. (1979) The neonatal blood count in health and disease. I. Reference values for neutrophilic cells. *Journal of Pediatrics* **95**, 89–98.

109 Marraro, G., Bonati, M., Ferrari, A. *et al.* (1994) Advantages of using perfluorcarbon (PFC) over saline solution for bronchoalveolar lavage (BAL) in experimental meconium aspiration in guinea pigs. *Pediatric Research* **35**, 343A.

110 Marraro, G., Bonati, M., Ferrari, A. *et al.* (1995) Perfluorocarbon (RIMAR) liquid lavage versus saline lavage

in experimental meconium inhalation guinea pig model. *Pediatric Research* **37**, 222A.

111 Matthews, T.G., Warshaw, J.B. (1979) Relevance of gestational age distribution of passage of meconium in utero. *Pediatrics* **64**, 30–31.

112 Mazor, M., Furman, B., Wiznitzer, A. *et al.* (1995) Maternal and perinatal outcome of patients with preterm labor and meconium-stained amniotic fluid. *Obstetrics and Gynecology* **86**, 830.

113 Merlob, P., Amir, J., Zaizov, R., Reisner, S.H. (1980) The differential leukocyte count in full-term newborn infants with meconium aspiration and neonatal asphyxia. *Acta Paediatrica Scandinavica* **69**, 779–780.

114 Meydanli, M.M., Dilbaz, B., Caliskan, E., Dilbaz, S., Haberal, A. (2001) Risk factors for meconium aspiration syndrome in infants born through thick meconium. *International Journal of Gynaecology and Obstetrics* **72**, 9–15.

115 Moses, D., Holm, B., Spitale, P. *et al.* (1991) Inhibition of pulmonary surfactant function by meconium. *American Journal of Obstetrics and Gynecology* **164**, 477–481.

116 Naeye, R.L., Letts, H.W. (1962) The effects of prolonged neonatal hypoxemia on the pulmonary vascular bed and heart. *Pediatrics* **30**, 902–906.

117 Narang, A., Nair, P.M., Bhakoo, O.N. *et al.* (1993) Management of meconium stained amniotic fluid: a team approach. *Indian Pediatrics* **30**, 9–14.

118 Narchi, H., Kulaylat, N. (1999) Is gastric lavage needed in neonates with meconium-stained amniotic fluid? *European Journal of Pediatrics* **158**, 315–317.

119 Nathan, L., Leveno, K.J., Carmody, T.J. *et al.* (1994) Meconium: a 1990s perspective on an old obstetric hazard. *Obstetrics and Gynecology* **83**, 329–332.

120 Newell, S.J., Booth, I.W., Morgan, M.E.I. *et al.* (1989) Gastro-oesophageal reflux in preterm infants. *Archives of Disease in Childhood* **64**, 780–786.

121 Newman, B. (1999) Imaging of medical diseases of the newborn lung: neonatal imaging. *Radiologic Clinics of North America* **37**, 1049–1065.

122 Nickerson, B.G. (1997) A test for recurrent aspiration in children. *Pediatric Pulmonology* **3**, 65–69.

123 Oelberg, D.G., Downey, S.A., Flynn, M. (1990) Bile salt-induced intracellular Ca^{++} accumulation in type II pneumocytes. *Lung* **168**, 297–308.

124 Ogawa, Y., Ohama, Y., Itakura, Y. *et al.* (1996). Bronchial lavage with surfactant solution for the treatment of meconium aspiration syndrome. *Journal of the Japanese Medical Society Biological – Interface* **26**(Suppl), 179–184.

125 Ohama, Y., Itakura, Y., Koyama, N. *et al.* (1994) Effect of surfactant lavage in a rabbit model of meconium aspiration syndrome. *Acta Paediatrica Japonica* **36**, 236–238.

126 Ohlsson, A., Cumming, W.A., Najjar, H. (1985) Neonatal aspiration syndrome due to vernix caseosa. *Pediatric Radiology* **15**, 193–195.

127 Paranka, M.S., Walsh, W.F., Stancombe, B.B. (1992) Surfactant lavage in a piglet model of meconium aspiration syndrome. *Pediatric Research* **31**, 625–628.

128 Pender, C.B. (1970) Respiratory distress in the newborn infant due to blood aspiration in infants delivered by cesarean section. *American Journal of Obstetrics and Gynecology* **106**, 711–717.

129 Peng, T.C.C., Gutcher, G.R., Van Dorsten, J.P. (1996) A selective aggressive approach to the neonate exposed to meconium-stained amniotic fluid. *American Journal of Obstetrics and Gynecology* **175**, 296–300.

130 Perlman, E.J., Moore, G.W., Hutchins, G.M. (1989) The pulmonary vasculature in meconium aspiration. *Human Pathology* **20**, 701–706.

131 Revak, S.D., Cochrane, C.G., Merritt, T.A. (1997) The therapeutic effect of bronchoalveolar lavage with KL4-Surfactant in animal models of meconium aspiration syndrome. *Pediatric Research* **41**, 265A.

132 Richey, S.D., Ramin, S.M., Bawdon, R.E. *et al.* (1995) Markers of acute and chronic asphyxia in infants with meconium-stained amniotic fluid. *American Journal of Obstetrics and Gynecology* **172**, 1212–1215.

133 Roberton, N.R.C. (1996) Aspiration syndromes. In Greenough, A., Milner, A. (eds), *Neonatal Respiratory Disorders*. London: Arnold, 313–333.

134 Roberts, J.D., Fineman, J.R., Motrin, F.C. *et al.* (1997) Inhaled nitric oxide and persistent pulmonary hypertension of the newborn. *New England Journal of Medicine* **336**, 605–610.

135 Rogers, M.S., Lau, T.K., Wang, C.C. *et al.* (1996) Amnioinfusion for the prevention of meconium aspiration during labour. *Australian and New Zealand Journal of Obstetrics and Gynaecology* **36**, 407–410.

136 Romero, R., Hanaoka, S., Mazor, M. *et al.* (1991) Meconium-stained amniotic fluid: a risk factor for microbial invasion of the amniotic cavity. *American Journal of Obstetrics and Gynecology* **164**, 859–861.

137 Saia, O.S., Gasparotto, G. (1982) Macroscopic hemoglobinuria in a neonate with massive blood aspiration. *Journal of Pediatrics* **101**, 446–447.

138 Schrama, A.J.J., de Beaufort, A.J., Sukul, Y.R.M. *et al.* (2001) Phospholipase A2 is present in meconium and inhibits the activity of pulmonary surfactant: an *in vitro* study. *Acta Paediatrica* **90**, 412–416.

139 Segal, M.L., Goetzman, B.W., Schick, J.B. (1980) Thrombocytopenia and pulmonary hypertension in the perinatal aspiration syndrome. *Journal of Pediatrics* **96**, 727–730.

140 Sepulveda, W.H., Gonzalez, C., Cruz, M.A., Rudolph, M.I. (1991) Vasoconstrictive effect of bile acids on isolated human placental corionic veins. *European Journal of Obstetrics & Gynecology and Reproductive Biology* **42**, 211–215.

141 Shabarek, F.M., Cocanour, C.S., Xue, H. *et al.* (1996) Meconium stimulates alveolar macrophage prostaglandin E2 production but not procoagulant activity. *Pediatric Research* **39**, 349A.

142 Shabarek, F.M., Xue, H., Lally, K.P. (1997) Human meconium stimulates murine alveolar macrophage procoagulant activity. *Pediatric Research* **41**, 267A.

143 Short, B.L. (1995) Neonatal ECMO: are indications changing? *International Journal of Artificial Organs* **18**, 562–564.

144 Soukka, H.R., Kääpä, O. (1997) Methylprednisolone modulates plasma endothelin-1 and atrial natriuretic peptide level in meconium aspiration-induced hypertensive lung injury. *Pediatric Research* **41**, 268A.

145 Soukka, H.R., Kääpä, P.O., Kero, P.O. (1995) Meconium aspiration induces non-hypoxic pulmonary vasoconstriction in pigs. *Pediatric Research* **37**, 351A.

146 Soukka, H.R., Kero, P.O., Kääpä, P.O. (1996) Biphasic increase in plasma endothelin concentration and pulmonary vascular resistance after meconium aspiration in pigs. *Pediatric Research* **39**, 359A.

147 Soukka, H.R., Halkola, L., Aho, H. *et al.* (1997) Methylprednisolone attenuates the pulmonary hypertensive response in porcine meconium aspiration. *Pediatric Research* **42**, 145–149.

148 Starks, G.C. (1980) Correlation of meconium stained amniotic-fluid,early intrapartum fetal pH and Apgar scores as predictors of perinatal outcome. *Obstetrics and Gynecology* **56**, 604–609.

149 Steer, P.J., Eigbe, F., Lissauer, T.J., Beard, R.W. (1989) Interrelationships among abnormal cardiotocograms in labor, meconium staining of amniotic fluid, arterial cord blood pH and Apgar scores. *Obstetrics and Gynecology* **74**, 715–719.

150 Sun, B., Cursedt, T., Robertson, B. (1993) Surfactant inhibition in experimental meconium aspiration. *Acta Paediatrica* **82**, 182–189.

151 Sun, B., Curstedt, T., Song, G., Robertson, B. (1993) Surfactant improves lung function and morphology in newborn rabbits with meconium aspiration. *Biology of the Neonate* **63**, 96–99.

152 The Neonatal Inhaled Nitric Oxide Study Group (1997) Inhaled nitric oxide in full-term and nearly full-term infants with hypoxic respiratory failure. *New England Journal of Medicine* **336**, 597–603.

153 Thureen, P.J., Hall, D.M., Hoffenberg, A. *et al.* (1997) Fatal meconium aspiration in spite of appropriate perinatal airway management: pulmonary and placental evidence of prenatal disease. *American Journal of Obstetrics and Gynecology* **176**, 967–975.

154 Tran, N., Lowe, C., Sivieri, E.M., Shaffer, T.H. (1980) Sequential effects of acute meconium obstruction on pulmonary function. *Pediatric Research* **14**, 34–38.

155 Trindale, O., Goldberg, R.N., Bancalari, E. *et al.* (1985) Conventional vs high frequency jet ventilation in a piglet model of meconium aspiration: comparison of pulmonary and hemodynamic effects. *Journal of Pediatrics* **107**, 115–120.

156 Truog, W.E., Lyrene, R.K., Standaert, T.A. *et al.* (1982) Effects of PEEP and tolazoline infusion on respiratory and inert gas exchange in experimental meconium aspiration. *Journal of Pediatrics* **100**, 284–290.

157 Tyler, D.C., Murphy, J., Cheney, F.W. (1978) Mechanical and chemical damage to lung tissue caused by meconium aspiration. *Pediatrics* **62**, 454–459.

158 UK Collaborative ECMO Group (1998) UK Collaborative ECMO Trial: follow-up to 1 year of age. *Pediatrics* **101**, E1.

159 UK Collaborative ECMO Trial Group (1996) UK Collaborative randomized trial of neonatal extracorporeal membrane oxygenation. *Lancet* **341**, 75–82.

160 Usta, I.M., Mercer, B.M., Aswad, N.J. *et al.* (1995) The impact of a policy of amnioinfusion for meconium aspiration syndrome. *Obstetrics and Gynecology* **85**, 237–241.

161 Vain, N., Szyld, E., Prudent, L., Wiswell, T.E. *et al.* (2002) Oro- and nasopharyngeal suction of meconium-stained neonates before delivery of their shoulders does not prevent meconium aspiration syndrome: results of the international, multicenter, randomized, controlled trial (RCT). *Pediatric Research* **51**, 379A.

162 Valencia, P., Sosa, R., Wyble, L. *et al.* (1993) Accuracy of admission chest x-ray (CXR) in the prediction of sickness severity in infants with meconium aspiration syndrome (MAS). *Clinical Research* **41**, 736A.

163 Walker, J. (1954) Fetal anoxia. *British Journal of Obstetrics and Gynaecology* **61**, 162–167.

164 Walsh-Sukys, M.C., Baeur, R.E., Cornell, D.J. *et al.* (1994) Severe respiratory failure in neonates: mortality and morbidity rates and neurodevelopmental outcome. *Journal of Pediatrics* **125**, 104–110.

165 Wen, T.S., Eriksen, N.L., Blanco, J.D. *et al.* (1993) Association of clinical intraamniotic infection and meconium. *American Journal of Perinatology* **10**, 438–442.

166 Wiswell, T.E. (1997) Meconium staining and the meconium aspiration syndrome. In Stevenson, D.K., Sunshine, P. (eds), *Fetal and Neonatal Brain Injury: Mechanisms, Management, and the Risks of Practice*, 2nd edition. Oxford: Oxford University Press, 539–563.

167 Wiswell, T.E. (2001) Advances in the treatment of the meconium aspiration syndrome. *Acta Paediatrica Supplementum* **436**, 28–30.

168 Wiswell, T.E., Bent, R.C. (1993) Meconium staining and the meconium aspiration syndrome. *Pediatric Clinics of North America* **40**, 955–981.

169 Wiswell, T.E., Fuloria, M. (1999) Management of meconium-stained amniotic fluid. *Clinics in Perinatology* **26**, 659–668.

170 Wiswell, T.E., Henley, M.A. (1992) Intratracheal suctioning, systemic infection, and the meconium aspiration syndrome. *Pediatrics* **89**, 203–206.

171 Wiswell, T.E., Tuggle, J.M., Turner, B.S. (1990) Meconium aspiration syndrome: have we made a difference? *Pediatrics* **85**, 715–721.

172 Wiswell, T.E., Foster, N.H., Slayter, M.V. *et al.* (1992) Management of a piglet model of the meconium aspiration syndrome with high frequency or conventional ventilation. *American Journal of Diseases of Children* **146**, 1287–1293.

173 Wiswell, T.E., Peabody, S.S., Davis, J.M. *et al.* (1994) Surfactant therapy and high frequency jet ventilation in management of a piglet model of meconium aspiration syndrome. *Pediatric Research* **36**, 494–500.

174 Wiswell, T.E., Popek, E., Barfield, W.D. *et al.* (1994) The effect of intraamniotic meconium on histologic findings over time in a fetal rabbit model. *Pediatric Research* **35**, 261A.

175 Wiswell, T.E., Gannon, C.M., Jacob, J. *et al.* (2000) Delivery room management of the apparently vigorous meconium stained neonate: results of the multicenter, international collaborative trial. *Pediatrics* **105**, 1–7.

176 Wiswell, T.E., Knight, G.R., Finer, N.N. *et al.* (2002) A multicenter, randomized, controlled trial comparing Surfaxin® (lucinactant) lavage with standard care for treatment of meconium aspiration syndrome (MAS). *Pediatrics* **109**, 1081–1087.

177 Wu, J.M., Yeh, T.F., Lin, Y.J. *et al.* (1995) Increases of leukotriene B4 (LTB4) and D4 (LTD4) and cardiohemodynamic changes in newborn piglets with meconium aspiration (MAS). *Pediatric Research* **37**, 357A.

178 Wu, J.M., Wang, J.N., Lin, Y.J. *et al.* (1997) The role of pulmonary inflammation in the development of pulmonary hypertension in newborn piglets with meconium aspiration syndrome (MAS). *Pediatric Research* **41**, 273A.

179 Wu, J.M., Yeh, T.F., Wang, J.Y. *et al.* (1999) The role of pulmonary inflammation in the development of pulmonary hypertension in newborn with meconium aspiration syndrome (MAS). *Pediatric Pulmonology Supplement* **18**, 205–208.

180 Yeh, T.F., Srinivasan, G., Harris, V., Pildes, R.S. (1977) Hydrocortisone therapy in meconium aspiration syndrome: a controlled study. *Journal of Pediatrics* **90**, 140–143.

181 Yeh, T.F., Harris, V., Srinivasan, G. *et al.* (1979) Roentgenographic findings in infants with meconium aspiration syndrome. *Journal of the American Medical Association* **242**, 60–65.

182 Yoder, B.A. (1994) Meconium-stained amniotic fluid and respiratory complications: impact of selective tracheal suction. *Obstetrics and Gynecology* **3**, 77–81.

183 Yuksel, B., Greenough, A., Gamsu, H.R. (1993) Neonatal meconium aspiration syndrome and respiratory morbidity during infancy. *Pediatric Pulmonology* **16**, 358–361.

184 Zagariya, A., Bhat, R., Uhal, B., Navale, S., Freidine, M., Vidyasagar, D. (2000) Cell death and lung cell histology in meconium aspirated newborn rabbit lung. *European Journal of Pediatrics* **59**, 819–826.

185 Ziadeh, S.M., Sunna, E. (2000) Obstetric and perinatal outcome of pregnancies with term labor and meconium stained amniotic fluid. *Archives of Gynecology and Obstetrics* **264**, 84–87.

24

Pleural effusions

ANNE GREENOUGH

PLEURAL EFFUSION

Incidence

The incidence of primary fetal hydrothorax has been estimated as one case per 15 000 pregnancies.[50] In one series,[49] 2.2 percent of admissions to the neonatal intensive care unit (NICU) had a pleural effusion.

Etiology

Pleural effusions diagnosed antenatally are frequently associated with chromosomal abnormalities, particularly trisomy 21,[26] or congenital abnormalities, including congenital heart disease and diaphragmatic hernia.[4,31,58] Right-sided diaphragmatic herniae have been associated with hydrothorax and ascites, the hydrothorax resulting from a fluid-filled peritoneal sac in the right side of the chest; this may occur in as many as 20 percent of CDH cases.[80] Two-thirds of fetal pleural effusions are diagnosed in the third trimester of pregnancy.[3] Sixty percent occur in male fetuses, 47 percent are bilateral and 53 percent have associated polyhydramnios.

In the neonatal period, isolated pleural effusions are uncommon; such effusions may be either a chylothorax or occur in association with infection, transient tachypnea of the newborn, persistent pulmonary hypertension of the newborn or heart failure. Congenital chylothorax is the most frequent cause of pleural effusion seen in the neonatal period.[75] Pleural effusions are more usually part of a generalized edematous state (hydrops fetalis) (see p. 468), although an isolated fetal pleural effusion may progress to generalized hydrops.[68] Possible mechanisms include diminished venous return, liver congestion, portal hypertension, congestive heart failure, loss of protein, interference with liver function and lymphatic obstruction in other areas.[31]

In one series,[49] infants first noted to have a small effusion after the second day of life were likely to have congenital heart disease. Meconium aspiration syndrome (MAS) was the most commonly associated respiratory disease. Approximately 9 percent of MAS cases have pleural effusions.[30,34,82] Pleural fluid collections are also seen in transient tachypnea of the newborn and congenital myotonic dystrophy.[18]

Rarely, pleural effusions result from trauma, for example nasogastric tube insertion causing a hypopharyngeal tear,[42] by direct erosion of the inferior vena cava by a total parenteral nutrition catheter into the pleural space,[4,48] or perforation of an intrathoracic vessel.[44] Hypopharyngeal tears are usually proximal to the cricopharyngeus muscle and will most commonly result in a fluid collection in the neck, which may block swallowing of saliva and simulate esophageal atresia.[29] If, however, the perforation communicates with the pleural space, a pleural effusion will result. Right-sided hydrothoraces in extremely low birthweight (ELBW) infants have been described secondary to retrograde passage of a central venous catheter into the lymphatic duct or erosion of the internal jugular vein.[40] A unilateral hydrothorax may also occur if a central venous catheter migrates into the pulmonary vasculature.[51] This may result in hyperosmotic endothelial damage, as the osmolarity of total parenteral nutrition is greater than 1000 mosmol/l.[51] Rarely, umbilical venous catheterization (UVC) has been associated with the development of bilateral pleural effusions.[76] The postulated mechanism was perforation of the inferior vena cava (IVC) wall by the UVC, but only as far as the adventitia and fluid then tracked along the sheath of the adventitia to enter the thorax. Pleural effusions may also develop in the postoperative period, most commonly noted following congenital diaphragmatic hernia (CDH) repair (p. 496).

Infection, either viral or bacterial, results in an inflammatory reaction and, particularly in the preterm infant, is associated with pleural thickening. Intrauterine cytomegalovirus, toxoplasmosis and rubella infections may all cause pleural effusions.[60] Adenovirus has been isolated from a massive pleural effusion diagnosed at birth.[56] Perinatal infection which results in a pleural effusion is usually due to group B streptococcus and is often associated with premature rupture of the membranes. It has been suggested that, in infants who have the radiological features of respiratory distress syndrome and pleural effusions, the diagnosis of group B streptococcal infection should be considered.[38,79] Perinatally acquired staphylococcal pneumonia can also be associated with pleural effusion.[41] Postnatally, the most common infectious agent to cause a pleural effusion is *Staphylococcus aureus*.

Clinical signs

Infants with large effusions present immediately at birth with failure to establish adequate respiration and are difficult to resuscitate. The underlying lung or lungs may be hypoplastic, as the pleural effusion will have acted as a space-occupying lesion restricting the development of the fetal lung.[16] In infants with pulmonary hypoplasia, there is an associated decreased pulmonary vascular bed and the infants may have persistent pulmonary hypertension of the newborn. On examination, the trachea and mediastinum will be shifted to the contralateral side and the ipsilateral thorax dull to percussion and the breath sounds absent. Active resuscitation may result in a pneumothorax or pneumomediastinum. Small effusions are asymptomatic and diagnosed incidentally on a chest radiograph. Large effusions developing later in the neonatal period will cause tachypnea and cyanosis and the infant will have chest wall retractions. Hydrothorax resulting from migration of a central venous catheter into the pulmonary vasculature presents with hypoxia and acute respiratory distress.[51]

Differential diagnosis

At birth the presentation may be similar to diaphragmatic hernia, but that condition may be differentiated by the presence of a scaphoid abdomen and bowel sounds in the chest. An effusion may also be mistaken for an eventration.[25] The chest radiograph appearance of a pleural effusion may be confused with atelectasis. Pleural thickening may be mistaken for a pleural effusion. On a chest radiograph, extrapleural effusions, resulting from an anastomotic leakage from an esophageal atresia repair when an extrapleural approach is used, may look like

fluid in the pleural space. Affected infants are at increased risk for developing a delayed esophageal stricture.[21]

Diagnosis

ANTENATAL

Pleural effusions can be detected by ultrasonography[19] and should be suspected in patients presenting with polyhydramnios.[61] The pleural effusion raises the intrathoracic pressure, interfering with swallowing and hence causes polyhydramnios.[60] This hypothesis is supported by the results of one study demonstrating a lack of dye in the gastrointestinal tract after intra-amniotic instillation of urograffin.[57] An alternative explanation is interference with redistribution of fetal lung fluid.[60] A thorough search must be made for ultrasonically detectable markers of fetal chromosomal abnormalities and fetal echocardiography should be undertaken. Massive pleural effusions may compromise the fetus by increasing intrapleural pressure, resulting in inversion of the diaphragm and obstruction of the venous return with compression of the heart leading to heart failure. Pleural effusions presenting antenatally can be associated with pulmonary hypoplasia.[16,59] This complication may be detected by ultrasonographic demonstration of a small, immobile lung, which is of abnormal contour.[3] The ratio of lung span to hemithorax diameter may be low. In one series of nine fetuses with fetal pleural effusions who all developed pulmonary hypoplasia, the mean ratio was 0.6 (range 0.44–0.77).[16] Unfortunately, no normal data were given and it is important to repeat such measurements after thoracocentesis, as the fetal lung can then expand.[68]

POSTNATAL

Large effusions may be demonstrated on chest radiography by a 'complete whiteout' of the affected side with depression of the diaphragm and shift of the mediastinum (Figure 24.1). Pleural fluid collects in the most dependent parts of the pleural space and thus, if the effusion is small, the fluid will move in position. A chest radiograph in the vertical position will show a fluid shift to the base of the pleural cavity.[8] Small effusions in the supine infant will present as a rim of fluid around the lateral chest wall and diaphragm (Figures 24.2 and 24.3). If the effusion is very small, it will cause only a loss of the costophrenic angle (Figure 24.4). If a lateral decubitus chest radiograph is taken, the fluid will lie on the dependent side. Following thoracocentesis, microscopy, culture and biochemical analysis can be useful to establish the diagnosis. If the effusion is due to infection, then the fluid obtained will have a high protein content, neutrophils and possibly organisms. Fluid should always be sent for cytology, a high lymphocyte content being indicative of a chylothorax.

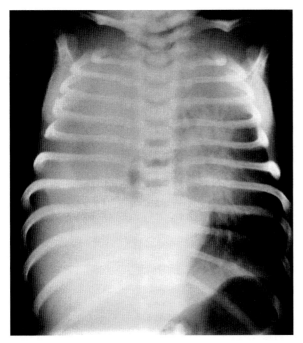

Figure 24.1 *Large unilateral pleural effusion with complete opacity of the right chest and mediastinal shift to the left.*

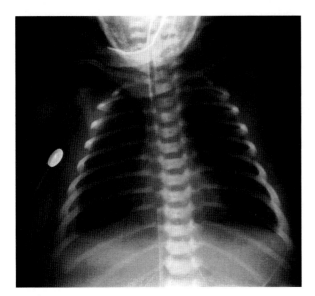

Figure 24.2 *Right-sided pleural effusion demonstrated by a rim of fluid around the lateral chest wall and diaphragm.*

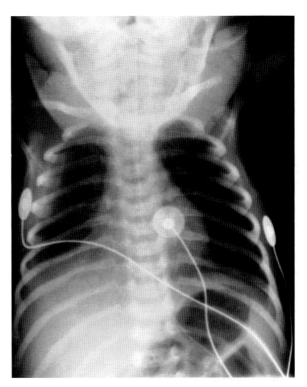

Figure 24.3 *Unilateral right-sided pleural effusion with a lamellar component tracking laterally; the patient is in the supine position.*

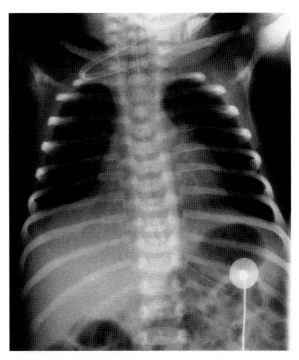

Figure 24.4 *Small right-sided pleural effusion with obliteration of the right hemidiaphragm. This is the same patient as in Figure 24.3 but the chest radiograph is taken in the erect position.*

Management

ANTENATAL

Spontaneous resolution of pleural fluid can occur, thus aggressive investigation or therapy should be delayed until it is clear at a follow-up scan there is no improvement.[31] Drainage can be achieved by thoracocentesis,[7,60] which may need to be repeated if there is recurrence or the effusion is large.[60] Alternatively, a thoracoamniotic shunt can be inserted (Figure 24.5).[10] The advantage of

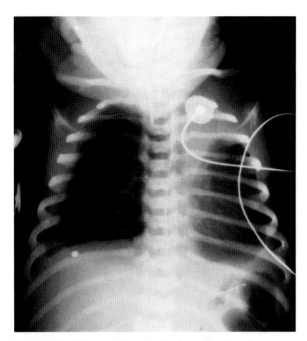

Figure 24.5 *Bilateral pleural effusions. The tip of a thoracoamniotic shunt is visible in the right chest overlying the hemidiaphragm. Collapse of the left upper lobe is present.*

this latter technique over thoracocentesis is that it can achieve chronic drainage[9] and thus may be more effective in permitting normal lung growth if inserted at a critical stage of gestation. Additional advantages are, first, that the diagnosis of an underlying lesion may become apparent only after effective decompression and the return of the mediastinum to its normal position, and second, the degree of pulmonary hypoplasia can be determined as severely affected lungs often fail to expand after shunting. To achieve continuous drainage, a pleuroamniotic shunt, a double-ended pigtail catheter, is inserted under local anesthetic under ultrasound guidance as an outpatient procedure. If the effusions are bilateral, pleuroamniotic shunts are inserted on both sides. Such procedures have resulted in chronic drainage of effusions and, in certain cases, resolution of associated hydrops.[9] The likely mechanism is that drainage of the effusion may reverse the distortion of the cardiac anatomy (brought about by the presence of the effusion) which had impaired heart function and brought about the hydropic state. The drains remain *in situ* until delivery when they are immediately clamped and removed. Some recommend drainage of intrauterine fetal pleural effusions only after assessment of the fetal lung.[31] If there is no expansion of the fetal lung after removal of fluid under pressure, this may indicate irreversible damage. If the lung expands to normal limits, then further intervention may not be necessary. If there is expansion, but the lung is still significantly small, hypoplasia will usually

worsen without intervention. Drainage is indicated if there is hydrops fetalis. Pleuroamniotic shunting rather than repeated thoracocenteses seems to give a better outcome.[31] Pleuroamniotic shunts have generally been inserted in the third trimester,[73] so it seems unlikely their presence will have influenced lung growth. Whether they affect outcome requires testing in a randomized controlled trial. Malpositioned pleuroamniotic shunts can cause permanent injury and scarring. Rarely, phrenic nerve palsy may occur, resulting in a permanently raised right hemidiaphragm postnatally.

AT BIRTH

Active and early resuscitation is needed for infants with large effusions; indeed it is recommended that such patients be intubated at birth.[61] Intubation and positive pressure ventilation is the preferred method of resuscitation as bag and mask resuscitation will not achieve the frequently required high pressures. If this fails to achieve adequate gas exchange, thoracocentesis should be attempted. After the infant has been turned onto the contralateral side, a 21 G butterfly needle, attached to a syringe, should be inserted via a Z-track 1 cm above the vertebral column, in between the fifth and sixth or sixth and seventh ribs. Alternatively, a silicone rubber catheter can be inserted under ultrasound guidance. Unless the infant is very edematous, fluid should be aspirated easily with the needle tip only 0.5 cm below the skin surface. Aspiration should continue only while fluid is obtained easily. In one series,[61] between 50 and 500 ml of fluid was obtained. All aspirated fluid should be sent for culture and biochemical analysis (see below). *Ex utero* intrapartum treatment (EXIT) has been used successfully in the management of an infant with large bilateral hydrothoraces.[63] The infant was delivered by cesarean section and, while temporary preservation of the fetoplacental circulation was maintained, bilateral thoracocenteses were simultaneously performed and more than 400 ml of fluid was drained. The cord was then clamped and the infant underwent elective intubation and ventilation.

POSTNATAL PERIOD

Large effusions should always be drained, not only to improve gas exchange, but also to establish the diagnosis. Until an infective etiology has been excluded, the infant should receive penicillin and gentamicin. Despite drainage, infants who have had severe bilateral congenital pleural effusions may be difficult to ventilate, as a paucity of alveoli may lead to respiratory failure and hypoventilation with carbon dioxide retention. Anecdotally, high-frequency oscillation has been used successfully in such cases.[46] Infants with pulmonary hypoplasia may also have PPHN.[14] Tolazoline was given with a good response in an affected prematurely born infant.[14]

Prognosis

MORTALITY

Fetal pleural effusions, if bilateral, are frequently associated with non-viable pulmonary hypoplasia.[11,16,59] Antenatally detected pleural effusions have a 15 percent mortality,[39] although if diagnosed prior to 32 weeks of gestation the neonatal death rate may be as high as 55 percent.[31] Large effusions can prevent effective resuscitation at birth. Part of the mortality associated with pleural effusion is from the underlying condition, for example diaphragmatic hernia. Infants with effusions due to infection, particularly group B streptococcus, usually die. In one series,[49] a 48 percent mortality rate was reported. Review of 82 cases from 31 separate reports[31] found a 37 percent neonatal death rate in 54 cases managed conservatively and a 32 percent neonatal death rate in the 24 who received intrauterine intervention. The high perinatal mortality rate was due to the development of non-immune hydrops, prematurity and pulmonary hypoplasia.

MORBIDITY

Spontaneous resolution of even bilateral fetal hydrothorax has been reported,[50,61,71] but this occurred in only five of 32 cases without other abnormalities. Effusions also resolve in the neonatal period without sequelae. The preterm delivery rate is high, occurring in between 25 and 66 percent of cases.[31] Prolonged pleural effusions increase the risk of chronic oxygen dependency. In one series,[49] infants with effusions which persisted for 3 days or more were at increased risk for requiring supplemental oxygen for more than 21 days.

CHYLOTHORAX

Chylothorax, first described in 1917,[62] is the most frequent etiology of an isolated fetal pleural effusion.[17,39] Indeed, it has even been suggested that chylothorax is the only antenatal diagnosis of a unilateral echo-free pleural effusion when the diaphragm is intact and fetal hydrops is absent.[54] One in 10 000 deliveries have a chylothorax and one in 2000 neonatal admissions may have a chylothorax.[75]

Pathophysiology

Development of the lymphatic system begins as early as the fifth week of fetal life. Lymph produced in the gut is collected in the cisterna chyli. The thoracic duct originates from the latter structure at the level of the second lumbar vertebrae in the midline and enters the thorax through the aortic hiatus. At the level of the fourth thoracic vertebra it crosses to the left and enters the junction of the left internal jugular and subclavian vein. There is a rich collateral network and thus ligation of the duct at any point in its course is feasible. In the gut, long-chain fatty acids pass into the lymph as chylomicrons after being re-esterified to triglycerides before entering the venous network, whereas medium-chain fatty acids (10 C or fewer) pass directly into the portal venous blood. An abnormality in the lymphatic system at the level of the thoracic duct below or above the fifth thoracic vertebrae may lead to a right- or left-sided chylothorax.[75] An anatomical cause of chylothorax has, however, only been recognized in a few cases. Lymph accumulation in the pleural cavity can result from overproduction. It may also result from a congenital fistula, brought about by a failure of some of the channels to connect with the major lymphatic network; this results in outflow of chyle into the pleural cavity.[75]

Etiology

Chylothorax may occur spontaneously or be associated with lymphedema due to congenitally abnormal lymph vessels as found in congenital lymphangiectasia,[36] Turner's or Noonan's syndrome and pulmonary lymphangiectasia. In pulmonary lymphangiectasia, the lungs show diffuse dilatation of the interlobular and subpleural lymphatics. In patients with chylothorax and extralobar pulmonary sequestration, a similar mechanism has been proposed.[22] It may also result from various congenital defects of the thoracic duct or trauma. Absence or atresia of the thoracic duct has been postulated.[70] Others have reported oozing with no apparent thoracic duct abnormality.[65] Trauma to the thoracic duct may occur at delivery by hyperextension of the spinal column and increased venous pressure during birth; this appears rare from postmortem data.[65] A chylothorax may occur following cardiac surgery (repair of coarctation of the aorta or ligation of a patent ductus arteriosus) or repair of a congenital posterolateral diaphragmatic hernia.[55] In the latter surgery, it seems probable that the diaphragmatic lymph channels are injured at operation when the sac is excised, but before the hernia repair. Chylothorax may be secondary to superior vena caval obstruction in patients undergoing total parenteral nutrition catheterization.[4] Congenital chylothorax has also been described in association with neonatal thyrotoxicosis secondary to maternal Graves' disease.[37] The postulated mechanism was heart failure secondary to tachyarrhythmia. In heart failure, chylothorax may be produced by an increase in lymph production secondary to an augmented pulmonary capillary filtration associated with an obstruction to lymphatic flow caused by increased pressure in the subclavian vein.[78]

Most cases of chylothorax are sporadic, but an X-linked recessive transmission has been suggested[67] and, as congenital chylothorax has been described in two consecutive female siblings, autosomal recessive inheritance has been suggested.[43] Congenital chylothorax has been reported with trisomy X[13] and in patients with trisomy 21;[74] the cause of the association remains unclear.

Clinical signs

Chylothorax is the most common form of pleural effusion in the fetus and neonates. It can cause hydrops by two possible mechanisms: by impairing venous return by cardiac and vena caval compression and/or loss of protein into the pleural space leading to generalized hypoproteinemia and edema.[83] Typically, the condition presents as a right-sided unilateral effusion in 60 percent of cases,[81] although occasionally it may be bilateral (Figure 24.6) and associated with gross hydrops. It is associated with foregut malformations and extralobar sequestration.[22] In 50 percent of cases, symptoms are present at birth, but they can also develop within the first week of life.[81]

The clinical features are those described under isolated pleural effusion. Persistent pulmonary hypertension associated with a bilateral chylothorax has been described.[14] In a chronic chylothorax, the daily chyle production may be higher than the circulating volume and so may be associated with hypovolemia, hypoalbuminemia, hyponatremia and weight loss caused by caloric loss.[77] The patients are immunocompromised, because of loss of lymphocytes and humoral antibodies.[53]

Diagnosis

The diagnosis of chylothorax may be suspected antenatally by ultrasonography[47] and subsequently confirmed by thoracocentesis.[7] In an unfed infant, the fluid obtained at thoracocentesis is clear and yellow and will contain large numbers of lymphocytes so that the infant may suffer from lymphopenia. The diagnosis of chylothorax is made in the presence of 20–50 leukocytes per high power field, with 90 percent being lymphocytes; the protein and electrolyte content are as in plasma.[64] It has been suggested that the sole finding of 80 percent or more lymphocytes in the pleural fluid is pathognomonic of chylothorax,[50] but the reliability of pleural fluid lymphocyte counts has been questioned.[23] The fluid should be analyzed by lipoprotein electrophoresis to identify the predominance of high-density lipoprotein.[54] If there is a chylothorax, a high triglyceride level (± 0.9 g/l) and a low cholesteral level (0.6 g/l) is found.[77] Once the infant is milk fed, the fluid will become chylous. After discontinuation of human milk or standard formula and administration of a medium-chain triglyceride formula, the chyle becomes clear and yellow again.[77] Chylothorax associated with superior vena cava (SVC) obstruction should be suspected in infants with swelling of the face, neck and upper extremities. Ultrasonography will confirm the presence of fluid in the chest and the position of the catheter tip. Doppler ultrasonography can identify the SVC obstruction. On the chest radiograph a chylothorax may present as a unilateral pleural effusion (Figure 24.6) or bilateral effusions with skin edema as part of a generalized hydropic process (Figure 24.7).

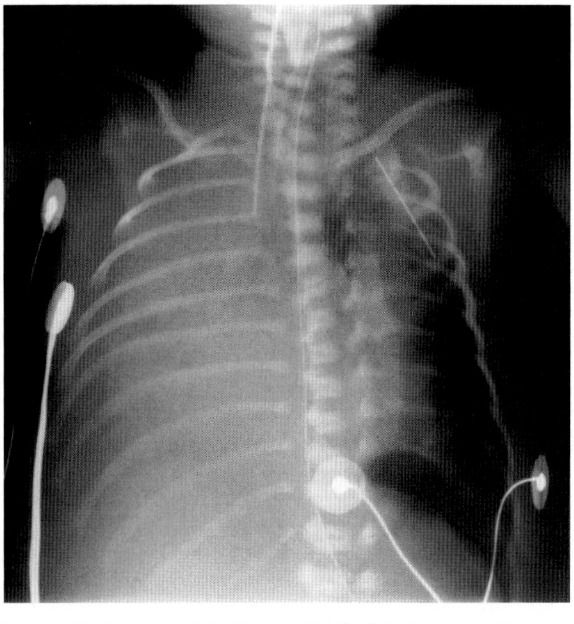

Figure 24.6 *Large chylothorax. A left-sided pneumothorax is present.*

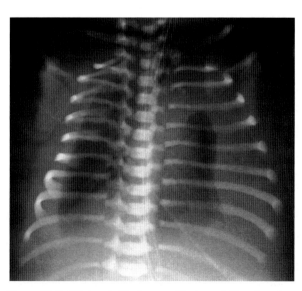

Figure 24.7 *Bilateral effusions and hydrops (skin edema) due to congenital chylothorax.*

Management

ANTENATAL

If the diagnosis is late in the third trimester, the infant will require immediate delivery with postpartum decompression or drainage prior to delivery. Chronic antenatal drainage by placement of a pleuroamniotic shunt is another option if the diagnosis is made early in the pregnancy (see p. 96).

POSTNATAL

Conservative

Frequently, a single thoracocentesis causes resolution of the chylothorax, as this will result in expansion of the lung and tamponade of the duct or defect, preventing further formation of pleural fluid. If, however, the chylothorax recurs, then a chest tube should be inserted and left in situ until drainage of fluid has ceased. Affected infants should also be changed to total parenteral nutrition[12] or a milk containing fat only in the form of medium-chain triglycerides.[32] Either maneuver reduces throughput in the leaking duct and will facilitate its healing.[17,28,45] Pregestemil or Pepti-Junior can be tried, but if enteral nutrition with such milks fails to control the chylothorax, a semi-elementary diet should be used and continued for at least 2 weeks after the fluid has disappeared. If this fails, then total parenteral nutrition should be used with complete withdrawal of enteral feeds.

Conservative management is associated with such complications as lymphopenia, hypoalbuminemia, hyponatremia and weight loss. Complications are most common in patients whose effusions required the longest drainage.[64] To compensate for the loss of lymphocytes and antibodies and reduce the risk of infection, a combination of equal volumes of fresh frozen plasma and pasteurized plasma solution (or albumin) should be administered.[77] Weekly intravenous immunoglobulins should also be given.[46]

Surgical

If, after 3 weeks, conservative management fails to reduce the leakage of chyle or there is reaccumulation of the chylothorax after relaxation of restricted enteral fat intake, then surgical intervention should be considered. An underlying lymphatic disorder is an indication for surgery early rather than late. Pleural abrasion, ligation of the thoracic duct and pleurodesis are possible options.[65] At thoracotomy, if the leak is small it can be repaired, but if the leak is large or repair is unsuccessful, ligation of the duct above and below the leak is required.[5] If a localized thoracic duct injury cannot be identified, pleurectomy is the surgical procedure of choice.[64] In ventilator-dependent infants, pleuroperitoneal shunts may be useful for persistent chylothoraces.[6] An alternative to surgical treatment is bilateral pleurodesis which has been achieved by injecting 50 ml of 50 percent dextrose into the pleural space.[46]

Prognosis

The mortality may be as high as 25 percent for a unilateral chylothorax and 60 percent for bilateral chylothoraces.[14]

HEMOTHORAX

Etiology

Penetration of the fetal thorax is a known complication of amniocentesis,[2,27] but fetal hemothorax is unusual.[2]

Postnatally, hemothorax results from trauma either at thoracic surgery for ligation of a patent ductus arteriosus (PDA) or damage to the arteries alongside the ribs from misplacement of a chest tube to drain a pneumothorax. Hemothorax has been described following central venous catheter placement, albeit usually in the 1–6 year-old age group.[33] Vascular injury to the subclavian artery, vein or superior vena cava were noted in most at operation. Clotting abnormalities very rarely present as an isolated hemothorax,[52,66] but can increase the amount of blood in the pleural space following trauma to the chest wall. Rare causes include spontaneous rupture of a PDA,[20] a tumour of the thymus and hypoprothrombinemia.[52] Arteriovenous malformations have also been incriminated.[1]

Diagnosis

The chest radiograph may demonstrate a whiteout; ultrasonography will confirm that this is due to fluid rather than a solid tumour such as a hamartoma or a teratoma. A radioisotope lung scan will identify if there is an underlying arteriovenous fistula.

Management

The hemothorax may be associated with catastrophic bleeding and urgent transfusion of blood and clotting factors are then required for resuscitation. Clotting abnormalities should be actively sought and promptly treated. If the hemothorax is the result of trauma to a large blood vessel, for example at chest tube insertion, then surgical intervention should be considered, providing it is possible to support the infant long enough for this to be feasible.

HYDROPS FETALIS

Hydrops fetalis is defined as generalized edema of the soft tissues in utero, with or without effusions. Non-immune hydrops (see below) occurs in one per 1500–4000 deliveries.

Pathophysiology

The pleural effusions associated with hydrops fetalis are due to heart failure.

Etiology

Hydrops fetalis may be classified as immune, that is if there is hematological evidence of isoimmunization, or non-immune of which there are over 70 etiological factors (Table 24.1).[24,35] Fetuses without anemia as the cause of the hydrops are more likely to exhibit pleural effusions, 87 percent in one series.[69] By contrast, only 20 percent of those with anemia as the cause of the hydrops had pleural effusions. Fetal pleural effusions develop into non-immune hydrops because of diminished venous return, liver congestion, portal hypertension, congestive heart failure, loss of protein, interference with liver function and lymphatic obstruction in other areas.

Diagnosis

ANTENATAL

Fetal chromosomal and cardiac abnormalities should be looked for by amniocentesis or cordocentesis and fetal echocardiography, respectively. Maternal blood should be screened for blood group, antibodies, the presence of fetal cells using the Kleihauer–Bekte test or evidence of possible infective causes such as toxoplasmosis or parvovirus.

Table 24.1 *The commoner causes of non-immune hydrops*

Hematological	*Cardiovascular*
Anemia	Congenital heart disease
Alpha-thalassemia	Arrhythmia
Fetomaternal hemorrhage	
Glucose 6-PD deficiency	
Pulmonary	*Chromosomal*
Diaphragmatic hernia	Turner's syndrome
Cystic adenomatoid	Trisomy 21, 18, 13
malformation	Translocation/Mosaic
Chylothorax	
Sequestration	
Renal	*Infective*
Congenital nephrosis	Parvovirus
	Cytomegalovirus
	Toxoplasmosis
Skeletal	*Neoplastic*
Achondroplasia	Teratoma
Achondrogenesis	Neuroblastoma
Metabolic	*Syndromal*
Gaucher's disease	Noonan

Fetal blood sampling is invaluable in such cases and allows determination of the fetal hemoglobin, electrophoresis and karyotype. A viral screen may also be performed to detect specific IgM or viral DNA. In cases where fetal anemia is suspected, Doppler ultrasound assessment of fetal blood flow velocities provides useful information. Increased velocities suggest anemia and suitable preparations may be made to perform fetal blood transfusion.

Prognosis

The development of hydrops is associated with a poor outcome. In one series,[15] there was a 100 percent mortality in hydropic infants who had persistent pleural effusions, but in another,[72] two-thirds of hydropic infants died regardless of whether an effusion persisted until birth.

REFERENCES

1 Aaron, B.L., Doohen, D.J. (1970) Spontaneous hemothorax in the newborn: another cause for respiratory distress. *Annals of Thoracic Surgery* **9**, 258–262.

2 Achiron, R., Zakut, H. (1986) Fetal hemothorax complicating amniocentesis – antenatal sonographic diagnosis. *Acta Obstetricia et Gynecologica Scandinavica* **65**, 869–870.

3 Adams, H., Jones, A., Hayward, C. (1988) The sonographic features and implications of fetal pleural effusions. *Clinical Radiology* **39**, 398–401.

4 Amodio, J., Abramson, S., Berdon, W. *et al.* (1987) Iatrogenic causes of large pleural fluid collections in the premature infant: ultrasonic and radiographic findings. *Pediatric Radiology* **17**, 104–108.

5 Andersen, E.A., Hertel, J., Pedersen, S.A., Sorensen, H.R. (1984) Congenital chylothorax: management by ligature of the thoracic duct. *Scandinavian Journal of Thoracic and Cardiovascular Surgery* **18**, 193–194.

6 Azizkhan, R.G., Canfield, J., Alford, B.A., Rodgers, B.M. (1983) Pleuroperitoneal shunts in the management of neonatal chylothorax. *Journal of Pediatric Surgery* **18**, 842–850.

7 Benacerraf, B.R., Frigoletto, F.D., Wilson, M. (1986) Successful midtrimester thoracentesis with analysis of the lymphocyte population in the pleural effusion. *American Journal of Obstetrics and Gynecology* **155**, 398–399.

8 Berg, H.v.d., Koppe, J.G. (1983) Respiratory insufficiency in the neonatal period due to chylothorax [in Dutch]. *Nederlands Tijdschrift voor Geneeskunde* **127**, 1948–1951.

9 Blott, M., Nicolaides, K.H., Greenough, A. (1988) Pleuroamniotic shunting for decompression of fetal pleural effusions. *Obstetrics and Gynecology* **71**, 798–800.

10 Booth, P., Nicolaides, K.H., Greenough, A., Gamsu, H.R. (1987) Pleuro-amniotic shunting for fetal chylothorax. *Early Human Development* **15**, 365–367.

11 Bovicilli, L., Rizzo, N., Orsini, L.F., Calderoni, P. (1981) Ultrasound real-time diagnosis of fetal hydrothorax and lung hypoplasia. *Journal of Clinical Ultrasound* **9**, 253–254.

12 Brodman, R.F., Zarelson, T.M., Schiebler, G.L. (1974) Treatment of congenital chylothorax. *Journal of Pediatrics* **85**, 516–520.

13 Cardoso, D., Tuna, M., Abrantes, M. *et al.* (2001) Congenital chylothorax associated with trisomy X. *European Journal of Pediatrics* **160**, 743.

14   Carmant, L., Le Guennec, J.C. (1989) Congenital chylothorax and persistent pulmonary hypertension of the neonate. *Acta Paediatrica Scandinavica* **78**, 789–792.

15   Castillo, R.A., Devoe, L.D., Hadi, H.A. *et al.* (1986) Nonimmune hydrops fetalis: clinical experience and factors related to a poor outcome. *American Journal of Obstetrics and Gynecology* **155**, 812–816.

16   Castillo, R.A., Devoe, L.D., Falls, G. *et al.* (1987) Pleural effusions and pulmonary hypoplasia. *American Journal of Obstetrics and Gynecology* **157**, 1252–1255.

17   Chernick, V., Reed, M.H. (1970) Pneumothorax and chylothorax in the neonatal period. *Journal of Pediatrics* **76**, 624–632.

18   Curry, C.J., Chopra, D., Finer, N.N. (1988) Hydrops and pleural effusions in congenital myotonic dystrophy. *Journal of Pediatrics* **113**, 555–557.

19   Defoort, P., Thiery, M. (1978) Antenatal diagnosis of congenital chylothorax by gray scale sonography. *Journal of Clinical Ultrasound* **6**, 47–48.

20   Dippel, W.F., Doty, D.B., Ehrenhaft, J.L. (1973) Tension hemothorax due to patent ductus arteriosus. *New England Journal of Medicine* **288**, 353–354.

21   Donnelly, L.F., Frush, D.P., Bisset, G.S. (1999) The appearance and significance of extrapleural fluid after esophageal atresia repair. *American Journal of Radiology* **172**, 231–233.

22   Dresler, S. (1981) Massive pleural effusion and hypoplasia of the lung accompanying extralobar pulmonary sequestration. *Human Pathology* **12**, 862–864.

23   Eddleman, K.A., Levine, A.B., Chitkara, U., Berkowitz, R.L. (1991) Reliability of pleural fluid lymphocyte counts in the antenatal diagnosis of congenital chylothorax. *Obstetrics and Gynecology* **78**, 530–532.

24   Etches, P.C. (1986) Hydrops fetalis. In Roberton, N.R.C. (ed.), *Textbook of Neonatology*. Edinburgh: Churchill Livingstone, 484–494.

25   Falade, A.G. (1992) Right diaphragmatic eventration simulating neonatal pleural effusion: a case report. *Annals of Tropical Paediatrics* **12**, 221–223.

26   Foote, K.D., Vickers, D.W. (1986) Congenital pleural effusion in Down's syndrome. *British Journal of Radiology* **59**, 609–610.

27   Galle, P.C., Meis, P.J. (1982) Complications of amniocentesis: a review. *Journal of Reproductive Medicine* **27**, 149–155.

28   Gershanik, J.J., Johnson, H.J., Riopel, D.A., *et al.* (1974) Dietary management of neonatal chylothorax. *Pediatrics* **53**, 400–403.

29   Girdany, B.R., Sieber, W.K., Osman, M.Z. (1969) Traumatic pseudodiverticulums of the pharynx in newborn infants. *New England Journal of Medicine* **280**, 237–240.

30   Gooding, C.A., Gregory, G.A. (1971) Roentgenographic analysis of meconium aspiration of the newborn. *Radiology* **100**, 131–135.

31   Hagay, Z., Reece, A., Roberts, A., Hobbins, J.C. (1993) Isolated fetal pleural effusion: a prenatal management dilemma. *Obstetrics and Gynecology* **81**, 147–152.

32   Hashim, S.A., Roholt, H.B., Babayan, V.K., Van Itallie, T.B. (1964) Treatment of chyluria and chylothorax with medium chain triglyceride. *New England Journal of Medicine* **270**, 756–761.

33   Hoeffel, J.C., Marcon, F., Worms, A.M. (1992) Diffuse pulmonary lymphangiectasis with heart defect discovered 4 months post-natally. *Padiatrie und Padologie* **27**, 25–27.

34   Hoffman, R.R., Campbell, R.E., Decker, J.P. (1974) Fetal aspiration syndrome. Clinical, roentgenologic and pathologic features. *American Journal of Roentgenology, Radium Therapy and Nuclear Medicine* **122**, 90–96.

35   Holzgreve, W., Holzgreve, B., Curry, C.J.R. (1985) Non-immune hydrops fetalis: diagnosis and management. *Seminars in Perinatology* **9**, 52–67.

36   Hunter, W.S., Becroft, D.M. (1984) Congenital pulmonary lymphangiectasis associated with pleural effusions. *Archives of Disease in Childhood* **59**, 278–279.

37   Ibrahim, H., Asamoah, A., Krouskop, R.W. *et al.* (1999) Congenital chylothorax in neonatal thyrotoxicosis. *Journal of Perinatology* **19**, 68–71.

38   Jacob, J., Edwards, D., Gluck, L. (1980) Early-onset sepsis and pneumonia observed as respiratory distress syndrome: assessment of lung maturity. *American Journal of Diseases of Children* **134**, 766–768.

39   Jaffa, A.J., Barak, S., Kaysar, N., Peyser, M.R. (1985) Antenatal diagnosis of bilateral congenital chylothorax with pericardial effusion. *Acta Obstetricia et Gynecologica Scandinavica* **64**, 455–456.

40   John, H., Seguin, M.D. (1992) Right-sided hydrothorax and central venous catheter in extremely low birthweight infants. *American Journal of Perinatology* **9**, 154–158.

41   Kanof, A., Epstein, B.S., Kraemer, B., Mauss, I. (1953) Staphylcoccal pneumonia and emphysema. *Pediatrics* **11**, 385–392.

42   Kassner, E.G., Baumstark, A., Balsam, D., Haller, J.O. (1977) Passage of feeding catheters into the pleural space: a radiographic sign of trauma to the pharynx and esophagus in the newborn. *American Journal of Roentgenology* **128**, 19–22.

43   King, P.A., Ghosh, A., Tang, M.H.Y., Lam, S.K. (1991) Recurrent congenital chylothorax. *Prenatal Diagnosis* **11**, 809–811.

44   Knight, L., Tobin, J.J., L'Heureux, P. (1974) Hydrothorax: a complication of hyperalimentation with radiologic manifestations. *Radiology* **111**, 693–695.

45   Kosloske, A.M., Martin, L.W., Schubert, W.K. (1974) Management of chylothorax in children by thoracentesis and medium-chain triglyceride feedings. *Journal of Pediatric Surgery* **9**, 365–371.

46   Kugelman, A., Gonen, R., Bader, D. (2000) Potential role of high-frequency ventilation in the treatment of severe congenital pleural effusion. *Pediatric Pulmonology* **29**, 404–408.

47   Ladreyt, J.P., Bourlon, J.P., Maillet-Robert, J. *et al.* (1987) [Neo-natal chylothorax: antenatal echographic diagnosis and favourable outcome]. [French]. *Pediatrie* **42**, 535–536.

48   Leipala, J.A., Petaja, J., Fellman, V. (2001) Perforation complications of percutaneous central venous catheters in very low birthweight infants. *Journal of Paediatrics and Child Health* **37**, 168–171.

49   Long, W.A., Lawson, E.E., Harned, H.S., Kraybill, E.N. (1984) Pleural effusion in the first days of life: a prospective study. *American Journal of Perinatology* **1**, 190–194.

50   Longaker, M.T., Laberge, J.M., Dansereau, J. *et al.* (1989) Primary fetal hydrothorax: natural history and management. *Journal of Pediatric Surgery* **24**, 573.

51   Madhavi, P., Jameson, R., Robinson, M.J. (2000) Unilateral pleural effusion complicating central venous catheterization. *Archives of Disease in Childhood Fetal and Neonatal Edition* **82**, F248–F249.

52   Mazzi, E., White, J.J., Nishida, H., Risemberg, H.M. (1977) Neonatal respiratory distress from hemothorax. *Pediatrics* **59** (Suppl 6), 1057–1058.

53   McWilliams, B., Fan, L., Murphy, S. (1981) Transient T-cell depression in postoperative chylothorax. *Journal of Pediatrics* **99**, 595–597.

54   Meizner, I., Carmi, R., Bar-Ziv, J. (1986) Congenital chylothorax – prenatal ultrasonic diagnosis and successful post partum management. *Prenatal Diagnosis* **6**, 217–221.

55   Mercer, S. (1986) Factors involved in chylothorax following repair of congenital posterolateral diaphragmatic hernia. *Journal of Pediatric Surgery* **21**, 809–811.

56 Meyer, K., Girgis, N., McGravey, V. (1985) Adenovirus associated with congenital pleural effusion. *Journal of Pediatrics* **107**, 433–435.

57 Murayama, K., Jimbo, T., Matsumoto, Y. *et al.* (1987) Fetal pulmonary hypoplasia with hydrothorax. *American Journal of Obstetrics and Gynecology* **157**, 119–120.

58 Nicolaides, K.H., Azar, G.B. (1990) Thoraco-amniotic shunting. *Fetal Diagnosis and Therapy* **5**, 153–164.

59 Peleg, D., Golichowski, A.M., Ragan, W.D. (1985) Fetal hydrothorax and bilateral pulmonary hypoplasia. Ultrasonic diagnosis. *Acta Obstetricia et Gynecologica Scandinavica* **64**, 451–453.

60 Petres, R.E., Redwine, F.O., Cruikshank, D.P. (1982) Congenital bilateral chylothorax. Antepartum diagnosis and successful intrauterine surgical management. *Journal of the American Medical Association* **248**, 1360–1361.

61 Pijpers, L., Reuss, A., Stewart, P.A., Wladimiroff, J.W. (1989) Noninvasive management of isolated bilateral fetal hydrothorax. *American Journal of Obstetrics and Gynecology* **161**, 330–332.

62 Pisek, G. (1917) Report of chylothorax. *Archives of Paediatrics* **34**, 929–937.

63 Prontera, W., Jaeggi, E.T., Pfizenmaier, M. *et al.* (2002) *Ex utero* intrapartum treatment (EXIT) of severe fetal hydrothorax. *Archives of Disease in Childhood Fetal and Neonatal Edition* **86**, F58–F60.

64 Puntis, J.W., Roberts, K.D., Handy, D. (1987) How should chylothorax be managed? *Archives of Disease in Childhood* **62**, 593–596.

65 Randolph, J.G., Gross, R.E. (1957) Congenital chylothorax. *Archives of Disease in Childhood* **74**, 405–419.

66 Ransome, O.J., Argent, A.C., Parbhoo, K.B., Delahunt, T. (1987) Haemothorax of the newborn – an unusual cause of respiratory distress. A case report. *South African Medical Journal* **71**, 463–464.

67 Reece, E.A., Lockwood, C.J., Rizzo, N. *et al.* (1987) Intrinsic intrathoracic malformations of the fetus: sonographic detection and clinical presentation. *Obstetrics and Gynecology* **70**, 627–632.

68 Roberts, A.B., Clarkson, P.M., Pattison, N.S. *et al.* (1986) Fetal hydrothorax in the second trimester of pregnancy: successful intra-uterine treatment at 24 weeks gestation. *Fetal Therapy* **1**, 20320–20329.

69 Saltzman, D.H., Frigoletto, F.D., Harlow, B.L. *et al.* (1989) Sonographic evaluation of hydrops fetalis. *Obstetrics and Gynecology* **74**, 106–111.

70 Sardet, A. (1981) Chylothorax in children and newborn infants [French]. *Archives Francaises de Pediatrie* **38**, 455.

71 Sherer, D.M., Abramowicz, J.S., Eggers, P.C., Woods, J.R.J. (1992) Transient severe unilateral and subsequent bilateral primary fetal hydrothorax with spontaneous resolution at 34 weeks' gestation associated with normal neonatal outcome. *American Journal of Obstetrics and Gynecology* **166**, 169–170.

72 Thompson, P.J., Greenough, A., Brooker, R. *et al.* (1993) Antenatal diagnosis and outcome in hydrops fetalis. *Journal of Perinatal Medicine* **21**, 63–67.

73 Thompson, P.J., Greenough, A., Nicolaides, K.H. (1993) Respiratory function in infancy following pleuro-amniotic function shunting. *Fetal Diagnosis Therapy* **8**, 79–83.

74 Turan, O., Canter, B., Ergenekon, E. *et al.* (2001) Chylothorax and respiratory distress in a newborn with trisomy 21. *European Journal of Pediatrics* **160**, 744–745.

75 van Aerde, J., Campbell, A., Smyth, J. *et al.* (1984) Spontaneous chylothorax in newborns. *American Journal of Diseases of Children* **138**, 961–964.

76 van Niekerk, M., Kalis, N.N., van der Merwe, P.-L. (1998) Cardiac tamponade following umbilical vein catheterisation in a neonate. *South African Medical Journal* **88** (Cardiovascular Suppl 2), C87–C90.

77 van Straaten, H.L., Gerards, L.J., Krediet, T.G. (1993) Chylothorax in the neonatal period. *European Journal of Pediatrics* **152**, 2–5.

78 Villena, V., de Pablo, A., Martin-Escribano, P. (1995) Chylothorax and chylous ascites due to heart failure. *European Respiratory Journal* **8**, 1235–1236.

79 Weller, M.H., Katzenstein, A.A. (1976) Radiological findings in group B streptococcal sepsis. *Radiology* **118**, 385–387.

80 Whittle, M.J., Gilmore, D.H., McNay, M.B. *et al.* (1989) Diaphragmatic hernia presenting *in utero* as a unilateral hydrothorax. *Prenatal Diagnosis* **9**, 115–118.

81 Yancy, W.S., Spock, A. (1967) Spontaneous neonatal pleural effusion. *Journal of Pediatric Surgery* **2**, 313–319.

82 Yeh, T.F., Harris, V., Srinivasan, G. *et al.* (1979) Roentgenographic findings in infants with meconium aspiration syndrome. *Journal of the American Medical Association* **242**, 60–63.

83 Zito, L., Keszler, M. (1989) Massive edema and bilateral pleural effusions in a newborn infant. *Annals of Allergy* **63**, 277–280.

Pulmonary hemorrhage

GRENVILLE F FOX

Pulmonary hemorrhage is recognized when large amounts of blood appear in the airway, usually associated with a sudden deterioration in the infant's clinical condition. Sometimes referred to as massive pulmonary hemorrhage, it should be distinguished from the relatively common occurrence of minor blood staining of respiratory secretions, occurring in ventilated infants secondary to trauma resulting from intubation or airway suction.

INCIDENCE

The overall incidence of pulmonary hemorrhage has been reported in a number of population studies and varies from 0.1 per 1000 live births in 1970[18] to 1.2 per 1000 in more recent series.[35] The apparent rise in incidence, seen in these and other studies over a similar time period, is likely to be explained by the increased number of infants surviving after extremely premature birth. Whereas earlier studies described pulmonary hemorrhage occurring predominantly in term infants,[11,29] more recently it has been found to be more common in preterm infants who have usually been treated with exogenous surfactant and often have a patent ductus arteriosus.[33] The incidence of pulmonary hemorrhage has been reported to be 11.9 percent in infants of birthweight less than 1500 g treated with surfactant,[51] 6.4 percent in infants of birthweight less than 1700 g,[33] and 9.5 percent in infants less than 30 weeks of gestation.[27]

PATHOLOGY

Postmortem examination findings in infants dying before 48 hours of age suggest that interstitial hemorrhage is common,[26] with pulmonary interstitial emphysema being associated with pulmonary hemorrhage in these infants.[70] As most have severe surfactant deficiency, other pathological findings include solid, gasless lungs which sink in water. The cut surface of the lung is a deep red or purple color and histological changes include necrosis and desquamation of pneumocytes with hyaline membrane formation.

In deaths after the first 48 hours of life, particularly after treatment with surfactant, intra-alveolar hemorrhage is more common.[52] This has been described as a form of fulminant lung edema, with leakage of red blood cells and capillary filtrate into the lungs,[66] hence the alternative name for pulmonary hemorrhage of hemorrhagic pulmonary edema. A more recent study has, however, demonstrated that massive bleeding may also be secondary to severe necrotizing tracheobronchitis.[70] Other findings at postmortem examination in the later deaths associated with pulmonary hemorrhage are those of severe chronic lung disease (CLD), which include airway inflammation and smooth muscle hypertrophy, along with enlargement and destruction of alveolar sacs.

PATHOPHYSIOLOGY

The mechanism of pulmonary hemorrhage has been studied in asphyxiated lambs and newborn humans.[1,2] It has been postulated that following a rise in pulmonary capillary pressure, there is an initial increase in interstitial fluid. Damage to the alveolar epithelium due to underlying lung disease or distention due to the increased interstitial fluid then causes this fluid to leak into the alveoli. In the early stages, only relatively small molecules

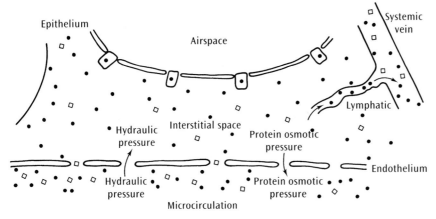

Figure 25.1 *Schematic diagram of the fluid compartments of the newborn lung and the variables that influence filtration of fluid in the pulmonary microcirculation. The small closed circles represent albumin molecules and the open squares represent globulin molecules.*[8]

such as albumin may leak, but if capillary endothelial and alveolar epithelial permeability become more marked, larger molecules and red blood cells also appear in the alveoli. This results in massive pulmonary hemorrhage and hence the alternative name of hemorrhagic pulmonary edema. The hematocrit of material suctioned from the airway of infants with pulmonary hemorrhage has been found to be below 10 percent in most cases, thus supporting the suggested hypothesis.[22] Increased lung microvascular pressure, reduced protein osmotic pressure, impaired lymphatic drainage and microvascular endothelial injury may all contribute to pulmonary edema in the newborn lung (Figure 25.1) (p. 391).[8]

Pulmonary edema and subsequent pulmonary hemorrhage may result from increased lung microvascular pressure, which most commonly arises due to a large left-to-right shunt from a patent ductus arteriosus in preterm infants. Myocardial dysfunction due to hypoxia or sepsis may exacerbate this, as may rapid infusion of colloid or crystalloid.[9] Experiments in newborn lambs have suggested that hypoxia further exacerbates pulmonary edema by increasing lymph flow.[7,13,55] In theory, increase in lung microvascular pressure is more likely in pulmonary hypoplasia with the reduced size of the pulmonary vascular bed. Excessive intravenous fat administration has been shown to increase pulmonary arterial pressure in sheep[48] and may also be associated with decreased lung function in adults[34] and worse pulmonary outcomes and pulmonary hypertension in neonates.[45,54] There is, however, no evidence that early administration of intravenous lipid increases the incidence of pulmonary hemorrhage or other adverse lung outcomes in prematurely born infants.[32]

Reduced protein osmotic pressure has been shown to increase pulmonary edema in experimental animals by increasing the transvascular filtration of fluid in the lung.[37,39,72] Contributory factors are prematurity, hydrops, excessive fluid intake and renal or gastrointestinal protein loss.[8]

Impaired lymphatic drainage from scar tissue in pulmonary interstitial emphysema or bronchopulmonary dysplasia,[64] or raised systemic venous pressure[53] may also increase pulmonary edema. Bacterial infections, *Pseudomonas*, *Escherichia coli* and *Streptococcus agalactiae*, have been shown to increase microvascular endothelial injury and contribute to pulmonary edema.[15,16,57] Oxygen toxicity also causes severe pulmonary edema by inducing microvascular endothelial injury.[7,14]

Surfactant inactivation can occur as a result of pulmonary hemorrhage. Holm and Notter, using a pulsating bubble apparatus in an *in vitro* rat lung model, demonstrated that hemoglobin, red cell membrane lipids and serum proteins increased surface tension and thereby decreased respiratory system compliance.[41] Further work with lavaged rabbit surfactant showed that different plasma proteins interfered with surfactant function to varying degrees, with fibrin monomers being particularly potent inhibitors. Fibrinogen had a less marked adverse effect on surfactant function, but was more potent than albumin.[61]

ETIOLOGY

Antenatal risk factors

Possible antenatal risk factors were examined in 91 infants who died of pulmonary hemorrhage and infants without pulmonary hemorrhage who died during the same period.[58] Breech delivery, but not antepartum hemorrhage, pre-eclampsia, cord prolapse or birth by elective cesarean section, was more common in the infants who died of pulmonary hemorrhage. Several studies have suggested that being small for gestational age increases the risk for pulmonary hemorrhage;[24,62] the association was shown to be independent of other variables by multivariate analysis in one study.[31] Multiple gestation and a lower 5-minute Apgar score have also been associated with an increased risk of pulmonary hemorrhage.[5] In a retrospective cohort study of infants with birthweight less than 1700 g, Garland *et al.* highlighted that pulmonary hemorrhage was also more common in infants whose mothers had received antibiotics in labor and in male infants.[33]

Pulmonary edema

Pulmonary hemorrhage has been noted where there are underlying contributory factors for the development of pulmonary edema, as detailed above. Hence, it has been described in newborn infants with perinatal asphyxia,[69] bacterial infection,[31,58] viral infection,[43] congenital heart disease,[26,58] hydrops secondary to rhesus hemolytic disease,[25,67] pulmonary hypoplasia[44] and hypothermia.[47]

Patent ductus arteriosus

The occurrence of pulmonary hemorrhage has been associated with patent ductus arteriosus and earlier treatment with surfactant, a poor response to surfactant and requirement for inotropic support. These factors are all known markers for illness severity and, when adjusted for this, only patent ductus arteriosus appeared to be independently associated with pulmonary hemorrhage.[33] In support of these findings, preterm infants with echocardiographic evidence of a large left-to-right shunt across a patent ductus arteriosus and high pulmonary blood flow were found to have a higher incidence of pulmonary hemorrhage.[27]

The role of prophylactic indomethacin in reducing pulmonary hemorrhage, however, remains unclear. A meta-analysis of prophylactic versus early symptomatic treatment for patent ductus arteriosus suggested that the incidence of pulmonary hemorrhage was reduced with prophylactic indomethacin [odds ratio (OR) 0.54; 95 percent confidence interval (CI) 0.30–0.96].[19] By contrast, in a large, multicenter, randomized, controlled trial of prophylactic indomethacin, no difference in the incidence of pulmonary hemorrhage between treatment and control groups was found.[60]

Exogenous surfactant

Treatment with surfactant increases left-to-right ductal shunting and pulmonary blood flow, increasing the likelihood of hemorrhagic pulmonary edema (pulmonary hemorrhage).[20] Many randomized, controlled trials of exogenous surfactant have demonstrated this increased risk in treated infants. It appears to be greatest in the smallest, most prematurely born infants. In one trial of a synthetic surfactant, involving infants with birthweights of 500–699 g, there was a sixfold increase in the incidence of pulmonary hemorrhage in those receiving surfactant.[65] A smaller increase in the incidence of pulmonary hemorrhage (1.9 percent versus 1.0 percent) has also been highlighted by analysis of five randomized, controlled trials involving the same synthetic surfactant given to infants with birthweights greater than 700 g. The incidence of autopsy confirmed pulmonary hemorrhage, however, was not increased in treated infants who died in those five trials.[70] Meta-analysis of the results of randomized, placebo-controlled trials of surfactant treatment showed a 3 percent incidence of pulmonary hemorrhage overall, but only trials reporting that complication were included.[56] The relative risk (RR) for pulmonary hemorrhage with surfactant treatment in those trials was 1.47 (95 percent CI 1.05–2.07). Logistic regression modelling suggested that synthetic surfactant and lower birthweight increased the risk of pulmonary hemorrhage. Since then, the risk of pulmonary hemorrhage with both rescue and prophylactic synthetic surfactant has been assessed in two Cochrane reviews. No significant difference was found between treatment and control groups for rescue surfactant treatment.[63] Four of the seven trials of prophylactic synthetic surfactant reported pulmonary hemorrhage as an outcome measure and meta-analysis found an increased risk in the treatment group (RR 3.28; 95 percent CI 1.5–7.16).[63] Overall, natural surfactant does not appear to increase the incidence of pulmonary hemorrhage, but many placebo-controlled trials have not reported this as an outcome.

Coagulation abnormalities

Disorders of coagulation may have an etiological role in pulmonary hemorrhage. Hemorrhagic disease of the newborn and hemophilia, however, have not been reported to be associated with pulmonary hemorrhage, although bleeding in other sites was found at autopsy in two-thirds of infants dying of pulmonary hemorrhage.[58] It has been suggested that this evidence of widespread bleeding is likely to be due to secondary disseminated intravascular coagulation (DIC) in most cases.[22] More recent evidence points to hypocoagulability as a risk factor for pulmonary hemorrhage. In infants less than 30 weeks of gestation, platelet counts and fibrinogen levels were reduced and prothrombin and partial thromboplastin times elevated in the first 12 hours after birth in infants who subsequently developed pulmonary hemorrhage compared to those who did not. There was also an increased number of infants with very low platelet counts and abnormal clotting times in the index cases compared to controls in the same study.[24]

Miscellaneous risk factors

Pulmonary hemorrhage has also been described during exchange transfusion,[36] induction of anesthesia,[30] neonatal tetanus[59] and in one infant with a urea cycle defect.[28] Meta-analyses suggest that early systemic corticosteroids have not been shown to alter the incidence of pulmonary hemorrhage in very low birthweight infants.[38] Other major antenatal and postnatal interventions that have been subjected to extensive randomized, controlled trials, such as maternal antenatal corticosteroids and early high-frequency oscillatory (HFO) or jet ventilation and nitric oxide, may, in theory, also influence the incidence of pulmonary hemorrhage. The vast majority of these trials, however, have not reported pulmonary hemorrhage as an outcome and therefore systematic reviews have been unable to assess any impact on incidence.[4,6,23,40]

CLINICAL SIGNS

Massive pulmonary hemorrhage usually presents with sudden clinical deterioration with poor perfusion, tachycardia, hypotension and worsening respiratory status, along with copious amounts of blood-stained fluid from the nostrils, mouth or endotracheal tube. However, frank bleeding from the airway may not occur, and in one series was found in only 42 percent of infants with an autopsy diagnosis of pulmonary hemorrhage.[58] A systolic cardiac murmur, full pulses, a wide pulse pressure and an active precordium indicating a patent ductus arteriosus, have been found in 60–68 percent of preterm infants with pulmonary hemorrhage.[33,35] A sudden deterioration of respiratory function often occurs with increased signs of respiratory distress, cyanosis, poor chest movement and fine crackles, indicative of pulmonary edema on chest auscultation. Preterm infants often become inactive, whereas term infants may become agitated due to sudden hypoxia. Pulmonary hemorrhage in preterm infants usually occurs in the first few days after birth. One series documented the mean age of the event was 3.1 days, with a range of 2 hours to 25 days.[34] Others have documented a similar time course.[12,68]

DIFFERENTIAL DIAGNOSIS

It is important to distinguish between local trauma, often secondary to endotracheal intubation or airway suction, and pulmonary hemorrhage. The former is usually associated with smaller amounts of bleeding and less clinical deterioration, which only occurs if there is airway or endotracheal tube blockage.

INVESTIGATION

Hematological

The hematocrit of pulmonary hemorrhage fluid has been found to be less than 10 percent in most cases, but the hemoglobin should be measured as this may fall considerably. Although coagulation studies have been found to be normal prior to pulmonary hemorrhage,[22] subsequent coagulation abnormalities are common[24] and secondary DIC can occur. Therefore, platelet counts and clotting times should be assessed in all cases.

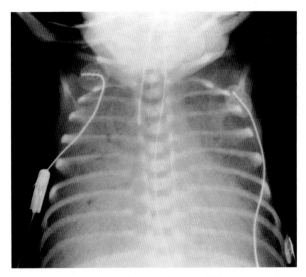

Figure 25.2 *Pulmonary haemorrhage – diffuse opacification and associated air bronchograms.*

Chest radiograph

Chest radiograph changes usually reflect the generalized nature of the condition throughout both lung fields, showing bilateral uniform opacification (often 'whiteout') with air bronchograms (Figure 25.2). This appearance is indistinguishable from severe surfactant deficiency and may be a reflection of the secondary surfactant deficiency that is known to occur following pulmonary hemorrhage.[41,61]

Bacteriology

As a high incidence of positive blood cultures has been found in infants with pulmonary hemorrhage,[31,58] an infection screen should be performed in all cases (p. 72).

Blood gases

Arterial blood gas analysis after pulmonary hemorrhage usually shows a severe deterioration of all parameters. Hypoxia and respiratory acidosis may be marked due to worsening gas exchange. A metabolic acidosis may also occur, secondary to the hypoxia and circulatory collapse due to massive blood and fluid loss.

MANAGEMENT

Initial resuscitation

Massive pulmonary hemorrhage is often an acute event associated with a dramatic deterioration in the infant's condition. Following a rapid initial assessment, immediate attention with an 'ABC' resuscitation sequence may be necessary. Particular attention should be given to vigorous airway suction, followed by positive pressure ventilation, cautious fluid administration and inotropic support as appropriate. Underlying possible etiological factors such as heart failure, patent ductus arteriosus, sepsis, anemia due to hemolytic disease of the newborn and coagulation abnormalities should be sought and treated as necessary.

Mechanical ventilation

Intermittent positive pressure ventilation is required in all infants with massive pulmonary hemorrhage. Studies in experimental animals with pulmonary edema have suggested that a high peak end expiratory pressure (PEEP) redistributes the fluid in the alveoli, improving gas exchange and ventilation perfusion mismatch, but does not reduce lung fluid.[17,42,46,53,71] A relatively high PEEP is usually used, but such a policy has not been tested in a randomized trial. It is not clear whether HFO has a role in the management of pulmonary hemorrhage (p. 172).

Surfactant

In vitro studies suggest pulmonary hemorrhage leads to surfactant inactivation due to 'contamination' with hemo-globin and red blood cell lipids.[41,61] Chest radiograph changes after pulmonary hemorrhage are compatible with this secondary surfactant deficiency (Figure 25.3a) and improve after surfactant administration (Figure 25.3b). Thus, although administration of exogenous surfactant is associated with the onset of pulmonary hemorrhage, further surfactant administration may be beneficial after the event. There are no randomized, controlled trials support-ing that policy, but one case series has suggested improved short-term outcomes in infants with pulmonary hemor-rhage treated with surfactant.[50] A further case report of a 5-month old infant who suffered a pulmonary hemor-rhage following abdominal surgery also suggests benefit.[49]

Physiotherapy/airway suction

Frequent endotracheal tube suction is required to pre-vent airway obstruction and endotracheal tube blockage, which may be common after pulmonary hemorrhage. Adequate humidification of ventilator gases may help prevent clotting of bloody secretions. Physiotherapy is not recommended immediately after pulmonary hemor-rhage (p. 242).

Fluid balance and diuretics

Fluid restriction is appropriate if signs of fluid overload, congestive cardiac failure or patent ductus arteriosus occur in infants with pulmonary hemorrhage. Echocardiography may be helpful in identifying intravascular fluid overload,

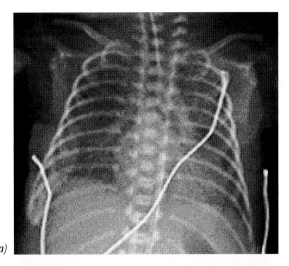

(a)

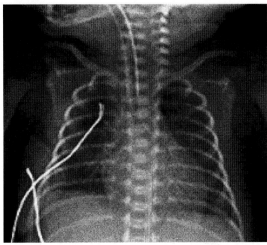

(b)

Figure 25.3 *(a) Chest radiograph of a preterm infant following pulmonary hemorrhage showing bilateral diffuse opacification of the lung fields. (b) The same infant following surfactant administration – note the decreased lung field opacification.*

which is manifested by dilatation of the left atrium, and sometimes the left ventricle. If, however, there are signs of intravascular fluid depletion because of massive blood loss, this should be resolved by blood transfusion. Blood transfusion may also be necessary if there is a decrease in hemoglobin levels due to massive blood loss with pul-monary hemorrhage. 'Loop' diuretics, such as frusemide, have a beneficial effect on respiratory function in pul-monary edema by decreasing lung lymph flow and improving ventilation–perfusion mismatch.[3,10] There is, however, no direct evidence that they are of benefit in pulmonary hemorrhage.

Closure of patent ductus arteriosus

It would seem logical to attempt to close a patent ductus arteriosus to prevent further pulmonary hemorrhage and other complications. Therefore, if there are clinical and/or echocardiographic signs of patent ductus arteriosus in infants with pulmonary hemorrhage, indomethacin or ibuprofen should be considered. Contraindications to starting these treatments include severe thrombocytopenia [$<20 \times 10^9$/l ($200\,000$/mm^3)] and renal failure. Surgical ligation of a patent ductus arteriosus should be considered if medical management fails or contraindications to medical treatment exist.

Coagulopathy

Pre-existing abnormalities of coagulation or secondary DIC, as a consequence of pulmonary hemorrhage, should be treated with platelet transfusion and fresh frozen plasma, as appropriate. This may help prevent further pulmonary hemorrhage or bleeding from other sites.

Antibiotics

Broad-spectrum antibiotics should be commenced after an infection screen has been performed, as bacterial sepsis is common in infants with pulmonary hemorrhage.[31,58]

PROGNOSIS

Mortality

Pulmonary hemorrhage has been regarded as a universally fatal condition,[29] but with the advent of positive pressure ventilation, reports emerged of improving survival.[21,67,69] Nowadays, pulmonary hemorrhage is a problem occurring predominantly in the sickest and most prematurely born infants. A relatively high mortality rate is expected in this group, and there is some evidence that this is increased in those with pulmonary hemorrhage. In a series of 94 very low birthweight infants who developed pulmonary hemorrhage after surfactant treatment, Pandit et al. found a significantly increased risk of mortality compared to matched controls who did not have pulmonary hemorrhage (38 percent versus 13 percent; OR 3.8, 95 percent CI 2.0–7.2).[51] Infants with pulmonary hemorrhage were graded mild, moderate or severe pulmonary hemorrhage according to the rise in the inspired oxygen concentration associated with the event. Not surprisingly, those with more severe pulmonary hemorrhage had the greatest risk of mortality. Other case–control studies have also documented a significantly increased mortality rate in infants with pulmonary hemorrhage.[5,12]

Morbidity

The incidence of short-term outcomes such as necrotizing enterocolitis (NEC), seizures, intraventricular hemorrhage (IVH), periventricular leukomalacia (PVL), retinopathy of prematurity (ROP) and CLD have been documented in a number of case–control studies, comparing those with pulmonary hemorrhage to matched controls. In the one study reporting the incidence of NEC in pulmonary hemorrhage cases compared to controls, no statistically significant differences were found.[68] This same study found an eightfold increase in the incidence of seizures in infants with pulmonary hemorrhage. Differences in the incidence of IVH in infants with pulmonary hemorrhage compared to matched controls have been analyzed in five case–control studies. In two of these studies,[5,12] no statistically significant increases in the incidence of IVH were identified. The other studies all found that the incidence of grade 3 and 4 IVH more than doubled in infants with pulmonary hemorrhage.[31,51,68] It is unclear whether pulmonary hemorrhage is directly associated with IVH or whether both are more likely to occur in the sickest infants, who are at risk of generalized bleeding. In two studies,[51,68] the incidence of PVL has been compared in infants surviving after pulmonary hemorrhage to controls in two studies and no statistically significant differences were found. There was no effect on the incidence of ROP in one study.[51]

Pandit et al. found that CLD was more common in infants surviving after moderate pulmonary hemorrhage (OR 6.2; 95 percent CI 1.6–25), but not significantly increased in mild or severe cases.[51] Although infants with pulmonary hemorrhage remained ventilator dependent for approximately the same time, they required supplementary oxygen until a mean corrected gestational age of 36 weeks compared to 34 weeks in controls.[51] The incidence of CLD and length of oxygen dependence, however, was not found to be significantly increased in one other study, but there was a trend towards worse outcomes in infants who survived pulmonary hemorrhage.[68] Long-term neurodevelopmental outcome has been assessed in two case–control studies;[51,68] no statistically significant differences were found between survivors of pulmonary hemorrhage and matched controls.

REFERENCES

1 Adamson, T.M., Boyd, R.D.H., Normand, I.C.S. et al. (1969) Haemorrhagic pulmonary oedema (massive pulmonary haemorrhage) in the newborn. Lancet 1, 494–495.

2 Adamson, T.M., Boyd, R.D.H., Hill, J.R. et al. (1970) Effect of asphyxia due to umbilical cord occlusion in the foetal lamb on a leakage of liquid from the circulation and permeability of lung capillaries to albumin. Journal of Physiology 207, 493–505.

3 Ali, J., Wood, L.D.H. (1983) Pulmonary vascular effects of frusemide on gas exchange in pulmonary edema. Journal of Applied Physiology 57, 160–167.

4 Barrington, K.J., Finer, N.N. (1999) Inhaled nitric oxide for respiratory failure in preterm infants (Cochrane review). In The Cochrane Library, Issue 4. Oxford: Update Software.

5 Bhandari, V., Gagnon, C., Hussain, N., Rosenkrantz, T. (1996) Pulmonary hemorrhage in neonates. *Pediatric Research* **39**, 196A.

6 Bhuta, T., Henderson-Smart, D.J. (2001) Update Software, Oxford.

7 Bland, R.D. (1980) Special considerations in oxygen therapy for infants and children. *American Review of Respiratory Disease* **122**, 45–54.

8 Bland, R.D. (1982) Edema formation in the newborn lung. *Clinics in Perinatology* **9**, 593–611.

9 Bland, R.D., Bressack, M.A. (1979) Lung fluid balance in awake newborn lambs with pulmonary edema from rapid intravenous infusion of isotonic saline. *Pediatric Research* **13**, 1037–1042.

10 Bland, R.D., McMillan, D.D., Bressack, M.A. (1978) Decreased pulmonary transvascular fluid filtration in awake newborn lambs after intravenous furosemide. *Journal of Clinical Investigation* **62**, 601–609.

11 Boothby, C.B., de Sa, D.J. (1973) Massive pulmonary haemorrhage in the newborn. *Archives of Disease in Childhood* **48**, 21–30.

12 Braun, K., Nielsen, H.C. (1996) Antecedents to neonatal pulmonary hemorrhage (PH) in the surfactant era. *Pediatric Research* **39**, 259A.

13 Bressack, M.A., Bland, R.D. (1980) Alveolar hypoxia increases lung fluid filtration in unanesthetized newborn lambs. *Circulation Research* **46**, 111–116.

14 Bressack, M.A., McMillan, D.D., Bland, R.D. (1979) Pulmonary oxygen toxicity: increased microvascular permeability to protein in unanaesthetized lambs. *Lymphology* **12**, 133–139.

15 Brigham, K.L., Woolverton, W.C., Staub, N.C. (1974) Reversible increase in pulmonary vascular permeability after *Pseudomonas aeruginosa* bacteremia in unanesthetized sheep. *Chest* **65**, 51S–54S.

16 Brigham, K.L., Bowers, R., Haynes, J. (1979) Increased sheep lung vascular permeability caused by *Escherichia coli* endotoxin. *Circulation Research* **45**, 292–297.

17 Caldini, P., Leith, J.D., Brennan, M.J. (1975) Effect of continuous positive-pressure ventilation (CPPV) on edema formation in dog lung. *Journal of Applied Physiology* **39**, 672–679.

18 Chamberlain, R., Chamberlain, G., Howlett, H., Claireaux, A. 1975: *British Births (1970)*. The First Week of Life, Chapter 4. London: William Heinemann Medical Books Ltd.

19 Clyman, R.I. (1996) Recommendations for the postnatal use of indomethacin: an analysis of four separate treatment strategies. *Journal of Pediatrics* **128**, 601–607.

20 Clyman, R.I., Jobe, A., Heymann, M. *et al.* (1982) Increased shunt through the patent ductus arteriosus after surfactant replacement therapy. *Journal of Pediatrics* **100**, 101–107.

21 Cole, A.P., Entress, A. (1974) Continuous positive airways pressure in infants. *Lancet* **1**, 505.

22 Cole, V.A., Normand, I.C.S., Reynolds, E.O.R., Rivers, R.P.A. (1973) Pathogenesis of hemorrhagic pulmonary edema and massive pulmonary hemorrhage in the newborn. *Pediatrics* **51**, 175–187.

23 Crowley, P.A. (1995) Antenatal corticosteroid therapy: a meta-analysis of the randomized trials, 1972 to 1994. *American Journal of Obstetrics and Gynecology* **173**, 322–335.

24 DeCarolis, M.P., Romagnoli, C., Cafforio, C. *et al.* (1998) Pulmonary hemorrhage in infants with gestational age of less than 30 weeks. *European Journal of Pediatrics* **157**, 1037–1038.

25 Ellis, M.I., Hey, E.N., Walker, W. (1979) Neonatal death in babies with rhesus isoimmunization. *Quarterly Journal of Medicine* **48**, 211–225.

26 Esterley, J.R., Oppenheimer, E.H. (1966) Massive pulmonary hemorrhage in the newborn. I. Pathologic considerations. *Journal of Pediatrics* **69**, 3–11.

27 Evans, N., Kluckow, M. (1999) High pulmonary blood flow and pulmonary hemorrhage. *Pediatric Research* **45**, 195A.

28 Farriaux, J.P., Ponte, C., Pollitt, R.J. *et al.* (1977) Carbamyl-phosphate-synthetase deficiency with neonatal onset of symptoms. *Acta Paediatrica Scandinavica* **66**, 529–534.

29 Fedrick, J., Butler, N.R. (1971) Certain causes of neonatal death, IV. Massive pulmonary haemorrhage. *Biology of the Neonate* **18**, 243–262.

30 Fenton, A.C., Tanner, M.S., Wandless, J.G. (1988) Pulmonary haemorrhage as a complication of neonatal anaesthesia. *Anaesthesia* **43**, 156–157.

31 Finlay, E.R., Subhedar, N.V. (2000) Pulmonary hemorrhage in preterm infants. *European Journal of Pediatrics* **159**, 870–871.

32 Fox, G.F., Wilson, D.C., Ohlsson, A. (1998) Effect of early versus late introduction of intravenous lipid to preterm infants on death and chronic lung disease (CLD) – results of meta-analyses. *Pediatric Research* **43**, 214A.

33 Garland, J., Buck, R., Weinberg, M. (1994) Pulmonary hemorrhage risk in infants with a clinically diagnosed patent ductus arteriosus: a retrospective cohort study. *Pediatrics* **94**, 719–723.

34 Greene, H.L., Hazlett, D., Demarec, R. (1976) Relationship between intralipid-induced hyperlipidemia and pulmonary function. *American Journal of Clinical Nutrition* **29**, 127–135.

35 Greenough, A., Morley, C.J., Roberton, N.R.C. (1999) Acute respiratory disease in the newborn. In Roberton, N.R.C., Rennie, J.M. (eds), *Textbook of Neonatology*. Edinburgh: Churchill Livingstone, 481–607.

36 Guaran, R.L., Drew, J.H., Watkins, A.M. (1992) Jaundice: clinical practice in 88,000 liveborn infants. *Australian and New Zealand Journal of Obstetrics and Gynaecology* **32**, 186–192.

37 Guyton, A.C., Lindsay, A.W. (1959) Effect of elevated left atrial pressure and decreased plasma protein concentration on the development of pulmonary edema. *Circulation Research* **7**, 649.

38 Halliday, H.L., Ehrenkranz, R.A. (2001) Update Software, Oxford.

39 Hazinski, T.A., Bland, R.D., Hansen, T.N. *et al.* (1986) Effect of hypoproteinemia on lung fluid balance in awake newborn lambs. *Journal of Applied Physiology* **61**, 1139–1148.

40 Henderson-Smart, D.J., Bhuta, T., Cools, F., Offringa, M. (2001) Update Software, Oxford.

41 Holm, B.A., Notter, R.H. (1987) Effects of hemoglobin and cell membrane lipids on pulmonary surfactant activity. *Journal of Applied Physiology* **63**, 603–610.

42 Hopewell, P.C., Murray, J.F. (1976) Effects of continuous positive-pressure ventilation and experimental pulmonary edema. *Journal of Applied Physiology* **40**, 568–574.

43 Hurley, R., Norman, A.P., Pryse-Davies, J. (1969) Massive pulmonary haemorrhage in the newborn associated with Coxsackie B virus infection. *British Medical Journal* **3**, 636–637.

44 Knox, W.F., Barson, A.J. (1986) Pulmonary hypoplasia in a regional perinatal unit. *Early Human Development* **14**, 33–42.

45 Lloyd, T.R., Boucek, M.M. (1986) Effect of Intralipid on the neonatal pulmonary bed: an echographic study. *Journal of Pediatrics* **108**, 130–133.

46 Malo, J., Ali, J., Wood, L.D.H. (1984) How does positive end expiratory pressure reduce intrapulmonary shunt in canine pulmonary edema? *Journal of Applied Physiology* **57**, 1002–1010.

47 Mann, T.P., Elliott, R.I.K. (1957) Neonatal cold injury due to accidental exposure to cold. *Lancet* **1**, 229–234.

48 McKeen, C.R., Brigham, K.L., Bowers, R.E., Harris, T.R. (1978) Pulmonary vascular effects of fat emulsion infusion in unanesthetized sheep. Prevention by indomethacin. *Journal of Clinical Investigation* **61**, 1291–1297.

49 Mikawa, K., Maekawa, N., Nishina, K. *et al.* (1994) Improvement of gas exchange following endobronchial instillation of an exogenous surfactant in an infant with respiratory failure by postoperative pulmonary haemorrhage. *Intensive Care Medicine* **20**, 58–60.

50 Pandit, P.B., Dunn, M.S., Colucci, E.A. (1995) Surfactant therapy in neonates with respiratory deterioration due to pulmonary hemorrhage. *Pediatrics* **95**, 32–36.

51 Pandit, P.B., O'Brien, K., Asztalos, E. *et al.* (1999) Outcome following pulmonary haemorrhage in very low birthweight neonates treated with surfactant. *Archives of Disease in Childhood* **81**, F40–F44.

52 Pappin, A., Shenker, N., Hack, M., Redline, R.W. (1994) Extensive intraalveolar pulmonary hemorrhage in infants dying after surfactant therapy. *Journal of Pediatrics* **124**, 621–626.

53 Pare, P.D., Warriner, B., Baile, E.M., Hogg, J.C. (1983) Reduction of pulmonary extravascular water with positive end expiratory pressure in canine pulmonary edema. *American Review of Respiratory Disease* **127**, 590–593.

54 Periera, G.R., Fox, W.W., Stanley, C.A. *et al.* (1980) Decreased oxygenation and hyperlipemia during intravenous fat infusions in premature infants. *Pediatrics* **66**, 26–30.

55 Raj, J.U., Hazinski, T.A., Bland, R.D. (1988) Effect of hypoxia on lung lymph flow in newborn lambs with left atrial hypertension. *American Journal of Physiology* **254**, H487–H493.

56 Raju, T.N.K., Langerberg, P. (1993) Pulmonary hemorrhage and exogenous surfactant therapy: a meta analysis. *Journal of Pediatrics* **123**, 603–610.

57 Rojas, J., Green, R.S., Hellerqvist, C.G. *et al.* (1981) Studies on group B beta-hemolytic Streptococcus. II. Effects on pulmonary hemodynamics and vascular permeability in unanesthetized sheep. *Pediatric Research* **15**, 899–904.

58 Rowe, S., Avery, M.E. (1966) Massive pulmonary hemorrhage in the newborn II. Clinical considerations. *Journal of Pediatrics* **69**, 12–20.

59 Salimpour, R. (1977) Cause of death in tetanus neonatorum: study of 233 cases with 54 necropsies. *Archives of Disease in Childhood* **52**, 587–594.

60 Schmidt, B., Davis, P., Moddemann, D. *et al.* (2001) Long term effects of indomethacin prophylaxis in extremely-low-birth-weight infants. *New England Journal of Medicine* **344**, 1966–1972.

61 Seeger, W., Stohr, G., Wolf, H.R.D., Neuhof, H. (1985) Alteration of surfactant function due to protein leakage: special interaction with fibrin monomer. *Journal of Applied Physiology* **58**, 326–338.

62 Sly, P.D., Drew, J.H. (1981) Massive pulmonary haemorrhage: a cause of sudden unexpected deaths in severely growth retarded infants. *Australian Paediatric Journal* **17**, 32–34.

63 Soll, R.F. (2001) Update Software, Oxford.

64 Stahlman, M.T., Cheatham, W., Gray, M.E. (1979) The role of air dissection in bronchopulmonary dysplasia. *Journal of Pediatrics* **95**, 878–885.

65 Stevenson, D., Walther, F., Long, W. *et al.* (1992) Controlled trial of a single dose of synthetic surfactant at birth in premature infants weighing 500–699 grams. *Journal of Pediatrics* **120**, S3–S12.

66 Strang, L.B. (1977) Haemorrhagic lung oedema and massive pulmonary haemorrhage. In Strang, L.B. (ed.), *Neonatal Respiration*. Oxford: Blackwell, 259.

67 Thomas, D.B. (1975) Survival after massive pulmonary haemorrhage in the neonatal period. *Acta Paediatrica Scandinavica* **64**, 825–829.

68 Tomaszewska, M., Stork, E.K., Friedman, H.G. *et al.* (1998) Pulmonary hemorrhage in VLBW (<1.5 kg) infants: correlates of death and neonatal and neurodevelopmental outcomes of survivors. *Pediatric Research* **43**, 230A.

69 Trompeter, R., Yu, V.Y., Aynsley-Green, A., Roberton, N.R.C. (1975) Massive pulmonary haemorrhage in the newborn infant. *Archives of Disease in Childhood* **50**, 123–127.

70 van Houten, J., Long, W., Mullett, M. *et al.* (1992) Pulmonary hemorrhage in premature infants after treatment with synthetic surfactant. An autopsy evaluation. The American Exosurf Neonatal Study Group I and The Canadian Exosurf Neonatal Study Group. *Journal of Pediatrics* **120**, S40–S44.

71 Woolverton, W.C., Brigham, K.L., Staub, N.C. (1978) Effect of positive pressure breathing on lung lymph flow and water content in sheep. *Circulation Research* **43**, 550–557.

72 Zarins, C.K., Rice, C.L., Peters, R.M., Virgilio, R.W. (1978) Lymph and pulmonary response to isobaric reduction in plasma oncotic pressure in baboons. *Circulation Research* **43**, 925–930.

Persistent pulmonary hypertension of the newborn

STEVEN H ABMAN AND JOHN P KINSELLA

Insights into the physiology and treatment of persistent pulmonary hypertension of the newborn (PPHN) begin with an understanding of normal development of the lung circulation and its changes immediately after birth (p. 62). Successful adaptation of the newborn to postnatal conditions requires a dramatic transition of the pulmonary circulation, from its high resistance state in utero to its low resistance state within minutes after birth. This fall in pulmonary vascular resistance (PVR) allows for the roughly eightfold rise in pulmonary blood flow at birth, thereby enabling the lung to assume its postnatal role in gas exchange. Several mechanisms contribute to the normal fall in PVR at birth. These include the establishment of a gas–liquid interface in the lung, increased oxygen tension, rhythmic distention of the lung (ventilation), and shear stress.[25,26,59,130,131] Birth-related stimuli cause vasodilation through changes in the production of vasoactive products, including increased release of potent vasodilators, including nitric oxide (NO) and prostacyclin (PgI$_2$), and decreased activity of endogenous vasoconstrictors, such as endothelin-1 (ET-1).[5,25,32,33,88,89,156] Within minutes of this vasodilator response, high pulmonary blood flow abruptly increases shear stress and distends the vasculature, causing a 'structural reorganization' of the vascular wall that includes flattening of the endothelium and thinning of smooth muscle cells and matrix.[12,58] Thus, the ability to accommodate this marked rise in blood flow requires rapid functional and structural adaptations to ensure the normal postnatal fall in PVR. Following this early period of pulmonary vasodilation, PVR continues to decrease over the next days to weeks of life due to vascular remodeling and growth in the normal infant.[59,130,131]

Some infants fail to achieve or sustain the normal decrease in PVR at birth, leading to severe respiratory distress and hypoxemia, which is referred to as persistent pulmonary hypertension of the newborn (PPHN). PPHN is not a single disease, but rather, it is a clinical syndrome that occurs in association with diverse neonatal cardiorespiratory disorders, such as meconium aspiration, sepsis, pneumonia, acute respiratory distress syndrome, asphyxia, congenital diaphragmatic hernia, lung hypoplasia, and others.[47,73,90,103,142,159] Although striking differences exist between these conditions, these disorders share common pathophysiological features, including high PVR leading to extrapulmonary right-to-left shunting of blood flow across the ductus arteriosus or foramen ovale. PPHN remains a major clinical problem, contributing significantly to high morbidity and mortality in both full-term and premature neonates.[106]

Although mechanisms that contribute to high PVR may vary between these diseases, the central hallmark of PPHN is abnormal pulmonary vasoreactivity with sustained elevation of PVR leading to hypoxemia due to extrapulmonary shunting. Mechanisms that cause severe pulmonary hypertension after birth are poorly understood, but can include abnormalities of pulmonary vascular tone, reactivity, growth and structure. PPHN represents the failure of postnatal adaptation of the lung circulation at birth; therefore, understanding the normal functional and structural development of the pulmonary circulation in utero and the mechanisms that contribute to pulmonary vasodilation at birth may provide insights into PPHN and its treatment.

PHYSIOLOGY OF THE DEVELOPING LUNG CIRCULATION (p. 62)

The fetal lung receives less than 8–10 percent of combined ventricular output, with most of the right ventricular output crossing the ductus arteriosus to the aorta. Pulmonary artery pressure and blood flow progressively increase with advancing gestational age, along with increasing lung vascular growth.[23] Despite this increase in vascular surface area, PVR actually increases with gestational age when corrected for lung or body weight. Thus, pulmonary vascular tone increases during late gestation, especially prior to birth. Studies of the human fetus support these physiological observations from fetal lambs.[63] Based on multiple Doppler ultrasound measurements that include assessments of fetal left and distal pulmonary artery velocity waveforms, Rasanen and coworkers[123] have demonstrated that fetal pulmonary artery impedance progressively decreases during the second and early part of the third trimester. Pulmonary artery vascular impedance does not decrease further during the latter stage of the third trimester.[63,123]

Mechanisms contributing to the high basal PVR in the fetus

These include low oxygen tension, low basal production of vasodilator products (such as PgI$_2$ and NO), increased production of vasoconstrictors (including ET-1 or leukotrienes), and altered smooth muscle cell reactivity (such as enhanced myogenic tone).[5,25,32,88,89,139,146,156] The pulmonary vasculature responds to vasoactive stimuli relatively early during development in the sheep fetus, but responsiveness to some stimuli increases during late gestation. For example, the pulmonary vasoconstrictor response to hypoxia, and vasodilation to increased fetal Po_2 and acetylcholine increase with gestation.[92,131] Human studies also suggest maturational changes in the fetal pulmonary vascular response to increased PaO_2.[123] Maternal hyperoxia did not increase pulmonary blood flow between 20 and 26 weeks of gestation, but increased PaO_2 caused pulmonary vasodilation in the 31–36-week gestation fetus. These findings suggest that, in addition to structural maturation and growth of the developing lung circulation, the vessel wall also undergoes functional maturation leading to enhanced vasoreactivity during fetal life.

Nitric oxide

MATURATIONAL CHANGES

Mechanisms that contribute to progressive changes in pulmonary vasoreactivity during development are unknown, but maturational changes in endothelial cell function, especially with regard to NO production, have been suggested.[1,2,6,10] NO is produced primarily by vascular endothelium during the conversion of L-arginine to L-citrulline by the enzyme, NO synthase (NOS).[61,99] Once produced, NO rapidly diffuses to underlying smooth muscle cells and causes vasodilation by stimulating soluble guanylate cyclase and increasing cGMP production. Elevated cGMP stimulates cGMP kinase, which then opens calcium-activated K$^+$-channels and causes membrane hyperpolarization. This lowers intracellular calcium in the smooth muscle cell by decreasing calcium entry through L-type channels and causes vasodilation. In some experimental settings, NO has been shown to directly stimulate K$^+$-channels or voltage-gated Ca^{2+}-channels independent of increased cGMP.[14] In some settings, NO has been shown to directly open calcium-activated K$^+$-channels.[20]

NOS expression and activity are affected by multiple factors, including oxygen tension, hemodynamic forces, hormonal stimuli (for example estradiol), paracrine factors (including vascular endothelial growth factor), substrate and cofactor availability, superoxide production (which inactivates NO), and others.[8,115–117,134] Lung endothelial NOS mRNA and protein are present in the early fetus and increase with advancing gestation *in utero* and during the early postnatal period in rats.[114,135] In fetal sheep, lung endothelial NOS mRNA, protein and activity increase markedly between 113 and 118 days (term is at 147 days).[55,116] The timing of this increase in lung endothelial NOS content coincides with the capacity to respond to endothelium-dependent vasodilator stimuli, such as oxygen and acetylcholine.[104,130,131] By contrast, fetal pulmonary arteries are already quite responsive to exogenous NO much earlier in gestation.[6,77] Overall, the ability of exogenous NO to dilate fetal pulmonary arteries is greater at less mature gestational ages; this contrasts with the responsiveness to vasodilator stimuli that require the endothelium to release endogenous NO. These findings suggest that the ability of the endothelium to produce or sustain production of NO in response to specific stimuli during maturation lacks the capacity of fetal pulmonary smooth muscle to relax to NO. This may account for clinical observations that extremely premature newborns are highly responsive to inhaled NO (p. 184).

VASCULAR RESPONSIVENESS TO NO

Vascular responsiveness to endogenous or exogenous NO is dependent upon several smooth muscle cell enzymes, including soluble guanylate cyclase, cGMP-specific (types V) phosphodiesterase (PDE$_5$), and cGMP kinase.[16,22,56,133] Several studies have shown that soluble guanylate cyclase, which produces cGMP in response to NO activation, is active before 70 percent of term gestation is completed in the ovine fetal lung.[6,77] Similarly, PDE$_5$, which limits cGMP-mediated vasodilation by hydrolysis and inactivation of cGMP, is also normally active *in utero*.[150,168]

Infusions of selective PDE_5 antagonists, including zaprinast, dipyridamole, E4021 and DMPPO, cause potent and sustained fetal pulmonary vasodilation. In the fetal lung, PDE_5 expression has been localized to vascular smooth muscle, and PDE_5 activity is high in comparison with the postnatal lung.[56] Thus, PDE_5 activity appears to play a critical role in pulmonary vasoregulation during the perinatal period, and must be accounted for in assessing responsiveness to endogenous NO and related vasodilator stimuli.

ROLE OF NO IN THE FETAL PULMONARY CIRCULATION

Vasoregulation

Functionally, the NO-cGMP cascade plays several important physiological roles in vasoregulation of the fetal pulmonary circulation.[8] These include modulation of basal PVR in the fetus,[5] mediating the vasodilator response to specific physiological and pharmacological stimuli[5,32] and opposing the strong myogenic tone in the normal fetal lung.[146] Studies in fetal lambs have demonstrated that intrapulmonary infusions of NO synthase inhibitors increase basal PVR by 35 percent.[5] Since inhibition of NO synthase increases basal PVR at least as early as three-quarters of completed gestation (112 days) in the fetal lamb, endogenous NOS activity appears to contribute to vasoregulation throughout late gestation.[77] NOS inhibition also selectively blocks pulmonary vasodilation to such stimuli as acetylcholine, oxygen, and shear stress in the normal fetus.[5,32,96,146] In addition, more recent studies have suggested that NO release plays an additional role in modulating high intrinsic or myogenic tone in the fetal pulmonary circulation. The myogenic response is commonly defined by the presence of increased vasoconstriction caused by acute elevation of intravascular pressure or 'stretch stress'.[98] Past *in vitro* studies demonstrated the presence of a myogenic response in sheep pulmonary arteries, and that fetal pulmonary arteries have greater myogenic activity than neonatal or adult arteries.[17,82] More recent studies of intact fetal lambs have demonstrated that high myogenic tone is normally operative in the fetus, and contributes to maintaining high PVR *in utero*.[4,10] In addition, studies[145] demonstrated that NOS inhibition further unmasks a potent myogenic response, suggesting that down-regulation of NOS, as observed in experimental models of pulmonary hypertension,[147,148] may further increase myogenic activity, increasing the risk for unopposed vasoconstriction in response to stretch stress at birth (p. 64).

Vascular growth and remodeling

The role of endogenous NO in the regulation of pulmonary vascular tone during late gestation is well established. Little is known, however, of its potential role in the pulmonary circulation during earlier stages of lung development. In addition to its effects on vascular tone, cell culture studies have also reported that NO influences vascular endothelial and smooth muscle cell growth *in vitro*. Since eNOS protein is present at a stage of lung development when blood flow is absent or minimal, it has been hypothesized that NO may potentially contribute to angiogenesis during early lung development.[55] Whether early eNOS expression implies a role in promoting vascular growth or is merely a marker of growing endothelial cells is unknown. Recent studies report conflicting data regarding the effects of eNOS activity in promoting new vessel formation in different experimental models of angiogenesis. Although NO can inhibit endothelial cell mitogenesis and proliferation, it has also been shown to mediate the angiogenic effects of substance P and vascular endothelial growth factor *in vitro*.[100,167] Growing bovine aortic endothelial cells in culture express greater eNOS mRNA and protein than confluent cells, but NOS inhibition does not affect their rate of proliferation *in vitro*.[15] NO has also been shown to decrease smooth muscle proliferation *in vitro*,[45,149] but NO may have biphasic, dose-dependent effects on fetal pulmonary artery smooth muscle cell growth. High doses of NO donors inhibit smooth muscle cell growth, but low doses cause paradoxical stimulation. Whether NO modulates smooth muscle cell growth *in vivo* remains controversial; one study reported the failure of chronic NOS inhibition to alter pulmonary vascular structure during late gestation in the fetal lamb.[44] Thus, although multiple studies have examined the role of NO in vascular growth and remodeling, its effects vary between experimental settings, and the effects of NO on angiogenesis and structure of the vessel wall are controversial.

OTHER VASODILATORS

Although other vasodilator products, including PgI_2, are released upon stimulation of the fetal lung (for example, increased shear stress), basal prostaglandin release appears to play a less important role than NO in fetal pulmonary vasoregulation. For example, cyclooxygenase inhibition has minimal affect on basal PVR and does not increase myogenic tone in the fetal lamb.[4,166] The physiological roles of other dilators, including adrenomedullin, adenosine and endothelium-derived hyperpolarizing factor (EDHF), are uncertain. EDHF is a short-lived product of cytochrome P_{450} activity that is produced by vascular endothelium, and has been found to cause vasodilation through activation of calcium-activated K^+-channels in vascular smooth muscle *in vitro*. K^+-channel activation appears to modulate basal PVR and vasodilator responses to shear stress and increased oxygen tension in the fetal lung, but whether this is partly related to EDHF activity is unknown.[145]

VASOCONSTRICTING AGENTS

Vasoconstrictors have long been considered as potentially maintaining high PVR *in utero*. Several candidate products, including lipid mediators (thromboxane A_2, leukotrienes C_4 and D_4, and platelet-activating factor) and ET-1, have been extensively studied. Thromboxane

A_2, a potent pulmonary vasoconstrictor that has been implicated in animal models of group B streptococcal sepsis, does not appear to influence PVR in the normal fetus. By contrast, inhibition of leukotriene production causes fetal pulmonary vasodilation;[139] however, questions have been raised regarding the specificity of the antagonists used in these studies. In light of the recent availability of newer and more selective inhibitors for the treatment of asthma, additional studies are needed. Similarly, inhibition of platelet-activating factor may influence PVR during the normal transition, but data from recent experimental studies are difficult to interpret due to extensive non-specific hemodynamic effects.

ET-1, a potent vasoconstrictor and co-mitogen that is produced by vascular endothelium, has been demonstrated to play a key role in fetal pulmonary vasoregulation.[21,65,165] PreproET-1 mRNA (the precursor to ET-1) was identified in fetal rat lung early in gestation, and high circulating ET-1 levels are present in umbilical cord blood. Although ET-1 causes an intense vasoconstrictor response *in vitro*, its effects in the intact pulmonary circulation are complex. Brief infusions of ET-1 cause transient vasodilation, but PVR progressively increases during prolonged treatment.[28] The biphasic pulmonary vascular effects during pharmacological infusions of ET-1 are explained by the presence of at least two different ET receptors. The ET B receptor, localized to the endothelium in the sheep fetus, mediates the ET-1 vasodilator response through the release of NO.[65] A second receptor, the ET A receptor, is located on vascular smooth muscle, and when activated, causes marked constriction. Although capable of both vasodilator and constrictor responses, ET-1 is more likely to play an important role as a pulmonary vasoconstrictor in the normal fetus. This is suggested in extensive fetal studies that have shown that inhibition of the ET A receptor decreases basal PVR and augments the vasodilator response to shear stress-induced pulmonary vasodilation.[66,68] Thus, ET-1 is likely to modulate PVR through the ET A and B receptors, but its predominant role is as a vasoconstrictor through stimulation of the ET A receptor.

MECHANISMS OF PULMONARY VASODILATION AT BIRTH

Minutes after delivery, the pulmonary artery pressure falls and blood flow increases in response to birth-related stimuli, such as ventilation, increased P_{O_2} and shear stress. These stimuli cause pulmonary vasodilation in part by increasing production of potent vasodilators, including NO and PgI_2. Pretreatment with the NO synthase inhibitor, nitro-L-arginine, attenuates pulmonary vasodilation after delivery by 50 percent in near-term fetal lambs.[5] These findings suggest that a significant part of the rise in pulmonary blood flow at birth may be directly related to

the acute release of NO. Each of the birth-related stimuli can independently stimulate NO release,[32] followed by vasodilation through cGMP kinase-mediated stimulation of K^+-channels.[34] Although the endothelial isoform of NO synthase (type III) has been presumed to be the major contributor of NO at birth, recent studies suggest that other isoforms [inducible (type II) and neuronal (type I)] may be important sources of NO release *in utero* and at birth as well.[24,121,122,137] Although early studies were performed in term animals, NO also contributes to the rapid decrease in PVR at birth in premature lambs, at least as early as 112–115 days of gestation.[77]

Other vasodilator products, including PgI_2, also modulate changes in pulmonary vascular tone at birth.[89,156] Rhythmic lung distention and shear stress stimulate both PgI_2 and NO production in the late gestation fetus, but increased oxygen tension triggers NO activity and overcomes the effects of prostaglandin inhibition at birth. In addition, the vasodilator effects of exogenous PgI_2 are blocked by NO synthase inhibitors, suggesting that NO modulates PgI_2 activity in the perinatal lung.[166] Adenosine release may also contribute to the fall in PVR at birth, but its actions may be partly through enhanced production of NO.[80] Thus, although NO does not account for the entire fall in PVR at birth, NOS activity appears important in achieving postnatal adaptation of the lung circulation. Transgenic eNOS knockout mice successfully make the transition at birth without evidence of PPHN.[42,143] This finding suggests that eNOS knockout mice may have adaptive mechanisms, such as a compensatory vasodilator mechanisms (such as upregulation of other NOS isoforms or dilator prostaglandins) or less constrictor tone. Interestingly, these animals are more sensitive to the development of pulmonary hypertension at relatively mild decreases in PaO_2,[42,143] and have higher neonatal mortality when exposed to hypoxia after birth. We speculate that isolated eNOS deficiency alone may not be sufficient for the failure of postnatal adaptation, but that decreased ability to produce NO in the setting of a perinatal stress (such as hypoxia, inflammation, hypertension, or upregulation of vasoconstrictors) may contribute to PPHN.

EXPERIMENTAL MODELS OF PPHN

Several experimental models have been studied to explore the pathogenesis and pathophysiology of PPHN.[142] Such models have included exposure to acute or chronic hypoxia after birth, chronic hypoxia *in utero*, placement of meconium into the airways of neonatal animals, sepsis and others. Although each model demonstrates interesting physiological changes that may be especially relevant to particular clinical settings, most studies examine only brief changes in the pulmonary circulation, and mechanisms underlying altered lung vascular structure and function of

PPHN are poorly understood. Clinical observations that neonates with severe PPHN who die during the first days after birth already have pathological signs of chronic pulmonary vascular disease suggest that intrauterine events may play an important role in this syndrome.[46,58,107] Adverse intrauterine stimuli during late gestation, such as abnormal blood flow, changes in substrate or hormone delivery to the lung, chronic hypoxia, chronic hypertension, inflammation or others, may potentially alter lung vascular function and structure, contributing to abnormalities of postnatal adaptation.

Chronic intrauterine stress

Several investigators have examined the effects of chronic intrauterine stresses, such as hypoxia or hypertension, in animals in order to attempt to mimic the clinical problem of PPHN. Whether chronic hypoxia alone can cause PPHN is controversial. Maternal hypoxia in rats had been reported to increase pulmonary vascular smooth muscle thickening in newborns,[49] but this observation has not been reproduced in maternal rats or guinea pigs in more extensive studies.[109] Animal studies, however, suggest that hypertension, due to either renal artery ligation or partial or complete closure of the ductus arteriosus, can cause structural and physiological changes which resemble features of clinical PPHN.[4,91,103]

Early ductal closure

Pulmonary hypertension induced by early closure of the ductus arteriosus in fetal lambs alters lung vascular reactivity and structure, causing the failure of postnatal adaptation at delivery, and providing an experimental model of PPHN.[4,103] In this model, partial closure of the ductus arteriosus acutely increases pulmonary artery pressure and flow, but after 1 hour, blood flow returns toward baseline values.[1] Over days, pulmonary artery pressure and PVR progressively increase, but flow remains low and PaO_2 is unchanged.[4] Thus, this model illustrates the effects of chronic intrauterine hypertension, but not high flow, on intrauterine lung vascular structure and function. Marked right ventricular hypertrophy and structural remodeling of small pulmonary arteries develops after 8 days of hypertension. After delivery, these lambs have persistent elevation of PVR despite mechanical ventilation with high oxygen concentrations.[4,103] Thus, physiological and structural studies suggest that this experimental model of PPHN mimics many of the abnormalities found in severe idiopathic PPHN in the human newborn.

Results from experimental models

To determine how chronic hypertension causes pulmonary vascular abnormalities in PPHN, our laboratory and others have studied endothelial and smooth muscle cell function in this experimental model. That chronic hypertension can alter NO production or activity was first suggested in physiological studies of pulmonary vasodilation of hypertensive and control lambs.[97] The pulmonary vasodilator responses to shear stress, acetylcholine and increased oxygen, which act in part by stimulating NO release, are impaired after chronic hypertension.[97,147] Interestingly, the pulmonary vascular response to acute changes in hemodynamic forces is dramatically altered after chronic hypertension. Acute increases in pressure and flow, which normally cause vasodilation, induce a paradoxical vasoconstrictor response, due to impaired NOS activity and an enhanced myogenic response.[147] Responsiveness to atrial natriuretic peptide, which causes vasodilation by directly increasing smooth muscle cGMP content independent of NO release by vascular endothelium, remains relatively intact. These findings further suggest that intrauterine hypertension impairs endothelial function, and decreases NO production. Subsequent molecular and biochemical studies have demonstrated that chronic pulmonary hypertension decreases lung eNOS mRNA and protein expression and total NOS activity.[136,157] Thus, these studies support the hypothesis that vascular injury *in utero* can decrease vasodilator responsiveness to birth-related stimuli by reducing lung eNOS content and NO production. Whether impaired NOS activity *in utero* also contributes to hypertensive structural remodeling of pulmonary arteries (including smooth muscle hypertrophy or hyperplasia) is uncertain.

Pulmonary vasodilation to endogenous NO is also dependent upon several other factors (p. 183), including smooth muscle soluble guanylate cyclase (sGC) and cGMP specific phosphodiesterase (type 5; PDE_5) activities.[31,57] Studies have examined sGC and PDE_5 activities after chronic DA closure in this experimental model of PPHN. Steinhorn and coworkers reported impaired sGC activity in hypertensive lambs, as reflected by decreased generation of cGMP and reduced vascular relaxation to NO stimulation *in vitro*.[140] In addition, Hanson and coworkers found marked elevation of lung PDE_5 activity, suggesting that rapid cGMP hydrolysis limits cGMP-dependent pulmonary vasodilation after chronic hypertension.[57] Thus, decreased lung eNOS protein and activity in the presence of decreased sGC and elevated PDE_5 activities limits the ability to sustain smooth muscle cGMP, favoring vasoconstriction and high PVR in experimental PPHN. These observations may have clinical implications regarding potential strategies for enhancing responsiveness to vasodilator therapy of PPHN.

Alterations of ET-1 may also contribute to the pathophysiology of PPHN. Circulating levels of ET-1, a potent vasoconstrictor and co-mitogen for vascular smooth muscle cell hyperplasia, are increased in human newborns with severe PPHN.[128] In the experimental model of PPHN due to compression of the ductus arteriosus in fetal sheep, lung ET-1 mRNA and protein content are markedly increased, and the balance of ET receptors are altered, favoring vasoconstriction.[70] Chronic inhibition of the ET A receptor attenuates the severity of pulmonary hypertension, decreases pulmonary artery wall thickening, and improves the fall in PVR at birth in this model.[69]

Thus, experimental studies have shown the important role of the NO-cGMP cascade and the ET-1 system in the regulation of vascular tone and reactivity of the fetal and transitional pulmonary circulation. In addition, abnormalities in these systems contribute to abnormal pulmonary vascular tone and reactivity in an experimental model of PPHN. Although inhaled NO therapy can dramatically improve oxygenation in sick neonates with severe PPHN and premature neonates with RDS, responsiveness is poor in some patients. Further studies of the NO-cGMP cascade may provide helpful insights into novel clinical strategies for more successful treatment of neonatal pulmonary vascular disease. In addition, since studies of vascular growth suggest important functions of NO in angiogenesis, we speculate that fetal NO production may contribute to normal lung vascular development. Mechanisms linking abnormal lung growth, the risk for pulmonary hypertension and regulation of the NO-cGMP cascade may have important therapeutic implications in the clinical setting.

PATHOGENESIS

PPHN is characterized by altered pulmonary vascular reactivity, structure, and in some cases, growth. Diseases associated with PPHN are often classified within one of three categories: maladaptation, that is, the vessels are presumably of normal structural but have abnormal vasoreactivity; excessive muscularization, i.e. there is increased smooth muscle cell thickness and increased distal extension of muscle to vessels which are usually non-muscular; and underdevelopment, i.e. there is lung hypoplasia associated with decreased pulmonary artery number.[46] This designation is imprecise, however, and high PVR in most patients likely involve overlapping changes among these categories. For example, neonates with congenital diaphragmatic hernia (CDH) are primarily classified as having vascular 'underdevelopment' due to lung hypoplasia, yet lung histology of fatal cases typically shows marked muscularization of pulmonary arteries and clinically, some patients respond to vasodilator therapy. Similarly, neonates with meconium aspiration often have clinical evidence of altered vasoreactivity, but often have muscularization at autopsy.[107] Thus, the failure to achieve a fall in PVR after birth can be due to abnormalities of vascular tone and reactivity, structure and growth.

Histological findings of structural vascular lesions are present in the lungs of neonates with fatal PPHN, even in those who die shortly after birth, suggesting that many cases of severe disease are associated with chronic intra-uterine stress. The exact intrauterine events that alter pulmonary vascular reactivity and structure are poorly understood, but experimental studies suggest that chronic hypertension due to either systemic hypertension due to renal artery ligation, single umbilical artery constriction, or other stresses, or partial closure of the ductus arteriosus, can mimic physiological and structural features of human PPHN. Recent experimental studies suggest that impaired vascular epidermal growth factor (VEGF) signaling during late gestation can cause fetal pulmonary hypertension with structural vascular remodeling, right ventricular hypertrophy, downregulation of endothelial NOS expression and impaired pulmonary vasodilation.[54] Interestingly, human neonates with PPHN have lower blood VEGF levels than controls.[86]

Epidemiological studies have demonstrated strong associations between PPHN and maternal smoking and ingestion of cold remedies that include aspirin or other non-steroidal anti-inflammatory products.[155] Since these agents can induce partial constriction of the ductus arteriorus, it is possible that hypertension due to ductus arteriosus narrowing contributes to PPHN. Other perinatal stresses, including placenta previa and abruption, and asymmetric growth restriction, are associated with PPHN;[163] however, most neonates who are exposed to these prenatal stresses do not develop PPHN. Circulating levels of L-arginine, the substrate for NO, are decreased in some newborns with PPHN, suggesting that impaired NO production may contribute to the pathophysiology of PPHN, as observed in experimental studies.[27,38,119] It is possible that genetic factors increase susceptibility for pulmonary hypertension. A recent study reported strong links between PPHN and polymorphisms of the carbamoyl phosphate synthase gene.[119] The importance of this finding, however, is uncertain and further work is needed in this area. Studies of adults with idiopathic primary pulmonary hypertension have identified abnormalities of bone morphogenetic protein receptor genes;[113] whether polymorphisms of genes for vasoactive substances, critical growth factors or other products increase the risk for some newborns to develop PPHN is unknown. Perinatal stress in selected patients with genetic risk factors may combine to increase susceptibility for severe pulmonary hypertension, as has been observed in an animal model of genetic pulmonary hypertension.[87]

PATHOPHYSIOLOGY

Not all term newborns with hypoxemic respiratory failure have PPHN-type physiology.[3,73] Hypoxemia in the newborn can be due to several mechanisms, including: extrapulmonary shunt, in which high pulmonary artery pressure at systemic levels leads to right-to-left shunting of blood flow across the PDA or patent foramen ovale (PFO); and intrapulmonary shunt or ventilation–perfusion mismatch, in which hypoxemia results from the lack of mixing of blood with aerated lung regions due to parenchymal lung disease, without the shunting of blood flow across the PDA and PFO. In the latter setting, hypoxemia is related to the amount of pulmonary arterial blood that perfuses non-aerated lung regions. Although PVR is often elevated in hypoxemic newborns without PPHN, high PVR does not contribute significantly to hypoxemia in these cases.

Several factors can contribute to high pulmonary artery pressure in patients with PPHN-type physiology. For example, high pulmonary artery pressure can be due to vasoconstriction or structural lesions that directly increase PVR. Changes in lung volume in neonates with parenchymal lung disease can also be an important determinant of PVR. For example, PVR increases at low lung volumes due to dense parenchymal infiltrate and poor lung recruitment, or with high lung volumes due to hyperinflation due to overdistention or gas trapping. Cardiac disease is also associated with PPHN.[124] High pulmonary venous pressure due to left ventricular dysfunction can also elevate pulmonary artery pressure (for example asphyxia or sepsis), causing right-to-left shunting, with little vasoconstriction. In this setting, enhancing cardiac performance and systemic hemodynamics may lower pulmonary artery pressure more effectively than achieving pulmonary vasodilation. Thus, understanding cardiopulmonary interactions is key to improving the outcome of PPHN.

CLINICAL SIGNS

The first reports of PPHN described term newborns with profound hypoxemia who lacked radiographic evidence of parenchymal lung disease and echocardiographic evidence of structural cardiac disease.[47,48,73,91] In these patients, hypoxemia was caused by marked elevations of PVR leading to right-to-left extrapulmonary shunting of blood across the patent ductus arteriosus (PDA) or foramen ovale (PFO) during the early postnatal period. Due to the persistence of high PVR and blood flow through these 'fetal shunts', the term 'persistent fetal circulation' was originally used to describe this group of patients.[48] Consequently, it was recognized that this physiological pattern can complicate the clinical course of neonates with diverse causes of hypoxemic respiratory failure. As a result, the term 'PPHN' has been considered as a syndrome, and is currently applied more broadly to include neonates that have a similar physiology in association with different cardiopulmonary disorders, such as meconium aspiration, sepsis, pneumonia, asphyxia, congenital diaphragmatic hernia, respiratory distress syndrome (RDS), and others. In many clinical settings, hypoxemic respiratory failure in term newborns is often presumed to be associated with PPHN-type physiology; however,

hypoxemic term newborns can lack echocardiographic findings of extrapulmonary shunting across the PDA or PFO.[138] Thus, PPHN should be reserved to neonates in whom extrapulmonary shunting contributes to hypoxemia and impaired cardiopulmonary function.

Clinically, PPHN is most often recognized in term or near term neonates, but clearly can occur in premature neonates as well.[7,106,161] PPHN is often associated with perinatal distress, such as asphyxia, low Apgar scores, meconium staining, and other factors; however, idiopathic PPHN often lacks signs of acute perinatal distress. PPHN often presents as respiratory distress and cyanosis within 6–12 hours of birth. Laboratory findings can include low glucose, hypocalcemia, hypothermia, polycythemia or thrombocytopenia. Radiographic findings are variable, depending upon the primary disease associated with PPHN. Classically, the chest radiograph in idiopathic PPHN is oligemic, may appear slightly hyperinflated, and lacks parenchymal infiltrates. In general, the degree of hypoxemia is often disproportionate to the severity of radiographic evidence of lung disease.

Diagnosis

PPHN is characterized by hypoxemia that is poorly responsive to supplemental oxygen. In the presence of right-to-left shunting across the PDA, 'differential cyanosis' is often present, which is defined by a difference in PaO_2 between right radial artery versus descending aorta values greater or equal to 10 mmHg (1.33 kPa), or an O_2 saturation gradient greater than 5 percent. Post-ductal desaturation can be found in ductus-dependent cardiac diseases, including hypoplastic left heart syndrome, critical aortic stenosis or interrupted aortic arch. The response to supplemental oxygen can help to distinguish PPHN from primary lung or cardiac disease.[40,41,120] Although supplemental oxygen traditionally increases PaO_2 more readily in lung disease than cyanotic heart disease or PPHN, this may not be obvious with more advanced parenchymal lung disease. Acute respiratory alkalosis induced by hyperventilation to achieve $PaCO_2$ less than 30 mmHg (4.0 kPa) and a pH greater than 7.50 may increase PaO_2 greater than 50 mmHg (6.65 kPa) in PPHN, but rarely in cyanotic heart disease.

Echocardiogram

The echocardiogram plays an essential diagnostic role. As stated above, not all term newborns with hypoxemia have PPHN physiology. Although high pulmonary artery pressure may be common, the diagnosis of PPHN is uncertain without evidence of bidirectional or predominant right-to-left shunting across the PFO or PDA. In addition to demonstrating the presence of PPHN physiology, the echocardiogram is critical for the evaluation of left ventricular function and diagnosis of anatomical

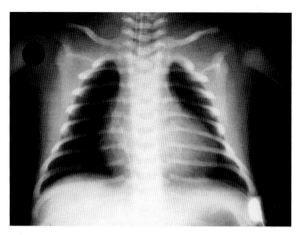

Figure 26.1 *Chest radiograph of an infant with PPHN, characterized by normal lung volumes and features of pulmonary vasoconstriction and oligemia.*

heart disease, including such 'PPHN mimics' as coarctation of the aorta, total anomalous pulmonary venous return, transposition of the great vessels, hypoplastic left heart syndrome, and others. Studies should carefully assess the predominant direction of shunting at the PFO as well as the PDA. For example, although right-to-left shunting at the PDA and PFO is typical for PPHN, predominant right-to-left shunting at the PDA but left-to-right shunt at the PFO may help to identify the important role of left ventricular dysfunction to the underlying pathophysiology.

Chest radiograph

In primary PPHN, the chest radiograph changes are often minimal (Figure 26.1). There may be a mild, non-specific decrease in lung markings only, but in some cases there is cardiomegaly, pulmonary vascular congestion and even pleural effusions.[110] In secondary PPHN, the radiograph appearances are those of the underlying disease.

MANAGEMENT

In general, management of the newborn begins with PPHN and includes the treatment and avoidance of hypothermia, hypoglycemia, hypocalcemia, anemia and hypovolemia; correction of metabolic acidosis; diagnostic studies for sepsis; serial monitoring of arterial blood pressure, pulse oximetry (pre- and post-ductal); and transcutaneous PCO_2, especially with the initiation of high-frequency oscillatory ventilation (HFOV) (p. 172).[29] Therapy includes aggressive management of systemic hemodynamics with volume and inotropes (dobutamine, dopamine, and milrinone), in order to enhance cardiac output and systemic O_2 transport. In addition, increasing systemic arterial pressure can improve oxygenation

in some cases by reducing right-to-left extrapulmonary shunting.

Respiratory support

The goal of mechanical ventilation is to improve oxygenation and to achieve 'optimal' lung volume to minimize the adverse effects of high or low lung volumes on PVR, while minimizing the risk for lung injury ('volutrauma'). Mechanical ventilation using inappropriate settings can produce acute parenchymal lung injury (ventilator-induced lung injury; VILI), causing pulmonary edema, decreased lung compliance and promoting lung inflammation due to increased cytokine production and lung neutrophil accumulation.[153] The development of VILI is an important determinant of clinical course and eventual outcome of newborns with hypoxemic respiratory failure, and postnatal lung injury worsens the degree of pulmonary hypertension.[118] Failure to achieve adequate lung volumes contributes to hypoxemia and high PVR in newborns with PPHN.[78,79] Some newborns with parenchymal lung disease with PPHN physiology improve oxygenation and decrease right-to-left extrapulmonary shunting with aggressive lung recruitment during HVOV,[79] or with an 'open lung approach' of higher positive end expiratory pressure (PEEP) with low tidal volumes, as more commonly utilized in older patients with acute respiratory distress syndrome (ARDS).[11,43]

Marked controversy and variability exists between centers regarding the use of hyperventilation to achieve alkalosis in order to improve oxygenation.[160] Past studies have clearly shown that acute hyperventilation can improve PaO_2 in neonates with PPHN, providing a diagnostic test and therapeutic strategy.[40,41] However, there are many issues with the use of hypocapnic alkalosis for prolonged therapy. Depending upon the ventilator strategy and underlying lung disease, hyperventilation is likely to increase VILI, and the ability to sustain decreased PVR during prolonged hyperventilation is unproven. Experimental studies suggest that the response to alkalosis is transient, and that alkalosis may paradoxically worsen pulmonary vascular tone, reactivity and permeability edema.[39,51,52,83,84,101] In addition, prolonged hyperventilation reduces cerebral blood flow and oxygen delivery to the brain, potentially worsening neurodevelopmental outcome.

Additional therapies

Use of infusions of sodium bicarbonate, surfactant therapy and the use of intravenous vasodilator therapy is also highly variable between centers.[160] Although surfactant may improve oxygenation in some lung diseases, such as meconium aspiration and RDS, a multicenter trial failed to show a reduction in extracorporeal membrane

Table 26.1 *Drugs used to cause pulmonary vasodilation*

Drug	Dose	Reference
Tolazoline	2 mg/kg stat 2 mg/kg/h	Stevenson et al.[144]
D-Tubocurarine	1 mg/kg prn	Hutchinson and Yu[64]
Chlorpromazine	0.2–0.8 mg/kg stat 0.03–0.2 mg/kg/h	Larsson et al.[85]
Sodium nitroprusside	0.5–6.0 μg/kg/min	Benitz et al.[18]
Prostacyclin	5–20 ng/kg/min	Kaapa et al.[71] Lock et al.[93]
Verapamil		Morett and Ortega[102]
Nifedipine		Dickstein et al.[37]
Acetylcholine		
Isoproterenol (isoprenaline)		Kulik and Lock[81]
Morphine		
Magnesium sulfate	200 mg/kg over 20–30 min 25–50 mg/kg/h	Abu-Osba et al.[9]

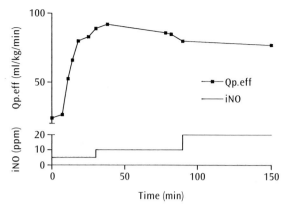

Figure 26.2 *The effect of inhaled nitric oxide (iNO) on effective pulmonary blood flow (Qp.eff) in a term infant with persistent pulmonary hypertension. A concentration of 5 ppm produces a rapid rise from 24 to >90 ml/kg/min (normal, 120–160 ml/kg/min). Raising the concentration to 10 and then 20 ppm had no additional effect.*

oxygenation (ECMO) utilization in newborns with PPHN.[94] The use of intravenous vasodilator drug therapy (Table 26.1), with agents such as tolazoline, magnesium sulfate, prostacyclin and sodium nitroprusside, is also controversial due to the non-selective effects of these agents on the systemic circulation.[53,144] Systemic hypotension worsens right-to-left shunting, may impair oxygen delivery and worsen gas exchange in patients with parenchymal lung disease. Tolazoline, which has both α-adrenergic and histaminergic effects, successfully improves oxygenation only in approximately 50 percent of patients. Magnesium sulfate, a calcium antagonist[13] which modulates vascular tone,[95] has been used successfully to treat the hypoxemia of PPHN.[9,95,152,164] During magnesium treatment, however, levels must be carefully monitored, as hypermagnesemia can cause central sedation, muscle relaxation, hyporeflexia and decreased excitability, as well as calcium and potassium disturbances. In a preclinical model, magnesium sulfate was less effective than inhaled nitric oxide.[132] The initial response to agents such as tolazoline are often transient, and they can have severe adverse effects (such as gastrointestinal hemorrhage and renal failure).[9,144] Side-effects have been reported in between 30 and 85 percent of patients.[151]

Endotracheal administration of vasodilators, including tolazoline, PGI_2 and sodium nitroprusside, may cause selective pulmonary vasodilation and minimize systemic hypotension.[19,35,158,170] Administration of aerosolized PGI_2 to two neonates with PPHN resulted in an improvement in their alveolar–arterial oxygen gradient.[19] It should be remembered, however, that the action of inhaled NO is restricted to the lung vasculature because of its immediate binding to hemoglobin; hence it is inactivated on entering the vascular compartment (see below). By contrast, high doses of aerosolized PGI_2 could spill over into the systemic circulation.[170] Thus, titration of the dose is critical if PGI_2 is to be a selective pulmonary vasodilator.

Nitric oxide (p. 183)

Inhaled nitric oxide (iNO) therapy at low doses (5–20 ppm) improves oxygenation and decreases the need for ECMO therapy in patients with diverse causes of PPHN (Chapter 23) (Figure 26.2).[30,36,75,76,79,111,112,125–127,162] Regulatory approval for the use of iNO therapy was based on the findings of large, multicenter randomized trials that demonstrated a reduction in the need for ECMO therapy in neonates with severe hypoxemia and PPHN.[30,111] Although clinical improvement during inhaled NO therapy occurs with many disorders associated with PPHN, not all neonates with acute hypoxemic respiratory failure and pulmonary hypertension respond to iNO. Several mechanisms may explain the clinical variability in responsiveness to iNO therapy. An inability to deliver NO to the pulmonary circulation due to poor lung inflation is the major cause of poor responsiveness. In some settings, administration of NO with HFOV has improved oxygenation more effectively than during conventional ventilation in the same patient.[74,79] In addition, poor NO responsiveness may be related to myocardial dysfunction or systemic hypotension, severe pulmonary vascular structural disease, and unsuspected or missed anatomical cardiovascular lesions (such as total anomalous pulmonary venous return, coarctation of the aorta, alveolar capillary dysplasia, and others). Another mechanism of poor responsiveness to inhaled NO may be altered smooth muscle cell responsiveness, and as described from animal studies and case reports, combined therapy with PDE_5 inhibitors may enhance the vasodilator response to iNO in some settings.[78,168,169] Recent experimental studies suggest that superoxide dismutase (SOD) treatment with iNO therapy may have an additive affect on lowering PVR in lambs with pulmonary hypertension.[141] Besides administering iNO as an inhalational agent, Moya et al.[105] have recently suggested that treatment with a unique gas, O-nitrosoethanol, may increase the endogenous pool of S-nitrosothiols in the airway and circulation, thereby providing a new treatment strategy for PPHN. Whether this strategy is more effective or will improve responsiveness in neonates who fail to respond to iNO therapy is unknown.

Finally, prolonged use of inhaled NO without resolution of disease should lead to a more extensive evaluation to determine whether previously unsuspected anatomic lung or cardiovascular disease is present (for example, pulmonary venous stenosis, alveolar capillary dysplasia, severe lung hypoplasia, or others).[50,62]

Extracorporeal membrane oxygenation (ECMO) (p. 179)

Although newer therapies, including HFOV and iNO, have led to a dramatic reduction in the need for ECMO therapy,[60,72,109] ECMO has been shown to be an effective rescue agent for severe PPHN.[154] Current patterns of ECMO use demonstrate persistent use in neonates with CDH and patients with severe hemodynamic instability, with less need for ECMO in meconium aspiration, RDS, idiopathic PPHN and other disorders.

REFERENCES

1 Abman, S.H., Accurso, F.J. (1989) Acute effects of partial compression of the ductus arteriosus on the fetal pulmonary circulation. American Journal of Physiology 257, H626–H634.

2 Abman, S.H., Accurso, F.J. (1991) Sustained fetal pulmonary vasodilation during prolonged infusion of atrial natriuretic factor and 8-bromo-guanosine monophosphate. American Journal of Physiology 260, H183–H192.

3 Abman, S.H., Kinsella, J.P. (1995) Inhaled NO for PPHN: the physiology matters. Pediatrics 96, 1147–1151.

4 Abman, S.H., Shanley, P.F., Accurso, F.J. (1989) Failure of postnatal adaptation of the pulmonary circulation after chronic intrauterine pulmonary hypertension in fetal lambs. Journal of Clinical Investigation 83, 1849–1858.

5 Abman, S.H., Chatfield, B.A., Hall, S.L. McMurtry, I.F. (1990) Role of endothelium-derived relaxing factor during transition of pulmonary circulation at birth. American Journal of Physiology 259, H1921–H1927.

6 Abman, S.H., Chatfield, B.A., Rodman, D.M. et al. (1991) Maturation-related changes in endothelium-dependent relaxation of ovine pulmonary arteries. American Journal of Physiology 260, L280–L285.

7 Abman, S.H., Kinsella, J.P., Schaffer, M.S., Wilkening, R.B. (1993) Inhaled nitric oxide therapy in a premature newborn with severe respiratory distress and pulmonary hypertension. Pediatrics 92, 606–609.

8 Abman, S.H., Kinsella, J.P., Parker, T.A., Storme, L., Le Cras, T.D. (1999) Physiologic roles of NO in the perinatal pulmonary circulation. In Weir, E.K., Archer, S.L., Reeves, J.T. (eds), Fetal and Neonatal Pulmonary Circulation. New York: Futura, 239–260.

9 Abu-Osba, Y., Galal, O., Manasra, K., Reijal, A. (1992) Treatment of severe persistent pulmonary hypertension of the newborn with magnesium sulphate. Archives of Disease in Childhood 67, 31–35.

10 Accurso, F.J., Alpert, B., Wilkening, R.B. et al. (1986) Time-dependent response of fetal pumonary blood flow to an increase in fetal oxygen tension. Respiratory Physiology 63, 43–52.

11 Acute Respiratory Distress Syndrome Network (2000) Ventilation with lower tidal volumes as compared with traditional tidal volumes for acute lung injury and the ARDS. New England Journal of Medicine 342, 1301–1308.

12 Allen, K., Haworth, S.G. (1986) Impaired adaptation of intrapulmonary arteries to extrauterine life in newborn pigs exposed to hypoxia. An ultrastructural study. Federation Proceedings 45, 879.

13 Altura, B.M., Altura, B.T. (1981) Magnesium ions and contraction of vascular smooth muscles: relationship to some vascular diseases. FASEB Journal 40, 2672–2679.

14 Archer, S.L., Huang, J.M.C., Hampl, V. et al. (1994) NO and cGMP cause vasorelaxation by activation of a charybdotoxin-sensitive K channel by cGMP-dependent protein kinase. Proceedings of the National Academy of Sciences of the United States of America 91, 7583–7587.

15 Arnal, J.-F., Yamin, J., Dockery, S., Harrison, D.G. (1994) Regulation of endothelial NO synthase mRNA, protein, and activity during cell growth. American Journal of Physiology 267, C1381–C1388.

16 Beavo, J.A., Reifsnyder, D.H. (1990) Primary sequence of cyclic nucleotide phosphodiesterase isozymes and the design of selective inhibitors. Trends in Pharmacological Sciences 11, 150–155.

17 Belik, J., Stephens, N. (1993) Developmental differences in vascular smooth muscle mechanics in pulmonary and systemic circulations. Journal of Applied Physiology 74, 682–687.

18 Benitz, W.E., Malachowski, N., Cotten, R.S., Stevenson, D.K., Ariagno, R.L., Sunshine, P. (1985) Use of sodium nitroprusside in neonates. Efficacy and safety. Journal of Pediatrics 106, 102–110.

19 Bindl, L., Fahnenstich, H., Peukert, U. (1994) Aerosolized prostacyclin for pulmonary hypertension in neonates. Archives of Disease in Childhood 71, F214–F216.

20 Bolotina, V.M., Najibi, S., Palacino, J.J. et al. (1994) NO directly activates calcium-dependent potassium channels in vascular smooth muscle. Nature 368, 850–853.

21 Boulanger, C., Luscher, T.F. (1990) Release of endothelin from the porcine aorta. Inhibition by endothelium-derived nitric oxide. Journal of Clinical Investigation 85, 587–590.

22 Braner, D.A., Fineman, J.R., Chang, R. et al. (1993) M and B 22948, a cGMP phosphodiesterase inhibitor, is a pulmonary vasodilator in lambs. American Journal of Physiology 264, H252–H258.

23 Burri, P.H. (1997) Structural aspects of prenatal and postnatal development and growth of the lung. In McDonald, J.A. (ed.), Lung Growth and Development. New York: Marcel Dekker, 1–36.

24 Bustamante, S.A., Pang, Y., Romero, S. *et al.* (1996) Inducible NOS and the regulation of central vessel caliber in the fetal rat. *Circulation* **94**, 1948–1953.

25 Cassin, S. (1987) Role of prostaglandins, thromboxanes and leukotrienes in the control of the pulmonary circulation in the fetus and newborn. *Seminars in Perinatology* **11**, 53–63.

26 Cassin, S., Dawes, G.S., Mott, J.C. *et al.* (1964) Vascular resistance of the foetal and newly ventilated lung of the lamb. *Journal of Physiology* **171**, 61–79.

27 Castillo, L., DeRojas-Walker, T., Yu, Y.M. *et al.* (1995) Whole body arginine metabolism and NO synthesis in newborns with persistent pulmonary hypertension. *Pediatric Research* **38**, 17–24.

28 Chatfield, B.A., McMurtry, I.F., Hall, S.L., Abman, S.H. (1991) Hemodynamic effects of endothelin-1 on the ovine fetal pulmonary circulation. *American Journal of Physiology* **261**, R182–R187.

29 Clark, R.H. (1994) High frequency ventilation. *Journal of Pediatrics* **124**, 661–670.

30 Clark, R.H., Kueser, T.J., Walker, M.W. *et al.* (2000) Low-dose inhaled NO treatment of PPHN. *New England Journal of Medicine* **342**, 469–474.

31 Cohen, A.H., Hanson, K., Morris, K. *et al.* (1996) Inhibition of cGMP-specific phosphodiesterase selectively vasodilates the pulmonary circulation in chronically hypoxic rats. *Journal of Clinical Investigation* **97**, 172–179.

32 Cornfield, D.N., Chatfield, B.A., McQueston, J.A. *et al.* (1992) Effects of birth-related stimuli on L-arginine-dependent pulmonary vasodilation in the ovine fetus. *American Journal of Physiology* **262**, H1474–H1481.

33 Cornfield, D.N., McQueston, J.A., McMurtry, I.F. *et al.* (1992) Role of ATP-sensitive K^+-channels in ovine fetal pulmonary vascular tone. *American Journal of Physiology* **263**, H1363–H1368.

34 Cornfield, D.N., Reeves, H.L., Tolarova, S. *et al.* (1996) Oxygen causes fetal pulmonary vasodilation through activation of a calcium-dependent potassium channel. *Proceedings of the National Academy of Sciences of the United States of America* **93**, 8089–8094.

35 Curtis, J., O'Neill, J.T., Pettett, G. (1993) Endotracheal administration of tolazoline in hypoxia-induced pulmonary hypertension. *Pediatrics* **92**, 403–408.

36 Davidson, D., Barefield, E.S., Katwinkel, J. *et al.* (1998) Inhaled NO for the early treatment of persistent pulmonary hypertension of the term newborn: a randomized double blinded placebo-controlled dose-response multicenter study. *Pediatrics* **101**, 325–334.

37 Dickstein, P.J., Trindade, O., Goldberg, R.N., Bancalari, E. (1984) The effect of calcium antagonists in hypoxic pulmonary hypertension in the piglet. *Pediatric Research* **18**, 1262–1265.

38 Dollberg, S., Warner, B.W., Myatt, L. (1994) Urinary nitrite and nitrate concentrations in patients with idiopathic PPHN and effect of ECMO. *Pediatric Research* **37**, 31–34.

39 Domino, K.B., Swenson, E.R., Hlastala, M.P. (1995) Hypocapnia-induced ventilation/perfusion mismatch: a direct CO_2 or pH mediated effect? *American Journal of Respiratory and Critical Care Medicine* **152**, 1534–1539.

40 Drummond, W.H., Peckam, G.J., Fox, W.W. (1977) The clinical profile of the newborn with persistent pulmonary hypertension. *Clinical Pediatrics* **16**, 335–341.

41 Drummond, W.H., Gregory, G., Heymann, M.A. *et al.* (1981) The independent effects of hyperventilation, tolazoline, and dopamine on infants with persistent pulmonary hypertension. *Journal of Pediatrics* **98**, 603–611.

42 Fagan, K.A., Fouty, B.W., Tyler, R.C. *et al.* (1999) The pulmonary circulation of mice with either homozygous or heterozygous disruption of endothelial NO synthase is hyper-responsive to chronic hypoxia. *Journal of Clinical Investigation* **103**, 291–299.

43 Feihl, F., Perret, C. (1994) Permissive hypercapnia. How permissive should we be? *American Journal of Respiratory and Critical Care Medicine* **150**, 1722–1737.

44 Fineman, J.R., Wong, J., Morin, F.C. *et al.* (1994) Chronic NO inhibition *in utero* produces persistent pulmonary hypertension in newborn lambs. *Journal of Clinical Investigation* **93**, 2675–2683.

45 Garg, U.C., Hassid, A. (1989) NO-generating vasodilators and 8-bromo-cGMP inhibit mitogenesis and proliferation of cultured rat vascular smooth muscle cells. *Journal of Clinical Investigation* **83**, 17744–17747.

46 Geggel, R.L., Reid, L.M. (1984) The structural basis of persistent pulmonary hypertension of the newborn. *Clinics in Perinatology* **3**, 525–549.

47 Gersony, W.M. (1984) Neonatal pulmonary hypertension: pathophysiology, classification and etiology. *Clinics in Perinatology* **11**, 517–524.

48 Gersony, W.M., Duc, G.V., Sinclair, J.C. (1969) 'PFC' syndrome (persistent fetal circulation). *Circulation* **40**(Suppl 3), 87.

49 Goldberg, S.J., Levy, R.A., Siassi, B. (1971) Effects of maternal hypoxia and hyperoxia upon the neonatal pulmonary vasculature. *Pediatrics* **48**, 528.

50 Goldman, A.P., Tasker, R.C., Haworth, S.G. *et al.* (1996) Four patterns of response to inhaled NO for PPHN. *Pediatrics* **98**, 706–713.

51 Gordon, J.B., Martinez, F.R., Keller, P.A. *et al.* (1993) Differing effects of acute and prolonged alkalosis on hypoxic pulmonary vasoconstriction. *American Review of Respiratory Disease* **148**, 1651–1656.

52 Gordon, J.B., Rehorst-Paea, L.A., Hoffman, G.M., Nelin, L.D. (1999) Pulmonary vascular responses during acute and sustained respiratory alkalosis or acidosis in intact newborn piglets. *Pediatric Research* **46**, 735–741.

53 Greenough, A. (1998) Therapeutic strategies in persistent pulmonary hypertension of the newborn. *Progress in Pediatric Cardiology* **9**, 69–72.

54 Grover, T.R., Parker, T.A., Zenge, J.P. *et al.* (2002) VEGF inhibition impairs endothelial function and causes pulmonary hypertension in the late gestation ovine fetus. *Circulation Research* (in press).

55 Halbower, A.C., Tuder, R.M., Franklin, W.A. *et al.* (1994) Maturation-related changes in endothelial NO synthase immunolocalization in the developing ovine lung. *American Journal of Physiology* **267**, L585–L591.

56 Hanson, K.A., Burns, F., Rybalkin, S.D. *et al.* (1995) Developmental changes in lung cGMP phosphodiesterase-5 activity, protein and message. *American Journal of Respiratory and Critical Care Medicine* **158**, 279–288.

57 Hanson, K.A., Beavo, J.A., Abman, S.H., Clarke, W.R. (1998) Chronic pulmonary hypertension increases fetal lung cGMP activity. *American Journal of Physiology* **275**, L931–L941.

58 Haworth, S.G., Reid, L.M. (1976) Persistent fetal circulation. Newly recognized structural features. *Journal of Pediatrics* **88**, 614–620.

59 Heymann, M.A., Soifer, S.J. (1989) Control of fetal and neonatal pulmonary circulation. In Weir, E.K., Reeves, J.T. (eds), *Pulmonary Vascular Physiology and Pathophysiology.* New York: Marcel Dekker, 33–50.

60 Hintz, S.R., Suttner, D.M., Sheehan, A.M. *et al.* (2000) Decreased use of neonatal ECMO: how new treatment modalities have affected ECMO utilization. *Pediatrics* **106**, 1339–1343.

61 Hobbs, A.J., Ignarro, L.J. (1996) NO-cGMP signal transduction system. In Zapol, W.M., Bloch, K. (eds), *Nitric Oxide and the Lung*. New York: Marcel Dekker, 1–57.

62 Holcomb, R.G., Tyson, R.W., Ivy, D.D. *et al.* (1999) Congenital pulmonary venous stenosis presenting as persistent pulmonary hypertension of the newborn. *Pediatric Pulmonology* **28**, 301–306.

63 Huhta, J.C., Rasanen, J. (1999) Maturational changes in the human pulmonary vascular resistance. In Weir, E.K., Archer, S.L., Reeves, J.T. (eds), *Fetal and Neonatal Pulmonary Circulation*. New York: Futura, 343–353.

64 Hutchinson, A.A., Yu, V.Y.H. (1980) Curare in the treatment of pulmonary hypertension as it occurs in the idiopathic respiratory distress syndrome. *Australian Journal of Paediatrics* **16**, 94–100.

65 Ivy, D.D., Abman, S.H. (1999) Role of endothelin in perinatal pulmonary vasoregulation. In Weir, E.K., Archer, S.L., Reeves, J.T. (eds), *Fetal and Neonatal Pulmonary Circulation*. New York: Futura, 279–302.

66 Ivy, D.D., Kinsella, J.P., Abman, S.H. (1994) Physiologic characterization of endothelin A and B receptor activity in the ovine fetal lung. *Journal of Clinical Investigation* **93**, 2141–2148.

67 Ivy, D.D., Kinsella, J.P., Abman, S.H. (1996) Endothelin blockade augments pulmonary vasodilation in the ovine fetal lung. *Journal of Applied Physiology* **81**, 2481–2487.

68 Ivy, D.D., Ziegler, J.W., Dubus, M.F. *et al.* (1996) Chronic intrauterine pulmonary hypertension alters endothelin receptor activity in the ovine fetus. *Pediatric Research* **39**, 335–342.

69 Ivy, D.D., Parker, T.A., Ziegler, J.W. *et al.* (1997) Prolonged endothelin A receptor blockade attenuates chronic pulmonary hypertension in the ovine fetus. *Journal of Clinical Investigation* **99**, 1179–1186.

70 Ivy, D.D., LeCras, T.D., Horan, M.P., Abman, S.H. (1998) Increased lung prepro-endothelin-1 and decreased endothelin B receptor gene expression after chronic pulmonary hypertension in the ovine fetus. *American Journal of Physiology* **274**, L535–L541.

71 Kaapa, P., Koivisto, M., Yukorkala, O., Kouvalainen, K. (1985) Prostacyclin in the treatment of neonatal pulmonary hypertension. *Journal of Pediatrics and Child Health* **28**, 429–431.

72 Kennaugh, J.M., Kinsella, J.P., Abman, S.H. *et al.* (1997) Impact of new treatments for neonatal pulmonary hypertension on ECMO use and outcome. *Journal of Perinatology* **17**, 366–369.

73 Kinsella, J.P., Abman, S.H. (1995) Recent developments in the pathophysiology and treatment of PPHN. *Journal of Pediatrics* **126**, 853–864.

74 Kinsella, J.P., Abman, S.H. (2000) Clinical approach to inhaled NO therapy in the newborn. *Journal of Pediatrics* **136**, 717–726.

75 Kinsella, J.P., Neish, S., Shaffer, E., Abman, S.H. (1992) Low dose inhalational nitric oxide in persistent pulmonary hypertension of the newborn. *Lancet* **340**, 819–820.

76 Kinsella, J.P., Neish, S.R., Ivy, D.D., Shaffer, E., Abman, S.H. (1993) Clinical responses to prolonged treatment of persistent pulmonary hypertension of the newborn. *Journal of Pediatrics* **123**, 103–108.

77 Kinsella, J.P., Ivy, D.D., Abman, S.H. (1994) Ontogeny of NO activity and response to inhaled NO in the developing ovine pulmonary circulation. *American Journal of Physiology* **267**, H1955–H1961.

78 Kinsella, J.P., Toriella, F., Ziegler, J.W., Ivy, D.D., Abman, S.H. (1995) Dipyridamole augmentation of the response to inhaled NO. *Lancet* **346**, 647–648.

79 Kinsella, J.P., Troug, W., Walsh, W. *et al.* (1997) Randomized multicenter trial of inhaled nitric oxide and high frequency oscillatory ventilation in severe PPHN. *Journal of Pediatrics* **131**, 55–62.

80 Konduri, G.G., Mital, S. (2000) Adenosine and ATP cause NO-dependent pulmonary vasodilation in fetal lambs. *Biology of the Neonate* **78**, 220–229.

81 Kulik, T.J., Lock, J.E. (1984) Pulmonary vasodilator therapy in persistent pulmonary hypertension of the newborn. *Clinics in Perinatology* **11**, 693–701.

82 Kulik, T.J., Evans, J.N., Gamble, W.J. (1988) Stretch-induced contraction in pulmonary arteries. *American Journal of Physiology* **255**, H1391–H1398.

83 Laffey, J.G., Kavanaugh, B.P. (2000) Biological effects of hypercapnia. *Intensive Care Medicine* **26**, 133–138.

84 Laffey, J.G., Engelberts, D., Kavanagh, B.P. (2000) Injurious effects of hypocapnic alkalosis in the isolated lung. *American Journal of Critical Care Medicine* **162**, 399–405.

85 Larsson, L.E., Ekstrom-Jodal, B., Hjalmarson, O. (1982) The effect of chlorpromazine in severe hypoxia in newborn infants. *Acta Paediatrica Scandinavica* **71**, 399–402.

86 Lassus, P., Turanlahti, M., Heikkila, P. *et al.* (2001) Pulmonary vascular endothelial growth factor and Flt-1 in fetuses, in acute and chronic lung disease, and in PPHN. *American Journal of Respiratory and Critical Care Medicine* **164**, 1981–1987.

87 Le Cras, T.D., Kim, D., Markham, N.E., Abman, S.H. (2000) Early abnormalities in pulmonary vascular development in the fawn-hooded rat. *American Journal of Respiratory Cell and Molecular Biology* **279**, L283–L291.

88 Leffler, C.W., Tyler, T.L., Cassin, S. (1978) Effect of indomethacin on pulmonary vascular response to ventilation of fetal goats. *American Journal of Physiology* **234**, H346–H351.

89 Leffler, C.W., Hessler, J.R., Green, R.S. (1984) Mechanism of stimulation of pulmonary prostacyclin synthesis at birth. *Prostaglandins* **28**, 877–887.

90 Levin, D.L., Heymann, M.A., Kitterman, J.A. *et al.* (1976) Persistent pulmonary hypertension of the newborn. *Journal of Pediatrics* **89**, 626–633.

91 Levin, D.L., Hyman, A.I., Heymann, M.A., Rudolph, A.M. (1978) Fetal hypertension and the development of increased pulmonary vascular smooth muscle: a possible mechanism for persistent pulmonary hypertension of the newborn infant. *Journal of Pediatrics* **92**, 265–269.

92 Lewis, A.B., Heymann, M.A., Rudolph, A.M. (1976) Gestational changes in pulmonary vascular responses in fetal lambs *in utero*. *Circulation Research* **39**, 536–541.

93 Lock, J.E., Olley, P.M., Coceani, F., Swyer, P.R., Rowe, R.D. (1979) Use of prostacyclin in persistent fetal circulation. *Lancet* **1**, 1343.

94 Lotze, A., Mitchel, B.R., Bulas, D. *et al.* (1998) Multicenter study of surfactant (beractant) use in the treatment of term infants with severe respiratory failure. *Journal of Pediatrics* **132**, 40–47.

95 Matthew, R., Altura, B.T., Altura, B.M. (1989) Strain differences in pulmonary hypertensive response to monocrotaline alkaloid and the beneficial effect of oral magnesium treatment. *Magnesium* **8**, 110–116.

96 McQueston, J.A., Cornfield, D.N., McMurtry, I.F., Abman, S.H. (1993) Effects of oxygen and exogenous L-arginine on endothelium-derived relaxing factor activity in the fetal pulmonary circulation. *American Journal of Physiology* **264**, H865–H871.

97 McQueston, J.A., Kinsella, J.P., Ivy, D.D., McMurtry, I.F., Abman, S.H. (1995) Chronic pulmonary hypertension *in utero* impairs endothelium-dependent vasodilation. *American Journal of Physiology* **268**, H288–H294.

98 Meininger, G.A., Davis, M.J. (1992) Cellular mechanisms involved in the vascular myogenic response. *American Journal of Physiology* **263**, H647–H659.

99 Moncada, S., Palmer, R.M.J., Higgs, E.A. (1991) Nitric oxide: physiology, pathophysiology, and pharmacology. *Pharmacological Reviews* **43**, 109–142.

100 Morbidelli, L., Chang, C.-H., Douglas, J.G. *et al.* (1996) NO mediates mitogenic effect of VEGF on coronary venular endothelium. *American Journal of Physiology* **270**, H411–H415.

101 Moreira, G.A., O'Donnell, D.C., Tod, M.L. *et al.* (1999) Discordant effects of alkalosis on elevated PVR and vascular reactivity in lamb lungs. *Critical Care Medicine* **27**, 1838–1842.

102 Morett, L.A., Ortega, R. (1987) Pulmonary hypertension in the fetus, the newborn and the child. *Clinics in Perinatology* **14**, 227–242.

103 Morin, F.C. (1989) Ligating the ductus arteriosus before birth causes persistent pulmonary hypertension in the newborn lamb. *Pediatric Research* **25**, 245–250.

104 Morin, F.C., Egan, E.A., Ferguson, W., Lundgren, C.E.G. (1988) Development of pulmonary vascular response to oxygen. *American Journal of Physiology* **254**, H542–H546.

105 Moya, M.P., Gow, A.J., McMahon, T.J. *et al.* (2001) S-nitrosothiol repletion by an inhaled gas regulates pulmonary function. *Proceedings of the National Academy of Sciences of the United States of America* **98**, 5792–5797.

106 Muraskas, J.K., Juretschke, L.J., Weiss, M.G., Bhola, M., Besinger, R.E. (2001) Neonatal-perinatal risk factors for the development of PPHN in preterm newborns. *American Journal of Perinatology* **18**, 87–91.

107 Murphy, J.D., Rabinovitch, M., Goldstein, J.D., Reid, L.M. (1981) The structural basis for PPHN infant. *Journal of Pediatrics* **98**, 962–967.

108 Murphy, J.D., Vawter, G., Reid, L.M. (1984) Pulmonary vascular disease in fatal meconium aspiration. *Journal of Pediatrics* **104**, 758–762.

109 Murphy, J.D., Aronovitz, M.J., Reid, L.M. (1986) Effects of chronic in utero hypoxia on the pulmonary vasculature of the newborn guinea pig. *Pediatric Research* **20**, 292–295.

110 Nielson, H.C., Riemenschneider, T.A., Jaffe, R.B. (1976) Persistent transitional circulation. *Radiology* **120**, 649–652.

111 Neonatal Inhaled NO Study Group (1997) Inhaled NO in full-term and nearly full-term infants with hypoxic respiratory failure. *New England Journal of Medicine* **336**, 597–604.

112 Neonatal Inhaled NO Study Group (2000) Inhaled NO in term and near-term infants: neurodevelopmental follow-up of the NINOS. *Journal of Pediatrics* **136**, 611–617.

113 Newman, J.H., Wheeler, L., Lane, K.B. *et al.* (2001) Mutation in the gene for bone morphogenetic protein receptor II as a cause of primary pulmonary hypertension in a large kindred. *New England Journal of Medicine* **345**, 367–371.

114 North, A.J., Star, R.A., Brannon, T.S. *et al.* (1994) NO synthase type I and type III gene expression are developmentally regulated in rat lung. *American Journal of Physiology* **266**, L635–L641.

115 Parker, T.A., Kinsella, J.P., Galan, H.L., Richter, G., Abman, S.H. (2000) Prolonged infusions of estradiol dilate the ovine fetal pulmonary circulation. *Pediatric Research* **47**, 89–96.

116 Parker, T.A., Le Cras, T.D., Kinsella, J.P., Abman, S.H. (2000) Developmental changes in endothelial NO synthase expression in the ovine fetal lung. *American Journal of Physiology* **278**, L202–L208.

117 Parker, T.A., Afshar, S., Kinsella, J.P. *et al.* (2001) Effects of chronic estrogen receptor blockade on the pulmonary circulation in the late gestation ovine fetus. *American Journal of Physiology Heart and Circulatory Physiology* **281**, H1005–H1014.

118 Patterson, K., Kapur, S.P., Chandra, R.S. (1988) PPHN: pulmonary pathologic effects. In Rosenberg, H.S., Bernstein, J. (eds), *Cardiovascular Diseases, Perspectives in Pediatric Pathology*. Basel: Karger, **12**, 139–154.

119 Pearson, D.L., Dawling, S., Walsh, W.F. *et al.* (2001) Neonatal pulmonary hypertension: urea cycle intermediates, NO production and carbamoyl phosphate synthetase function. *New England Journal of Medicine* **344**, 1932–1938.

120 Peckham, G.J., Fox, W.W. (1978) Physiologic factors affecting pulmonary artery pressure in infants with persistent pulmonary hypertension. *Journal of Pediatrics* **93**, 1005–1010.

121 Rairigh, R., Le Cras, T.D., Ivy, D.D. *et al.* (1998) Role of inducible nitric oxide synthase in regulation of pulmonary vascular tone in the late gestation ovine fetus. *Journal of Clinical Investigation* **101**, 15–21.

122 Rairigh, R.L., Parker, T.A., Ivy, D.D. *et al.* (2001) Role of inducible nitric oxide synthase in the transition of the pulmonary circulation at birth. *Circulation Research* **88**, 721–726.

123 Rasanen, J., Wood, D.C., Debbs, R.H. *et al.* (1998) Reactivity of the human fetal pulmonary circulation to maternal hyperoxygenation increases during the second half of pregnancy: a randomized study. *Circulation* **97**, 257–262.

124 Riemenschneider, T.A., Nielson, H.C., Ruttenberg, H.D., Jaffe, R.B. (1976) Disturbances of the transitional circulation: spectrum of pulmonary hypertension and myocardial dysfunction. *Journal of Pediatrics* **89**, 622–625.

125 Roberts, J.D., Polaner, D.M., Lang, P., Zapol, W.M. (1992) Inhaled nitric oxide in persistent pulmonary hypertension of the newborn. *Lancet* **340**, 818–819.

126 Roberts, J.D., Kinsella, J.P., Abman, S.H. (1996) Inhaled NO in neonatal pulmonary hypertension and severe RDS: experimental and clinical studies. In Zapol, W.M., Bloch, K. (eds), *Nitric Oxide and the Lung*. New York: Marcel Dekker, 333–363.

127 Roberts, J.D., Fineman, J.R., Morin, F.C. *et al.* (1997) Inhaled NO and PPHN. *New England Journal of Medicine* **336**, 605–610.

128 Rosenberg, A.A., Kennaugh, J., Koppenhafer, S.L. *et al.* (1993) Increased immunoreactive endothelin-1 levels in persistent pulmonary hypertension of the newborn. *Journal of Pediatrics* **123**, 109–114.

129 Rosenberg, A.A., Kennaugh, J.M., Moreland, S.G. *et al.* (1997) Longitudinal follow-up of a cohort of newborn infants treated with inhaled NO for persistent pulmonary hypertension. *Journal of Pediatrics* **131**, 70–75.

130 Rudolph, A.M. (1979) Fetal and neonatal pulmonary circulation. *Annual Review of Physiology* **41**, 383–395.

131 Rudolph, A.M., Heymann, M.A., Lewis, A.B. (1977) Physiology and pharmacology of the pulmonary circulation in the fetus and newborn. In Hodson, W. (ed.), *Development of the Lung*. New York: Marcel Dekker, 497–523.

132 Ryan, C.A., Finer, N.N., Barrington, K.J. (1994) Effects of magnesium sulphate and nitric oxide in pulmonary hypertension induced by hypoxia in newborn piglets. *Archives of Disease in Childhood* **71**, F151–F155.

133 Sanchez, L.S., Del La Monte, S.M., Filippov, G. *et al.* (1998) Cyclic GMP binding cGMP-specific phosphodiesterase gene expression is regulated during rat pulmonary development. *Pediatric Research* **43**, 163–168.

134 Shaul, P.W. (1999) Regulation of endothelial NO synthase expression in developing lung. In Weir, E.K., Archer, S.L., Reeves, J.T. (eds), *Fetal and Neonatal Pulmonary Circulation*. New York: Futura, 261–278.

135 Shaul, P.W., Farrar, M.A., Magness, R.R. (1993) Pulmonary endothelial NO production is developmentally regulated in the fetus and newborn. *American Journal of Physiology* **265**, H1056–H1063.

136 Shaul, P.W., Yuhanna, I.S., German, Z. *et al.* (1997) Pulmonary endothelial NO synthase gene expression is decreased in fetal lambs with pulmonary hypertension. *American Journal of Physiology* **272**, L1005–L1012.

137 Sherman, T.S., Chen, Z., Yuhanna, I.S. *et al.* (1999) NO synthase isoform expression in the developing lung epithelium. *American Journal of Physiology* **276**, L383–L390.

138 Skinner, J.R., Hunter, S., Hey, E.N. (1996) Hemodynamic features at presentation in PPHN and outcome. *Archives of Disease in Childhood* **74**, F26–F32.

139 Soifer, S.J., Loitz, R.D., Roman, C. *et al.* (1985) Leukotriene end organ antagonists increase pulmonary blood flow in fetal lambs. *American Journal of Physiology* **249**, H570–H576.

140 Steinhorn, R.H., Russell, J.A., Morin, F.C. (1995) Disruption of cGMP production in pulmonary arteries isolated from fetal lambs with pulmonary hypertension. *American Journal of Physiology* **268**, H1483–H1489.

141 Steinhorn, R.H., Albert, G., Swartz, D.D. *et al.* (2001) Recombinant human superoxide dismutase enhances the effect of inhaled NO in persistent pulmonary hypertension. *American Journal of Respiratory and Critical Care Medicine* **164**, 834–839.

142 Stenmark, K.R., Abman, S.H., Accurso, F.J. (1989) Etiologic mechanisms of persistent pulmonary hypertension of the newborn. In Weir, E.K., Reeves, J.T. (eds), *Pulmonary Vascular Physiology and Pathophysiology*. New York: Marcel Dekker, 335.

143 Steudel, W., Scherrer-Crosbie, M., Bloch, K.D. *et al.* (1998) Sustained pulmonary hypertension and right ventricular hypertrophy after chronic hypoxia in mice with congenital deficiency of NOS III. *Journal of Clinical Investigation* **101**, 2468–2477.

144 Stevenson, D.K., Kasting, D.S., Darnall, R.A. *et al.* (1979) Refractory hypoxemia associated with neonatal pulmonary disease: the use and limitations of tolazoline. *Journal of Pediatrics* **95**, 595–599.

145 Storme, L., Rairigh, R.L., Parker, T.A. *et al.* (1999) Potassium channel blockade attenuates shear stress-induced pulmonary vasodilation in the ovine fetus. *American Journal of Physiology* **276**, L220–L228.

146 Storme, L., Rairigh, R.L., Parker, T.A. *et al.* (1999) *In vivo* evidence for a myogenic response in the ovine fetal pulmonary circulation. *Pediatric Research* **45**, 425–431.

147 Storme, L., Rairigh, R.L., Parker, T.A. *et al.* (1999) Acute intrauterine pulmonary hypertension impairs endothelium-dependent vasodilation in the ovine fetus. *Pediatric Research* **45**, 575–581.

148 Storme, L., Parker, T.A., Kinsella, J.P., Rairigh, R.L., Abman, S.H. (2002) Chronic hypertension impairs flow-induced vasodilation and augments the myogenic response in fetal lung. *American Journal of Respiratory Cell and Molecular Biology* **282**, L56–L66.

149 Thomae, K.R., Nakayama, D.K., Billiar, T.R. *et al.* (1996) Effect of NO on fetal pulmonary artery smooth muscle growth. *Journal of Surgical Research* **270**, H411–H415.

150 Thusu, K.G., Morin, F.C., Russell, J.A. *et al.* (1995) The cGMP phosphodiesterase inhibitor zaprinast enhances the effect of NO. *American Journal of Respiratory and Critical Care Medicine* **152**, 1605–1610.

151 Tiefenbrunn, L.J., Riemenschneider, T.A. (1986) Persistent pulmonary hypertension of the newborn. *American Heart Journal* **111**, 564–572.

152 Tolsa, J.F., Cotting, J., Sekarski, N., Payot, M., Micheli, J.L., Calame, A. (1995) Magnesium sulphate as an alternative and safe treatment for severe persistent pulmonary hypertension of the newborn. *Archives of Disease in Childhood* **72**, F184–F187.

153 Tremblay, L., Valenza, F., Ribeiro, S.P. *et al.* (1997) Injurious ventilator strategies increase cytokines and c-fos mRNA expression in an isolated rat lung model. *Journal of Clinical Investigation* **99**, 944–952.

154 UK Collaborative ECMO Trial Group (1996) UK Collaborative randomized trial of neonatal ECMO. *Lancet* **348**, 75–82.

155 Van Marter, L.J., Leviton, A., Allred, E.N. *et al.* (1996) PPHN and smoking and aspirin and nonsteroidal antiinflammatory drug consumption during pregnancy. *Pediatrics* **97**, 658–663.

156 Velvis, H., Moore, P., Heymann, M.A. (1991) Prostaglandin inhibition prevents the fall in pulmonary vascular resistance as the result of rhythmic distension of the lungs in fetal lambs. *Pediatric Research* **30**, 62–67.

157 Villamor, E., Le Cras, T.D., Horan, M. *et al.* (1997) Chronic hypertension impairs endothelial NO synthase in the ovine fetus. *American Journal of Physiology* **16**, L1013–L1020.

158 Walmrath, D., Schneider, T., Pilch, J., Grimminger, F., Seeger, W. (1993) Aerosolized prostacyclin in adult respiratory distress syndrome. *Lancet* **342**, 961–962.

159 Walsh, M.C., Stork, E.R. (2001) PPHN: rational therapy based on pathophysiology. *Clinics in Perinatology* **28**, 609–627.

160 Walsh-Sukys, M.C., Tyson, J.E., Wright, L.L. *et al.* (2000) PPHN in the era before NO: practice variation and outcomes. *Pediatrics* **105**, 14–20.

161 Walther, F.J., Bender, F.J., Leighton, J.O. (1992) Persistent pulmonary hypertension in premature neonates with severe RDS. *Pediatrics* **90**, 899–904.

162 Wessel, D.L., Adatia, I., van Marter, L.J. *et al.* (1997) Improved oxygenation in a randomized trial of inhaled NO for PPHN. *Pediatrics* **100**, E7.

163 Williams, M.C., Wyble, L.E., O'Brien, W.F. *et al.* (1998) PPHN and asymmetric growth restriction. *Obstetrics and Gynecology* **91**, 336–341.

164 Wu, T.J., Teng, R.J., Yau, K.I.T. (1995) Persistent pulmonary hypertension in the newborn treated with magnesium sulphate in premature neonates. *Pediatrics* **96**, 472–474.

165 Yanagisawa, M., Masaki, T. (1989) Endothelin: a novel endothelium derived peptide. Pharmacological activities, regulation and possible roles in cardiovascular control. *Biochemical Pharmacology* **38**, 1877–1883.

166 Zenge, J.P., Rairigh, R.L., Grover, T.R. *et al.* (2001) NO and prostaglandins modulate the pulmonary vascular response to hemodynamic stress in the late gestation fetus. *American Journal of Respiratory Cell and Molecular Biology* **281**, L1157–L1163.

167 Ziche, M., Morbidelli, L., Masini, E. *et al.* (1994) NO mediates angiogenesis *in vivo* and endothelial cell growth and migration *in vitro* promoted by substance P. *Journal of Clinical Investigation* **94**, 2036–2044.

168 Ziegler, J.W., Ivy, D.D., Fox, J.J. *et al.* (1995) Dipyridamole, a cGMP phosphodiesterase inhibitor, causes pulmonary vasodilation in the ovine fetus. *American Journal of Physiology* **269**, H473–H479.

169 Ziegler, J.W., Ivy, D.D., Wiggins, J.W., Kinsella, J.P., Clarke, W.R., Abman, S.H. (1998) Hemodynamic effects of dipyridamole and inhaled NO in children with severe pulmonary hypertension. *American Journal of Respiratory and Critical Care Medicine* **158**, 1388–1395.

170 Zobel, G., Dacar, D., Rod, L.S., Friehs, I. (1995) Inhaled nitric oxide versus inhaled prostacyclin and intravenous vs inhaled prostacyclin in acute respiratory failure in pulmonary hypertension in piglets. *Pediatric Research* **38**, 198–204.

27

Respiratory presentation of cardiac disease

EDWARD BAKER

INTRODUCTION

A common dilemma for the clinician is the differentiation of cardiac and respiratory disease. Acquired heart failure in children tends to be recognized late, since in its early stages it is often mistaken for respiratory disease. This is perhaps not surprising since the pulmonary and cardio-vascular systems are so closely inter-related. Abnormalities of the heart inevitably affect pulmonary function just as abnormalities of the lungs will affect cardiac function.

Cardiac disease in children, at least in the developed world, principally results from congenital abnormalities. Functional abnormalities are brought about by structural defects in the heart or major vessels. The pulmonary effects of these defects can broadly be classified into those that lead to an increase and those that lead to a decrease in the pulmonary blood flow. Structural defects can also lead to obstruction of the pulmonary venous return to the heart. Structural abnormalities of the great arteries can compress the trachea or bronchial tree. While structural defects of the heart predominate, purely functional defects, such as reduced myocardial contractility, can occur and may also cause reduction of pulmonary perfusion or functional pulmonary venous obstruction.

CONDITIONS WITH AN INCREASED PULMONARY BLOOD FLOW

The commoner congenital heart defects, for example ventricular septal defects and patent ductus arteriosus, cause an increased pulmonary blood flow. Beyond the neonatal period, the pulmonary vascular resistance is much lower than the systemic vascular resistance so any communication between the systemic and pulmonary circulations will lead to a left-to-right shunt.[7,23] Large shunts at ventricular or great artery level which are associated with very high pulmonary blood flows present with early-onset heart failure. The magnitude of a left-to-right shunt is usually expressed as the ratio of the pulmonary to systemic blood flow (Q_p/Q_s). A Q_p/Q_s of 3 or greater is typically found in an infant presenting in heart failure with a left-to-right shunt.

Clinical presentation

HEART FAILURE

Ventricular septal defects typically present in the neonatal period, or soon after, as the pulmonary vascular resistance falls. The magnitude of the left-to-right shunt depends upon two factors: the physical size of the defect and the relationship between the pulmonary and systemic vascular resistances. When the defect is restrictive, small enough to allow a pressure difference between the left and right sides of the circulation, the pulmonary artery pressure will decrease as the pulmonary vascular resistance falls. The magnitude of the left-to-right shunt and therefore the likelihood of clinical heart failure is principally determined by the physical size of the defect. Isolated defects in the atrial septum also lead to left-to-right shunt and an increased pulmonary blood flow. In these though, it is the compliance of the right and left ventricles, rather than the vascular resistances, that determines the size of the shunt. Even the largest atrial septal defect can only cause an equalization of the pressures in the two atria. It will not cause pulmonary hypertension as large ventricular septal defects do. Shunts at atrial level tend to develop gradually as the compliance of the right ventricle increases during infancy. This gradual increase in the magnitude of the shunt means that despite the development of high pulmonary blood flows, such patients do not usually exhibit signs of heart failure until there is secondary myocardial decompensation. In typical atrial septal defects this does not happen until well into adult life.[5]

Heart failure in infants presents with tachypnea or dyspnea with feeding. Reduced lung compliance leads to subcostal and intercostal recession.[23] Venous congestion of the mucosa or an increase in peribronchial fluid may cause airways obstruction, retention of secretions and precipitate infections. Other features of heart failure in infants are tachycardia and fluid retention manifested by hepatomegaly and increased weight. Occasionally infants appear particularly pale and may show excess sweating.

An increase in the pulmonary blood flow leads to a rise in the left atrial pressure. Together these lead to increased water in the interstitium of the lungs. This causes an increase in the resistance of small airways and an increase in pulmonary vascular resistance. Left-to-right shunts may lead to retention of carbon dioxide and an increase in the alveolar–arterial oxygen gradient. If there is pulmonary hypertension, this together with the high blood flow will lead to reduced lung compliance.[4] This combination also has a profound effect on the development of the pulmonary vasculature.[11]

Diagnosis

On the chest radiograph, the high pulmonary blood flow may lead to visible enlargement of the pulmonary vessels, both veins and arteries (Figure 27.1). The pulmonary vascular tree appears engorged and extends well out into the lung periphery. In infants with heart failure, this may be accompanied by hyperinflation of the lungs. Evidence of pulmonary plethora can coexist with arterial desaturation in patients with bidirectional shunting. Chest radiographs are, however, a relatively insensitive way of detecting left-to-right shunts, and interpretation is by necessity subjective. However, cardiomegaly is a constant feature if heart failure is present (Figure 27.2). Heart failure is manifest in the lung fields by the onset of haziness as interstitial fluid accumulates. This haziness makes the hilar vessels less distinct. If this progresses, the buildup of interstitial fluid progresses to pulmonary edema and the hilar vessels are obscured (Figure 27.3).[23]

Management

In the child with heart failure, it is often difficult to determine to what extent any lung pathology is secondary to the heart disease. There is no easy solution to this. Heart disease and lung disease can, and often do, coexist. Vigorous treatment of the heart failure is essential, but care has to

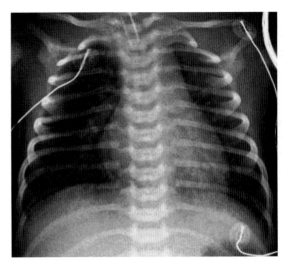

Figure 27.1 *Pulmonary plethora in an infant with a hypoplastic left heart. The pulmonary vessels are enlarged and distinct. There is fluid in the horizontal fissure.*

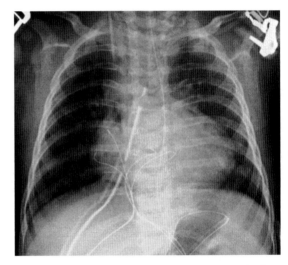

Figure 27.2 *Early pulmonary edema in a post-operative patient. There is general haziness over the lung fields. Linear septal shadows (Kerley B lines) are seen in the lower part of the lungs.*

be exercised. Excessive use of diuretics, for example, can have deleterious effects if there is undiagnosed lung pathology.

DESATURATION DUE TO BIDIRECTIONAL SHUNTING

Truncus arteriosus and complex pulmonary atresia are examples of defects with bidirectional shunting. Typically they present with a high pulmonary blood flow from a net left-to-right shunt, but their anatomy is such that there will also always be an element of right-to-left shunting. So despite the evidence of a high pulmonary blood flow, they will always have a degree of arterial desaturation.

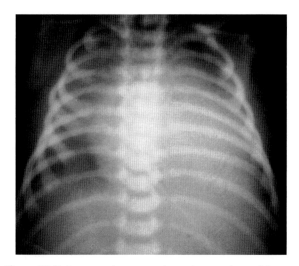

Figure 27.3 *Severe pulmonary edema in a patient with hypoplastic left heart syndrome. There is severe pulmonary venous obstruction and the haziness obscures all the pulmonary vascular markings.*

A similar situation occurs in some cases of transposition of the great arteries, where there is a ventricular septal defect. Because of the connections, such infants will always be centrally cyanosed, even if they have a very high pulmonary blood flow.

PULMONARY HYPERTENSION

A large communication at great artery or ventricular level causes an equalization of pressures on the two sides of the circulation. This means that pressures will be at systemic levels in the right heart and pulmonary circulation. This pulmonary hypertension has an effect on the normal maturation of the pulmonary vasculature. The normal fall in the pulmonary vascular resistance is delayed and the smooth muscle of the pulmonary arterioles persists to a greater extent than normal. Pulmonary vascular resistance does fall, but slowly, reaching a nadir after several months. Even at its lowest it is maintained at higher levels than normal.[11,23] As the pulmonary vascular resistance falls, the pulmonary blood flow increases, but the pulmonary artery pressure remains high. Apart from the hemodynamic effect of a large ventricular or great artery shunt, pulmonary hypertension may occur secondary to chronic lung disease.

Diagnosis

This is often made echocardiographically. The right ventricle is hypertrophied and hypertensive in the absence of any structural obstruction to the right ventricular outflow. The right ventricular systolic pressure can usually be estimated from the maximum velocity of a tricuspid regurgitant jet.[2] Where there is a ventricular septal defect or patent ductus arteriosus, Doppler interrogation will show the maximum velocity of blood flow across the defect. From this the pressure gradient between the two sides of the circulation can be estimated and the pulmonary artery pressure inferred.[17] It is unusual to need any further investigation to confirm the diagnosis, but catheterization may be needed if the estimates of the pulmonary vascular resistance are required.

Management

The pulmonary vascular resistance in an infant with cardiac disease and increased muscularization of their arterioles can be very labile. Pulmonary hypertensive crises can occur in which the pulmonary vascular resistance increases and there is an acute fall in the pulmonary blood flow. Postoperatively, once any septal defect is closed this may lead to a critical fall in the systemic output. Hypoxia, hypercapnia, and acidosis increase the pulmonary vascular resistance. This means that the first-line treatment must be maintaining adequate ventilation, with a low $PaCO_2$ and high FiO_2 essential. Acidosis should be treated and, if necessary, inotropes that tend to reduce pulmonary vascular resistance can be used (sodium nitroprusside or phosphodiesterase inhibitors such as enoximone).[12] Pulmonary vasodilators are not likely to be effective if these steps have not been taken. Nitric oxide is a powerful endogenous pulmonary vasodilator, produced in the vascular endothelium. Apart from its inotropic effects, sodium nitroprusside is a donor of nitric oxide and has a strong pulmonary vasodilator effect, as does exogenous nitric oxide.[20] Prostacyclin (epoprostenol, PGI_2) is an effective pulmonary vasodilator that acts directly on the vascular smooth muscle cells by increasing cAMP. It has an additive effect to that of nitric oxide.[13]

PULMONARY VASCULAR DISEASE

Pulmonary hypertension, caused by a large communication at great artery or ventricular level, causes early changes in the distribution of smooth muscle in the pulmonary arterioles. This has a protective effect, limiting the fall in pulmonary vascular resistance and the magnitude of the pulmonary blood flow. The mechanisms that control this process are not fully understood, but it appears to be mediated by the vascular endothelium.[26] The key hemodynamic determinant of the process seems to be increased pulmonary artery pressure, rather than increased pulmonary blood flow, but it is known that both hypoxia and increased flow will exacerbate the increase in pulmonary vascular resistance.[8] If these hemodynamic substrates persist, the changes to the smooth muscle will progress. The increase in smooth muscle in the media extends more peripherally into the smaller arterioles. After about 1 year of age this is followed by proliferation of the intima in the peripheral arterioles. This change is progressive and is followed by intimal fibrosis. Intimal thickening and fibrosis, together with a further increase in the muscularization of the arterioles, leads to a gradual and eventually an inexorable rise in the pulmonary vascular resistance.[11]

Untreated large defects at ventricular or great artery level most typically lead to pulmonary vascular disease. In the majority it only becomes irreversible after the first year, but the time course is variable. Where the defect coexists with hypoxia, such as truncus arteriosus, the progression of pulmonary vascular disease appears to be accelerated. Rarely, infants seem to be born with pulmonary vascular disease; indeed, they may never lower their pulmonary vascular resistance sufficiently to develop clinical evidence of a left-to-right shunt. These infants present a high risk for corrective surgery.

Management

Treatment of established pulmonary vascular disease is often based upon the response of the measured pulmonary vascular resistance to therapy during cardiac catheterization. Patients are usually anticoagulated and may respond symptomatically to nocturnal oxygen therapy, oral vasodilators, such as nifedipine, or intravenous therapy with prostacyclin.[27]

CONDITIONS WITH A REDUCED PULMONARY BLOOD FLOW

Less common congenital cardiac malformations may cause obstructions to the flow of blood to the lungs and lead to a reduced overall pulmonary blood flow.

Tetralogy of Fallot

Most common of these is the tetralogy of Fallot, where a combination of sub-pulmonary, pulmonary valve and sometimes supravalve pulmonary stenosis and a large ventricular septal defect creates a net right-to-left shunt. Arterial desaturation is the key clinical finding and the severity of this depends upon the magnitude of pulmonary blood flow. The physical obstruction to the right ventricular outflow tract is fixed, but the pulmonary blood flow is variable and this is why the degree of cyanosis varies. The magnitude of the net right-to-left shunt depends upon the relationship between the fixed resistance to flow to the lungs and the systemic vascular resistance. Reduction of the systemic vascular resistance causes an increase in the shunt and a fall in the pulmonary blood flow. In cases with severe pulmonary stenosis, the level of arterial saturation can depend critically on the systemic vascular resistance. This is the cause of so-called hypercyanotic spells in this condition.[1]

Pulmonary stenosis

Pulmonary valve stenosis by itself does not lead to a fall in the pulmonary blood flow, unless there is an associated septal defect. In so-called critical pulmonary stenosis of the newborn, severe pulmonary stenosis leads to right-to-left shunting through the foramen ovale. Neonates with a critically low pulmonary blood flow are dependent on the ductus arteriosus to maintain an adequate pulmonary perfusion. This is often the case with pulmonary atresia; however, in one type of pulmonary atresia, where there is a coexistent ventricular septal defect, there may be major collateral arteries extending from the anterior wall of the descending aorta or occasionally from other systemic arteries to supply the intrapulmonary arteries at or near the hilum. The relationship between these major collateral arteries and bronchial arteries has not been fully established, but characteristically the collateral arteries have no independent course within the lung parenchyma. These major collaterals are extremely varied in their morphology and distribution. Typically they are between two and six in number and can supply all or part of the pulmonary vascular bed of one or both lungs. They may coexist with central pulmonary arteries, which are often severely hypoplastic. The collateral arteries may contain stenoses that limit the blood flow and pressure transmitted to the pulmonary vascular bed. This is not consistent and in these patients the distribution of pulmonary perfusion is very complex. Parts of the pulmonary vascular bed may receive a high flow at high pressure while other parts of the same lung may be hypoperfused.[14]

Ebstein's malformation

Ebstein's malformation (dysplasia of the tricuspid valve) is characterized by cardiomegaly, even though the pulmonary blood flow is often reduced by the obstruction at tricuspid valve level. In the neonate, the combination of massive cardiomegaly and central cyanosis is characteristic of this condition. This massive cardiac enlargement is present in fetal life and can lead to pulmonary hypoplasia. Indeed, in those that present in the neonatal period the degree of respiratory insufficiency is often the principal determinant of survival.[6]

Clinical presentation

Typically the patient with a low pulmonary blood flow presents with central cyanosis due to arterial desaturation. The hyperoxia, or nitrogen washout, test is a sensitive way of detecting a right-to-left shunt. Cyanotic heart disease, severe respiratory disease and persistent pulmonary hypertension can all cause right-to-left shunts in neonates.

Diagnosis

A hyperoxia test is occasionally of value if it is uncertain whether a structural heart anomaly is present. When challenged with a high level of inspired oxygen, patients with right-to-left shunts will only occasionally be able to raise their arterial PO_2 above 20 kPa (150 mmHg), and will certainly not raise it above 27 kPa (203 mmHg).[14]

CHEST RADIOGRAPH

Chest radiographs in patients with low pulmonary blood flow will generally show oligemia. The size of the heart will be variable, depending on the underlying cardiac anomaly.

PULMONARY VENOUS ANOMALIES

Anomalous connections of the pulmonary veins are usually divided into infracardiac, cardiac and supracardiac. The situation is more complicated than this, as the connection can be mixed with different veins draining to different sites. If all the veins drain anomalously, they usually all drain to the same site. One of the key features that determines the clinical presentation is the extent to which the anomalous anatomy leads to obstruction of the pulmonary venous drainage. Supracardiac connection can be to either the innominate vein, the superior vena cava or, occasionally, the azygous vein or a persistent left superior vena cava. In each case the four pulmonary veins form a confluence behind the left atrium, which is drained by an ascending vertical vein. The presence of obstruction is variable. If the vertical vein drains to the innominate vein, it may pass anterior to the left pulmonary artery or between the left pulmonary artery and left bronchus. In the latter case it will be obstructed. A vertical vein draining to the right superior vena cava may likewise be obstructed as it passes between the right pulmonary artery and carina.

Cardiac drainage of anomalous pulmonary veins is most commonly to the coronary sinus, when obstruction is rare. Infracardiac drainage is the most consistently associated with severe obstruction. In this case, the pulmonary venous confluence is drained by a descending vein that passes through the diaphragm to join the portal venous system or, rarely, the inferior vena cava. The descending vein may be obstructed as it passes through the diaphragm, but principally obstruction occurs at the level of the ductus venosus.[10]

Anomalous pulmonary venous drainage will cause a bidirectional shunt. The connection itself causes a left-to-right shunt, while a right-to-left shunt, usually through a patent foramen ovale, is needed to maintain the systemic circulation.

PULMONARY VENOUS OBSTRUCTION

Obstruction of the pulmonary venous drainage causes pulmonary venous hypertension.

Clinical presentation

Severe obstructed total anomalous pulmonary venous drainage, will lead to the onset of pulmonary edema within a few hours of birth. In less severe cases, the presentation may be delayed for a few days or weeks. In the infant with obstructed anomalous pulmonary veins, respiratory distress and hypoxia are the two dominant clinical features. The expected features of heart failure – hepatomegaly, cardiomegaly and cardiac murmurs – are usually absent.

Differential diagnosis

It is often difficult to clinically differentiate obstructed pulmonary veins from respiratory disease or from persistent pulmonary hypertension in the newborn.

Diagnosis

Affected infants will fail the hyperoxia test, showing they have a right-to-left shunt. This is one of the most valuable indications for this test.

CHEST RADIOGRAPH

The chest radiograph of the newborn infant with severely obstructed pulmonary veins is highly characteristic. The heart is not enlarged, but pulmonary edema is manifested as a 'ground-glass' pattern in the lung fields (Figure 27.4). This pattern may be mistaken for respiratory distress syndrome. The uniform nature of the pattern of pulmonary edema and the absence of an air bronchogram support the diagnosis of obstructed anomalous pulmonary veins.[16]

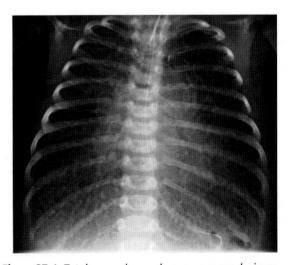

Figure 27.4 *Total anomalous pulmonary venous drainage. There is pulmonary edema with a characteristic "ground glass" pattern throughout the lung fields.*

PULMONARY EDEMA

Pulmonary edema occurs when there is leakage of fluid from pulmonary capillaries into the interstitium and alveoli. The amount of fluid leaking from the pulmonary capillaries depends upon a balance between the pulmonary capillary pressure and plasma oncotic pressure. The plasma oncotic pressure is normally around 25 mmHg, higher than the pulmonary capillary pressure, about 7–12 mmHg. Normally any fluid is drained by the lymphatic system. Fluid accumulates if the lymphatic system is overloaded. Excess fluid may leak if the pulmonary capillary pressure rises higher than the plasma oncotic pressure, or if there is disruption of the normally impermeable connective tissue and cellular barriers between the vascular space and the lung interstitium. Initially any excess fluid builds up in the interstitium. If the fluid accumulation increases, it will eventually disrupt the alveolar membrane. Fluid then fills the alveoli themselves, giving the clinical picture of pulmonary edema. There is some evidence that in preterm infants this happens at lower pulmonary capillary pressures than normal.[23]

Etiology

Pulmonary edema can be caused by several different mechanisms. It may be secondary to increased pulmonary capillary pressure. This is often secondary to cardiac disease. The increased pressure may be caused by obstruction of the pulmonary veins as in the severe forms of total anomalous pulmonary venous drainage. It can also occur where there is stenosis of normally draining pulmonary veins. Other congenital causes are cor triatriatum (divided left atrium), supravalve mitral membrane, congenital mitral stenosis and hypoplasia of the left ventricle. A rare condition, pulmonary veno-occlusive disease, may be associated with congenital heart defects or may occur in isolation later in childhood. Its etiology is unclear, but it may be seen after treatment with cytotoxic drugs or bone marrow transplantation.

Left atrial hypertension can also be present when the left ventricular function is reduced. It can occur in all forms of left ventricular dysfunction including dilated cardiomyopathy, but it is particularly seen where there is diastolic dysfunction as may occur in restrictive forms of cardiomyopathy, constrictive pericarditis and cardiac tamponade. Cardiac arrhythmias, particularly tachyarrhythmias, are important causes of acute onset of heart failure and pulmonary edema in infants. They are usually well tolerated in older children, but in infants they can rapidly cause a critical increase in left atrial pressure. An increase in the circulating volume will increase the left atrial pressure and can, if severe, cause pulmonary edema in a healthy child. However, volume-induced pulmonary edema is much more likely when the volume load coexists with either structural or functional obstruction of the pulmonary venous drainage.

Pulmonary edema may also be secondary to altered capillary permeability. This mechanism operates in acute respiratory deficiency syndrome (ARDS), near drowning, septicemia, and following aspiration or inhalation of toxic chemicals. It may be caused or made worse by decreased oncotic pressure when there is hypoalbuminemia. Pulmonary edema can be caused by abnormalities of the pulmonary lymphatic drainage. It may also occur in a variety of other circumstances, where the mechanism is not well understood. These include high altitude pulmonary edema, neurogenic pulmonary edema, pulmonary embolism, after an anesthetic or extubation, and following cardiopulmonary bypass.[18,21]

Clinical presentation

Pulmonary edema is recognized from the clinical picture of profound respiratory distress, pulmonary crepitations and evidence of reduced cardiac output. The infant with pulmonary edema is tachycardic, pale, sweaty, and has poor volume peripheral pulses.

Diagnosis

The chest radiograph appearances are characteristic (Figure 27.2). There is perihilar shadowing obscuring the vascular structures. Linear septal shadows (Kerley B lines) may be seen in the lower part of the lungs.[4] In the most severe cases, there may be fluid visible in the horizontal and oblique fissures and pericardial effusions may be present.

Cardiac causes of pulmonary edema can usually be diagnosed from the echocardiogram or electrocardiogram. The one structural cause that may be difficult to identify is congenital stenosis of normally connected pulmonary veins. This may be detected by careful Doppler interrogation of the veins, or may require cardiac catheterization or magnetic resonance imaging for diagnosis.

Management

Diuretic treatment, typically with frusemide, will lower the circulating volume and reduce the obvious clinical manifestations of pulmonary edema. However, this may be at the expense of critically lowering the cardiac output. Treatment of the underlying structural or functional cause is fundamental. Positive pressure ventilation is valuable in the emergency stabilization of a patient with pulmonary edema.[25]

VASCULAR RINGS AND ABSENT PULMONARY VALVE

The great arteries and major airways are closely related anatomically. Anomalies in the former can lead to compression of the airways. These anomalies are often referred to as vascular rings.

Double aortic arch

The most ring-like is a double aortic arch. The ascending aorta divides into two. The right branch gives rise to the right common carotid and subclavian arteries and the left to the left common carotid and subclavian arteries. The two arches come together posteriorly, forming a single descending aorta. Together they form a complete ring around the trachea and esophagus. Such a complete ring almost always causes significant obstruction to both the trachea and esophagus.

CLINICAL PRESENTATION

Characteristically infants with a double aortic arch present with stridor, usually in the first few months after birth. The onset of symptoms is often insidious. There may be a history of recurrent respiratory infections and sometimes wheezing dominates the clinical picture. The stridor is more inspiratory rather than expiratory. Dysphagia is usually not the presenting symptom.[15]

Other vascular rings

However, vascular rings are very varied. There may be interruption of part of one of the two aortic arches. A fibrous band may replace the interrupted segment, so that the possibility of compression is still present. Indeed, most vascular rings can be viewed as a double aortic arch with a segment missing. If there is no continuity of one of the arches, compression can still occur because of the presence of a ductus arteriosus, which may be left-, right-sided, or bilateral. This together with the pulmonary arteries can form an effective vascular ring. An example of this is a right-sided aortic arch with a left-sided ductus arteriosus. The left duct (or ligamentum) passes from the left subclavian artery to the left pulmonary artery. This unusual defect, particularly, causes compression of the left main bronchus. The so-called 'ductal sling' occurs when an anomalous ductus connects the right pulmonary artery with a left-sided descending aorta. The anomalous duct passes over the right main bronchus and between the trachea and esophagus to reach the aorta. This causes compression principally of the right main bronchus and also to some extent the trachea.[3]

A more common defect is an aberrant right subclavian artery and left aortic arch. The right subclavian artery originates from the descending aorta and crosses the midline posterior to the esophagus. This defect may sometimes cause dysphagia, but rarely causes any airway compression and is often asymptomatic.

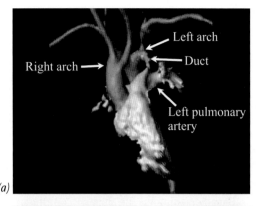

(a)

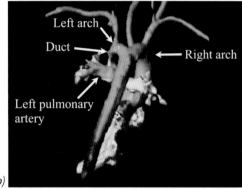

(b)

Figure 27.5(a) and (b) *Magnetic resonance angiogram images of a double aortic arch. The right arch is complete and the left arch is interrupted. Compression is brought about by the left sided duct and the left pulmonary artery.*

DIAGNOSIS

Some vascular rings may be apparent on chest radiographs, but this is not a reliable finding. Cross-sectional echocardiography can demonstrate the vascular anatomy well in neonates and young infants. Fiberoptic bronchoscopy can be of value to demonstrate the site of airway compression, but confirmation of the anatomy is best achieved by magnetic resonance scanning (Figure 27.5). This is particularly valuable as it allows simultaneous imaging of the vascular structures and the airways. There is no longer any place for the traditional barium swallow or invasive angiography.

MANAGEMENT

Not all vascular rings require surgical division, but where there is significant airway compression this is generally undertaken. Double aortic arches usually require surgery in early infancy. Division of a vascular ring usually results in some immediate symptomatic improvement, but a degree of airway obstruction often persists. This usually resolves with time.

Pulmonary sling

Occasionally an anomaly is seen in which the left pulmonary artery arises distally from the right pulmonary artery. It passes over the right main bronchus and then between the trachea and esophagus to reach the left lung. This anomaly is often known as 'pulmonary sling'. This may occur in isolation or associated with other cardiac anomalies such as tetralogy of Fallot, coarctation or ventricular septal defect. A pulmonary sling almost always leads to compression of the right main bronchus and the trachea.

CLINICAL PRESENTATION

Clinical findings are similar to those with other vascular rings. Usually symptoms of airway compression are present from the neonatal period.

DIAGNOSIS

Often the chest radiograph appearances are asymmetrical with hyperinflation of the right lung. Diagnosis should be readily apparent echocardiographically.

MANAGEMENT

Surgical repair should usually be undertaken early and requires cardiopulmonary bypass. That being so, it is usually combined with the repair of any underlying cardiac pathology.[9]

Absent pulmonary valve syndrome

Compression of the airways by the pulmonary arteries is a dominant feature in a condition known as absent pulmonary valve syndrome. This cardiac anomaly is usually regarded as a form of the tetralogy of Fallot, although clinically it is very distinct. The valve is not truly absent, but it is rudimentary. As a result there is a combination of severe pulmonary stenosis and severe regurgitation. This is associated with gross dilation of the pulmonary arteries.

CLINICAL PRESENTATION

These children present in the neonatal period and usually respiratory features predominate. There is inspiratory and expiratory stridor. They have evidence of both lobar collapse and emphysema.

COR PULMONALE

Chronic diseases of the lungs may themselves lead to changes in the pulmonary vasculature and pulmonary hypertension, with inevitable effects on the right ventricle. This can occur with chronic lung disease following neonatal lung disease, bronchopulmonary dysplasia, cystic fibrosis, severe scoliosis, pulmonary hypoplasia and thoracic dystrophy. The right ventricle is hypertrophied

because of the pressure load it has to sustain. The course of the condition depends on the progress of the pulmonary hypertension. Rapidly progressive pulmonary hypertension will lead to early right ventricular failure. A more insidious rise in the pulmonary artery pressure can be sustained by the right ventricle for many years. Right ventricular failure is eventually heralded by the onset of hemodynamically important tricuspid regurgitation or cardiac arrhythmias.[24]

Hypercapnia, caused by obstructive sleep apnea or congenital central hypoventilation syndrome, is an additional cause of cor pulmonale in young children. The former is particularly associated with Down syndrome and this may be the explanation for the increased incidence of pulmonary hypertension in these patients. It is also seen in a myriad of other conditions such as Pierre Robin syndrome, congenital myopathy and cleft palate. While these patients may have echocardiographic or electrocardiographic evidence of right ventricular hypertrophy, they do not usually present with evidence of right heart failure. Respiratory symptoms predominate. Usually the pulmonary hypertension is reversible once the upper airway obstruction has been resolved.[19,22]

REFERENCES

1 Baker, E.J. (2002) Tetralogy of Fallot with pulmonary atresia. In Anderson, R.H., Baker, E.J., Macartney, F.J. *et al.* (eds), *Paediatric Cardiology*. London: Churchill Livingstone, 1251–1279.

2 Berger, M., Haimowitz, A., Van Tosh, A. *et al.* (1985) Quantitative assessment of pulmonary hypertension in patients with tricuspid regurgitation using continuous wave Doppler ultrasound. *Journal of the American College of Cardiology* **6**, 359–365.

3 Binet, J.P., Conso, J.F., Losay, J. *et al.* (1978) Ductus arteriosus sling: report of a newly recognised anomaly and its surgical correction. *Thorax* **33**, 72–75.

4 Bush, A. (2002) Lung function and exercise testing. In Anderson, R.H., Baker, E.J., Macartney, F.J. *et al.* (eds), *Paediatric Cardiology*. London: Churchill Livingstone, 593–620.

5 Campbell, M.J. (1970) Natural history of atrial septal defect. *British Heart Journal* **32**, 820–826.

6 Celermajer, D.S., Cullen, S., Sullivan, I.D. *et al.* (1992) Outcome in neonates with Ebstein's anomaly. *Journal of the American College of Cardiology* **19**, 1041–1046.

7 Fineman, J.R., Soifer, S.J., Heymann, M.A. (1995) Regulation of pulmonary vascular tone in the perinatal period. *Annual Review of Physiology* **57**, 115–134.

8 Gibbs, J.S. (2001) Recommendations on the management of pulmonary hypertension in clinical practice. *Heart* **86**, 1–13.

9 Gikonyo, B.M., Jue, K.L., Edwards, J.E. (1989) Pulmonary vascular sling: report of seven cases and review of the literature. *Pediatric Cardiology* **10**, 81–89.

10 Haworth, S.G. (1982) Total anomalous pulmonary venous return. Prenatal damage to pulmonary vascular bed and extrapulmonary pulmonary veins. *British Heart Journal* **48**, 513–524.

11 Haworth, S.G. (1987) Pulmonary vascular disease in ventricular septal defect: structural and functional considerations in lung biopsies from 85 patients, with outcomes of intra-cardiac repair. *Journal of Pathology* **152**, 157–168.

12 Haworth, S.G. (2002) The pulmonary circulation. In Anderson, R.H., Baker, E.J., Macartney, F.J. *et al.* (eds), *Paediatric Cardiology*. London: Churchill Livingstone, 57–93.

13 Hermon, M., Golej, J., Burda, G. *et al.* (1999) Intravenous prostacyclin mitigates inhaled nitric oxide rebound effect: A case control study. *Artificial Organs* **23**, 975–978.

14 Jones, R.W., Baumer, J.H., Joseph, M.C., Shinebourne, E.A. (1976) Arterial oxygen tension and response to oxygen breathing in differential diagnosis of congenital heart disease in infancy. *Archives of Disease in Childhood* **51**, 667–673.

15 Lincoln, J.C., Deverall, P.B., Stark, J. *et al.* (1969) Vascular anomalies compressing the oesophagus and trachea. *Thorax* **24**, 295–306.

16 Lucas, R.V.J., Adams, P.J., Anderson, R.C. *et al.* (1961) Total anomalous pulmonary venous connection to the portal venous system: a cause of pulmonary venous obstruction. *American Journal of Roentgenology* **86**, 561–575.

17 Murphy, D.J.J., Judomirsky, A., Hutha, J.C. (1986) Continuous wave Doppler in children with ventricular septal defect: non-invasive estimation of interventricular pressure gradient. *American Journal of Cardiology* **57**, 428–432.

18 Patterson, C.E., Lum, H. (2001) Update on pulmonary edema: the role and regulation of endothelial barrier function. *Endothelium* **8**, 75–105.

19 Perkin, R.M., Downey, R.R., Macquarrie, J. (1999) Sleep-disordered breathing in infants and children. *Respiratory Care Clinics of North America* **5**, 395–426.

20 Roberts, J.D., Zapol, W.M. (2000) Inhaled nitric oxide. *Seminars in Perinatology* **24**, 55–58.

21 Robin, E.D., Cross, C.E., Zelis, R. (1973) Pulmonary edema. *New England Journal of Medicine* **239**, 288–292.

22 Rosen, C.L. (1996) Obstructive sleep apnea syndrome (OSAS) in children: diagnostic challenges. *Sleep* **December**, S274–S277.

23 Rudolph, A.M. (2001) *Congenital Diseases of the Heart: Clinical-Physiological Considerations*. New York: Futura.

24 Sie, K.C., Perkins, J.A., Clarke, W.R. (1997) Acute right heart failure due to adenotonsillar hypertrophy. *International Journal of Pediatric Otorhinolaryngology* **41**, 53–58.

25 Uejima, T. (2001) General pediatric emergencies. Acute pulmonary edema. *Anesthesiology Clinics of North America* **19**, 383–389, viii.

26 Wong, J., Vanderford, P.A., Fineman, J.R., Soifer, S.J. (1994) Developmental effects of endothelin-1 on the pulmonary circulation in sheep. *Pediatric Research* **36**, 394–401.

27 Wood, P. (2002) Attacks of deeper cyanosis and loss of consciousness (syncope) in Fallot's tetralogy. *British Heart Journal* **20**, 282–286.

28

Acute respiratory distress syndrome

ANNE GREENOUGH

Acute respiratory distress syndrome (ARDS) follows a catastrophic pulmonary or non-pulmonary event. The term ARDS is used because of the similarities to the abnormalities suffered by prematurely born neonates with RDS (p. 245). ARDS can result from many lung injuries (see below). It is important to consider this diagnosis in infants with severe hypoxemia, so that appropriate management is undertaken.

PATHOLOGY

The pathological features of ARDS are typically described as passing through three overlapping phases – an inflammatory or exudative phase, a proliferative phase and lastly a fibrotic phase.[1] Early in the course of ARDS there is polymorphonuclear leukocyte infiltration, endothelial swelling, interstitial and alveolar edema with type 1 pneumocyte destruction and hyaline membrane formation. Subsequently, type II cell hyperplasia, dense fibrosis centered on alveolar ducts and interstitial emphysema occur.

PATHOPHYSIOLOGY

There is increased permeability of the alveolar-capillary membrane to both fluid and solutes. This results in edema in the alveoli and interstitial space, which reduces compliance and functional residual capacity and increases the physiological dead space. The associated ventilation–perfusion mismatch and the large intrapulmonary shunt result in hypoxemia.[8] In bronchoalveolar lavage (BAL) fluid, lung surfactant has been found to be abnormal, with decreased phosphatidylcholine and phophatidylglycerol.[6]

This reflects direct injury to the type II cells with decreased synthesis, release or processing of surfactant.[10] In addition, the increase in permeability results in plasma proteins entering the alveolar hypophase, which inhibit the surface properties of surfactant.[10] The mechanisms of surfactant inhibition are competitive adsorption and interfacial shielding, chemical degradation of surface apoproteins and phospholipids, surface film fluidization or disruption, subphase binding of surfactant components and alterations in the subphase surfactant aggregates.[3] With the exception of chemical degradation, all of the inhibitory mechanisms can be overcome by raising the surfactant concentration (see below). Administration of surfactants containing higher concentrations of the surfactant proteins A, B and C are likely to be most effective in ARDS, as they are more resistant to inactivation.[15]

ARDS can result from acute lung injury due to a number of causes. These include asphyxia, meconium aspiration, shock, sepsis and disseminated intravascular coagulation.

CLINICAL SIGNS

Infants with ARDS are severely hypoxemic and have an acute onset of diffuse pulmonary infiltrates of non-cardiac origin on their chest radiograph (see below).

MONITORING

Chest radiograph

The chest radiograph demonstrates diffuse pulmonary infiltrates (Figure 28.1), with an appearance similar to

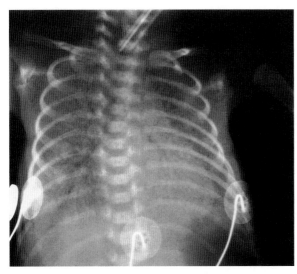

Figure 28.1 *Chest radiograph of an infant with ARDS demonstrating new diffuse pulmonary infiltrates.*

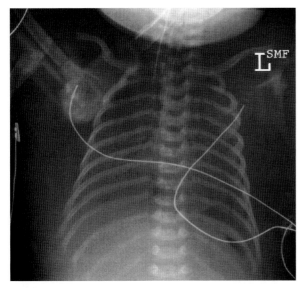

Figure 28.2 *Chest radiograph of an infant with severe hypoxemia. The infant has chest wall edema and severe pulmonary edema as demonstrated by a 'whiteout' on the chest radiograph. The infant developed ARDS following sepsis; he had a good response to HFO.*

RDS (p. 253). In severe cases there may be a complete 'whiteout' (Figure 28.2).

MANAGEMENT

Surfactant administration can improve oxygenation and is most effective if given early[9] and in larger doses than used in RDS (see above).[11] Surfactant dysfunction, however, is only one of the many abnormalities in ARDS, thus even complete normalization of surfactant activity would not be expected to restore lung function to normal. In addition, it is more difficult to deliver adequate doses of surfactant to the alveoli of patients with ARDS compared to those with RDS, in whom pulmonary edema is not a prominent feature.[3] In adults and children with ARDS,[2] prone positioning is associated with improved oxygenation, analogous to that seen in infants with RDS.

The level of positive end expiratory pressure should be increased. In ARDS, because of the decreased lung compliance, the functional residual capacity (FRC) can fall below the closing volume and gas trapping occurs during normal tidal breathing. PEEP can reverse this and increase the FRC. Increasing the PEEP level may further increase oxygenation by increasing the mean airway pressure (p. 158). Excess PEEP, however, will cause alveolar overdistention, increase the alveolar dead space and have detrimental effects on cardiac function. The optimum PEEP level is that which results in maximum tissue oxygen delivery with the lowest inspired oxygen concentration and allowing the inspired oxygen concentration to be reduced to 40–50 percent while maintaining the PaO_2 at greater than 80 mmHg.[7] High-volume strategy HFO can also improve oxygenation,[5] particularly in those infants who had a positive response to PEEP elevation during conventional ventilation (p. 175). High-frequency jet ventilation has also been used with success.[14] Inhaled nitric oxide (iNO) can enhance pulmonary gas exchange with concomitant hemodynamic stabilization in neonates with ARDS. In one series,[4] the most effective dose of iNO was 20 ppm.

PROGNOSIS

Mortality

Despite the advent of new treatment modalities, the mortality of ARDS remains high,[13] particularly in those who are severely hypoxic.[12] The mortality rate is also increased in patients who develop secondary infection or do not respond to elevation of their PEEP level.

Morbidity

There is a high incidence of acute complications, including air leaks and infection. The long-term pulmonary outcome of infants who have had ARDS has not been documented in large series.

REFERENCES

1 Bellingan, G.J. (2000) The pulmonary physician in critical care. The pathogenesis of ALI/ARDS. *Thorax* **57**, 540–546.
2 Curley, M.A., Thompson, J.E., Arnold, J.H. (2000) The effects of early and repeated positioning in paediatric patients with acute lung injury. *Chest* **118**, 156–163.

3 Davis, J.M., Notter, R.H. (1994) Lung surfactant replacement for neonatal abnormalities other than primary respiratory distress syndrome. In Boyton, B.R., Carlo, W.A., Jobe, A.H. (eds), *New Therapies for Neonatal Respiratory Failure*. Cambridge: Cambridge University Press.

4 Demirakca, S., Dotsch, J., Knothe, C. *et al*. (1996) Inhaled nitric oxide in neonatal and paediatric acute respiratory distress syndrome: dose response, prolonged inhalation and weaning. *Critical Care Medicine* **24**, 1913–1919.

5 Giffin, F., Greenough, A. (1994) ARDS-type disease in children: modern respiratory management. *Intensive Care Britain*, 3rd edition. London: Greycoat Publishing, 28–31.

6 Hallman, M., Spragg, R.G., Harell, J.H. (1982) Evidence of lung surfactant abnormality in respiratory failure. Study of bronchoalveolar lavage phospholipids, surface activity, phospholipase and activity and plasma myoinositol. *Journal of Clinical Investigation* **70**, 673–683.

7 Holbrook, P.R., Taylor, G., Pollack, M.M. *et al*. (1980) Adult respiratory distress syndrome in children. *Pediatric Clinics of North America* **27**, 677–685.

8 Lamy, M., Fallat, R.J., Koeniger, E. *et al*. (1976) Pathological features and mechanisms of hypoxemia in adult respiratory distress syndrome. *American Review of Respiratory Disease* **114**, 267–284.

9 Marraro, G.A., Luchetti, M., Galassini, E.M., Abbiati, G. (1999) Natural surfactant supplementation in ARDS in pediatric age. *Minerva Anestesiologica* **65**, 92–97.

10 Nicholas, T.E., Doyle, I.R., Bersten, A.D. (1997) Surfactant replacement therapy in ARDS: white knight or noise in the system? *Thorax* **52**, 195–197.

11 Ogawa, Y., Shimizu, H., Ikatura, Y. *et al*. (1999) Functional pulmonary surfactant deficiency and neonatal respiratory disorders. *Pediatric Pulmonology* **18**, 175–177.

12 Paret, G., Ziv, T., Augarten, A. *et al*. (1999) Acute respiratory distress syndrome in children: a ten year experience. *Israel Medical Association Journal* **1**, 149–153.

13 Pfenninger, J. (1996) Acute respiratory distress syndrome (ARDS) in neonates and children. *Paediatric Anaesthesia* **6**, 173–181.

14 Pfenninger, J., Tschaeppeler, M., Wagner, B.P. *et al*. (1991) The paradox of the adult respiratory distress syndrome in neonates. *Pediatric Pulmonology* **10**, 18–24.

15 Taeusch, H.W., Keough, K.M. (2001) Inactivation of pulmonary surfactant and the treatment of acute lung injuries. *Pediatric Pathology and Molecular Medicine* **20**, 519–536.

29

Bronchopulmonary dysplasia

ILENE RS SOSENKO AND EDUARDO BANCALARI, with introduction by ANNE GREENOUGH

INTRODUCTION

Anne Greenough

The term bronchopulmonary dysplasia (BPD) has been used to encompass all infants who are oxygen dependent at 28 days of age in association with an abnormal chest radiograph appearance. As many affected infants are born at very early gestations, it is not unexpected that they should remain oxygen dependent for the first few weeks after birth. As a consequence, some authors have used an alternative criteria to diagnose BPD, that is oxygen dependence at a postconceptional age of 36 weeks.[11] Some[135] had suggested that the diagnosis of BPD should only be made in infants with severe disease and who fulfilled the historical Northway criteria (Figures 29.1, 29.2, 29.3).[135] In this chapter the term BPD will be used according to the National Institutes of Health (NIH) workshop consensus (p. 40) and distinctive forms of CLD described subsequently in recognition that the forms of chronic respiratory distress are particularly diagnosed in Europe and Japan.

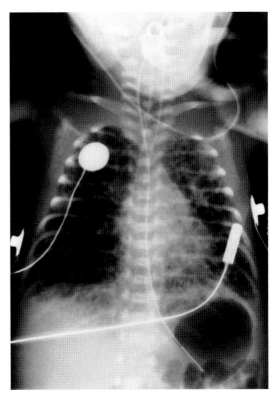

Figure 29.2 *BPD stage 3 (Northway classification). There are cystic abnormalities throughout both lung fields.*

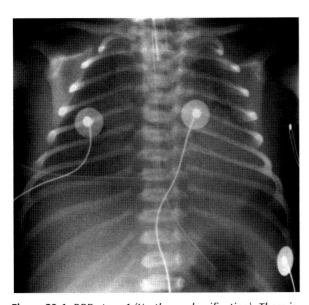

Figure 29.1 *BPD stage 1 (Northway classification). There is diffuse opacification of both lungs.*

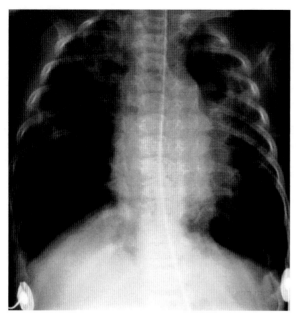

Figure 29.3 *BPD stage 4 (Northway classification). There are gross cystic abnormalities particularly in the bases, hyperinflation and interstitial changes.*

BRONCHOPULMONARY DYSPLASIA

Bronchopulmonary dysplasia (BPD) was first described by Northway and colleagues in 1967 and continues to be a major complication in premature infants who require prolonged mechanical ventilation.[135] The increasing survival of these extremely low birthweight infants has resulted in an incidence of BPD that varies among institutions, with a range between 15 and 50 percent of all infants weighing less than 1500 g at birth.[11,94,142,146,192] Since its original description, the understanding of this chronic lung process has increased, and most recently, the concept, terminology, pathophysiology, clinical course and even the clinical approach to BPD are currently being redefined.

The natural course of severe RDS in the premature infant was altered in the 1960s by the introduction of the ability to manage these infants with mechanical ventilation. As a result of receiving mechanical ventilation, smaller and sicker infants were able to survive. Many of the survivors, however, were left with the sequelae of chronic lung damage. Northway and colleagues named this process bronchopulmonary dysplasia (BPD) and attributed the chronic lung damage to multiple injuries to the immature lung. The original group of infants described had all been born prematurely, had severe RDS, and required prolonged mechanical ventilation with high airway pressures and high inspired oxygen concentrations. The progression of their clinical and radiographic course culminated in severe respiratory failure with hypoxemia and hypercapnia, often with cor pulmonale,

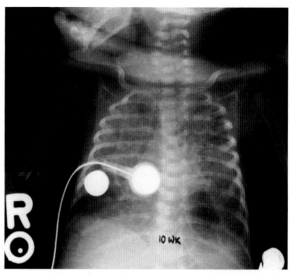

Figure 29.4 *Chest radiograph demonstrating hyperinflation with non-homogeneity of the pulmonary tissues.*

and a chest radiograph demonstrating increased density due to fibrosis, enlarged and emphysematous alveolar areas juxtaposed with areas of collapse (Figure 29.4).[135]

Although much less commonly seen in recent years, this severe form of chronic lung damage usually follows severe respiratory failure due to severe RDS, pneumonia, lung hypoplasia and meconium aspiration syndrome. These infants require mechanical ventilation with high airway pressures and inspired oxygen concentrations during the first days after birth, and frequently their course is complicated by pulmonary interstitial emphysema.[12,13] They may also manifest other complications such as persistent patent ductus arteriosus (PDA) with associated left ventricular failure and pulmonary edema[125] and nosocomial infections, which may contribute to the progression in severity of their lung damage.[73] Despite all therapeutic efforts, these infants frequently remain oxygen and ventilator dependent for prolonged periods of time. Mortality rates for this severe form of chronic lung damage have been reported to be 30–40 percent, with most deaths occurring during the first year after birth, secondary to respiratory failure and intercurrent infections.[86] Follow-up studies of survivors have shown that their pulmonary function may remain abnormal for years, even though the infants may be asymptomatic.[19] Infants with severe BPD also have neurodevelopmental sequelae and impaired growth curves.[23,134,194]

Since the introduction of antenatal steroids, postnatal surfactant therapy and modern respiratory care, the severe clinical presentation of BPD has become much less common in recent years and has been replaced by a milder clinical course. This milder form of chronic disease is often found in small premature infants who survive after prolonged mechanical ventilation. Many of these infants initially present with no RDS or mild RDS that responds rapidly to surfactant therapy, and instead require prolonged mechanical ventilation because of apnea and poor respiratory effort.[152] Thus, these infants have not been exposed to high airway pressures or inspired oxygen concentrations, although they, too, may have been adversely affected by the development of nosocomial infections and PDA, both of which have been identified as important pathogenetic factors.[73] This milder form of illness is often referred to as chronic lung disease (CLD) (Figure 29.5).

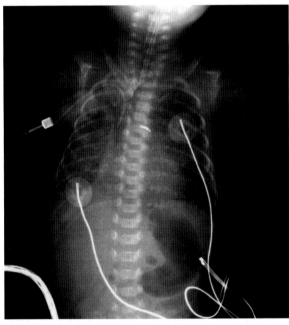

Figure 29.5 *Chest radiograph from an infant with mild BPD. The radiograph demonstrates diffuse haziness only.*

Terminology

Most recently, an NIH-sponsored workshop on BPD was convened to review terminology, definition and current understanding of the process of BPD. When deciding on terminology, the consensus of this workshop was to refer to this disease process as BPD, readopting the name utilized in the older literature, rather than the term CLD, to distinguish this distinct neonatal lung process from the various chronic lung illnesses seen in later life.[104] In addition to readopting the term BPD, a more extensive definition was proposed, which delineates severity (mild, moderate, severe) and distinguishes between infants of less than 32 weeks and greater than 32 weeks of gestational age in terms of diagnostic criteria (Table 29.1).

The reported incidence of BPD varies widely, due not only to differences in patient susceptibility and management, but also to differences in BPD definition. With the adaptation of the new, more extensive definition, more current and precise incidence figures will likely be forthcoming. Other factors responsible for differences in reported incidence include differences in the base population from which incidence is calculated, as well as the indications for mechanical ventilation and the survival rate of ventilated infants. With increasing survival of extremely premature infants, the number of patients at risk for developing BPD increases. The incidence of BPD in infants with RDS who receive mechanical ventilation is closely related to both birthweight and gestational age. BPD is exceedingly uncommon in infants born at greater than 32 weeks of gestation (Figure 29.6). Analysis of the effect of exogenous surfactant therapy on BPD outcome suggests that although surfactant therapy for RDS decreases mortality, it does not appear to independently affect the incidence of BPD. When, however, both

Table 29.1 *Definition of bronchopulmonary dysplasia*

Gestational age	<32 weeks	≥32 weeks
Time point of assessment	36 weeks PMA or discharge to home, whichever comes first Treatment with oxygen >21% for at least 28 days PLUS:	28 days but <56 days postnatal age or discharge to home, whichever comes first
Mild BPD	Breathing room air at 36 weeks PMA or discharge, whichever comes first	Breathing room air by 56 days postnatal age or discharge, whichever comes first
Moderate BPD	Need for >21% but <30% oxygen at 36 weeks PMA or discharge, whichever comes first	Need for >21% but <30% oxygen at 56 days postnatal age or discharge, whichever comes first
Severe BPD	Need for ≥30% oxygen and/or positive pressure (PPV) or positive pressure (PPV or NCPAP) at 36 weeks PMA or discharge, whichever comes first	Need for ≥ 30% oxygen and/or NCPAP at 56 days postnatal age or discharge, whichever comes first

BPD, bronchopulmonary dysplasia; NCPAP, nasal continuous positive airway pressure; PMA, postmenstrual age; PPV, positive pressure ventilation.

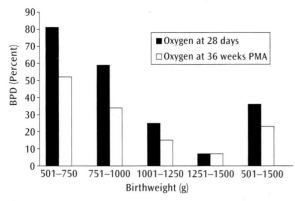

Figure 29.6 *Incidence of BPD (percentage of total births) in the NICHD neonatal research network from January 1995 to December 1996.*

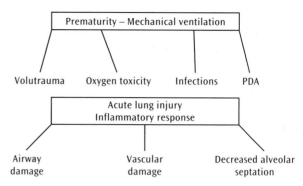

Figure 29.7 *Pathogenesis of BPD.*

endpoints, death and BPD, are analyzed in relation to surfactant administration, the number of infants surviving without BPD has been found to be increased.[40,95,103,115,160]

Pathology

In general, the pathology that has been described for BPD represents the most severe form of chronic lung damage, since those infants with milder forms of BPD rarely die and thus are under-represented in published series of BPD pathology. Macroscopically, the lungs of infants dying of severe BPD are firm, heavy and dark in color, with a grossly abnormal appearance, showing emphysematous areas alternating with areas of collapse. Histologically, the lungs show areas of emphysema, with abnormal alveoli that have coalesced into larger cystic areas, surrounded by areas of atelectasis. Widespread bronchial and bronchiolar mucosal hyperplasia and metaplasia reduce the lumen in many small airways and may interfere with mucus transport.[149] In addition, there is interstitial edema and an increase in fibrous tissue with focal thickening of the basal membrane separating capillaries from alveolar spaces. Lymphatics may be dilated and torturous. There may be vascular evidence of pulmonary hypertension, such as medial muscle hypertrophy, elastic degeneration, and reduction in the branching of the pulmonary vascular bed. The heart may show evidence of right ventricular hypertrophy, and at times left ventricular hypertrophy as well.[125] Infants dying with severe BPD show a marked reduction in the number of alveoli and capillaries, with a reduction in the gas exchange surface area.[38,97,122] Whereas infants who have mild BPD at time of death have diffuse, milder lung injury, with only mild or moderate alveolar septal fibrosis, lack of severe airway epithelial lesions and a normal appearing vascular bed, they, nonetheless, still show evidence of inhibition of acinar development.[97]

Pathogenesis

Many factors, alone or in combination, have been implicated in the pathogenesis of BPD (Figure 29.7). As BPD occurs almost exclusively in premature infants who have received mechanical ventilation with positive pressure, prematurity and barotrauma/volutrauma have been implicated as crucial factors in BPD pathogenesis.[178] Other factors that may play an important role in BPD pathogenesis include oxygen toxicity, inflammation (alone or associated with infection), pulmonary edema resulting from a PDA or excess fluid administration, increased airway resistance and nutritional factors.

PREMATURITY

BPD is presently almost exclusively a problem for the extremely premature infant, occurring rarely in infants of greater than 32 weeks of gestation. The prevalence of BPD in mechanically ventilated infants is inversely related to gestational age and birthweight. One explanation for this vulnerability of the very preterm infant may be the immaturity of lung development. At 24 weeks of gestation the lung is in the canalicular stage of development, which progresses to the sacccular stage by 30 weeks. Thus, it is likely that premature birth and lifesaving therapeutic interventions could disrupt the normal progression of lung development occurring during this crucial developmental period, producing an interruption and/or disruption in the development of alveoli, resulting in significant sequelae.[37]

BAROTRAUMA/VOLUTRAUMA

As most premature infants who develop BPD have received prolonged mechanical ventilation and because of the frequent association between pulmonary interstitial emphysema and BPD (p. 319), it is likely that acute barotrama/volutrauma secondary to positive pressure ventilation plays an important role in the pathogenesis of BPD. It is uncertain whether the presence of an endotracheal tube also contributes to BPD pathogenesis, perhaps by hindering the drainage of bronchial secretions, thereby increasing the risk of pulmonary infections. It is also unclear whether high peak inspiratory pressures associated with mechanical ventilation have a causal effect on the chronic lung damage seen with BPD or whether high pressures are required once lung damage has already occurred. In fact, no significant differences in the incidence of BPD have been found between infants ventilated with low pressures and prolonged inspiration and those ventilated with higher pressures and shorter inspiration. Studies in preterm experimental animals, however, have demonstrated a damaging effect of high airway pressure and high tidal volume in the surfactant-deficient lung. Only a few breaths with excessive tidal volumes, given prior to surfactant replacement, are required to produce a decrease in lung compliance.[18,195] Thus experimental evidence suggests that excessive tidal volumes can damage the lung and initiate the inflammatory cascade.

Similar to the uncertainty about peak inspiratory pressure having a causal effect on BPD or being a result of the disease process, it is also difficult to determine whether the duration of assisted ventilation and oxygen therapy has a separate pathogenetic role in BPD or is merely a marker of the initial severity of the underlying lung disease. The more severe the underlying lung disease, the higher the ventilator and oxygen settings and the longer time required for assisted ventilation.

OXYGEN TOXICITY

Pulmonary oxygen toxicity is considered a major factor in the pathogenesis of BPD.[59,164] The toxicity is felt to be caused by an increased production of cytotoxic oxygen free radicals, which overwhelm the antioxidant defenses in the capillary endothelial cells and the alveolar epithelial cells of the lung. These oxygen free radicals, including the superoxide radical, hydrogen peroxide (hydrogen peroxide is not technically a free radical, but additional free radicals are produced from it), hydroxyl radical and singlet oxygen, are formed from the univalent reduction of molecular oxygen. They can subsequently react with intracellular constituents, including membrane lipids, resulting in chain reactions that can result in cell destruction.[59]

The premature infant, emerging from a relatively hypoxic intrauterine milieu, with oxygen tensions of 20–30 mmHg, encounters an extrauterine environment at birth, which consists of a several-fold increase in oxygen tension. Multiple lines of experimental and epidemiological evidence suggest that the premature newborn is poorly equipped to handle this postnatal increase in oxygen exposure, particularly in relation to incomplete development and inadequate responsiveness of the pulmonary antioxidant enzyme system, consisting of superoxide dismutase, catalase, glutathione peroxidase and the complex glutathione-redox enzymes.[61] In addition, there is interruption at birth of the transplacental delivery of the secondary, chemical system of lung antioxidants, including such substances as glutathione, selenium and other trace metals, vitamins E and C, and ceruloplasmin.[170]

Although many body tissues can be injured by sufficiently high concentrations of oxygen, the lung appears most vulnerable, not due to an increase in inherent tissue sensitivity, but due to its large surface area of type I and II cells which are in direct contact with inspired gases. The precise concentration of oxygen that is toxic to the lung is unknown, and likely depends on a large number of variables, including degree of lung maturation, the nutritional, endocrine and inflammatory status of the infant, and the duration of exposure of oxygen alone and in combination with other pathogenetic factors. A specific safe level of inspired oxygen has not been established; in fact, any concentration in excess of room air may increase the risk of lung damage when administered over a prolonged period of time. Results from the trial exploring the effect of supplemental therapeutic oxygen for prethreshold retinopathy of prematurity (STOP-ROP) demonstrated that providing even modest increases in inspired oxygen concentrations after the first several weeks after birth for at least 2 weeks (to maintain pulse oximetry values of 96–99 percent) produced increases in markers of BPD severity, suggesting a worse pulmonary status.[183]

The pulmonary pathological changes produced in experimental animals as a result of oxygen toxicity are somewhat non-specific, and consist of atelectasis, edema, alveolar hemorrhage, inflammation, fibrin deposition, and thickening and hyalinization of alveolar membranes.[49,59] In addition, there is early damage to capillary endothelium, with plasma leak into interstitial and alveolar spaces. Pulmonary surfactant may be inactivated, further producing atelectasis. Type I alveolar lining cells are injured early, and bronchiolar and tracheal ciliated cells are also vulnerable to damage by oxygen.[21] It is unclear what role alveolar macrophages play in this pathological process. Exposure to a high oxygen concentration, however, does result in an influx of polymorphonuclear leukocytes containing proteolytic enzymes and produces impairment of the antiprotease lung defense system. These factors may contribute to the pathology of pulmonary oxygen toxicity via proteolytic damage of structural elements in alveolar walls.[27] An important additional pathological feature of pulmonary oxygen toxicity is lung growth arrest and a decrease in branching morphogenesis in the lung.[37] Exposure to high oxygen concentrations results in reduction of ciliary movements in cultured neonatal respiratory epithelium, suggesting that loss of mucociliary function secondary to high oxygen may contribute to the development of BPD.[20] It is presumed that cellular pathological processes similar to those described in experimental animals also occur in human infants.

INFECTION AND INFLAMMATION

Evidence has been mounting to support a role for infection and inflammation in the pathogenesis of BPD. This appears to be the case, particularly in very small infants who ultimately develop BPD after receiving prolonged mechanical ventilation for poor respiratory effort rather than because of severe underlying lung disease. Studies have shown that the occurrence of nosocomial infections in these infants is associated with a marked increase in the risk of developing BPD.[152] This is even more pronounced when the infection occurs simultaneously with a PDA.[73]

Increased levels of IgM in infants who go on to develop BPD suggest a possible role for prenatally acquired infections, such as prenatal adenovirus, in the pathogenesis of BPD.[44] Postnatal infection appears to play an important role as well, since cytomegalovirus infection after birth has been associated with an increased incidence of BPD, and respiratory syncytial virus infection is a major cause of deterioration and rehospitalization in infants with established BPD.[158] The evidence of an association between *Ureaplasma urealyticum* tracheal colonization and the development of BPD in very low birthweight (VLBW) infants has been inconsistent.[33,91,93,139,197] Striking, however, has been the increasing evidence that maternal infections, specifically chorioamnionitis, are associated with an increased risk of BPD. Several inflammatory cytokines were found to be in higher concentrations in fetal cord blood and in the amniotic fluid of mothers who delivered infants who subsequently developed BPD.[200,213]

Apart from specific infections, there is increasing evidence suggesting that inflammation plays a major role in the pathogenesis of BPD. The inflammatory response can be triggered not only by prenatal or postnatal infections, but also by a number of non-infectious factors, including oxygen free radicals, positive pressure ventilation, ventilation with excessive tidal volume, and increased pulmonary blood flow due to a PDA.[148] A significant increase in inflammatory cells, eicosanoids and various cytokines has been reported in airways of infants who go on to develop BPD.[83,177] Among the markers of inflammation found in high concentrations in tracheobronchial secretions in these infants are neutrophils, macrophages, leukotrienes, platelet activating factor (PAF), IL-6, IL-8, and tumor necrosis factor (TNF).[26,127,137,171,175,196,199] An increase in cytokine concentration has been found as early as the first days after birth in some infants, supporting the hypothesis that the inflammatory process may start before or shortly after birth. The increased concentration of inflammatory mediators may be responsible for the bronchoconstriction, vasoconstriction and increased vascular permeability characteristic of these infants.[83] Studies have shown increased desmosine excretion in urine during the first week after birth in some infants developing BPD, indicating increased elastin degradation resulting from lung inflammation and injury.[27] By contrast, higher concentrations of fibronectin have been reported in tracheal lavage fluid of infants with BPD, which may promote the development of interstitial fibrosis seen in some patients.[66] The potential role of inflammation in the pathogenesis of BPD is supported by the reported beneficial effects of steroids and possibly sodium cromoglycate in some infants.[10,45,47,174]

Chronic gastroesophageal reflux may be present in infants with BPD, and may exacerbate or maintain inflammatory lung damage and interstitial fibrosis, thereby contributing to a decompensation of lung function.[96,165]

PULMONARY EDEMA AND PATENT DUCTUS ARTERIOSUS

Clinical evidence has demonstrated that infants with RDS who receive greater fluid intake or do not have a diuretic phase in early life have a higher incidence of BPD.[172,190] One explanation for this may be that high fluid intake increases the incidence of PDA, which then produces increased pulmonary blood flow, an increase in interstitial lung fluid and causes a decrease in pulmonary compliance.[15,24,67] This decreased pulmonary compliance, combined with an increased airway resistance, may prolong the requirement for mechanical ventilation with high inspiratory pressures and inspired oxygen concentrations, thereby increasing the risk of BPD. In addition, the increased pulmonary blood flow can induce neutrophil margination and activation in the lung and contribute to the progression of the inflammatory cascade.[193] These inter-related factors could explain the strong association between the duration of the PDA and the increased risk of BPD.[73,126,152]

Additional evidence of the role that pulmonary edema may play in the pathogenesis of BPD comes from the predisposition of infants with established BPD to fluid accumulation in their lungs. Why this occurs is not entirely understood, but likely explanations include functional alternations in pulmonary vascular resistance, low plasma oncotic pressure, increased capillary permeability and impaired lymphatic drainage, all of which favor the extravascular accumulation of fluid. Pulmonary vascular resistance may be elevated because of hypercapnia, hypoxemia, reduced pulmonary vascular bed, and may even be secondary to the left ventricular dysfunction seen in some infants with chronic respiratory failure. Plasma oncotic pressure may be low due to decreased plasma protein content resulting from the poor nutritional state seen in some of these infants. Capillary permeability may be elevated due to the effects of high inspired oxygen concentration, volutrauma or infection on the capillary endothelium. Another factor that may contribute to increased lung water in infants with BPD is the increased plasma levels of vasopressin in some infants, with a reduced urine output and decrease in free water clearance.[92,113,116] With multiple factors contributing to the abnormal accumulation of lung fluid in infants with BPD, lung function is further compromised, perpetuating a cycle in which more aggressive respiratory support is required, thereby resulting in additional lung injury.

INCREASED AIRWAY RESISTANCE

Infants who subsequently develop BPD have increased pulmonary resistance from the first week after birth; therefore, it is possible that airway obstruction may play a significant role in the pathogenesis of BPD.[71,130] Increased airway resistance can alter the time constant of different regions of the lung, impair distribution of the inspired gas, and thereby favor uneven lung expansion. The airway obstruction may be secondary to bronchiolar epithelial hyperplasia and metaplasia and mucosal edema, and may also relate to pulmonary edema secondary to PDA or fluid overload. These infants may also have bronchoconstriction resulting from smooth muscle hypertrophy and even a familial predisposition.[132] Other possible factors producing increased airway resistance in infants with BPD include the inflammatory mediators such as leukotrienes and PAF which have been found in high concentrations in the airways of infants with BPD. Finally, tracheobronchomalacia, which may be present in some infants with severe BPD, can produce marked airway obstruction, particularly during periods of agitation and increased intrathoracic pressure.[123,124,129]

OTHER FACTORS

Several miscellaneous factors have been proposed as having a pathogenetic role in BPD. One of these factors is a genetic predisposition to abnormal airway reactivity, since there have been reports of a stronger family history of asthma in infants with BPD.[132] Vitamin A deficiency has been proposed to play a role, because of evidence that infants who develop BPD have lower vitamin A levels than those who recover without chronic lung damage.[162] This possible association is supported by the similarities between some of the airway epithelial changes observed both in BPD and in vitamin A deficiency and by the recent clinical evidence that vitamin A administration in the first weeks after birth affords some degree of protection against BPD.[161,188] Another factor suggested to play a role in the development of BPD is early adrenal insufficiency, because infants with lower cortisol levels in the first week after birth have an increased incidence of lung inflammation and BPD and early treatment with low dose hydrocortisone increases survival without BPD.[198,201]

Clinical presentation

Once lung damage has occurred, infants can require mechanical ventilation and supplementary oxygen for several weeks or months, sometimes years. An increasing number of small infants have mild respiratory disease, which initially requires ventilation with low pressures and low oxygen concentrations. This is often followed by a few days with minimal or no supplementary oxygen requirement (the so-called 'honeymoon' period). After a few days or weeks of mechanical ventilation, these infants may show progressive deterioration in lung function, an increase in their ventilatory or oxygen requirements, accompanied by signs of respiratory failure and then ultimately develop BPD. This deterioration is frequently triggered by a bacterial or viral infection or heart failure secondary to a PDA.[73]

The clinical progression of infants who survive with BPD is a slow, but steady improvement in both lung function and chest radiographic appearances, with gradual weaning from mechanical ventilation and supplementary oxygen. Chest retractions and tachypnea frequently persist long after extubation, with crackles and bronchial sounds on lung auscultation. Many infants demonstrate lobar or migratory segmental atelectasis (Figure 29.8), as a result of retained secretions and airway obstruction.

Infants with more severe BPD may evolve into progressive respiratory failure and even death as a result of more severe lung damage, pulmonary hypertension resulting in cor pulmonale, with signs of right heart failure including cardiomegaly, hepatomegaly and fluid retention or intercurrent infections. These more severely affected infants may also develop severe airway damage with bronchomalacia, which can lead to significant airway obstruction, particularly during episodes of agitation and increased intrathoracic pressure.[124,129] Sudden episodes of severe cyanosis with wheezing may occur, at such times the infants are difficult to ventilate even when an anesthesia bag and high pressure are used. Spontaneous desaturations occur frequently in ventilated infants with BPD.[52] In one series, whereas spontaneous desaturations to an oxygen saturation of less than 90 percent occurred for 4–5 percent of the time in infants with acute lung disease, they occurred for 27.1 percent of the time in the chronic patients. The number of more severe desaturations (oxygen saturation of less than 80 percent) was also significantly greater in the BPD group.[52] Some of these infants may develop anastomoses between the systemic and pulmonary circulations, which may aggravate their pulmonary hypertension.[74] Acute pulmonary infection, either bacterial or viral, frequently complicates the course of BPD and in many cases is the precipitating cause of death in infants with severe lung damage.[86] Currently, this severe pattern of BPD disease accounts for less than a fourth of all the infants with BPD at our institution.

Often infants with BPD have difficulty in taking oral feeds, as a result of their respiratory failure, and may require nasogastric or orogastric feeding. Due to the

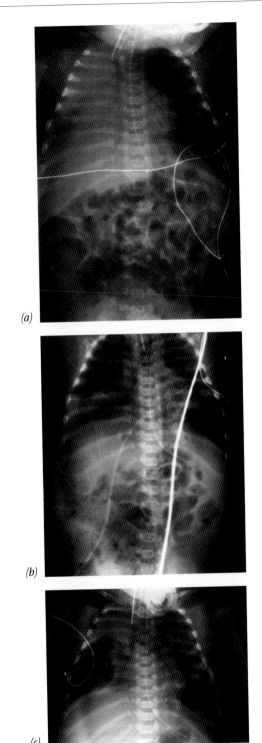

(a)

(b)

(c)

Figures 29.8 *A series of chest radiographs demonstrating the pattern of lobar collapse which can complicate prolonged ventilation for BPD. (a) This chest radiograph demonstrates that the right lung is collapsed and there is hyperinflation of the left lung. (b) This radiograph demonstrates collapse of the middle lobe and to a lesser extent the right lower lobe. (c) This radiograph demonstrates that the right upper lobe is now collapsed and there are areas of both segmental atelectasis and hyperinflation of both lungs.*

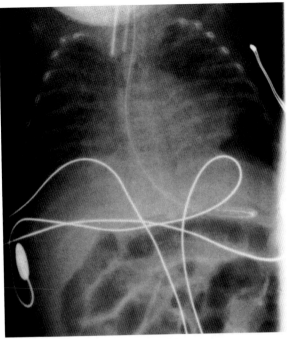

Figure 29.9 *Chest radiograph of an infant with BPD demonstrating demineralization of the ribs.*

chronic hypoxia and higher energy expenditure required by their increased work of breathing, weight gain in these infants is usually below normal, even when receiving appropriate caloric intake for their age. In addition, a tendency toward fluid retention and pulmonary edema may necessitate fluid restriction as well as diuretic therapy, further limiting the calories that can be provided and compromising weight gain.

Osteopenia is a frequent complication of CLD (Figure 29.9) and as a consequence rib (Figure 29.10) and other (Figure 29.11) fractures are not uncommon.[173] Calcium is deposited in the bones in the last 2 months of gestation and, typically, infants with BPD are born prior to this time. In addition, solutions for parenteral alimentation are low in calcium and vitamin D and the infants may be undergoing treatment with diuretics, which are potent calciurics.

Differential diagnosis

The diagnosis of BPD is based on the clinical course and chest radiograph changes, but these are not specific for any given etiology, hence other specific etiologies must be considered in the differential diagnosis. These include viral, fungal or bacterial infections, congenital heart disease, such as total anomalous pulmonary venous return, pulmonary lymphangiectasia, chemical pneumonitis resulting from recurrent aspiration, cystic fibrosis, idiopathic pulmonary fibrosis, surfactant protein B deficiency and Wilson–Mikety syndrome (p. 414).

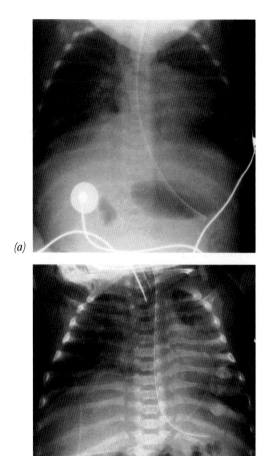

(a)

(b)

Figures 29.10 *(a) Chest radiograph of a BPD infant demonstrating demineralization of the ribs and rib fractures on the right. (b) Chest radiograph demonstrating healing rib fractures on the left.*

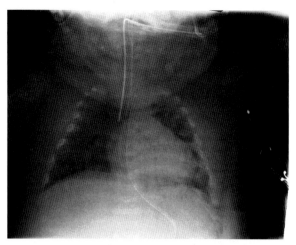

Figure 29.11 *Severe changes of metabolic bone disease with generalized osteopenia and pathological fractures. There is a pathological fracture of the right humerus.*

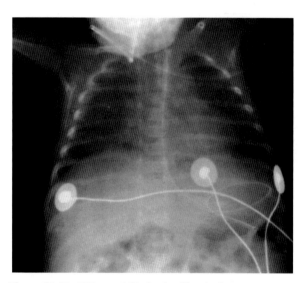

Figure 29.12 *CLD type I (Hyde classification).*

Diagnosis

The diagnosis is made using clinical and chest radiograph appearance manifestations, which are not specific.[53] With rare exceptions, BPD is preceded by the use of intermittent positive pressure ventilation early in life. The indications for mechanical ventilation can include respiratory failure from RDS, pneumonia, other forms of lung pathology or poor respiratory effort. When mechanical ventilation and oxygen dependence begin to extend beyond 10–14 days, the development of BPD is suspected.

RADIOLOGY

Radiographic confirmation, which typically does not develop until later in the course, includes hyperinflation and non-homogeneity of pulmonary tissues, with finer or coarser densities extending to the periphery, with or without cystic translucencies in the more severe forms of BPD (Figure 29.3). In milder forms, the radiographic changes are less severe, revealing mainly diffuse haziness (Figure 29.1). Those chest radiograph appearances have previously been termed type II (Figure 29.3) and type I (Figure 29.12) CLD, respectively.[99] Only a clinical course that is compatible with BPD and a chest radiograph picture showing chronic pulmonary involvement enables the assignment of this diagnosis with some degree of consistency.

Monitoring

RADIOGRAPHY

A variety of chest radiograph scoring systems have been developed to predict and/or monitor the progress of

Table 29.2 *Simple chest radiograph scoring system[78]*

	0	1	2	3	4
Degree of expansion*	<14	14–16	>16		
Fibrosis/interstitial shadows** (absent/present)	Absent	1 zone	2 zones	3 zones	4 zones
Cystic elements***	Absent	Small	Multiple/large		

*Number of posterior ribs visible above the diaphragm bilaterally.
**Focal areas of linear or nodular density within a zonal basis (chest divided into the right upper and lower and the left upper and lower zones).
***Lucent intraparenchymal lesions with a well circumscribed margin.

BPD.[53,187,217] More recently, a simplified system has been developed (Table 29.2).[78] Using this system it was possible to differentiate between those who were and were not oxygen dependent at 36 weeks PCA[78] and to predict recurrent respiratory symptoms at 6 months corrected age.[185] Others have also demonstrated that the chest radiograph appearance can predict long-term outcome.[143] Use of a system in which changes of opacification and hyperinflation/emphysema were scored, demonstrated that the chest radiographic appearance can be predictive of which infants will respond to dexamethasone.[159] Eighty percent of responders to dexamethasone had opacification on their chest radiograph, whereas seven of eight infants with emphysema and 80 percent of infants with a mixed picture of emphysema and consolidation were non-responders.[159] Infants with BPD frequently develop osteopenia of prematurity (p. 514). Chest radiographs should be carefully examined for the presence of rib fractures (Figure 29.10).

TRANSCUTANEOUS OXYGEN AND OXYGEN SATURATION

Chronic, even intermittent, hypoxia increases pulmonary vascular resistance, leading to pulmonary hypertension and right heart failure in infants with BPD. Transcutaneous oxygen (TcO_2) monitoring significantly underestimates arterial PaO_2 in infants with BPD.[90,153] Pulse oximetry offers major advantages over transcutaneous measurements in the management of infants with BPD, as the sensors do not require calibration and are unheated, thus will not cause skin burns.[169] The minimum oxygen saturation level at which to maintain infants with BPD is disputed (p. 411).

PULMONARY FUNCTION

As a result of the structural alterations of their lungs, infants with BPD demonstrate disruption of pulmonary function. Minute ventilation is usually increased. This is accomplished with a smaller tidal volume and higher respiratory rate due to lower lung compliance. There is an increase in dead space ventilation, which in part explains their alveolar hypoventilation and CO_2 retention. Airway

resistance and airway reactivity are markedly increased, resulting in a decreased dynamic compliance.[30,68,81] Lung compliance may also be decreased because of fibrosis, overdistention, collapse of lung parenchyma, or a decreased concentration of surfactant.[35] The high resistance and decreased compliance thereby result in a markedly increased work of breathing. FRC is initially low or normal. In cases of severe BPD, FRC may increase later due to abnormalities in distribution of ventilation, reflecting small airway involvement.[71] In infants with mild BPD, the distribution of inspired gas is usually normal as measured by nitrogen clearance delay.[204]

Most infants with severe BPD have marked hypoxemia and hypercapnia. The hypoxemia is mainly due to a combination of ventilation–perfusion mismatch and to alveolar hypoventilation. The oxygen requirement decreases with time as the disease improves, but may increase during feedings, physical activity, agitation, or episodes of lung infection or pulmonary edema. The hypercapnia in infants with severe BPD is secondary to alveolar hypoventilation and to an increased alveolar–arterial CO_2 gradient caused by mismatch of ventilation and perfusion and increased alveolar dead space. The chronic hypercapnia and respiratory acidosis in infants with BPD results in an increased serum bicarbonate concentration, which attempts to compensate for the respiratory acidosis. The diuretics frequently employed in the management of infants with BPD tend to exaggerate this increase in base.

CARDIOVASCULAR STATUS

Infants with BPD may develop pulmonary hypertension; this is indicated on clinical examination by a single heart sound and possibly the murmur of tricuspid regurgitation. Electrocardiograms should be performed routinely once a week, as this will give an indirect assessment of the severity of right ventricular hypertension secondary to pulmonary artery hypertension. Echocardiography is also a useful non-invasive assessment of right ventricular pressure. Increased right ventricular pressure is indicated by the contour of the interventricular septum, which becomes straightened as the right ventricular pressure increases until it exceeds the systemic pressure, resulting in bowing of the septum into the left ventricle. Cardiac catheterization of infants with CLD is not routinely indicated, but does allow assessment of the responsiveness of the pulmonary vascular bed to potential vasodilators (p. 380).

BLOOD PRESSURE

It has been suggested that a high proportion (40 percent) of infants with BPD develop systemic hypertension.[1] The mechanism may be a renal complication of prolonged umbilical arterial catheterization or renal damage due to nephrocalcinosis. Although the hypertension is frequently transient and responds well to antihypertensive medication, it may result in left ventricular hypertrophy or even cerebrovascular hemorrhage. Hypertensive infants on home oxygen required a longer duration of home oxygen and a greater proportion died (36 versus 1 percent) than those who were not hypertensive.[6] Thus, close blood pressure monitoring is recommended even at follow-up of BPD infants. Blood pressure elevation also occurs in infants with less severe disease, but this does appear to be mild and not associated with clinical abnormalities.[55]

RENAL FUNCTION

Infants with BPD are prone to nephrocalcinosis and should have regular renal ultrasounds. This complication is particularly common in BPD infants receiving maintenance diuretic therapy, but other risk factors include renal candidiasis, a family history of renal stones, parental nutrition and oliguria.

Prophylaxis

Strategies to prevent BPD focus on eliminating or reducing the multiplicity of factors known to contribute to lung injury (Table 29.3). Since lung immaturity is the main predisposing factor in the pathogenesis of BPD, prevention of BPD should start prenatally by attempting to prolong pregnancy as much as possible. When preterm birth is imminent, administration of antenatal steroids has been found to reduce the incidence and severity of RDS and the subsequent development of BPD.[191]

RESPIRATORY SUPPORT

Strict attention should be given to the application of mechanical ventilation and oxygen therapy, with a goal of minimizing volutrauma from exposure to high airway pressures[70] and minimizing oxygen toxicity from exposure to high inspired oxygen concentrations. Surfactant replacement therapy in infants with RDS improves the respiratory course, usually enabling successful mechanical ventilation with low inspiratory pressures and oxygen

Table 29.3 *Potential strategies to prevent BPD*

Established
Prolongation of pregnancy
Minimizing volutrauma and the duration of mechanical ventilation
Minimizing oxygen toxicity
Prevention/aggressive management of pre- and postnatal infections
Avoidance of excessive fluid administration
Prompt PDA closure
Nutritional intervention

Investigational
Exogenous administration of antioxidant enzymes
Induction of cytochrome P_{450} system
Gene therapy/genetic manipulation

---

concentrations.[40,95,103,115,160] The use of positive end expiratory pressure (PEEP) is critical, because insufficient PEEP is associated with marked increase in ventilator-associated lung damage. Ventilation at high frequencies may not reduce BPD in infants (p. 172), but data from experimental animals suggest that this ventilation modality may reduce lung injury.[7,41,69,100,102,150,186] There is an increased risk of BPD in infants exposed to prenatal and postnatal infections; as a consequence prevention and aggressive management of these infections should play a preventative role in BPD.

FLUID BALANCE

Attention to fluid administration with avoidance of excessive fluid intake is important in the prevention of BPD.[190] Furthermore, since lung injury is associated with capillary damage and increased water permeability, infants with developing BPD demonstrate a predisposition for pulmonary edema. Fluid administration in these infants should be restricted to the minimal intake necessary to keep a normal fluid and electrolyte balance while supplying necessary calories for growth. Randomized trials of fluid restriction versus 'normal' maintenance fluid volumes, however, have failed to highlight that fluid restriction reduces the incidence of BPD.[114] Diuretics, specifically loop diuretics, may be necessary, not only to increase renal water losses, but also to improve pulmonary fluid balance and reduce interstitial lung water, independent from their renal effects.[16] Evidence that the presence of a PDA is associated with an increased risk of BPD suggests that prompt closure of a PDA, using prostaglandin inhibitors or by surgical ligation, may be important in reducing the risk and/or severity of BPD.[43,73,126]

NUTRITION

Attention to nutritional issues may be crucial in BPD prevention (p. 216). There is considerable experimental evidence that undernutrition and, in particular, an insufficiency in dietary protein may increase the vulnerability of the preterm infant to oxidant lung injury and the development of BPD.[50] Dietary provision of lipid, particularly polyunsaturated fatty acids, in addition to preventing essential fatty acid deficiency may also play a role in preventing or reducing the severity of BPD, although animal and human data are conflicting. Whether early administration of intralipid plays any protective function against BPD is yet to be determined.[170] Meta-analysis of the results of clinical trials failed to show a protective effect of early administration of intralipid,[58] but it is possible that these findings are explained by the toxicity of lipid peroxidation products within the lipid preparation. The manufacturing process has recently been modified to markedly reduce the levels of lipid hydroperoxides within some intralipid preparations, so it is possible that future investigations may show a protective role for early intralipid administration against BPD. Additional nutrients, including those that may increase intracellular glutathione (such as sulfur-containing amino acids), inositol to serve as substrate for surfactant, selenium and other trace minerals to function as essential cofactors for the pulmonary antioxidant enzymes, and vitamin A, may provide added protection to the premature infants against the development of BPD.[170] Epidemiological evidence has shown that premature infants who subsequently develop BPD have lower plasma levels of vitamin A within the first month after birth. Subsequent clinical trials in preterm infants with severe RDS have shown that vitamin A administration reduced the incidence and severity of BPD.[98,147,161,163,188]

FUTURE DIRECTIONS

Future directions in BPD prevention may include exogenous administration of specific antioxidants, such as superoxide dismutase,[48,155,180] or inducers of the cytochrome P_{450} system. Initial controlled clinical trials of human recombinant copper/zinc superoxide dismutase instilled in the trachea of premature infants have shown reduction in tracheal injury markers, but no differences in BPD. Other possibilities may include gene therapy or genetic manipulation and strategies for maturing the preterm lung that have greater selectivity and fewer adverse effects than glucocorticoids.

Management

Management strategies for BPD infants are based on avoiding, as much as possible, some of the proposed causative factors for producing chronic lung damage. These include mechanical ventilation, high oxygen concentrations, excess fluid administration, PDA and lung infection.

MECHANICAL VENTILATION

Mechanical ventilation should only be used when clearly indicated in infants with BPD and lung overdistention avoided. This strategy involves using the lowest peak airway pressure necessary to obtain adequate ventilation, with inspiratory times of at least 0.3 seconds and with flow rates between 5 and 10 l/min. When shorter inspiratory times and high flow rates are used, there may be an exaggeration of the maldistribution of inspired gas, whereas longer inspiratory times may increase the risk of alveolar rupture and cardiovascular side-effects. The use of end expiratory pressure between 4 and 6 cmH$_2$O enables the use of a minimum oxygen concentration to keep the PaO_2 above 50 mmHg. In infants with severe airway obstruction, often due to bronchomalacia, the use of higher levels of PEEP (5–8 cmH$_2$O) may reduce expiratory airway resistance and improve alveolar ventilation.[144]

Tracheostomy

Many infants with BPD require prolonged ventilation. Chronic use of either an oral or nasal endotracheal tube can be associated with cosmetic problems due to mechanical deformation of soft tissues (p. 155). Although tracheostomy avoids such problems and makes nursing of an increasingly active infant easier, tracheostomies are not without problems and may not be closed for a number of years in this population. One policy is to restrict their use to infants who remain fully ventilated at 3 months of age.

Weaning

Mechanical ventilation in infants with BPD should be used for as short a duration as possible, as this strategy reduces the risk of volutrauma and infection. Weaning ventilator-dependent infants with BPD is extremely difficult, so it must be accomplished gradually. Allowing permissive hypercapnia (p. 158), that is elevated $PaCO_2$ values in the 50s or 60s (mmHg), providing the pH is within acceptable limits, facilitates this weaning process. When the infant is able to maintain an acceptable PaO_2 and $PaCO_2$ with low peak inspiratory pressures (in the range of 15–18 cmH$_2$O or lower) and an inspired oxygen concentration lower than 0.3–0.4, the ventilator rate should be gradually reduced to allow the infant to perform an increasing proportion of the minute ventilation. To facilitate weaning and eventual extubation in small infants, aminophylline or caffeine can be used as a respiratory stimulant during the weaning period,[77] although this may be less successful when used in infants older than 1 month.[154] When the infant demonstrates the ability to maintain acceptable blood gas values after several hours on low ventilator rates (20 breaths/min) with low ventilator pressures, it is prudent to give a trial of extubation. Chest physiotherapy and even direct endotracheal suctioning may be necessary, because of the possibility of airway obstruction and lung collapse secondary to retained secretions following extubation. In a randomized trial,[34] there was no difference overall in the reintubation rate following extubation to either headbox or nasal CPAP. Nevertheless, anecdotally, small infants benefit from the use of nasal CPAP for a period of time following extubation to stabilize their respiratory function.

SUPPLEMENTARY OXYGEN

The approach to supplementary oxygen therapy in infants with BPD is a complex one. On the one hand, it is necessary to reduce the inspired oxygen concentration as quickly as tolerated, to avoid pulmonary oxygen toxicity. On the other hand, it is crucial to maintain the PaO_2 at a level which provides adequate tissue oxygenation and avoids the pulmonary hypertension and cor pulmonale that can result from chronic hypoxemia[2,89] and the episodes of increased airway resistance which can result from acute hypoxemia.[181,182] It is recommended that the PaO_2 be maintained above 50–55 mmHg to prevent the above effects of hypoxemia. This may require an increase in the inspired oxygen concentration during periods of feeding, bathing, or agitation when oxygen consumption is increased.[166] Pulse oximetry offers the most reliable means of assessing oxygenation in these infants, and enables the assessment of oxygenation not just at rest, but also during activity. Supplementary oxygen should be administered to infants with BPD to maintain their oxygen saturation level at least at 92 percent, although some would suggest the minimum level should be 95 percent (p. 225).

Infants with BPD may have increased metabolic demands associated with low arterial oxygen tension.[205] Therefore, the maintenance of a relatively normal blood hemoglobin concentration by either blood transfusions and/or administration of recombinant erythropoietin is an important part of therapy for infants with BPD.

In infants with severe BPD, oxygen therapy may be required for several months or even years. Some of these babies may be discharged on home oxygen therapy, which can offer a better environment for a growing infant and a cost savings, but which requires the proper family and home environment to ensure the oxygen therapy is administered safely and successfully (p. 190).

FLUID MANAGEMENT AND DIURETIC THERAPY

Poor fluid tolerance is a characteristic of most infants with BPD. These infants have difficulty tolerating an excessive or even, in some cases, a normal fluid intake. This is manifested by a tendency to accumulate excessive interstitial fluid in the lung, which can result in deterioration of pulmonary function and a worsening of hypoxemia, hypercapnia and ventilator dependency.[92,116] Fluid management of infants with BPD involves limiting water and salt intake to the minimum required to provide adequate fluid for metabolic needs and adequate calories for growth.[42,179]

Diuretics may be necessary when increased lung water persists, despite fluid restriction. Infants with BPD respond to diuretics with a rapid improvement in lung compliance and decrease in resistance, but without necessarily improving blood gas measurements.[4,56,106,111,136] Complications of chronic diuretic therapy include hypokalemia, hyponatremia, metabolic alkalosis, hypercalciuria with nephrocalcinosis and hypochloremia.[107] Some of these side-effects may be reduced by using either alternate day therapy with furosemide[156] or thiazide diuretics.

NUTRITION

The appropriate nutritional support for BPD infants is crucial for lung growth, as well as somatic growth and the development of all organ systems, but is a process fraught with difficulties in such complex infants. Provision of adequate calories is confounded by the relatively high caloric requirements required for growth (sometimes as high as 150–160 kcal/kg) and the inability of many of these infants to handle a high fluid intake.[119] Infants with BPD have a high resting oxygen consumption, partially related to their increased work of breathing.[205,210] Dietary management of these infants can be further complicated by the fact that excessive glucose intake can increase their carbon dioxide production, further compromising respiratory function.[218] In addition, feeding difficulties are common in these infants, including sucking and swallowing problems. They may also suffer from gastroesophageal reflux, often requiring medical and occasionally surgical management. Yet, inadequate nutrition in infants with BPD can potentially delay somatic growth, the repair and development of new alveoli (thereby delaying successful weaning from mechanical ventilation), and make these infants more prone to infection and oxygen toxicity.[62] An aggressive approach to nutrition, therefore, should be taken in infants with BPD, with the goal of supplying parenteral and/or oral caloric intake adequate for growth. High calorie formulas or breast milk with supplementation with human milk fortifier enable the intake of calories to be maximized, while fluid intake can be restricted to prevent pulmonary edema and even congestive heart failure in severe cases of BPD.[29] Another way to improve caloric density without increasing fluid intake significantly is to supplement formula or breast milk with medium chain triglyceride (MCT) oil, glucose polymers and/or rice cereal. If for any reason, enteral nutrition is precluded for even a brief time, parenteral alimentation with glucose, amino acids and fat should be given, until the infant is able to tolerate enteral feedings. The adequacy of nutrition should be closely monitored, using growth charts for weight, head circumference and height. Other means of assessing growth include arm anthropometry to determine muscle mass and fat deposits and measurement of serum albumin levels.

Infants with BPD often manifest signs of rickets, with rib fractures on routine chest roentgenograms (Figure 29.10), together with generalized bone demineralization (Figure 29.9). This is due to inadequate calcium, phosphorus and vitamin D intake during prolonged parenteral nutrition, the calciuria resulting from chronic diuretic therapy and from glucocorticoid therapy. Administration of extra calcium and vitamin D may prevent or improve rickets in these infants. Several specific nutrients may be important in terms of BPD prevention or repair. These include polyunsaturated fatty acids, vitamin A, trace elements such as copper, zinc, magnesium and selenium, and sulfur-containing amino acids (p. 218).[170]

PHARMACOLOGICAL THERAPY

Bronchodilator therapy

Infants with severe BPD have airway smooth muscle hypertrophy and airway hyperreactivity. In order to avoid bronchoconstriction in these infants, maintenance of adequate oxygenation is crucial, as hypoxia can increase their airway resistance. Bronchodilators, most of them β-agonists, administered by inhalation, have been shown to reduce airway resistance in infants with BPD.[28,72,108,110] Their effect, however, is short-lived and often associated with cardiovascular side-effects (for example tachycardia, hypertension and possible arrhythmias). As a consequence, their use should be limited to the management of acute exacerbations of airway obstruction. A metered dose inhaler (MDI) and spacer device is the preferred method of administration rather than by nebulization. In certain infants, nebulized bronchodilator can cause an initial paradoxical deterioration in lung function, as demonstrated by an increase in airways resistance;[216] this can be avoided by using an MDI and the same degree of subsequent bronchodilation achieved. Use of nebulized therapy should be restricted to hospitalized infants and those undergoing careful monitoring with supplementary oxygen readily available.

The methylxanthine family of bronchodilators (aminophylline and caffeine) were previously a mainstay of chronic BPD therapy, but are now used much less frequently. These drugs have been shown to reduce airway resistance in BPD infants and have other potential beneficial effects, including respiratory stimulation, a mild diuretic effect, and improvement in respiratory muscle contractility.[46,109,154] They do, however, have many side-effects; as a consequence their use should be limited to specific, severe cases where clear benefit has been demonstrated.

Sodium cromoglycate has been used in an attempt to reduce airway resistance, because of the increased concentration of leukotrienes in bronchial secretions of infants with BPD. Its use in established BPD has been associated with a clinical improvement and a reduction in the inspired oxygen concentration and ventilator pressures.[174] Experience is too limited to recommend widespread use.[174] At follow-up, however, it does reduce symptoms and the need for additional bronchodilator therapy and improves lung function in symptomatic VLBW infants, when administered via an MDI and simple spacer device.[215]

Pulmonary vasodilators

Infants with severe BPD may develop pulmonary hypertension. Oxygen therapy is felt to be the most effective means of reducing pulmonary hypertension in these infants.[89] The pulmonary vascular resistance is very sensitive to changes in alveolar P_{O_2} in BPD infants; it is crucial therefore to provide these infants with adequate oxygenation at all times, including at times of sleeping, feeding, crying and physical activity. Inhaled nitric oxide can be used to reduce pulmonary vascular resistance in infants with BPD and severe pulmonary hypertension (p. 183). The advantage of nitric oxide therapy is that it causes pulmonary vasodilatation without producing systemic dilatation, thereby potentially improving ventilation–perfusion matching in the lung.[14] The calcium channel blocker nifedipine can cause a decrease in pulmonary vascular resistance in BPD infants with severe pulmonary hypertension and cor pulmonale but this is associated with systemic vasodilatation and depression of myocardial function, which limit its usefulness.[25,105]

Corticosteroid therapy

The use of corticosteroids in the treatment of BPD is controversial with regard to the risk–benefit ratio and long-term efficacy. The rationale for corticosteroid use is based on the evidence that inflammation is an important pathogenetic factor in BPD.[211] Studies have examined whether there could be a potential role for exogenous administration of corticosteroids during the early stages of the disease to reduce its progression or during the later stages to improve respiratory outcome. Several reports have shown that corticosteroid compared to placebo administration results in a rapid improvement in lung function, facilitating weaning from the ventilator.[8,10,45,145] It has not yet been established that these acutely observed improvements in respiratory status translate into decreased morbidity, mortality or length of hospital stay. The optimal age of treatment, dose schedule and duration of therapy remain to be identified.[9,17,88,138,140]

Corticosteroids may produce beneficial effects by a number of different mechanisms. They appear to enhance production of surfactant and antioxidant enzymes, decrease bronchospasm, pulmonary and bronchial edema and fibrosis, improve vitamin A status, and decrease inflammatory cells and mediators in the lung.[82,112,203] The side-effects of corticosteroid therapy are well recognized, including hyperglycemia, arterial hypertension, increased proteolysis, masking signs of infection, adrenocortical suppression, somatic and lung growth suppression, and hypertrophic cardiomyopathy.[5,54,60,101,138,176,177,184,189,206] Most alarming are recent follow-up data demonstrating that infants who received short or prolonged steroid therapy have worse neurological outcome compared to controls.[22,133,141,212] Those results have caused cautionary flags to be raised in relation to the use of corticosteroid therapy in BPD. Recent recommendations include that systemic corticosteroids should only be used after the first several weeks after birth and reserved for infants who show clear evidence of progressive pulmonary damage, remain oxygen and ventilator dependent, and whose clinical status suggests they might be capable of tolerating a trial of extubation in response to a corticosteroid course. The duration of therapy should be limited to the minimum needed for efficacy.

Preliminary data suggest that providing steroids to the ventilator-dependent infant by inhalation, rather than by the systemic route, may induce beneficial effects on the lung with minimum side-effects.[36,39,120] The data, however, are not conclusive enough to recommend their routine use in infants with BPD.[57,84,128]

CONTROL OF INFECTION

Infants with BPD risk serious setbacks if infected with bacterial, fungal or even viral agents.[214] It is crucial that measures be in place to prevent pulmonary nosocomial infections, including meticulous hand washing before handling the airway, maintaining sterility of respiratory equipment and isolation from individuals with respiratory infection. In addition, these infants require close monitoring for early signs of infection, including the periodic collection of tracheal secretions for culture and Gram stain, and obtaining a full blood count, blood culture and chest radiograph if pneumonia is suspected. Often the quality or quantity of secretions indicate the possibility of infection, but it can be difficult to distinguish between true infection and airway colonization (p. 73). Overtreatment with antibiotics, however, should be avoided to prevent emergence of more virulent organisms. Antibiotics should be selected according to the sensitivity of the implicated organisms and continued until the infection is eradicated.

INFANT STIMULATION AND PARENTAL SUPPORT

Infants with BPD may require respiratory support for several months and thereby be deprived of normal parental stimulation. These infants often show developmental delays, which may be compounded by gross neurological handicap. Thus, a well-organized program of infant stimulation, including physiotherapy, speech and occupational therapy, may help such infants to achieve their maximum potential. Progress should be monitored by serial developmental evaluations and emphasis placed on areas where delay is evident.

Parents of infants with BPD experience serious emotional trauma in dealing with the realities of prematurity, the intensive care environment, repeated life-threatening illnesses and separation from their infant, as well as the possibility of a chronic lung disorder. In addition, they lose considerable control of their child to the hospital staff, particularly in areas related to medical care. For these reasons, parental participation in various aspects of their infant's care is crucial to the development of the child and the establishment of an appropriate parent–infant attachment. Parents, therefore, should be encouraged to visit frequently and to participate in the day-to-day care of their child. Continuing parental support from medical personnel, social services and parent support groups is essential during prolonged hospitalization and the complexities of follow-up care.[51,85]

OUTCOME

The outcome of BPD has improved in recent years, as the majority of affected infants manifest a milder pathological process and experience better management. Mortality from BPD is low and is usually the result either of sepsis or overwhelming infection or severe respiratory failure associated with pulmonary hypertension and cor pulmonale.

Infants with BPD are at high risk for lower respiratory tract infections during the first year after birth and rehospitalization for episodes of wheezing suggestive of bronchiolitis or asthma are common during the first 2 years.[131] Infection with respiratory syncytial virus (RSV) can result in prolonged hospitalization and even death in these infants. (Review of a BPD cohort demonstrated that on average three (0–20) readmissions were required during the first 2 years after birth[80] the readmission rate was approximately doubled in those being discharged home on supplementary oxygen.[79] Infants who had had at least one admission for proven RSV infection compared to the other BPD infants, required more frequent and longer admissions to the general pediatric wards and intensive care units, more outpatient attendances and GP consultations for respiratory-related disorders and a higher total cost of care.[80]) RSV prophylaxis is, therefore, an important aspect of care both before and after hospital discharge (p. 295).[86]

Studies at follow-up have demonstrated that infants with a history of severe BPD have abnormal pulmonary function, even after they become asymptomatic.[19,87] A high incidence of obstructive airway disease has been described in a small group of BPD survivors at 8 years of age.[168] Follow-up of the original cohort of infants with BPD described by Northway demonstrated that at 18 years of age, the young adults had evidence of airway obstruction and hyperactivity and hyperinflation.[134] The ultimate clinical consequences of these findings remain to be determined, but the results of most long-term studies suggest that, with growth and time, pulmonary function tends to normalize, especially in the more recent groups with milder forms of BPD.

Infants with severe BPD have more neurodevelopmental sequelae when compared to infants without BPD, this in part related to associated risk factors in addition to the presence of BPD. In addition, BPD infants have transient impairment in growth.[23,121,122,167,194] Infants with BPD have been reported to have an increased risk for sudden infant death, but evidence for this finding is not conclusive.[3,75,207]

OTHER FORMS OF CHRONIC LUNG DISEASE

Anne Greenough

It is disputed whether there are distinct forms of CLD or infants with chronic supplementary oxygen requirements should rather be classified simply according to the severity of their disease. Distinctive clinical presentations and chest radiograph appearances, have been recognised. In the USA these are now recognised as BPD, but elsewhere distinctive forms of chronic respiratory distress are still recognised.

Respiratory insufficiency

Wung *et al.* described a lung disease which occurred in very small infants, usually of birthweight less than 1000 g, and which appeared to be due to immaturity.[209] The infants initially had either no respiratory problems or only mild RDS and had not required ventilation. Their illness was characterized by apnea and bradycardia and their prognosis was good, with the disease mainly resolving before discharge. The chest radiograph was characterized by diffuse haziness, streaky infiltrates with small cystic areas and a small chest. Respiratory insufficiency syndrome (RIS) was described by Carlsson and Svenningsen[32] and occurred in infants less mature than 32 weeks of gestational age. Signs in infants with RIS usually developed early, with the initial apnea occurring in the period 2–72 hours post-delivery. More than 50 percent required ventilation, but 76 percent survived. Rhodes *et al.*[151] described a group of nine infants out of 150 ventilated for idiopathic RDS, who had a radiological appearance of diffuse haziness with loss of identifiable lung markings occurring at 5–15 days, but which was not associated with clinical signs or symptoms nor increased oxygen needs; these changes disappeared in 1–5 days.

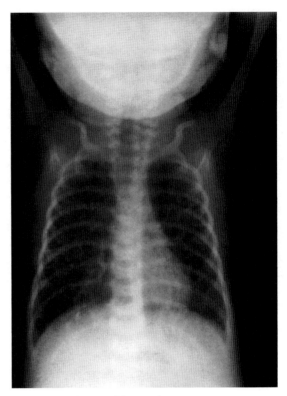

Figure 29.13 *Wilson–Mikity syndrome.*

Chronic pulmonary insufficiency of prematurity

This diagnosis has been used for infants who were previously healthy and then presented with respiratory symptoms, frequent apnea and a requirement for supplementary oxygen, at 4–7 days of age. The symptoms persisted for 2–4 weeks.[118] The chest radiograph demonstrates small volume lungs with a hazy opacification in a perihilar distribution and is distinct from that seen in BPD and Wilson–Mikity syndrome (Figures 29.13 and 29.14). Affected infants frequently required supplementary oxygen and CPAP to treat worsening hypoxemia and apnea. Antibiotics should only be given to treat secondary infection. The mortality is between 10 and 20 percent. The infants have slowly progressive atelectasis, hypoxemia and hypercapnia, but recovery is usually complete by 6 weeks of age.

Wilson–Mikity syndrome

This form of chronic respiratory distress usually affects infants of less than 32 weeks of gestational age.[208] There is equal male and female distribution. The infants have no respiratory problems in the first week after birth and the diagnosis is made when progressive respiratory failure develops during the second week.

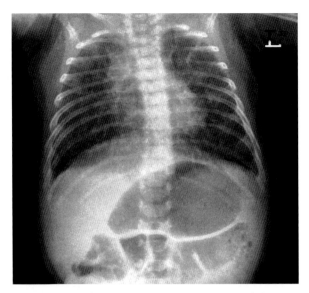

Figure 29.14 *Chest radiograph of a 2-month-old infant with Wilson–Mikity syndrome. Note the widespread changes and hyperinflation.*

ETIOLOGY

Burnard suggested that the only consistent etiological association of this condition was a low gestational age, typically less than 32 completed weeks of gestation.[31] Others have suggested it represents a functional and anatomical immaturity of the airways[157] or repeated aspiration. Fujimura *et al.* reported high plasma IgM levels on the first day after birth in infants with Wilson–Mikity syndrome.[63] The same group have found a high incidence of chorioamnionitis in mothers of infants with Wilson–Mikity syndrome but not with other forms of CLD;[64] this was associated with a raised cord blood IgM, suggesting intrauterine infection. The mean polymorphonuclear leukocyte elastase–proteinase inhibitor complex (PMN elastase-α-P1) has been found to be significantly elevated in tracheal aspirates from affected infants compared to those with BPD or respiratory distress in whom BPD did not develop.[65] It was postulated the PMN elastase-α-P1 was elevated by intrauterine inflammation and then caused lung injury resulting in postnatal pulmonary emphysema consistent with the Wilson–Mikity syndrome.

CLINICAL SIGNS

There is an insidious onset of cyanosis, tachypnea and retraction which persists for several months. The clinical characteristics of the illness include: a premature infant less than a month old, insidious onset of hyperpnea and cyanosis, later, dyspnea, especially on effort. The infant frequently has an overexpanded chest, wheezing and coughing but there are no rales unless heart failure occurs

and no fever unless infection intervenes. Such infants have intrapulmonary shunting and maldistribution of ventilation and perfusion,[117] pulmonary hypertension is detected at cardiac catheterization and can be confirmed by angiocardiography. The increased pulmonary vascular resistance is unresponsive to oxygen, suggesting permanent damage to the pulmonary capillary bed.

DIAGNOSIS

The diagnosis is made from the characteristic clinical course and the chest radiograph.

Chest radiograph

The changes, diffuse small bilateral cystic translucencies, affect both lungs and initially, unlike BPD, are more marked in the upper zones (Figure 29.13). There is a diffuse fine reticular pattern infiltrating the lung fields, interspersed with areas of emphysematous cysts. As the disease progresses the cysts coalesce and marked hyperinflation is a prominent feature (Figure 29.14).

MANAGEMENT

Infants with Wilson–Mikity syndrome frequently require an increased inspired oxygen concentration, but not mechanical ventilation. Indeed ventilation should, if possible, be avoided as this, as in other forms of CLD, may result in a deterioration in the clinical course.

PROGNOSIS

There is a tendency to cor pulmonale and a variable effect on general growth. Symptoms may persist for many months and abnormal lung function test results, suggesting persistent small airway damage, have been found in survivors even at 8–10 years of age. Respiratory infections are increased in the first year after birth. The usual tendency is for the pulmonary disease to resolve, but death may occur due to cardiac failure, respiratory failure or infection.

Lung function

Longitudinal studies of pulmonary function have revealed affected infants have a low compliance and a high resistance and TGV. These abnormalities only improve at or after the onset of clinical recovery.[157] Air trapping was demonstrated in these infants in association with episodes of clinical deterioration.

REFERENCES

1 Abman, S.H., Accurso, F.J., Koops, B.L. (1984) Experience with home oxygen in the management of infants with bronchopulmonary dysplasia. *Clinical Pediatrics (Philadelphia)* **23**, 471–476.

2 Abman, S.H., Wolfe, R.R., Accurso, F.J. *et al.* (1985) Pulmonary vascular response to oxygen in infants with severe bronchopulmonary dysplasia. *Pediatrics* **75**, 80–84.

3 Abman, S.H., Burchell, M.F., Shaffer, M.S. *et al.* (1989) Late sudden unexpected deaths in hospitalized infants with bronchopulmonary dysplasia. *American Journal of Disease in Childhood* **143**, 815–819.

4 Albersheim, S.G., Solimano, A.J., Sharma, A.K. *et al.* (1989) Randomized double blind controlled trial of long term diuretic therapy for bronchopulmonary dysplasia. *Journal of Pediatrics* **115**, 615–620.

5 Alkalay, A.L., Pomerance, J.J., Puri, A.R. *et al.* (1990) Hypothalamic-pituitary-adrenal axis function in very low birth weight infants treated with dexamethasone. *Pediatrics* **86**, 204–210.

6 Anderson, A.H., Warady, B.A., Daily, D.K. *et al.* (1993) Systemic hypertension in infants with severe bronchopulmonary dysplasia: associated clinical factors. *American Journal of Perinatology* **10**, 190–193.

7 Anonymous (1989) High-frequency oscillatory ventilation compared with conventional mechanical ventilation in the treatment of respiratory failure in preterm infants. The HIFI Study Group. *New England Journal of Medicine* **320**, 88–93.

8 Anonymous (1991) Dexamethasone therapy in neonatal chronic lung disease. An international placebo controlled trial. Collaborative Dexamethasone Trial Group. *Pediatrics* **88**, 421–427.

9 Arias-Camison, J.M., Lau, J., Cole, C.H. *et al.* (1999) Meta-analysis of dexamethasone therapy started in the first 15 days of life for prevention of chronic lung disease in premature infants. *Pediatr Pulmonol* **28**, 167–174.

10 Avery, G.B., Fletcher, A.B., Kaplan, M., Bruda, M.S. (1985) Controlled trial of dexamethasone in respirator-dependent infants with bronchopulmonary dysplasia. *Pediatrics* **75**, 106–111.

11 Avery, M.E., Tooley, W.H., Keller, J.B. *et al.* (1987) Is chronic lung disease in low birth weight infants preventable? A survey of eight centers. *Pediatrics* **79**, 26–30.

12 Bancalari, E., Gerhardt, T. (1986) Bronchopulmonary dysplasia. *Pediatric Clinics of North America* **33**, 1–23.

13 Bancalari, E., Abdenour, G.E., Feller, R., Cannon, J. (1979) Bronchopulmonary dysplasia: clinical presentation. *Journal of Pediatrics* **95**, 819–823.

14 Banks, B.A., Seri, I., Ischiropoulos, H. *et al.* (1999) Changes in oxygenation with inhaled nitric oxide in severe bronchopulmonary dysplasia. *Pediatrics* **103**, 610–618.

15 Bell, E.F., Warburton, D., Stonestreet, B., Oh, W. (1980) Effect of fluid administration on the development of symptomatic patent ductus arteriosus and congestive heart failure in premature infants. *New England Journal of Medicine* **302**, 598–604.

16 Berner, M.E., Teague, W.G.J., Scheerer, R.G. *et al.* (1989) Furosemide reduces lung fluid filtration in lambs with lung microvascular injury from air emboli. *Journal of Applied Physiology* **67**, 1990–1996.

17 Bhuta, T., Ohlsson, A. (1998) Systematic review and meta-analysis of early postnatal dexamethasone for prevention of chronic lung disease. *Archives of Disease in Childhood Fetal and Neonatal Edition* **79**, F26–F33.

18 Björklung, L.J., Ingimarsson, J., Curstedt, T. *et al.* (1997) Manual ventilation with a few large breaths at birth compromises the therapeutic effect of subsequent surfactant replacement in immature lambs. *Pediatric Research* **42**, 348–355.

19 Blayney, M., Kerem, E., Whyte, H., O'Brodovich, H. (1991) Bronchopulmonary dysplasia: improvement in lung function between 7 and 10 years of age. *Journal of Pediatrics* **118**, 201–206.

20 Boat, T.F. (1979) Studies of oxygen toxicity in cultured human neonatal respiratory epithelium. *Journal of Pediatrics* **95**, 916–919.

21 Boat, T.F., Kleinerman, J.I., Fanaroff, A.A. *et al.* (1973) Toxic effects of oxygen on cultured human neonatal respiratory epithelium. *Pediatric Research* **7**, 607–615.

22 Bos, A.F., Martijn, A., van Asperen, R.M. *et al.* (1998) Qualitative assessment of general movements in high risk preterm infants with chronic lung disease requiring dexamethasone therapy. *Journal of Pediatrics* **132**, 300–306.

23 Bozynski, M.E., Nelson, M.N., Matalon, T.A. *et al.* (1987) Prolonged mechanical ventilation and intracranial hemorrhage: impact on developmental progress through 18 months in infants weighing 1,200 grams or less at birth. *Pediatrics* **79**, 670–675.

24 Brown, E.R., Stark, A., Sosenko, I. *et al.* (1978) Bronchopulmonary dysplasia: possible relationship to pulmonary edema. *Journal of Pediatrics* **92**, 982–984.

25 Brownlee, J.R., Beekman, R.H., Rosenthal, A. (1988) Acute hemodynamic effects of nifedipine in infants with bronchopulmonary dysplasia and pulmonary hypertension. *Pediatric Research* **24**, 186–190.

26 Bruce, M.C., Martin, R.J., Boat, T.F. *et al.* (1982) Proteinase inhibitors and inhibitor inactivation in neonatal airways secretions. *Chest* **81**, 44S.

27 Bruce, M.C., Wedig, K.E., Jentoft, N. *et al.* (1985) Altered urinary excretion of elastin cross-links in premature infants who develop bronchopulmonary dysplasia. *American Review of Respiratory Disease* **131**, 568–572.

28 Brundage, K.L., Mohsini, K.G., Froese, A.B., Fisher, J.T. (1990) Bronchodilator response to ipratropium bromide in infants with bronchopulmonary dysplasia. *American Review of Respiratory Disease* **142**, 1137–1142.

29 Brunton, J.A., Saigal, S., Atkinson, S.A. (1998) Growth and body composition in infants with bronchopulmonary dysplasia up to 3 months corrected age: a randomized trial of a high-energy nutrient enriched formula fed after hospital discharge. *Journal of Pediatrics* **133**, 340–345.

30 Bryan, M.H., Hardie, M.J., Reilly, B.J. *et al.* (1973) Pulmonary function studies during the first year of life in infants recovering from respiratory distress syndrome. *Pediatrics* **52**, 169–178.

31 Burnard, E.D. (1966) The pulmonary syndrome of Wilson and Mikity and respiratory function in very small premature infants. *Pediatric Clinics of North America* **13**, 999–1016.

32 Carlsson, J., Svenningsen, N.W. (1975) Respiratory insufficiency syndrome (RIS) in preterm infants with gestational age of 32 weeks and less. *Acta Paediatrica Scandinavica* **64**, 813–821.

33 Cassell, G.H., Waites, K.B., Crouse, D.T. *et al.* (1988) Association of *Ureaplasma urealyticum* infection of the lower respiratory tract with chronic lung disease and death in very low birthweight infants. *Lancet* **2**, 240–244.

34 Chan, V., Greenough, A. (1993) Randomized trial of methods of extubation in acute and chronic respiratory distress. *Archives of Disease in Childhood* **68**, 570–572.

35 Clement, A., Masliah, J., Housset, B. *et al.* (1987) Decreased phosphatidyl choline content in bronchoalveolar lavage fluids of children with bronchopulmonary dysplasia: a preliminary investigation. *Pediatric Pulmonology* **3**, 67–70.

36 Cloutier, M.M., McLellan, N. (1993) Nebulized steroid therapy in bronchopulmonary dysplasia. *Pediatric Pulmonology* **15**, 111–116.

37 Coalson, J.J. (2000) Pathology of chronic lung disease of early infancy. In Bland, R.J., Coalson, J.J. (eds), *Chronic Lung Disease in Early Infancy.* New York: Marcel Dekker, 85–124.

38 Coalson, J.J., Winter, V., deLemos, R.A. (1995) Decreased alveolarization in baboon survivors with bronchopulmonary dysplasia. *American Journal of Respiratory and Critical Care Medicine* **152**, 640–646.

39 Cole, C.H., Colton, T., Shah, B.L. *et al.* (1999) Early inhaled glucocorticoid therapy to prevent bronchopulmonary dysplasia. *New England Journal of Medicine* **340**, 1005–1010.

40 Collaborative European Multicenter Study Group (1990) Surfactant replacement therapy for severe neonatal respiratory distress syndrome: an international randomized clinical trial. *Pediatrics* **82**, 683–690.

41 Cools, F., Offringa, M. (1999) Meta-analysis of elective high frequency ventilation in preterm infants with respiratory distress syndrome. *Archives of Disease in Childhood Fetal and Neonatal Edition* **80**, F15–F20.

42 Costarino, A.T.J., Gruskay, J.A., Corcoran, L. *et al.* (1992) Sodium restriction versus daily maintenance replacement in very low birth weight premature neonates: a randomized, blind therapeutic trial. *Journal of Pediatrics* **120**, 99–106.

43 Cotton, R.B., Stahlman, M.T., Bender, H.W. *et al.* (1978) Randomized trial of early closure of symptomatic patent ductus arteriosus in small preterm infants. *Journal of Pediatrics* **93**, 647–651.

44 Couroucli, X.I., Welty, S.E., Ramsay, P.L. *et al.* (2000) Detection of micro-organisms in the tracheal aspirates of preterm infants by polymerase chain reaction: association of adenovirus infection with bronchopulmonary dysplasia. *Pediatric Research* **47**, 225–232.

45 Cummings, J.J., D'Eugenio, D.B., Gross, S.J. (1989) A controlled trial of dexamethasone in preterm infants at high risk for bronchopulmonary dysplasia. *New England Journal of Medicine* **320**, 1505–1510.

46 Davis, J.M., Bhutani, V.K., Stefano, J.L. *et al.* (1989) Changes in pulmonary mechanics following caffeine administration in infants with bronchopulmonary dysplasia. *Pediatric Pulmonology* **6**, 49–52.

47 Davis, J.M., Sinkin, R.A., Aranda, V. *et al.* (1990) Drug therapy for bronchopulmonary dysplasia. *Pediatric Pulmonology* **8**, 117–125.

48 Davis, J.M., Richter, S.E., Biswas, S. *et al.* (2000) Long-term follow-up of premature infants treated with prophylactic intratracheal recombinant human CuZn superoxide dismutase. *Journal of Perinatology* **20**, 213–216.

49 Deneke, S.M., Fanburg, B.L. (1980) Normobaric oxygen toxicity of the lung. *New England Journal of Medicine* **303**, 76–86.

50 Deneke, S.M., Lynch, B.A., Fanburg, B.L. (1985) Effect of low protein diets or feed restriction on rat lung glutathione and oxygen toxicity. *Journal of Nutrition* **115**, 726–732.

51 Donn, S. (1982) Cost-effectiveness of home management of bronchopulmonary dysplasia. *Pediatrics* **70**, 330–331.

52 Durand, M., McEvoy, C., Macdonald, K. (1992) Spontaneous desaturations in intubated very low birth weight infants with acute and chronic lung disease. *Pediatric Pulmonology* **13**, 136–142.

53 Edwards, D.K., Dyer, W.M., Northway, W.H.J. (1977) Twelve years' experience with bronchopulmonary dysplasia. *Pediatrics* **59**, 839–846.

54 Ellington, B., McBride, J.T., Stokes, D.C. (1990) Effects of corticosteroids on postnatal lung and airway growth in the ferret. *Journal of Applied Physiology* **68**, 2029–2033.

55 Emery, E.F., Greenough, A. (1993) Blood pressure levels at follow-up of preterm infants with and without chronic lung disease. *Journal of Perinatal Medicine* **21**, 377–383.

56 Engelhardt, B., Elliott, S., Hazinski, T.A. (1986) Short- and long-term effects of furosemide on lung function in infants with bronchopulmonary dypslasia. *Journal of Pediatrics* **109**, 1034–1039.

57 Fok, T.F., Lam, K., Dolovich, M. *et al.* (1999) Randomised controlled study of early use of inhaled corticosteroid in preterm infants with respiratory distress syndrome. *Archives of Disease in Childhood Fetal and Neonatal Edition* **80**, F203–F208.

58 Fox, G.F., Wilson, D.C., Ohlsson, A. (1998) Effect of early versus late introduction of intravenous lipid to preterm infants on death and chronic lung disease (CLD) – results of meta-analyses. *Pediatric Research* **43**, 214A.

59 Frank, L. (1985) Effects of oxygen on the newborn. *Federation Proceedings* **44**, 2328–2334.

60 Frank, L. (1991) The use of dexamethasone in premature infants at risk for bronchopulmonary dysplasia or who already have developed chronic lung disease: a cautionary note. *Pediatrics* **88**, 413–416.

61 Frank, L., Sosenko, I.R. (1987) Development of lung antioxidant enzyme system in late gestation. Possible implications for the prematurely born infant. *Journal of Pediatrics* **110**, 9–14.

62 Frank, L., Sosenko, I.R. (1988) Undernutrition as a major contributing factor to the pathogenesis of bronchopulmonary dysplasia. *American Review of Respiratory Disease* **138**, 725–729.

63 Fujimura, M., Takeuchi, T., Ando, M. *et al.* (1983) Elevated immunoglobulin M levels in low birthweight neonates with chronic respiratory insufficiency. *Early Human Development* **9**, 27–32.

64 Fujimura, M., Takeuchi, T., Kitajima, H., Nakayama, M. (1989) Chorioamnionitis and serum IgM in Wilson-Mikity syndrome. *Archives of Disease in Childhood* **64**, 1379–1383.

65 Fujimura, M., Kitajima, H., Nakayama, M. (1993) Increased leukocyte elastase of the tracheal aspirate at birth and neonatal pulmonary emphysema. *Pediatrics* **92**, 564–569.

66 Gerdes, J.S., Yoder, M.C., Douglas, S.D. *et al.* (1986) Tracheal lavage and plasma fibronectin: relationship to respiratory distress syndrome and development of bronchopulmonary dysplasia. *Journal of Pediatrics* **108**, 601–606.

67 Gerhardt, T., Bancalari, E. (1980) Lung compliance in newborns with patent ductus arteriosus before and after surgical ligation. *Biology of the Neonate* **38**, 96–105.

68 Gerhardt, T., Hehre, D., Feller, R. *et al.* (1987) Serial determination of pulmonary function in infants with chronic lung disease. *Journal of Pediatrics* **110**, 448–456.

69 Gerhardt, T., Reifenberg, L., Goldberg, R.N., Bancalari, E. (1989) Pulmonary function in preterm infants whose lungs were ventilated conventionally or by high frequency oscillation. *Journal of Pediatrics* **115**, 121–126.

70 Gerstmann, D.R., deLemos, R.A., Coalson, J.J. *et al.* (1988) Influence of ventilatory technique on pulmonary baroinjury in baboons with hyaline membrane disease. *Pediatric Pulmonology* **5**, 82–91.

71 Goldman, S.L., Gerhardt, T., Sonni, R. *et al.* (1983) Early prediction of chronic lung disease by pulmonary function testing. *Journal of Pediatrics* **102**, 613–617.

72 Gomez-Del Rio, M., Gerhardt, T., Hehre, D. *et al.* (1986) Effect of a beta-agonist nebulization on lung function in neonates with increased pulmonary resistance. *Pediatric Pulmonology* **2**, 287–291.

73 Gonzalez, A., Sosenko, I.R.S., Chandar, J. *et al.* (1996) Influence of infection on patent ductus arteriosus and chronic lung disease in premature infants weighing 1000 g or less. *Journal of Pediatrics* **128**, 470–478.

74 Goodman, G., Perkin, R.M., Anas, N.G. *et al.* (1988) Pulmonary hypertension in infants with bronchopulmonary dysplasia. *Journal of Pediatrics* **112**, 67–72.

75 Gray, P.H., Rogers, Y. (1994) Are infants with bronchopulmonary dysplasia at risk for sudden infant death syndrome? *Pediatrics* **93**, 774–777.

76 Greenough, A. (1990) Personal practice. Bronchopulmonary dysplasia. Early diagnosis, prophylaxis and treatment. *Archives of Disease in Childhood* **65**, 1082–1088.

77 Greenough, A., Elias-Jones, A., Pool, J., Morley, C.J. (1985) The therapeutic actions of theophylline in preterm ventilated infants. *Early Human Development* **12**, 15–22.

78 Greenough, A., Kavvadia, K., Johnson, A.H. *et al.* (1999) A simple chest radiograph score to predict chronic lung disease in prematurely born infants. *British Journal of Radiology* **72**, 530–533.

79 Greenough, A., Alexander, J., Burgess, S. *et al.* (2001) Home oxygen status on rehospitalisation and primary care requirements of chronic lung disease infants. *Archives of Disease in Childhood* **85**, 463–468.

80 Greenough, A., Boorman, J., Alexander, J. *et al.* (2001) Health care utilisation of CLD infants related to hospitalisation for RSV infection. *Archives of Disease in Childhood* **85**, 463–468.

81 Greenspan, J.S., DeGiulio, P.A., Bhutaniv, K. (1989) Airway reactivity as determined by a cold air challenge in infants with bronchopulmonary dysplasia. *Journal of Pediatrics* **114**, 452–454.

82 Groneck, P., Reuss, D., Goetze-Speer, B., Speer, C.P. (1993) Effects of dexamethasone on chemotactic activity and inflammatory mediators in tracheobronchial aspirates of preterm infants at risk for chronic lung disease. *Journal of Pediatrics* **122**, 938–944.

83 Groneck, P., Götze-Speer, B., Oppermann, M. *et al.* (1994) Association of pulmonary inflammation and increased microvascular permeability during the development of bronchopulmonary dysplasia: a sequential analysis of inflammatory mediators in respiratory fluids of high risk preterm neonates. *Pediatrics* **93**, 712–718.

84 Groneck, P., Goetze-Speer, B., Speer, C.P. (1999) Effects of inhaled beclomethasone compared to systemic dexamethasone on lung inflammation in preterm infants at risk of chronic lung disease. *Pediatric Pulmonology* **27**, 383–387.

85 Groothuis, J.R., Rosenberg, A.A. (1987) Home oxygen promotes weight gain in infants with bronchopulmonary dysplasia. *American Journal of Diseases in Children* **141**, 992–995.

86 Groothuis, J.R., Gutierrez, K.M., Lauer, B.A. (1988) Respiratory syncytial virus infection in children with bronchopulmonary dysplasia. *Pediatrics* **82**, 199–203.

87 Gross, S.J., Iannuzzi, D.M., Kveselis, D.A., Anbar, R.D. (1999) Effect of preterm birth on pulmonary function at school age: a prospective controlled study. *Journal of Pediatrics* **133**, 188–192.

88 Halliday, H.L. (1999) Clinical trials of postnatal corticosteroids: inhaled and systemic. *Biology of the Neonate* **76**, 29–40.

89 Halliday, H.L., Dumpit, F.M., Brandy, J.P. (1980) Effects of inspired oxygen on echocardiographic assessment of pulmonary vascular resistance and myocardial contractility in bronchopulmonary dysplasia. *Pediatrics* **65**, 536–540.

90 Hamilton, P.A., Whitehead, M.D., Reynolds, E.O.R. (1985) Underestimation of arterial oxygen tension by transcutaneous electrode with increasing age in infants. *Archives of Disease in Childhood* **60**, 1162–1165.

91 Hannaford, K., Todd, D.A., Jeffery, H. *et al.* (1999) Role of *Ureaplasma urealyticum* in lung disease of prematurity. *Archives of Disease in Childhood Fetal and Neonatal Edition* **81**, F162–F167.

92 Hazinski, T.A., Blalock, W.A., Engelhardt, B. (1988) Control of water balance in infants with bronchopulmonary dysplasia: role of endogenous vasopressin. *Pediatric Research* **23**, 86–88.

93 Holtzman, R.B., Hageman, J.R., Yogev, R. (1989) Role of *Ureaplasma urealyticum* in bronchopulmonary dysplasia. *Journal of Pediatrics* **114**, 1061–1063.

94 Horbar, J.D., McAuliffe, T.L., Adler, S.M. *et al.* (1988) Variability in 28-day outcomes for very low birth weight infants: an analysis of 11 neonatal intensive care units. *Pediatrics* **82**, 554–559.

95 Horbar, J.D., Wright, L.L., Soll, R.F. (1993) A multicenter randomized trial comparing two surfactants for the treatment of neonatal respiratory distress syndrome. *Journal of Pediatrics* **123**, 757–766.

96 Hoyoux, C.I., Forget, P., Lambrechts, L. *et al.* (1985) Chronic bronchopulmonary disease and gastroesophageal reflux in children. *Pediatr Pulmonol* **1**, 149–153.

97 Husain, A.N., Siddiqui, N.H., Stocker, J.T. (1998) Pathology of arrested acinar development in postsurfactant bronchopulmonary dysplasia. *Human Pathology* **29**, 710–717.

98 Hustead, V.A., Gutcher, G.R., Anderson, S.A. *et al.* (1984) Relationship of vitamin A (retinol) status to lung disease in the preterm infant. *Journal of Pediatrics* **105**, 610–615.

99 Hyde, I., English, E.R., Williams, J.A. (1989) The changing pattern of chronic lung disease of prematurity. *Archives of Disease in Childhood* **64**, 448–451.

100 Imai, Y., Kawano, T., Miyasaka, K. *et al.* (1994) Inflammatory chemical mediators during conventional ventilation and during high frequency oscillatory ventilation. *American Journal of Respiratory and Critical Care Medicine* **150**, 1550–1554.

101 Israel, B.A., Sherman, F.S., Guthrie, R.D. (1993) Hypertrophic cardiomyopathy associated with dexamethasone therapy for chronic lung disease in preterm infants. *American Journal of Perinatology* **10**, 307–310.

102 Jackson, J.C., Truog, W.E., Standaert, T.A. *et al.* (1994) Reduction in lung injury after combined surfactant and high-frequency ventilation. *American Journal of Respiratory and Critical Care Medicine* **150**, 534–539.

103 Jobe, A.H. (1993) Pulmonary surfactant therapy. *New England Journal of Medicine* **328**, 861–868.

104 Jobe, A.H., Bancalari, E. (2001) Bronchopulmonary dysplasia. NICHD-NHLBI-ORD Workshop. *American Journal of Respiratory and Critical Care Medicine* **163**, 1723–1729.

105 Johnson, C.E., Beekman, R.H., Kostyshak, D.A. *et al.* (1991) Pharmacokinetics and pharmacodynamics of nifedipine in children with bronchopulmonary dysplasia and pulmonary hypertension. *Pediatric Research* **29**, 500–503.

106 Kao, L.C., Warburton, D., Sargent, C.W. *et al.* (1983) Furosemide acutely decreases airway resistance in chronic bronchopulmonary dysplasia. *Journal of Pediatrics* **103**, 624–629.

107 Kao, L.C., Warburton, D., Cheng, M.H. *et al.* (1984) Effect of oral diuretics on pulmonary mechanics in infants with chronic bronchopulmonary dysplasia: results of a double-blind crossover sequential trial. *Pediatrics* **74**, 37–44.

108 Kao, L.C., Warburton, D., Platzker, A.C.G., Keens, T.G. (1984) Effect of isoproterenol inhalation on airways resistance in chronic bronchopulmonary dysplasia. *Pediatrics* **73**, 509–514.

109 Kao, L.C., Durand, D.J., Dhillias, B.L., Nickerson, B.G. (1987) Oral theophylline and diuretics improve pulmonary mechanics in infants with bronchopulmonary dysplasia. *Journal of Pediatrics* **111**, 439–444.

110 Kao, L.C., Durand, D.J., Nickerson, B.G. (1989) Effects of inhaled metaproterenol and atropine on the pulmonary mechanics of infants with bronchopulmonary dysplasia. *Pediatric Pulmonology* **6**, 74–80.

111 Kao, L.C., Durand, D.J., McCrea, R.C. *et al.* (1994) Randomized trial of long-term diuretic therapy for infants with oxygen-dependent bronchopulmonary dysplasia. *Journal of Pediatrics* **124**, 772–781.

112 Kari, M.A., Heinonen, K., Ikonen, R.S. *et al.* (1993) Dexamethasone treatment in preterm infants at risk for bronchopulmonary dysplasia. *Archives of Disease in Childhood* **68**, 566–569.

113 Kavvadia, V., Greenough, A., Dimitriou, G., Forsling, M.L. (2000) A comparison of arginine vasopressin levels and fluid balance in the perinatal period in infants who did and did not develop chronic oxygen dependency. *Biology of the Neonate* **78**, 86–91.

114 Kavvadia, V., Greenough, A., Dimitriou, G., Hooper, R. (2000) Randomized trial of fluid restriction in ventilated very low birthweight infants. *Archives of Disease in Childhood* **83**, F91–F96.

115 Kendig, J.W., Notter, R.H., Cox, C., *et al.* (1988) Surfactant replacement therapy at birth: final analysis of a clinical trial and comparisons with similar trials. *Pediatrics* **82**, 756–762.

116 Kojima, T., Fukuda, Y., Hirata, Y. *et al.* (1990) Changes in vasopressin, atrial natriuretic factor and water homeostasis in the early stage of bronchopulmonary dysplasia. *Pediatric Research* **27**, 260–263.

117 Krauss, A.N., Levin, A.R., Grossman, H., Auld, P.A.M. (1970) Physiologic studies on infants with Wilson-Mikity syndrome. *Journal of Pediatrics* **77**, 27–36.

118 Krauss, A.N., Klain, D.B., Auld, P.A.M. (1975) Chronic pulmonary insufficiency of prematurity (CPIP). *Pediatrics* **55**, 55–58.

119 Kurzner, S.I., Garg, M., Bautista, D.B. *et al.* (1988) Growth failure in bronchopulmonary dysplasia: elevated metabolic rates and pulmonary mechanics. *Journal of Pediatrics* **112**, 73–80.

120 LaForce, W.R., Brudno, D.S. (1993) Controlled trial of beclomethasone dipropionate by nebulization in oxygen- and ventilator-dependent infants. *Journal of Pediatrics* **122**, 285–288.

121 Maisels, S.J., Rivers, A., Hack, M. (1986) Growth and development of preterm infants with respiratory distress syndrome and bronchopulmonary dysplasia. *Pediatrics* **77**, 345–352.

122 Margraf, L.R., Tomashefski, J.F., Bruce, M.C., Dahms, B.B. (1991) Morphometric analysis of the lung in bronchopulmonary dysplasia. *American Review of Respiratory Disease* **143**, 391–400.

123 McCoy, K.S., Bagwell, C.E., Wagner, M. *et al.* (1992) Spirometric and endoscopic evaluation of airway collapse in infants with bronchopulmonary dysplasia. *Pediatric Pulmonology* **14**, 23–27.

124 McCubbin, M., Frey, E.E., Wagener, J.S. *et al.* (1989) Large airway collapse in bronchopulmonary dysplasia. *Journal of Pediatrics* **114**, 304–307.

125 Melnick, G., Pickoff, A.S., Ferrer, P.L. *et al.* (1980) Normal pulmonary vascular resistance and left ventricular hypertrophy in young infants with bronchopulmonary dysplasia: an echocardiographic and pathologic study. *Pediatrics* **66**, 589–596.

126 Merritt, T.A., Harris, J.P., Roghmann, K., *et al.* (1981) Early closure of patent ductus arteriosus in very-low-birth weight infants: a controlled trial. *Journal of Pediatrics* **99**, 281–286.

127 Merritt, T.A., Cochrane, C.G., Holcomb, K. *et al.* (1983) Elastase and alpha-1 protease inhibitor activity in tracheal aspirates during RDS: the role of inflammation and pathogenesis of bronchopulmonary dysplasia. *Journal of Clinical Investigation* **72**, 656–666.

128 Merz, U., Kusenbach, G., Hausler, M. *et al.* (1999) Inhaled budesonide in ventilator dependent preterm infants: a randomized, double-blind pilot study. *Biology of the Neonate* **75**, 46–53.

129 Miller, R.W., Woo, P., Kellman, R.K., Slagle, T.S. (1987) Tracheobronchial abnormalities in infants with bronchopulmonary dysplasia. *Journal of Pediatrics* **111**, 779–782.

130 Motoyama, E.K., Fort, M.D., Klesh, K.W. *et al.* (1987) Early onset of airway reactivity in premature infants with bronchopulmonary dysplasia. *American Review of Respiratory Disease* **136**, 50–57.

131 Myers, M.G., McGuinness, G.A., Lachenbrugh, P.A. *et al.* (1986) Respiratory illnesses in survivors of infant respiratory distress syndrome. *American Review of Respiratory Disease* **133**, 1011–1018.

132 Nickerson, B.G., Taussig, L.M. (1980) Family history of asthma in infants with bronchopulmonary dysplasia. *Pediatrics* **65**, 1140–1144.

133 Noble-Jamieson, C.M., Regev, R., Silverman, M. (1989) Dexamethasone in neonatal chronic lung disease: pulmonary effects and intracranial complications. *European Journal of Pediatrics* **148**, 365–367.

134 Northway, W.H., Moss, R.B., Carlisle, K.B. *et al.* (1990) Late pulmonary sequelae of bronchopulmonary dysplasia. *New England Journal of Medicine* **323**, 1793–1799.

135 Northway, W.H.J., Rosan, R.C., Porter, D.Y. (1967) Pulmonary disease following respiratory therapy of hyaline membrane disease: bronchopulmonary dysplasia. *New England Journal of Medicine* **276**, 357–368.

136 O'Donovan, B.H., Bell, E.F. (1989) Effects of furosemide on body water compartments in infants with bronchopulmonary dysplasia. *Pediatric Research* **26**, 121–124.

137 Ogden, B.E., Murphy, S.A., Saunders, G.C. *et al.* (1984) Neonatal lung neutrophils and elastase/proteinase imbalance. *American Review of Respiratory Disease* **130**, 817–821.

138 Ohlsson, A., Calvert, S.A., Hosking, M., *et al.* (1992) Randomized controlled trial of dexamethasone treatment in very-low-birth-weight infants with ventilator-dependent chronic lung disease. *Acta Paediatr* **81**, 751–756.

139 Ollikainen, J., Hiekkaniemi, H., Korppi, M., *et al.* (1993) *Ureaplasma urealyticum* infection associated with acute respiratory insufficiency and death in premature infants. *Journal of Pediatrics* **122**, 756–760.

140 O'Shea, T.M., Kothadia, J.M., Klinepeter, K.L. *et al.* (1993) Follow-up of preterm infants treated with dexamethasone for chronic lung disease. *American Journal of Diseases in Children* **147**, 658–661.

141 O'Shea, T.M., Kothadia, J.M., Klinepeter, K.L. *et al.* (1999) Randomized placebo controlled trail of a 42-day tapering course of dexamethasone to reduce the duration of ventilator dependency in very low birthweight infants: outcome of study participants at one-year adjusted age. *Pediatrics* **104**, 15–21.

142 Palta, M., Gabbert, D., Weinstein, M., Peters, M. (1991) Multivariate assessment of traditional risk factors for chronic lung disease in very low birth weight neonates. The newborn lung project. *Journal of Pediatrics* **119**, 285–292.

143 Palta, M., Sadek, M., Barnet, J.H. *et al.* (1998) Evaluation of criteria for chronic lung disease in surviving very low birthweight infants. *Journal of Pediatrics* **132**, 57–63.

144 Pantich, H.B., Allen, J.L., Alpert, B.E., Schidlow, D.V. (1994) Effects of CPAP on lung mechanics in infants with acquired tracheobronchomalacia. *American Journal of Respiratory and Critical Care Medicine* **150**, 1341–1346.

145 Papile, L.-A., Tyson, J.E., Stoll, B.J. *et al.* (1998) A multicenter trial of two dexamethasone regimens in ventilator-dependent premature infants. *New England Journal of Medicine* **338**, 1112–1118.

146 Parker, R.A., Lindstrom, D.P., Cotton, R.B. (1992) Improved survival accounts for most, but not all, of the increase in bronchopulmonary dysplasia. *Pediatrics* **90**, 663–668.

147 Pearson, E., Bose, C., Snidow, T. *et al.* (1992) Trial of vitamin A supplementation in very low birth weight infants at risk for bronchopulmonary dysplasia. *Journal of Pediatrics* **121**, 420–427.

148 Pierce, M.R., Bancalari, E. (1995) The role of inflammation in the pathogenesis of bronchopulmonary dysplasia. *Pediatric Pulmonology* **19**, 371–378.

149 Reid, L. (1979) Bronchopulmonary dysplasia: pathology. *Journal of Pediatrics* **95**, 836–841.

150 Rettwitz-Volk, W., Veldman, A., Roth, B. *et al.* (1998) A prospective, randomized, multicenter trial of high frequency oscillatory ventilation compared with conventional ventilation in preterm infants with respiratory distress syndrome receiving surfactant. *Journal of Pediatrics* **132**, 249–254.

151 Rhodes, P.G., Hall, R.T., Leonidas, J.C. (1975) Chronic pulmonary disease in neonates with assisted ventilation. *Pediatrics* **55**, 788–795.

152 Rojas, M.A., Gonzalez, A., Bancalari, E. *et al.* (1995) Changing trends in the epidemiology and pathogenesis of neonatal chronic lung disease. *Journal of Pediatrics* **126**, 605–610.

153 Rome, E.S., Stork, E.K., Carlo, W.A. (1984) Limitations of transcutaneous PO_2 and PCO_2 monitoring in infants with bronchopulmonary dysplasia. *Pediatrics* **74**, 217–220.

154 Rooklin, A.R., Moomjian, A.S., Shutack, J.G. *et al.* (1979) Theophylline therapy in bronchopulmonary dysplasia. *Journal of Pediatrics* **95**, 882–885.

155 Rosenfeld, W., Evans, H., Concepcion, L. *et al.* (1984) Prevention of bronchopulmonary dysplasia by administration of bovine superoxide dismutase in preterm infants with respiratory distress syndrome. *Journal of Pediatrics* **105**, 781–785.

156 Rush, M.G., Engelhardt, B., Parker, R.A., *et al.* (1990) Double-blind, placebo-controlled trial of alternate-day furosemide therapy in infants with chronic bronchopulmonary dysplasia. *Journal of Pediatrics* **117**, 112–118.

157 Saunders, R.A., Milner, A.D., Hopkin, I.E. (1978) Longitudinal studies of infants with the Wilson-Mikity syndrome. *Biology of the Neonate* **33**, 90–99.

158 Sawyer, M.H., Edwards, D.K., Spector, S.A. (1987) Cytomegalovirus infection and bronchopulmonary dysplasia in premature infants. *American Journal of Diseases of Children* **141**, 303–305.

159 Schrod, L., Neuhaus, T., Horwitz, A.E., Speer, C.P. (2001) The effect of dexamethasone on respirator-dependent very-low-birthweight infants is best predicted by chest X-ray. *Pediatric Radiology* **31**, 332–338.

160 Schwartz, R.M., Luby, A.M., Scanlon, J.W., *et al.* (1994) Effect of surfactant on morbidity, mortality, and resource use in newborn infants weighing 500 to 1500g. *New England Journal of Medicine* **330**, 1476–1480.

161 Shenai, J.P. (1999) Vitamin A supplementation in very low birth weight neonates: rationale and evidence. *Pediatrics* **104**, 1369–1374.

162 Shenai, J.P., Chytil, F., Stahlman, M.T. (1985) Vitamin A status of neonates with bronchopulmonary dysplasia. *Pediatric Research* **19**, 185–189.

163 Shenai, J.P., Kennedy, K.A., Chytil, F., Stahlman, M.T. (1987) Clinical trial of vitamin A supplementation in infants susceptible to bronchopulmonary dysplasia. *Journal of Pediatrics* **111**, 269–277.

164 Shennan, A.T., Dunn, M.S., Ohlsson, A. *et al.* (1988) Abnormal pulmonary outcomes in premature infants: prediction from oxygen requirement in the neonatal period. *Pediatrics* **82**, 527–532.

165 Sindel, B.D., Maisels, M.J., Ballantine, T.V. (1989) Gastroesophageal reflux to the proximal esophagus in infants with bronchopulmonary dysplasia. *American Journal of Diseases of Children* **143**, 1103–1106.

166 Singer, L., Martin, R.J., Hawkins, S.W. *et al.* (1992) Oxygen desaturation complicates feeding in infants with bronchopulmonary dysplasia after discharge. *Pediatrics* **90**, 380–384.

167 Skidmore, M.D., Rivers, A., Hack, M. (1990) Increased risk of cerebral palsy among very low-birthweight infants with chronic lung disease. *Developmental Medicine and Child Neurology* **32**, 325–332.

168 Smyth, J.A., Tabachnik, E., Duncan, W.J. *et al.* (1981) Pulmonary function and bronchial hyperreactivity in long-term survivors of bronchopulmonary dysplasia. *Pediatrics* **68**, 336–340.

169 Solimano, A.J., Smyth, J.A., Mann, T.K. *et al.* (1986) Pulse oximetry advantages in infants with bronchopulmonary dysplasia. *Pediatrics* **78**, 844–849.

170 Sosenko, I.R.S., Kinter, M.T., Roberts, R.J. (2000) Nutritional issues in chronic lung disease of premature infants. In Bland, R.J., Coalson, J.J. (Eds.), *Chronic Lung Disease in Early Infancy.* New York, NY: Marcel Dekker Inc, 285–296.

171 Speer, C.P., Ruess, D., Harms, K. *et al.* (1993) Neutrophil elastase and acute pulmonary damage in neonates with severe respiratory distress syndrome. *Pediatrics* **91**, 794–799.

172 Spitzer, A.R., Fox, W.W., Delivoria-Papadopoulos, M. (1981) Maximum diuresis – a factor in predicting recovery from respiratory distress syndrome and the development of bronchopulmonary dysplasia. *Journal of Pediatrics* **98**, 476–479.

173 Steichen, J.J., Gratton, T.L., Tsang, R.C. (1980) Osteopenia of prematurity: the cause and possible treatment. *Journal of Pediatrics* **96**, 528–534.

174 Stenmark, K.R., Eyzaguine, M., Remigio, L. *et al.* (1985) Recovery of platelet activating factor and leukotrienes from infants with severe bronchopulmonary dysplasia: clinical improvement with cromolyn treatment. *American Review of Respiratory Disease* **131**, 236A.

175 Stenmark, K.R., Eyzaguirre, M., Westcott, J.Y. *et al.* (1987) Potential role of eicosanoids and PAF in the pathophysiology of bronchopulmonary dysplasia. *American Review of Respiratory Disease* **136**, 770–772.

176 Stoll, B.J., Temprosa, M., Tyson, J.E., *et al.* (1999) Dexamethasone therapy increases infection in very low birth weight infants. *Pediatrics* **104**, E63.

177 Strauss, A., Brakin, M., Norris, K., *et al.* (1992) Adrenal responsiveness in very-low-birth-weight infants treated with dexamethasone. *Developmental Pharmacology and Therapeutics* **19**, 147–154.

178 Taghizadeh, A., Reynolds, E.O.R. (1976) Pathogenesis of bronchopulmonary dysplasia following hyaline membrane disease. *American Journal of Pathology* **82**, 241–257.

179 Tammela, O.K.T., Kovisto, M.E. (1992) Fluid restriction for preventing bronchopulmonary dysplasia? Reduced fluid intake during the first weeks of life improves the outcome of low birthweight infants. *Acta Paediatrica Scandinavica* **81**, 207–212.

180 Tanswell, A.K., Freeman, B.A. (1987) Liposome-entrapped antioxidant enzymes prevent lethal O_2 toxicity in the newborn rat. *Journal of Applied Physiology* **63**, 347–352.

181 Tay-Uyboco, J.S., Kwiatkowski, K., Cates, D.B. *et al.* (1989) Hypoxic airway constriction in infants of very low birth weight recovering from moderate to severe bronchopulmonary dysplasia. *Journal of Pediatrics* **115**, 456–459.

182 Teague, W.G., Pian, M.S., Heldt, G.P., Tooley, W.H. (1988) An acute reduction in the fraction of inspired oxygen increases airway constriction in infants with chronic lung disease. *American Review of Respiratory Disease* **137**, 861–865.

183 The STOP-ROP Multicenter Study Group. (2000) Supplemental therapeutic oxygen for prethreshold retinopathy of prematurity (STOP-ROP): a randomized, controlled trial. I. Primary outcomes. *Pediatrics* **105**, 295–310.

184 Thibeault, D.W., Heimes, B., Rezaiekhaligh, M., *et al.* (1993) Chronic modifications of lung and heart development in glucocorticoid-treated newborn rats exposed to hyperoxia or room air. *Pediatric Pulmonology* **16**, 81–88.

185 Thomas, M., Greenough, A., Johnson, A. *et al.* (2003) Frequent wheeze at follow-up of very preterm infants – which factors are predictive? *Archives of Disease in Childhood* (in press).

186 Thome, U., Kossel, H., Lipowsky, G. *et al.* (1999) Randomized comparison of high-frequency ventilation with high-rate intermittent positive pressure ventilation in preterm infants with respiratory failure. *Journal of Pediatrics* **135**, 39–46.

187 Toce, S.S., Farrell, P.M., Leavitt, L.A. *et al.* (1984) Clinical and roentgenographic scoring systems for assessing bronchopulmonary dysplasia. *American Journal of Diseases in Children* **138**, 581–585.

188 Tyson, J.E., Wright, L.L., Oh, W. *et al.* (1999) Vitamin A supplementation for extremely-low-birth-weight infants. *National Institute of Child Health and Human Development Neonatal Research Network* **340**, 1962–1968.

189 Van Goudoever, J.B., Wattimena, V.P., Carnielli, V.P. *et al.* (1994) Effect of dexamethasone on protein metabolism in infants with bronchopulmonary dysplasia. *J Pediatr* **124**, 112–118.

190 van Marter, L.J., Leviton, A., Allred, E.N. *et al.* (1990) Hydration during the first days of life and the risk of bronchopulmonary dysplasia in low birth weight infants. *Journal of Pediatrics* **116**, 942–949.

191 van Marter, L.J., Leviton, A., Kuban, K.C.K. *et al.* (1990) Maternal glucocorticoid therapy and reduced risk of bronchopulmonary dysplasia. *Pediatrics* **86**, 331–336.

192 van Marter, L.J., Pagano, M., Alfred, E.N. *et al.* (1992) Rate of bronchopulmonary dsyplasia as a function of neonatal intensive care practices. *Journal of Pediatrics* **120**, 938–946.

193 Varsila, E., Hallman, M., Venge, P., Andersson, S. (1995) Closure of patent ductus arteriosus decreases pulmonary myeloperoxidase in premature infants with respiratory distress syndrome. *Biology of the Neonate* **67**, 167–171.

194 Vohr, B.R., Bell, E.F., Oh, W. (1982) Infants with bronchopulmonary dysplasia: growth pattern and neurologic and developmental outcome. *American Journal of Diseases of Children* **136**, 443–447.

195 Wada, K., Jobe, A.H., Ikegami, M. (1997) Tidal volume effects on surfactant treatment responses with the initiation of ventilation in preterm lambs. *Journal of Applied Physiology* **83**, 1054–1061.

196 Walti, H., Tordet, C., Gerbaut, L. *et al.* (1989) Persistent elastase/proteinase inhibitor imbalance during prolonged ventilation of infants with BPD: evidence for the role of nosocomial infections. *Pediatric Research* **26**, 351–355.

197 Wang, E.E.L., Frayha, H., Watts, J. *et al.* (1988) Role of ureaplasma urealyticum and other pathogens in the development of chronic lung disease of prematurity. *Pediatric Infectious Disease Journal* **7**, 547–551.

198 Watterberg, K.L., Scott, S.M. (1995) Evidence of early adrenal insufficiency in babies who develop bronchopulmonary dysplasia. *Pediatrics* **95**, 120–125.

199 Watterberg, K.L., Carmichael, D.F., Gerdes, J.S. *et al.* (1994) Secretory leukocyte protease inhibitor and lung inflammation in developing bronchopulmonary dysplasia. *Journal of Pediatrics* **125**, 264–269.

200 Watterberg, K.L., Demers, L.M., Scott, S.M., Murphy, S. (1996) Chorioamnionitis and early lung inflammation in infants in whom bronchopulmonary dysplasia develops. *Pediatrics* **97**, 210–215.

201 Watterberg, K.L., Gerdes, J.S., Gifford, K.L., Lin, H.M. (1999) Prophylaxis against early adrenal insufficiency to prevent chronic lung disease in premature infants. *Pediatrics* **104**, 1258–1263.

202 Watterberg, K.L., Scott, S.M., Backstrom, C. *et al.* (2000) Links between early adrenal function and respiratory outcome in preterm infants: airway inflammation and patent ductus arteriosus. *Pediatrics* **150**, 320–324.

203 Watts, C.L., Bruce, M.C. (1992) Effect of dexamethasone therapy on fibronectine and albumin levels in lung secretions of infants with bronchopulmonary dysplasia. *Journal of Pediatrics* **121**, 597–607.

204 Watts, J.L., Ariagno, R.L., Brady, J.P. (1977) Chronic pulmonary disease in neonates after artificial ventilation: distribution of ventilation and pulmonary interstitial emphysema. *Pediatrics* **60**, 273–281.

205 Weinstein, M.R., Oh, W. (1981) Oxygen consumption in infants with bronchopulmonary dysplasia. *Journal of Pediatrics* **99**, 958–961.

206 Werner, J.C., Sicard, R.E., Hansen, T.W.R. *et al.* (1992) Hypertrophic cardiomyopathy associated with dexamethasone therapy for bronchopulmonary dysplasia. *Journal of Pediatrics* **120**, 286–291.

207 Werthammer, J., Brown, E.R., Neff, R.K., Taeusch, H.W.J. (1982) Sudden infant death syndrome in infants with bronchopulmonary dysplasia. *Pediatrics* **69**, 301–304.

208 Wilson, M.G., Mikity, V.G. (1960) A new form of respiratory disease in premature infants. *American Journal of Diseases of Children* **99**, 489–499.

209 Wung, J.T., Koons, A.H., Driscoll, J.M., James, L.S. (1979) Changing incidence of bronchopulmonary dysplasia. *Journal of Pediatrics* **95**, 845–847.

210 Yeh, T.F., McClenan, D.A., Ajayi, O.A., Pildes, R.S. (1989) Metabolic rate and energy balance in infants with bronchopulmonary dysplasia. *Journal of Pediatrics* **114**, 448–451.

211 Yeh, T.F., Lin, Y.L., Lin, C.H. *et al.* (1997) Early postnatal (<12 hours) dexamethasone therapy for prevention of BPD in preterm infants with RDS: a two-year follow-up study. *Pediatric Research* **41**, 118A.

212 Yeh, T.F., Lin, Y.J., Huang, C.C. *et al.* (1998) Early dexamethasone therapy in preterm infants: a follow-up study. *Pediatrics* **101**, E7.

213 Yoon, B.H., Romero, R., Jun, J.K. *et al.* (1997) Amniotic fluid cytokines (interleukin-6, tumor necrosis factor-alpha, interleukin-1β and interleukin-8) and the risk for the

development of bronchopulmonary dysplasia. *American Journal of Obstetrics and Gynecology* **177**, 825–830.

214 Yüksel, B., Greenough, A. (1992) Acute deteriorations in neonatal chronic lung disease. *European Journal of Pediatrics* **151**, 697–700.

215 Yüksel, B., Greenough, A. (1992) Inhaled sodium cromoglycate for preterm children with respiratory symptoms at follow-up. *Respiratory Medicine* **86**, 131–134.

216 Yüksel, B., Greenough, A., Green, S. (1991) Paradoxical response to nebulized ipratropium bromide in preterm infants asymptomatic at follow-up. *Respiratory Medicine* **85**, 189–194.

217 Yüksel, B., Greenough, A., Karani, J., Page, A. (1991) Chest radiograph scoring system for use in preterm infants. *British Journal of Radiology* **64**, 1015–1018.

218 Yunis, K.A., Oh, W. (1989) Effects of intravenous glucose loading on oxygen consumption, carbon dioxide production, and resting energy expenditure in infants with bronchopulmonary dysplasia. *Journal of Pediatrics* **115**, 127–132.

30

Apnea and bradycardia of prematurity

JALAL M ABU-SHAWEESH, TERRY M BAIRD AND RICHARD J MARTIN

Idiopathic apnea of prematurity continues to be an extremely common disorder and a major source of morbidity in the growing number of premature infants who require neonatal intensive care. Apnea of prematurity has been associated with poor developmental outcome in school-age children, although a cause and effect relationship is difficult to establish.

Apnea of prematurity has been defined as cessation of breathing for between 10 and 30 seconds' duration.[8,20,43,48,63,66,77] Shorter episodes of apnea may also be accompanied by significant bradycardia or hypoxia.[15] Brief respiratory pauses of less than 10 seconds in duration can occur in conjunction with startles, movement, defecation or swallowing during feeding. These short pauses are self-limited and not typically associated with bradycardia or hypoxemia.[134] Prolonged desaturation episodes have been reported in the absence of apnea or bradycardia, both in healthy preterm infants[107,112,127] and more frequently in infants with chronic lung disease (p. 405).[125] These episodes might represent obstructive apnea, hypoventilation or intrapulmonary right-to-left shunting.[112,125] The significance of such episodes is unclear; however, recurrent hypoxemia has been associated with retinopathy of prematurity,[12] necrotizing entercolitis[18] and periventricular leukomalacia.[135]

CLASSIFICATION OF APNEA

Apnea is traditionally classified into three categories based on the presence or absence of obstruction of the upper airways. These include central, obstructive and mixed apneas. Central apnea is characterized by total cessation of inspiratory efforts with no evidence of obstruction. In obstructed apnea, the infant tries to breathe against an obstructed upper airway resulting in chest wall motion without nasal airflow throughout the entire apnea. Mixed apnea consists of obstructed respiratory efforts usually following central pauses (Figure 30.1) and is probably the most common type of apnea. The contribution of obstruction to apnea was first described by Thach and Stark,[134] who observed that the frequency of apnea increased when the premature infant's neck was flexed. Subsequently, upper airway obstruction was found to accompany apnea even in the absence of neck flexion.[33,99] The site of obstruction in the upper airways is mostly in the pharynx; however, it may also occur at the larynx, and possibly both sites. Mixed apneas are the most common type of apnea in small premature infants and account for more than half of all apneas, followed in decreasing frequency by central and obstructive apnea.

Periodic breathing

Periodic breathing is characterized by regular cycles of breathing of 10–18 seconds' duration, interrupted by pauses of at least 3 seconds in duration, this pattern recurring for at least 2 minutes.[117] Although periodic breathing has been considered a benign respiratory pattern for which no treatment is required,[39] it shares some characteristics with apnea of prematurity. Both disorders tend to decline in frequency with advancing postconceptional age and with administration of theophylline.[9,65,71,76,106] The respiratory pauses in both can be preceded by a decline

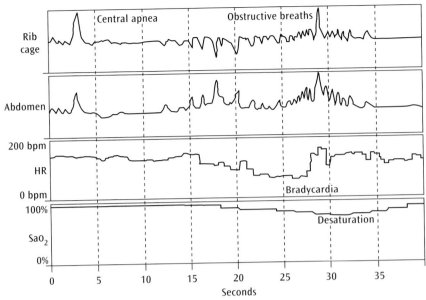

Figure 30.1 *Characteristic mixed apnea of approximately 20 seconds' duration commencing with a central component and prolonged by obstructed inspiratory efforts. In the absence of simultaneous measurement of rib cage and abdominal motion as occurs during routine impedance monitoring of chest wall motion, the obstructed inspiratory efforts would not be recognized. As noted in this tracing, bradycardia and desaturation are secondary to the cessation of effective ventilation during the mixed apnea. (Reproduced with permission from Miller, M.J., Fanaroff, A.A., Martin, R.J. (2001) Respiratory disorders in preterm and term infants. In Fanaroff, A.A., Martin, R.J. (eds),* Neonatal-Perinatal Medicine, *7th edn. Philadelphia: Harcourt.)*

in tidal volume and a decrease in respiratory frequency, indicating a decrease in central neural output.[97] Obstructive breaths at the level of the pharynx can precede the onset of respiratory cycles in both disorders.[97] Important differences, however, exist between the two disorders. During periodic breathing the respiratory pauses appear to be self-limited, and ventilation does continue, albeit in cyclic fashion. By contrast, infants with prolonged apnea may fail to reinitiate ventilation entirely or do so ineffectively. In addition, the respiratory pauses during apnea are associated with swallowing movements which are not observed during periodic breathing. Periodic breathing can be resolved with an increase in environmental oxygen,[39] but as the disorder is benign and does not result in significant bradycardia or desaturation, this is not clinically indicated. Periodic breathing is not a precursor to significant apnea.[15]

EPIDEMIOLOGY

The incidence of apnea of prematurity is inversely related to gestational age.[94] The incidence was found to be 19 percent for infants weighing between 1250 and 1750 g, 70 percent for infants between 1001 and 1250 g, and 84 percent for infants less than 1000 g.[7,94] There appears to be a relationship between the time of appearance of apnea of prematurity and the presence of lung disease. Carlo *et al.*[21]

have shown that the onset of apnea may occur on the first day after birth in infants without RDS but the peak frequency of apnea may be on day 7 in infants with RDS. Barrington and Finer demonstrated that apnea occurred on the first day after birth in all healthy preterm infants investigated.[16] The precise incidence of apnea obviously depends on the diagnostic criteria employed; nevertheless, both the frequency and duration of apnea decrease between 1 and 20 weeks postnatal age.[80]

Recent evidence suggests that some full-term infants have apnea in the first month after birth. In a study that included at-risk and healthy term control infants on home monitors,[114] apnea exceeding 20 seconds was detected in 43 percent of healthy term infants.

PATHOPHYSIOLOGY

Apnea of prematurity is thought to be secondary to immaturity of brainstem centers that regulate breathing. This immaturity in regulation of breathing is also manifested by immaturity in the respiratory responses to hypoxia, hypercapnia and an exaggerated inhibitory response to stimulation of airway receptors (Figure 30.2). Although a cause and effect relationship has not been documented for disturbed control of breathing and the occurrence of apnea in preterm infants, strong associations are very well established. Histologically, immaturity of the preterm

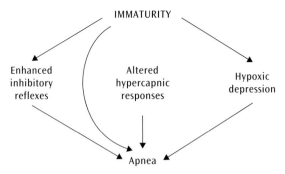

Figure 30.2 *Proposed pathophysiological mechanisms predisposing or leading to apnea of prematurity.*

brain is manifested by a decreased number of synaptic connections, dendritic arborizations and poor mylenization.[69,123] Henderson-Smart and coworkers reported that auditory evoked responses are longer in infants with apnea than in matched preterm controls, indicating delay in brainstem conduction time.[60] Furthermore, multiple inhibitory neurotransmitters and neuromodulators have been implicated in the pathogenesis of disturbances of breathing, both at the peripheral and central chemoreceptors; these include dopamine, adenosine, endorphins, GABA and prostaglandins (p. 38) and may be upregulated in early life.

Ventilatory responses to hypercapnia and hypoxia

The ventilatory response to CO_2 has been shown to increase with advancing postnatal[41,75,119] and gestational[41,75] age in prematurely born human infants. The breathing response to CO_2 in preterm infants is impaired when compared to term neonates or adults.[41,75,119] This difference is both quantitative and qualitative. Whereas term neonates and adults increase their ventilation through an increase in both tidal volume and frequency, preterm infants were not able to increase frequency in response to CO_2.[75,102,119] Several mechanisms have been proposed to explain this attenuation in the hypercapnic ventilatory response to CO_2 exhibited by premature newborns of various species. Possibilities include differences in the mechanical properties of the lung or central integration of chemoreceptor or other neuronal signals and/or lack of maturation in the peripheral or central chemoreceptors. Krauss *et al.* characterized simultaneous improvement in lung compliance and increasing postconceptional age in parallel with maturation of the hypercapnic response in infants.[75] Frantz *et al.* confirmed that the ventilatory responses to CO_2 are decreased in premature infants and, by measuring end expiratory occlusion pressures, suggested that decreased respiratory center sensitivity contributed to this phenomenon.[41] In vagotomized, intubated, and ventilated rats, the hypercapnic ventilatory response

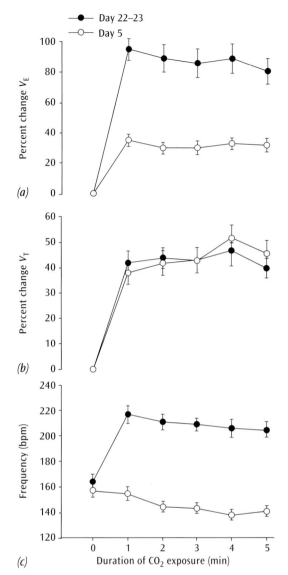

Figure 30.3 *Effect of 5-min exposure to 5 percent CO_2 on V_E (a), tidal volume (V_T) (b), and frequency (c) at 5 and 22–23 days of age in unrestrained rats. Values are means $\pm$ se. Hypercapnia caused a significantly greater increase in V_E at 22–23 days compared with 5 days. Percentage increase in V_T was similar at the two ages. Frequency decreased significantly from baseline at 5 days, whereas it increased significantly from baseline at 22–23 days. Open circles indicate 5-day-old and closed circles indicate 22–23-day-old animal.* (Reproduced with permission from Abu-Shaweesh, J.M., Dreshaj, I.A., Thomas, A. et al. (1999) Changes in respiratory timing induced by hypercapnia in maturing rats. Journal of Applied Physiology **87**, 484–490)

is impaired in newborn rats relative to adult rats, signifying a central origin for such response (Figure 30.3).[1]

The hypercapnic breathing response in preterm infants with apnea is impaired to a greater extent when compared with non-apneic controls.[35,43,117] Gerhardt and Bancalari[43] and others documented that the CO_2 response in preterm infants with apnea was shifted to the right and had a lower slope than in infants without apnea. At the same level of CO_2 and for the same degree of change in alveolar CO_2, babies with apnea had lower minute ventilation. Pulmonary mechanics, respiratory frequency and dead space volume were similar between the two groups, indicating a central origin for this disturbed breathing in preterm infants with apnea.[43] These data indicate a central origin for the attenuated CO_2 response in preterm babies, in particular in those with apnea. A cause and effect relationship between apnea of prematurity and the attenuated response to CO_2, however, has not been clearly established, and both might simply represent facets of a decreased respiratory drive.

The hypoxic ventilatory response has been well characterized in newborn (especially preterm) infants. On exposure to hypoxia, neonates have an initial increase in ventilation that lasts 1–2 minutes, followed by a decline in breathing to below baseline ventilation.[26,118] This late decline has been traditionally termed hypoxic ventilatory depression (Figure 30.4). The initial increase in ventilation is believed to be secondary to stimulation of peripheral chemoreceptors, primarily in the carotid body. In preterm human infants, the late decrease in ventilation is mainly secondary to a decrease in frequency while the increase in tidal volume is relatively sustained. The origin of the late depression is not well understood.

Several theories have been postulated to explain hypoxic ventilatory depression, including a decrease in $PaCO_2$ secondary to the initial hyperventilation or decrease in cerebral blood flow, a decrease in metabolism,[3] and hypoxia-mediated central depression of ventilation.[26] Exposure to a combination of CO_2 and hypoxia did not prevent the late respiratory depression, suggesting that a decrease in $PaCO_2$ is not the origin of this hypoxic depression.[115] Multiple neurotransmitters have been implicated as mediators for hypoxic depression including adenosine, endorphins and γ-aminobutyric acid (GABA). The use of blockers for these neurotransmitters such as methylxanthines for adenosine, naloxone for endorphins and bicuculline for GABA have successfully prevented the late hypoxic depression and caused a sustained ventilatory response. Furthermore, the depressive response to hypoxia is diminished by experimental lesions in the upper brainstem and midbrain of fetal lambs,[46] indicating the presence of descending inhibitory tracts that contribute to hypoxic ventilatory depression. Consistent with these findings is the observation that a progressive decrease in inspired oxygen concentration causes a significant flattening of carbon dioxide responsiveness in preterm infants.[120]

Hypoxic ventilatory depression has been implicated as underlying apnea of prematurity;[117] however, recent data do not support this hypothesis. Hypoxia does not appear to precede episodes of apnea, and in most occasions the infants start with a normal PaO_2 prior to the occurrence

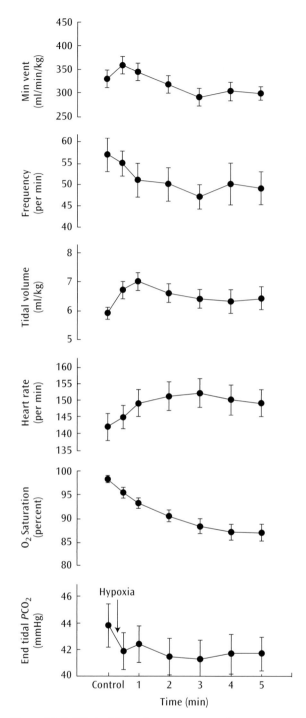

Figure 30.4 *Effect of hypoxic exposure on minute ventilation (Min vent), frequency, tidal volume, heart rate, O_2 saturation and end tidal PCO_2 in 12 preterm infants of 2–3 weeks postnatal age. Five-minute exposure to 15 percent O_2 caused a transient increase in minute ventilation at 1–2 minutes followed by a decrease to below baseline at 5 minutes. While the tidal volume exhibited sustained increase above baseline, frequency decreased significantly with the hypoxic exposure. (Reproduced with permission from Martin, R.J., DiFiore, J.M., Jana, L. et al. (1998) Persistence of the biphasic ventilatory response to hypoxia in preterm infants.* Journal of Pediatrics **132**, 960–964.)

of apnea.[63] Although supplemental oxygen is successful in preventing periodic breathing, it has no role for treating apnea of prematurity in the absence of hypoxemia. Furthermore, hypoxic ventilatory depression persists in healthy preterm infants at the time of hospital discharge at around 33–36 weeks postconceptional age, at a time where there may not be clinically significant apnea.[88] In addition, the biphasic ventilatory response to hypoxia is not unique to apneic infants. Once hypoxia occurs, however, it might aggravate apnea and result in delayed recovery from apnea.

Upper airway and lung afferents

Stimulation of the laryngeal mucosa, either chemically (by water, ammonium chloride or acidic solutions) or mechanically, causes inhibition of breathing and apnea in humans and animals.[55,79,110,132] This reflex-induced apnea is mediated through the superior laryngeal nerve, as bilateral sectioning of the superior laryngeal nerve (SLN) abolishes laryngeal stimulation-induced apnea.[47,55,81] The reflex apnea has been shown to be associated with contraction of the thyroarytenoid muscle, causing closure of the glottis and swallowing movements, signifying active stimulation of expiratory related brainstem centers.

There appears to be a maturational change in reflex-induced apnea. Chemical stimulation of the larynx in newborn piglets caused respiratory arrest, while older piglets do not express a similar response.[47,81] Maturation of the laryngeal inhibitory reflex is also common to a wide variety of other animals including dogs, monkeys, sheep and cats.[93,122,131,132] Preterm infants also appear to express such an exaggerated inhibitory reflex as they elicit prolonged apnea in response to instilling saline in the oropharynx.[110] The mechanisms underlying such a maturational change in reflex-induced apnea are not known; however, they do not seem to be related to changes in laryngeal receptors,[56] changes in central synaptic connections, or maturation of the carotid body.[38] It has been shown that hypercapnia increases while hypocapnia decreases the threshold for SLN stimulation-induced apnea.[78,84] Cooling of the ventromedullary surface, a technique used to decrease central chemosensitivity by inhibiting synaptic transmission at this site, decreased the threshold for laryngeal stimulation-induced apnea.[84] Theophylline, which stimulates respiratory neural output, has been shown to block SLN stimulation-induced apnea.[81] It seems, therefore, that the exaggerated reflex-induced apnea seen in newborn infants and animals is related to decreased central neural output or a dominance of inhibitory pathways. Furthermore, blocking $GABA_A$ receptors resulted in complete abolition of SLN stimulation-induced apnea in piglets (Figure 30.5).

Reflex-induced apnea has been implicated as an underlying mechanism in apnea of prematurity[110] and gastroesophageal reflux-induced apnea.[79,91] Swallows were found to be much more common during apnea than during comparable periods of interrupted sleep.[90] Furthermore, swallowing during respiratory pauses is unique to apnea and does not occur during periodic breathing.[95] In addition, Kianicka et al.[72] and Renolleau et al.[116] described spontaneous apneas associated with contraction of the thyroarytenoid muscle and swallowing movements in fetal and preterm lambs. These observations may suggest a common origin for apnea of prematurity and reflex-induced apnea.

Lung afferents play an important role in regulating respiratory timing and may play a role in apnea of prematurity. Stimulation of pulmonary stretch receptors, via increasing lung volume, causes shortening of inspiratory time, prolongation of expiratory time, or both.[27,62,87] This reflex, known as the Hering–Breuer reflex, is mediated through the vagus nerve (p. 42).[62] Preterm infants seem to be more dependent than term infants on the Hering–Breuer reflex to regulate breathing frequency. Olinsky et al.[103] used airway occlusion to estimate the contribution of stretch receptors to respiratory timing in term and preterm infants. Preterm infants had more prolongation of inspiratory time following occlusion than term infants, signifying that in preterm infants the Hering–Breuer reflex is more active and contributes to their higher respiratory frequency.[103] The purpose of such an exaggerated reflex may be to prevent full emptying of the lung and maintain adequate lung volume at end expiration. The Hering–Breuer reflex, however, was found to be weak in infants of 32 weeks gestation, increasing in strength at 36–38 weeks and decreasing thereafter.[19] The Hering–Breuer deflation reflex is also activated on deflation of the lung and results in inspiratory augmentation.[62] Hannam and colleagues found that, unlike term infants, preterm infants responded to the deflation reflex by their shortening inspiratory time.[54] Preterm infants also had short apneas during chest compression that were mostly central in origin, and infants with apnea had even greater shortening of inspiratory time. Such data indicate that on deflation of the lung, as during an apnea, preterm infants were less likely to initiate breathing and tended to have respiratory pauses.

Upper airway muscles

The prominence of mixed apnea has led to comparative analysis of upper airway versus chest wall muscle responses to chemoreceptor stimulation. Upper airway muscles, such as the alae nasi, genioglossus, and posterior cricoarytenoid (laryngeal abductor), typically have their onset and peak of phasic activity prior to corresponding events in the diaphragm.[22] This presumably serves to ensure upper airway patency at peak inspiratory flow. In response to hypercapnic exposure in piglets, there was a relatively linear

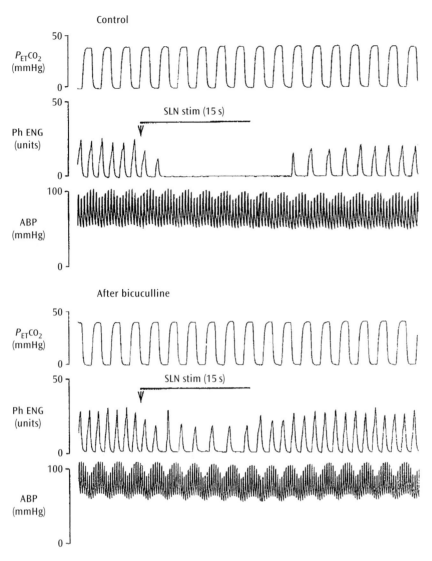

Figure 30.5 *Phrenic nerve electrogram (ENG) and $P_{ET}CO_2$ in response to superior laryngeal nerve stimulation (SLN) before (top) and after (bottom) intercisternal administration of $GABA_A$ receptor blocker bicuculline. SLN stimulation before bicuculline caused apnea that persisted beyond the duration of the stimulation. The same level of stimulation after bicuculline administration caused a decrease in phrenic nerve amplitude and frequency but failed to produce apnea. ABP, arterial blood pressure.* (Reproduced with permission from Abu-Shaweesh, J.M., Dreshaj, I.A., Haxhiu, M.A. et al. (2001) GABAergic mechanisms are involved in superior laryngeal nerve stimulation-induced apnea. Journal of Applied Physiology **90**, 1570–1576.)

increase in diaphragm activation.[22] By contrast, genioglossus and alae nasi exhibited a higher threshold and activities only began to increase at a significantly higher level of CO_2.[23] It is possible that during hypercapnia, as occurs during apnea, an initial increase in diaphragm, but not upper airway activation, superimposed upon collapsed pharyngeal or laryngeal structures, might predispose to the obstructed inspiratory efforts that characterize mixed apnea. In premature infants, non-invasive measurements have demonstrated that the diaphragm EMG of obstructed inspiratory efforts is low.[42] However, at resolution of apnea, both diaphragm and upper airway activities are increased. It therefore appears that decrease in diaphragm activity is common to both central and mixed apnea, although collapse or closure of the upper airway may prolong the episode and its consequences.

Neurotransmitters and neuromodulaters

There are limited data regarding the balance of excitatory and inhibitory neurotransmitters in the genesis of apnea of prematurity. For obvious reasons, invasive studies cannot be performed in newborn infants and there is no optimal animal model for apnea of prematurity. Therefore, most studies on the relationship of neurotransmitters to respiratory control are related to the effect of these substances, or their inhibitors, on the breathing responses to hypoxia, hypercapnia, and reflex apnea in animals and to a lesser extent in neonates. The most widely studied inhibitory neurotransmitters in relation to disturbances in control of breathing include adenosine, γ-aminobutyric acid (GABA), prostaglandin and endorphins.

Adenosine is a product of adenosine triphosphate (ATP) that is present in various portions of the brain and cerebrospinal fluid (CSF).[101,105] Adenosine is known to depress neural function,[34] and analogs of adenosine have been shown to decrease respiration in neonatal rabbits and pigs.[28,58,121] The involvement of adenosine in hypoxic ventilatory depression is suggested by the observation that hypoxia increases adenosine in the interstitial fluid of the brain as well as the CSF and plasma in newborn piglets.[101,105] Furthermore, adenosine antagonists reversed hypoxic depression in anesthetized newborn piglets.[28] The role of adenosine in apnea of prematurity is suggested by the ability of adenosine antagonists, the xanthine derivatives theophylline and caffeine, to decrease the incidence of apnea of prematurity. The exact mechanism and location of action of adenosine as well as the interaction of adenosine with other neurotransmitters, however, remain to be identified.

GABA is the major inhibitory neurotransmitter in the CNS. Its involvement in the control of breathing is suggested by the ability of exogenous GABA to inhibit breathing and cause apnea in animals.[57,64] Both structural and functional differences in GABA$_A$ receptors have been observed during development.[24,73,86] GABA$_A$ receptors are hetero-oligomers assembled from different subunits.[124] During embryonic and early postnatal development, the 'mix' of GABA$_A$ receptor subunits differs from that in adults.[73,86] Furthermore, Xia and Haddad[139] demonstrated that the newborn rat brainstem has a much higher GABA$_A$ receptor density than does the adult brainstem. GABA has been implicated in the attenuated ventilatory responses to hypoxia, hypercapnia and reflex-induced apnea in piglets. GABA antagonist was able to prevent the hypoxic depression induced by repeated hypoxia and prevent apnea induced by hypoxia in newborn piglets.[98] Blocking GABA$_A$ receptors also prevents the decrease in breathing frequency in response to CO_2 in newborn rats.[1] Administration of bicuculline, a GABA$_A$ receptor blocker, both systematically and intracisternally was able to prevent the reflex-induced apnea originating from superior laryngeal nerve stimulation in newborn piglets.[2] Therefore, GABA has the potential to play a key role in the vulnerability of preterm infants to disturbed breathing including apnea of prematurity.

Endorphins have been widely studied in the control of breathing. Exogenous endorphin and encephalin analogs produced a consistent decrease in respiration in fetal and neonatal animals.[49,89] Administration of endorphin antagonists to adult subjects, however, had no effect on their breathing.[40] Endorphin levels are elevated in the human neonate at birth.[137] Although β-endorphin is increased in neonatal piglets, this effect is confined to the plasma and does not involve the CSF or respiratory-related regions.[100] Endogenous opioids, however, were found to modulate the hypoxic ventilatory response in newborn infants and animals.[29,50] Furthermore, naloxone produced an improvement in apnea and periodic breathing in infants in whom β-endorphin-like immunoreactivity in the CSF was elevated.[104] Although these data support a role for opioids in respiratory control in the neonates, the effect of anesthesia in such studies and the interaction of opioids with other inhibitory neurotransmitters need to be clarified. Opioid antagonists are not used routinely in the treatment of apnea of prematurity.

Infusion of PGE$_1$ produces respiratory depression in 12 percent of infants during treatment for congenital

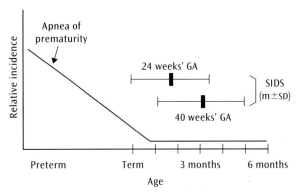

Figure 30.6 *Schematic representation of the timing of sudden infant death syndrome (SIDS) in term (40 weeks' gestation) and very preterm (24 weeks' gestation) infants, in relation to the decline in incidence of apnea of prematurity. It would appear that apnea has largely resolved by 44 weeks' post-conceptional age, which is prior to the peak incidence of SIDS at all gestational ages (GA). (Reproduced with permission from Miller, M.T., Fanaroff, A.A., Martin, R.J. (2001) Respiratory disorders in preterm and term infants. In Fanaroff, A.A., Martin, R.J. (eds),* Neonatal-Perinatal Medicine, *7th edn. Philadelphia: Harcourt.)*

heart disease.[83] PGE$_1$ also decreases and indomethacin enhances phrenic activity in newborn piglets.[85] Hammerman and Zangen described a case of apnea of prematurity that was resistant to conventional management but responded to treatment with indomethacin.[53]

Clinical resolution of apnea

Apnea of prematurity requiring intervention generally resolves by about 37–40 weeks postconceptional age.[96] In the most premature infants, however, apnea may persist beyond this age, especially episodic desaturation and bradycardia associated with short respiratory pauses.[32] Eichenwald *et al.* described, in a group of infants of 24–28 weeks gestational age, that apnea and bradycardia frequently persisted beyond 36 weeks postconceptional age and in infants of 24 weeks of gestation beyond 40 weeks postconceptional age.[37] The persistence of these episodes of apnea and the accompanying bradycardia is frequently a cause for prolonged hospitalization.

The CHIME group have looked at the incidence of cardiorespiratory events at home in at-risk infants, that is those for whom a monitor would be prescribed; this includes preterm infants and siblings of SIDS infants, as well as a control group of asymptomatic term neonates. Their findings suggest that the incidence of cardiorespiratory events in preterm infants is greater than that in term infants until about 43 weeks postconceptional age (Figure 30.6).[114] Beyond that period, within the power of that clinical trial, there was no longer a significant

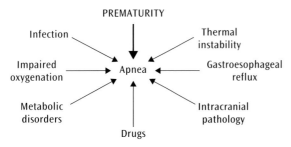

Figure 30.7 *Some diverse factors known to precipitate development of apneic episodes in predisposed preterm infants. (Reproduced with permission from Martin, R.J., Miller, M.J., Carlo, W.A. (1986) Pathogenesis of apnea in preterm infants.* Journal of Pediatrics ***107***, 738.)*

increased number of events in the preterm infants. This has likely implications for the duration of home monitoring when this is prescribed.

CLINICAL ASSOCIATIONS

Although typically idiopathic, other disorders are associated with or lead to apnea. Before concluding that apnea in a preterm infant is due to immature respiratory control, a number of potential causes should be ruled out (Figure 30.7). Central nervous system problems, including intracranial bleed, congenital malformations and hydrocephalus, can precipitate apnea in the preterm infant. Infections (sepsis, meningitis) are common in preterm infants and sometimes present with unstable breathing patterns. Anemia, another frequent problem in preterm infants, can also be associated with apnea. Joshi et al.[67] showed that blood transfusions improved irregular breathing patterns in preterm infants. While clinical practice has moved away from using blood transfusion as treatment for apnea, Joshi's study supported the notion that mild hypoxic respiratory depression may contribute to apnea. Additional factors that may precipitate apnea include metabolic disorders, especially hypoglycemia and hypocalcemia, temperature instability and drugs such as opiates and magnesium.

Gastroesophageal reflux (GER) was first associated with apnea when Herbst et al.[61] suggested it might be related to the 'near miss' sudden infant death syndrome (SIDS). It has further been suggested that while breathing abnormalities are more frequent when an infant is sleeping, apnea during waking periods might be more likely to be due to GER.[128] The possibility of GER precipitating apnea has also been extended to the preterm newborn.[5] Although apnea and GER often are seen in the same infant, the timing of reflux in relation to apneic events suggest the relationship is more coincidental than causal. Furthermore, although reflux of gastric contents to the larynx induces reflex apnea, there is no clear evidence that treatment of reflux will affect frequency of apnea in most preterm infants.

TREATMENT

The management of apnea should be tailored toward choosing an appropriate treatment for the particular patient. Attention should be directed toward excluding secondary pathologies that might be accompanied by apnea (Figure 30.2). Most minor episodes of apnea can be successfully resolved with stimulation. Once the frequency and severity of such episodes is high enough to require vigorous stimulation or bag and mask ventilation or cause prolonged desaturation episodes, additional treatment should be instituted.

Pharmacological treatment

The methylxanthines theophylline and caffeine are the pharmacological agents most commonly used for the treatment of apnea. Initiation of such therapy often occurs routinely prior to initial extubation of very preterm infants (p. 161) which results in extremely widespread use of this therapy in such infants. Theophylline (1,3-dimethylxanthine) is available in both oral and intravenous preparations. The intravenous form of theophylline is its ethylenediamine tetraacetic acid salt, aminophylline. Theophylline was first reported for use in apnea of prematurity in 1973,[76] and aminophylline was used shortly thereafter.[17] Initial reports emphasized increased respiratory center output[44] and enhanced diaphragmatic contractility[11] as mechanisms of action.

Caffeine (1,3,7-trimethylxanthine) is naturally occurring in many plants, and appears naturally or is added to many beverages such as coffee. Caffeine has also been shown to decrease apnea in preterm infants.[9] It is available as caffeine citrate, for both oral and intravenous use. Early studies suggested that caffeine was effective in infants who were non-responders to theophylline. This finding, however, may have been an artifact of study design, as the use of caffeine was reserved for those infants who did not respond to an initial course of theophylline. Caffeine, however, does have advantages over theophylline and may be a preferable alternative for a number of reasons. It has a higher therapeutic index, making toxicity less of a concern. Also, a once-a-day dosing is possible because of its longer half-life.[10] Both methylxanthines have been shown to reduce apnea episodes and the use of intermittent positive pressure ventilation (IPPV) in preterm infants.[59]

Methylxanthines are thought to stimulate central neural output to the respiratory muscles, probably via antagonism of adenosine receptors; however, the precise site of action and mechanism(s) whereby apnea is decreased have not been determined. Theophylline exhibits a prolonged half-life in premature newborns when compared with more mature newborns, children, or adults. There are two metabolic pathways for the elimination of theophylline: through hydroxylation or demethylation. These pathways, however, are underdeveloped in the premature infant and elimination progresses by a slower pathway of methylation to caffeine, which itself is biologically active. Disposition can be highly variable. Serum concentrations of methylxanthines may not be entirely predictable based on dosage and vary considerably from infant to infant. Serum concentrations of theophylline should be monitored whenever aminophylline or theophylline is used. Due to the higher therapeutic index of caffeine, serum concentrations of caffeine are less critical and are not usually followed, except in the absence of clinical response or evidence of toxicity. A recent report suggests the use of saliva for therapeutic drug monitoring may be valuable,[31] but this is still under investigation.

The treatment of apneic episodes with methylxanthines is not without hazards. Side-effects of theophylline include hyperactivity, tachycardia, cardiac dysrhythmias, feeding intolerance, and seizures. Mild diuresis is caused by all methylxanthines. The clinician should be aware of possible drug–drug interactions when dosing methylxanthines. Concomitant administration of medications that affect liver function and those whose clearance depend on the cytochrome P_{450} should alert the clinician to the need for close monitoring of therapeutic effects and toxic side-effects.

Doxapram is a respiratory stimulant that is typically used in addition to a methylxanthine.[14,113] In two head-to-head trials (both involving small numbers of infants) it was shown to be effective, but not better for the reduction of apnea in preterm infants. Doxapram may also have some benefits when added to an infant's regimen in refractory cases.[36,108] Side-effects include poor tolerance of the oral preparation and a report of second-degree heart block in a small number of preterm infants.[30]

Non-pharmacological treatment

Some infants continue to have clinically troublesome apnea while on methylxanthines. Continuous positive airway pressure (CPAP) is a relatively safe and effective treatment for such infants. CPAP is thought to decrease the frequency of apnea by increasing functional residual capacity (FRC) and stabilizing oxygenation and/or by splinting the upper airway with positive pressure (p. 150). Apnea frequently involves an obstructive component; therefore, CPAP is effective in infants whose episodes are precipitated or prolonged by pharyngeal obstruction. Typically, relatively low CPAP levels of 3–5 cmH$_2$O are used. The main disadvantage of nasal CPAP is that it may become cumbersome over a prolonged period secondary to nasal breakdown and interference with gavage feeding. Recently, use of a nasal cannula flow in which CPAP can be delivered with flows exceeding 1 l/min has been suggested as an equivalent treatment modality.[129]

Inhalation of a low concentration of CO_2 has also been proposed as a safe and effective treatment. In 10 preterm infants, exposure to 1 hour of a low concentration of CO_2 ranging from 0.5 percent to 1.5 percent was associated with significant decrease in apnea, and improved oxygenation.[6] These data are, however, too limited to recommend this method of therapy at this time.

For severe and refractory apnea, endotracheal intubation and artificial ventilation may be needed. Minimal ventilator settings should be used to allow for spontaneous ventilatory efforts, and to minimize the risk of barotrauma.

Role of home monitoring

Most preterm infants have resolved their apnea and bradycardia by the time they are ready for hospital discharge. For a subset of infants, however, the persistence of apnea and bradycardia may delay their discharge from hospital. In infants in whom cardiorespiratory events require intervention, the common practice of delaying discharge until the infant is event free for 5–7 days is widely accepted. For infants in whom apnea and bradycardia events resolve spontaneously, it is possible that a shorter episode-free period prior to discharge may be sufficient. Such events frequently persist until a postconceptional age of around 43 weeks.

Home cardiorespiratory monitoring may offer an alternative to a prolonged hospital stay in selected infants. One of the roles of home apnea monitoring may include the monitor functioning as a therapeutic device, not simply an alarm mechanism. It has been suggested that the alarm may not only alert the caregivers, but may also arouse the infant sufficiently to terminate an event, although this hypothesis has never been rigorously tested. Home monitoring is probably indicated in the small number of infants who are discharged on oxygen or xanthine therapy. Diagnostic pneumograms prior to discharge are of limited value in deciding who needs a home monitor; however, when used in a selective manner, they may aid in the characterization of events (that is determining whether they are central or obstructive) and serve a useful educational role. In those infants for whom a home monitor is prescribed, this can usually be discontinued by 42–44 weeks postconceptional age. While persistence of apnea and bradycardia until 42–44 weeks is widely recognized, there is no evidence that this is a risk factor for SIDS. The peak incidence for SIDS is several weeks later even in the most preterm infants (see below).

OUTCOME

Physiological consequences of apnea

Cessation of breathing is usually accompanied by multiple ventilatory and cardiovascular consequences. Both hypoxia and hypercapnia accompany prolonged apnea.[94] Transcutaneous PO_2 (TcO_2) in preterm infants was observed to start decreasing 8 seconds after the onset of apnea and continued to drop 26 seconds after the establishment of respiratory effort.[63] The decrease in TcO_2 has been found to be directly related to the duration of apnea and the initial TcO_2,[63,68] and to be significantly greater in obstructive than in central apnea.[68]

The cardiovascular consequences of apnea include changes in heart rate, blood pressure and pulse pressure. Bradycardia may begin within 1.5–8 seconds after the onset of apnea,[63,136] and is most often sinus in character. Hiatt et al.[63] did not find a correlation between the change in heart rate associated with apnea and the duration of apnea or the degree of hypoxemia. Henderson-Smart noted a significant correlation between the decrease in oxygen saturation and heart rate and postulated that bradycardia during apnea might be related to hypoxic stimulation of the carotid body chemoreceptors,[136] especially in the absence of lung inflation (Figure 30.8). The changes in blood pressure during apnea seem to be related to the change in heart rate. In mild and moderate bradycardia, heart rate 80–120 bpm, there was an increase in pulse pressure secondary to a decrease in diastolic pressure with and without increase in systolic blood pressure.[45,109] With more severe bradycardia (heart rate $<$ 80 bpm), both systolic and diastolic blood pressures decreased. The blood pressure returned to normal with initiation of spontaneous breathing, unless intervention was needed.[109]

The changes in cerebral blood flow velocity (CBFV) during apnea are similar to those in blood pressure. During mild and moderate bradycardia, the diastolic CBFV decreased with no change in systolic velocity; however, during severe bradycardia, the CBFV decreased further, usually to the extent that no or minimal diastolic flow could be detected, together with a decrease in systolic CBFV.[109] Therefore, in infants without adequate cerebrovascular autoregulation, cerebral perfusion may decrease to very low levels during prolonged apnea and might potentially exacerbate hypoxic-ischemic brain injury in susceptible premature infants.

Sudden infant death syndrome

Apnea has long been suspected as a final common pathway involved in the unexpected death of an infant. It has been suggested that sudden infant death syndrome (SIDS) must result from either cardiac or respiratory arrest, and that respiratory arrest is the more likely cause.[52] Although

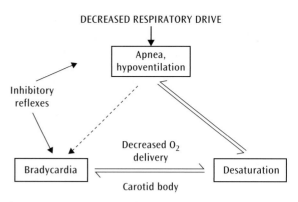

Figure 30.8 *Proposed physiological mechanisms whereby apnea induces reflex bradycardia. This may occur secondary to hypoxemia in the absence of lung inflation or via stimulation of upper airway inhibitory afferents. (Reproduced with permission from Martin, R.J., Fanaroff, A.A. (1998) Neonatal apnea, bradycardia or desaturation: does it matter? Journal of Pediatrics* **132***, 758.)*

the pauses in breathing that constitute apnea of prematurity are not the equivalent of respiratory arrests, the relationship between apnea and SIDS is somewhat more complicated.

The term SIDS was given to the constellation of clinical findings of a sudden unexpected death in a previously well infant, in the 1960s. A few years later, the first suggestion that prolonged apnea might be related to SIDS was published.[130] Although subsequent events proved both the facts and the logic of the observations in that report were flawed, the relationship between breathing abnormalities and SIDS is still being investigated. Infants who are born prematurely have a higher incidence of apnea, and also a higher incidence of SIDS. Premature birth was first proposed as a risk factor for SIDS by Adelson and Kinney in 1956;[4] however, the coexistence of the two conditions in premature infants does not necessarily imply cause and effect.

Much effort has been devoted to identifying the breathing patterns that might either be predictive of SIDS, or shed some light on the pathophysiology of a specific breathing abnormality in these infants. Most of these studies have involved infants who came to medical attention with clinical signs of altered breathing. The research has largely focused on infants who had had a 'near-miss' or acute life-threatening events (ALTEs). Suspected abnormalities have included prolonged sleep apnea[51] and excessive periodic breathing.[70] In one of the largest series, Southall et al.[126] reported on term and preterm infants in whom prospective cardiorespiratory recordings were made. When the recordings of infants who went on to die of SIDS were analyzed, there were no cases exhibiting prolonged apnea. This finding suggests that prolonged apnea is not a predictor of subsequent SIDS, although it leaves unanswered the question of apnea playing a role in the terminal event. One remarkable report has documented apparent continued breathing during a sudden and unexpected death.[92] The finding that SIDS rates have decreased following an education program to encourage supine sleeping position[138] lends support to the idea that airway obstruction or asphyxiation may cause some of these deaths.

Although numerous abnormalities in breathing and other physiological parameters have been reported, the majority of infants who die of SIDS are not identified as abnormal in any way prior to their death. It is currently thought that a number of problems comprise the deaths that in the past were labeled SIDS. A small percentage of these deaths may include such things as undetected metabolic disease, homicide (lethal Munchausen by proxy), and cardiac arrhythmia. It is likely, however that many are due to factors relating to the respiratory system, such as airway occlusion problems, abnormalities in arousal and disorders of respiratory control.

Effect on long-term outcome

The long-term effects of apnea, with or without bradycardia, on the preterm infant are not clear. It has long been suspected that apneic episodes may be associated with neurodevelopmental delay,[13] but separating the consequences of premature birth from the effects of apnea of prematurity has proven difficult. These infants often have multiple problems during the course of their hospital stay, many of which, including sepsis and intraventricular hemorrhage (IVH), are also suspected of contributing to poor neurodevelopmental outcome. In one series amongst infants born weighing less than 750 g,[133] factors that predicted poor school-age outcomes included chronic lung disease and apnea of prematurity. In an attempt to answer this question, Cheung et al.[25] followed 124 very low birth weight (VLBW) infants to 24 months of age to evaluate the relationship between predischarge apnea and subsequent neurodevelopmental outcome. They found that the duration of artificial ventilation and the grade of IVH were independent predictors of neurodevelopmental outcome, and that mean oximetry desaturation and frequency of predischarge apnea correlated with mental and motor developmental scores. Although several other studies have found no difference in outcome of infants with apnea,[74,82] it would seem prudent to suspect that the recurrent hypoxia experienced by these infants may affect their neural development.

ACKNOWLEDGMENT

This work was supported by NIH Grant #HL 62527. We thank Ms Cecily Lewis for secretarial support.

REFERENCES

1 Abu-Shaweesh, J.M., Dreshaj, I.A., Thomas, A. et al. (1999) Changes in respiratory timing induced by hypercapnia in maturing rats. *Journal of Applied Physiology* **87**, 484–490.

2 Abu-Shaweesh, J.M., Dreshaj, I.A., Haxhiu, M.A. et al. (2001) GABAergic mechanisms are involved in superior laryngeal nerve stimulation-induced apnea. *Journal of Applied Physiology* **90**, 1570–1576.

3 Adamsons, K., Jr (1959) Breathing and the thermal environment in young rabbits. *Journal of Physiology* **149**, 144.

4 Adelson, L., Kinney, E.R. (1956) Sudden and unexpected death in infancy and childhood. *Pediatrics* **17**, 663–697.

5 Ajuriaguerra, M., Radvanyi-Bouvet, M.-F., Houn, C. et al. (1991) Gastroesophegeal reflux and apnea in prematurely born infants during wakefulness and sleep. *American Journal of Diseases of Children* **145**, 1132–1136.

6 Al-Aif, S., Alvaro, R., Manfreda, J. et al. (2001) Inhalation of low (0.5 percent – 1.5 percent) CO_2 as a potential treatment for apnea of prematurity. *Seminars in Perinatology* **25**, 100–106.

7 Alden, E.R., Mandelkorn, T., Woodrum, D.E. et al. (1972) Morbidity and mortality of infants weighing less than 1000 grams in an intensive care nursery. *Pediatrics* **50**, 40–49.

8 Aranda, J.V., Turmen, T. (1979) Methylxanthines in apnea of prematurity. *Clinical Perinatology* **6**, 87–108.

9 Aranda, J.V., Gorman, W., Bergsteinsson, H. et al. (1977) Efficacy of caffeine in treatment of apnea in the low-birthweight infant. *Journal of Pediatrics* **90**, 467–472.

10 Aranda, J.V., Cook, C.E., Gorman, W. et al. (1979) Pharmacokinetic profile of caffeine in the premature newborn infant with apnea. *Journal of Pediatrics* **94**, 663–668.

11 Aubier, M., DeTroyer, A., Sampson, M. et al. (1981) Aminophylline improves diaphragmatic contractility. *New England Journal of Medicine* **305**, 249–252.

12 Avery, G.B., Glass, P. (1988) Retinopathy of prematurity: what causes it? *Clinics in Perinatology* **15**, 917–928.

13 Bacola, E., Behrle, F.C., De Schweinitz, L. et al. (1966) Perinatal and environmental factors in late neurologic sequelae. I. Infants having birth weight under 1500 grams. *American Journal of Diseases of Children* **112**, 359–368.

14 Bairam, A., Faulon, M., Monin, P., Vert, P. (1992) Doxapram for the initial treatment of idiopathic apnea of prematurity. *Biology of the Neonate* **61**, 209–213.

15 Barrington, K.J., Finer, N.N. (1990) Periodic breathing and apnea in preterm infants. *Pediatric Research* **27**, 118–121.

16 Barrington, K., Finer, N. (1991) The natural history of the appearance of apnea of prematurity. *Pediatric Research* **29**, 372–375.

17 Bednarek, F.J., Roloff, D.W. (1976) Treatment of apnea of prematurity with aminophylline. *Pediatrics* **58**, 335–339.

18 Beeby, P.J., Jeffery, H. (1992) Risk factors for necrotizing enterocolitis: the influence of gestational age. *Archives of Disease in Childhood* **67**, 432–435.

19 Bodegard, G., Schwieler, G.H., Skoglund, S., Zetterstrom, R. (1969) Control of respiration in newborn babies. I. The development of the Hering–Breur inflation reflex. *Acta Paediatrica Scandinavica* **58**, 567–571.

20 Boros, S.J., Reynolds, J.W. (1976) Prolonged apnea of prematurity: treatment with continuous distending pressure delivered by nasopharyngeal tube. *Clinical Pediatrics (Philadelphia)* **15**, 123–134.

21 Carlo, W.A., Martin, R.J., Versteegh, F.G. et al. (1982) The effect of respiratory distress syndrome on chest wall

movements and respiratory pauses in preterm infants. *American Review of Respiratory Disease* **126**, 103–107.

22 Carlo, W.A., Martin, R.J., Abboud, E.F. *et al.* (1983) Effect of sleep state and hypercapnia on alae nasi and diaphragm EMGs in preterm infants. *Journal of Applied Physiology* **54**, 1590–1596.

23 Carlo, W.A., Martin, R.J., DiFiore, J.M. (1988) Differences in CO_2 threshold of respiratory muscles in preterm infants. *Journal of Applied Physiology* **65**, 2434–2439.

24 Cherubini, E., Gaiarsa, J.L., Ben-Ari, Y. (1991) GABA: an excitatory transmitter in early postnatal life. *Trends in Neuroscience* **14**, 515–519.

25 Cheung, P., Barrington, K.J., Finer, N.N., Robertson, C.M.T. (1999) Early childhood neurodevelopment in very low birth weight infants with predischarge apnea. *Pediatric Pulmonology* **27**, 14–20.

26 Cross, K.W., Oppe, T.E. (1952) The effect of inhalation of high and low concentration of oxygen on the respiration of the premature infant. *Journal of Physiology* **117**, 38.

27 Cross, K.W., Klaus, M., Tooley, W.H., Weisser, K. (1960) The response of the newborn baby to inflation of the lung. *Journal of Physiology* **151**, 551–565.

28 Darnall, R.A., Bruce, R.D. (1987) Effects of adenosine and xanthine derivatives on breathing during acute hypoxia in the anesthetized newborn piglet. *Pediatric Pulmonology* **3**, 110–116.

29 De Boeck, C., Van Reempts, P., Rigatto, H., Chernick, V. (1984) Naloxone reduces decrease in ventilation induced by hypoxia in newborn infants. *Journal of Applied Physiology* **56**, 1507–1511.

30 DeVilliers, G.S., Walele, Van Der Merwe, P.-L., Kalis, N.N. (1998) Second-degree atrioventricular heart block after doxapram administration. *Journal of Pediatrics* **133**, 149–150.

31 DeWildt, S.N., Kerkvliet, K.T., Wezenberg, M.G. *et al.* (2001) Use of saliva in therapeutic drug monitoring of caffeine in preterm infants. *Therapeutic Drug Monitoring* **23**, 250–254.

32 Di Fiore, J.M, Arko, M.K., Miller, M.J. *et al.* (2001) Cardiorespiratory events in preterm infants referred for apnea monitoring studies. *Pediatrics* **108**, 1304–1308.

33 Dransfield, D.A., Spitzer, A.R., Fox, W.W. (1983) Episodic airway obstruction in premature infants. *American Journal of Diseases of Children* **137**, 441–443.

34 Dunwiddie, T.V. (1985) The physiological role of adenosine in the central nervous system. *International Review of Neurobiology* **27**, 63–139.

35 Durand, M., Cabal, L.A., Gonzalez, F. *et al.* (1985) Ventilatory control and carbon dioxide response in preterm infants with idiopathic apnea. *American Journal of Diseases of Children* **139**, 717–720.

36 Eyal, F., Alpan, G., Sagi, E. *et al.* (1985) Aminophylline versus doxapram in idiopathic apnea of prematurity: a double-blind controlled study. *Pediatrics* **75**, 709–713.

37 Eichenwald, E.C., Aina, A., Stark, A.R. (1997) Apnea frequently persists beyond term gestation in infants delivered at 24 to 28 weeks. *Pediatrics* **100**, 354–359.

38 Fagenholz, S.A., Lee, J.C., Downing, S.E. (1979) Laryngeal reflex apnea in the chemodenervated newborn piglet. *American Journal of Physiology* **237**, R10–R14.

39 Fenner, A., Schalk, U., Hoenicke, H. *et al.* (1973) Periodic breathing in premature and neonatal babies: incidence, breathing pattern, respiratory gas tension, response to changes in the composition of ambient air. *Pediatric Research* **7**, 174–183.

40 Fleetham, J.A., Clarke, H., Dhingra, S. *et al.* (1980) Endogenous opiates and chemical control of breathing in humans. *American Review of Respiratory Disease* **121**, 1045–1049.

41 Frantz, I. D. III, Adler, S.M., Thach, B.T., Taeusch, H.W. Jr. (1976) Maturational effects on respiratory responses to carbon dioxide in premature infants. *Journal of Applied Physiology* **41**, 41–45.

42 Gauda, E.B., Miller, M.J., Carlo, W.A. *et al.* (1989) Genioglossus and diaphragm activity during obstructive apnea and airway occlusion in infants. *Pediatric Research* **26**, 583–587.

43 Gerhardt, T., Bancalari, E. (1984) Apnea of prematurity: 1. Lung function and regultion of breathing. *Pediatrics* **74**, 58–62.

44 Gerhardt, T., McCarthey, J., Bancalari, E. (1979) Effect of aminophylline on respiratory center activity and metabolic rate in premature infants with idiopathic apnea. *Pediatrics* **63**, 537–542.

45 Girling, D.J. (1972) Changes in heart rate, blood pressure, and pulse pressure during apnoeic attacks in newborn babies. *Archives of Diseases in Childhood* **47**, 405–410.

46 Gluckman, P.D., Johnston, B.M. (1987) Lesions in the upper lateral pons abolish the hypoxic depression of breathing in unanesthetized fetal lambs *in utero*. *Journal of Physiology* **382**, 373–383.

47 Goding, G.S., Richardson, M.A., Trachy, R.E. (1987) Laryngeal chemoreflex: anatomic and physiologic study by use of the superior laryngeal nerve in the piglet. *Otolaryngology – Head & Neck Surgery* **97**, 28–38.

48 Grisemer, A.N. (1990) Apnea of prematurity; current management and nursing implications. *Pediatric Nursing* **16**, 606–611.

49 Grunstein, M.M., Grunstein, J.S. (1982) Maturational effect of enkephalin on respiratory control in newborn rabbits. *Journal of Applied Physiology* **53**, 1063–1070.

50 Grunstein, M.M., Hazinski, T.A., Schlueter, M.A. (1981) Respiratory control during hypoxia in newborn rabbits: implied action of endorphins. *Journal of Applied Physiology* **51**, 122–130.

51 Guilleminault, C., Ariagno, R., Souquet, M., Dement, W.C. (1976) Abnormal polygraphic findings in near-miss sudden infant death. *Lancet* **1**, 1326.

52 Guntheroth, W.G. (1995) Final pathways: Apnea. In *Crib Death: the Sudden Infants Death Syndrome*. Aromonk, NY: Futura.

53 Hammerman, C., Zangen, D. (1993) Indomethacin and apnea of prematurity. *Critical Care Medicine* **21**, 154–155.

54 Hannam, S., Ingram, D.M., Milner, A.D. (1998) A possible role for the Hering–Breuer deflation reflex in apnea of prematurity. *Journal of Pediatrics* **132**, 35–39.

55 Harding, R. (1984) Function of the larynx in the fetus and newborn. *Annual Review of Physiology* **46**, 645–659.

56 Harding, R., Johnson, P., McClelland, M.E. (1978) Liquid-sensitive laryngeal receptors in the developing sheep, cat, and monkey. *Journal of Physiology* **277**, 409–422.

57 Hedner, T., Hedner, J., Bergman, B., Iversen, K., Honason, J. (1983) Effects of GABA and some GABA analogues on respiratory regulation in the preterm rabbit. *Biology of the Neonate* **43**, 134–145.

58 Hedner, T., Hedner, J., Bergman, B., Mueller, R.A., Jonason, J. (1985) Characterization of adenosine-induced respiratory depression in the preterm rabbit. *Biology of the Neonate* **47**, 323–332.

59 Henderson-Smart, D.J., Steer, P. (2000) Methylxanthine treatment for apnea in preterm infants. *Cochrane Database System Review.* Rev 2, CD0000140.

60 Henderson-Smart, D.J., Pettigrew, A.G., Campbell, D.J. (1983) Clinical apnea and brainstem neural function in preterm infants. *New England Journal of Medicine* **308**, 353.

61 Herbst, J.J., Book , L.S., Bray, P.F. (1978) Gastroesophageal reflux in the 'near miss' sudden infant death syndrome. *Journal of Pediatrics* **92**, 73.

62 Hering, E., Breuer, J. (1868) Die Selbststeurung der Athmung durch den nervus vagus. *Sitzungsbericht der Kaiserlichen Akademie der Wissenshaften in Wien* **57**, 672–677.

63 Hiatt, I.M., Hegyi, T., Indyk, L. *et al.* (1981) Continuous monitoring of PO_2 during apnea of prematurity. *Journal of Pediatrics* **98**, 288–291.

64 Holzer, P., Hagmuller, K. (1979) Transient apnea after systemic injection of GABA in the rat. *Naunyn-Schmiedebergs Archives of Pharmacology* **308**, 55–60.

65 Hoppenbrouwers, T., Hedgman, J.E., Harper, R.M. *et al.* (1977) Polygraphic studies of normal infants during the first six months of life: III. Incidence of apnea and periodic breathing. *Pediatrics* **60**, 418–425.

66 Jones, R.A. (1982) Apnoea of immaturity. 1. A controlled trial of theophylline and face mask continuous positive airways pressure. *Archives of Diseases in Childhood* **57**, 761–765.

67 Joshi, A., Gerhardt, T., Shandloff, P., Bancalari, E. (1987) Blood transfusion effect on the respiratory pattern of preterm infants. *Pediatrics* **80**, 79–84.

68 Kahn, A., Blum, D., Waterschoot, P. *et al.* (1982) Effects of obstructive sleep apneas on transcutaneous oxygen pressure in control infants, siblings of sudden infant death syndrome victims and near miss infants: comparison with the effects of central sleep apneas. *Pediatrics* **70**, 852.

69 Kattwinkel, J. (1977) Neonatal apnea: pathogenesis and therapy. *Journal of Pediatrics* **90**, 342–347.

70 Kelly, D.H., Shannon, D.C. (1979) Periodic breathing in infants with near-miss sudden infant death syndrome. *Pediatrics* **63**, 355–360.

71 Kelly, D.H., Shannon, D.C. (1981) Treatment of apnea and excessive periodic breathing in the full term infant. *Pediatrics* **68**, 183–186.

72 Kianicka, I., Diaz, V., Dorion, D., Praud, J.P. (1998) Coordination between glottic adductor muscle and diaphragm EMG activity in fetal lambs *in utero. Journal of Applied Physiology* **84**, 1560–1565.

73 Killisch, I., Dotti, C.G., Laurie, D.J. *et al.* (1991) Expression patterns of $GABA_A$ receptor subtypes in developing hippocampal neurons. *Neuron* **7**, 927–936.

74 Koons, A.H. (1992) Neurodevelopmental outcome in infants with apnea. *New England Journal of Medicine* **89**, 688–690.

75 Krauss, A.N., Klain, D.B., Waldman, S., Auld, P.A.M. (1965) Ventilatory response to carbon dioxide in newborn infants. *Pediatric Research* **9**, 46–50.

76 Kuzemko, J.A., Paala, J. (1973) Apnoeic attacks in the newborn treated with aminophyline. *Archives of Disease in Childhood* **48**, 404.

77 Lagercrantz, H., Rane, A., Tunell, R. (1980) Plasma concentration-effect relationship of theophylline in treatment of apnea in preterm infants. *European Journal of Clinical Pharmacology* **18**, 65–68.

78 Lawson, E.E. (1982) Recovery from central apnea: effect of stimulus duration and end-tidal CO_2 partial pressure. *Journal of Applied Physiology* **53**, 105–109.

79 Leape, L.L., Holder, T.M., Franklin, J.D. *et al.* (1977) Respiratory arrest in infants secondary to gastro-esophageal reflux. *Pediatrics* **60**, 924–928.

80 Lee, D., Caces, R., Kiatkowski, K. *et al.* (1987) Developmental study on types and frequency distribution of short apnea (3 to 15 seconds) in term and preterm infants. *Pediatric Research* **22**, 344.

81 Lee, J.C., Stoll, B.G., Downing, S.E. (1977) Properties of the laryngeal chemoreflex in neonatal piglets. *American Journal of Physiology* **233**, R30–R36.

82 Levitt, G.A,. Mushin, A., Bellman, S., Harvey, D.R. (1988) Outcome of preterm infants who suffered neonatal apnoeic attacks. *Early Human Development* **16**, 235–243.

83 Lewis, A.B., Freed, M.D., Heymann, M.A. *et al.* (1981) Side effects of therapy with prostaglandin E1 in infants with critical congenital heart disease. *Circulation* **64**, 893–898.

84 Litmanovitz, I., Dreshaj, I.A., Miller, M.J. *et al.* (1994) Central chemosensitivity affects respiratory muscle responses to laryngeal stimulation in the piglet. *Journal of Applied Physiology* **76**, 403–408.

85 Long, W.A. (1988) Prostaglandins and control of breathing in newborn piglets. *Journal of Applied Physiology* **64**, 409–418.

86 MacLennan, A.J., Brecha, N., Khrestchatisky, M. *et al.* (1991) Independent cellular and ontogenetic expression of mRNAs encoding three α-polypeptides of the rat $GABA_A$ receptor. *Neuroscience* **43**, 369–380.

87 Martin, R.J., Okken, A., Katona, P.G., Klaus, M.H. (1978) Effect of lung volume on expiratory time in the newborn infant. *Journal of Applied Physiology* **45**, 18.

88 Martin, R.J., DiFiore, J.M., Jana, L. *et al.* (1998) Persistence of the biphasic ventilatory response to hypoxia in preterm infants. *Journal of Pediatrics* **132**, 960–964.

89 McMillen, I.C., Walker, D.W. (1986) Effect of β-endorphin on fetal breathing movements in sheep. *Journal of Applied Physiology* **61**, 1005–1011.

90 Menon, A.P., Schefft, G.L., Thach, B.T. (1984) Frequency and significance of swallowing during prolonged apnea in infants. *American Review of Respiratory Disease* **130**, 969.

91 Menon, A.P., Schefft, G.L., Thach, B.T. (1985) Apnea associated with regurgitation in infants. *Journal of Pediatrics* **106**, 625.

92 Meny, R.G., Carroll, J.L., Carbone, M.T., Kelly, D.H. (1994) Cardiorespiratory recordings from infants dying suddenly and unexpectedly at home. *Pediatrics* **93**, 44–49.

93 Miller, A.J. (1976) Characterization of the postnatal development of superior laryngeal nerve fibers in the postnatal kitten. *Journal of Neurobiology* **7**, 483–494.

94 Miller, H.C., Behrle, F., Snell, N. (1959) Severe apnea and irregular respiratory rhythms among premature infants. A clinical and laboratory study. *Pediatrics* **23**, 676.

95 Miller, M.J., Difiore, J.M. (1995) A comparison of swallowing during apnea and periodic breathing in premature infants. *Pediatric Research* **37**, 796.

96 Miller, M.J., Martin, R.J. (1998) Pathophysiology of apnea of prematurity. In Polin, R.A., Fox, W.W. (eds), *Fetal and Neonatal Physiology*. Philadelphia: W.B. Saunders, 1129–1143.

97 Miller, M.J., Carlo, W.A., DiFiore, J.M. *et al.* (1988) Airway obstruction during periodic breathing in premature infants. *Journal of Applied Physiology* **64**, 2496–2500.

98 Miller, M.J., Haxhiu, M.A., Haxhiu-Poskurica, B. *et al.* (2000) Recurrent hypoxic exposure and reflex responses during development in the piglet. *Respiration Physiology* **123**, 51–61.

99 Milner, A.D., Boon, A.W., Saunders, R.A. *et al.* (1980) Upper airway obstruction and apnea in preterm infants. *Archives of Disease in Childhood* **55**, 22.

100 Moss, I.R., Inman, J.G. (1989) Proopiomelanocortin opioids in brain, CSF, and plasma of piglets during hypoxia. *Journal of Applied Physiology* **66**, 2280–2286.

101 Moss, I.R., Runold,M., Dahlin, J. *et al.* (1987) Respiratory and neuroendocrine responses of piglets to hypoxia during postnatal development. *Acta Physiologica Scandinavica* **131**, 533–541.

102 Noble, L.M., Carlo, W.A., Miller, M.J., DiFiore, J.M., Martin, R.J. (1987) Transient changes in expiratory time during

hypercapnia in premature infants. *Journal of Applied Physiology* **62**, 1010–1013.

103 Olinsky, A., Bryan, M.H., Bryan, A.C. (1974) Influence of lung inflation on respiratory control in neonates. *Journal of Applied Physiology* **36**, 426–429.

104 Orlowski, J.P. (1986) Cerebrospinal fluid endorphins and the infant apnea syndrome. *Pediatrics* **78**, 233–237.

105 Park, T.S., Van Wylen, D.G., Rubio, R., Berne, R.M. (1987) Increased brain interstitial fluid adenosine concentration during hypoxia in newborn piglets. *Journal of Cerebral Blood Flow and Metabolism* **7**, 178–183.

106 Parmelee, A.H., Stein, E., Harris, M.A. (1972) Maturation of respiration in prematures and young infants. *Neuropediatrics* **3**, 294–304.

107 Peabody, J.L., Gregory, G.A., Willis, M.M. *et al.* (1979) Failure of conventional monitoring to detect apnea resulting in hypoxemia. *Birth Defects* **15**, 276–284.

108 Peliowski, A., Finer, N. (1990) A blinded, randomized, placebo-controlled trial to compare theophylline and doxapram for the treatment of apnea of prematurity. *Journal of Pediatrics* **116**, 648–653.

109 Perlman, J.M., Volpe, J.J. (1985) Episodes of apnea and bradycardia in the preterm newborn: impact on cerebral circulation. *Pediatrics* **76**, 333.

110 Pickens, D.L., Schefft, D., Thach, B.T. (1988) Prolonged apnea associated with upper airway protective reflexes in apnea of prematurity. *American Review of Respiratory Disease* **137**, 113–118.

111 Poets, C.F., Samuels, M.P., Southall, D.P. (1992) Potential role of intrapulmonary shunting in the pathogensis of hypoxemic episodes in infants and young children. *Pediatrics* **90**, 385–391.

112 Poets, C.F., Stebbens, V.A., Richard, D., Southall, D.P. (1995) Prolonged episodes of hypoxemia in preterm infants undetectable by cardiorespiratory monitors. *Pediatrics* **95**, 860–863.

113 Poets, C.F., Darraj, S., Bohnhorst B. (1999) Effect of doxapram on episodes of apnoea, bradycardia and hypoxaemia in preterm infants. *Biology of the Neonate* **76**, 207–213.

114 Ramanathan, R., Corwin, M.J., Hunt, C.E. *et al.* (2001) Cardiorespiratory events recorded on home monitors: comparison of healthy infants with those at increased risk for SIDS. *Journal of the American Medical Association* **285**, 2199–2207.

115 Rehan, V., Haider, A.Z., Alvaro, R.E. *et al.* (1996) The biphasic ventilatory response to hypoxia in preterm infants is not due to a decrease in metabolism. *Pediatric Pulmonology* **22**, 287–294.

116 Renolleau, S., Letourneau, P., Niyonsenga, T., Praud, J.P., Gagne, B. (1999) Thyroarytenoid muscle electrical activity during spontaneous apneas in preterm lambs. *American Journal of Respiratory and Critical Care Medicine* **159**, 1396–1404.

117 Rigatto, H., Brady, U.P. (1972) Periodic breathing and apnea in preterm infants: 1. Evidence of hypoventilation possibly due to central respiratory depression. *Pediatrics* **50**, 202–218.

118 Rigatto, H., Brady, J.P., De La Torre Verduzco, R. (1975) Chemoreceptor reflexes in preterm infants: 1. The effect of gestational and postnatal age on the ventilatory response to inhalation of 100 percent and 15 percent oxygen. *Pediatrics* **55**, 604–613.

119 Rigatto, H., Brady, J.P., De La Torre Verduzco, R.T. (1975) Chemoreceptor reflexes in preterm infants II. The effects of gestational and postnatal age on the ventilatory response to inhaled carbon dioxide. *Pediatrics* **55**, 614–620.

120 Rigatto, H., De La Torre Verduzco, R., Gates, D.B. (1975) Effects of O_2 on the ventilatory response to CO_2 in preterm infants. *Journal of Applied Physiology* **39**, 896–899.

121 Runold, M., Lagercrantz, H., Fredholm, B.B. (1986) Ventilatory effect of an adenosine analogue in unanaesthetized rabbits during development. *Journal of Applied Physiology* **61**, 255–259.

122 Sasaki, C.T. (1979) Development of laryngeal function: etiologic significance in the sudden infant death syndrome. *Laryngoscope* **89**, 1964–1982.

123 Schulte, F.J. (1977) Apnea. *Clinics in Perinatology* **4**, 65–76.

124 Seeburg, P.H., Wisden, W., Verdoorn, T.A. *et al.* (1990) The GABA$_A$ receptor family: molecular and functional diversity. *Cold Spring Harbor Symposium on Quantitative Biology* **55**, 29–40.

125 Singer, L., Martin, R.J., Hawkins, S.W. *et al.* (1992) Oxygen desaturation complicates feedings in infants with bronchopulmonary dysplasia after discharge. *Pediatrics* **90**, 380–384.

126 Southall, D.P. *et al.* (1983) Identification of infants destined to die unexpectedly during infancy: evaluation of predictive importance of prolonged apnoea and disorders of cardiac rhythm or conduction. *British Medical Journal (Clinical Research Edition)* **286**, 1092–1096.

127 Spear, M.L., Stefano, J.L., Spitzer, A.R. (1992) Prolonged apnea and oxyhemoglobin desaturation in asymptomatic premature infants. *Journal of Pediatric Pulmonology* **13**, 151–154.

128 Spitzer, A.R., Boyle, J.T., Tuchman, D.N., Fox, W.W. (1984) Awake apnea associated with gastroesophageal reflux: a specific clinical syndrome. *Journal of Pediatrics* **104**, 200–205.

129 Sreenan, C., Lemke, R.P., Hudson-Mason, A., Osiovich, H. (2001) High-flow nasal cannulae in the management of apnea of prematurity: a comparison with conventional nasal continuous positive airway pressure. *Pediatrics* **107**, 1081–1083.

130 Steinschneider, A. (1972) Prolonged apnea and the sudden infant death syndrome: clinical and laboratory observations. *Pediatrics* **50**, 646–654.

131 Storey, A.T., Johnson, P. (1975) Laryngeal water receptors initiating apnea in the lamb. *Experimental Neurology* **47**, 42–55.

132 Sutton, D., Taylor, E.M., Lindeman, R.C. (1978) Prolonged apnea in infant monkeys resulting from stimulation of superior laryngeal nerve. *Pediatrics* **61**, 519–527.

133 Taylor, H.G., Klein, N., Schatschneider, C., Hack, M. (1998) Predictors of early school age outcomes in very low birth weight children. *Journal of Developmental and Behavioral Pediatrics* **19**, 235–243.

134 Thach, B.T., Stark, A.R. (1979) Spontaneous neck flexation and airway obstruction during apneic spells in preterm infants. *Journal of Pediatrics* **94**, 275.

135 Volpe, J.J. (1992) Brain injury in the premature infant–current concept of pathogenesis and prevention. *Biology of the Neonate* **62**, 231–242.

136 Vyas, H., Milner, A.D., Hopkin, I.E. (1981) Relationship between apnoea and bradycardia in preterm infants. *Acta Paediatrica Scandinavica* **70**, 785–790.

137 Wardlaw, S.L., Stark, R.I., Baxi, L., Frantz, A.G. (1979) Plasma beta-endorphin and beta-lipotropin in the human fetus at delivery: correlation with arterial pH and pO_2. *Journal of Clinical Endocrinology and Metabolism* **49**, 888–891.

138 Willinger, M., Hoffman, H.J., Wu, K.-T. *et al.* (1998) Factors associated with the transition to non-prone sleep positions of infants in the United States: the National Infant Sleep Position Study. *Journal of the American Medical Association* **280**, 329–335.

139 Xia, Y., Haddad, G.G. (1992) Ontogeny and distribution of GABA$_A$ receptors in rat brainstem and rostral brain regions. *Neuroscience* **49**, 973–989.

31

Neonatal upper airway obstruction

DAVID ALBERT

When a neonate develops upper airway obstruction, simple measures such as suction may be all that is required. If this fails, an oral airway or intubation may be needed. Once the neonate is stabilized, the cause of the obstruction should be investigated using the experience of other specialists and an array of highly technological investigative techniques. Occasionally, intubation is either not possible, or does not relieve the obstruction, demanding a rapid response from whoever is available to help. Rarely, and very worryingly, even an emergency tracheostomy may fail to relieve the obstruction due to low tracheobronchial pathology. Airway obstruction may also occur after extubation of the intubated neonate or develop in the first few days or weeks.

CLINICAL SITUATIONS

Antenatal diagnosis of high airway obstruction

Routine prenatal ultrasonography should demonstrate large obstructing masses such as cervical teratoma (p. 92),[57,59] cystic hygroma[105] and rhabdomyosarcoma,[106] the anatomy of which can be further defined using magnetic resonance imaging.[22,62] Even in the absence of a mass, airway obstruction can be inferred, as with the tracheal dilatation and enlarged lungs seen in laryngeal atresia.[20,38] Polyhydramnios may occur with obstructing lesions, reflecting impaired fetal swallowing.

Forewarned should be forearmed, with resources mobilized and management discussed before the infant is born. Holinger described the successful airway management of an affected case in 1985,[59] and Catalano reported a tracheotomy with intact maternal–fetal circulation, possibly the first such extrauterine surgical procedure.[22] Since then the term CHAOS has been used to describe antenatally diagnosed congenital high airway obstruction. The term 'OOPS' (operation on placental support)[105] has been replaced by the more acceptable EXIT procedure (*ex utero* intrapartum treatment).[20,38,73] The multispecialty team usually involves neonatologists, obstetricians, anesthetists and ENT surgeons with other specialties involved, depending on the results of the ultrasound and magnetic resonance imaging (MRI). At a planned cesarean section the airway can be established with expert intubation[108] or occasionally a tracheostomy is performed if intubation is not possible.[20,38] Extracorporeal membrane oxygenation can be made available,[68] but intubation or tracheostomy is faster and preferable. Resection of an obstructing mass is usually delayed until the infant is stable.[68]

Unexpected airway obstruction at birth

NASOPHARYNGEAL

In the absence of antenatal diagnosis, the unfortunate clinician is presented unexpectedly with a neonate with airway obstruction. Choanal atresia is the commonest cause of true nasal obstruction. Occasionally, neonates referred with a diagnosis of choanal atresia, on the basis of inability to pass a suction catheter, have normal CT appearances. Presumably in these neonates the suction catheter's passage is impeded by a tortuous route around the turbinates. Pyriform aperture stenosis, mid-nasal stenosis and choanal stenosis are less common causes. These nasal causes of obstruction will be relieved by an oral airway as will nasopharyngeal masses such as nasopharyngeal teratomas.

LARYNGEAL

Airway obstruction relieved by intubation

Airway obstruction relieved by intubation but not an oral airway, implies obstruction at the laryngeal level. The obstruction can result from dynamic causes such as severe laryngomalacia and vocal cord palsy. Displaceable lesions such as laryngeal polyps and masses will also be relieved by intubation. In laryngeal stenosis, it may be possible to force the tip of a small shouldered tube through the stenosis as a temporary measure to secure the airway. Some units now advocate using a laryngeal mask[47] for neonatal resuscitation, which has the advantage that a tight stenosis will not be worsened by attempts at intubation. Very rarely, in laryngeal atresia with a low tracheoesophageal fistula, it may be possible to ventilate the neonate, though on closer examination the tube is actually in the esophagus with ventilation via the fistula. Intubation is possible with low tracheal and bronchial obstruction, but does not relieve the problem.

Intubation is impossible

Time is at a premium and the neonatologist is faced with a real challenge. If adequate ventilation is not possible with a laryngeal mask or a very fine endotracheal tube, a decision has to be made to open into the trachea. Cricothyroid membrane or tracheal needle puncture may be the best option for a neonatologist, but it is not easy in an emergency situation without previous experience. The neonate needs to be placed straight with the neck extended over a roll. The first and second fingers of the left hand are placed either side of the trachea and the needle inserted vertically and very strictly in the midline until air can be aspirated. It is difficult to palpate cricoid and thyroid cartilages in a neonate and it is more important to remain midline rather than worry about the level. Further and larger needles can be inserted above or below the first. Open tracheostomy in an emergency is again difficult, even for an experienced surgeon unless he has current experience of neonatal tracheostomy. The neonate needs to be placed straight with their neck extended. A long vertical, but strictly midline incision with careful palpation of the trachea should avoid drifting off the midline, which is the main danger.

Laryngeal lesions such as congenital webs or subglottic stenosis will be bypassed with a tracheostomy, but low lesions such as tracheal stenosis and tracheobronchial malacia will not.

TRACHEOBRONCHIAL

The risk with low tracheobronchial obstruction is that neither intubation nor tracheostomy will relieve the obstruction, although positive pressure will tend to improve malacia and, to a lesser extent, stenosis. An extended (long) tracheostomy will physically support tracheomalacia but not carinal malacia or bronchomalacia. A most difficult situation occurs if a tracheostomy is attempted for tapering long-segment tracheal stenosis. Not only is it not possible to insert a normal neonatal size tracheostomy tube, but the tracheostomy itself severely limits the therapeutic options for surgical reconstruction of the stenosis.

Airway obstruction developing shortly after birth

Laryngomalacia typically presents over the first couple of days. Immediate stridor should alert one to the possibility of other causes such as vocal cord palsy or static lesions such as laryngeal web,[9,10,84] cyst[112] and stenosis.[20,51,117] Laryngomalacia[24,48,100] is the commonest cause of 'congenital stridor', but it is by no means the only cause. Unfortunately, the two terms are often used synonymously and the neonate is often labelled with 'congenital stridor' as a diagnosis rather than a description. Other possible diagnoses, such as vocal cord palsy, then tend to be ignored. Subglottic hemangiomas[8,25,46,96,101] usually develop progressively in the first few months, later than most other neonatal causes of airway obstruction.

Airway obstruction at extubation

Post-extubation laryngeal edema can be predicted if there is no leak around an appropriate size tube. In these circumstances, corticosteroids can be given pre-extubation and CPAP and epinephrine (adrenaline) nebulizers should be available. Despite such treatment, some neonates require reintubation because of stridor, recession and airway compromise. It is often better to leave the neonate intubated for a period and avoid repeated attempts at extubation, which merely compound the problem with further laryngeal damage. Graham has written on the concept of formal reintubation, which may be helpful by allowing the laryngeal mucosa to recover.[53] If extubation fails despite a period of 'laryngeal rest', then an endoscopic examination should be performed to diagnose the cause and to treat endoscopically simple lesions, such as vocal cord granulations. These often wrap around the tube and, once the infant is extubated, look like 'seal flippers'. Subglottic cysts are the other easily remediable cause and can be lasered or removed with careful forceps dissection. If there are no discrete lesions, but merely a diffuse subglottic and glottic edema, then consideration needs to be given to a cricoid split, a single-stage laryngeal reconstruction or a tracheostomy (p. 442). A tracheostomy will be required before definitive treatment for other causes of obstruction, such as a congenital laryngeal web or severe tracheobronchomalacia.

DIAGNOSIS

History

When presented with a neonate who has failed extubation, the otolaryngologist needs to glean as much information as possible from the neonatologist to try to distinguish the possible causes for failed extubation. Key to this is the intubation history. Subglottic stenosis is not always associated with prolonged intubation[50,52] and a history of a traumatic, emergency intubation may be more relevant. Shouldered endotracheal tubes[16] with the shoulder passed through the glottis can cause damage, as can oversized tubes placed to improve ventilation or airway patency.[30] Lack of an initial air leak around the tube or any tightness on intubation may suggest a narrow subglottis either associated with prematurity, Down syndrome,[103] or as part of the normal range.[30]

In neonates who present with stridor at birth, the obstetric history is relevant as traumatic labor is responsible for 20 percent of vocal cord palsy.[28] Stridor occurring immediately after delivery should always raise suspicions of a vocal cord palsy. Any diurnal or other variation can help identify the cause, laryngomalacia typically being better with the neonate at rest and asleep, but made worse by crying, feeding and when distressed. Airway obstruction with the neonate supine can occur with a pedunculated laryngeal mass, but more often is due at least in part to a degree of supralaryngeal obstruction such as micrognathia and resultant tongue base occlusion. Improvement in the airway with crying occurs in gross nasal obstruction such as bilateral choanal atresia.

It is important to ask about other abnormal signs. These include apneas, cyanosis, a hoarse cry and feeding difficulties. Apneas with cyanosis are typical of severe tracheobronchomalacia and are sometimes termed 'dying spells'. Hoarseness clearly suggests a laryngeal lesion, such as a laryngeal web or vocal cord palsy.

Feeding is closely connected with breathing, particularly in the neonate, and an accurate picture of the feeding pattern must be obtained. Aspiration suggests a vocal cord palsy, tracheoesophageal fistula, or, rarely, a cleft larynx with recurrent chest infections usually accompanying significant aspiration. Regurgitation is common in neonates and by itself may not represent significant gastroesophageal reflux.

General medical inquiry may explain a vocal cord palsy occurring as a result of neurological disease or cardiac surgery or may suggest vascular compression associated with congenital cardiac disease. Finally, the parents should be asked about the presence of any birthmarks, as they may be associated with a subglottic hemangioma.

Examination

Typically, inspiratory stridor is due to an extrathoracic obstruction in the larynx or high trachea with bronchial obstruction producing an expiratory stridor (Figure 31.1). Biphasic stridor can occur with obstruction anywhere in the tracheobronchial tree. Expiratory stridor may be absent but a prolonged expiratory phase may be present, indicating an intrathoracic obstruction (Figure 31.2). The characteristic sound of stridor, even in a common condition such as laryngomalacia, is so variable as to be of little diagnostic use on its own. Laryngomalacia is said to have a 'musical quality', vocal cord palsy a 'breathy quality' and the cough in tracheomalacia to be 'barking'. The site of the abnormal vibration can rarely be tracked down with the aid of a stethoscope because of the variable transmission of sound through the thorax. Auscultation is, however, useful to detect heart murmurs and wheeze.

Subcostal, intercostal and suprasternal recession may occur separately or together and may also be associated with see-saw respiration. The severity of recession is a better indicator of the severity of airway compromise than the degree of stridor, which can paradoxically become less obvious as obstruction worsens due to the diminishing airflow.

If a supralaryngeal component is suspected, nasal patency should be assessed with a mirror, a wisp of cotton wool or using the bell end of a stethoscope. Conscious assessment should be made of jaw and tongue size.

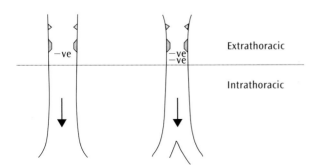

Figure 31.1 *Inspiratory stridor with an extrathoracic obstruction.*

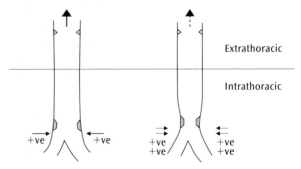

Figure 31.2 *Expiratory stridor with an intrathoracic obstruction.*

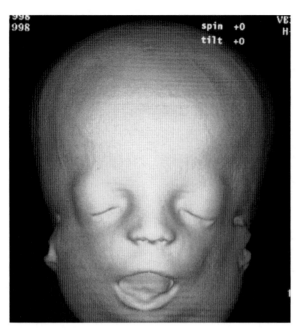

Figure 31.3 *Treacher–Collins syndrome – three-dimensional reconstruction.*

Both stridor and recession will vary as the infant rests, cries and sleeps but it is rare to be able to demonstrate a similar repeatable change with position. Observing the child feeding is very valuable, particularly if poor feeding or aspiration are significant features in the history.

Imaging

The most appropriate imaging technique will depend on the suspected site of neonatal airway obstruction. For nasal lesions, a CT scan identifies abnormalities such as choanal atresia,[86] choanal stenosis,[107] vestibular stenosis[64,97] and pyriform aperture stenosis.[3,18,63,93] It is important that the nasal cavity is sucked clear of secretions prior to the examination, to avoid a spurious diagnosis of membranous choanal atresia.[67] MRI should also be employed to demonstrate possible intracranial connections in suspected encephalocele, meningocele and nasal glioma,[92,119] as CT alone can be misleading. Three-dimensional reconstructions of the cranial CTs are used to plan craniofacial reconstructions and give a clear appreciation of the midface and mandibular deficiency that predisposes to airway compromise (Figure 31.3). In the pharynx, an MRI is particularly useful for vascular lesions such as hemangioma and lymphangioma. Lesions within the laryngotracheobronchial tree, such as stenosis, are sometimes visible on a plain chest x-ray or a penetrated filtered (Cincinnati) view. The current resolution of CT and MRI scans[56,115,116] does not usually give sufficiently high definition to fully characterize a stenotic segment,[17] even if software is used to reconstruct the image three-dimensionally. For extrinsic lesions, particularly vascular

compression, an MRI is the investigation of choice. Video-fluoroscopy is an excellent way of demonstrating tracheomalacia and can be combined with a contrast swallow looking for vascular compression[5,54] and aspiration. Bronchography is now much safer, with the introduction of non-ionic contrast media. It is particularly useful for the lower airway demonstrating tracheobronchial stenosis and malacia. Echocardiography can be used to screen for vascular compression, demonstrating most but not all abnormal vasculature as well as coincidental or symptomatic congenital heart disease.

Gastroesophageal reflux is very common in neonates. It may, however, be the result, rather than the cause of airway obstruction, and be the consequence of the magnitude of the negative intrathoracic pressures generated. The role of a pH study is, therefore, rather limited, unless more complex studies measuring upper esophageal or pharyngeal pH are available.[29]

Ultrasound can be used to demonstrate vocal cord palsy with reasonable accuracy and complement the endoscopic findings. Transcutaneous electromyography (EMG) is helpful in adults, especially if the nerve has been severed. In the pediatric situation, the nerve is usually intact and action potentials can be identified, even in the presence of an established bilateral cord palsy. Technical problems have limited the use of EMG in children even under the controlled conditions of anesthetized endoscopy.

Endoscopy

Neonatal airway endoscopy has to be safe, as well as providing accurate diagnostic information. To achieve these objectives, a full range of specialized pediatric endoscopy equipment and a high level of experience in the endoscopist, anesthesiologist and nursing staff must be available. An inadequate evaluation will need to be repeated. If in doubt, refer to a center with sufficient experience to perform a single comprehensive and definitive evaluation. A systematic approach will provide a diagnosis in most cases.

AWAKE FLEXIBLE LARYNGOSCOPY[12]

This has the advantage over conventional rigid endoscopy under anesthesia of interfering less with dynamic conditions. The introduction of ultra-thin endoscopes,[4,36,89] with good optics and a diameter of less than 2 mm, has allowed neonates to be endoscoped without the need for a general anesthetic. Endoscopy without general anesthesia is less controlled than with anesthesia, but in selected cases is safe with an experienced endoscopist. Laryngomalacia can usually be distinguished from vocal cord palsy, however if the collapse from laryngomalacia is severe, it is sometimes not possible to visualize the glottis and exclude a coexisting cord palsy. Lesions below the glottis are not well visualized and it is important to be aware that other lesions coexist in approximately 5 percent of patients. Awake flexible laryngoscopy should, therefore, be viewed as a screening procedure.

RIGID LARYNGOTRACHEOBRONCHOSCOPY

This is performed under general anesthesia and is still the investigation of choice for all complex airway lesions. It is a highly technical procedure and the whole team (surgeon, anesthetist and nursing staff) need to fully understand the equipment to perform the examination safely and to optimize the assessment. Ideally, the same surgeon, anesthetist and nurse should routinely work together and be used to dealing with neonates. Most units now use spontaneous ventilation, as this is not only safer, but also allows a dynamic assessment of the airway. Spontaneous ventilation is facilitated by topical anesthesia of the larynx and trachea. This prevents coughing without needing a level of anesthesia that prevents spontaneous breathing. The lidocaine (lignocaine) dose must be carefully measured, as the preparations used in adults can easily result in overdosage.[1,104] Ideally, intubation is avoided as this allows the larynx to be examined without any intubation artifacts. In the intubated neonate who is being examined for failed extubation, it is often helpful to apply topical epinephrine to the glottis around the endotracheal tube, so that when the tube is removed there is a better airway and thus more time for a careful examination. Examinations should be recorded on videotape to provide a permanent record to facilitate subsequent management.

The larynx

The larynx is examined first with a microscope or rigid endoscope, checking for cysts, webs and a posterior laryngeal cleft. The arytenoid movement is checked passively with a probe, as cricoarytenoid fixation can mimic a vocal cord palsy. The time available for the examination will depend on the airway. In an infant breathing spontaneously with a normal airway and normal lung function, anesthesia can be maintained solely by the use of inhalational agents with the endotracheal tube withdrawn into the pharynx. In others, the time available may be very limited and it is essential to be prepared to perform a rigid ventilating bronchoscopy at any stage. If there is significant subglottic stenosis, an ultra-fine telescope passed through the laryngoscope will cause less trauma than a bronchoscope.

Trachea and bronchi

These are examined using an appropriate size bronchoscope, unless stenosis is suspected (Figure 31.4). Neonates pose particular problems if manipulation of the airway is required.[61,75] The main bronchi, the carina, the trachea and the subglottis should all be systematically examined and videographs or digital images recorded. Tracheomalacia can be observed with a small bronchoscope withdrawn from the area in question and without positive airways

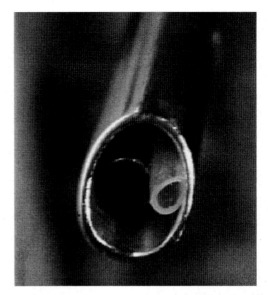

Figure 31.4 *Neonatal bronchoscope with Storz–Hopkins telescope and fine sucker.*

pressure to avoid splinting. The ratio of cartilage to trachealis is significant in determining the type of malacia and if an aortopexy is likely to be successful.

Dynamic assessment of the larynx on recovery from anesthesia

This examination aims to demonstrate the vocal cord movement and any laryngeal collapse (laryngomalacia). Typically this can be achieved by withdrawing the bronchoscope to just behind the tip of the epiglottis. This affords a good view of the vocal cords and arytenoids; as a consequence cord palsy and the common posterior form of laryngomalacia can be excluded. If anterior collapse of the epiglottis is suspected, however, a 30 or 70° telescope should be used. The anesthetist should call the phase of respiration to check for paradoxical vocal cord movements caused by the cords being sucked in passively on inspiration by the negative airways pressure created by the airflow. With active cord movement, the cords abduct on inspiration due to the action of the posterior cricoarytenoid muscle.

TREATMENT

Nasopharyngeal airway obstruction

This can be improved medically with saline, suction and topical steroids, although the dose and duration of topical steroids in neonates needs to be carefully monitored. Vasoconstrictor nose drops such as 0.5 percent ephedrine also need to be used with care. Nasal airways can either be purpose-made prongs or a shortened endotracheal tube with the end sitting in the nasopharynx or oropharynx.

Such airways act as stents, maintaining an airway through a narrow edematous nasal cavity or posteriorly placed palate or tongue base. Surgical options in the nose include endoscopic choanal surgery to address choanal atresia, and open operations such as lateral rhinotomy and external rhinoplasty to remove nasal masses such as nasal gliomas.

Laryngeal airway obstruction

This can sometimes be bypassed by intubation, but otherwise will usually require endoscopic or open laryngeal surgery. These techniques are used as initial treatments to avoid tracheostomy if possible. Endoscopic treatment of the neonatal larynx requires considerable experience of both the surgeon and anesthetist, as well as specialized equipment. Damage to the delicate vocal fold can produce dysphonia, which is difficult to correct. Endoscopic procedures commonly used in neonates include resection of small subglottic cysts and removal of cord granulomas. The CO_2 laser can vaporize small lesions without bleeding, but must be used carefully in the subglottis to avoid causing stenosis. Aryepiglottic trimming for larygomalacia removes a small wedge of the aryepiglottic mucosa on each side to prevent the forward prolapse of the posterior larynx and arytenoids, which is typical of the condition. Open surgery on the neonatal larynx is usually for developing subglottic stenosis and consists of a cricoid split or immediate laryngeal reconstruction using rib cartilage. Surgery is followed by a period of elective intubation prior to planned extubation with concurrent corticosteroid administration.

Tracheostomy

Tracheostomy is used to bypass laryngeal or tracheal obstruction that can not be dealt with by endoscopic or open surgery. It is also used if the infant requires long-term ventilation or to support physically an area of tracheomalacia. Neonatal tracheostomy has particular risks because of the small dimensions. The tube is more likely to block than in an older child and is also more likely to become displaced. There is a narrow margin between the tube tip being past the carina and tending to come out of the stoma. Tracheostomy is usually conducted intubated and under general anesthesia with the infant supine. Rigorous hemostasis is ensured with microbipolar diathermy forceps (Figure 31.5). A vertical incision is made through the third and fourth tracheal rings with stay sutures placed either side of the incision (Figure 31.6). The correct tube length should be checked on the operating table by listening to the right lung with the infant's head flexed. It is important to use a large enough tube to allow ventilation without a significant leak. A 'fairly' tight fit of the tracheostomy tube into the trachea also minimizes air escape and facilitates ventilation. Postoperatively a chest

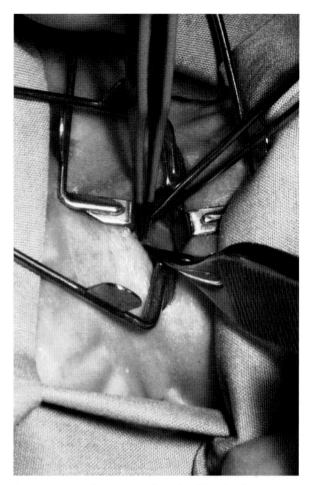

Figure 31.5 *Tracheostomy using microbiopolar forceps.*

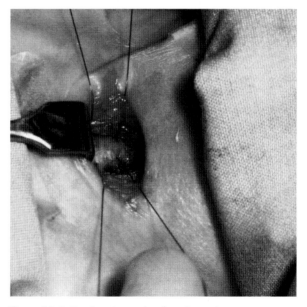

Figure 31.6 *Tracheostomy showing stay sutures.*

radiograph should be performed to check the tube length and exclude a pneumothorax, which rarely can occur from puncturing the lung apex or, in neonates, from high pressure ventilation. Tube dislodgment and blockage remain the most important late complications and are responsible for the mortality of 1–2 percent. There is now a move to avoid neonatal tracheostomy, with tracheostomy now only being used after a failure of initial surgery.

SPECIFIC CONDITIONS

Nasal conditions

Neonates are obligate or at least preferential nasal breathers and will become cyanosed rather than open their mouth to breathe. Neonatal rhinitis is a common condition with nasal obstruction from increased secretions and mucosal edema.[109] It is usually due to allergy or non-specific infection although occasionally a swab will show a specific infection such as *Chlamydia* (p. 291).[102]

The nasal dimensions are smaller than normal in choanal stenosis, choanal atresia, mid nasal stenosis and vestibular stenosis.[31] The site and extent of narrowing can be estimated by passing a catheter or assessed accurately with a CT scan. Choanal atresia can be unilateral or bilateral and isolated or associated with other congenital abnormalities such as in CHARGE syndrome (**c**oloboma of the iris and retina, **h**eart disease, **a**tresia choanae, **r**etarded growth, **g**enital hypoplasia, **e**ar defects).[85]

Nasal tumors include gliomas, nasal dermoids, encephaloceles, meningoceles, lipomas, fibromas and nasolacrimal duct cysts.[92] Treatment is surgical once an intracranial connection has been excluded radiologically.[92] Hemangiomas can be observed and may eventually need plastic surgery if resolution is not complete.

Nasopharyngeal and oral conditions

The physical size of a large tongue, macroglossia, or a small mouth, microstomia, can cause oropharyngeal airway obstruction alongside the tongue retrusion seen with micrognathia and the poor nasopharyngeal airway in maxillary hypoplasia. The common **craniofacial syndromes** causing obstruction include Pierre Robin,[21,39,66,83,110] hemifacial microsomia and Crouzon's. The hairy polyp or nasopharyngeal teratoma derives from two germinal layers, ectoderm and mesoderm,[23] and requires simple surgical excision.[71,82,113]

Laryngeal conditions

LARYNGOMALACIA

Laryngomalacia is most commonly due to the forward prolapse of the posterior supraglottic structures:[24,48,100] the arytenoid cartilages and the aryepiglottic folds. Anatomically the aryepiglottic fold is found to be shorter, tending to pull the arytenoids forward to the tongue base.

The supraglottic collapse on inspiration increases with increasingly negative airways pressures from increased airflow. The stridor is therefore worse on crying and feeding, but tends to be better when the child is at rest. If it is associated with severe failure to thrive, the short aryepiglottic fold can be divided.[48,69,76,91,94,96,111]

VOCAL CORD PALSY

This is the second most common cause of neonatal stridor, accounting for 10 percent of all congenital laryngeal anomalies.[27,60] It presents within the first month after birth with stridor, cyanosis, apneas and feeding difficulties. Flexible fiberoptic endoscopy is a good initial investigation. It should be followed by rigid endoscopy to allow manual palpation of the cords, to distinguish true paralysis from cricoarytenoid joint fixation.[37] Laryngeal ultrasound is improving with better scanners, smaller probe sizes and more experience.[49] Many neonates, especially those with unilateral cord palsy, will cope without intubation or a tracheostomy. Reported tracheotomy rates vary from 0 to 36 percent for unilateral vocal cord palsy[28,98] and from 0 to 73 percent for bilateral cases.[28,88] In the absence of an obvious cause such as birth trauma or cardiac surgery, a neurological opinion should be sought to exclude hydrocephalus, congenital hypotonia, Mobius syndrome, cerebral palsy, arthrogryposis multiplex congenita, leukodystrophy, hypoxic encephalopathy and Charcot–Marie–Tooth disease. Spontaneous recovery does occur, being more likely in unilateral cases (70 percent) than bilateral (80 percent).[37,98]

CONGENITAL SUBGLOTTIC STENOSIS

This is due to a thickened elliptical cricoid cartilage,[58] occasionally with a trapped first tracheal ring. The stenosis can be truly subglottic or involve the vocal cords as in a congenital laryngeal web, which almost always has a significant anterior subglottic component.[55] The stridor and recession in a significant stenosis may be quite unremarkable if airflow is reduced. This is a trap for the unwary, as any attempt at intubation can cause edema and rapid airway obstruction.

ACQUIRED SUBGLOTTIC STENOSIS

If this occurs as the result of neonatal intubation (Figure 31.7), it is treated conservatively at first with corticosteroids and then a planned extubation after a period of laryngeal rest.[53] Minor lesions such as granulations and cysts are then excluded (Figure 31.8). Developing soft stenosis (Figure 31.9) can be relieved with a cricoid split. The split is achieved via an external incision and opens the larynx anteriorly from just beneath the vocal cords to the first tracheal rings. The gap produced in the cricoid is not great and it may be that the operation owes its success to decompression as much as releasing the

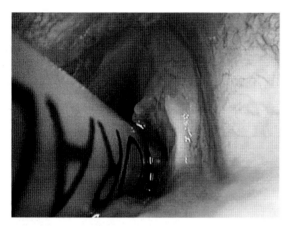

Figure 31.7 *Intubation trauma.*

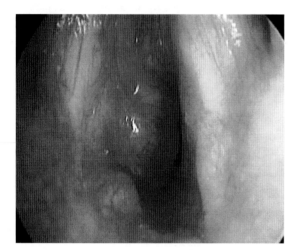

Figure 31.8 *Subglottic cyst following neonatal intubation.*

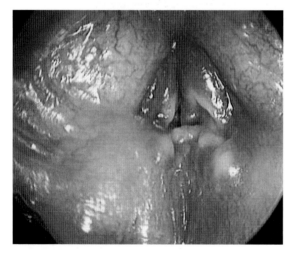

Figure 31.9 *Glottic edema and ulceration following neonatal intubation.*

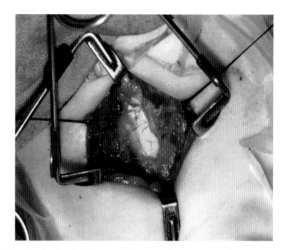

Figure 31.10 *Single-stage laryngeal reconstruction showing graft in place.*

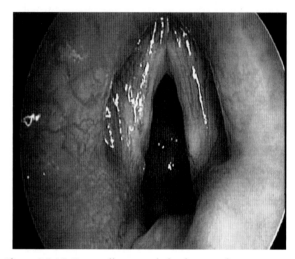

Figure 31.11 *Severe discrete subglottic stenosis following neonatal intubation.*

reconstruction (Figure 31.10), leaving the neonate intubated at the end of the procedure. The complication rate of immediate reconstruction in neonates is higher than in single-stage laryngeal reconstruction in older children,[15] but it may avoid tracheostomy, which also has a higher complication rate in neonates. In complex neonates with poor cardiorespiratory function or multiple congenital anomalies, a tracheostomy and laryngeal reconstruction after an interval is preferable,[2,7,11,33,77,78] as in children with established severe stenosis (Figure 31.11).

Tracheobronchial conditions

TRACHEAL AGENESIS

Tracheal agenesis comprises a group of rare and uniform anomalies that are characterized by the absence or atresia of all or part of the trachea.[90] Several systems of classification have been proposed.[42,45] After delivery all neonates

integrity of the cricoid ring. The neonate is intubated for 2–5 days, after which extubation is successful in 70 percent.[6,34,35,99] If the stenosis is found to be firm at endoscopy, augmentation is required with costal cartilage. This can be achieved in the neonate with an **immediate** laryngeal

display respiratory distress, as well as an absent or weak cry. Attempts at intubation reveal an absent glottic or subglottic opening and an inability to intubate the infant. Confusion may arise by esophageal intubation, which may allow relatively adequate ventilation in the short term. Stabilization may also be achieved by bag and mask ventilation.[70] Tracheal agenesis is frequently associated with other anomalies, including cardiac and vertebral anomalies, radial ray defects and duodenal and anal atresia.[41] Laryngoscopy, bronchoscopy and esophagoscopy can confirm the diagnosis. If there is any doubt about the infant's anatomy, neck exploration should be undertaken to ensure that a tracheal remnant for tracheostomy does not exist.[70] A temporary airway can be provided by intubation of the esophagus. Several attempts have been made at definitive repair, but there are no long-term survivors.

TRACHEAL STENOSIS

This can be isolated or affect the whole length of the trachea, often with abnormal or complete tracheal rings. Both tracheostomy and intubation should be avoided if possible and the neonate transferred to a center with experience of these complex and difficult anomalies. Surgical options include grafting with pericardium or cartilage as well as resection or tracheoplasty. Postoperative stenosis or collapse can be supported with endoscopically placed expanding metal stents, which are dilated with an endoscopic balloon.[13,44,114]

TRACHEOMALACIA

Tracheomalacia is an abnormal collapse of the trachea which, when severe, can produce symptoms of airway obstruction with expiratory stridor, cough and cyanotic attacks.[43] Unexplained respiratory distress on the neonatal intensive care unit may be due to tracheomalacia and with the myriad of other possible causes can often be missed.[40,74] Primary or intrinsic malacia is due to an abnormality in the wall of the airway; secondary malacia is due to extrinsic compression, often vascular.[74,80] An aberrant innominate artery compresses the right anterior trachea just above the carina. A double aortic arch surrounds the trachea and main bronchi, producing concentric or triangular-shaped compression at endoscopy. A pulmonary artery sling compresses the right main bronchus, often to the extent that the lumen of the right main bronchus is occluded. Vascular anomalies are demonstrated on echocardiograph and MRI.[115] Mild primary tracheomalacia usually requires no treatment as the disease is self-limiting over 1–2 years and resolves without surgery.[65] Aortopexy was initially used in tracheomalacia associated with tracheoesophageal fistula,[32,81] but has also been used for primary tracheomalacia.[74,80] An extended tracheostomy tube[120] will effectively support mid-tracheal tracheomalacia but is less effective for low tracheal and bronchial collapse.

BRONCHOMALACIA

Bronchomalacia is the equivalent collapse in the bronchi (see above). Occasionally bronchomalacia can be improved with a suspension procedure,[72] though this is less established than aortopexy. Carinal tracheomalacia and severe bronchomalacia can be supported with CPAP from a standard home CPAP machine as used in obstructive sleep apnea.[95,118] The device can be used nasally with a close fitting mask or via a tracheostomy tube. Internal stents support the area of collapse well but suffer from migration, extrusion and localized reactions including granulations and frank infections. Both siliconized plastic and expandable metal stents have been used with success. The expandable metal stents are difficult to insert even using an introducer and need to expand at just the right point in the lumen once released.[1,14,19,44,79] Balloon dilatation can be used to further increase the lumen to accommodate future growth.[79]

SUMMARY

Unless mild, self-limiting or easily reversed with simple measures, neonatal airway obstruction requires urgent referral to a specialist center.

REFERENCES

1 Amitai, Y., Zylber Katz, E., Avital, A. *et al.* (1990) Serum lidocaine concentrations in children during bronchoscopy with topical anesthesia. *Chest* **98**, 1370–1373.

2 April, M.M., Marsh, B.R. (1993) Laryngotracheal reconstruction for subglottic stenosis. *Annals of Otology, Rhinology and Laryngology* **102**, 176–181.

3 Arlis, H., Ward, R.F. (1992) Congenital nasal pyriform aperture stenosis. Isolated abnormality vs developmental field defect. *Archives of Otolaryngology – Head and Neck Surgery* **118**, 989–991.

4 Arnold, J.E. (1989) Advances in pediatric flexible bronchoscopy. *Otolaryngology Clinics of North America* **22**, 545–551.

5 Backer, C., Ilbawi, M., Idriss, F., De Leon, S. (1989) Vascular anomalies causing tracheoesophageal compression. *Journal of Thoracic and Cardiovascular Surgery* **97**, 725–731.

6 Bagwell, C.E., Marchildon, M.B., Pratt, L.L. (1987) Anterior cricoid split for subglottic stenosis. *Journal of Pediatric Surgery* **22**, 740–742.

7 Bailey, C.M., Clary, R.A., Pengilly, A., Albert, D.M. (1995) Voice quality following laryngotracheal reconstruction. *International Journal of Pediatric Otorhinolaryngology* **32**, S93–S95.

8 Bailey, C.M., Froehlich, P., Hoeve, H.L. (1998) Management of subglottic haemangioma. *Journal of Laryngology and Otology* **112**, 765–768.

9 Benjamin, B. (1983) Chevalier Jackson Lecture. Congenital laryngeal webs. *Annals of Otology, Rhinology and Laryngology* **92**, 317–326.

10 Benjamin, B., Mair, E.A. (1991) Congenital interarytenoid web. *Archives of Otolaryngology Head and Neck Surgery* **117**, 1118–1122.

11 Berkowitz, R.G. (1995) Paediatric laryngotracheal reconstruction: Melbourne experience at the Royal Children's Hospital. *Australia and New Zealand Journal of Surgery* **65**, 650–653.

12 Berkowitz, R.G. (1998) Neonatal upper airway assessment by awake flexible laryngoscopy. *Annals of Otology, Rhinology and Laryngology* **107**, 75–80.

13 Boothroyd, A.E., Edwards, R., Petros, A.J., Franks, R. (1995) The expandable metal stent for tracheal obstruction. *Archives of Disease in Childhood* **72**, 435–436.

14 Bousamra, M., Tweddell, J.S., Wells, R.G. *et al.* (1996) Wire stent for tracheomalacia in a five-year-old girl. *Annals of Thoracic Surgery* **61**, 1239–1240.

15 Brenner, K.E., Oca, M.J., Donn, S.M. (2000) Congenital choanal atresia in siblings. *Journal of Perinatology* **20**, 443–444.

16 Brewis, C., Pracy, J.P., Albert, D.M. (1999) Localized tracheomalacia as a complication of the Cole tracheal tube. *Paediatric Anaesthesia* **9**, 531–533.

17 Brody, A.S., Kuhn, J.P., Seidel, F.G., Brodsky, L.S. (1991) Airway evaluation in children with use of ultrafast CT: pitfalls and recommendations. *Radiology* **178**, 181–184.

18 Brown, O.E., Myer, C.M., Manning, S.C. (1989) Congenital nasal pyriform aperture stenosis. *Laryngoscope* **99**, 86–91.

19 Bugmann, P., Rouge, J.C., Berner, M. *et al.* (1994) Use of Gianturco Z stents in the treatment of vascular compression of the tracheobronchial tree in childhood. A feasible solution when surgery fails. *Chest* **106**, 1580–1582.

20 Bui, T.H., Grunewald, C., Frenckner, B. *et al.* (2000) Successful EXIT (*ex utero* intrapartum treatment) procedure in a fetus diagnosed prenatally with congenital high-airway obstruction syndrome due to laryngeal atresia. *European Journal of Pediatric Surgery* **10**, 328–333.

21 Caouette Laberge, L., Bayet, B., Larocque, Y. (1994) The Pierre Robin sequence: review of 125 cases and evolution of treatment modalities. *Plastic and Reconstructive Surgery* **93**, 934–942.

22 Catalano, P.J., Urken, M.L., Alvarez, M. *et al.* (1992) New approach to the management of airway obstruction in 'high risk' neonates. *Arch Otolaryngol Head Neck Surg* **118**, 306–309.

23 Chakravarti, A., Vishwakarma, S.K., Arora, V.K., Singh, I. (1998) Dermoid (hairy polyp) of the nasopharynx. *Indian Journal of Pediatrics* **65**, 473–476.

24 Chandra, R.K., Gerber, M.E., Holinger, L.D. (2001) Histological insight into the pathogenesis of severe laryngomalacia. *International Journal of Pediatric Otorhinolaryngology* **61**, 31–38.

25 Choa, I.D., Smith, M.C.F., Evans, J.N.G., Bailey, C.M. (1986) Subglottic haemangioma in children. *Journal of Laryngology and Otology* **100**, 447–454.

26 Choi, S.S., Zalzal, G.H. (2000) Changing trends in neonatal subglottic stenosis. *Otolaryngology Head and Neck Surgery* **122**, 61–63.

27 Cohen, S.R., Eavey, R.D., Desmond, M.S., May, B.C. (1977) Endoscopy and tracheotomy in the neonatal period. A 10-year review. *Annals of Otology, Rhinology and Laryngology* **86**, 577–583.

28 Cohen, S.R., Geller, K.A., Birns, J.W., Thompson, J.W. (1982) Laryngeal paralysis in children: a long-term retrospective study. *Annals of Otology, Rhinology and Laryngology* **91**, 417–424.

29 Conley, S.F., Werlin, S.L., Beste, D.J. (1995) Proximal pH-metry for diagnosis of upper airway complications of gastroesophageal reflux. *Journal of Otolaryngology* **24**, 295–298.

30 Contencin, P., Narcy, P. (1993) Size of endotracheal tube and neonatal acquired subglottic stenosis. Study Group for Neonatology and Pediatric Emergencies in the Parisian Area.

Archives of Otolaryngology – Head and Neck Surgery **119**, 815–819.

31 Contencin, P., Gumpert, L., Sleiman, J. *et al.* (1999) Nasal fossae dimensions in the neonate and young infant: a computed tomographic scan study. *Archives of Otolaryngology – Head and Neck Surgery* **125**, 777–781.

32 Corbally, M.T., Spitz, L., Kiely, E. *et al.* (1993) Aortopexy for tracheomalacia in oesophageal anomalies. *European Journal of Pediatric Surgery* **3**, 264–266.

33 Cotton, R.T., O'Connor, D.M. (1995) Paediatric laryngotracheal reconstruction: 20 years' experience. *Acta Otorhinolaryngologica Belgica* **49**, 367–372.

34 Cotton, R.T., Seid, A.B. (1980) Management of the extubation problem in the premature child; and anterior cricoid split as an alternative to tracheostomy. *Annals of Otology, Rhinology and Laryngology* **89**, 508–511.

35 Cotton, R.T., Myer, C.M.I., Bratcher, G.O., Fitton, C.M. (1988) Anterior cricoid split, 1977–1987. Evolution of a technique. *Archives of Otolaryngology – Head and Neck Surgery* **114**, 1300–1302.

36 de Blic, J., Delacourt, C., Scheinmann, P. (1991) Ultrathin flexible bronchoscopy in neonatal intensive care units. *Archives of Disease in Childhood* **66**, 1383–1385.

37 de Gaudemar, I., Roudaire, M., Francois, M., Narcy, P. (1996) Outcome of laryngeal paralysis in neonates: a long term retrospective study of 113 cases. *International Journal of Pediatric Otorhinolaryngology* **34**, 101–110.

38 DeCou, J.M., Jones, D.C., Jacobs, H.D., Touloukian, R.J. (1998) Successful ex utero intrapartum treatment (EXIT) procedure for congenital high airway obstruction syndrome (CHAOS) owing to laryngeal atresia. *Journal of Pediatric Surgery* **33**, 1563–1565.

39 Deegan, P.C., McGlone, B., McNicholas, W.T. (1995) Treatment of Robin sequence with nasal CPAP. *Journal of Laryngology and Otology* **109**, 328–330.

40 Duncan, S., Eid, N. (1991) Tracheomalacia and bronchopulmonary dysplasia. *Annals of Otology, Rhinology and Laryngology* **100**, 856–858.

41 Evans, J.A., Greenberg, C.R., Erdile, L. (1999) Tracheal agenesis revisited: analysis of associated anomalies. *American Journal of Medical Genetics* **82**, 415–422.

42 Faro, R.S., Goodwin, C.D., Organ, C.H.J. *et al.* (1979) Tracheal agenesis. *Annals of Thoracic Surgery* **28**, 295–299.

43 Filler, R.M., de Fraga, J.C. (1994) Tracheomalacia. *Seminars in Thoracic and Cardiovascular Surgery* **6**, 211–215.

44 Filler, R.M., Forte, V., Fraga, J.C., Matute, J. (1995) The use of expandable metallic airway stents for tracheobronchial obstruction in children. *Journal of Pediatric Surgery* **30**, 1050–1055.

45 Floyd, J., Campbell, D.C., Dominy, D.E. (1962) Agenesis of the trachea. *American Review of Respiratory Disease* **86**, 557–560.

46 Froehlich, P., Stamm, D., Floret, D., Morgon, A. (1995) Management of subglottic haemangioma. *Clinics in Otolaryngology* **20**, 336–339.

47 Gandini, D., Brimacombe, J.R. (1999) Neonatal resuscitation with the laryngeal mask airway in normal and low birth weight infants. *Anesthesia and Analgesia* **89**, 642–643.

48 Garabedian, E.N., Roger, G., Denoyelle, F., Triglia, J.M. (1997) Severe laryngomalacia: surgical indications and results. *Pediatric Pulmonology* **Supplement 16**, 292.

49 Garel, C., Contencin, P., Polonovski, J.M. *et al.* (1992) Laryngeal ultrasonography in infants and children: a new way of investigating. Normal and pathological findings. *International Journal of Pediatric Otorhinolaryngology* **23**, 107–115.

50 Gould, S.J. (1988) The pathology of neonatal endotracheal intubation and its relationship to subglottic stenosis. *Journal of Laryngology and Otology* **Supplement 17**, 3–7.

51 Gould, S.J., Graham, J.M. (1985) Acquired subglottic stenosis in neonates. *Clinics in Otolaryngology* **10**, 299–302.

52 Gould, S.J., Graham, J. (1989) Long term pathological sequelae of neonatal endotracheal intubation. *Journal of Laryngology and Otology* **103**, 622–625.

53 Graham, J.M. (1994) Formal reintubation for incipient neonatal subglottic stenosis. *Journal of Laryngology and Otology* **108**, 474–478.

54 Han, M.T., Hall, D.G., Manche, A., Rittenhouse, E.A. (1993) Double aortic arch causing tracheoesophageal compression. *American Journal of Surgery* **165**, 628–631.

55 Hisa, Y., Tatemoto, K., Toyoda, K. *et al.* (1989) [A case of congenital laryngeal web with subglottic stenosis]. *Nippon Jibiinkoka Gakkai Kaiho* **92**, 1394–1398.

56 Hofmann, U., Hofmann, D., Vogl, T. *et al.* (1991) Magnetic resonance imaging as a new diagnostic criterion in paediatric airway obstruction. *Progress in Pediatric Surgery* **27**, 221–230.

57 Holinger, L.D., Birnholz, J.C. (1987) Management of infants with prenatal ultrasound diagnosis of airway obstruction by teratoma. *Annals of Otology, Rhinology and Laryngology* **96**, 61–64.

58 Holinger, L.D., Oppenheimer, R.W. (1989) Congenital subglottic stenosis: the elliptical cricoid cartilage. *Annals of Otology, Rhinology and Laryngology* **98**, 702–706.

59 Holinger, L.D., Birnholz, J.C., Bruce, D.R., Rabin, D.N. (1985) Management of an infant with prenatal ultrasound diagnosis of upper airway obstruction. *International Journal of Pediatric Otorhinolaryngology* **10**, 263–270.

60 Holinger, P.H., Brown, W.T. (1967) Congenital webs, cysts, laryngocoeles and other anomolies of the larynx. *Annals of Otology, Rhinology and Laryngology* **76**, 744–752.

61 Holmes, D.K. (1995) Expanding the envelope of neonatal endoscopic tracheal and bronchial surgery. *Southern Medical Journal* **88**, 571–574.

62 Hubbard, A.M., Crombleholme, T.M., Adzick, N.S. (1998) Prenatal MRI evaluation of giant neck masses in preparation for the fetal exit procedure. *American Journal of Perinatology* **15**, 253–257.

63 Hui, Y., Friedberg, J., Crysdale, W.S. (1995) Congenital nasal pyriform aperture stenosis as a presenting feature of holoprosencephaly. *International Journal of Pediatric Otorhinolaryngology* **31**, 263–274.

64 Jablon, J.H., Hoffman, J.F. (1997) Birth trauma causing nasal vestibular stenosis. *Archives of Otolaryngology – Head and Neck Surgery* **123**, 1004–1006.

65 Jacobs, I.N., Wetmore, R.F., Tom, L.W. *et al.* (1994) Tracheobronchomalacia in children. *Archives of Otolaryngology – Head and Neck Surgery* **120**, 154–158.

66 Judge, B., Hamlar, D., Rimell, F.L. (1999) Mandibular distraction osteogenesis in a neonate. *Archives of Otolaryngology – Head and Neck Surgery* **125**, 1029–1032.

67 Kearns, D.B., Wickstead, M., Choa, D.I. *et al.* (1988) Computed tomography in choanal atresia. *Journal of Laryngology and Otology* **102**, 414–418.

68 Kelly, M.F., Berenholz, L., Rizzo, K.A. *et al.* (1990) Approach for oxygenation of the newborn with airway obstruction due to a cervical mass. *Annals of Otology, Rhinology and Laryngology* **99**, 179–182.

69 Kelly, S.M., Gray, S.D. (1995) Unilateral endoscopic supraglottoplasty for severe laryngomalacia. *Archives of Otolaryngology – Head and Neck Surgery* **121**, 1351–1354.

70 Kerschner, J., Klotch, D.W. (1997) Tracheal agenesis: a case report and review of the literature. *Otolaryngology Head and Neck Surgery* **116**, 123–128.

71 Kochanski, S.C., Burton, E.M., Seidel, F.G. *et al.* (1990) Neonatal nasopharyngeal hairy polyp: CT and MR appearance. *Journal of Computerized Assisted Tomography* **14**, 1000–1001.

72 Kosloske, A.M. (1991) Left mainstem bronchopexy for severe bronchomalacia. *Journal of Pediatric Surgery* **26**, 260–262.

73 Larsen, M.E., Larsen, J.W., Hamersley, S.L. *et al.* (1999) Successful management of fetal cervical teratoma using the EXIT procedure. *Journal of Maternal and Fetal Medicine* **8**, 295–297.

74 Lassaletta, L., Eire, P.F., Carrero, C. *et al.* (1993) [Neonatal tracheomalacia. Study of 3 cases treated with aortopexy+] Traqueomalacia neonatal. Estudio de tres casos tratados con aortopexia. *Cirugia Pediatrica* **6**, 79–83.

75 Lindahl, H., Rintala, R., Malinen, L. *et al.* (1992) Bronchoscopy during the first month of life. *Journal of Pediatric Surgery* **27**, 548–550.

76 Loke, D., Ghosh, S., Panarese, A., Bull, P.D. (2001) Endoscopic division of the ary-epiglottic folds in severe laryngomalacia. *International Journal of Pediatric Otorhinolaryngology* **60**, 59–63.

77 Lusk, R.P., Gray, S., Muntz, H.R. (1991) Single-stage laryngotracheal reconstruction. *Archives of Otolaryngology – Head and Neck Surgery* **117**, 171–173.

78 Lusk, R.P., Kang, D.R., Muntz, H.R. (1993) Auricular cartilage grafts in laryngotracheal reconstruction. *Annals of Otology, Rhinology and Laryngology* **102**, 247–254.

79 Mair, E.A., Parsons, D.S., Lally, K.P. (1990) Treatment of severe bronchomalacia with expanding endobronchial stents. *Archives of Otolaryngology – Head and Neck Surgery* **116**, 1087–1090.

80 Malone, P.S., Kiely, E.M. (1990) Role of aortopexy in the management of primary tracheomalacia and tracheobronchomalacia. *Archives of Disease in Childhood* **65**, 438–440.

81 Matute de Cardenas, J.A., Cuadros Garcia, J., Portela Casalod, E., Berchi Garcia, F.J. (1992) [Treatment of tracheomalacia by aortopexy] Tratamiento de la traqueomalacia mediante aortopexia. *Anales Espanoles de Pediatria* **36**, 228–231.

82 McShane, D., el Sherif, I., Doyle Kelly, W. *et al.* (1989) Dermoids ('hairy polyps') of the oro-nasopharynx. *Journal of Laryngology and Otology* **103**, 612–615.

83 Mecklem, D., Brimacombe, J.R., Yarker, J. (1995) Glossopexy in Pierre Robin sequence using the laryngeal mask airway. *Journal of Clinical Anesthesiology* **7**, 267–269.

84 Milczuk, H.A., Smith, J.D., Everts, E.C. (2000) Congenital laryngeal webs: surgical management and clinical embryology. *International Journal of Pediatric Otorhinolaryngology* **52**, 1–9.

85 Morgan, D., Bailey, M., Phelps, P. *et al.* (1993) Ear-nose-throat abnormalities in the CHARGE association. *Archives of Otolaryngology – Head and Neck Surgery* **119**, 49–54.

86 Morgan, D.W., Bailey, C.M. (1990) Current management of choanal atresia. *International Journal of Paediatric Otorhinolaryngology* **19**, 1–13.

87 Morgan, D.W., Evans, J.N. (1990) Developmental nasal anomalies. *Journal of Laryngology and Otology* **104**, 394–403.

88 Murty, G.E., Shinkwin, C., Gibbin, K.P. (1994) Bilateral vocal fold paralysis in infants: tracheostomy or not? *Journal of Laryngology and Otology* **108**, 329–331.

89 Nussbaum, E. (1994) Usefulness of miniature flexible fiberoptic bronchoscopy in children. *Chest* **106**, 1438–1442.

90 O'Neill, D., Morecroft, J.A., Gibson, A.T. *et al.* (1999) Unusual case of tracheal agenesis. *Pediatric and Developmental Pathology* **2**, 176–179.

91 Prescott, C.A. (1991) The current status of corrective surgery for laryngomalacia. *American Journal of Otolaryngology* **12**, 230–235.

92 Puppala, B., Mangurten, H.H., McFadden, J. *et al.* (1990) Nasal glioma. Presenting as neonatal respiratory

distress. Definition of the tumor mass by MRI. *Clinics in Pediatrics (Philadelphia)* **29**, 49–52.

93 Ramadan, H., Ortiz, O. (1995) Congenital nasal pyriform aperture (bony inlet) stenosis. *Otolaryngology Head and Neck Surgery* **113**, 286–289.

94 Reddy, D.K., Matt, B.H. (2001) Unilateral vs. bilateral supraglottoplasty for severe laryngomalacia in children. *Archives of Otolaryngology – Head and Neck Surgery* **127**, 694–699.

95 Reiterer, F., Eber, E., Zach, M.S., Muller, W. (1994) Management of severe congenital tracheobronchomalacia by continuous positive airway pressure and tidal breathing flow–volume loop analysis. *Pediatric Pulmonology* **17**, 401–403.

96 Remacle, M., Bodart, E., Lawson, G. *et al.* (1996) Use of the CO_2-laser micropoint micromanipulator for the treatment of laryngomalacia. *European Archives of Otorhinolaryngology* **253**, 401–404.

97 Rombaux, P., Hamoir, M., Francois, G. *et al.* (2000) Congenital nasal pyriform aperture stenosis in newborn: report on three cases. *Rhinology* **38**, 39–42.

98 Rosin, D.F., Handler, S.D., Potsic, W.P. *et al.* (1990) Vocal cord paralysis in children. *Laryngoscope* **100**, 1174–1179.

99 Seid, A.B., Canty, T.G. (1985) The anterior cricoid split procedure for the management of subglottic stenosis in infants and children. *Journal of Pediatric Surgery* **20**, 388–390.

100 Shah, U.K., Wetmore, R.F. (1998) Laryngomalacia: a proposed classification form. *International Journal of Pediatric Otorhinolaryngology* **46**, 21–26.

101 Sherrington, C.A., Sim, D.K., Freezer, N.J., Robertson, C.F. (1997) Subglottic haemangioma. *Archives of Disease in Childhood* **76**, 458–459.

102 Shinkwin, C.A., Gibbin, K.P. (1995) Neonatal upper airway obstruction caused by chlamydial rhinitis. *Journal of Laryngology and Otology* **109**, 58–60.

103 Shott, S.R. (2000) Down syndrome: analysis of airway size and a guide for appropriate intubation. *Laryngoscope* **110**, 585–592.

104 Sitbon, P., Laffon, M., Lesage, V. *et al.* (1996) Lidocaine plasma concentrations in pediatric patients after providing airway topical anesthesia from a calibrated device. *Anesthesia and Analgesia* **82**, 1003–1006.

105 Skarsgard, E.D., Chitkara, U., Krane, E.J. *et al.* (1996) The OOPS procedure (operation on placental support): *in utero* airway management of the fetus with prenatally diagnosed tracheal obstruction. *Journal of Pediatric Surgery* **31**, 826–828.

106 Skelton, V.A., Goodwin, A. (1999) Perinatal management of a neonate with airway obstruction caused by

rhabdomyosarcoma of the tongue. *British Journal of Anaesthesia* **83**, 951–955.

107 Tadmor, R., Ravid, M., Millet, D., Leventon, G. (1984) Computed tomographic demonstration of choanal atresia. *American Journal of Neuroradiology* **5**, 743–745.

108 Tanaka, M., Sato, S., Naito, H., Nakayama, H. (1994) Anaesthetic management of a neonate with prenatally diagnosed cervical tumour and upper airway obstruction. *Canadian Journal of Anaesthesia* **41**, 236–240.

109 Tolley, N.S., Ford, G., Commins, D. (1992) The management of neonatal rhinitis. *International Journal of Pediatric Otorhinolaryngology* **24**, 253–260.

110 Tomaski, S.M., Zalzal, G.H., Saal, H.M. (1995) Airway obstruction in the Pierre Robin sequence. *Laryngoscope* **105**, 111–114.

111 Toynton, S.C., Saunders, M.W., Bailey, C.M. (2001) Aryepiglottoplasty for laryngomalacia: 100 consecutive cases. *Journal of Laryngology and Otology* **115**, 35–38.

112 Triglia, J.M., Portaspana, T., Cannoni, M., Pech, A. (1991) Subglottic cyst in a newborn. *Journal of Laryngology and Otology* **105**, 222–223.

113 Van Haesendonck, J., Van de Heyning, P.H., Claes, J. *et al.* (1990) A pharyngeal hairy polyp causing neonatal airway obstruction: a case study. *International Journal of Pediatric Otorhinolaryngology* **19**, 175–180.

114 Vinograd, I., Klin, B., Brosh, T. *et al.* (1994) A new intratracheal stent made from nitinol, an alloy with 'shape memory effect'. *Journal of Thoracic and Cardiovascular Surgery* **107**, 1255–1261.

115 Vogl, T., Wilimzig, C., Bilaniuk, L.T. *et al.* (1990) MR imaging in pediatric airway obstruction. *Journal Computerized Assisted Tomography* **14**, 182–186.

116 Vogl, T., Wilimzig, C., Hofmann, U. *et al.* (1991) MRI in tracheal stenosis by innominate artery in children. *Pediatric Radiology* **21**, 89–93.

117 Walner, D.L., Loewen, M.S., Kimura, R.E. (2001) Neonatal subglottic stenosis – incidence and trends. *Laryngoscope* **111**, 48–51.

118 Weigle, C.G. (1990) Treatment of an infant with tracheobronchomalacia at home with a lightweight, high-humidity, continuous positive airway pressure system. *Critical Care Medicine* **18**, 892–894.

119 Yeoh, G.P., Bale, P.M., de Silva, M. (1989) Nasal cerebral heterotopia: the so-called nasal glioma or sequestered encephalocele and its variants. *Pediatric Pathology* **9**, 531–549.

120 Zinman, R. (1995) Tracheal stenting improves airway mechanics in infants with tracheobronchomalacia. *Pediatric Pulmonology* **19**, 275–281.

32

Pulmonary agenesis and hypoplasia

ANNE GREENOUGH

PULMONARY AGENESIS

Pulmonary agenesis is associated with failure of respiratory development beyond the carina. Bilateral pulmonary agenesis results when this occurs at the stage of the single respiratory bud in the embryonic phase. If the bud develops on one side only, unilateral pulmonary agenesis occurs (Figure 32.1) and the trachea runs into a sole bronchus with no carina. If an airway 'stump' is present, then the condition is called pulmonary aplasia. The pulmonary artery is always absent and there is agenesis of both sympathetic and parasympathetic plexuses with usually a lack of parietal pleura.[27] Lesions occur on the left in 70 percent of cases and equally in males and females. Lobar agenesis and aplasia are rarer than complete absence of one lung and usually affect the right upper and middle lobes together.[51,99]

Etiology

Pulmonary agenesis has been observed in monozygotic twins[51] and in rats after the mother was deprived of vitamin A.[124] Bilateral pulmonary agenesis is extremely rare and may occur in association with anencephaly.[88]

Diagnosis

The chest radiograph demonstrates a small, opaque hemithorax with narrowed intercostal spaces (Figure 32.1), ipsilateral cardiomediastinal shift and an intact diaphragm in pulmonary agenesis. A penetrated film may reveal the absence of the carina or a blind-ending bronchus. At bronchoscopy narrowing of the bronchus may be seen. Echocardiography or pulmonary angiography will demonstrate absence of the ipsilateral pulmonary vessel.

Differential diagnosis

This includes 'lung' atelectasis as a result of bronchial obstruction, diaphragmatic hernia, cystic adenomatoid malformation and sequestration.

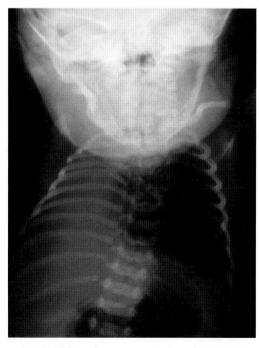

Figure 32.1 *Right pulmonary agenesis and vertebral anomalies.*

Presentation

Most patients present in the neonatal period with signs of respiratory distress. Associated anomalies are common, particularly with ipsilateral lesions.[35] These include cardiovascular abnormalities, particularly patent ductus arteriosus and hemivertebrae (Figure 32.1),[35] ipsilateral facial anomalies, including hemiatrophy, abnormal ears and facial paralysis, ipsilateral limb abnormalities and anomalies of the gastrointestinal tract (including tracheoesophageal fistulae, duodenal atresia, annular pancreas, malrotation and imperforate anus) and defects of the urogenital system (ipsilateral absence of the kidney or ovary). Unusually, the presentation will be of severe respiratory distress in childhood.[41] In those who present late, there is flattening of the chest on the affected side with impaired movement on inspiration.

Management

Prevention and prompt treatment of respiratory infections are essential. Prophylaxis against respiratory syncytial virus (RSV) infection should be considered. Correction of any associated anomalies may be required.

Prognosis

The mortality rate in patients with an absent right lung is 75 percent, but may be as low as 25 percent if the left lung is absent. The difference in mortality is explained by the higher frequency of associated cardiovascular anomalies with right lung absence, but it may also relate to the inadequacy of lung function and higher probability of pulmonary hypertension in patients who only have a left lung.[63] Patients with associated hemivertebrae develop scoliosis and rib anomalies.

PULMONARY HYPOPLASIA

Pulmonary hypoplasia is incomplete development of the lung so that it is smaller in weight and volume and there is a reduced number of airway branches, alveoli, arteries and veins. Pulmonary hypoplasia may be primary or secondary to conditions that impair lung growth. It is the commonest single abnormality found at postmortem, being present in 15–20 percent of early neonatal deaths.[121] In fetuses, infants and young children (18 weeks of gestation to 2 years of age), pulmonary hypoplasia was found in 26 percent of cases and considered to be the immediate cause of death in 22 percent.[54] The exact incidence of the condition, however, is unknown as it is likely to be underreported in survivors due to the coexistence of other conditions such as RDS.

Primary pulmonary hypoplasia

Pulmonary hypoplasia usually occurs in association with other major malformations. The most commonly associated anomalies are of the renal and urinary tract and then diaphragmatic hernia or eventration. In Page and Stocker's series of 77 cases of pulmonary hypoplasia,[82] 67 had other associated major malformations including diaphragmatic and renal anomalies, chromosomal disorders, extralobar pulmonary sequestration, severe musculoskeletal disorders and isolated right-sided lesions. Other anomalies found in association with pulmonary hypoplasia include exomphalos, hydrops fetalis and trisomy 18 and 21.[86] Some 'idiopathic' pulmonary hypoplasias may have a genetic basis as there are occasional occurrences of this condition in twins and families.[17,66] Only infants without associated abnormalities can be considered to have idiopathic pulmonary hypoplasia.[59,68] Idiopathic pulmonary hypoplasia was diagnosed in eight out of 1377 consecutive neonatal intensive care unit (NICU) admissions;[104] two of these cases survived.

CLINICAL SIGNS

Infants with pulmonary hypoplasia usually have respiratory problems in the labor suite. Their non-compliant lungs means they are difficult to resuscitate, requiring high peak inflating pressures. This requirement for aggressive ventilation often persists into the neonatal period. Not surprisingly, pneumothorax is a common complication. Hypoxia, acidosis and persistent pulmonary hypertension (PPHN) are common features. Pulmonary hypoplasia should be suspected in an infant with a persisting respiratory acidosis (pH < 7.25, $PCO_2 > 50$ mmHg) despite high pressure ventilation, particularly if this is in association with a chest radiograph demonstrating small volume, clear lung fields. The clinical presentation is often complicated by coexisting RDS, as affected infants may deliver prematurely. Infants with mild pulmonary hypoplasia, however, may only suffer a persistent raised respiratory rate.[3]

Unilateral hypoplasia may be associated with displacement of the mediastinum and/or poor development of the affected side (Figure 32.2). Affected infants have less respiratory distress than those with bilateral hypoplasia and frequently do not require mechanical ventilation in the neonatal period.

Secondary pulmonary hypoplasia

Secondary pulmonary hypoplasia is more common. It is due to a variety of abnormalities, which can be broadly categorized as disorders resulting in reduction of intrathoracic space, fetal breathing movements (FBM) or amniotic fluid volume.

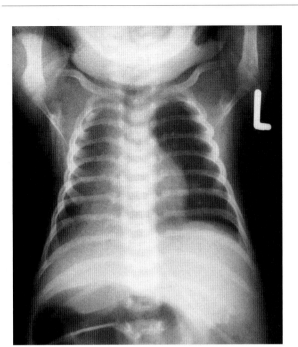

Figure 32.2 *Unilateral pulmonary hypoplasia of the right lung.*

PATHOLOGY

External examination may reveal the features of disorders associated with abnormal lung growth, for example the short limbs of skeletal dysplasia or the dysmorphic facial appearance of Potter's syndrome. Not infrequently, however, the infant will appear completely normal. When resuscitation has been attempted, pulmonary hypoplasia may be complicated by pneumothorax; even at post-mortem this is best detected by chest radiograph. When the thorax is opened, poorly grown hypoplastic lungs are usually very apparent, although they may be missed.[96] More objective confirmation of pulmonary hypoplasia can be obtained by calculating the lung to bodyweight ratio (Tables 32.1 and 32.2). The ratio should be >0.015 in infants less than 28 weeks of gestation and >0.012 in infants of 28 weeks of gestation or greater.[123] These ratios, however, can be distorted by postnatal survival, or coexisting pathology such as inhaled amniotic fluid or pulmonary hemorrhage and edema, which can increase the lung weight. Pulmonary hypoplasia may also be diagnosed by a low alveolar count using morphometric methods.[91] The radial alveolar count is a more reliable criterion of pulmonary hypoplasia than the lung:bodyweight ratio. Histological sections of lung are examined and radial alveolar counts made according to the line intersect method of Emery and Mithal.[30] A perpendicular line is drawn from a terminal bronchiole to the nearest septal division or pleural surface and the number of alveolar septae intersected by the line are counted. A radial alveolar count ≤4.1 (75 percent of the mean normal count) is diagnostic of pulmonary hypoplasia.[6]

Table 32.1 *Lung weight related to gestational age and crown–rump length**

Gestational age (weeks)	Crown–rump (cm)	Lungs combined (g)
20	18.3 ± 2.2	11.5 ± 2.9
21	19.1 ± 1.2	12.9 ± 2.8
22	20.0 ± 1.3	14.4 ± 4.3
23	20.8 ± 1.9	15.9 ± 4.9
24	21.6 ± 1.4	17.4 ± 5.9
25	22.5 ± 1.6	19.0 ± 5.3
26	23.3 ± 1.9	20.6 ± 6.3
27	24.2 ± 2.5	22.1 ± 9.7
28	25.0 ± 1.7	23.7 ± 10.0
29	25.9 ± 2.8	25.3 ± 12.6
30	26.7 ± 3.3	26.9 ± 20.3
31	27.6 ± 3.8	28.5 ± 13.2
32	28.4 ± 9.5	30.2 ± 19.0
33	29.3 ± 3.3	31.8 ± 13.5
34	30.1 ± 4.3	33.5 ± 16.5
35	30.9 ± 2.0	35.2 ± 20.5
36	31.8 ± 3.9	36.9 ± 17.5
37	32.6 ± 5.0	38.7 ± 22.9
38	33.5 ± 3.2	40.6 ± 17.1
39	34.3 ± 1.9	42.6 ± 14.9
40	35.2 ± 2.8	44.6 ± 22.7
41	36.0 ± 3.1	46.8 ± 26.2
42	36.9 ± 2.4	49.1 ± 14.6

*Data expressed as mean ± SD.
Compiled October 1, 1988, by C.J. Sung and D.B. Singer with 1975–1984 data from Women and Infants' Hospital, Providence, RI.

Table 32.2 *Lung weight related to body weight**

Body weight (g)	Lungs combined (g)
100–200	9.6 ± 0.7
201–300	11.1 ± 2.4
301–400	12.6 ± 4.3
401–500	14.1 ± 4.4
501–600	15.6 ± 4.8
601–700	17.1 ± 6.9
701–800	18.6 ± 8.0
801–900	20.1 ± 7.3
901–1000	21.6 ± 7.8
1001–1250	23.1 ± 9.6
1251–1500	26.9 ± 14.6
1501–1750	30.7 ± 16.8
1751–2000	34.5 ± 21.4
2001–2250	38.3 ± 20.0
2251–2500	42.2 ± 15.0
2501–2750	46.1 ± 13.2
2751–3000	50.0 ± 13.7
3001–3250	53.9 ± 20.4
3251–3500	57.9 ± 15.4
3501–3750	61.8 ± 11.8
3751–4000	65.8 ± 18.8
4001–4500	69.8 ± 7.0

*Data expressed as mean ± SD.
Compiled October 1, 1988, by C.J. Sung and D.B. Singer with 1975–1984 data from Women and Infants' Hospital, Providence, RI.

In pulmonary hypoplasia due to congenital acinar dysplasia the lungs show normal bronchial development, but each lobule contains a terminal bronchiole-like structure from which there are multiple cystic outpouchings lined by a bronchial type of epithelium, but no alveoli. This seems to be a primary maldevelopment of the lungs.[97] In trisomy 21 there are reduced numbers of alveoli and a smaller alveolar surface area.[24]

Microscopy and biochemistry

Despite the diverse causes of pulmonary hypoplasia, the lung pathology falls into two major subgroups: hypoplasia associated with oligohydramnios (OH lungs) and hypoplasia associated with other conditions, including primary hypoplasia (non-OH lungs).[119] Both subgroups show a reduction in the total DNA content, reflecting the reduction in cell numbers[120] and the radial alveolar count[30] and decrease air space size in comparison to reference ranges. Non-OH lungs are poorly grown, but maturation is normal for gestation. By contrast, OH lungs show both poor lung growth and retarded maturation; this delay in maturation affects both epithelium and interstitial matrix proteins. The disturbance in epithelial maturation is shown by morphometric data, suggesting a failure of type I pneumocyte differentiation in OH lungs, but the proportion of type II cells is similar to that found in controls.[43,44] The concentration of disaturated phosphatidylcholine, which reflects surfactant enzyme maturation, is reduced in OH but not non-OH lungs. This suggests that, although there is a normal proportion of type II pneumocytes in OH lungs, there is some functional impairment. By light microscopy the interstitial defect is best seen in late gestation. At that stage, elastin is normally readily detectable in septal crests, but is absent or very reduced in OH lungs.[43] More detailed studies have suggested that there is also a disturbance in the development of collagen.[42] The exact significance of the differences in maturation between the two groups is not fully understood but does suggest that the mechanisms producing abnormal lung growth may be fundamentally different. Wigglesworth et al. suggested that the maturational arrest which occurs in pulmonary hypoplasia may be specifically related to failure of fetal lung fluid retention.[123] Other studies,[52,91] however, have not shown a difference in the structure or maturity of hypoplastic lungs secondary to renal agenesis or dysplasia compared to those with other types of malformations.

ETIOLOGY

Reduction in intrathoracic space

This can result from small chest syndromes (Figures 32.3 and 32.4) (particularly asphyxiating thoracic dystrophy), tumors of the thorax (including cystic adenomatoid malformation of the lung; CAM),[81] (p. 466), congenital diaphragmatic hernia (CDH)[5] (Chapter 34) and pleural effusions (p. 355).[19,20] Rarely, thoracic compression can

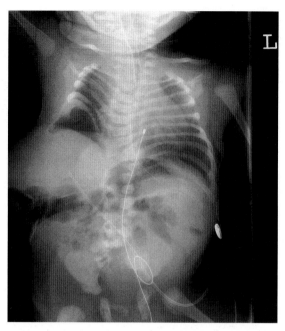

Figure 32.3 *Right pulmonary hypoplasia in association with absent ribs, vertebral abnormalities and lumbar hernia (costovertebral syndrome).*

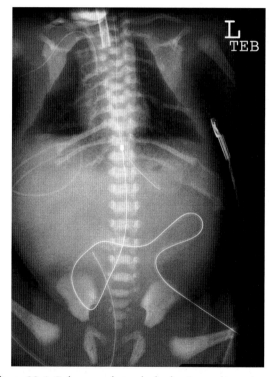

Figure 32.4 *Pulmonary hypoplasia due to cerebrocosto mandibular syndrome.*

result from tumors outside the chest, for example a huge cystic hygroma or teratoma (Figure 32.5).

Abnormal lung growth can be produced experimentally by limiting the intrathoracic space by producing a diaphragmatic hernia,[90] or placing a space-occupying balloon within the thorax.[45] This results in an overall

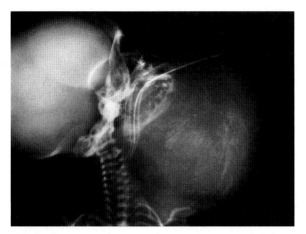

Figure 32.5 *Large teratoma of the neck led to thoracic compression* in utero *resulting in bilateral pulmonary hypoplasia.*

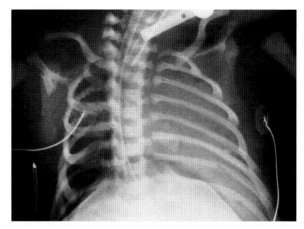

Figure 32.6 *Right pulmonary hypoplasia. The infant also has a gastroschisis and a silo is in place.*

reduction in bronchial and vascular branching and in alveolar development. Re-establishment of the normal amount of intrathoracic space antenatally induces the lungs to start growing again.[46] Infants with anterior abdominal wall defects (AWD) can have abnormal lung growth, as indicated by reduced chest wall widths and lung areas on chest radiography of infants with giant exomphalos.[50] In addition, stillbirths with exomphalos have been noted to have small chests.[40] Fetuses with AWD will, *in utero*, have a reduction in viscera in the upper part of the abdominal cavity and hence an inadequate framework for chest wall development. Thus one explanation for the associated abnormal lung growth in fetuses with AWDs is restriction by external compression; alternatively, FBM may be reduced.

Intrathoracic compression by pleural effusions may explain the association of hydropic fetuses due to rhesus isoimmunization and pulmonary hypoplasia. It has, however, also been suggested that an immune mechanism may operate. Chamberlain *et al.* demonstrated a significant positive correlation between the degree of fetal anemia and the reduction in lung weight.[20] Analysis of the lungs of six affected fetuses demonstrated reduction in airway number, suggesting growth had been arrested before the sixteenth week of gestation. At that early stage, the spleen and liver would not be enlarged and thus the abnormalities could not be explained by compression. In addition, lung function abnormalities at follow-up were significantly related to the severity of rhesus isoimmunization, as indicated by the need for early intrauterine transfusion. Infants who had required an intrauterine intravascular transfusion prior to, but not after, 22 weeks of gestation had low lung volumes.[126]

Reduction in FBM

Selective destruction of the upper cervical cord between the lower medulla and the level of the phrenic nucleus results in cessation of FBM[121,122] and arrested lung growth

and development. This occurred without atrophy of the diaphragm, thus excluding a thoracic compression mechanism. Cessation or reduction of FBM may be responsible for the abnormal lung growth seen in certain neurological abnormalities or neuromuscular disease presenting *in utero*, for example, Werdig–Hoffman disease[26] and myotonic dystrophy.[104,116] There is, however, considerable debate regarding the relevance of absent FBM in other conditions that are associated with abnormal lung growth, for example oligohydramnios resulting from premature rupture of the membranes (PROM).[15,71] Oligohydramnios may impair lung growth by a thoracic compression mechanism.[73] It has also been suggested that the prolonged thoracic compression could impair FBM. Compared to controls, 43 patients with PPROM had significantly fewer FBM in the first 2 weeks following membrane rupture.[94] Absence of FBM, however, is not an invariable association of oligohydramnios.[15] Adzick *et al.* demonstrated in an animal model that the effects of reduction in FBM and amniotic fluid volume had additive effects in producing severe lung disease.[2]

It has been suggested that the quality rather than the quantity of FBM may be more relevant to lung growth. In animals, the amplitude of pressure changes of FBM are an important determinant of lung growth.[61] Reduced strength of FBM, particularly in conditions that affect diaphragmatic function, for example CDH[33] and anterior abdominal wall defects (Figure 32.6),[113] has also been implicated in resulting in abnormal lung growth in humans. *In utero* the majority of the abdominal contents of infants with gastroschisis or exomphalos are outside the abdominal cavity. The low intra-abdominal pressure will impair diaphragmatic function and the ability of a fetus to generate FBM. In addition, diaphragmatic dysfunction may be further aggravated by a structural defect; both diaphragmatic hernia and eventration are common in association with anterior abdominal wall defects.[50,103] Postmortem studies[34] and studies in piglets[89] have indicated diaphragmatic function *per se* is an important determinant of lung growth. In addition, destruction of the spinal cord at the level of phrenic nucleus results in diaphragmatic atrophy and this is associated with greater retardation of lung growth than occurs when the phrenic nucleus is spared.[121] Phrenic nerve agenesis and diaphragmatic amyoplasia are associated with a marked reduction in the number of bronchial branches; that abnormality is due to interference with lung development prior to 16 weeks of gestation.

Reduction in amniotic fluid volume

Experimental production of oligohydramnios, by chronic drainage of amniotic fluid[70,73] or urinary tract obstruction,[47] is associated with the development of pulmonary hypoplasia. The importance of amniotic fluid volume in determining lung growth is further demonstrated by the finding that saline infusion, given to restore normal amniotic fluid volume after experimental urinary tract obstruction, results in less hypoplasia of the lungs.[73]

Reduction in amniotic fluid volume can result from a decrease in production of amniotic fluid due to fetal renal abnormalities – classically Potter's syndrome (Figure 32.7) or uteroplacental insufficiency.[87] It has been suggested that in renal agenesis, factors other than reduced amniotic fluid volume may be responsible for the abnormal lung growth – for example, a reduced proline production by the kidney.[52] In pulmonary hypoplasia associated with oligohydramnios not due to renal agenesis, however, hydroxyproline levels can be high.[84] In addition, pulmonary hypoplasia was only found in infants dying perinatally with urinary tract malformations if there had been fetal anuria.[84]

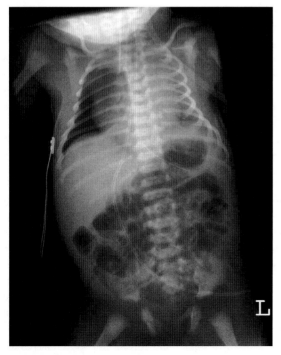

Figure 32.7 *Pulmonary hypoplasia due to Potter's syndrome.*

Loss of amniotic fluid following prolonged premature rupture of the membranes (PPROM)[11–13,125] or amniocentesis has also been associated with pulmonary hypoplasia or at least lung function abnormalities suggestive of abnormal lung growth.[111] The timing of onset of the oligohydramnios in pregnancies complicated by PPROM is critical. Pulmonary hypoplasia only occurs if the onset of membrane rupture is prior to 26 weeks of gestation.[77] Gestational age at premature membrane rupture and oligohydramnios are independent risk factors for pulmonary hypoplasia development.[57,115] The incidence of pulmonary hypoplasia following PPROM in the second trimester (i.e. before 28 weeks of gestation) may be as high as 28 percent.[115] Abnormal lung development, however, is not an invariable consequence of early-onset oligohydramnios. In one cohort,[12] 23 percent of patients who had membrane rupture prior to 20 weeks of gestation had no clinical signs suggestive of pulmonary hypoplasia.

Several groups have reported findings which suggest that if a small volume of amniotic fluid is removed, as occurs at amniocentesis, at a critical stage, lung growth can be adversely affected.[4,69,111,118] Following both first and second trimester amniocentesis, an excess of infants with lung function abnormalities in the neonatal period and early infancy have been reported. Unexplained respiratory difficulties at birth lasting for more than 24 hours and a requirement for oxygen therapy occurred in 30 of 2428 infants following second trimester amniocentesis, but only nine controls.[4] Tabor *et al.*,[106] in a prospective randomized trial, reported that, compared to controls, the occurrence of neonatal RDS and pneumonia was more than doubled in infants whose mothers had undergone amniocentesis at a mean of 16.4 weeks of gestation. First trimester amniocentesis has also been associated with an excess of neonatal problems. NICU admissions of 278 infants whose mothers had undergone early amniocentesis (EA), 262 whose mothers had undergone chorion villus sampling (CVS) and 264 controls whose mothers had undergone no invasive procedures were reviewed. Nineteen EA, eight CVS and five controls required NICU admission; nine EA, one CVS and four controls suffered respiratory problems.[39] In addition, infants whose mothers had undergone EA had more abnormal perinatal lung function than controls.[127] At follow-up, 31 percent of 439 EA infants, 22 percent of 453 CVS infants and 17 percent of 435 controls were symptomatic at 1 year (EA versus controls, and EA versus CVS, $P < 0.01$).[38] Amniocentesis in the monkey (*Macaca fascicularis*) caused changes in the fetal lungs, regardless of the amount of fluid removed and even if the membranes were simply punctured and no fluid removed.[53] The explanation could be leakage of amniotic fluid continuing for some time after the procedure. Alteration in fetal activity following the procedure is an alternative explanation. Manning *et al.*[65] documented a significant fall in FBM 24–48 hours after amniocentesis and attributed this to the increase in uterine activity known to occur after amniocentesis.[100] It is also possible that chronic amniotic fluid drainage which could occur after PPROM or amniocentesis might affect lung growth by influencing fetal lung fluid.[75] It has been suggested that in oligohydramnios, the extrinsic compression of the fetal thorax squeezed out lung liquid; this, however, seems unlikely as in oligohydramnios amniotic fluid pressures have been demonstrated to be below or at the limit of the normal range.[76] Fetal lung fluid is produced by an active transport process,[80] which fills the fetal lung to a volume similar to that of the postnatal functional residual capacity (FRC). There is controversy regarding the mechanisms which maintain fetal lung volume; the larynx and upper airway act as a sphincter.[1] In addition, the magnitude of the alveolar amniotic pressure gradient may be important. Nicolini et al.[76] postulated that in oligohydramnios, pulmonary hypoplasia results from excess loss of lung liquid because of the reduction in amniotic pressure and hence an increase in the alveolar–amniotic pressure gradient.

CLINICAL SIGNS

The clinical signs are similar to those seen with primary pulmonary hypoplasia. In addition, affected infants frequently have associated congenital anomalies, diaphragmatic hernia/eventration, anterior abominal defect (Figure 32.5), congenitally dislocated hip and/or talipes (following PPROM or Potter's syndrome). They may have the features of neuromuscular diseases such as Werdig–Hoffman disease or congenital dystrophia myotonica.

DIFFERENTIAL DIAGNOSIS

The 'dry lung syndrome' has been described following oligohydramnios due to premature rupture of the membranes.[67] Affected infants are difficult to resuscitate, requiring high peak inflating pressures; the requirement for high pressures continues, usually during the next 48 hours, after which time the infants make a spontaneous recovery.[62] No lung function data were reported, but as all the infants were successfully extubated, it seems unlikely they had significant pulmonary hypoplasia.[62] Their condition was ascribed to functional compression due to the oligohydramnios and the spontaneous recovery suggested no structural abnormality was present. Sakai et al. suggested that oligohydramnios may cause bronchospasm as, following oligohydramnios, they were unable to ventilate an infant, despite using mean airway pressure of 30 cmH$_2$O, until 1 ml of epinephrine was instilled into the trachea 10 times over a 30-minute period.[98] An alternative explanation is that the infant suffered collapse of small bronchi and bronchioli and instillation of liquid into the trachea distended the collapsed airways.[62]

DIAGNOSIS

Antenatal: ultrasound examination

Fetal anomaly scan Unilateral pulmonary agenesis is evidenced by mediastinal displacement by the hypertrophied normal lung, which herniates across the midline. On ultrasound examination, abnormalities commonly associated with pulmonary hypoplasia can be identified, for example pleural effusion and CDH.

Assessment of amniotic fluid volume Retrospective studies of premature rupture of the membranes have suggested the risk for pulmonary hypoplasia is increased if rupture occurred at an early gestational age resulting in severe oligohydramnios.[108] In a prospective study of patients with second trimester premature rupture of the membranes,[115] gestational age at the time of premature membrane rupture and the occurrence of oligohydramnios were found to be independent predictors of pulmonary hypoplasia. In a subsequent prospective study,[57] sequential assessment of amniotic fluid volume demonstrated premature rupture of the membranes of greater than 14 days' duration with severe oligohydramnios (<1 cm vertical pocket constituting severe oligohydramnios) significantly predicted pulmonary hypoplasia. The initial amniotic fluid index (AFI) at membrane rupture and the average AFI are also predictors of pulmonary hypoplasia.[125] An AFI less than the fifth percentile for gestational age or an AFI ≤5.0 cm regardless of gestational age are poor predictors of adverse outcome, defined as a requirement for a cesarean section because of fetal distress or an infant with low Apgar scores in high-risk parturients.[22]

Assessment of the fetal thorax Reference ranges of fetal chest growth related to gestational age have been established. There is dispute, however, whether the relationship of chest circumference to gestational age is linear[23,77] or quadratic.[32] Fetuses from high-risk pregnancies should be plotted on such reference ranges.[102] In one series,[32] seven of eight fetuses with pulmonary hypoplasia associated with oligohydramnios had chest circumferences below the normal range. It has been suggested that fetal lung length measurements are superior to fetal chest circumference measurements in the identification of pulmonary hypoplasia.[93] Fetal lung length was below the 95 percent prediction intervals in 11 of 12 fetuses with pulmonary hypoplasia but in only eight of the 12 where the chest circumference was outside the reference range. Although such measurements have been found to be highly reproducible,[78] if there are space-occupying lesions within the thorax the fetus may have pulmonary hypoplasia with a chest circumference within the normal range. The thoracic to abdominal circumference ratio is a gestational age-independent index and can be used to predict pulmonary hypoplasia.[60] This ratio is predictive in fetuses of women with PROM for more than 2 days, but less so in those patients with congenital anomalies.[79] The thoracic area to heart ratio [(thoracic area − heart area/thoracic area) × 100] may also be a useful predictor, particularly as the ratio is relatively constant throughout gestation.[117] Three-dimensional ultrasound can also be used to serially measure fetal lung volumes.[7] Reference intervals for fetal lung growth have been derived using three-dimensional ultrasound, fetal lung growth was demonstrated to increase in a non-linear way with gestation.[7] Fetal lung volume may also be assessed by echoplanar magnetic resonance imaging (EPIMRI).[8] The advantage of EPIMRI is that images are acquired in milliseconds, overcoming previous problems encountered due to fetal motion.[55]

Fetal breathing movements Initial data suggested that the absence of FBM might be a very accurate predictor of pulmonary hypoplasia in pregnancies complicated by PPROM.[14] Others have found FBM to be unusual in pregnancies with oligohydramnios following PROM regardless of outcome.[57,101] It has subsequently been suggested the reliability of the absence of FBM in predicting pulmonary hypoplasia depends on the definition of FBM used.[14,71] If brief periods of respiratory efforts which could be gasping are considered to be FBM, then absence of FBM is no longer an accurate predictor. In addition, a single ultrasound examination is insufficient to allow confident prediction.[15] There is disagreement whether, in pregnancies complicated by PPROM, the absence of FBM is a better predictor of pulmonary hypoplasia than the chest circumference.[16,93] In other conditions associated with pulmonary hypoplasia, the persistent presence of FBM is not necessarily reassuring. For example, fetuses with CDH may have FBM and fatal pulmonary hypoplasia (K.H. Nicolaides and A. Greenough, unpublished observations). A lack of perinasal fluid flow during breathing activity may predict pulmonary hypoplasia in CDH infants,[33] but nasal fluid flow must be interpreted according to the fetus' gestational age.[36]

Van Eyck *et al.* have suggested the degree of modulation of fetal ductal blood flow velocity by FBM after maternal glucose loading may be a more sensitive predictor of neonatal lung performance than FBM.[114] Ductal blood flow in the fetal lamb is modulated by lung expansion and this results from an opening of the pulmonary vascular bed with subsequent reduced shunting of right ventricular output through the ductus arteriosus. Increased pulmonary perfusion occurs with advancing gestational age, reflecting developing pulmonary vasculature; in pulmonary hypoplasia, this will be reduced and the pulmonary vascular resistance raised. In 50 normal fetuses an exponential increase in breathing related ductal blood flow velocity modulation was observed between 25 and 38 weeks. Three of 13 cases with oligohydramnios due to PPROM developed pulmonary hypoplasia; two of the cases had a downward trend in ductal blood flow velocity

modulation, whereas all cases with normal ductal flow had normal lung function.[114]

Postnatal

Lung function measurements Infants with pulmonary hypoplasia have small volume, non-compliant lungs.[95] The lung volume abnormality can be demonstrated by measurement of FRC using a helium gas dilution technique or plethysmographic measurement of thoracic gas volume. Such measurements are particularly useful at follow-up to determine the growth of the lung.[109]

Chest radiograph The chest wall is disproportionately small with respect to the abdomen; sometimes the ribs appear crowded (Figure 32.8). The lung fields are clear unless there is coexisting RDS. Pneumothorax or other forms of air leak will often be seen on the chest radiograph. Infants with dry lung syndrome may appear on their initial chest radiograph to have pulmonary hypoplasia, sequential radiographs (Figure 32.9), however, demonstrate increasing lung volume as the infant's clinical condition improves.

MANAGEMENT

Antenatal

Thoracoamniotic shunting Chronic relief of thoracic compression, as can be achieved by thoracoamniotic shunting,[109] is undertaken to facilitate subsequent lung growth and ease of resuscitation. Thoracoamniotic shunting was initially described to decompress a large cyst in a fetus with CAM type I.[74] The cyst was drained into the amniotic cavity by use of a double-pigtailed catheter. The infant had normal lung function at follow-up.[12] Antenatally diagnosed pleural effusions can also be

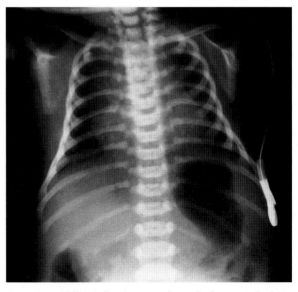

Figure 32.8 *Bilateral pulmonary hypoplasia. Note the low thoracic:abdominal ratio.*

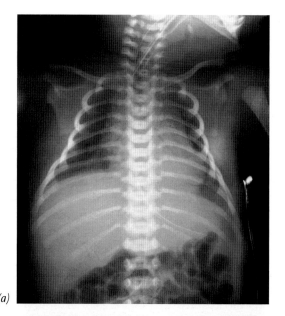

(a)

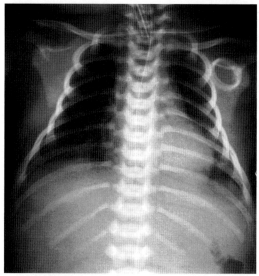

(b)

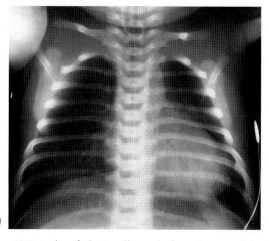

(c)

Figure 32.9 *Series of chest radiographs from the same infant taken over a 48-hour period. (a) Apparently hypoplastic lungs with horizontal ribs. (b) The subsequent film demonstrates clearing of lung fluid. (c) Normal lung inflation.*

chronically drained by a thoracoamniotic shunt. Follow-up lung function studies of infants who had undergone that procedure demonstrated lung volumes within the reference range in the majority.[112] Many fetuses in whom pleural effusions are diagnosed antenatally have other congenital abnormalities or chromosomal disorders;[11] a careful fetal anomaly scan including an echocardiograph is therefore essential before thoracoamniotic shunting is undertaken. Thoracoamniotic shunting has usually been undertaken in the third trimester of pregnancy. In the absence of a randomized trial, it is not possible to confidently conclude this procedure improves lung growth.

Repair of diaphragmatic hernia Although experimentally the pulmonary hypoplasia associated with CDH can be reversed by *in utero* repair, very few human fetuses have successfully undergone this procedure (p. 96).[48]

Experimental tracheal ligation (p. 96) Obstruction of the upper respiratory tract as occurs in laryngeal atresia results in larger than normal lungs.[18] When lung hypoplasia is secondary to a surgically produced diaphragmatic hernia, tracheal ligation can result in sufficient lung growth to return herniated abdominal organs to the abdominal cavity.[29] Following tracheal ligation, the lungs are larger than those of controls, there is an increased DNA content but a normal DNA:total protein ratio, which indicates that the increased size is due, at least in part, to cellular proliferation. In addition, there are changes in the pulmonary circulation.[29,105] Biochemical analyses, however, have not shown that tracheal ligation increases lung maturity.[49] There is a decrease in surfactant concentration, which is the result of a decreased number and degeneration of type II pneumocytes.[28] The loss of type II pneumocytes is dependent on the duration of tracheal ligation. Tracheal ligation for more than 2 weeks is associated with irreversible damage of the type II pneumocytes.[28] In addition, the density of cells expressing surfactant protein C substantially decreases even after 1 week of tracheal ligation.[85] It takes at least a week of tracheal ligation in human fetuses for lung growth to be evident on ultrasound examination. The gestation at which tracheal ligation commences appears also to be important; there is greater lung growth at a later than an earlier gestation, possibly due to the greater accumulation of lung liquid in older fetuses.[56] Tracheal ligation does not simply cause lung growth as a result of increased pressure by the retained lung liquid. Replacement of the lung liquid by saline following tracheal ligation is not associated with lung growth, indicating that growth factors (including insulin-like growth factor 1, insulin-like growth factor 2 and epidermal growth factor) in the lung liquid must have a crucial role.[83] Antenatal tracheal occlusion has been performed in fetuses with CDH in whom the prognosis has been predicted to be extremely poor (p. 96).

Prophylaxis

Preterm, premature rupture of the membranes is not a contraindication to antenatal administration of dexamethasone.[25] It is therefore important, maternal infection having been excluded, to institute prophylaxis to reduce the likelihood of further compromise to an infant with poor lung growth by the development of RDS.

Postnatal

If pulmonary hypoplasia or dry lung syndrome is anticipated,[67] it is essential that an experienced pediatrician attends the delivery. It is important to adequately inflate the lungs and this may require high peak pressures. Structural limb deformities in association with difficulties in obtaining good chest wall expansion are an ominous sign and it is our experience that the majority of affected infants are impossible to resuscitate.

Once on the neonatal unit, every attempt must be made to try and reduce the peak pressure, but not at the expense of impairing oxygenation or the development of a respiratory acidosis. Low-pressure, fast-rate ventilation or high-frequency oscillation (HFO) can be helpful in some babies, although, infants with pulmonary hypoplasia whose oxygen did not improve after 6 hours on HFO had a poor prognosis.[21] ECMO would usually be contraindicated (see Chapter 19). Pulmonary vasodilators are useful for coexisting PPHN, but care must be taken to avoid hypotension. Nitric oxide does not improve the outcome of infants with CDH (p. 493). Anecdotal evidence suggests surfactant administration may be helpful in infants with CDH, although there are concerns that surfactant might increase the susceptibility to pneumothorax in the presence of asymmetrical lung pathology. Surfactant should not be withheld if there is coexisting RDS. Corticosteroid administration may facilitate weaning but there are concerns such treatment would further impair lung growth (Chapter 34). Home oxygen therapy may allow early discharge,[37] but parents need to be counseled regarding the likely duration of the oxygen therapy. Every attempt should be made to reduce further compromise to the lungs; complete immunization is essential and RSV prophylaxis should be considered. In the future, heart–lung transplant may be a viable option for affected infants.

PROGNOSIS

Mortality

The reported prevalence of *in utero* death in pregnancies complicated by second trimester PROM ranges from 10 to 25 percent.[115] The likely cause is fetal hypoperfusion secondary to cord compression.[115] Infants with Potter's syndrome, Potter's facies (large low-set ears, prominent epicanthic folds and a flattened nose) and postural limb defects, die in the neonatal period. There is also a 100 percent mortality rate in infants with the oligohydramnios syndrome (pulmonary hypoplasia, abnormal facies and limb abnormalities) due to PPROM.[13] The perinatal survival rate when rupture of the membrane occurs between 14 and 19 weeks of gestation is 40 percent,[31] although an overall perinatal mortality rate of 54 percent has been reported if PROM occurs between 15 and 28 weeks.[125]

Infants with pulmonary hypoplasia who remain on high-pressure ventilation and high inspired oxygen concentrations at the end of the first week despite use of a pulmonary vasodilator are in an extremely bad prognostic group. It is our experience that such infants rarely go home and, if they do, only with home oxygen therapy and they die in the first 2 years following infection and/or worsening pulmonary hypertension. Parents need, therefore, realistic counseling.

Morbidity

Infants born following oligohydramnios suffer limb abnormalities as a result of compression, but the incidence is very variable. In one series,[12] 27 percent of survivors of PPROM of at least 1 week's duration had compressive limb abnormalities; all responded to passive physiotherapy. Yet, in another series,[57] 80 percent (12 of 15) infants born after oligohydramnios of longer than 14 days' duration had skeletal deformations. Infants who have been exposed to oligohydramnios following PROM also suffer from long-term respiratory problems. It has been suggested that survivors are at increased risk of bronchopulmonary dysplasia,[9,10,72,107] but this has been disputed.[110] Recurrent respiratory symptoms can occur. Follow-up of survivors of PPROM of at least 1 week's duration, some of whom were born prematurely and required ventilation, demonstrated 24 percent had recurrent episodes of wheezing and coughing occurring at least once a week.[110] That abnormality related significantly to very premature delivery and requirement for ventilation in the neonatal period. In another series, symptomatic chronic lung disease occurred in 22 percent of the PROM infants and 9 percent of the controls.[58] Abnormalities demonstrated on lung function testing in infants born following PPROM, however, appear uncommon. Serial measurements of FRC in 22 infants over the first 2 years after birth demonstrated the mean FRC at all ages studied was within the normal range[109] and, although there was a scatter of values, only two infants had an FRC below the normal range. By contrast, neurological or developmental deficits are common. Long-term follow-up demonstrated 28 percent of infants born after preterm rupture of the membranes prior to 26 weeks of gestation had major neurological or developmental deficits.[92] Others have reported the incidence of such deficits at 3 months to 6 years of follow-up may be as high as 32–52 percent.[9,64,72]

Lung function abnormalities have been demonstrated in the perinatal period in infants whose mothers had undergone antenatal invasive procedures. Vyas *et al.* demonstrated the mean crying vital capacity in 10 infants following amniocentesis was 24.3 ml/kg,[118] which was significantly lower than in 10 controls, being 31.3 ml/kg. The same group also demonstrated dynamic compliance to be reduced following second trimester amniocentesis.[69] Similarly, following first trimester amniocentesis or chorion villus sampling, perinatal lung function abnormalities have been described, the abnormalities being worse after amniocentesis.[127] Outside the neonatal period, abnormalities have also been reported. Measurement of FRC at a median age of 5 months (range 0.25–24) in 159 children whose mothers had undergone early amniocentesis (EA), 168 chorion villus sampling (CVS) and 165 whose mothers had undergone no invasive procedures (controls) demonstrated that the FRCs of the EA and the CVS groups were significantly higher than the controls.[38] A symptom questionnaire completed by 439 EA mothers, 453 CVS and 435 controls, when their infants were 1 year of age, revealed that significantly more of the EA and CVS groups were symptomatic; 31 percent of EA infants, 22 percent of the CVS infants and 17 percent of the controls.[38] AWD infants also have been demonstrated to have lung function abnormalities at follow-up[113] as do CDH infants (see Chapter 34).

REFERENCES

1 Adams, F.H., Desilets, D.T., Towers, B. (1967) Control of flow of fetal lung liquid at the laryngeal outlet. *Respiration Physiology* **2**, 302–309.

2 Adzick, N.S., Harrison, M.R., Glick, P.L. *et al.* (1984) Experimental pulmonary hypoplasia and oligohydramnios: relative contributions of lung fluid and fetal breathing movements. *Journal of Pediatric Surgery* **19**, 658–665.

3 Aiton, N.R., Fox, G.F., Hannam, S. *et al.* (1996) Pulmonary hypoplasia presenting as persistent tachypnoea in the first few months of life. *British Medical Journal* **312**, 1149–1150.

4 Anonymous. (1978) An assessment of the hazards of amniocentesis. Report to the Medical Research Council by their Working Party on Amniocentesis. *British Journal of Obstetrics and Gynaecology* **85**(Suppl 2), 1–41.

5 Areechon, W., Reid, L. (1963) Hypoplasia of lung with congenital diaphragmatic hernia. *British Medical Journal* **1**, 230–233.

6 Askenazi, S.S., Perlman, M. (1979) Pulmonary hypoplasia: lung weight and radial alveolar count as criteria of diagnosis. *Archives of Disease in Childhood* **54**, 614–618.

7 Bahmaie, A., Hughes, S.W., Clark, T.H. *et al.* (2000) Serial fetal lung volume measurement using three-dimensional ultrasound. *Ultrasound in Obstetrics and Gynecology* **16**, 154–158.

8 Baker, P.N., Johnson, I.R., Gowland, P.A. *et al.* (1994) Estimation of fetal lung volume using echo-planar magnetic resonance imaging. *Obstetrics and Gynecology* **83**, 951–954.

9 Bengtson, J.M., VanMarter, L.J., Barss, V.A. *et al.* (1989) Pregnancy outcome after premature rupture of the membranes at or before 26 weeks' gestation. *Obstetrics and Gynecology* **73**, 921–927.

10 Beydoun, S.N., Yasin, S.Y. (1986) Premature rupture of the membranes before 28 weeks: conservative management. *American Journal of Obstetrics and Gynecology* **155**, 471–479.

11 Blott, M., Greenough, A. (1988) Dry lung syndrome after oligohydramnios. *Archives of Disease in Childhood* **63**, 863–864.

12 Blott, M., Greenough, A. (1988) Neonatal outcome following prolonged rupture of the membranes. *Archives of Disease in Childhood* **63**, 1146–1150.

13 Blott, M., Greenough, A. (1988) Oligohydramnios in the second trimester of pregnancy, fetal breathing and normal lung growth. *Early Human Development* **17**, 37–40.

14 Blott, M., Greenough, A., Nicolaides, K.H. *et al.* (1987) Fetal breathing movements as a predictor of favourable pregnancy outcome after oligohydramnios due to membrane rupture in second trimester. *Lancet* **2**, 129–131.

15 Blott, M., Greenough, A., Nicolaides, K.H. (1990) Fetal breathing movements in pregnancies complicated by premature membrane rupture in the second trimester. *Early Human Development* **21**, 41–48.

16 Blott, M., Greenough, A., Nicolaides, K.H., Campbell, S. (1990) The ultrasonographic assessment of the fetal thorax and fetal breathing movements in the prediction of pulmonary hypoplasia. *Early Human Development* **21**, 143–151.

17 Boylan, P., Howe, A., Gearty, J., O'Brien, N.G. (1977) Familial pulmonary hypoplasia. *Irish Journal of Medical Science* **146**, 179–180.

18 Carmel, J.A., Friedman, F., Adams, F.H. (1965) Fetal tracheal ligation and lung development. *American Journal of Diseases of Children* **109**, 452–456.

19 Castillo, R.A., Devoe, L.D., Falls, G. *et al.* (1987) Pleural effusions and pulmonary hypoplasia. *American Journal of Obstetrics and Gynecology* **157**, 1252–1255.

20 Chamberlain, D., Hislop, A., Hey, E., Reid, L.S.O. (1977) Pulmonary hypoplasia in babies with severe rhesus isoimmunisation: a quantitative study. *Journal of Pathology* **122**, 43–52.

21 Chan, V., Greenough, A., Gamsu, H.R. (1994) High frequency oscillation for preterm infants with severe respiratory failure. *Archives of Disease in Childhood* **70**, F44–F46.

22 Chauhan, S.P., Hendrix, N.W., Morrison, J.C. *et al.* (1997) Intrapartum oligohydramnios does not predict adverse peripartum outcome among high-risk parturients. *American Journal of Obstetrics and Gynecology* **176**, 1130–1138.

23 Chitkara, U., Rosensera, J., Chervenak, F.A. *et al.* (1987) Prenatal sonographic assessment of the fetal thorax: normal values. *American Journal of Obstetrics and Gynecology* **156**, 1069–1074.

24 Cooney, T.P., Thurlbeck, W.M. (1982) Pulmonary hypoplasia in Down's syndrome. *New England Journal of Medicine* **307**, 1170–1173.

25 Crowley, P., Chalmers, I., Keirse, M. (1990) The effects of corticosteroid administration before preterm delivery: an overview of the evidence from controlled trials. *British Journal of Obstetrics and Gynaecology* **97**, 11–25.

26 Cunningham, M., Stocks, J. (1978) Werdnig-Hoffmann disease. The effects of intrauterine onset on lung growth. *Archives of Disease in Childhood* **53**, 921–925.

27 de la Rue, J., Palhas, H., Abelanet, R., Choriette, G. (1959) Les bronchopneumopathies congenitales. *Bronches* **9**, 114.

28 De Paepe, M.E., Papadakis, K., Johnson, B.D., Luks, F.I. (1998) Fate of the type II pneumocyte following tracheal occlusion in utero: a time-course study in fetal sheep. *Virchows Archiv* **432**, 7–16.

29 DiFiore, J.W., Fauza, D.O., Slavin, R. *et al.* (1994) Experimental fetal tracheal ligation reverses the structural and physiological effects of pulmonary hypoplasia in congenital diaphragmatic hernia. *Journal of Pediatric Surgery* **29**, 248–257.

30 Emery, J.L., Mithal, A. (1960) The number of alveoli in the terminal respiratory unit of man during late intrauterine life and childhood. *Archives of Disease in Childhood* **35**, 544–547.

31 Farooqi, A., Holmgren, P.A., Engberg, S., Serenius, F. (1998) Survival and 2-year outcome with expectant management of second-trimester rupture of membranes. *Obstetrics and Gynecology* **92**, 895–901.

32 Fong, K., Ohlsson, A., Zalev, A. (1988) Fetal thoracic circumference: a prospective cross-sectional study with real time ultrasound. *American Journal of Obstetrics and Gynecology* **158**, 1154–1159.

33 Fox, H.E., Badalian, S.S., Trimor-Tritsch, I.E. *et al.* (1993) Fetal upper respiratory tract function in cases of antenatally diagnosed congenital diaphragmatic hernia: preliminary observations. *Ultrasound in Obstetrics and Gynecology* **3**, 164–167.

34 Goldstein, J.D., Reid, L.M. (1980) Pulmonary hypoplasia resulting from phrenic nerve agenesis and diaphragmatic amyoplasia. *Journal of Pediatrics* **97**, 282–287.

35 Graf, J.L., Gibbs, D.L., Adzick, N.S., Harrison, M.R. (1997) Fetal hydrops after in utero tracheal occlusion. *Journal of Pediatric Surgery* **32**, 214–216.

36 Greenough, A. (1993) Fetal respiratory activity and pulmonary hypoplasia. *Ultrasound in Obstetrics and Gynecology* **3**, 159–162.

37 Greenough, A., Hird, M.F., Gamsu, H.R. (1991) Home oxygen therapy following neonatal intensive care. *Early Human Development* **26**, 29–35.

38 Greenough, A., Yüksel, B., Naik, S. *et al.* (1997) First trimester invasive procedures: effects on symptom status and lung volume in very young children. *Pediatric Pulmonology* **24**, 415–422.

39 Greenough, A., Yüksel, B., Naik, S., Nicolaides, K.H. (1997) Invasive antenatal procedures and requirement for NICU admission. *European Journal of Pediatrics* **156**, 550–552.

40 Griscom, N.T., Driscoll, S.G. (1980) Radiography of stillborn fetuses and infants dying at birth. *American Journal of Roentgenology* **134**, 485–489.

41 Güven, S., Koyutürk, Y., Cerrah Celayir, A. *et al.* (2001) An unusual cause of respiratory distress: unilateral agenesis. *Archives of Disease in Childhood* **84**, F197.

42 Haidar, A., Wigglesworth, J.S., Krausz, T. (1990) Type IV collagen in developing human lung: a comparison between normal and hypoplastic fetal lungs. *Early Human Development* **21**, 175–180.

43 Haidar, A., Ryder, T., Wigglesworth, J.S. (1991) Failure of elastin development in hypoplastic lungs associated with oligohydramnios: an electronmicroscopic study. *Histopathology* **18**, 471–473.

44 Haidar, A., Ryder, T.A., Wigglesworth, J.S. (1991) Epithelial cell morphology and airspace size in hypoplastic human fetal lungs associated with oligohydramnios. *Pediatric Pathology* **11**, 839–850.

45 Harrison, M.R., Jester, J.A., Ross, N.A. (1980) Correction of congenital diaphragmatic hernia in utero. I. The model: intrathoracic balloon produces fatal pulmonary hypoplasia. *Surgery* **88**, 174–182.

46 Harrison, M.R., Bressack, M.A., Churg, A.M., de Lorimier, A.A. (1980) Correction of congenital diaphragmatic hernia *in utero*. II. Simulated correction permits fetal lung growth with survival at birth. *Surgery* **88**, 260–268.

47 Harrison, M.R., Ross, N., Noall, R., de Lorimier, A.A. (1983) Correction of congenital hydronephrosis in utero. I. The model: fetal urethral obstruction produces hydronephrosis and pulmonary hypoplasia in fetal lambs. *Journal of Pediatric Surgery* **18**, 247–256.

48 Harrison, M.R., Adzick, N.S., Flake, A.W. *et al.* (1993) Correction of congenital diaphragmatic hernia in utero. VI Hard earned lessons. *Journal of Pediatric Surgery* **28**, 1411–1418.

49 Hedrick, M.H., Estes, J.M., Sullivan, K.M. *et al.* (1994) Plug the lung until it grows (PLUG): a new method to treat congenital diaphragmatic hernia in utero. *Journal of Pediatric Surgery* **29**, 612–617.

50 Hershenson, M.B., Brouillette, R.T., Klemka, C. *et al.* (1985) Respiratory insufficiency in newborns with abdominal wall defects. *Journal of Pediatric Surgery* **20**, 348–353.

51 Hislop, A., Reid, L. (1974) Growth and development of the respiratory system – anatomical development. In Davis, J.A., Dobbings, J. (eds.), *Scientific Foundations of Paediatrics*. London: W. Heinemann, 214.

52 Hislop, A., Hey, E., Reid, L. (1979) The lungs in congenital bilateral renal agenesis and dysplasia. *Archives of Disease in Childhood* **54**, 32–38.

53 Hislop, A., Fairweather, D.V.I., Blackwell, R.J., Howard, S. (1984) The effect of amniocentesis and drainage of amniotic fluid on lung development of *Macaca fascicularis*. *British Journal of Obstetrics and Gynaecology* **91**, 835–842.

54 Husain, A.N., Hessel, R.G. (1993) Neonatal pulmonary hypoplasia: an autopsy study of 25 cases. *Pediatric Pathology* **13**, 475–484.

55 Johnson, I.R., Sterling, M.K., Blamire, A.M. *et al.* (1990) Study of the internal structure of the human fetus *in utero* by echoplanar magnetic resonance imaging. *American Journal of Obstetrics and Gynecology* **163**, 601–607.

56 Keramidaris, E., Hooper, S.B., Harding, R. (1996) Effect of gestational age on the increase in fetal lung growth following tracheal obstruction. *Experimental Lung Research* **22**, 283–298.

57 Kilbride, H.W., Yeast, J., Thibeault, D.W. (1996) Defining limits of survival: lethal pulmonary hypoplasia after midtrimester premature rupture of membranes. *American Journal of Obstetrics and Gynecology* **175**, 675–681.

58 Kurkinen-Raty, M., Koivisto, M., Jouppila, P. (1998) Perinatal and neonatal outcome and late pulmonary sequelae in infants born after preterm premature rupture of membranes. *Obstetrics and Gynecology* **92**, 408–415.

59 Langer, R., Kaufman, H.J. (1986) Primary (isolated) bilateral pulmonary hypoplasia: a comparative study of radiologic findings and autopsy results. *Pediatric Radiology* **16**, 175–179.

60 Lauria, M.R., Gonik, B., Romero, R. (1995) Pulmonary hypoplasia: pathogenesis, diagnosis and antenatal prediction. *Obstetrics and Gynecology* **86**, 466–475.

61 Liggins, G.C., Vilos, G.A., Campos, G.A. *et al.* (1981) The effect of bilateral thoracoplasty on lung development in fetal sheep. *Journal of Developmental Physiology* **3**, 275–282.

62 Losa, M., Kind, C. (1998) Dry lung syndrome: complete airway collapse mimicking pulmonary hypoplasia? *European Journal of Pediatrics* **157**, 935–938.

63 Lukas, D.S., Dotter, C.T., Sternberg, I. (1953) Agenesis of the lung and patent ductus arteriosus with reversal of flow. *New England Journal of Medicine* **249**, 107.

64 Major, C.A., Kitzmiller, J.L. (1990) Perinatal survival with expectant management of midtrimester rupture of membranes. *American Journal of Obstetrics and Gynecology* **163**, 838–844.

65 Manning, F.A., Platt, L.D., Lemay, M. (1977) Effect of amniocentesis on fetal breathing movements. *British Medical Journal* **ii**, 1582–1583.

66 Marechal, M., Gillerot, Y., Chef, R. (1984) L'hypoplasia pulmonaire. A propos d'une observation chez des jumeaux. *Journal de Gynecologie, Obstetrique et Biologie de la Reproduction* **13**, 897–902.

67 McIntosh, N. (1988) Dry lung syndrome after oligohydramnios. *Archives of Disease in Childhood* **63**, 190–193.

68 Mendelsohn, G., Hutchins, G.M. (1977) Primary pulmonary hypoplasia: report of a case with polyhydramnios. *American Journal of Diseases of Children* **131**, 1220–1223.

69 Milner, A.D., Hoskyns, E.W., Hopkins, I.E. (1992) The effects of mid trimester amniocentesis on lung function in the perinatal period. *European Journal of Pediatrics* **151**, 458–460.

70 Moessinger, A.C., Fewell, J.E., Stark, R.I. *et al.* (1986) Lung hypoplasia and breathing movements following oligohydramnios in fetal lambs. In Jones, C.T., Nathanielsz, P.W. (eds), *Physiological Development of the Fetus and Newborn*. London: Academic Press, 293–298.

71 Moessinger, A.C., Fox, H.E., Higgins, A. *et al.* (1987) Fetal breathing movements are not a reliable predictor of continued lung development in pregnancies complicated by oligohydramnios. *Lancet* **2**, 1297–1300.

72 Moretti, M., Sibai, B.M. (1988) Maternal and perinatal outcome of expectant management of premature rupture of membranes in the midtrimester. *American Journal of Obstetrics and Gynecology* **159**, 390–396.

73 Nakayama, D.K., Glick, P.L., Harrison, M.R. *et al.* (1983) Experimental pulmonary hypoplasia due to oligohydramnios and its reversal by relieving thoracic compression. *Journal of Pediatric Surgery* **18**, 347–353.

74 Nicolaides, K.H., Blott, M., Greenough, A. (1987) Chronic drainage of fetal pulmonary cyst. *Lancet* **1**, 618.

75 Nicolini, U., Fisk, N.M., Rodeck, C.H. *et al.* (1989) Low amniotic pressure in oligohydramnios – is this the cause of pulmonary hypoplasia? *American Journal of Obstetrics and Gynecology* **161**, 1098–1101.

76 Nicolini, U., Fisk, N.M., Talbert, D.G. *et al.* (1989) Intrauterine manometry: technique and application to fetal pathology. *Prenatal Diagnosis* **9**, 243–254.

77 Nimrod, C., Davies, D., Iuanicui, S. *et al.* (1986) Ultrasound prediction of pulmonary hypoplasia. *Obstetrics and Gynecology* **68**, 495–498.

78 Nimrod, C., Nicholson, S., Davies, D. *et al.* (1988) Pulmonary hypoplasia testing in clinical obstetrics. *American Journal of Obstetrics and Gynecology* **158**, 277–280.

79 Ohlsson, A., Fong, K., Rose, T. *et al.* (1992) Prenatal ultrasonic prediction of autopsy-proven pulmonary hypoplasia. *American Journal of Perinatology* **9**, 334–337.

80 Olver, R.E., Strang, L.B. (1974) Ion fluxes across the pulmonary epithelium and the secretion of lung liquid in the foetal lamb. *Journal of Physiology* **241**, 327–357.

81 Ostor, A.G., Fortune, D.W. (1978) Congenital cystic adenomatoid malformation of the lung. *American Journal of Clinical Pathology* **70**, 595–604.

82 Page, D.V., Stocker, J.T. (1982) Anomalies associated with pulmonary hypoplasia. *American Review of Respiratory Disease* **125**, 216–221.

83 Papadakis, K., Luks, F.I., De Paepe, M.E. *et al.* (1997) Fetal lung growth after tracheal ligation is not solely a pressure phenomenon. *Journal of Pediatric Surgery* **32**, 347–351.

84 Perlman, M., Levin, M. (1974) Fetal pulmonary hypoplasia, anuria, and oligohydramnios: clinicopathologic observations and review of the literature. *American Journal of Obstetrics and Gynecology* **118**, 1119–1123.

85 Piedboeuf, B., Laberge, J.M., Ghitulescu, G. *et al.* (1997) Deleterious effect of tracheal obstruction on type II pneumocytes in fetal sheep. *Pediatric Research* **41**, 473–479.

86 Porter, H.J. (1999) Pulmonary hypoplasia. *Archives of Disease in Childhood Fetal and Neonatal Edition* **81**, F81–F83.

87 Potter, E.L. (1946) Bilateral renal agenesis. *Journal of Pediatrics* **29**, 68–76.

88 Potter, E.L. (1952) Pulmonary pathology of the fetus and the newborn. In *Advances in Pediatrics*, vol. IV. Chicago: Chicago Year Book Medical.

89 Price, M.R., Galantowicz, M.E., Stolar, C.J. (1992) Mechanical forces contribute to neonatal lung growth: the influence of altered diaphragm function in piglets. *Journal of Pediatric Surgery* **27**, 376–381.

90 Pringle, K.C., Turner, J.W., Schofield, J.C., Soper, R.T. (1984) Creation and repair of diaphragmatic hernia in the fetal lamb: lung development and morphology. *Journal of Pediatric Surgery* **19**, 131–140.

91 Reale, F.R., Esterly, J.R. (1973) Pulmonary hypoplasia: a morphometric study of the lungs of infants with diaphragmatic hernia, anencephaly, and renal malformations. *Pediatrics* **51**, 91–96.

92 Rib, D.M., Sherer, D.M., Woods, J.R. (1993) Maternal and neonatal outcome associated with prolonged premature rupture of membranes below 26 weeks' gestation. *American Journal of Perinatology* **10**, 369–373.

93 Roberts, A.B., Mitchell, J.M. (1990) Direct ultrasonographic measurement of fetal lung length in normal pregnancies and pregnancies complicated by prolonged rupture of membranes. *American Journal of Obstetrics and Gynecology* **163**, 1560–1566.

94 Roberts, A.B., Goldstein, I., Romero, R., Hobbins, J.C. (1991) Fetal breathing movements after preterm premature rupture of membranes. *American Journal of Obstetrics and Gynecology* **164**, 821–825.

95 Ross Russell, R.I., Greenough, A., Chan, V. *et al.* (1992) Diaphragmatic hypoplasia in association with hypoplastic lungs. *Pediatric Pulmonology* **13**, 181–183.

96 Rushton, I. (1991) West Midlands Perinatal Mortality Survey (1987) An audit of 300 perinatal autopsies. *British Journal of Obstetrics and Gynaecology* **98**, 624–627.

97 Rutledge, J.C., Jensen, P. (1986) Acinar dysplasia: a new form of pulmonary maldevelopment. *Human Pathology* **17**, 1290–1293.

98 Sakai, T., Igarashi, Y., Aiba, S. *et al.* (1994) New interpretation and management of dry lung syndrome: a case report. *Acta Paediatrica Japonica* **36**, 510–514.

99 Salzberg, A.M. (1983) Malformations of the lower respiratory tract. In Kendig, I., Chernick, V. (eds), *Disorders of the Respiratory Tract in Children*. Philadelphia: W.B. Saunders, 169.

100 Schwarz, R.H. (1975) Amniocentesis. *Clinics in Obstetrics and Gynecology* **18**, 1–22.

101 Sival, D.A., Visser, G.H., Prechtl, H.F. (1992) Fetal breathing movements are not a good indicator of lung development after premature rupture of membranes and oligohydramnios – a preliminary study. *Early Human Development* **28**, 133–143.

102 Songster, G.S., Gray, D.L., Crane, J.P. (1989) Prenatal prediction of lethal pulmonary hypoplasia using ultrasonic fetal chest circumference. *Obstetrics and Gynecology* **73**, 261–266.

103 Stringel, G., Filler, R.M. (1979) Prognostic factors in omphalocele and gastroschisis. *Journal of Pediatric Surgery* **14**, 515–519.

104 Swischuk, L.E., Richardson, C.J., Nichols, M.M., Ingman, M.J. (1979) Primary pulmonary hypoplasia in the neonate. *Journal of Pediatrics* **95**, 573–578.

105 Sylvester, K.G., Rasanen, J., Kitano, Y. *et al.* (1998) Tracheal occlusion reverses the high impedance to flow in the fetal pulmonary circulation and normalizes its physiological response to oxygen at full term. *Journal of Pediatric Surgery* **33**, 1071–1075.

106 Tabor, A., Madsen, M., Obel, E.B. *et al.* (1986) Randomised controlled trial of genetic amniocentesis in 4604 low risk women. *Lancet* **1**, 1287–1293.

107 Taylor, J., Garite, T.J. (1984) Premature rupture of membranes before fetal viability. *Obstetrics and Gynecology* **64**, 615–620.

108 Thibeault, D.W., Beatty, E.C., Hall, R.T. *et al.* (1985) Neonatal pulmonary hypoplasia with premature rupture of fetal membranes and oligohydramnios. *Journal of Pediatrics* **107**, 273–277.

109 Thompson, P., Greenough, A., Nicolaides, K.H. (1992) Longitudinal assessment of infant lung function following pregnancies complicated by prolonged and preterm rupture of the membranes. *European Journal of Pediatrics* **151**, 455–457.

110 Thompson, P.J., Greenough, A., Nicolaides, K.H. (1990) Chronic respiratory morbidity following prolonged and preterm rupture of the membranes. *Archives of Disease in Childhood* **65**, 878–880.

111 Thompson, P.J., Greenough, A., Nicolaides, K.H. (1992) Lung volume measured by functional residual capacity in infants following first trimester amniocentesis or chorion villus sampling. *British Journal of Obstetrics and Gynaecology* **99**, 479–482.

112 Thompson, P.J., Greenough, A., Nicolaides, K.H. (1993) Respiratory function in infancy following pleuro-amniotic function shunting. *Fetal Diagnosis Therapy* **8**, 79–83.

113 Thompson, P.J., Greenough, A., Nicolaides, K.H., Dykes, E. (1993) Impaired respiratory function in infants with anterior abdominal wall defects. *Journal of Pediatric Surgery* **28**, 664–666.

114 van Eyck, J., van der Mooren, K., Wladimiroff, J.W. (1990) Ductus arteriosus flow velocity modulation by fetal breathing movements as a measure of fetal lung development. *American Journal of Obstetrics and Gynecology* **163**, 558–566.

115 Vergani, P., Ghidini, A., Locatelli, A. *et al.* (1994) Risk factors for pulmonary hypoplasia in second-trimester premature rupture of the membranes. *American Journal of Obstetrics and Gynecology* **170**, 1359–1364.

116 Vilos, G.A., McLeod, W.J., Carmichael, L. *et al.* (1984) Absence or impaired response of fetal breathing to intravenous glucose is associated with pulmonary hypoplasia in congenital myotonic dystrophy. *American Journal of Obstetrics and Gynecology* **148**, 558–562.

117 Vintzileos, A.M., Campbell, W.A., Rodis, J.F. *et al.* (1989) Comparison of six different ultrasonographic methods for predicting lethal fetal pulmonary hypoplasia. *American Journal of Obstetrics and Gynecology* **161**, 606–612.

118 Vyas, H., Milner, A.D., Hopkins, I.E. (1982) Amniocentesis and fetal lung development. *Archives of Disease in Childhood* **57**, 627–628.

119 Wigglesworth, J.S. (1987) Pathology of the lung in the fetus and neonate, with particular reference to problems of growth and maturation. *Histopathology* **11**, 671–689.

120 Wigglesworth, J.S., Desai, R. (1981) Use of DNA estimation for growth assessment in normal and hypoplastic fetal lungs. *Archives of Disease in Childhood* **56**, 601–605.

121 Wigglesworth, J.S., Desai, R. (1982) Is fetal respiratory function a major determinant of perinatal survival? *Lancet* **i**, 264–267.

122 Wigglesworth, J.S., Winston, R.M., Bartlett, K. (1977) Influence of the central nervous system on fetal lung development. Experimental study. *Archives of Disease in Childhood* **52**, 965–967.

123 Wigglesworth, J.S., Desai, R., Guerrini, P. (1981) Fetal lung hypoplasia: biochemical and structural variations and their possible significance. *Archives of Disease in Childhood* **56**, 606–615.

124 Wilson, J.G., Warskam, J. (1949) Aortic arch and cardiac anomalies in the offspring of vitamin A deficient rats. *American Journal of Anatomy* **85**, 113.

125 Winn, H.N., Chen, M., Amon, E. *et al.* (2000) Neonatal pulmonary hypoplasia and perinatal mortality in patients with midtrimester rupture of amniotic membranes – a critical analysis. *American Journal of Obstetrics and Gynecology* **281**, 1638–1644.

126 Yüksel, B., Greenough, A., Nicolaides, K.H. (1994) Abnormalities of lung volume at follow up following antenatal rhesus iso-immunization. *Acta Paediatrica* **83**, 498–500.

127 Yüksel, B., Greenough, A., Naik, S., Nicolaides, K.H. (1997) Perinatal lung function and invasive antenatal procedures. *Thorax* **52**, 181–184.

33

Abnormalities of lung development

ANNE GREENOUGH AND MARK DAVENPORT

There are three abnormal anatomical and bronchial tree arrangements:

- situs inversus
- right isomerism (mirror imagery) (two morphologically right lungs)
- left isomerism (two morphologically left lungs).[105]

Right isomerism may be associated with asplenia (Ivemark's syndrome) and left isomerism with polysplenia.[101] Both left and right isomerism may be associated with malrotation of abdominal viscera and congenital heart disease.[44,101] The morphology of the bronchial tree is defined as the length of the main bronchus before the take-off of the upper lobe bronchus, the relation between the pulmonary artery and the upper lobe bronchus and the number of lobes in the lungs.[26,44,101,166] Atrial situs and bronchial situs are normally identical.[26] Left bronchial isomerism with normal atrial arrangement is extremely rare, but has been described as presenting with steroid-resistance airflow obstruction.[22]

SEQUESTRATION

Pulmonary sequestrations usually consist of intrathoracic, occasionally intra-abdominal, pulmonary parenchymal tissue, which have no connection either to the parent tracheobronchial tree or the pulmonary vascular supply. They were first described in 1861 by Rokitansky as 'accessory pulmonary lobes'. Pryce later recognized this abnormality as pulmonary sequestration and described a 'disconnected' (dislocated/ectopic) bronchopulmonary mass of cyst with an anomalous systemic artery supply

derived either from the abdominal or thoracic aorta.[136] Three variants were highlighted:[137]

- an abnormal artery to normally connected lung;
- an abnormal artery to a sequestered mass and adjacent normal lung;
- an abnormal artery confined to the sequestered mass.

It was subsequently suggested that those atypical forms of sequestration represent variants of a single primary complex of bronchovascular anomalies – the sequestration spectrum.[151] More recently, Clements and Warner have proposed that these abnormalities would be more appropriately described by the term 'malinosculation'.[35] Malinosculation describes the establishment of (abnormal) communications by means of small openings or anastomoses and this condition is applied especially to the establishment of such communications between already existing blood vessels or other tubular structures. Clements and Warner further suggested that the abnormalities should be classified according to the four components of the lesions, the tracheobronchial airway, the arterial supply, the venous drainage and the lung parenchyma.[35] In such a classification, tracheobronchopulmonary malinosculation would encompass any lesion with disruption of the normal airway and communication at any level from the trachea to the alveolus; this would include tracheal stenosis, bronchogenic cysts, congenital cystic adenomatoid malformation (CCAM) and lobar emphysema. The latter conditions can be associated with anomalies of venous drainage and lung parenchyma. Arterial pulmonary malinosculation would refer to an aberrant systemic arterial supply to an area of otherwise normal lung; bronchoarterial pulmonary malinosculation would describe an abnormality of both the bronchopulmonary airway and the arterial blood supply to an area of lung. Sequestrations, lung cysts with an aberrant systemic artery supply and congenital cystic bronchiectasis would thus be included in the bronchoarterial pulmonary malinosculation group.

Intra- and extralobar sequestrations

Traditionally, sequestrations are divided into intralobar, in which the lesion lies within the pleural cavity and in close contact with normal lung, and extralobar, in which the segment is more distal and lies within a pleura of its own. Extralobar sequestrations may represent a secondary and more caudal development from the primitive foregut, which is then sealed off and migrates caudally as the lung grows.

Intralobar sequestrations may have a different etiology from extralobar sequestrations as, when presenting in childhood, have pathological findings of chronic inflammation, leading to the hypothesis that they are an acquired lesion.[64,79,181] Findings of recent studies, however, tend to support a congenital origin.[27,103,127] Laurin and Hagerstrand reviewed seven children with intralobar sequestration and identified pre-existing chest radiograph abnormalities in six during infancy.[103] Sequestrations may maintain the original systemic connections to the dorsal aorta and hence the term accessory lobe may be used. In 75 percent of cases, the anomalous artery arises from the aorta whereas the artery may also originate from the subclavian, intercostal, phrenic, internal thoracic, celiac trunk or left gastric arteries.[50] Venous drainage in intralobar sequestration is usually via the pulmonary vein;[61] venous drainage in the extralobar type is to the systemic circulation usually the azygos, hemiazygos or caval veins.[61] In pulmonary sequestration, venous return to the portal vein rarely occurs.[88,168] In some individuals, the sequestered lobe and associated normal lung have an abnormal venous drainage into the inferior vena cava, which produces a characteristic chest radiograph appearance, the Scimitar syndrome (Figure 33.1). Eighty-five percent of sequestrations affect the lower lobe, with the majority on the left. Extralobar sequestrations are most commonly located between the lower lobe and diaphragm, but can be paracardiac, mediastinal, infracardiac, infradiaphragmatic and abdominal[59,158] and are often associated with diaphragmatic hernia. Extralobar sequestrations are usually left-sided, but rarely may be bilateral.[208]

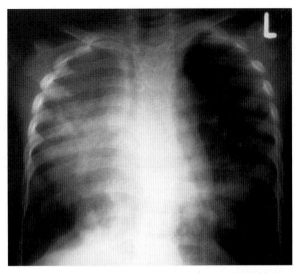

Figure 33.1 *Scimitar syndrome. Opacification of the right upper and middle lobe. The abnormal venous drainage into the inferior vena cava can be seen in the lower right half of the chest.*

percent are homogeneous, 33 percent non-homogeneous and 37 percent cystic. Hybrid cases of bronchopulmonary sequestration with CCAM histology have been reported.[27,47,115,210] The occurrence of CCAM and pulmonary sequestration in the same patient reflect similar embryological origins of these lesions. CCAM arises from failure of the pulmonary mesenchyme to induce normal bronchoalveolar differentiation and sequestration from an aberrant outpouching of the foregut. Theoretically, an aberrant lung bud in the presence of abnormal mesenchyme might lead to a combination of CCAM and sequestration. Alternatively, dilated bronchiolar-like airspaces within a sequestration might result from obstruction to the drainage of fluid in the sequestered lung.[27] There have now been many reports describing extralobar sequestrations that contain histological elements of CCAM. The outcome of these hybrid lesions depends primarily on the size of the mass and the secondary physiological derangement,[120] but also on their location, intra-abdominal lesions usually being asymptomatic.[180] Extralobar sequestrations with histological features of CCAM have been reported in association with diaphragmatic hernias and occasionally as intra-abdominal masses with an intact diaphragm.[7,58] Mostly the histological features are those of Stocker type 2 lesions (p. 467)[58] and striated muscle cells are particularly prominent.[59]

Pathophysiology

The affected lobe is cystic with airless alveoli, respiratory epithelium and cartilage supplied by a systemic artery. Subpleural lymphatics can be prominent and in some cases may mimic pulmonary lymphangiectasia. Twenty-five

Clinical signs

There is a male predominance (76 percent) in extralobar, but not in intralobar sequestrations. Only 20 percent of infants with an intralobar sequestration present with respiratory distress in the neonatal period. Occasionally intralobar sequestration causes heart failure due to massive arteriovenous shunting.[167] Later modes of presentation include secondary infection, pneumonia, pleural effusion and empyema. Hemopytysis may occur, but usually only in older children with longstanding disease. Aneurysm formation and, rarely, rupture of the anomalous artery can occur.[150] Extralobar sequestration is rarely symptomatic in the neonatal period, but may be incidentally found at operation to repair a congenital diaphragmatic defect.

Intralobar sequestrations are rarely associated with other defects, in approximately 10 percent of cases. By contrast, extrapulmonary anomalies have been documented in up to 59 percent of cases of extralobar sequestration. The commonest associated malformations are diaphragmatic hernia,[158] congenital heart disease,[21,158] megacolon[158] and vertebral defects. In addition, in intralobar sequestration, skeletal,[85] renal and cerebral anomalies have been described. Isolated examples of familial occurrence have been recorded.[1]

Differential diagnosis

Intralobar bronchopulmonary sequestration, in which there is an unexpanded portion of the lung with no tracheobronchial connection and a systemic arterial supply, may be mistaken for a cystic adenomatoid malformation of the lung, although cystic adenomatoid malformation can be found in sequestered lung (p. 466).[125] Antenatally, lobar sequestration may also be mistaken for tumors.[27] Right-sided diaphragmatic hernias containing the right hepatic lobe may be mistaken for lobar sequestration. Small sequestrations, however, are occasionally associated with right-sided CDH (p. 488). Bronchial cysts and intestinal duplications, renal and adrenal masses in the presence of small basal subdiaphragmatic extralobar forms of pulmonary sequestration, should also be considered in the differential diagnosis.[154,203]

Diagnosis

ANTENATAL

Ultrasonically, the abnormal lung appears as an echogenic intrathoracic or intra-abdominal mass. It may be triangular with high ultrasound density and of cystic quality early in pregnancy, but later may become of low density and filled with fluid, so difficult to distinguish from the surrounding parenchyma.[13] Doppler ultrasound is useful as it shows the characteristic vascular abnormality and confirms the diagnosis.[152] Fifty percent of cases have an associated pleural effusion and in 50 percent of cases mediastinal shift has been described. Polyhydramnios is a frequent complication. Extralobar sequestration has been more commonly diagnosed than intralobar sequestration.

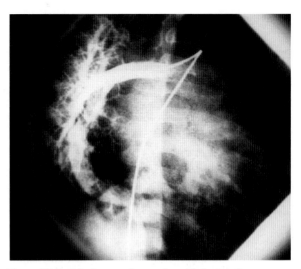

Figure 33.2 *Scimitar syndrome. Same infant as in Figure 32.1. A pulmonary arteriogram demonstrates abnormal pulmonary arterial distribution and the typical abnormal pulmonary venous drainage to the inferior vena cava below the diaphragm.*

Such lesions require postnatal investigation. The low incidence of fetal intralobar sequestration suggests that some of these lesions may be acquired after birth,[79] possibly as a result of infection.[64,181] Many sequestrations, like CCAM, 'appear to' resolve *in utero*.[13,171]

POSTNATAL

The diagnosis should be suspected if a dense lesion is seen on the posteromedial part of the left or, less frequently, right lower zone on chest radiograph (Figure 33.1). Extralobar sequestration is usually seen as a dense triangular or ball-like lesion close to the diaphragm. Arteriography is necessary to define the systemic supply (Figures 33.2 and 33.3). CT scans may also be useful in establishing the diagnosis.[41,175] MRI imaging can also provide useful information (p. 104).[88]

Management

ANTENATAL

Thoracocentesis has been undertaken,[201] but, despite resolution of the hydrops in one case, the infant died postnatally. Drainage of polyhydramnios may improve survival as polyhydramnios is associated with a poor prognosis.[13]

POSTNATAL

Excision is recommended once the infant becomes symptomatic, even if this is in the neonatal period. Such lesions are likely to produce problems due to local compression, infection and may lead to heart failure because of arteriovenous shunting. In the Scimitar syndrome, the abnormal venous drainage affects the normal lung as well as the sequestrated area; thus it is important to identify the Scimitar vein and implant this in the left atrium.[81] Failure to recognize the effect of the abnormal venous drainage on the normal lung can result in complete pulmonary venous ligation with potentially fatal consequences, such as massive pulmonary hemorrhage.[5,81] Surgery is also indicated if there has been an antenatal complication or antenatal treatment has been required. Similarly, postnatal problems such as intrathoracic bleeding, infection or hemoptysis indicate the need for surgical treatment. Surgery, however, should only be undertaken after assessing the size and caliber of the arterial supply; small sequestrations with a poor blood supply may be left in place and carefully monitored.[13] Surgical excision should always be conservative, sparing the surrounding normal parenchyma. This can be accomplished conventionally via a thoracotomy or using thoracoscopic-assisted minimally invasive techniques.[55] Alternatives to surgery include arterial embolization by an interventional radiologist or ligation of the supplying artery through thoracoscopy.[199]

Some have suggested a conservative approach to small lesions with a demonstrably poor blood supply,[13] but this is not accepted by the majority of clinicians. A few cases of apparent spontaneous resolution have been reported. Garcia-Pena reported two cases of imaged lesions suggestive of sequestration which had disappeared when investigated some years later.[63]

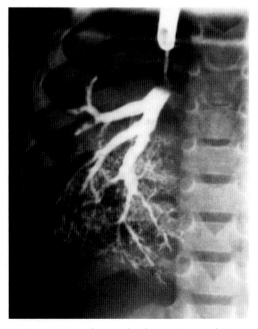

Figure 33.3 *Same patient as in Figures 33.1 and 33.2. Bronchogram showing absence of the right upper and middle lobe bronchus. The patient has unilateral pulmonary hypoplasia with associated Scimitar syndrome.*

Pulmonary hypertension is a common cause of mortality in sequestration, as with other major pulmonary malformations.[41,159] Extracorporeal membrane oxygenation (ECMO) (p. 179) can be a useful adjunctive therapy for affected patients.

Prognosis

This condition in the past had a poor prognosis, because of the associated pulmonary hypoplasia. Fifty percent of fetuses diagnosed antenatally in one series died;[48] all but one of the cases had mediastinal shift and pleural effusions. Currently, however, the prognosis for antenatally diagnosed lesions is good. Some cases do not become apparent until later in life,[205] the individual presenting with repeated chest infections or hemorrhage or associated malformations.[158,180] Generally, however, those diagnosed outside the neonatal period have a good prognosis following surgical excision.

CONGENITAL CYSTIC ADENOMATOID MALFORMATION (CCAM) OF LUNG

This condition was first described in the German literature by Stoek[184] and in the English literature by Ch'in and Tang.[31] CCAM consists of a mass of cysts lined by proliferating bronchial or cuboidal epithelium with intervening normal portions of lung (Table 33.1). CCAM is divided into three types: type I multiple large thin walled cysts, type II multiple even spaced cysts and type III bulky firm mass with even small spaced cysts (Table 33.2). The most widely used histopathological classification of CCAM now defines five variants (types 0–4) (Table 33.3),[179] type 0 being invariably fatal. CCAMs may simply be divided into

Table 33.1 *Histological features of CCAM[99]*

- Adenomatoid increase of terminal respiratory structures. Manifested by various size cysts, variably lined by cuboidal to ciliated pseudostratified columnar (bronchial type) epithelium or a single layered cuboidal epithelium
- Polypoid configuration of the mucosa
- Increased amounts of elastic tissue in the walls of the cystic portions
- Absence of cartilaginous plates in the cystic parenchyma
- Mucogenic cells lining the cyst wall or alveolar-like structures
- Absence of inflammation
- Striated muscle cells appear to be a frequent component (up to 20 percent). Their origin is obscure, as this is not a normal cell line within lung tissue, either during pre or postnatal life[59]

microcystic (cysts <5 mm) or macrocystic (>5 mm).[2] Cha et al.[28] analyzed the histopathology of 11 fetal lung resection specimens. Only pseudoglandular and canalicular type were described; both had variable cystic and solid components. The larger cysts were lined by pseudostratified ciliated columnar epithelium. The solid areas consisting of packed tubules, resembled the pseudoglandular stage of lung development; those consisting of round or branching alveolar duct-like spaces resembled the canalicular stage. The relationship between such cases and postnatal categories remains to be defined. Extralobar sequestrations with histological features of CCAM have been reported (p. 465).[37,119,202] Synchronous cases of CCAM and extralobar sequestrations have been reported (Figure 33.4).[29] It is also not uncommon for CCAM-affected lobes to have an accessory vascular supply, the hallmark of extralobar sequestration. Usually, only one lobe is affected. The defect is almost always restricted to one lung, but the other may be hypoplastic. Bilateral and multilobar disease has been reported.[196] Antenatal diagnosis appears to have markedly increased the incidence of this condition, as only 200 cases were described up to 1986 but a further 250 by 1991.

Table 33.2 *Types of CCAM*

Type I	Small number of large cysts with thick smooth muscle and elastic tissue wall, relatively normal alveoli are seen between and adjacent to these cysts and mucous glands may be present
Type II	Numerous smaller cysts (<1 cm in diameter) with a thin muscular coat beneath the ciliated columnar epithelium. The area between the cyst is occupied by large alveolar-like structures: the lesion blends with normal parenchyma. Often associated with other malformations, these include renal agenesis, Potter's syndrome[96] and bile duct hypoplasia[62]
Type III	Solid mass of bronchiolar microcysts occupies the entire lobe or lobes and are composed of regularly spaced bronchiole-like structures separated by masses of cuboidal epithelium-lined alveolar-like structures

Pathogenesis

This remains unclear, but it is likely to be due to a failure of normal interaction between the mesenchymal and epithelial elements during early (less than 10 weeks of gestation) fetal life. This results in developmental arrest and lack of maturation of both components. Experiments using transgenic mice have shown that defects in mesenchyme-derived keratinocyte growth factor (KGF) expression can lead to the formation of pulmonary cystic lesions. The results of other studies, however, suggest that the increase in cell proliferation typically seen in CCAM does not seem to be related to changes in KGF expression. Cangiarella et al.[25]

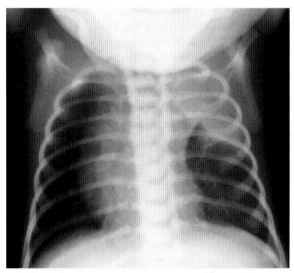

Figure 33.4 *Chest radiograph demonstrating an extralobar sequestration and a CCAM. Note the absence of air bronchograms in the left upper lobe and the left upper lobe density due to the CCAM. There is also an extrapulmonary configuration with an unusual solid subpleural radio-opaque mass, simulating a pleural-based mass; this was the sequestered lobe. At thoracotomy a sequestered lung segment distinct vascular pedicle arising from the intrathoracic vessels was found. In addition in the left upper lobe apex there was a cystic adenomatoid type II.*

Table 33.3 *Modified Stocker classification of CCAM*

Type	Macroscopic features	Microscopic features	Frequency (percent)
0	Hypoplastic, solid lung	Bronchial-like structures lined by pseudostratified tall columnar epithelium with goblet cells. Abundant cartilage	1–3
1	Multiple, usually large (>1 cm), thin-walled cysts	Cysts lined by ciliated pseudostratified epithelium polypoid projections. Mucinous cells present. Focal cartilage only.	75
2	Multiple, smaller (<1 cm) cysts	Cysts lined by cuboidal columnar ciliated epithelium. No mucinous cells present	20
3	Solid or dense multicystic (<2 mm)	'Adenomatoid' proliferation of bronchiole-like tubules	1–3
4	Large peripheral cyst(s)	Cysts lined by flattened epithelial cells (type 1 pneumocytes)	1–3

studied epithelial and mesenchymal proliferation kinetics in a series of nine infants. Both elements exhibited increased cellular proliferation compared to that seen in age-matched controls, but vascular development appeared lower than normal. Those findings suggest that focal developmental asynchrony could explain some of the observed features.

Clinical signs

Males and females are equally affected and there is no evidence of a familial tendency. Twenty percent of cases have associated congenital malformations.[183] Approximately 25 percent of patients are stillborn, they are usually hydropic and are most likely to have CCAM type III. Those stillborn or dying in the immediate neonatal period often have hypoplasia of the remainder of the lung(s).[131]

Fifty percent of the liveborn patients are preterm. Some are hydropic and there may be a history of polyhydramnios. Polyhydramnios may be due to decreased fetal swallowing, the consequence of esophageal compression by the mass,[49] or there may be increased fetal lung liquid production by the abnormal tissue.[96] The increased lung liquid production may result from mediastinal shift, caval obstruction and alteration of venous return to the heart. Affected infants can develop symptoms of respiratory distress immediately after birth, or the onset may not be for days or weeks. Neonatal cystic lung disease can be associated with the development of persistent pulmonary hypertension of the newborn (PPHN), as seen in infants with CDH.[27,142] The PPHN may be so severe, the infant requires ECMO.[142]

CCAM is now frequently diagnosed prior to birth – polyhydramnios being the indication for ultrasonography and a prenatal marker for CCAM.[73] Some antenatally diagnosed lesions, although when first seen are causing mediastinal shift, may regress and even disappear during the third trimester of pregnancy.[108,155,174] The mechanism of this regression is not known, but possibilities include growth of the surrounding lung tissue while the CCAM remains stable, rapid growth of the CCAM, causing it to outgrow its blood supply and involute, and spontaneous correction of the underlying bronchial obstruction.[108,117] Even those in whom the lesion is still present after delivery may be asymptomatic in the neonatal period.[124,144,153] The natural history of such lesions, however, is uncertain, as in the past the majority of affected patients underwent lobectomy in early infancy.[124,144,153]

Prior to routine antenatal diagnosis, children with CCAM presented with recurrent bronchitis or were discovered as an incidental finding when examined for another problem.[144] Adult cases have been diagnosed, mass lesions being discovered on a chest radiograph.[8,138] Other presentations include recurrent infection,[11,15,75] pneumothoraces,[75,133] hemoptysis[30] and mycetoma.[133] Very rarely,[135,156] adults present with slowly progressive dyspnea associated with diffuse multicystic lung disease. Although large-scale studies are lacking, it has been suggested that CCAM is a premalignant condition.[165] There are case reports of cystic lung disease and various lung malignancies, in particular: bronchoalveolar carcinoma,[14,89,145] rhabdomyosarcoma,[122,164,195] pulmonary blastoma and other mesenchymal malignancies.[176] The youngest reported case is a 15-month-old girl who developed diffuse rhabdomyosarcoma in a Stocker type 1 CCAM.[164]

Differential diagnosis

This includes pulmonary sequestration,[48] bronchogenic and enteric cysts,[78] cystic teratoma,[67] laryngeal atresia[200] and brain heterotopia.[68] Laryngeal obstruction may also give rise to a prenatal appearance similar to CCAM.[32] Postnatally, the most common confusion is with CDH.[75,144] The two conditions can be differentiated either by screening diaphragmatic movement or by passing a nasogastric tube into the stomach prior to the radiograph; a barium swallow is rarely necessary. CCAM in association with CDH has been described.[75] The differential diagnosis of cystic lung disease in adults includes bronchiectasis, postinflammatory pneumatoceles, bullous disease and cavitating lung infection.[135] Less commonly, other congenital lesions, such as sequestration, bronchopulmonary foregut anomalies and bronchogenic cysts are encountered.[83]

Diagnosis

ANTENATAL

The diagnosis of CCAM relies on the demonstration of a solid or cystic, non-pulsatile intrathoracic tumor. Microcystic disease results in a striking hyperechogenicity of the affected lung tissue, allowing easy diagnosis of the condition. In macrocystic disease, single or multiple cystic spaces may be seen with the thorax. This condition may be confused with CDH.[93,124] The hyperechogenicity, which facilitates diagnosis in later gestation, is obvious as early as 16 weeks[23,192] and is thought to represent fluid accumulation in small cystic spaces. That process is insufficiently advanced in very early pregnancy to cause a distinct alteration in the ultrasonic appearance of the lungs. Both microcystic and macrocystic disease may be associated with deviation of the mediastinum or the development of hydrops. In bilateral disease, the heart may be severely compressed, although not deviated. Hydrops may result from venocaval obstruction or cardiac compression due to extreme mediastinal shift. Hypoplasia of the non-affected lung may be due to compression by the expanding tumor or the development of pleural effusions, both of which results in a reduction of the effective intrathoracic volume.

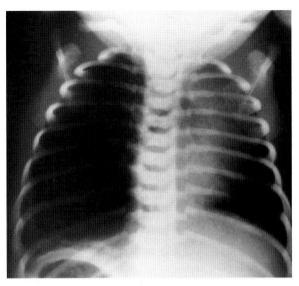

Figure 33.5 *Cystic adenomatoid malformation of the lung. Large cyst in lower right half of chest causing mediastinal shift and compression of adjacent normal lung.*

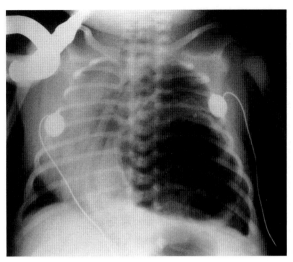

Figure 33.6 *Congenital cystic adenomatoid malformation of the lung. Classical appearance with mediastinal displacement.*

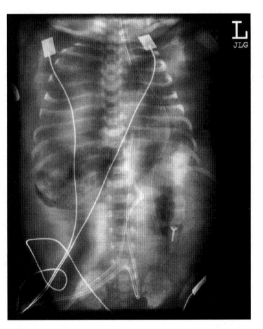

Figure 33.7 *Infant with CCAM affecting the whole of the right lung. The chest radiograph demonstrates mediastinal displacement to the left. Hemorrhage into the CCAM has obscured the cystic appearance. The position of the right hemidiaphragm is indicated by a rim of free air.*

Eight-six percent of 132 cases of antenatally diagnosed CCAM were unilateral and 58 percent were macrocystic.[192] CCAM was left sided in 51 percent, right sided in 35 percent and bilateral in 14 percent of the fetuses. Polyhydramnios was present in 35 percent of cases and hydrops in 43 percent. There were additional malformations in 11 percent of the fetuses, including exomphalos, congenital heart disease and renal anomalies. Additional malformations were more common if the lesion was bilateral rather than unilateral (28 percent versus 10 percent) and microcystic rather than macrocystic (18 percent versus 8 percent). In a recent series,[198] 43 percent had right-sided lesions and 4 percent had bilateral lesions of 51 fetuses in whom cystic lesions were diagnosed antenatally. Thirty-one percent were macrocystic, 59 percent microcystic and 10 percent mixed. Mediastinal shift was present in 41 percent and hydrops in 12 percent of fetuses. Sixty-seven percent of infants underwent surgical resection, 59 percent had CA, 22 percent pulmonary sequestration and 19 percent hybrid CCAM/sequestration.

POSTNATAL

The chest radiograph shows a focal cystic area either in a segmental or lobar distribution which may be causing mediastinal shift (Figures 33.5 and 33.6). Hemorrhage into the CCAM may obscure the diagnosis (Figure 33.7); ultrasound and CT scan (Figure 33.8) are then useful in determining the amount of normal lung and the position of the diaphragm and excluding a congenital diaphragmatic hernia. In some cases the chest radiograph appearance is normal or may only show a localized area of delayed lung fluid resorption (Figure 33.9a), but abnormalities may still be detected using ultrafast high resolution Imitron

computerized tomography scanning (Figure 33.9b).[92] It is important postnatally to seek an anomalous blood supply in patients who have congenital lung lesions, even if antenatally color flow Doppler studies have failed to identify a systemic arterial blood supply. Postnatally, systemic vessels arising directly from the aorta have been demonstrated; in some cases[27] they frequently are hybrid abnormalities, that is bronchopulmonary sequestrations with CCAM histology. The hybrid cases suggest a similar embryological origin for CCAM and bronchopulmonary sequestration

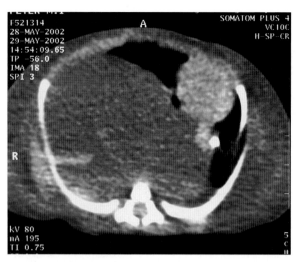

Figure 33.8 *CT scan of the infant in Figure 33.7 showing small amounts of normal right and left lung.*

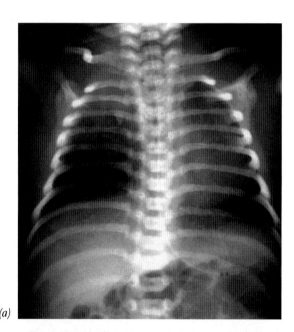

(a)

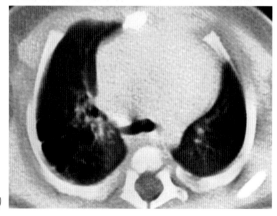

(b)

Figure 33.9 *(a) CXR demonstrating delayed resolution of lung fluid. (b) CT scan at 1 month demonstrating a CCAM.*

(p. 464). CCAM arises from failure of pulmonary mesenchyme to induce normal bronchoalveolar differentiation and sequestration from an aberrant outpouching of the developing foregut.[178] Theoretically, an aberrant lung bud, in the presence of abnormal mesenchyme, might lead to a combination of CCAM and sequestration. Alternatively, dilated bronchiolar airspaces with a sequestration might lead to a combination of CCAM and sequestration.[27] There are now several reports of CCAM that have a systemic arterial supply. Pathologically these were type II or III CCAM and in all but one case the lesion arose in a lower lobe. Similarly, there have been several reports of extra-lobar sequestrations that contain histological elements of CCAM; in all but one this was a type II CCAM.[27]

Management

ANTENATAL

It has been suggested that termination should only be advised if hydrops develops at a pre-viable stage of the pregnancy and the fetus is not a candidate for antenatal therapy.[115] Other indications for termination include severe associated malformations and chromosomal abnormalities.[143] Polyhydramnios is associated with premature delivery, thus repeated amniocenteses may improve prognosis as in twin–twin transfusion syndrome.[157] Antenatal therapy for CCAM has been directed at relieving thoracic compression and reducing the likelihood of pulmonary hypoplasia. If a large unilateral pulmonary cyst is causing mediastinal shift with compression of the contralateral lung or non-immune hydrops, thoracoamniotic shunting or fetal surgery may be considered. Fetal thoracoamniotic catheters have been used to drain a large cyst present in a CCAM,[34] with a good outcome.[126] Open fetal surgery may also be considered with resection of CCAM with microcystic lesions.[73,130] The development of non-immune hydrops may be an indication for open fetal surgery;[98] four of six cases so treated survived. Removing the mass lesion reverses the caval compression, the likely cause of the hydrops.[147] Fetal lobectomy was undertaken at 21–29 weeks of gestation in 13 hydropic fetuses. Pregnancy continued in eight fetuses with subsequent hydrops resolution, *in utero* lung growth and neonatal survival.[3] Five of six fetuses with a very large solitary cyst underwent thoracoamniotic shunting and survived.[3] Criteria for open fetal surgery include diagnosis at less than 30 weeks of gestation, a massive tumor with mediastinal shift and evolution of fetal hydrops.[57]

POSTNATAL

Infants with CCAM, like CDH infants (p. 486) have life-threatening mediastinal shift and pulmonary hypertension. High-frequency oscillatory ventilation (HFOV) has been used in such cases to achieve perioperative stabilization.[148]

The treatment of asymptomatic disease is controversial,[92,115,192] but generally early intervention has been recommended because of the increased risk of infection,[144,202] pneumothorax[153] and reports of malignant change.[190,195] Intervention should be considered within the first year after birth to utilize the maximal growth potential of the remaining lung tissue.

The surgical techniques used depend on the extent of the disease and intention of obtaining complete eradication.[23] Single or multiple lobectomy, single or multiple segmentectomy with or without lobectomy, non-anatomical resection, unroofing of the most bulky cysts and pneumonectomy have been employed. A potential advantage of unroofing of the cyst is that it may decompress underlying lung tissue and permit expansion of normal lung, which might otherwise have been resected. The disadvantage is that there is a high recurrence rate.[114] Limited resection rather than lobectomy has been advocated, as in some patients the CCAM may only involve an anatomical subdivision of a lobe. Some have suggested embolization,[143] particularly for small lesions with a vascular pedicle; embolization interrupted the vascular flow. Surgical lobectomy is usually undertaken and is possible in more than 90 percent of cases. Multiple lobectomies, multiple segmentectomies, non-anatomical resections and pneumonectomies (Figure 33.10) have all been described.[114] Each technique carries risk, although sublobar segmentectomy can be useful if the disease is well defined; it has a higher risk of postoperative air leaks from transected lung tissue. The greatest complications occur with pneumonectomy. These complications include the right pneumonectomy syndrome, twist of the bronchial axis, mediastinal shift

with consequent rotation and compression and kinking of vessels leading to life-threatening cardiac events.[185] Insertion of a silastic prosthesis, which is expansible by means of injections of saline solution, has been used to prevent such problems.[95] If surgery is contemplated, radical removal of the lesion is favored,[23,89,124] although the recurrence rate may be low, occurring only in one of 11 patients and that patient having undergone a partial cystectomy.[114] Malignant change can occur in the remaining lesion.[89] Bronchoalveolar carcinoma was reported in an 11-year-old evaluated for chest pain; as an infant she had had an incomplete resection of a type I CCAM.[89]

Prognosis

The outcome of antenatally diagnosed lesions appears variable.[56,66,153,155,174] Antenatal improvement in the disease with decrease in the size of the tumor, return of a deviated mediastinum to its normal position or resolution of polyhydramnios has been described.[192] We recently reviewed our series of antenatally diagnosed intrathoracic cystic lesions.[198] Fifty-five fetuses were diagnosed with a cystic lung lesion in a 5-year period up to 1990. Forty-eight (94 percent) of the fetuses were born alive. There were two intrauterine deaths and one termination of pregnancy. The fetus that was terminated had bilateral cystic lung disease and associated renal anomalies and the two intrauterine deaths occurred at 22 and 28 weeks of gestation. All three fetuses were hydropic at presentation. Thirty-two infants (67 percent) were treated by surgical resection.

There have been very few reports of lung function at follow-up of children who have undergone surgical excision of a CCAM. In one series,[60] despite on average 20 percent of their lungs had been removed, the children had spirometry values which were 90 percent of predicted.

PROGNOSTIC FACTORS (TABLE 33.4)

Polyhydramnios is a poor prognostic sign, increased amniotic fluid volume was present in 33 percent of surviving fetuses, but in 67 percent of those who subsequently died *in utero* or in the postnatal period. Mediastinal shift is a poor marker of pulmonary hypoplasia in CCAM, being present in 54 percent of all cases and in 55 percent of surviving infants in one series.[192] Microcystic disease[182]

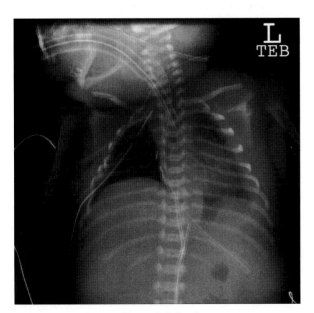

Figure 33.10 *Chest radiograph following a pneumonectomy for a CCAM, which involved the whole of the right lung (see Figures 33.7 and 33.8). The mediastinum remains displaced to the left.*

Table 33.4 *CCAM: predictors of outcome*

Accurate	Inaccurate
Good prognosis:	CCAM:chest ratio[115]
No hydrops	Mediastinal shift[115]
Regression[115]	Location of CCAM[115,192]
Amniotic fluid volume	Antenatal age at diagnosis[115]
normal or reduced[192]	
Macrocystic disease[2,192]	

and hydrops[2,131] have been associated with a worse prognosis.[2,72,131,192] In one series,[115] no hydropic fetus survived. It has been suggested that serial antenatal measurements of the lung–thorax (L/T) transverse-area ratio may be useful in the diagnosis of cystic lung disease and help to predict postnatal respiratory conditions.[88] A low ratio was associated with fatal outcome in some cases and a requirement for ventilation after birth, only 15 fetuses (8-month CCAM) were studied. Predictably, patients diagnosed postnatally have a better outcome.[71,72,74]

CONGENITAL LUNG CYSTS

Congenital lung cysts represent an anomalous development of the bronchopulmonary system. One classification divides them into bronchogenic (that is, derived from the trachea or main bronchi and lying outside the lungs), alveolar and combined forms.[38] They may lie outside the normal lung structure (extrapulmonary), or within it (intrapulmonary). The cysts, whether single or multiple, tend to be limited to one lung and are not associated with cystic disease elsewhere in the body. They affect males and females equally and do not show any familial tendency. Bronchogenic cysts vary in size from a small lesion at the periphery of the lung to involving a complete lobe. They are typically located near the carina, but may be located within the lung parenchyma or below the diaphragm. Bronchogenic cysts are found in five major locations within the thorax:[109]

- 51 percent in the carinal region
- 9 percent in the right paratracheal region
- 14 percent in the paresophageal region
- 9 percent in the hilar region
- 7 percent other locations: pericardial, retrosternal and paravertebral.

Atresia of an airway leads to development of a fluid-filled cyst. The position of the cyst within the branching pattern and its histological features indicate the time at which development occurred. A cyst formed early in gestation from the foregut is likely to contain histological features consistent with its enteric origin.[186] The airway epithelium contributes to lung liquid and may even differentiate into goblet cells which produce mucus. These secretions are then trapped in the cyst. Bronchogenic cysts contain respiratory epithelium, mucous glands, cartilage, elastic tissue and smooth muscle.

Bronchogenic cysts are rare in the newborn period,[41,46] only four cases presenting as neonatal respiratory distress being reported by 1999.[162] Overall, their prevalence is reported to be between 0.04 and 0.06 percent.[146] Other mediastinal cystic lesions include enteric duplication cysts, pericardial cysts, benign cystic teratomas, dermoid cysts, thymic cysts and mediastinal meningoceles. Associated

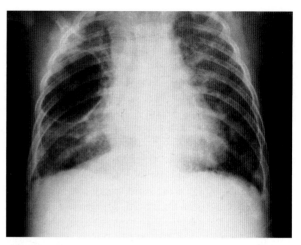

Figure 33.11 *Lung cyst developing in chronic lung disease in right upper lobe causing compression of adjacent lung.*

anomalies are common with enteric cysts and include spina bifida and hemivertebrae.

Differential diagnosis

Bronchogenic cysts can be diagnosed antenatally. They need to be distinguished from other bronchopulmonary foregut malformations, including neurenteric cysts, which originate from the notochord and are associated with vertebral body anomalies. The cyst walls contain neural and gastrointestinal elementals. Gastroenteric duplication cysts result from failure of vacuolation of the primitive solid esophagus. These cysts involve the middle or posterior esophagus and contain gastrointestinal mucosa.[170] They are usually located to the right of midline.[173] Bronchial atresia may result from an early vascular insult to the developing bronchus.[112] The lung distal to the atretic segment appears echogenic and mass-like with anechoic and hypoechoic areas.[173] The diagnosis is usually established from the chest radiograph appearance (Figures 33.11–33.15). The lesion, however, must be differentiated from congenital lobar emphysema, acquired cysts complicating pulmonary interstitial emphysema (PIE) (Figure 33.12a) and bronchopulmonary dysplasia (BPD). The latter two conditions can be distinguished by the history. Delayed clearance of lung fluid from the affected lesion apparent on the initial chest radiographs is very suggestive of congenital lobar emphysema.

Diagnosis

Routine radiography is sufficient in 88 percent of cases but, because of the cystic nature of the lesion, ultrasound and CT scans are usually employed.[188] On chest radiographs bronchogenic cysts may appear as homogenous water-density shadows or air–fluid levels.[188] Intrapulmonary bronchogenic cysts are usually sharply defined, solitary,

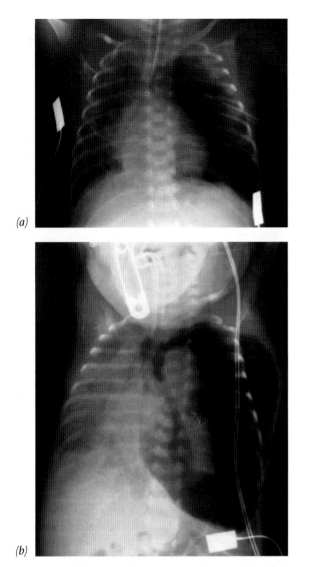

(a)

(b)

Figure 33.12 *(a) Acquired lung cyst in left lung, chest drain in situ. (b) Same patient as in (a). Left tension pneumothorax secondary to rupture of the cyst, subcutaneous air is also present.*

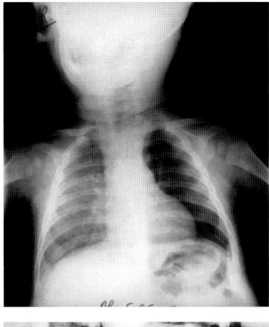

(a)

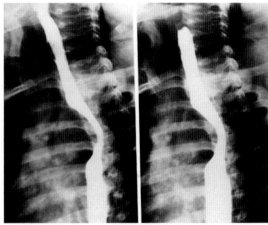

(b)

Figure 33.13 *(a) Bronchogenic cyst causing compression of the left main bronchus and hypoventilation of the left lung. (b) Barium swallow. Indentation demonstrating position of the bronchogenic cyst.*

non-calcified, round or oval opacities and confined to a single lobe. Barium swallow may show an indentation of the esophagus (Figure 33.13b).

Clinical signs

Congenital lung cysts sometimes produce symptoms in the immediate neonatal period, although many do not present until later in infancy when they become infected or are found by chance on a chest radiograph taken for other reasons. Intrapulmonary cysts tend to produce symptoms as a result of distention of the cyst, as gas gains free access on inspiration but its exit is obstructed during expiration. Distention of the cyst causes compression of the contralateral lung. Rarely, PPHN may complicate the neonatal course.[142] Although lung cysts can lead to

pneumothorax, by rupture into the pleura, this usually occurs later; however, it has been reported in a premature infant in the neonatal period with fatal consequences.[162]

Location of the cyst is important in determining the clinical presentation. Centrally located bronchogenic cysts can produce symptoms in the neonatal period due to compression of the trachea or main bronchi. The airway compression causes coughing and wheezing, particularly at times when the baby is crying and, if severe, may produce respiratory distress at rest. The majority lie in the region of the carina and can produce lobar emphysema.[65] Cysts located in the periphery usually present with infection or hemorrhage later in life or remain asymptomatic. Ten percent of bronchogenic cysts are recognized at birth, an additional 14 percent during infancy and 54 percent after the age of 15 years.[146]

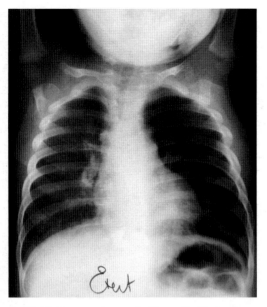

Figure 33.14 *Same patient as in Figure 33.12 showing more obvious changes of asymmetrical aeration when seen 8 months later with hypoventilation of the left lung.*

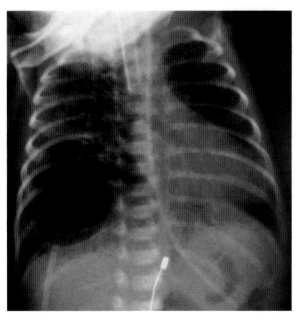

Figure 33.15 *Dominant interstitial lung cyst developed in association with pulmonary interstitial emphysema.*

OTHER MEDIASTINAL CYSTS

Enteric duplication cysts present according to their site and size, whether they are infected, and the contents of the cyst. Gastric cysts present early with the acidic contents provoking autodigestion, inflammatory ulceration or perforation. Hemoptysis, hematemesis and melena may also be presenting features.

Management

Rarely, antenatal diagnosis and treatment by thoraco-amniotic shunting has been reported.[45,126,139] Antenatal thoracocentesis may result only in transient spontaneous resolution, the affected infant still developing severe respiratory failure postnatally, requiring surgical intervention. Congenital intrapulmonary cysts, unlike acquired cysts, do not show spontaneous regression. They often seem to have check valves, which lead to their progressive enlargement producing compressive symptoms.[111] It is recommended that all cysts should be resected, as even those that are asymptomatic will later produce problems as a result of infection or compression.

ACQUIRED PULMONARY CYSTS

Acquired cysts may occur as a result of infection[24] or trauma from mechanical ventilation resulting in interstitial emphysema (Figures 33.11, 33.12 and 33.15) or bronchopulmonary dysplasia.[9,10,116] Unusually, an acquired cyst may be the sequelae of barotrauma and deep suctioning during conventional mechanical ventilation,[97] the suction catheter resulting in repeated trauma to the bronchial walls.

CONGENITAL LOBAR EMPHYSEMA

Congenital lobar emphysema is a rare cause of respiratory distress in the neonatal period, with an incidence of approximately 1 in 90 000. Males are affected twice as frequently as females.[123] Congenital lobar emphysema affects the upper lobes in 80 percent of cases. The left upper lobe is most frequently affected (43 percent of cases), then the right middle lobe is involved in 32 percent of cases and the right upper lobe in 20 percent.[118] Rarely, both the left upper and right middle lobes are affected;[52] bilateral involvement occurs in less than 20 percent of cases.[76,123] Associated congenital heart disease, patent ductus arteriosus[16,104] and Fallot's tetralogy with a right aortic arch[90] or vascular anomalies occur in 12–14 percent of patients.[141]

Pathophysiology

Congenital lobar emphysema may be the result of hyperinflation due to a 'ball valve mechanism'. This can be brought about by intraluminal mucous and inflammatory exudate,[123,191] or bronchostenosis, bronchial torsion, diffuse bronchial thickening obstructing mucosal flaps, cartilaginous septae and bronchial atresia.[177] Extraluminal compression by bronchogenic cysts, teratomas, neuroblastomas and mediastinal cysts and abnormal vessels can also cause congenital lobar emphysema. Congenital deficiency of bronchial cartilage is the most common cause of congenital lobar emphysema. In at least half of the reported cases, focal, patchy or diffuse reduction in bronchial cartilage has been described.[17,107] This results in an abnormally flaccid bronchial wall that narrows or collapses on expiration. Localized bronchomalacia and hence lobar emphysema is also reported in the acquired lobar emphysema (ALE) seen in some patients with BPD.[10] Although most congenital lobar emphysema patients have no evidence of preceding or concurrent respiratory tract infection, a small percentage of cases are thought to be secondary to acute bronchitis or bronchiolitis. In sporadic cases, a primary parenchymal abnormality has been shown to produce congenital lobar emphysema.

Pathology

The affected lobe or lung is diffusely distended and pale in color and is virtually without perfusion or ventilation. There may be almost total collapse of the unaffected lobes on the ipsilateral side and compression of the contralateral lung due to gross mediastinal shift.

Clinical signs

Approximately one-third of patients are symptomatic at birth and nearly half are symptomatic in the first few days of life.[20] Such infants are more likely to have severe symptoms which are progressive; occasionally there is a rapid deterioration resulting in respiratory failure and death. Infants present with an increasing respiratory rate, dyspnea and recession. Cyanosis occurs in 50 percent of cases and is more obvious on exertion, such as crying. An expiratory wheeze may be audible, but the most striking finding is a reduction in the breath sounds over the affected side. Hyperinflation can be present, particularly marked on the affected side, and there may be signs of mediastinal shift and displacement of the liver down into the abdomen. Pneumothorax, however, is rare.[132] Only 5 percent of cases present after 6 months of age and tend to have milder symptoms with less likelihood of progression. Rarely, congenital lobar emphysema has been discovered as an incidental finding in an older child or adult.

Differential diagnosis

The major differential diagnosis is ALE.[39,116] ALE is usually found in a preterm infant as a complication of respiratory distress syndrome (RDS), PIE, BPD and intensive respiratory support. In contrast to congenital lobar emphysema, ALE more commonly affects the middle and lower lobes.

The large cystic lesions of CCAM type I could be mistaken for congenital lobar emphysema, but will not have

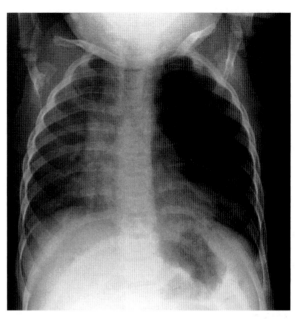

Figure 33.16 *Congenital emphysema of left upper lobe.*

the typical lobar distribution. The condition will be easily differentiated from a pneumothorax, as lung markings are present. Gross unilateral pulmonary hypoplasia or agenesis can produce a similar picture with mediastinal shift, but affected infants rarely present with severe neonatal respiratory distress and can be further differentiated by the presence of breath sounds in the radiotranslucent area.

Diagnosis

The chest radiograph will demonstrate marked hyperinflation and hyperlucency of the affected lobe,[132] with compression of the ipsilateral unaffected lobes and gross mediastinal shift (Figure 33.16). Initially, however, the presentation may be with an opaque lobe; bronchial obstruction results in delayed clearance of fetal lung liquid.[42,177] An alternative appearance is a diffuse reticular pattern representing distended lymphatic channels filled with fetal lung fluid.[6] The fluid is gradually cleared over the first few days; after this, the affected segment or lobe is hyperlucent. The affected lobe is often markedly expanded, resulting in separation of the ipsilateral ribs, shift of the heart and mediastinum and compressive atelectasis of the surrounding lobes. The sternum may be bowed forward and the heart posteriorly displaced on a lateral view.[100] An inspiratory:expiratory sequence of radiographs demonstrates gas trapping in the affected portion of the lung.[177] Occasionally it is necessary to proceed to a ventilation–perfusion (*V/Q*) scan; this will demonstrate grossly reduced ventilation and perfusion compared to the unaffected lobes. *V/Q* scintigraphy can facilitate decisions regarding management, as it may demonstrate that the affected lobe has more function than predicted from the plain films or CT and the compressed lobes may be functioning normally.[91] Such information should encourage conservative management. The morphological abnormality is more closely defined by CT scanning,[110] CT of the thorax demonstrating stretched, attenuated and separated vessels within the hyperlucent, expanded lobe.[132] It is also helpful in excluding an intrathoracic mass or vascular ring as a cause of the congenital lobar emphysema. A barium swallow is also helpful in excluding a vascular ring and other causes of infantile respiratory distress such as a tracheoesophageal fistula.

Management

Congenital lobar emphysema presenting with relatively mild symptoms or found coincidentally on radiograph later in infancy may be treated conservatively. Ten-year follow-up of five infants with mild symptoms did not reveal them to have an increased incidence of pulmonary infection or experience sudden deterioration from rapid massive distention or rupture of the emphysematous lobe.[51] There are a number of reports of successful conservative management of patients with congenital lobar emphysema.[91,163,177] Surgery should be limited to those patients who have persistent or progressive severe respiratory distress unresponsive to medical management.[177] Infants with significant respiratory distress in the neonatal period are likely to get progressively worse and, as the mortality rate is very high without treatment, early lobectomy should be undertaken. Selective intubation of the main stem bronchus results in collapse of the lobe, but there is deterioration following removal of the endotracheal tube. Bronchoscopy and removal of mucus or other debris from the airway occasionally relieves symptoms, but this is a hazardous procedure in a baby who has severe respiratory distress and is cyanosed when not receiving additional oxygen. If the patient requires surgical resection, the anesthesia in such cases requires special expertise.[135] Endobronchial intubation and gentle ventilation with 100 percent oxygen may be a better alternative to spontaneous bilateral lung ventilation, as it requires less deep anesthesia with the attendant risk of hypoxia. Nitrous oxide is contraindicated. If overinflation of the emphysematous lobe occurs, it can be allowed to herniate through an emergency thoracostomy incision.[69] Hyperinflation can be prevented by endobronchial intubation and one-lung anesthesia, which also provides better surgical exposure. Others have suggested that the compressed non-emphysematous lung tissue does not easily re-expand to fill the space of the resected lung following lobectomy and lung volume reduction surgery may be a better option.[161]

Prognosis

In the absence of associated congenital heart disease, the mortality rate is less than 5 percent. Following lobectomy, occasionally infants develop hyperinflation of a further lobe or segment in the subsequent weeks, with resultant attacks of coughing and wheezing over the next months. Results from long-term studies are usually encouraging, indicating compensatory lung growth with only minor reductions in vital capacity being noted 5–12 years after resection.[43] In other series, the patients had vital capacities of 90 percent of that predicted for height, normal working capacities and normal alveolar gas exchange even during intense exercise.[60] Other data, however, have suggested that, although there may be good compensatory growth of the lung parenchyma, growth of the airways may be less satisfactory.[113] Eighteen subjects investigated at the age of 8–30 years had evidence of airways obstruction, with a reduction in FEV_1, FEV_1/FVC, maximum mid-expiratory flow rate and specific conductance.[51] Others reporting 10–20-year follow-up of patients who had undergone lobectomy have also reported lung function abnormalities including reduction in airway conductance and forced expiratory volume. In addition, the incidence of chronic bronchitis and asthma may be increased.[40,172]

CONGENITAL PULMONARY LYMPHANGIECTASIS

Congenital pulmonary lymphangiectasis (CPL) was first described in 1896. In CPL, there is cystic dilatation of the pulmonary lymphatics and obstruction to their drainage. The condition is usually, but not always, bilateral. It is commoner in boys than girls with a ratio of 1.8:1. Rarely, a genetic component has been suggested.[82,160] Of three siblings with non-immune hydrops fetalis, CPL was diagnosed in two.[128]

Noonan et al. suggested affected infants can be subdivided into three groups:[129]

- Infants in whom the pulmonary lymphangiectasis is part of a generalized lymphangiectasis. These babies usually present with hydrops fetalis and, if they survive, develop malabsorption and hemihypertrophy. In four cases superior deviation of the QRS axis in the frontal plane of the electrocardiograms and moderate to severe valvular pulmonary stenosis was also found.[77]
- The pulmonary lymphangiectasis is associated with congenital heart disease. This is the largest group. Total anomalous pulmonary venous drainage and hypoplastic left heart in which there was an element of pulmonary venous obstruction are the most common associations. The dilation of the lung lymphatics is secondary to abnormal pulmonary venous flow. It has, however, also been described in patients with pulmonary stenosis, atrial septal defects[12] and ventricular septal defects and in one case of atrial fibrillation.[53]

- The generalized lymphangiectasis arises primarily as a developmental defect of the lung. This has been reported to occur in association with Noonan's and Turner's syndromes.

Pathophysiology

The lymphatic channels grow into the lung buds at 9 weeks of fetal life; the lymphatics originate as spaces within the lung bud and then fuse to form channels. CPL may represent a failure of fusion to occur, leading to cystic dilatation. The lungs are large, firm and heavy and distend poorly. There are dilated lympathics underneath the pleural surfaces with cystic dilatation of the lymphatics throughout the lung tissue. It has been postulated that CPL is due to a developmental error in which the normal regression of connective tissue elements fails to occur after the sixteenth week of life.[102]

The pulmonary lymphatics consist of:

- pleural lymphatics that give origin to the perivenous lymphatics
- peribronchial lymphatics that reach the hilium
- anastomatic channels that join the peribronchial and perivenous channels together.[194]

The lymphatics of the lungs have valves that direct the flow of lymph from the hilum.[193] From the hila, lymph is carried to the bronchomediastinal trunk. The internal mammary trunks drain the anterior parietal pleura, anterior peritoneal and pleural diaphragmatic surfaces. The thoracic duct drains the posterior pleura, posterior peritoneal, the pleural diaphragmatic surfaces and the infradiaphragmatic part of the body.[77] The thoracic duct and left internal mammary chain drain into the left subclavian vein and the right mammary into the right subclavian vein. The trunks can terminate directly into the veins, but usually there are many anastomotic channels to the neighboring lymphatics.[149] Pulmonary lymphangiectasia may be the result of dilation and ectasia of the pulmonary lymphatics due to incompetent valves or agenesis or interruption of the thoracic duct,[12] with establishment of collateral pathways through the diaphragm and parietal pleura to the internal mammary chain.[77]

Clinical signs

Most patients develop severe respiratory distress at birth or soon after (early-onset CPL). The lungs are stiff and, as a consequence, there is marked recession and grunting. The infants are cyanosed. Occasionally there may be associated pleural effusions[82,84,207] and pneumothorax.[169] Impairment of lymphatic drainage may lead to the production of pleural fluid. Unilateral, localized pulmonary lymphangiectasis has also mimicked congenital lobar

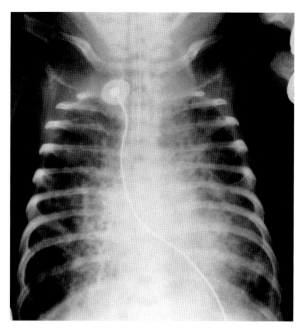

Figure 33.17 *Congenital pulmonary lymphangiectasia with evidence of perihilar interstitial lymphatic infiltration.*

emphysema, due to alveolar rupture and replacement of the fluid with air.[209] Late onset of CPL primarily causes pulmonary symptoms that develop after complaint-free days or months.[82,197]

Differential diagnosis

Roentgenographic differential diagnosis includes wet lung syndrome, respiratory distress syndrome, aspiration syndrome, pulmonary hemorrhage, intrauterine infection, pneumonia, aspiration pneumonia, Wilson–Mikity syndrome and bronchopulmonary dysplasia.[70] Rarely, CPL may present as a fluid-filled lobar mass,[106] then the differential diagnosis includes a fluid-filled CLE, a CCAM or a large fluid-filled lung cyst.

Diagnosis

The chest radiograph is rarely diagnostic (Figure 33.17). It can appear normal or show a fine interstitial pattern as in transient tachypnea, the ground-glass appearance of RDS or prominent interstitial lymphatics and Kerley G lines. In others, the radiograph shows acute or chronic pneumonia, overexpansion, atelectasis or lobar hyperinflation (presumed to be caused by secondary dissection of air along the dilated lymphatics) simulating congenital lobar emphysema.[209] As with other congenital pulmonary abnormalities, there may be delayed resolution of lung fluid (Figure 33.18). CT examinations may reveal areas of ground-glass opacity predominantly in the subpleural and

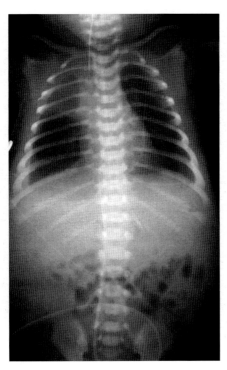

Figure 33.18 *Delayed resolution of lung fluid in an infant with pulmonary lymphangiectasia due to Noonan's syndrome.*

perihilar areas. In children with CPL, increased interstitial markings decrease over time and increased hyperinflation is associated with persistent patchy areas of ground-glass opacity.[33] The diagnosis is usually only made at thoracotomy and lung biopsy.

Prognosis

Infants who present with severe respiratory symptoms in the immediate neonatal period and have bilateral disease almost always die, because of hypoxemia and the rapid development of myocardial insufficiency.[19] Some babies have survived for a few months.[86,134] Patients with late-onset CPL have survived into childhood.[204] Reports of children with CPL who lived past infancy include 14 patients developing symptoms after infancy and two children who developed symptoms in infancy; five had disease localized to one or two lobes and seven others had Noonan's syndrome.[33] Review of the reported cases and their own[33] suggested that children with Noonan's syndrome or localized disease may have a better chance of survival, than do children with bilateral involvement. Localized disease has been reported in three adolescents (aged 13, 16 and 19 years).[197] The malformation had appeared as localized fluid matter found incidentally on chest radiographs.

In children who do survive, multiple respiratory symptoms including pneumonia and frequent airway infections have been reported.[128] In one series of five survivors,[18] the symptomatology and frequency of admissions diminished over time. Symptoms included progressive respiratory distress, chronic cough, recurrent pneumonia, bronchial asthma and choking. Pulmonary function results compatible with restrictive and obstructive disease in one case were reported.[204]

Management

Localized disease that is symptomatic may respond favorably to surgery.[106] In an adult of 22 years of age, oral corticosteroids administration was associated with almost complete resolution of pleural and pericardial effusion associated with CPL.[94]

PULMONARY ALVEOLAR PROTEINOSIS

This rare condition can produce chronic respiratory symptoms in the neonatal period.[36] The cause is unknown, but the progressive respiratory distress and cyanosis are due to increasing lung stiffness resulting from the accumulation of lipoprotein staining positively with periodic acid Schiff (PAS) in the alveoli. The lipoprotein is related to surfactant. It may be derived from the proliferation and then breakdown of type II pneumocytes, defective clearance of the lipoprotein derived from the normal breakdown of type II pneumocytes by alveolar macrophages resulting in accumulation. This accumulation is not associated with inflammation or pulmonary fibrosis.

For a discussion, see surfactant protein B deficiency (p. 20).

Clinical signs

Affected infants are tachypneic and progressively cyanosed. They fail to thrive, often having diarrhea and vomiting.

Diagnosis

The chest radiograph shows a fine pattern of alveolar edema in a perihilar distribution, similar to that seen in pulmonary edema but without associated cardiomegaly. IgA levels may be reduced. In some infants alveolar macrophage activity is defective. The diagnosis is made at lung biopsy.

Management

Pulmonary lavage is the only form of treatment which appears to have any effect; despite this, however, most infants die after a number of weeks or months.

IMMOTILE CILIA SYNDROME

Although this condition classically produces upper and lower respiratory symptoms later in infancy and early childhood, it can cause secretion retention and pneumonia in the immediate neonatal period.[140,206] The overall incidence is approximately one per 16 000 deliveries.

Pathophysiology

The primary defect is abnormal or absent ciliary function. A lack or partial lack of dynein arms on the outer microtubular doublets was first demonstrated by electron microscopy.[4] Subsequently, other defects have been found, including a defect in radial spoke linkages,[187] absence of central tubules and even the total absence of all cilia on the respiratory tract cells. A further group of patients have been identified who have ciliary dysfunction and yet normal ciliary ultrastructure on electron microscopy. The specific abnormality appears identical in affected subjects from any one family.

Although cilial abnormalities have been identified as early as the seventh week of gestation,[121] there is no evidence that the respiratory tract incurs damage during fetal life as a result of ciliary dysfunction. It has been postulated that alignment of the heart and gastrointestinal tract is determined by ciliary function and this would explain the presence of dextrocardia (Figure 33.19) and situs inversus in 50 percent of the patients with immotile cilia syndrome.

Clinical signs

Ciliary dysfunction leads to sputum retention with areas of atelectasis and pneumonia. Tachypnea, recession, rales and rhonchi on auscultation and often cyanosis may develop within the first 24 hours of life.[206] Mucoid nasal discharge has also been described.[80] Fifty percent of affected infants will have dextrocardia and/or cyanosis. Some will also have a positive family history (autosomal recessive inheritance).

Diagnosis

This is made by assessing ciliary function and ultrastructure. A superficial epithelial biopsy can be obtained by passing a bronchial biopsy brush via the nares to the nasopharyngeal space and then gently withdrawing and twisting the brush. The cells are transferred to a small quantity of saline and examined under a light microscope with a stage which is heated to 37°C. It is relatively easy to see whether the cilia are immotile or have poorly coordinated beating. More subtle functional changes can only be identified if the ciliary beat rate is measured, either with electronic counting devices or by strobing

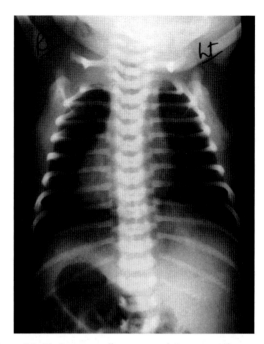

Figure 33.19 *Dextrocardia as part of Kartagener's syndrome.*

techniques. Electron microscopic studies will provide further supportive evidence in the majority of cases.

Management

Antibiotics are required for acute infective episodes and regular chest physiotherapy is required throughout the child's life.

Prognosis

Outside the neonatal period, the infants have recurrent upper respiratory tract infections with sinusitis and otitis media. A third develop bronchiectasis secondary to lower respiratory tract infections and sputum retention. If an aggressive approach to therapy is adopted, however, the majority of children thrive. Follow-up of patients at 21–43 years demonstrated all but one to have a normal working capacity,[54] but there was evidence of small airways disease and a tendency to hyperinflation in the majority.

REFERENCES

1 Abuhamad, A.Z., Bass, T., Katz, M.E., Heyl, P.S. (1996) Familial recurrence of pulmonary sequestration. *Obstetrics and Gynecology* **87**, 843–845.

2 Adzick, N.S., Harrison, M.R., Glick, P.L. *et al.* (1985) Fetal cystic adenomatoid malformation: prenatal diagnosis and natural history. *Journal of Pediatric Surgery* **20**, 483–488.

3 Adzick, N.S., Harrison, M.R., Crombleholme, T.M. *et al.* (1998) Fetal lung lesions: management and outcome. *American Journal of Obstetrics and Gynecology* **179**, 884–889.

4 Afzelius, B.A. (1976) A human syndrome caused by immotile cilia. *Science* **193**, 317–321.

5 Alivizatos, P., Cheatle, T., de-Leval, M., Stark, J. (1985) Pulmonary sequestration complicated by anomalies of pulmonary venous return. *Journal of Pediatric Surgery* **20**, 76–79.

6 Allen, R.P., Taylor, R.L., Reiquam, C.W. (1966) Congenital lobar emphysema with dilated septal lymphatics. *Radiology* **86**, 929–931.

7 Aulicino, M.R., Reis, E.D., Dolgin, S.E. *et al.* (1994) Intra-abdominal pulmonary sequestration exhibiting congenital cystic adenomatoid malformation. Report of a case and review of the literature. *Archives of Pathology and Laboratory Medicine* **118**, 1034–1037.

8 Avitabile, A.M., Greco, M.A., Hulnick, D.H., Ferner, H.D. (1984) congenital cystic adenomatoid malformation of the lung in adults. *American Journal of Surgical Pathology* **8**, 193–202.

9 Azizkhan, R., Lacey, S., Wood, R. (1990) Acquired symptomatic bronchial stenosis in infants: successful management using argon laser. *Journal of Pediatric Surgery* **25**, 19–24.

10 Azizkhan, R.G., Grimmer, D.L., Askin, F.B. *et al.* (1992) Acquired lobar emphysema (overinflation): clinical and pathological evaluation of infants requiring lobectomy. *Journal of Pediatric Surgery* **27**, 1145–1152.

11 Bale, P.M. (1979) Congenital cystic malformation of the lung: a form of congenital bronchiolar ('adenomatoid') malformation. *American Journal of Clinical Pathology* **71**, 411–420.

12 Baltaxe, H.A., Lee, J.G., Ehlers, K.H., Engle, M.A. (1975) Pulmonary lymphangiectasia demonstrated by lymphangiography in two patients with Noonan's syndrome. *Radiology* **115**, 149–153.

13 Becmeur, F., Horta-Geraud, P., Donato, L., Sauvage, P. (1998) Pulmonary sequestrations: prenatal ultrasound diagnosis, treatment and outcome. *Journal of Pediatrics* **33**, 492–496.

14 Benjamin, D.R., Cahill, J.L. (1991) Bronchioloalveolar carcinoma of the lung and congenital cystic adenomatoid malformation. *American Journal of Clinical Pathology* **95**, 889–892.

15 Benning, T.L., Godwin, J.D., Roggli, V.L., Askin, F.B. (1987) Cartilaginous variant of congenital adenomatoid malformation of the lung. *Chest* **92**, 514–516.

16 Berlinger, N.T., Porto, D.P., Thompson, T.R. (1987) Infantile lobar emphysema. *Annals of Otology, Rhinology and Laryngology* **96**, 106–111.

17 Binet, J.P., Wezelof, C., Fredet, J. (1962) Five cases of lobar emphysema in infancy: importance of bronchial malformation and value of postoperative steroid therapy. *Diseases of the Chest* **41**, 126–129.

18 Bouchard, S., Di Lorenzo, M., Youssef, S. *et al.* (2000) Pulmonary lymphangiectasia revisited. *Journal of Pediatric Surgery* **35**, 796–800.

19 Brown, M.D., Reidbord, H.E. (1967) Congenital pulmonary lymphangiectasis. *American Journal of Diseases of Children* **114**, 654–657.

20 Buckner, D.M. (1978) Congenital lobar emphysema. *Clinics in Perinatology* **5**, 105–113.

21 Buntain, W.L., Woolley, M.M., Mahour, G.H. *et al.* (1977) Pulmonary sequestration in children: A twenty-five year experience. *Surgery* **81**, 413–420.

22 Bush, A. (1999) Left bronchial isomerism, normal atrial arrangement and bronchomalacia mimicking asthma: a new syndrome? *European Respiratory Journal* **14**, 475–477.

23 Cacciari, A., Ceccarelli, P.L., Pilu, G.L. *et al.* (1997) A series of 17 cases of congenital cystic adenomatoid malformation of the lung: management and outcome. *European Journal of Pediatric Surgery* **7**, 87–89.

24 Campbell, P.W.I., Stokes, D.C. (1994) Pneumonia. In Loughlin, G.M., Eigen, H. (eds.), *Respiratory Disease in Children*. Baltimore: Williams and Wilkins, 351–372.

25 Cangiarella, J., Greco, M.A., Askin, F. *et al.* (1995) Congenital cystic adenomatoid malformation of the lung: insights into the pathogenesis utilizing quantitative analysis of vascular marker CD34 (QBEND-10) and cell proliferation marker MIB-1. *Modern Pathology* **8**, 913–918.

26 Caruso, G., Becker, A.E. (1979) How to determine atrial situs? Considerations initiated by 3 cases of absent spleen with discordant anatomy between bronchi and atria. *British Heart Journal* **41**, 559–567.

27 Cass, D.L., Crombleholme, T.M., Howell, L.J. *et al.* (1997) Cystic lung lesions with systemic arterial blood supply: a hybrid of congenital cystic adenomatoid malformation and bronchopulmonary sequestration. *Journal of Pediatric Surgery* **32**, 986–990.

28 Cha, I., Adzick, N.S., Harrison, M.R., Finkbeiner, W.E. (1997) Fetal congenital cystic adenomatoid malformations of the lung: a clinicopathologic study of eleven cases. *American Journal of Surgical Pathology* **21**, 537–544.

29 Chandran, H., Upadhyay, V., Pease, P.W. (2000) Congenital cystic adenomatoid malformation and extralobar sequestration occurring independently in the ipsilateral hemithorax. *Pediatric Surgery International* **16**, 102–103.

30 Chen, K.T. (1985) Congenital cystic adenomatoid malformation of the lung and pulmonary tumorlets in an adult. *Journal of Surgical Oncology* **30**, 106–108.

31 Ch'in, K.Y., Tang, M.Y. (1949) Congenital adenomatoid malformation of one lobe of a lung with general anasarca. *Archives of Pathology* **48**, 221–229.

32 Choong, K.K.L., Turdinger, B., Chow, C., Osburn, R.A. (1992) Fetal laryngeal obstruction: sonographic detection. *Ultrasound in Obstetrics and Gynecology* **2**, 357–359.

33 Chung, C.J., Fordham, L.A., Barker, P., Cooper, L.L. (1999) Children with congenital pulmonary lymphangiectasia: after infancy. *American Journal of Roentgenology* **173**, 1583–1588.

34 Clark, S.L., Vitale, D.J., Minton, D.S. *et al.* (1987) Successful fetal therapy for cystic adenomatoid malformation associated with second trimester hydrops. *American Journal of Obstetrics and Gynecology* **157**, 294–295.

35 Clements, B.S., Warner, J.O. (1987) Pulmonary sequestration and related congenital bronchopulmonary-vascular malformations: nomenclature and classification based on anatomical and embryological considerations. *Thorax* **42**, 401–408.

36 Coleman, M., Dehner, L.P., Sibley, R.K. *et al.* (1980) Pulmonary alveolar proteinosis: an uncommon cause of chronic neonatal respiratory distress. *American Review of Respiratory Disease* **121**, 583–586.

37 Conran, R.M., Stocker, J.T. (1999) Extralobar sequestration with frequently associated congenital cystic adenomatoid malformation, type 2: report of 50 cases. *Pediatric and Developmental Pathology* **2**, 454–463.

38 Cooke, F.N., Blades, B. (1952) Cystic disease of the lung. *Journal of Thoracic and Cardiovascular Surgery* **23**, 546–556.

39 Cooney, D.R., Menke, J.A., Allen, J.E. (1977) Acquired lobar emphysema. A complication of respiratory distress in premature infants. *Journal of Pediatric Surgery* **12**, 897–904.

40 Cooper, J.D., Trulock, E.P., Triantafillou, A.N. *et al.* (1995) Bilateral pneumectomy (volume reduction) for chronic

obstructive pulmonary disease. *Journal of Thoracic and Cardiovascular Surgery* **109**, 106–116; discussion 116–109.

41 Coran, A.G., Drongowski, R. (1994) Congenital cystic disease of the tracheobronchial tree in infants and children. *Archives of Surgery* **129**, 521–527.

42 Corbet, D.P., Washington, J.E. (1971) Respiratory obstruction in the newborn and excess pulmonary fluid. *American Journal of Roentgenology, Radium Therapy and Nuclear Medicine* **112**, 18–22.

43 De Muth, G.R., Sloan, H. (1966) Congenital lobar emphysema: long term effects and sequelase in treated cases. *Surgery* **59**, 601–607.

44 Deanfield, J.E., Leanage, R., Strooband, K. *et al.* (1980) Use of high kilovoltage filtered beam radiographs for detection of bronchial situs in infants and young children. *British Heart Journal* **44**, 577–583.

45 Dembinski, J., Kaminski, M., Schild, R. *et al.* (1999) Congenital intrapulmonary bronchogenic cyst in the neonate – perinatal management. *American Journal of Perinatology* **16**, 509–514.

46 Di Lorenzo, M., Collin, P.P., Vaillancourt, R., Duranceau, A. (1989) Bronchogenic cysts. *Journal of Pediatric Surgery* **24**, 988–991.

47 Dibden, L.J., Fischer, J.D., Zuberbuhler, P.C. (1986) Pulmonary sequestration and congenital cystic adenomatoid malformation in an infant. *Journal of Pediatric Surgery* **21**, 731–733.

48 Dolkart, L.A., Reimers, F.T., Helmuth, W.V. *et al.* (1992) Antenatal diagnosis of pulmonary sequestration: a review. *Obstetrical and Gynecological Survey* **47**, 515–520.

49 Donn, S.M., Martin, J.N., White, S.J. (1981) Antenatal ultrasound findings in cystic malformation. *Pediatric Radiology* **10**, 180–182.

50 Donovan, C.B., Edelman, R.R., Vrachliotis, T.G. *et al.* (1994) Bronchopulmonary sequestration with R angiographic evaluation. A case report. *Angiology* **45**, 239–244.

51 Eigen, H., Lemen, R.J., Waring, W.W. (1976) Congenital lobar emphysema: long term evaluation of surgically and conservatively treated children. *American Review of Respiratory Disease* **113**, 823–831.

52 Ekkelkamp, S., Vos, A. (1987) Successful surgical treatment of a newborn with bilateral congenital lobar emphysema. *Journal of Pediatric Surgery* **22**, 1001–1002.

53 Estlin, E.J., Bennett, M.K., Skinner, J.R. *et al.* (1998) Atrial fibrillation with neonatal pulmonary lymphangiectasia. *Acta Paediatrica* **87**, 1304–1306.

54 Evander, E., Arborelisu, M., Jonson, B. *et al.* (1983) Lung function and bronchial reactivity in six patients with immotile cilia syndrome. *European Journal of Respiratory Disease* **127**(Suppl), 137–143.

55 Ferro, M.M., Siedman, L., Feldstein, V.A. *et al.* (2000) Minimally invasive resection of prenatally diagnosed thoracic and abdominal pulmonary sequestrations. *Pediatric Endoscopic and Innovative Techniques* **4**, 137–141.

56 Fine, C., Adzick, N.S., Doubilet, P.M. (1988) Decreasing size of congenital cystic adenomatoid malformation in utero. *Journal of Ultrasound in Medicine* **7**, 405–408.

57 Flake, A.W., Howell, L.J. (1998) Fetal surgery. In Stringer, M.D., Mouriquand, P.D.E., Oldham, K.T., Howard, E.R. (eds), *Pediatric Surgery and Urology: Long Term Outcomes.* London: W.B. Saunders, 797–805.

58 Fraggetta, F., Cacciaguerra, S., Nash, R., Davenport, M. (1998) Intra-abdominal pulmonary sequestration associated with congenital cystic adenomatoid malformation of the lung: just an unusual combination of rare pathologies? *Pathology, Research and Practice* **194**, 209–211.

59 Fraggetta, F., Davenport, M., Magro, G. *et al.* (2000) Striated muscle cells in non-neoplastic lung tissue: a clinicopathologic study. *Human Pathology* **31**, 1477–1481.

60 Frenckner, B., Freyschuss, U. (1982) Pulmonary function after lobectomy for congenital lobar emphysema and congenital cystic adenomatoid malformation. A follow-up study. *Scandinavian Journal of Thoracic and Cardiovascular Surgery* **16**, 293–298.

61 Gamillscheg, A., Beitzke, A., Smolle-Juttner, F.M. *et al.* (1996) Extralobar sequestration with unusual arterial supply and venous drainage. *Pediatric Cardiology* **17**, 57–59.

62 Garcia, H., Heidl, G., Stohr, G. (1988) Congenital cystic adenomatoid malformation of the lung associated with bile duct hypoplasia. *Pathology, Research and Practice* **183**, 771–777.

63 Garcia-Pena, P., Lucaya, J., Hendry, G.M. *et al.* (1998) Spontaneous involution of pulmonary sequestration in children: a report of two cases and review of the literature. *Pediatric Radiology* **28**, 266–270.

64 Gebauer, P.W., Mason, C.B. (1959) Intralobar pulmonary sequestration associated with anomalous pulmonary vessels: a nonentity. *Chest* **35**, 282–291.

65 Gerami, S., Richardson, R., Harrington, B., Pate, J.W. (1969) Obstructive emphysema due to mediastinal bronchogenic cysts in infancy. *Journal of Thoracic and Cardiovascular Surgery* **58**, 432–436.

66 Glaves, J., Baker, J.L. (1983) Spontaneous resolution of maternal hydramnios in congenital cystic adenomatoid malformation of the lung. *British Journal of Obstetrics and Gynaecology* **90**, 1065–1068.

67 Golladay, E.S., Mollitt, D.L. (1984) Surgically correctable fetal hydrops. *Journal of Pediatric Surgery* **19**, 59–62.

68 Gonzalez-Crussi, F., Boggs, J.D., Raffersperger, J.G. (1980) Brain heterotopia in the lungs: a rare cause of respiratory disease in the newborn. *American Journal of Clinical Pathology* **73**, 281–285.

69 Gupta, R., Singhal, S.K., Rattan, K.N., Chhabra, B. (1998) Management of congenital lobar emphysema with endobronchial intubation and controlled ventilation. *Anesthesia and Analgesia* **86**, 71–73.

70 Gwinn, J.L., Lee, F.A., Underberg, J.T. (1973) Radiological case of the month. Pulmonary lymphangiectasia. *American Journal of Diseases of Children* **126**, 199–200.

71 Haller, J.A., Golladay, E.S., Pickard, L.R. *et al.* (1979) Surgical management of lung bud anomalies: lobar emphysema, bronchogenic cyst, cystic adenomatoid malformation and intralobar pulmonary sequestration. *Annals of Thoracic Surgery* **28**, 33–43.

72 Halloran, L.G., Silverberg, S.G., Salzberg, A.M. (1972) Congenital cystic adenomatoid malformation of the lung. *Archives of Surgery* **104**, 715–719.

73 Harrison, M.R., Adzick, N.S., Jennings, R.W. *et al.* (1990) Antenatal intervention for congenital cystic adenomatoid malformation. *Lancet* **336**, 965–967.

74 Hartenberg, A., Brewer, W.H. (1983) Cystic adenomatoid malformation: identification by sonography. *American Journal of Roentgenology* **140**, 693–694.

75 Heij, H.A., Ekkelkamp, S., Vos, A. (1990) Diagnosis of congenital cystic adenomatoid malformation of the lung in newborn infants and children. *Thorax* **45**, 122–125.

76 Hendren, W.H., McKee, D.M. (1966) Lobar emphysema of infancy. *Journal of Pediatric Surgery* **1**, 24–39.

77 Hernandez, R.J., Stern, A.M., Rosenthal, A. (1980) Pulmonary lymphangiectasis in Noonan syndrome. *American Journal of Roentgenology* **134**, 75–80.

78 Hobbins, J.C., Grannum, P.A., Berkowitz, R.L. *et al.* (1979) Ultrasound in the diagnosis of congenital anomalies. *American Journal of Obstetrics and Gynecology* **134**, 331–345.

79 Holder, P.D., Langston, C. (1986) Intralobar pulmonary sequestration (a nonentity?). *Pediatric Pulmonology* **2**, 147–153.

80 Holmes, L.B., Blennerhassett, J.B., Auston, K.F. (1968) A reappraisal of Kartagener's syndrome. *American Journal of Medical Science* **255**, 13–28.

81 Horcher, E., Helmer, F. (1987) Scimitar syndrome and associated pulmonary sequestration: a report of a successfully corrected use. *Progress in Pediatric Surgery* **21**, 107–111.

82 Huber, A., Schranz, D., Blaha, I. *et al.* (1991) Congenital pulmonary lymphangiectasia. *Pediatric Pulmonology* **10**, 310–313.

83 Hulnick, D.H., Nardick, D.P., McCauley, D.I. *et al.* (1984) Late presentation of congenital cystic adenomatoid malformation of the lung. *Radiology* **151**, 569–573.

84 Hunter, W.S., Becroft, D.M. (1984) Congenital pulmonary lymphangiectasis associated with pleural effusions. *Archives of Disease in Childhood* **59**, 278–279.

85 Iwa, T., Watnabe, Y. (1979) Unusual combination of pulmonary sequestration and funnel chest. *Chest* **76**, 314–316.

86 Javett, S.N., Webster, I., Braudo, J.L. (1963) Congenital dilatation of the pulmonary lymphatics. *Pediatrics* **31**, 416–419.

87 Kamata, S., Ishikawa, S., Usui, N. *et al.* (1999) Clinical significance of the lung/thorax transverse-area ratio in fetuses with cystic lung disease. *Pediatric Surgery International* **15**, 470–474.

88 Kamata, S., Sawai, T., Nose, K., *et al.* (2000) Extralobar pulmonary sequestration with venous drainage to the portal vein: a case report. *Pediatric Radiology* **30**, 492–494.

89 Kaslovsky, R.A., Purdy, S., Dangman, B.C. *et al.* (1997) Bronchoalveolar carcinoma in a child with congenital cystic adenomatoid malformation. *Chest* **112**, 548–551.

90 Keller, M.S. (1983) Congenital lobar emphysema with tracheal bronchus. *Journal of the Canadian Association of Radiologists* **34**, 306–307.

91 Kennedy, C.D., Habibi, P., Matthew, D.J., Gordon, I. (1991) Lobar emphysema: long term imaging follow-up. *Radiology* **180**, 189–193.

92 Khakoo, G.A., Jawad, J.H., Bush, A. *et al.* (1993) Conservative management of fetal lung lesions. *Early Human Development* **35**, 55–63.

93 King, S.J., Pilling, D.W., Walkinshaw, S. (1995) Fetal echogenic lung lesions: prenatal ultrasound diagnosis and outcome. *Pediatric Radiology* **25**, 208–210.

94 Kirchner, J., Jacobi, V., Schneider, M., Wagner, R. (1997) Primary congenital pulmonary lymphangiectasia – a case report. *Wiener Klinische Wochenschrift* **109**, 922–924.

95 Kosloske, A.M., Williamson, S.L. (1992) An expandable prosthesis for stabilization of the infant mediastinum following pneumonectomy. *Journal of Pediatric Surgery* **27**, 1521–1522.

96 Krous, H.F., Harper, P.E., Perlman, M. (1980) Congenital cystic adenomatoid malformation in bilateral renal agenesis. Its mitigation of Potter's syndrome. *Archives of Pathology and Laboratory Medicine* **104**, 368–370.

97 Kugelman, A., Weinger-Abend, M., Miselevich, I., Bader, D. (1997) Acquired pulmonary cyst in the newborn infant. *Pediatric Pulmonology* **24**, 295–301.

98 Kuller, J.A., Yankowitz, J., Goldberg, J.D. *et al.* (1992) Outcome of antenatally diagnosed cystic adenomatoid malformation. *American Journal of Obstetrics and Gynecology* **167**, 1038–1041.

99 Kwittken, J., Reiner, L. (1962) Congenital cystic adenomatoid malformation of the lung. *Pediatrics* **30**, 759–768.

100 Lacquet, L.K., Lacquet, A.M. (1977) Congenital lobar emphysema. *Progress in Pediatric Surgery* **10**, 307–322.

101 Landing, B.H., Lawrence, T.K., Payne, C.V., Wells, T.R. (1971) Bronchial anatomy in syndromes with abnormal visceral situs, abnormal spleen and congenital heart disease. *American Journal of Cardiology* **28**, 456–462.

102 Laurence, K.M. (1955) Congenital pulmonary cystic lymphangiectasis. *Journal of Pathology and Bacteriology* **70**, 325–333.

103 Laurin, S., Hagerstrand, I. (1999) Intralobar bronchopulmonary sequestration in the newborn – a congenital malformation. *Pediatric Radiology* **29**, 174–178.

104 Leape, L.L., Longino, L. (1964) Infantile lobar emphysema. *Pediatrics* **34**, 246–251.

105 Lee, P., Bush, A., Warner, J.O. (1991) Left bronchial isomerism associated with bronchomalacia, presenting with intractable wheeze. *Thorax* **46**, 459–461.

106 Li, Y.W., Snow, J., Smith, W.L., Franken, E.A., Jr (1985) Localized pulmonary lymphangiectasia. *American Journal of Roentgenology* **145**, 269–270.

107 Lincoln, J.C.R., Stark, J., Subramanian, S. (1971) Congenital lobar emphysema. *Annals of Surgery* **173**, 55–59.

108 MacGillivray, T.E., Harrison, M.R., Goldstein, R.B., Adzick, N.S. (1993) Disappearing fetal lung lesions. *Journal of Pediatric Surgery* **28**, 1321–1324.

109 Maier, H.C. (1948) Bronchogenic cysts of mediastinum. *Annals of Surgery* **127**, 476–502.

110 Markowitz, R.I., Mercurio, M.R., Vahjen, G.A. *et al.* (1989) Congenital lobar emphysema. The role of CT and V/Q scan. *Clinical Pediatrics (Philadelphia)* **28**, 19–23.

111 Mather, E.A., Hogg, J.I., Miller, A.R. (1995) Covert bronchogenic cyst as a cause of life-threatening cardiopulmonary impairment. *Postgraduate Medical Journal* **71**, 369–371.

112 McAlister, W.H., Wright, J.R., Crane, J.P. (1987) Mainstem bronchial atresia: intrauterine sonographic diagnosis. *American Journal of Roentgenology* **148**, 364–366.

113 McBride, J.T., Wohl, M.E.B., Strieder, D.J. (1980) Lung growth and airway function after lobectomy in infancy for congenital lobar emphysema. *Journal of Clinical Investigation* **66**, 962–967.

114 Mentzer, S.J., Filler, R.M., Phillips, J. (1992) Limited pulmonary resections for congenital cystic adenomatoid malformation of the lung. *Journal of Pediatric Surgery* **27**, 1410–1413.

115 Miller, J.A., Corteville, J.E., Langer, J.C. (1996) Congenital cystic adenomatoid malformation in the fetus: natural history and predictors of outcome. *Journal of Pediatric Surgery* **31**, 805–808.

116 Miller, K.E., Edwards, D.K., Hilton, S. *et al.* (1981) Acquired lobar emphysema in premature infants with bronchopulmonary dysplasia: an iatrogenic disease? *Pediatric Radiology* **138**, 589–592.

117 Moerman, P., Fryns, J.P., Vandenberghe, K. *et al.* (1992) Pathogenesis of congenital cystic adenomatoid malformation of the lung. *Histopathology* **21**, 315–321.

118 Monin, P., Didier, F., Vert, P. *et al.* (1979) Giant lobar emphysema: neonatal diagnosis. *Pediatric Radiology* **8**, 259–260.

119 Morin, C., Filiatrault, D., Russo, P. (1989) Pulmonary sequestration with histologic changes of cystic adenomatoid malformation. *Pediatric Radiology* **19**, 130–132.

120 Morin, L., Crombleholme, T.M., D'Alton, M.E. (1994) Prenatal diagnosis and management of fetal thoracic lesions. *Seminars in Perinatology* **18**, 228–253.

121 Moscoso, G.J., Driver, M., Codd, J., Whimster, W.R. (1988) The morphology of ciliogenesis in the developing fetal human respiratory epithelium. *Pathology, Research and Practice* **183**, 403–411.

122 Murphy, J.J., Blair, G.K., Fraser, G.C. *et al.* (1992) Rhabdomyosarcoma arising within congenital pulmonary cysts: report of three cases. *Journal of Pediatric Surgery* **27**, 1364–1367.

123 Murray, G.F. (1967) Congenital lobar emphysema. *Surgery, Gynecology and Obstetrics* **124**, 611–615.

124 Neilson, I.R., Russo, P., Laberge, J.M. *et al.* (1991) Congenital adenomatoid malformation of the lung: current management and prognosis. *Journal of Pediatric Surgery* **26**, 975–981.

125 Ng, K.J., Hasan, N., Gray, E.S. *et al.* (1994) Intralobar bronchopulmonary sequestration: antenatal diagnosis. *Thorax* **49**, 379–380.

126 Nicolaides, K.H., Azar, G.B. (1990) Thoraco-amniotic shunting. *Fetal Diagnosis and Therapy* **5**, 153–164.

127 Nicolette, L.A., Kosloske, A.M., Bartow, S.A., Murphy, S. (1993) Intralobar pulmonary sequestration: a clinical and pathological spectrum. *Journal of Pediatric Surgery* **28**, 802–805.

128 Njolstad, P.R., Reigstad, H., Westby, J., Espeland, A. (1998) Familial non-immune hydrops fetalis and congenital pulmonary lymphangiectasia. *European Journal of Pediatrics* **157**, 498–501.

129 Noonan, J.A., Walters, L.R., Reeves, J.T. (1970) Congenital pulmonary lymphangiectasis. *American Journal of Obstetrics and Gynecology* **148**, 314–318.

130 Obwegeser, R., Deutinger, J., Bernaschek, G. (1993) Fetal pulmonary cyst treated by repeated thoracocentesis. *American Journal of Obstetrics and Gynecology* **169**, 1622–1624.

131 Ostor, A.G., Fortune, D.W. (1978) Congenital cystic adenomatoid malformation of the lung. *American Journal of Clinical Pathology* **70**, 595–604.

132 Pardes, J.G., Auh, Y.H., Blomquist, K. *et al.* (1983) CT diagnosis of congenital lobar emphysema. *Journal of Computer Assisted Tomography* **7**, 1095–1097.

133 Patz, E.F.J., Muller, N.L., Swensen, S.J., Dodd, L.G. (1995) Congenital cystic adenomatoid malformation in adults: CT findings. *Journal of Computer Assisted Tomography* **19**, 361–364.

134 Pernot, C., Bernard, C., Hoeffel, J.C. *et al.* (1984) Diffuse pulmonary lymphangiectasia of late disclosure associated with cardiomegaly. *Archives Francaises de Pediatrie* **41**, 617–622.

135 Plit, M.L., Blott, J.A., Lakis, N. *et al.* (1997) Clinical, radiographic and lung function features of diffuse congenital cystic adenomatoid malformation of the lung in an adult. *European Respiratory Journal* **10**, 1680–1682.

136 Pryce, D.M. (1946) Lower accessory pulmonary artery with intralobar sequestration of lung: a report of seven cases. *Journal of Pathology* **58**, 457–467.

137 Pryce, D.M., Holmes, S.T., Blair, L.G. (1947) Intralobar sequestration of lung associated with an abnormal pulmonary artery. *British Journal of Surgery* **35**, 18–29.

138 Pulpeiro, J.R., Lopez, I., Sotelo, T. *et al.* (1987) Congenital cystic adenomatoid malformation of the lung in a young adult. *British Journal of Radiology* **60**, 1128–1130.

139 Rahmani, M.R., Filler, R.M., Shuckett, B. (1995) Bronchogenic cyst occurring in the antenatal period. *Journal of Ultrasound in Medicine* **14**, 971–973.

140 Ramet, J., Byloos, J., Delree, M. *et al.* (1986) Neonatal diagnosis of the immotile cilia syndrome. *Chest* **90**, 138–140.

141 Raynor, A.C., Capp, M.P., Sealy, W.C. (1967) Lobar emphysema of infancy: diagnosis, treatment and etiological aspects. *Annals of Thoracic Surgery* **4**, 374–385.

142 Rescorla, F.J., West, K.W., Vane, D.W. *et al.* (1990) Pulmonary hypertension in neonatal cystic lung disease: survival following lobectomy and ECMO in two cases. *Journal of Pediatric Surgery* **25**, 1054–1056.

143 Revillon, Y., Jan, D., Plattner, V. *et al.* (1993) Congenital cystic adenomatoid malformation of the lung: prenatal management and prognosis. *Journal of Pediatric Surgery* **28**, 1009–1011.

144 Ribet, M., Pruvot, F.R., Dubos, J.P. *et al.* (1990) Congenital cystic adenomatoid malformation of the lung. *European Journal of Cardiothoracic Surgery* **4**, 403–406.

145 Ribet, M.E., Copin, M.C., Soots, J.G., Gosselin, B.H. (1995) Bronchoalveolar carcinoma and congenital cystic adenomatoid malformation. *Annals of Thoracic Surgery* **60**, 1126–1128.

146 Ribet, M.E., Copin, M.C., Gosselin, B.H. (1996) Bronchogenic cysts of the lung. *Annals of Thoracic Surgery* **61**, 1636–1640.

147 Rice, H.E., Estes, J.M., Hedrick, M.H. *et al.* (1994) Congenital cystic adenomatoid malformation: a sheep model of fetal hydrops. *Journal of Pediatric Surgery* **29**, 692–696.

148 Rossi, R., Tjan, T.D., Hentschel, R. *et al.* (1998) Successful perioperative management of congenital cystic adenomatoid malformation of the lung by high frequency oscillatory ventilation – report of two cases. *Klinische Padiatrie* **210**, 94–96.

149 Rouviere, H. (1983) *Anatomy of the Human Lymphatic System.* Ann Arbor: Edward Bros.

150 Rubin, E.M., Garcia, H., Horowitz, M.D., Guerra, J.J.J. (1994) Fatal massive haemoptysis secondary to intralobar sequestration. *Chest* **106**, 954–955.

151 Sade, R.M., Clouse, M., Ellis, F.H. (1974) The spectrum of pulmonary sequestration. *Annals of Thoracic Surgery* **18**, 644–655.

152 Sakala, E.P., Perrot, W.S., Grube, G.L. (1994) Sonographic characteristics of antenatally diagnosed extralobar pulmonary sequestration and congenital cystic adenomatoid malformation. *Obstetrics and Gynecology* **49**, 647–655.

153 Saltzman, D.H., Adzick, N.S., Benacerraf, B.R. (1988) Fetal cystic adenomatoid malformation of the lung: apparent improvement in utero. *Obstetrics and Gynecology* **71**, 1000–1002.

154 Samuel, M., Burge, D.M. (1996) Extralobar intra-abdominal pulmonary sequestration. *European Journal of Pediatric Surgery* **6**, 107–109.

155 Sands, R.H., Lilford, R.J. (1992) Hyperechogenic areas detected in fetal chest at routine ultrasound examination. *Prenatal Diagnosis* **12**, 79–82.

156 Sarnelli, R., Pistolesi, M., Petruzzeli, S. *et al.* (1986) Fatal peripheral airway cystic disease in a young woman. *American Journal of Medicine* **80**, 541–544.

157 Saunders, N.J.S.G., Snijders, R.S.M., Nicolaides, K.H. (1992) Therapeutic amniocentesis in twin–twin transfusion syndrome appearing in the second trimester of pregnancy. *American Journal of Obstetrics and Gynecology* **166**, 820–824.

158 Savic, B., Birtel, F.J., Tholen, W. *et al.* (1979) Lung sequestration: report of seven cases and review of 540 published cases. *Thorax* **34**, 96–101.

159 Schwartz, M.Z., Ramachandran, P. (1997) Congenital malformations of the lung and mediastinum – a quarter century of experience from a single institution. *Journal of Pediatric Surgery* **32**, 44–47.

160 Scott-Emuakpor, A.B., Warren, S.T., Kapur, S. *et al.* (1981) Familial occurrence of congenital pulmonary lymphangiectasis. Genetic implications. *American Journal of Diseases of Children* **135**, 532–534.

161 Shafei, H., Al-Ebrahim, K. (1997) Lung volume reduction for congenital lobar emphysema. *European Journal of Cardiothoracic Surgery* **12**, 327–328.

162 Shah, D.S., Lala, R., Rajegowda, B., Bhatia, J. (1999) Bronchogenic cyst and its progress in a premature infant. *Journal of Perinatology* **19**, 150–152.

163 Shannon, D.C., Todres, I.D., Moylan, F.M. (1977) Infantile lobar hyperinflation: expectant treatment. *Pediatrics* **59**, 1012–1018.

164 Shariff, S., Thomas, J.A., Shetty, N., D'Cunha, S. (1988) Primary pulmonary rhabdomyosarcoma in a child, with a review of literature. *Journal of Surgical Oncology* **38**, 261–264.

165 Sheffield, E.A., Addis, B.J., Corrin, B., McCabe, M.M. (1987) Epithelial hyperplasia and malignant change in congenital lung cysts. *Journal of Clinical Pathology* **40**, 612–614.

166 Shinebourne, E.A., Macartney, F.J., Anderson, R.H. (1976) Sequential chamber localisation the logical approach to diagnosis in congenital heart disease. *British Heart Journal* **38**, 327–340.

167 Sholler, G.F., Whight, C.M., Nunn, G.R. (1985) Pulmonary sequestration in a newborn mimicking cardiac disease: a trap for diagnosis. *Australian Paediatric Journal* **21**, 279–280.

168 Shuford, W.H., Sybers, R.G. (1969) Bronchopulmonary sequestration with venous drainage to the portal vein. *American Journal of Roentgenology, Radium Therapy and Nuclear Medicine* **106**, 118–120.

169 Siegal, A., Katsenstein, M., Wolach, B. (1985) Neonatal pneumothorax, a rare complication of pulmonary cystic lymphangiectasis. *European Journal of Respiratory Disease* **66**, 153–157.

170 Siffring, P.A., Forrest, T.S., Hill, W.C. (1989) Fetal prenatal sonographic diagnosis of bronchopulmonary foregut malformations. *Journal of Ultrasound in Medicine* **8**, 277–280.

171 Sintzoff, S.A., Avni, E.F., Rocmans, P. *et al.* (1991) Pulmonary sequestration-like anomaly presenting as a spontaneously resolving mass. *Pediatric Radiology* **21**, 143–144.

172 Sloan, H. (1953) Lobar obstruction emphysema in infancy treated by lobectomy. *Journal of Thoracic Surgery* **26**, 1.

173 Sohaey, R., Zwiebel, W.J. (1996) The fetal thorax: noncardiac chest anomalies. *Seminars in Ultrasound* **17**, 34–50.

174 Sonek, J.D., Foley, M.R., Iams, J.D. (1991) Spontaneous regression of a large intrathoracic fetal lesion before birth. *American Journal of Perinatology* **8**, 41–43.

175 Spinetta, G., Montrucchio, E., Franchi, M. *et al.* (1987) Computerized tomography in pulmonary sequestration. *Acta Biomedica de L'Ateno Parmanse* **58**, 117–123.

176 Stephanopoulos, C., Catsaras, M.R. (1963) Myxosarcoma complicating a cystic hamartoma of the lung. *Thorax* **18**, 144–145.

177 Stigers, K.B., Woodring, J.H., Kanga, J.F. (1992) The clinical and imaging specrum of findings in patients with congenital lobar emphysema. *Pediatric Pulmonology* **14**, 160–170.

178 Stocker, J.T. (1986) Sequestrations of the lung. *Seminars in Diagnostic Pathology* **3**, 106–121.

179 Stocker, J.T. (1994) Congenital and developmental diseases. In Dail, D.H., Hammar, S.P. (eds), *Pulmonary Pathology*. New York: Springer-Verlag, 155–190.

180 Stocker, J.T., Kagan-Hallet, K. (1979) Extralobar pulmonary sequestration. Analysis of 15 cases. *American Journal of Clinical Pathology* **72**, 917–925.

181 Stocker, J.T., Malczak, H.T. (1956) A study of pulmonary ligament arteries: relationship to intralobar sequestration. *Chest* **86**, 611–620.

182 Stocker, J.T., Madewell, J.E., Drake, R.M. (1977) Congenital cystic adenomatoid malformation of the lung: classification and morphologic spectrum. *Human Pathology* **8**, 155–171.

183 Stocker, J.T., Drake, R.M., Madewell, J.E. (1978) Cystic and congenital lung disease in the newborn. *Pediatric Pathology* **4**, 93–99.

184 Stoek, O. (1897) Ueber Angeborene Blasige Missbildung der Lunge. *Wiener Klinische Wochenschritt* **10**, 25–30.

185 Stolar, C., Berdon, W., Reyes, C. *et al.* (1988) Right pneumonectomy syndrome: a lethal complication of lung resection in a newborn with cystic adenomatoid malformation. *Journal of Pediatric Surgery* **23**, 1180–1183.

186 Stringer, M.D., Dinwiddie, R., Hall, C.M., Spitz, L. (1993) Foregut duplication cysts: a diagnostic challenge. *Journal of the Royal Society of Medicine* **86**, 174–175.

187 Sturgess, J.M., Thompson, M.W., Lzegledy-Nady, E., Turner, J.A. (1986) Genetic aspects of immotile cilia syndrome. *American Journal of Medical Genetics* **25**, 149–160.

188 Suen, H.C., Mathisen, D.J., Grillo, H.C. *et al.* (1993) Surgical management and radiological characteristics of bronchogenic cysts. *Annals of Thoracic Surgery* **55**, 476–481.

189 Tapper, D., Schuster, S., McBride, J. *et al.* (1980) Polyalveolar lobe: anatomic and physiologic parameters and their relationship to congenital lobar emphysema. *Journal of Pediatric Surgery* **15**, 931–937.

190 Thilenius, O.G., Ruschhaupt, D.G., Replogle, R. *et al.* (1983) Spectrum of pulmonary sequestration: association with anomalous pulmonary venous drainage in infants. *Pediatric Cardiology* **4**, 97–103.

191 Thompson, J., Forfar, J.O. (1958) Regional obstructive emphysema in infancy. *Archives of Disease in Childhood* **33**, 97–102.

192 Thorpe-Beeston, J.G., Nicolaides, K.H. (1994) Cystic adenomatoid malformation of the lung: prenatal diagnosis and outcome. *Prenatal Diagnosis* **14**, 677–688.

193 Trapnell, D.H. (1963) The peripheral lymphatics of the lung. *British Journal of Radiology* **36**, 660–672.

194 Trapnell, D.H. (1970) The anatomy of the lymphatics of the lungs and chest wall. *Thorax* **25**, 255–256.

195 Ueda, K., Gruppo, R., Unger, F. (1977) Rhabdomysarcoma of lung arising in congenital cystic adenomatoid malformation of the lungs. *Cancer* **40**, 383–388.

196 Uroz-Tristan, J., Cabrera-Roca, G., Wiehoff-Neumann, A. *et al.* (1998) Bilateral and multilobar cystic adenomatoid malformation of the lung. *European Journal of Pediatric Surgery* **8**, 364–367.

197 Wagenaar, S.S., Swierenga, J., Wagenvoort, C.A. (1978) Late presentation of primary pulmonary lymphangiectasis. *Thorax* **33**, 791–795.

198 Warne, S., Davenport, M., Cacciaguerra, S. *et al.* (2000) presented to the British Association of Paediatric Surgeons.

199 Watine, O., Mensier, E., Delecluse, P., Ribet, M. (1994) Pulmonary sequestration treated by video-assisted thoracoscopic resection. *European Journal of Cardiothoracic Surgery* **8**, 155–156.

200 Watson, W.J., Thorp, J.M., Miller, M.C. *et al.* (1990) Prenatal diagnosis of laryngeal atresia. *American Journal of Obstetrics and Gynecology* **163**, 1456–1457.

201 Weiner, C., Varner, M., Pringle, K. *et al.* (1986) Antenatal diagnosis and palliative treatment of nonimmune hydrops fetalis secondary to pulmonary extralobar sequestration. *Obstetrics and Gynecology* **68**, 275–280.

202 Wesley, J.R., Heidelberger, K.P., DiPietro, M.A. *et al.* (1986) Diagnosis and management of congenital cystic disease of the lung in children. *Journal of Pediatric Surgery* **21**, 202–207.

203 White, J., Chan, Y.F., Neuberger, S., Wilson, T. (1994) Prenatal sonographic detection of intra-abdominal extralobar pulmonary sequestration: report of three cases and literature review. *Prenatal Diagnosis* **14**, 653–658.

204 White, J.E., Veale, D., Fishwick, D. *et al.* (1996) Generalised lymphangiectasia: pulmonary presentation in an adult. *Thorax* **51**, 768.

205 White, J.J., Donahoo, J.S., Ostrow, P.T., Murphy J., Haller J.A. Jr. (1974) Cardiovascular and respiratory manifestations of pulmonary sequestration in childhood. *Annals of Thoracic Surgery* **18**, 286–294.

206 Whitelaw, A., Evans, A., Corrin, B. (1981) Immotile cilia syndrome: a new cause of neonatal respiratory distress. *Archives of Disease in Childhood* **56**, 432–435.

207 Wilson, R.H., Duncan, A., Hume, R., Bain, A.D. (1985) Prenatal pleural effusion associated with congenital pulmonary lymphangiectasia. *Prenatal Diagnosis* **5**, 73–76.

208 Wimbish, K.J., Agha, F.P., Brady, T.M. (1983) Bilateral pulmonary sequestration: computed tomographic appearance. *American Journal of Roentgenology* **140**, 689–690.

209 Wockel, W., Heller, K., Volmer, I. (1986) Congential unilateral pulmonary lymphangiectasis. *Deutsche Medzinische Wochenschrift* **111**, 264–267.

210 Zangwill, B.C., Stocker, J.T. (1993) Congenital cystic adenomatoid malformation within an extralobar pulmonary sequestration. *Pediatric Pathology* **13**, 309–315.

34

Abnormalities of the diaphragm

ANNE GREENOUGH AND MARK DAVENPORT

EMBRYOLOGY

The diaphragm develops first as the septum transversum, which is a sheet of mesodermal tissue separating the thoracic cavity and the stalk of the yolk sac. This initially lies opposite the primitive cervical vertebrae and, as a consequence, the phrenic nerves are derived from the third, fourth and fifth cervical segments. The septum, however, is incomplete, with two large posterolateral canals in which the lung buds initially form. The primitive diaphragm then migrates caudally, creating the potential pleural space. The pleuroperitoneal canals are closed by the development of the pleuropericardial folds. The folds develop first as small ridges and, by the seventh week of intrauterine life, fuse with the septum transversum and the mesentery of the abdominal cavity. Primitive muscle cells then migrate in from the body wall to form the muscular part of the diaphragm.

This normal embryological process may not occur leading to a variety of congenital abnormalities:

- failure of development of the septum transversum – agenesis of the diaphragm
- failure of closure of the pleuroperitoneal canal to fuse with the septum transversum – congenital posterolateral diaphragmatic hernia (Bochdalek)
- failure of the development of the retrosternal segment of the septum transversum – congenital anterior diaphragmatic hernia (Morgagni)
- failure of the migration of primitive muscle cells – eventration of the diaphragm.

The most common form of congenital diaphragmatic hernia (CDH) has been assumed to result from failure of the pleuroperitoneal canals to close at the end of the embryonic period, the eighth gestational week[62] and that compression of gut entering the thoracic cavity through the defect causes lung hypoplasia. Results from scanning electron microscopy and the nitrofen rat CDH model, however, have contradicted those assumptions.[73] Measurement of the pleuroperitoneal openings demonstrated none was of sufficient dimensions to permit gut loops to herniate.[87,88] Nitrofen (2,4-di-chloro-phenyl-p-nitrophenyl ether) is a teratogen which, when administered to rats causes disturbed diaphragmatic development at a timing equivalent to the early embryonic period.[86] Nitrofen may also interfere with early lung development, before and separate from causing aberrant diaphragm development.[82] Nitrofen negatively influenced branching morphogenesis of the lung and resulted in attenuation of epithelial cell differentiation and cell proliferation. In a murine model, nitrofen-induced pulmonary hypoplasia existed with or without diaphragmatic hernia.[23] As a consequence, Keijzer et al.[82] have proposed a dual hit hypothesis, pulmonary hypoplasia in CDH infants resulting from two insults, one affecting both lungs before diaphragm development and the other the ipsilateral lung after defective diaphragm development. The second insult affects the ipsilateral lung only at a later stage, when the herniated abdominal organs interfere with fetal breathing movements, resulting in greater impairment of the development of the ipsilateral lung. Studies with the nitrofen model[77] have suggested CDH might be due to primary disturbance of pulmonary growth into the pleuroperitoneal canal, thereby disturbing the growth of the post-hepatic mesenchymal plate, the main origin of the diaphragm.

DIAPHRAGMATIC HERNIA

Diaphragmatic hernia may be found as an isolated abnormality or associated with certain syndromes: de Lange, DiGeorge, Ehlers–Danlos, Marfan's syndrome, anencephaly sequence and in certain chromosomal abnormalities, particularly trisomies 13 and 18. There have been reports of families with a higher incidence of CDH, suggesting that a genetic defect is in part responsible for some CDH cases.[38,158]

The incidence of congenital diaphragmatic hernia (CDH) is reported to be between one per 2200–5500 live-births,[17,29,58,59] or 0.08–0.45 per 1000 live births.[92] CDH accounts for approximately 10 percent of all major congenital anomalies. The male to female ratio is between 0.67 and 0.77.[17,33]

Posterolateral (Bochdalek) diaphragmatic hernia

This is the commonest type of hernia, accounting for 85–95 percent of cases; the incidence is one per 2000–3500 deliveries. Eighty-five percent are left sided and 5 percent are bilateral (Figure 34.1). The commonest contents of a left-sided hernia are stomach, bowel and spleen and of a right-sided hernia, liver and gallbladder.

PATHOPHYSIOLOGY

Lung growth is compromised with hypoplasia of the lung on the ipsilateral side, but there may also be hypoplasia of

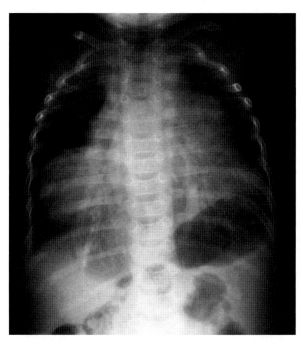

Figure 34.1 *Abnormal mediastinal configuration due to bilateral diaphragmatic herniae. There is air-filled bowel centrally in an intrathoracic position.*

the contralateral lung, even though it is considerably larger than the ipsilateral lung.[50] In both lungs, there is a marked reduction in the number of bronchial generations and a proportional decrease in the number of arterial vessels.[11] These abnormalities are usually more pronounced in the ipsilateral lung. The reduction in airway number is mainly in the non-cartilaginous airways, suggesting a general arrest of growth at 12–14 weeks of gestation.[85] As a result of the reduced airway number, the alveolar number is reduced, but the number per acinus may or may not be decreased. In one series, alveoli were immature in structure.[50] The medial muscle of the pulmonary arterioles is increased with abnormal extension of muscle into arterioles at the acinar level.[49] In addition, the external diameter of the arteries is decreased.[85] There is a significant increase in medial, adventitial and total wall thickness in pulmonary arteries with an external diameter of less than 200 μm.[138] These structural abnormalities may result in increased pulmonary vascular resistance.[14] Significantly raised levels of vascular endothelial growth factor (VEGF), an endothelial cell-specific mitogen, have been found in lung specimens.[137] VEGF was detected mainly in the bronchial epithelium and the medial smooth muscle cells of large and small pulmonary arteries. The increased levels of VEGF, especially in the small, pressure-regulating pulmonary arteries, were suggested to point to a potential role in vascular remodeling and that it may reflect an unsuccessful attempt by the developing fetus to increase the pulmonary vascular bed in the hypoplastic lungs to alleviate the associated pulmonary hypertension. The degree of hypoplasia tends to be less marked when the right diaphragm is involved. The migration of the abdominal contents into the thorax is associated with a 20 percent prevalence of malrotation and poor development of the abdominal cavity.

The lung of CDH infants may also be immature as well as hypoplastic. Fetuses at term have low amniotic fluid L:S ratios (p. 256)[71] and low levels of surfactant protein A and saturated phosphatidylcholine have also been reported (p. 15).[109] The concentration of dipalmitoyl phosphatidylcholine (DPPC) was significantly lower in the ipsilateral as compared to the contralateral lung and to age-matched controls.[110] Others, however, have reported no significant differences in the concentrations of surfactant phospholipids in the bronchoalveolar lavage fluid of CDH infants compared to controls.[75] Such conflicting results suggest that the amniotic fluid L:S ratio may not reflect lung maturity in CDH.[75]

CLINICAL SIGNS

The time of onset and severity of symptoms depend on the degree of pulmonary hypoplasia. The infant may present with respiratory distress immediately at birth and be difficult to resuscitate. The baby will often be cyanosed in air, dyspneic and tachypneic, often with an associated tachycardia. The diagnosis should be suspected in all infants in whom the cardiac impulse is abnormally sited. Breath sounds are absent over the involved side, the chest is barrel-shaped and the abdomen may be scaphoid. Bowel sounds will not be heard over the affected side of the chest for some hours. Persistent pulmonary hypertension is common in infants with CDH, affecting 46 percent of one series,[14] 18 of 21 affected babies dying.

Some infants present later, but in the first few days of life as the herniated bowel fills with air, compressing the lung and causing respiratory distress. Right-sided lesions may present even later, herniation of abdominal contents into the thorax may only occur after birth with the onset of breathing. In some cases this may be associated with group B streptococcal sepsis.[7] Delayed-onset right-sided CDH following early sepsis with obstructive jaundice has also been described.[47] The proportion of late-presenting CDHs varies from 5 to 30 percent of reported series, although only half will first present outside of infancy.[115] The symptoms at late presentation in one series[115] were vomiting and abdominal pain. Young CDH children presenting late usually have respiratory symptoms: dyspnea, wheezing, repeated respiratory infections and cough. The older children have gastrointestinal complaints: abdominal pain and vomiting. Rarely they may present with intestinal obstruction,[99] with or without gangrene or perforation of the obstructed bowel or torsion of the spleen.[13,121,156] If the spleen accompanies the stomach into the intrathoracic space, then the herniated spleen can cause hypertension[130] and undergo intra-abdominal or intrathoracic torsion.[13,121,156] The herniated spleen can be detected as a paravertebral mass on the chest radiograph; the exact location of the spleen can be detected by radionucleid scanning.[13,28] Exceptionally, diagnosis can be delayed into adulthood[39] and there are reports of presentation in pregnancy.[89] The outcome in patients with late presentation is generally good, although failure to make the diagnosis and provide timely treatment can result in death in children[18] and adults.[22]

DIFFERENTIAL DIAGNOSIS

Cystic adenomatoid malformation of the lung, lung leiomyosarcoma and mediastinal cystic teratomas may be confused antenatally with congenital diaphragmatic hernia (CDH).[61] In the labor suite, it can be difficult to differentiate between bronchogenic cysts, hemangiomas and lymphangiomas and CDH. Postnatally cystic adenomatoid malformation of the lung may be mistaken for a CDH. Such cases may be correctly diagnosed by an intrathoracic contrast study or computerized tomography (CT). Right-sided diaphragmatic hernia can be confused with segmental collapse or pleural effusion. Where there is initial confusion regarding the diagnosis, the correct diagnosis of CDH can be established by the use of ultrasound, by the position of the nasogastric tube or a barium meal. Only in extreme cases is a chest CT scan required.

DIAGNOSIS

Antenatal

Diaphragmatic hernia may be diagnosed by routine ultrasonography in the second and third trimester. The ultrasound findings include herniated abdominal viscera visualized at the level of the four-chamber view of the heart. This is usually accompanied by mediastinal shift away from the side of herniation. A right-sided hernia may be harder to diagnose because of the similar echogenicity of the lung and liver tissue, but the condition may be suspected by the presence of mediastinal shift or hydrothorax.[163] The diagnosis may be confirmed by recognition of branching portal venous structures or the gallbladder within the thorax.

Polyhydramnios is a common associated finding but is rarely observed before 24 weeks of gestation.[9] It is thought to be due either to esophageal compression decreasing swallowing or reduced absorption of fluid by the hypoplastic lungs. Glick et al.[51] hypothesized that the associated polyhydramnios in cases of CDH may be due to an increase in a pulmonary growth factor synthesized by the fetal kidney; however, this substance has yet to be identified.

The incidence of associated abnormalities reported antenatally is considerably higher than that reported in the literature by pediatric surgeons and considerably lower than those reported in postmortem studies.[1,17,33,123,140] In a series of 79 cases of CDH diagnosed at the Harris Birthright Research Centre (King's College Hospital) between 1986 and 1992, only 38 (48 percent) of fetuses were found to have an isolated diaphragmatic defect. Seventeen (22 percent) had chromosomal abnormalities (trisomy 18 being the commonest chromosomal defect) and 24 (30 percent) had major associated defects including congenital heart disease, exomphalos, renal, brain and spinal anomalies. Analysis of the medical and autopsy records of 301 CDH patients presenting at two institutions over a 23-year period demonstrated 33 percent to have one or more associated anomaly.[97] These included cardiac, skeletal, gastrointestinal, genitourinary and pulmonary (including lobar sequestration, p. 463) anomalies. Multiple anomalies occurred in 10 percent of patients with right-sided hernias and 7.3 percent of left-sided. Cardiac abnormalities were associated with 10 percent of right-sided and 8.5 percent of left-sided diaphragmatic hernias. Hypoplastic left heart syndrome was only seen in patients with left-sided hernias. Although this association only occurred in five of the patients, extrapolating from the results of nitrofen administration to pregnant rats,[4] this suggests that different mechanisms might underlie the formation of left- and right-sided hernias in rats. Losty et al.[97] have speculated that the association of hypoplastic left heart syndrome with left-sided CDH in humans could also have implications for correlated patterns of development of the diaphragm and heart during embryogenesis.

As a consequence of the high incidence of associated anomalies, it is essential when CDH is diagnosed antenatally, that fetal karyotyping and expert ultrasound examination of the fetus (in particular the heart) should be undertaken. These investigations should be performed even in the third trimester of pregnancy, because knowledge that the fetus is chromosomally and otherwise structurally normal allows the parents, obstetrician, pediatrician and surgeon to discuss the appropriate mode, place and timing of delivery. If the fetus is found to be chromosomally abnormal, obstetric intervention such as a cesarean section may be avoided.

POSTNATAL INVESTIGATIONS

Chest radiograph

A chest radiograph taken immediately after birth will show a large, opaque, space occupying mass on the affected side (Figure 34.2) and mediastinal shift (Figure 34.3). With increasing postnatal age, swallowed gas reaches the displaced bowel in the chest. CDH infants are at high risk of pneumothorax and this may complicate the classical chest radiograph appearance of a left-sided CDH (Figure 34.4). The diagnosis may be missed if the chest radiograph is taken with the baby in the erect position, as this will occasionally allow the bowel to slip back into the

abdominal cavity. Right-sided hernias are more difficult to diagnose, as the liver prevents other abdominal contents herniating into the chest. The abdominal gas pattern on the right side may appear higher than usual and the lower edge of the liver more horizontal.

Postoperative changes Postoperatively the diaphragm will be taut and is displaced downwards (Figure 34.5a). The mediastinum will usually remain displaced to the contralateral side. Inititally there is a 'vacuum' on the affected side, but if a chest drain is not inserted this will fill with fluid. This fluid will gradually resorb over days or even weeks (Figure 34.5b). Loculated collection of fluid postoperatively can indicate a rare single pleural pericardial sac (Figure 34.6).

Prediction of pulmonary hypoplasia Goodfellow et al.[53] examined retrospectively the chest and abdominal radiographs of 50 neonates with CDH and found that 20 of 34 (59 percent) with an intrathoracic position of the stomach died, whereas 15 of 16 (945) where this was not the case survived. Cloutier et al.[26] used the postoperative chest radiograph appearance to classify infants into three groups according to the degree of pulmonary hypoplasia: none or mild hypoplasia; moderate to severe hypoplasia; very severe hypoplasia. The presence of large diaphragmatic defects or intrathoracic stomachs usually meant more severe hypoplasia on the postoperative chest radiograph, as did antenatal diagnosis and polyhydramnios – but none of these factors precluded survival. Eight out of nine patients survived, in spite of apparently very severe hypoplasia being diagnosed from their postoperative chest radiograph. Saifuddin and Arthur examined both pre- and postoperative chest radiographs.[132] They found preoperatively that a contralateral pneumothorax, absence

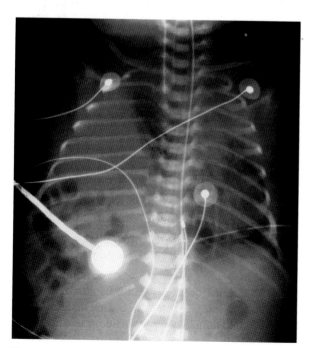

Figure 34.2 *Right-sided diaphragmatic hernia. Herniated liver and bowel are occupying the hemithorax. There is major mediastinal displacement to the left; there is a left pneumothorax and a chest drain in situ.*

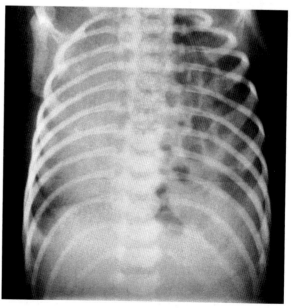

Figure 34.3 *Classical left diaphragmatic hernia with characteristic intrathoracic mediastinal shift.*

of contralateral aerated lung and an intrathoracic site for the stomach were all associated with a poor prognosis. Identification of an ipsilateral aerated lung was associated with survival in all cases. Postoperatively, a low lung area on the chest radiograph, determined by computer-assisted analysis, has been suggested to indicate a poor outcome (death or oxygen dependency at 28 days).[36]

Other investigations

Barium contrast studies are rarely required in the neonatal period. Fluoroscopic examination will document the absence of normal diaphragmatic excursion. Ultrasonography or a radionuclide liver scan usually indicates that the liver is excessively high and partially in the defect. For suspected right-sided lesions, induction of a diagnostic pneumoperitoneum with nitrous oxide and the

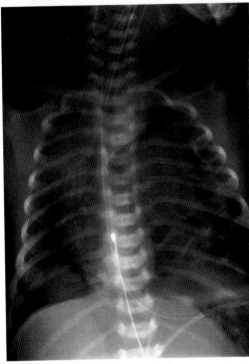

(a)

(b)

Figure 34.4 (a) Left-sided CDH; note mediastinal shift as evidenced by position of the nasogastric tube. (b) Twelve hours later free air has developed.

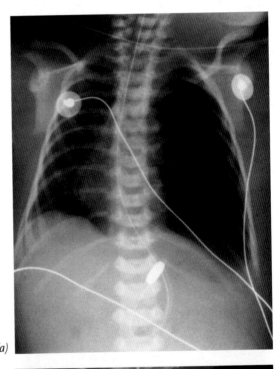

(a)

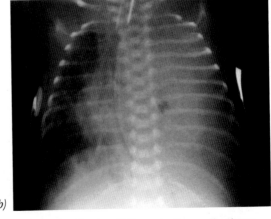

(b)

Figure 34.5 (a) Following CDH repair, the mediastinum is more central. The hypoplastic left underlying lung is demonstrated within the air-filled thorax. (b) The same infant 48 hours later; there remains mediastinal shift and increased opacity throughout the left lung, representing fluid.

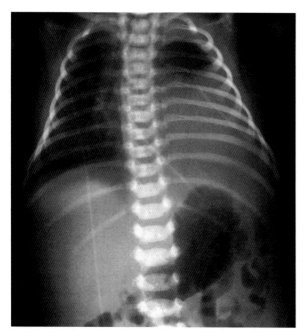

Figure 34.6 *Chest radiograph of an infant post-CDH repair demonstrating abnormal configuration of the cardiac silhouette with absence of the pericardium. There is fluid in the left pleural space overlying the apex. This unusual appearance is due to the absence of the normal pleuropericardial interface.*

demonstration of a small pneumothorax on the right side proves the existence of a diaphragmatic defect, but should rarely be necessary. In late-presenting CDH, contrast roentgenograms of the upper gastrointestinal tract, barium enemas or both may be necessary to confirm the diagnosis. The herniated abdominal contents can reduce spontaneously through the defect and the presence of a normal chest radiograph and contrast roentgenogram does not rule out the diagnosis.[8] Chest CT or MRI can be useful, oral contrast material demonstrating herniation of the stomach.

MONITORING

These babies need an arterial line for continuous blood pressure monitoring and frequent blood gas sampling. This can be an umbilical arterial catheter, although others prefer to place a line in the right radial artery as right-to-left ductal shunting may be significant.[135] Transcutaneous oxygen tension ($TcPO_2$) gives guidance regarding pre- and post-ductal oxygenation trends. Central venous pressure should be measured either via the umbilical or internal jugular vein, aiming to maintain a pressure of 5–10 cmH$_2$O above the mid-axillary baseline.

MANAGEMENT

Antenatal steroids should be given in CDH infants who are expected to deliver prior to 34 weeks of gestation. In the

nitrofen rat model of CDH, antenatal steroids reversed many of the histological and biochemical markers of immaturity.[148] In a lamb model, glycogen and protein DNA levels were increased in the contralateral lung with significant improvements in oxygenation and dynamic compliance.[134] In a preclinical model (New Zealand rabbit) intra-amniotic surfactant or dexamethasone administration was associated with less pulmonary hypoplasia in CDH infants.[151] Antenatal betamethasone also has been found to have beneficial effects on pulmonary vasculature in an experimental CDH model, including downregulation of the expression of endothelin receptors in vascular smooth muscle rat cells.[112]

Antenatal repair

Experimentally, the pulmonary hypoplasia associated with CDH is reversible.[2,60] As a consequence, attempts have been made at *in utero* repair of CDH in ongoing pregnancies.[57,62,63] Between 1989 and 1991, 61 patients were referred to Harrison *et al.* for consideration of *in utero* repair.[64] This was attempted in 14 cases, who had severe isolated lesions diagnosed prior to 24 weeks of gestation. All had left-sided herniae with significant contralateral mediastinal shift and normal karyotypes confirmed by amniocentesis or percutaneous umbilical blood sampling. The outcome was variable; five fetuses died intraoperatively from technical problems related to reduction of incarcerated liver and uterine contractions, nine patients were successfully repaired. Only four of the other nine patients survived, two others delivered prematurely and died and three died *in utero* within 48 hours of the repair. The four survivors required a median of approximately 3 weeks of respiratory support and three had an interval fundal plication. Key to the success of the procedure seemed to be choosing cases who would be amenable to *in utero* surgery. This particularly required preoperative assessment of the extent of liver herniation. This was determined by color Doppler evaluation of the umbilical vein; if the umbilical vein was deviated far to the left, the liver was usually in the left chest, but if the course of the sinus venosus remained below where the diaphragm should be, then the herniated liver was amenable to surgery. If, however, the sinus venosus was well up in the chest, this indicated the entire liver was torqued into the chest and could not be reduced without compromising umbilical blood flow. This particularly applied to right-sided hernia when, on repair, both the sinus venosus and inferior vena cava would be kinked. Further experience of such cases has also resulted in modifications to the surgical procedure.[64] The subcostal incision which is usually employed postnatally, if used alone antenatally provides insufficient exposure for severe defects and needs to be combined with a thoracotomy incision. Measures have to be taken to reduce uterine disruption and amniotic fluid leakage; this can be achieved by all-layer stay sutures, fibrin glue and a two-layer closure. The major obstacle to successful repair, however, remains an inability to manage premature labor induced by the hysterotomy and fetal surgery.[67]

Attempts to further develop *in utero* surgery have been based on the discovery that obstructing the normal egress of fetal lung fluid enlarged fetal lungs, reducing herniated viscera and accelerating lung growth in experimental models. The effect is believed to be secondary to increased lung fluid retention and elevated tracheal pressure; in experimental CDH models, a pressure of 4 mmHg was documented compared to 0 mmHg in the controls.[68] It is surprising that such a small increase in pressure would cause a change in lung development. It seems more likely that it is a combination of the volume of fluid and growth factors in the fluid and pressure.[153] Modulation of local growth factors occur via airspace receptor stimulation,[35] the increase in lung fluid pressure stimulating a local growth factor cascade. Controlled tracheal obstruction *in utero* also reverses the increased muscularization of the pulmonary arteries,[35] but it may delay pulmonary maturation as measured by surfactant production.[119]

Temporary tracheal occlusion by internal plugs or external clips at 25–28 weeks of gestation has been applied in human fetuses with CDH and liver herniation.[41,70,142] Currently, techniques range from an open dissection of the fetal neck through a hysterotomy and application of a clip to achieve complete tracheal occlusion, to video-assisted fetal endoscopic manipulation of a detachable balloon within the trachea through a hysterotomy port without opening the uterus.[142] Clearly, at the time of birth, whatever the nature of the tracheal occlusion, it needs to be reversed and a technique of maintenance of feto-placental circulation during delivery was also developed to facilitate this. Initially termed the EXIT (*ex utero* intra-partum treatment) procedure,[96] it allows for manipulation of the trachea, removal of the occluding clip or balloon and safe intubation while the fetoplacental circulation is still intact. It can be extended for periods of up to 1 hour. Flake *et al.*[41] described the results for 15 fetuses where such a tracheal clip had been applied within the second trimester. Although the technique was associated with restitution of lung growth in a subset and a mean period of *in utero* occluded lung growth of 38 days, overall the results were poor, with only five (33 percent) survivors. Studies in fetal sheep have suggested that, although tracheal occlusion restored most aspects of lung structure to normal in fetuses with lung hypoplasia, there was altered alveolar development.[32] Animals sacrificed 8 weeks after birth, which had tracheal occlusion for the 10 days prior to delivery, had reduced alveolar numbers and surface area. The presence of fewer, larger alveoli may predispose to respiratory complications in later life. In fetal sheep, tracheal occlusion by a balloon-tipped catheter resulted in marked changes to the epithelium and cartilage of the trachea. The ciliated cells were absent from the trachea.[32] Similar morphological abnormalities in tracheal structure have been reported when latex balloons[68] or foam plugs[66] were used to obstruct the fetal trachea. These intratracheal devices may result in persistent tracheal injury at the site of the obstruction, due to mechanical stretching or compression of the tracheal wall.

In the labor ward

Infants who require resuscitation should be intubated. It is important to avoid resuscitation using a face mask and T-piece or bag and mask system as this will cause gaseous distention of the herniated bowel, increasing respiratory embarrassment. It is desirable, because of the high risk of pneumothorax (which increases mortality), to keep the inflation pressures below 30 cmH$_2$O and instead to achieve adequate gas ventilation by employing fast ventilator rates. Swallowing is to be avoided; thus paralysis with a neuromuscular blocking agent, such as pancuronium, is advocated in the labor suite. A nasogastric tube should be passed as soon as possible and suctioned continuously to reduce the amount of gas in the herniated bowel.

Preoperative stabilization

Infants with CDH should be transferred to the intensive care unit as soon as possible, where they should be carefully assessed for the presence of other congenital abnormalities and stabilized. Surfactant administration may be helpful, but should be given cautiously and slowly. Sudden and, on occasion, irreversible deterioration, such that immediate cannulation for extracorporeal membrane oxygenation (ECMO) to survive was required,[40] has been described in CDH infants given a full dose of surfactant.

It has previously been assumed that infants with CDH required immediate postoperative repair, in the hope that removal of bowel from the thorax and closure of the diaphragmatic defect would lead to improvements in gas exchange through expansion of the ipsilateral lung. Lung function measurements have shown that the reverse is true, that is lung compliance is reduced postoperatively,[133] making ventilation more difficult. The postoperative compliance changes may be due to aggregate stresses of anatomical repair and postoperative alterations in water and sodium balance.[171] A period of preoperative stabilization is now recommended, although a randomized trial of early (within 6 hours) and delayed (at 96 hours or greater) surgical repair did not demonstrate any significant difference in mortality, ECMO requirement or the occurrence of bleeding complications, but only 32 infants were included.[114] Numerous anecdotal series have highlighted that preoperative stabilization appears to reduce mortality[19,20,45,69,90] and the need for ECMO.[171] Nakayama *et al.*[111] reported only six of 13 infants undergoing emergency closure survived, compared to eight of nine who had had their operation deliberately delayed for 2–11 days while severe hypoxemia was corrected.

Prolonged stabilization for more than 48 hours using high-frequency oscillatory ventilation (HFOV) or ECMO, however, does not appear to improve survival in high-risk patients with CDH.[80,168] Continuous non-invasive whole body plethysmographic monitoring of ten infants with CDH demonstrated that their vascular and pulmonary function undergo the same changes as the normal transitional circulation, but over a much more protracted time course.[107] Although unstable initially, the infants had improved gas exchange, compliance and minute ventilation, while the mechanical work of breathing and supplementary oxygen requirement decreased. Deviations from the norm may identify high-risk patients and the failure to stabilize a patient before surgical repair may indicate an infant who has overwhelming pulmonary hypoplasia incompatible with life.[143] It has been suggested that the key during preoperative stabilization is to avoid overdistention;[171] pulmonary vascular resistance has been shown to be augmented by increased distending pressures with and without hypoxemia.[94] In addition, an increase in arterial pressure has been demonstrated as the parenchyma pressure increases and the lung is stretched.[100] In addition, overdistention results in volutrauma and may interfere with systemic venous return. During a period of preoperative stabilization with conservative management, partial reduction of the hernia and mediastinal shift can occur.[131]

Ventilatory support

CDH infants require paralysis and analgesics such as fentanyl (3–10 μg/kg/h) (p. 316). Avoidance of painful stimuli and adequate analgesia may reduce the risk of persistent pulmonary hypertension of the newborn (PPHN). Where possible, peak inspiratory pressures should be limited to 20–25 cmH$_2$O. Rates of 60–80/min with an inspiratory time of 0.3–0.5 seconds and a sufficiently high inspired oxygen concentration to produce an arterial oxygen level of at least 8 kPa (60 mmHg) are preferred. The aim is to achieve a $PaCO_2$ of 5–5.5 kPa (37.59– 41.35 mmHg) and a pH of at least 7.30. Positive end expiratory pressure is kept low, but sufficient to achieve maximum alveolar ventilation; in some babies 3–5 cmH$_2$O of PEEP will raise PaO_2 to acceptable levels. HFOV has been used to successfully achieve preoperative stabilization.[105]

Surgical management

Where possible, the diaphragmatic defect is closed after correction of any bowel malrotation and reduction of the hernia. Many patients will have malrotation of the cecum and this needs to be treated by adequate fixation of the restored bowel. Where the defect is large, chest wall muscle or a synthetic patch may be needed to close the defect. It has been suggested that requirement for a patch is a bad prognostic sign.[133] In some infants the abdominal cavity is poorly formed and cannot accommodate the bowel; then only skin closure is attempted and the ventral hernia repaired at a later date. Chest drains may be used, particularly in the ipsilateral thorax; some units also insert a drain prophylactically into the contralateral side in an attempt to avoid the catastrophic deterioration that occurs with the development of a pneumothorax. The underwater seal should be at atmospheric pressure and never placed on suction because of the hazard of the shift of mediastinal structures.[25] Others advocate avoidance of a chest tube, unless there is active bleeding or a pneumothorax.[171] The ipsilateral lung is smaller than the contralateral lung and the pleural space seeks to be obliterated. The ipsilateral lung is unable to fill the space immediately and it passively fills with fluid. A chest tube prolongs this process, but also, by allowing the mediastinum to swing to the ipsilateral side, causes undue stretch and overdistention.[171] We do not use chest drains.

Postoperative care

Fluid retention secondary to antidiuretic hormone secretion is relatively common.[129] Blood and plasma infusions, however, are often necessary to maintain a mean arterial blood pressure of at least 35 mmHg. The left lung may expand relatively rapidly in the first few postoperative days; this would indicate that the ipsilateral lung was atelectatic rather than hypoplastic. Such infants wean rapidly from ventilation postoperatively. More usually the space initially becomes filled with fluid and lung growth occurs slowly over weeks. Such infants may be hypoxic postoperatively or become hypoxic after a postoperative honeymoon period of good oxygenation lasting 12–24 hours. In many infants, this will be due to severe hypoplasia, affecting both the ipsilateral and contralateral lungs.

Pulmonary hypertension

Pulmonary hypertension is present in approximately 50 percent of patients.[14] There is an important, but small, subset of CDH infants who, after early survival, suffer from recurrent pulmonary hypertension.[144] It is likely such infants probably never truly achieved normal pulmonary vasculature and succumb to the consequences of untreatable pulmonary hypertension secondary to severe pulmonary hypoplasia. Previously, some infants were helped by pulmonary vasodilators, such as tolazoline[11,19,95,149] or sodium nitroprusside, but it is essential to maintain systemic blood pressure with inotrope support (p. 209). Tolazoline in one series was not an effective vasodilator and resulted in a significant drop in blood pressure.[14] By contrast, in one series prostacyclin was noted to be an effective vasodilator but, as its use did not affect overall outcome, it was suggested it should be used as a bridge to ECMO.[14] Inhaled nitric oxide (iNO; p. 183) has also been used to improve oxygenation in infants with CDH, but may not improve long-term outcome (p. 9). A randomized, double blind multicenter study failed to demonstrate that in 53 term and near-term infants with CDH and hypoxemic respiratory failure unresponsive to conventional therapy, iNO therapy reduced the need for ECMO or death.[152] In addition, there was no significant improvement in oxygenation nor reduction in the oxygenation index associated with iNO treatment.

Refractory hypoxia on maximum conventional ventilation may be susceptible to jet ventilation,[44] but, although the short-term oxygenation is improved, long-term jet ventilation has not been consistently successful.[11] ECMO has also been used as respiratory support in infants with CDH,[91,118,125] but it does not improve outcome (p. 179).[160] Adventitial thinning of pulmonary arteries with an external diameter of less than 200 μm has been noted in CDH infants who received ECMO and, as a consequence, postulated to be one of the mechanisms by which ECMO alters PPHN in CDH cases.[138] In one series,[118] however, although ECMO was associated with 35 percent survival in 26 patients with a predicted mortality of 100 percent, overall the survival rate of CDH infants in that institution was unchanged. Others have reported an unchanged survival rate since ECMO became available.[83] Fifty-nine percent of 2627 CDH infants treated with ECMO and reported to the Neonatal ECMO Registry of the Extracorporeal Life Support Organization (ELSO) by July 1997 had survived. A minimum lung volume of 45 percent of the value predicted for age-matched controls is required for survival in ECMO-treated infants.[154] It must also be remembered the mortality rate of ECMO-treated CDH infants is positively biased as it ignores those suffering intrauterine demise, too premature for ECMO, or dying before ECMO could be started.[65] ECMO also is expensive, the cost per survivor in the non-ECMO group was US$98 000 compared to US$365 000 in ECMO-treated individuals.[104] Intratracheal pulmonary ventilation (ITPV) has been used to wean infants with CDH who could not be successfully weaned from ECMO because of uncontrollable hypercapnia. During ITPV, a reverse thrust catheter, developed by Koslobow, is used. This incorporates a continuous flow of humidified gas through a reverse Venturi catheter positioned at the distal end of the endotracheal tube.[169] Results from an animal model have suggested external thoracic vibration may also aid treatment of PPHN in CDH.[98] PLV in animal models[166] has been shown to improve gas exchange and pulmonary mechanics and in CDH infants[122,165] to allow effective delivery of nitric oxide to reduce pulmonary hypertension. It may also be a method of stimulating lung growth over a few days (Chapter 33).[173]

PROGNOSIS

Prediction of outcome

Antenatally Survival is influenced by a number of factors including gestation at diagnosis,[65] presence of polyhydramios,[37] site of the stomach,[16] presence or absence of abdominal viscera in the chest cavity[147] and whether the hernia is isolated or associated with other anomalies.[150] In one series,[150] 40 of 64 infants who died during resuscitation and stabilization before surgery had associated anomalies compared to only four of 52 who survived till operation. Survival is higher in left-sided than right-side

or bilateral lesions.[48] Mediastinal shift, defined as being significant if the heart was found to be entirely in either hemisphere created by an imaginary line between the sternum and the spine in a transverse section of the fetal thorax, did not prove to be a useful prognostic feature in a series of 36 cases of antenatally diagnosed CDH.[155]

In neonates with isolated CDH, the primary determinant of survival is the presence of pulmonary hypoplasia and persistent pulmonary hypertension of the newborn. A variety of features detected by antenatal ultrasound have been proposed to indicate pulmonary hypoplasia (Table 34.1). Adzick *et al.*[1] suggested that polyhydramnios may be a useful predictor of likely poor prognosis. They surveyed the records of surgeons and obstetricians in the USA and Canada and reported neonatal death in 89 percent of cases of CDH when polyhydramnios was present and 45 percent of cases when the amniotic fluid volume was normal. Polyhydramnios, however, may be a relatively late manifestation of the disease and its value has been disputed.[136,155] The majority of antenatally diagnosed cases of diaphragmatic hernia are noted to have an intrathoracic stomach and it has not proved to be a useful predictor of neonatal survival.[155] It is possible that this discrepancy exists because smaller hernias, not associated with intrathoracic stomachs, are less readily detected antenatally and yet are associated with an improved outcome.

The relationship between fetal breathing movements and pulmonary hypoplasia has aroused considerable controversy. This may in part be explained by the differing definitions that have been used[56,106] and that the many factors that affect breathing movements may not be similarly accounted for in the different studies, for example gestational age, glucose levels and diurnal rhythm.[55] In fetuses with CDH, absent fetal breathing movements do not necessarily equate with pulmonary hypoplasia.[43,155] Fox and colleagues investigated fetal upper respiratory tract function in fetuses with CDH, using color Doppler ultrasound.[43] Color Doppler imaging of fetal breathing-related nasal and oropharyngeal fluid flow confirmed

Table 34.1 *Antenatal prediction of pulmonary hypoplasia*

Predictor	Reference
Early antenatal diagnosis	Harrison *et al.*[65]
Polyhydramnios	Dommergues *et al.*[37]
Intrathoracic stomach	Burge *et al.*[16]
Mediastinal shift	Thorpe-Beeston *et al.*[155]
Reduced fetal breathing movements	Thorpe-Beeston *et al.*[155]
Upper respiratory tract function – reduced nasal fluid flow	Fox *et al.*[43]
Abnormal chest circumference	Bahlmann *et al.*[6]
Ventricular asymmetry	Sharland *et al.*[136]

that fetal breathing movements prompt a fluid movement between the amniotic sac and fetal airway. Of five fetuses with CDH, one had no breathing-related nasal or oropharyngeal color flow and died from pulmonary hypoplasia. It was suggested that the absence of flow may prove to be a useful marker for the prenatal prediction of pulmonary hypoplasia. In another small study of six fetuses, color Doppler studies to visualize the fluid displacement in the trachea generated by fetal breathing movements was useful in predicting CDH outcome.[79] The tracheal volume flow was significantly lower in those with a lethal outcome. Larger studies must be awaited before this may be confirmed.

Measurement of the chest circumference has been suggested as a method of predicting pulmonary hypoplasia,[42] although its value in predicting pulmonary hypoplasia in CDH has yet to be established. Sonographic measurement of the traverse thoracic diameter, sagittal thoracic diameter, fetal lung diameters at the level of the four chamber view and lung/thoracic circumference ratio in one series of 19 infants with CDH enabled the diagnosis of pulmonary hypoplasia to be made in all infants who died postnatally.[6] Perhaps the promising ultrasonographic marker is the ventricular ratio. Sharland and colleagues studied the left-to-right ventricular ratio in 33 cases of CDH;[136] 73 percent of the survivors in this group had a left/right ventricular ratio within the normal range, whereas the majority of non-survivors (83 percent) had a reduced ratio. It was suggested that examination of the fetal heart may be helpful in distinguishing cases likely to be associated with a poor outcome, although the cause for the underdeveloped left heart is uncertain.

Postnatal (**Table 34.2**) Severe hypoxia (AaDO$_2$ > 500 mmHg) unresponsive to therapy prior to surgery is a bad prognostic sign,[124] as is a pH less than 7.0. Carbon dioxide retention unresponsive to hyperventilation with high ventilator pressures and rates was also associated with a high mortality rate (90 percent).[12] Bohn et al.[11] subsequently demonstrated that if hyperventilation could produce PaCO$_2$ levels of <5.5 kPa (41.35 mmHg) and the product of mean airway pressure and ventilator rate was less than 1000, the survival rate was good (86 percent), but if the PaCO$_2$ exceeded 5.5 kPa and the mean airway pressure–ventilator rate product was in excess of 1000, there was 100 percent mortality in the 13 infants studied. Johnston et al.[78] evaluated the accuracy of different predictors of pulmonary hypoplasia in CDH. In their series they found that the postductal PaO$_2$ (<70 mmHg) was a better predictor of survival than Bohn's ventilation CO$_2$ index. Both that group[78] and Redmond et al.[125] report evidence which suggests that the PaO$_2$ and ventilation index of Bohn should not be used to deny a patient access to ECMO. Others have also demonstrated the best preoperative PaCO$_2$ to be an independent predictor of survival; when combined with the ventilation index, birthweight and Apgar score at 5 minutes, it had 94 percent sensitivity and 82 percent specificity in predicting outcome on conventional treatment.[83] Comparison of parameters derived from infants' best preoperative ventilatory and blood gas data in the first 24 hours after birth revealed that an oxygenation index (MAP × FiO$_2$/PaO$_2$) of <0.08 predicted a 94 percent chance of survival, with a sensitivity of 96 percent and a specificity of 95 percent.[116] Similarly, a modified ventilation index (PIP × RR × CO$_2$/1000) of <40 predicted a 91 percent chance of survival, with a sensitivity of 94 percent and a specificity of 86 percent.[116] Others have suggested that RR × PCO$_2$ × FiO$_2$ × MAP/PaO$_2$ × 6000, using the arterial blood gas measured within a few hours of admission, is a superior predictor, being 100 percent predictive for mortality and 85 percent predictive of survival.[117] Lung function data may also facilitate accurate prediction of survival. A low tidal volume (<4 ml/kg) has been associated with poor outcome.[159]

Table 34.2 *Postnatal predictors of poor outcome*

Predictor	Reference
Short term	
Abdominal viscera in the chest cavity	Stringer et al.[147]
Requirement for a patch	Sakai et al.[133]
AaDO$_2$ > 500 mmHg unresponsive to therapy	Raphaely and Downes[124]
pH < 7.0	Raphaely and Downes[124]
High CO$_2$ unresponsive to hyperventilation	Bohn et al.[12]
MAP × ventilator rate > 1000 and a PaCO$_2$ > 5.5 kPa (41.35 mmHg)	Bohn et al.[11]
MAP × FiO$_2$/PaO$_2$ < 0.08	Norden et al.[116]
PIP × RR × CO$_2$/1000 < 40	Norden et al.[116]
RR × PCO$_2$ × FiO$_2$ × MAP/PaO$_2$ × 6000	Numanoglu et al.[117]
Tidal volume < 4 ml/kg	Tracy et al.[159]
Long term	
Large defect – worst outcome at one year	D'Agostino et al.[30]
ECMO requirement	McGaren et al.[102]; Stolar et al.[145]

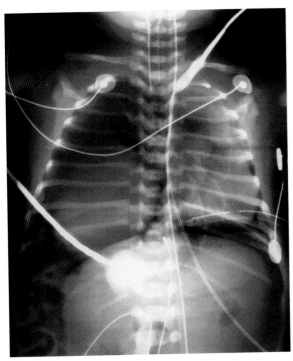

Figure 34.7 *Diaphragmatic hernia with herniated liver and colon in the right hemithorax. There is an associated pneumoperitoneum and left pneumothorax.*

The presence of a large shunt through the patent ductus arteriosus or foramen ovale postoperatively also carried a bad prognosis.[12] Pneumothorax is increased in infants with CDH (Figure 34.7), when it occurs it worsens the prognosis.

SHORT-TERM PROGNOSIS

The survival of CDH infants is approximately 60 percent (95 percent CI 55–65 percent).[92] Systematic review of 51 studies including 2980 patients revealed a mortality rate amongst prenatally diagnosed patients of 75.6 percent.[141] Termination of pregnancy was opted for in 46.9 percent of cases with associated major malformations and in only 10.3 percent of isolated CDH cases. Amongst infants referred to a treatment center, the visible mortality was 44.6 percent (range 9.3–79 percent), the mortality rate was higher in right compared to left CDH infants (65.2 percent versus 47.1 percent). Pooled hidden postnatal mortality rate (deaths before admittance to a treatment center) in population-based studies was 34.9 percent. Infants who present within 6 hours of birth have the highest mortality – approximately 50 percent.[101] By contrast, infants who survive 24 hours prior to diagnosis have a mortality rate of less than 10 percent.

The postoperative course of infants with CDH can be complicated by ipsilateral pleural effusion, in approximately one-third of cases.[132] After removal of the herniated viscera as the air in the cavity is absorbed if the lung does not fully expand or there is no compensatory mediastinal shift, fluid may accumulate to fill the resulting space. Alternately, a chylothorax may develop.[24,81] In one series,[81] effusions developed in all 22 infants who underwent surgery and six of the eight, who required drainage, had a chylothorax. Drainage was undertaken because of evidence of cardiorespiratory embarrassment and mediastinal shift. Although only a mean of 8 days of thoracocentesis was required, the infants were maintained on a medium chain triglyceride (MCT) formula for a mean of 81 days. The infants who had a chylothorax had a worse outcome in that they had a significantly longer supplementary oxygen requirement and hospital stay. No risk factors for chylothorax development could be identified. The appropriate management of a chylothorax remains controversial. Surgical ligation has been recommended if the volume of chylous drainage is greater than 15 ml/kg/day.[146] Others have suggested 100 ml/kg/day should be the criterion.[120] Spontaneous resolution, however, has occurred with even high losses.[81,103] A further indication for surgery has been a prolonged requirement for drainage, that is for longer than 7–9 days.[164] Again, however, spontaneous resolution can occur when drainage has been required for 17 days.[81]

Some patients have pulmonary hypertension which persists beyond the neonatal period. In one series, the pulmonary hypertension had resolved in six of seven patients by 12 months, the remaining infant died at 13 months.[76] Demonstration of pulmonary hypertension by echocardiography at 2 months was predictive of this condition.

Long-term prognosis

CDH infants frequently undergo further surgical intervention. Reherniation occurs in 22 percent of cases and is more likely if a patch is required.[161] Fundoplication may be needed for infants with severe gastroesophageal reflux. Up to 40 percent of survivors have bronchopulmonary dysplasia.[108] Those who required ECMO are particularly likely to suffer symptomatic BPD. Compensatory lung growth following postnatal repair of CDH appears to be associated with alveolar overdistension.[72] In another report,[157] the ipsilateral lung of two CDH survivors dying at 8 and 64 months of age of non-pulmonary causes were found to contain fewer, albeit larger, alveoli. Amongst survivors evidence of persisting low lung volumes as well as other lung function abnormalities has been found. Wohl *et al.*[170] demonstrated vital capacity and total lung capacity to be normal, but forced expiratory volume mildly reduced in 19 patients aged between 6 and 18 years, as has previously been reported.[21] Others have found evidence of air trapping during adolescence, the residual volume and FRC tending to be elevated.[46] Comparison of CDH patients of age 7–18 years to age-matched controls with CDH or pulmonary hypoplasia who underwent similar neonatal treatment revealed the CDH patients to have evidence of mild airway obstruction and increased airway hyper-responsiveness to metacholine.[74] Ventilation–perfusion studies have shown that although ventilation to the ipsilateral lung is often normal at 6–18 years of age, perfusion is decreased,[34] consistent with a persistent reduction in the number of branches or generations of pulmonary arteries on the affected side.[126] Infants requiring the longest duration of ventilation had the greatest disparity in ventilation–perfusion scan to the ipsilateral lung.[172] Some studies have suggested these abnormalities are not associated with persisting symptoms,[46,170] but others[172] reported that exercise tolerance and oxygen consumption are significantly reduced, with only 50 percent describing sufficient stamina to take part in sports.

The postnatal development of the lung is also modified by the growth of the axial skeleton and the rib cage. The lifelong disparity in the size of the hemithoraces of patients with CDH and an increased incidence of pectus abnormalities may be related to an increased incidence of scoliosis. Chest asymmetry has been reported in 48–74 percent of cases, scoliosis in 10–27 percent and pectus abnormalities in approximately 20 percent of cases.[144] The potentially progressive nature of these skeletal abnormalities mandates lifelong pulmonary evaluation and early intervention.[144]

Foregut dysmotility (esophageal ectasia, gastroesophageal reflux, delayed gastric emptying) is an important source of morbidity in CDH survivors. These problems particularly occur in left-sided hernias and may be related to translocation of the stomach into the chest with kinking and obstruction of the gastroesophageal junction. The kinking may cause ectasia; this is supported by the frequent finding of CDH with polyhydramnios.[144] The diaphragmatic defect can also compromise the contribution of the esophageal hiatus to a competent lower esophageal sphincter. Frequent non-rotation of the stomach (mesoaxial and organoaxial) and the midgut may account for malpositioning of the stomach. It has been suggested that all CDH infants have some degree of foregut dysmotility.[144] In most series, however, only those with symptoms have been investigated. In a population who had vomiting, aspiration, failure to thrive or recurrent pneumonia, 62 percent were shown to have gastroesophageal reflux.[84] Gastroesophageal reflux may occur in between 43 percent[40] and 89 percent[161] of infants who required ECMO. Significant gastroesophageal reflux was significantly correlated to an intra-thoracic stomach, prenatal diagnosis, prolonged mechanical ventilation and hospitalization,[84] as well as a very large defect requiring prosthetic repair.[139] Right-sided defects are more likely to require prosthetic closure and may be more prone to severe foregut dysmotility/gastroesophageal reflux.[113] Feeding difficulties[40] and growth failure are common at follow-up of CDH infants, particularly in those who required ECMO.[161] Fifty percent of infants were less than the fifth percentile for weight at both 1 and 2 years.[161]

There remains genuine concern that the techniques associated with increasing the survival of infants with

Table 34.3 *Pentalogy of Cantrell*

Anterior diaphragmatic hernia
Supraumbilical omphalocele
Bifid lower sternum
Pericardial hernia, containing a cardiac diverticulum
Intracardiac anomaly

borderline CDH will increase the incidence of long-term neurological handicap. One study of selected high-risk long-term survivors, not treated with ECMO, found major neurological handicap in 2 of 23 children, although there was no clear relationship between poor outcome and measured indices of hypoxia and acidosis during the neonatal period.[31]

CDH infants who required ECMO have greater morbidity than infants who had other conditions and were treated with ECMO; lower motor and cognitive scores at 1 year and persisting hypotonicity in 75 percent of cases.[10,102,145] More ECMO survivors required gastrostomy tube placement (50 versus 16 percent) and more needed Nissen's fundoplication (42 versus 12 percent).[102] A high prevalence (60 percent) of sensorineural hearing loss has been reported in CDH survivors with or without ECMO requirement.[127] In one study, ECMO survivors who had a bilateral hearing loss had greater impairment of high frequencies than low frequencies.[93] In the same series,[93] HFO survivors had similar hearing loss, which was also progressive. These data suggest those infants who experience severe oxygen deprivation are at increased risk of hearing loss.[93]

Anterior diaphragmatic hernia (Morgagni)

Unusually, viscera may herniate through the foraminae of Morgagni, which lie anteriorly on either side of the sternal attachment. Morgagni herniae represent only 1–2 percent of CDH cases. These herniae are usually right-sided and then most commonly involve the liver and omentum, producing a mass close to the heart in the right anterior mediastinum. Anterior diaphragmatic hernia may be seen as part of the rare pentalogy of Cantrell (Table 34.3).

MANAGEMENT

Anterior herniae are usually asymptomatic in the neonatal period, but when coincidentally found on chest radiograph, they should be repaired, as strangulation of the abdominal organs can occur.

EVENTRATION OF THE DIAPHRAGM

This may be a primary abnormality, failure of the migration of primitive muscle cells into the central portion of the diaphragm, or a secondary condition as a consequence of phrenic nerve absence when the diaphragm is replaced by a fibrous sheet. It is usually unilateral, affecting the left side more than the right, but it may be bilateral.[128] It can be one feature of a generalized condition such as congenital myotonic dystrophy. Eventrations differ from herniae in that they must have a large base, that is, involvement of the entire hemidiaphragm. If one portion of the hemidiaphragm is normal in location and muscular thickness, but another portion bulges into the chest, that is a hernia.[27] In addition, an eventration possesses three layers: peritoneum, thinned out diaphragm and pleura.

Clinical signs

Severe eventration presents in the neonatal period with respiratory distress, tachypnea and cyanosis from birth and evidence of mediastinal shift away from the affected side. The ipsilateral lung may be hypoplastic. Localized lesions may produce few or no symptoms. Paradoxical motion, as in diaphragmatic paralysis, is usually absent.

Differential diagnosis

The differential diagnosis is of a paralyzed diaphragm, as a result of an acquired phrenic nerve injury, but in such cases there will be a history of birth trauma classically with Erb's palsy or surgery (p. 524).

Diagnosis

Elevation of the affected diaphragm will be apparent on the chest radiograph (Figure 34.8). Synchronous diaphragmatic movements are present in those less severely affected, but in those with either extensive lesions or phrenic nerve palsies, the diaphragm may show minimal motion while breathing or the motion may be paradoxical with the diaphragm rising with inspiration and falling with expiration.

Management

Infants who are asymptomatic, but identified by chance from the radiograph or with relatively mild symptoms, do not require intervention in the neonatal period. Those with dyspnea and cyanosis in the neonatal period need surgical plication.[52,162] Successful outcome has also been reported with plication for bilateral eventration.[128]

DIAPHRAGMATIC PARALYSIS

Etiology

This can occur as a result of birth trauma, usually after a breech delivery and, although occasionally is bilateral, is usually unilateral and on the right. There is excessive

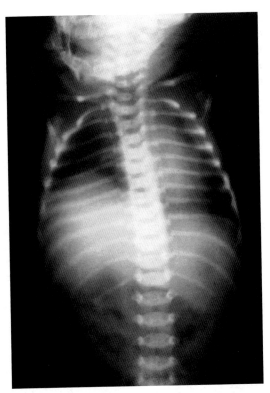

Figure 34.8 *Diaphragmatic eventration in a neonate with congenital myotonic dystrophy. Note: the elevated and abnormal configured right diaphragm. The infant's gracile ribs are illustrated.*

stretching of C3 to C5 nerve roots in the neck. Diaphragmatic paralysis may also result from phrenic nerve trauma at thoracic operation, such as ligation of patent ductus arteriosus, creation of a systemic pulmonary shunt or repair of a tracheoesophageal fistula. Rarely, it has been described following insertion of a chest tube to drain a tension pneumothorax (p. 318).[27,167] It may also occur following antenatal insertion of a pleuroamniotic shunt (p. 93).

Clinical signs

The usual presentation is with respiratory distress, but in cases of bilateral paralysis there is cyanosis and poor respiratory effort necessitating mechanical ventilation. The diaphragm is an especially important respiratory muscle in the newborn, particularly during active sleep when the intercostals are inhibited. Other signs of birth trauma may be present; in particular there is frequently an associated Erb's palsy. Indeed, any infant who is noted to have an Erb's palsy should undergo diaphragmatic screening.

Diagnosis

This is suggested on the chest radiograph if the right hemidiaphragm is two intercostal spaces higher than the left (Figure 34.9) or if the left hemidiaphragm is one intercostal space higher than the right.[54] There may be associated basal atelectasis and, on fluoroscopy or ultrasound examination, the involved diaphragm shows either limited or paradoxical movement.[5]

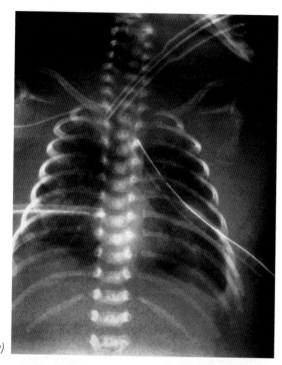

(a)

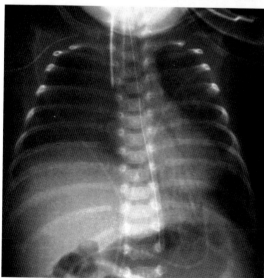

(b)

Figure 34.9 *(a) Chest radiograph demonstrating intercostal catheters which had drained bilateral pleural effusions. (b) A subsequent chest radiograph demonstrates elevation of the right hemidiaphragm secondary to phrenic nerve injury from intercostals drain insertion. (Reproduced with permission from Williams, O., Greenough, A., Rafferty, G.F. (2003) Extubation failure due to phrenic nerve injury.* Archives of Disease in Childhood, *88, F72–F73.[167])*

Management

Management is similar whether the lesion is the result of birth trauma or post-thoracotomy. Nasal continuous positive airways pressure can be useful particularly if there is associated atelectasis.[15] If both hemidiaphragms are paralyzed, prolonged mechanical ventilation is necessary.[3] Usually recovery is over 2 weeks, but improvement can occur for up to 2 months. Once no further improvement is expected and the patient cannot be weaned from mechanical ventilation then surgical plication of the diaphragm should be performed.

REFERENCES

1 Adzick, N.S., Harrison, M.R., Glick, P.L. *et al.* (1985) Diaphragmatic hernia in the fetus: prenatal diagnosis and outcome in 94 cases. *Journal of Pediatric Surgery* **20**, 357–361.

2 Adzick, N.S., Outwater, K., Harrison, M.R. *et al.* (1985) Correction of congenital diaphragmatic hernia in utero. IV. An early gestational fetal lamb model for pulmonary vascular morphometric analysis. *Journal of Pediatric Surgery* **20**, 673–680.

3 Aldrich, T.K., Heran, J.H., Rochester, D.F. (1980) Bilateral diaphragmatic paralysis in the newborn infant. *Journal of Pediatrics* **97**, 988.

4 Alles, A.J., Losty, P.D., Donahoe, P.K. *et al.* (1995) Embryonic cell death patterns in rats with nitrofen-induced congenital diaphragmatic hernia. *Journal of Pediatric Surgery* **30**, 353–360.

5 Ambler, R., Gruenewald, S., John, E. (1985) Ultrasound monitoring of diaphragm activity in bilateral diaphragmatic paralysis. *Archives of Disease in Childhood* **60**, 170.

6 Bahlmann, F., Merz, E., Hallermann, C. *et al.* (1999) Congenital diaphragmatic hernia: ultrasonic measurement of fetal lungs to predict pulmonary hypoplasia. *Ultrasound in Obstetrics and Gynecology* **14**, 162–168.

7 Banagale, R.C., Watters, J.H. (1983) Delayed right-sided diaphragmatic hernia following group B Streptococcal infection. *Human Pathology* **14**, 67–69.

8 Battu, P., D'Cruz, I.A., Holman, M., Locksmith, J.P. (1992) Noninvasive imaging of a retrocardiac spleen. Unusual component of paraesophageal diaphragmatic hernia. *Chest* **101**, 1159–1160.

9 Benacerraf, B.R., Adzick, N.S. (1987) Fetal diaphragmatic hernia: Ultrasound diagnosis and clinical outcome in 19 cases. *American Journal of Obstetrics and Gynecology* **156**, 573–576.

10 Bernbaum, J., Schwartz, I.P., Gerdes, M. *et al.* (1995) Survivors of extracorporeal membrane oxygenation at 1 year of age: the relationship of primary diagnosis with health and neurodevelopmental sequelae. *Pediatrics* **96**, 907–913.

11 Bohn, D., Tamura, M., Perrin, D. *et al.* (1987) Ventilatory predictors of pulmonary hypoplasia in congenital diaphragmatic hernia, confirmed by morphologic assessment. *Journal of Pediatrics* **111**, 423–431.

12 Bohn, D.J., James, I., Filler, R.M. *et al.* (1984) The relationship between $PaCO_2$ and ventilation parameters in predicting survival in congenital diaphragmatic hernia. *Journal of Pediatric Surgery* **19**, 666–671.

13 Bohrer, J.V. (1940) Torsion of the wandering spleen. *Annals of Surgery* **111**, 416–424.

14 Bos, A.P., Tibboel, D., Koot, V.C.M. *et al.* (1993) Persistent pulmonary hypertension in high-risk congenital diaphragmatic hernia patients: incidence and vasodilator therapy. *Journal of Pediatric Surgery* **28**, 1463–1465.

15 Bucci, G., Marzetti, G., Preece-Bucci, S. *et al.* (1974) Phrenic nerve palsy treated by continuous positive airways pressure breathing by nasal cannula. *Archives of Disease in Childhood* **49**, 230–232.

16 Burge, D.M., Atwell, J.D., Freeman, N.V. (1989) Could the stomach site help predict outcome in babies with left sided congenital diaphragmatic hernia diagnosed antenatally? *Journal of Pediatric Surgery* **24**, 567–569.

17 Butler, N., Claireaux, A.E. (1962) Congenital diaphragmatic hernia as a cause of perinatal mortality. *Lancet* **i**, 659–663.

18 Byard, R.W., Bohn, D.J., Wilson, G. *et al.* (1990) Unsuspected diaphragmatic hernia: a potential cause of sudden and unexpected death in infancy and early childhood. *Journal of Pediatric Surgery* **25**, 1166–1168.

19 Cartlidge, P.H., Mann, N.P., Kapila, L. (1986) Preoperative stabilization in congenital diaphragmatic hernia. *Archives of Disease in Childhood* **61**, 1226–1228.

20 Charlton, A.J., Bruce, J., Davenport, M. (1991) Timing of surgery in congenital diaphragmatic hernia. *Anaesthesia* **46**, 820–823.

21 Chatrath, R.R., El-Shafie, M., Jones, R.S. (1971) Fate of hypoplastic lungs after repair of congenital diaphragmatic hernia. *Archives of Disease in Childhood* **46**, 633–638.

22 Chui, P.P., Tan, C.T. (1993) Sudden death due to incarcerated Bochdalek hernia in an adult. *Annals of the Academy of Medicine, Singapore* **22**, 57–60.

23 Cilley, R.E., Zgleszewski, S.E., Krummel, T.M., Chinoy, M.R. (1997) Nitrofen dose-dependent gestational day-specific murine lung hypoplasia and left-sided diaphragmatic hernia. *American Journal of Physiology* **272**, L362–371.

24 Claris, O., Besnier, S., Lapillonne, A. *et al.* (1996) Chylothorax following surgical repair of congenital diaphragmatic hernia in five neonates. *Prenatal and Neonatal Medicine* **1**, 94–96.

25 Cloutier, R., Fournier, L., Levasseur, L. (1983) Reversion of fetal circulation in congenital diaphragmatic hernia: a preventable postoperative complication. *Journal of Pediatric Surgery* **18**, 551–559.

26 Cloutier, R., Allard, V., Fournier, L. *et al.* (1993) Estimation of lungs' hypoplasia on postoperative chest X-rays in congenital diaphragmatic hernia. *Journal of Pediatrics* **28**, 1086–1089.

27 Collins, D.L. (1980) Diaphragmatic hernia. In Holder, T.M., Ashcraft, K.W. (eds), *Pediatric Surgery*. Philadelphia, PA: W.B. Saunders, 227–240.

28 Coren, M.E., Rosenthal, M., Bush, A. (1997) Congenital diaphragmatic hernia misdiagnosed as tension pneumothorax. *Pediatric Pulmonology* **24**, 119–121.

29 Crane, J.P. (1979) Familial congenital diaphragmatic hernia: prenatal diagnostic approach and analysis of twelve families. *Clinical Genetics* **116**, 244–252.

30 D'Agostino, J.A., Bernbaum, J.C., Gerdes, M. *et al.* (1995) Outcome for infants with congenital diaphragmatic hernia requiring extracorporeal membrane oxygenation: the first year. *Journal of Pediatric Surgery* **30**, 10–15.

31 Davenport, M., Rivlin, E., D'Souza, S.W., Bianchi, A. (1992) Delayed surgery for congenital diaphragmatic hernia: neurodevelopmental outcome in later childhood. *Archives of Disease in Childhood* **67**, 1353–1356.

32 Davey, M.G., Hooper, S.B., Cock, M.L., Harding, R. (2001) Stimulation of lung growth in fetuses with lung hypoplasia leads to altered postnatal lung structure in sheep. *Pediatric Pulmonology* **32**, 267–276.

33 David, T.J., Illingworth, C.A. (1976) Diaphragmatic hernia in the south-west of England. *Journal of Medical Genetics* **13**, 253–262.

34 Delepoulle, F., Martinot, A., Leclerc, F. *et al.* (1991) Long-term outcome of congenital diaphragmatic hernia. A study of 17 patients. *Archives Francaises de Pediatrie* **48**, 703–707.

35 DiFiore, J.W., Fauza, D.O., Slavin, R. *et al.* (1994) Experimental fetal tracheal ligation reverses the structural and physiological effects of pulmonary hypoplasia in congenital diaphragmatic hernia. *Journal of Pediatric Surgery* **29**, 248–257.

36 Dimitriou, G., Greenough, A., Davenport, M., Nicolaides, K.H. (2000) Prediction of outcome by computer assisted analysis of lung area on the chest radiograph of infants with congenital diaphragmatic hernia. *Journal of Pediatric Surgery* **35**, 489–493.

37 Dommergues, M., Louis-Sylvestre, C., Mandelbrot, L. *et al.* (1996) Congenital diaphragmatic hernia: can prenatal ultrasonography predict outcome? *American Journal of Obstetrics and Gynecology* **174**, 1377–1381.

38 Enns, G.M., Cox, V.A., Goldstein, R.B. *et al.* (1998) Congenital diaphragmatic defects and associated syndromes, malformations, and chromosome anomalies: a retrospective study of 60 patients and literature review. *American Journal of Medical Genetics* **79**, 215–225.

39 Erhardt, A., Aker, S., Saleh, A. *et al.* (2002) A seropneumothorax? *Lancet* **359**, 578.

40 Finer, N.N., Tierney, A., Etches, P.C. *et al.* (1998) Congenital diaphragmatic hernia: developing a protocolized approach. *Journal of Pediatric Surgery* **33**, 1331–1337.

41 Flake, A.W., Crombleholme, T.M., Johnson, M.P. *et al.* (2000) Treatment of severe congenital diaphragmatic hernia by fetal tracheal occlusion: clinical experience with fifteen cases. *American Journal of Obstetrics and Gynecology* **183**, 1059–1066.

42 Fong, K., Ohlsson, A., Zalev, A. (1988) Fetal thoracic circumference: a prospective cross-sectional study with real time ultrasound. *American Journal of Obstetrics and Gynecology* **158**, 1154–1159.

43 Fox, H.E., Badalian, S.S., Trimor-Tritsch, I.E. *et al.* (1993) Fetal upper respiratory tract function in cases of antenatally diagnosed congenital diaphragmatic hernia: preliminary observations. *Ultrasound in Obstetrics and Gynecology* **3**, 164–167.

44 Fox, W.W., Duara, S. (1983) Persistent pulmonary hypertension in the neonate. Diagnosis and management. *Journal of Pediatrics* **103**, 505–514.

45 Frenckner, B., Ehren, H., Granholm, T. *et al.* (1997) Improved results in patients who have congenital diaphragmatic hernia using preoperative stabilization, extracorporeal membrane oxygenation, and delayed surgery. *Journal of Pediatric Surgery* **32**, 1185–1189.

46 Freyschuss, V., Hannergren, K., Frenckner, B. (1984) Lung function after repair of congenital diaphragmatic hernia. *Acta Paediatrica Scandinavica* **73**, 589–593.

47 Garcia-Munoz, F., Santana, C., Reyes, D. *et al.* (2001) Early sepsis, obstructive jaundice and right-sided diaphragmatic hernia in the newborn. *Acta Paediatrica* **90**, 96–98.

48 Geary, M.P., Chitty, L.S., Morrison, J.J. *et al.* (1998) Perinatal outcome and prognostic factors in prenatally diagnosed congenital diaphragmatic hernia. *Ultrasound in Obstetrics and Gynecology* **12**, 107–111.

49 Geggel, R., Murphy, J., Langleben, D. *et al.* (1985) Congenital diaphragmatic hernia. Arterial structural changes and persistent pulmonary hypertension after surgical repair. *Journal of Pediatrics* **107**, 457–464.

50 George, K., Cooney, T., Chiou, B., Thurlbeck, W. (1987) Hypoplasia and immaturity of the terminal lung unit (acinus)

in congenital diaphragmatic hernia. *American Review of Respiratory Disease* **136**, 947–950.

51 Glick, P.L., Siebert, J.R., Benjamin, D.R. (1990) Pathophysiology of congenital diaphragmatic hernia: I. Renal enlargement suggests feedback modulation by pulmonary derived renotropins – a unifying hypothesis to explain pulmonary hypoplasia, polyhydramnios and renal enlargement in the fetus/newborn with congenital diaphragmatic hernia. *Journal of Pediatric Surgery* **25**, 492–495.

52 Goldstein, J.D., Reid, L.M. (1980) Pulmonary hypoplasia resulting from phrenic nerve agenesis and diaphragmatic amyoplasia. *Journal of Pediatrics* **97**, 282–287.

53 Goodfellow, T., Hyde, I., Burge, D.M., Freeman, N.O. (1987) Congenital diaphragmatic hernia: the prognostic significance of the site of the stomach. *British Journal of Radiology* **60**, 993–995.

54 Greene, W., L'Heureux, P., Hunt, C.E. (1975) Paralysis of the diaphragm. *American Journal of Diseases in Children* **129**, 1402–1405

55 Greenough, A. (1993) Fetal respiratory activity and pulmonary hypoplasia. *Ultrasound in Obstetrics and Gynecology* **3**, 159–162.

56 Greenough, A., Blott, M., Nicolaides, K.H., Campbell, S. (1988) Interpretation of fetal breathing movements in oligohydramnios due to membrane rupture. *Lancet* **i**, 182–183.

57 Harrison, M.R. (1990) The fetus with a diaphragmatic hernia: pathophysiology, natural history and surgical management. In Harrison, M.R., Golbus, M.S., Filly, R.A. (eds), *The Unborn Patient. Fetal Diagnosis and Treatment*. Philadelphia, PA: W.B. Saunders, 295–319.

58 Harrison, M.R., de Lorimier, A.A. (1981) Congenital diaphragmatic hernia. *Surgical Clinics of North America* **61**, 1023–1033.

59 Harrison, M.R., Bjordal, R.I., Langmark, I., Knutrud, O. (1978) Congenital diaphragmatic hernia: the hidden mortality. *Journal of Pediatric Surgery* **13**, 227–230.

60 Harrison, M.R., Bressack, M.A., Churg, A.M., DeLorrimer, A.A. (1980) Correction of congenital diaphragmatic hernia in utero. II. Simulated correction permits fetal lung growth with survival at birth. *Surgery* **88**, 260–268.

61 Harrison, M.R., Adzick, N.S., Wakayama, D.K., de Lorimier, A.A. (1986) Fetal diaphragmatic hernia: pathophysiology, natural history and outcome. *Clinical Obstetrics and Gynecology* **29**, 490–501.

62 Harrison, M.R., Adzick, N.S., Longaker, M.T. *et al.* (1990) Successful repair in utero of a fetal diaphragmatic hernia after removal of viscera from the left thorax. *New England Journal of Medicine* **322**, 1522–1525.

63 Harrison, M.R., Langer, J.C., Adzick, N.S. *et al.* (1990) Correction of congenital diaphragmatic hernia in utero. V. Initial clinical experience. *Journal of Pediatric Surgery* **25**, 47–57.

64 Harrison, M.R., Adzick, N.S., Flake, A.W., Jennings, R.W. (1993) The CDH two-step: a dance of necessity. *Journal of Pediatric Surgery* **28**, 813–816.

65 Harrison, M.R., Adzick, N.S., Estes, J.M., Howell, L.J. (1994) A prospective study of the outcome for fetuses with diaphragmatic hernia. *Journal of the American Medical Association* **271**, 382–384.

66 Harrison, M.R., Adzick, N.S., Flake, A.W. *et al.* (1996) Correction of congenital diaphragmatic hernia in utero VIII: Response of the hypoplastic lung to tracheal occlusion. *Journal of Pediatric Surgery* **31**, 1339–1348.

67 Harrison, M.R., Adzick, N.S., Bullard, K.M. *et al.* (1997) Correction of congenital diaphragmatic hernia *in utero*. VII: a prospective trial. *Journal of Pediatric Surgery* **32**, 1637–1642.

68 Hashim, E., Laberge, J.-M., Chen, M.-F., Quillen, E.W. (1995) Reversible tracheal obstruction in the fetal sheep: effects on tracheal fluid pressure and lung growth. *Journal of Pediatric Surgery* **30**, 1172–1177.

69 Hazebroek, R.W.J., Tibboel, L.D., Bos, A.P. *et al.* (1988) Congenital diaphragmatic hernia: impact of pre-operative stabilization. A pre-operative pilot study in 13 patients. *Journal of Pediatric Surgery* **23**, 1139–1146.

70 Hedrick, M.H., Estes, J.M., Sullivan, K.M. *et al.* (1994) Plug the lung until it grows (PLUG): a new method to treat congenital diaphragmatic hernia in utero. *Journal of Pediatric Surgery* **29**, 612–617.

71 Hisanaga, S., Shimokawa, H., Kashiwabara, Y. *et al.* (1984) Unexpectedly low lecithin/sphingomyelin ratio associated with fetal diaphragmatic hernia. *American Journal of Obstetrics and Gynecology* **149**, 905–906.

72 Hislop, A., Reid, L. (1976) Persistent hypoplasia of the lung after repair of congenital diaphragmatic hernia. *Thorax* **31**, 450–455.

73 Hunt, J., Baston, B. (2000) Airway nitrogen oxide measurements in asthma and other pediatric respiratory diseases. *Journal of Pediatrics* **137**, 14–20.

74 Ijsselstijn, H., Tibboel, D., Hop, W.J.C. *et al.* (1997) Long-term pulmonary sequelae in children with congenital diaphragmatic hernia. *American Journal of Respiratory and Critical Care Medicine* **155**, 174–180.

75 Ijsselstijn, H., Zimermann, L.J.I., Bunt, J.E.H. *et al.* (1998) Prospective evaluation of surfactant composition in bronchoalveolar lavage fluid of infants with congenital diaphragmatic hernia and of age-matched controls. *Critical Care Medicine* **26**, 573–580.

76 Ionoco, J.A., Cilley, R.E., Mager, D.T. *et al.* (1999) Postnatal pulmonary hypertension after repair of congenital diaphragmatic hernia: predicting risk and outcome. *Journal of Pediatric Surgery* **34**, 349–353.

77 Iritani, I. (1984) Experimental study on embryogenesis of congenital diaphragmatic hernia. *Anatomy and Embryology* **169**, 133–139.

78 Johnston, P.W., Liberman, R., Gangitano, E., Vogt, J. (1990) Ventilation parameters and arterial blood gases as a prediction of hypoplasia in congenital diaphragmatic hernia. *Journal of Pediatric Surgery* **25**, 496–499.

79 Kalache, K.D., Chaoui, R., Hartung, J. *et al.* (1998) Doppler assessment of tracheal fluid flow during fetal breathing movements in cases of congenital diaphragmatic hernia. *Ultrasound in Obstetrics and Gynecology* **12**, 27–32.

80 Kamata, S., Usui, N., Ishikawa, S. *et al.* (1998) Prolonged pre-operative stabilization using high-frequency oscillatory ventilation does not improve the outcome in neonates with congenital diaphragmatic hernia. *Pediatric Surgery International* **13**, 542–546.

81 Kavvadia, V., Greenough, A., Davenport, M. *et al.* (1998) Chylothorax after repair of congenital diaphragmatic hernia – risk factors and morbidity. *Journal of Pediatric Surgery* **33**, 500–502.

82 Keijzer, R., Liu, J., Deimling, J. *et al.* (2000) Dual-hit hypothesis explains pulmonary hypoplasia in the nitrofen model of congenital diaphragmatic hernia. *American Journal of Pathology* **156**, 1299–1306.

83 Keshen, T.H., Gursoy, M., Shew, S.B. *et al.* (1997) Does extracorporeal membrane oxygenation benefit neonates with congenital diaphragmatic hernia. Application of a predictive equation. *Journal of Pediatric Surgery* **32**, 818–822.

84 Kieffer, J., Sapin, E., Berg, A. *et al.* (1995) Gastroesophageal reflux after repair of congenital diaphragmatic hernia. *Journal of Pediatric Surgery* **30**, 1330–1333.

85 Kitagawa, M., Hislop, A.A., Boyden, E.A., Reid, L. (1971) Lung hypoplasia in congenital diaphragmatic hernia: a quantitative study of airway, artery and alveolar development. *British Journal of Surgery* **58**, 342–346.

86 Kluth, D., Tenbrinck, R., von Ekesparre, M. *et al.* (1993) The natural history of congenital diaphramatic hernia and pulmonary hypoplasia in the embryo. *Journal of Pediatric Surgery* **28**, 456–463.

87 Kluth, D., Kaestner, M., Tibboel, D., Lambrecht, W. (1995) Rotation of the gut: fact or fantasy? *Journal of Pediatric Surgery* **30**, 448–453.

88 Kluth, D., Tander, B., von Ekesparre, M., *et al.* (1995) Congenital diaphragmatic hernia: the impact of embryological studies. *Pediatric Surgery International* **10**, 16–22.

89 Kurzel, R.B., Naunheim, K.S., Schwartz, R.A. (1988) Repair of symptomatic diaphragmatic hernia during pregnancy. *Obstetrics and Gynecology* **71**, 869–871.

90 Langer, J.C., Filler, R.M., Bohn, D.J. *et al.* (1988) Timing of surgery for congenital diaphragmatic hernia: is emergency operation necessary? *Journal of Pediatric Surgery* **23**, 731.

91 Langham, M.R., Krummel, T.M., Bartlett, R.H. *et al.* (1987) Mortality with extracorporeal membrane oxygenation following repair of congenital diaphragmatic hernia in 93 infants. *Journal of Pediatric Surgery* **22**, 1150–1154.

92 Langham, M.R., Kays, D.W., Ledbetter, D.J. *et al.* (1996) Congenital diaphragmatic hernia: epidemiology and outcome. *Clinics in Perinatology* **23**, 671–688.

93 Lasky, R.E., Wiorek, L., Becker, T.R. (1998) Hearing loss in survivors of neonatal extracorporeal membrane oxygenation (ECMO) therapy and high frequency oscillatory (HFO) therapy. *Journal of the American Academy of Audiology* **9**, 47–58.

94 Levine, G., Boyd, G., Milstern, G. (1992) Influence of airway state on hemodynamics of the pulmonary circulation in newborn lambs. *Pediatric Research* **31**, 1869.

95 Levy, R.J., Rosenthal, A., Freed, M.D. *et al.* (1977) Persistent pulmonary hypertension in a newborn with congenital diaphragmatic hernia: successful management with tolazoline. *Pediatrics* **60**, 740–742.

96 Liechty, K.W., Crombleholme, T.M., Flake, A.W. *et al.* (1997) Intrapartum airway management for giant fetal neck masses: the EXIT (ex utero intrapartum treatment) procedure. *American Journal of Obstetrics and Gynecology* **177**, 870–874.

97 Losty, P.D., Vanama, K., Rintala, R.J. *et al.* (1998) Congenital diaphragmatic hernia – does the side of the defect influence the incidence of associated malformations? *Journal of Pediatric Surgery* **33**, 507–510.

98 Major, D., Cloutier, R., Fournier, L. *et al.* (1993) A new method of treatment for pulmonary hypertension in congenital diaphragmatic hernia: experimental study in cats. *Journal of Pediatric Surgery* **28**, 1090–1092.

99 Malone, P.S., Brain, A.J., Kiely, E.M., Spitz, L. (1989) Congenital diaphragmatic defects that present late. *Archives of Disease in Childhood* **64**, 1542–1544.

100 Mansell, A.L., McAteer, A.L., Pipkin, A.C. (1993) Maturation of interdependence between extra-alveolar arteries and lung parenchyma in piglets. *Circulation Research* **71**, 701–710.

101 Marshall, A., Sumner, E. (1982) Improved prognosis in congenital diaphragmatic hernia. Experience of 62 cases over a two-year period. *Journal of the Royal Society of Medicine* **75**, 607.

102 McGaren, E.D., Mallik, K., Rodgers, B.M. (1997) Neurological outcome is diminished in survivors of congenital diaphragmatic hernia requiring extracorporeal

membrane oxygenation. *Journal of Pediatric Surgery* **32**, 1216–1220.

103 Mercer, S. (1986) Factors involved in chylothorax following repair of congenital posterolateral diaphragmatic hernia. *Journal of Pediatric Surgery* **21**, 809–811.

104 Metkus, A.P., Esserman, L., Sola, A. *et al.* (1995) Cost per anomaly: what does a diaphragmatic hernia cost? *Journal of Pediatric Surgery* **30**, 226–230.

105 Miguet, D., Claris, O., Lapillonne, A. *et al.* (1994) Preoperative stabilization using high-frequency oscillatory ventilation in the management of congenital diaphragmatic hernia. *Critical Care Medicine* **22**, S77–S82.

106 Moessinger, A.C., Fox, H.E., Higgins, A. *et al.* (1987) Fetal breathing movements are not a reliable predictor of continued lung development in pregnancies complicated by oligohydramnios. *Lancet* **2**, 1297–1300.

107 Moffitt, S.T., Schulze, K.F., Sahni, R. *et al.* (1995) Preoperative cardiorespiratory trends in infants with congenital diaphragmatic hernia. *Journal of Pediatric Surgery* **30**, 604–611.

108 Molenaar, J.C., Bos, A.P., Hazebroek, F.W.J., Tibboel, D. (1991) Congenital diaphragmatic hernia. What defect? *Journal of Pediatric Surgery* **26**, 248–251.

109 Moya, F.R., Thomas, V.L., Romaguera, J. *et al.* (1995) Fetal lung maturation in congenital diaphragmatic hernia. *American Journal of Obstetrics and Gynecology* **173**, 1401–1405.

110 Nakamura, Y., Yamamoto, I., Fukuda, S., Hashimoto, T. (1991) Pulmonary acinar development in diaphragmatic hernia. *Archives of Pathology and Laboratory Medicine* **115**, 372–376.

111 Nakayama, D.K., Motoyama, E.K., Tagge, E.M. (1991) Effect of preoperative stabilization on respiratory system compliance and outcome in newborn infants with congenital diaphragmatic hernia. *Journal of Pediatrics* **118**, 793–799.

112 Nambi, P., Pullen, M., Wu, H.L. *et al.* (1992) Dexamethasone down-regulates the expression of endothelin receptors in vascular smooth muscle cells. *Journal of Biological Chemistry* **267**, 19555–19559.

113 Narwal, S., DeFelice, A.R., Stolar, C.J.H., *et al.* (1995) Severe gastroesophageal reflux and increased ECMO need in infants with right as opposed to left-sided congenital diaphragmatic hernia. *Journal of Pediatric Gastroenterology and Nutrition* **21**, 335.

114 Nio, M., Haase, G., Kennaugh, J. *et al.* (1994) A prospective randomized trial of delayed versus immediate repair of congenital diaphragmatic hernia. *Journal of Pediatric Surgery* **29**, 618–621.

115 Nitecki, S., Bar-Maor, J.A. (1992) Late presentation of Bochdalek hernia: our experience and review of the literature. *Israel Journal of Medical Sciences* **28**, 711–714.

116 Norden, M.A., Butt, W., McDougall, P. (1994) Predictors of survival for infants with congenital diaphragmatic hernia. *Journal of Pediatric Surgery* **29**, 1442–1447.

117 Numanoglu, A., Morrison, C., Rode, H. (1998) Prediction of outcome in congenital diaphragmatic hernia. *Pediatric Surgery International* **13**, 564–568.

118 O'Rourke, P., Lillehei, C.W., Crone, R.K., Vacanti, J.P. (1991) The effect of extracorporeal membrane oxygenation on the survival of neonates with high risk congenital diaphragmatic hernia: 45 cases from a single institution. *Journal of Pediatric Surgery* **26**, 147–152.

119 O'Toole, S.J., Sharma, A., Karamanoukian, H.L. *et al.* (1996) Tracheal ligation does not correct the surfactant deficiency associated with congenital diaphragmatic hernia. *Journal of Pediatric Surgery* **31**, 546–550.

120 Paes, M.L., Powell, H. (1994) Chylothorax: an update. *British Journal of Hospital Medicine* **151**, 482–490.

121 Phillpott, J.W., Cumming, W.A. (1994) Torsion of the spleen: an unusual presentation of congenital diaphragmatic hernia. *Pediatric Radiology* **24**, 150–151.

122 Pranikoff, T., Gauger, P.G., Hirschl, R.B. (1996) Partial liquid ventilation in newborn patients with congenital diaphragmatic hernia. *Journal of Pediatric Surgery* **31**, 613–618.

123 Puri, P., Gorman, F. (1984) Lethal non-pulmonary anomalies associated with congenital diaphragmatic hernia: implications for early intrauterine surgery. *Journal of Pediatric Surgery* **19**, 29–32.

124 Raphaely, R.C., Downes, J.J. (1973) Congenital diaphragmatic hernia: prediction of survival. *Journal of Pediatric Surgery* **8**, 815–823.

125 Redmond, C., Haton, J., Calix, J. *et al.* (1987) A correlation of pulmonary hypoplasia, mean airway pressure and survival in congenital diaphragmatic hernia treated with extracorporeal membrane oxygenation. *Journal of Pediatric Surgery* **22**, 1143–1149.

126 Reid, I.S., Hutcherson, R.J. (1976) Long term follow-up of patients with congenital diaphragmatic hernia. *Journal of Pediatric Surgery* **11**, 939.

127 Robertson, C.M., Cheung, P.Y., Haluschak, M.M. *et al.* (1998) High prevalence of sensorineural hearing loss among survivors of neonatal congenital diaphragmatic hernia. Western Canadian ECMO Follow-up Group. *American Journal of Otology* **19**, 730–736.

128 Rodgers, B.M., Hawks, P. (1986) Bilateral congenital eventration of the diaphragm: successful surgical management. *Journal of Pediatric Surgery* **21**, 858–864.

129 Rowe, M.I., Smith, D.S., Chev, H. (1988) Inappropriate fluid response in congenital diaphragmatic hernia: first report of a frequent occurrence. *Journal of Pediatric Surgery* **23**, 1147–1157.

130 Roy, D.V., Pattison, C.W., Townsend, E.R. (1988) Splenic herniation. Case report. *Scandinavian Journal of Thoracic and Cardiovascular Surgery* **22**, 83–85.

131 Ryan, C.A., Finer, N.N., Phillips, H., Ainsworth, W. (1995) Radiological decompression of bowel gas and return of mediastinal shift in congenital diaphragmatic hernia: a signal for surgical repair? *Journal of Pediatric Surgery* **30**, 538–542.

132 Saifuddin, A., Arthur, R. (1993) Congenital diaphragmatic hernia – a review of pre- and postoperative chest radiology. *Clinical Radiology* **47**, 104–110.

133 Sakai, H., Tamura, M., Hosokawa, Y. *et al.* (1987) Effect of surgical repair on respiratory mechanics in congenital diaphragmatic hernia. *Journal of Pediatrics* **111**, 432–438.

134 Schnitzer, J.J., Hedrick, H.L., Pacheco, B.A. *et al.* (1996) Prenatal glucocorticoid therapy reverses pulmonary immaturity in congenital diaphragmatic hernia in fetal sheep. *Annals of Surgery* **224**, 430–439.

135 Schumacher, R.E., Farrell, P.M. (1985) Congenital diaphragmatic hernia. A major remaining challenge in neonatal respiratory care. *Perinatology Neonatology* **9**, 29.

136 Sharland, G.K., Lockhart, S.M., Heward, A.J., Allan, L.D. (1992) Prognosis in fetal diaphragmatic hernia. *American Journal of Obstetrics and Gynecology* **166**, 9–13.

137 Shehata, S.M.K., Mooi, W.J., Okazaki, T. *et al.* (1999) Enhanced expression of vascular endothelial growth factor in lungs of newborn infants with congenital diaphragmatic hernia and pulmonary hypertension. *Thorax* **54**, 427–431.

138 Shehata, S.M.K., Sharma, H.S., van der Staak, F.H. *et al.* (2000) Remodeling of pulmonary arteries in human congenital diaphragmatic hernia with or without extracorporeal membrane oxygenation. *Journal of Pediatric Surgery* **35**, 208–215.

139 Sigalet, D.L., Nguyen, L.T., Adolph, V. *et al.* (1994) Gastroesophageal reflux associated with large diaphragmatic hernias. *Journal of Pediatric Surgery* **29**, 1262–1265.

140 Simson, J.N.L., Eckstein, H.B. (1985) Congenital diaphragmatic hernia: a 20-year experience. *British Journal of Surgery* **72**, 733–736.

141 Skari, H., Bjornland, K., Haugen, G. *et al.* (2000) Congenital diaphragmatic hernia: a meta-analysis of mortality factors. *Journal of Pediatric Surgery* **35**, 1187–1197.

142 Skarsgard, E.D., Meuli, M., VanderWall, K.J. *et al.* (1996) Fetal endoscopic tracheal occlusion ('Fetendo-PLUG') for congenital diaphragmatic hernia. *Journal of Pediatric Surgery* **31**, 1335–1338.

143 Stolar, C., Dillon, P., Reyes, C. (1988) Selective use of extracorporeal membrane oxygenation in the management of congenital diaphragmatic hernia. *Journal of Pediatric Surgery* **23**, 207–211.

144 Stolar, C.J.H. (1996) What do survivors of congenital diaphragmatic hernia look like when they grow up? *Seminars in Pediatric Surgery* **5**, 275–279.

145 Stolar, C.J.H., Crisafi, M.A., Driscoll, Y.T. (1995) Neurocognitive outcome for neonates treated with extracorporeal membrane oxygenation: are infants with congenital diaphragmatic hernia different? *Journal of Pediatric Surgery* **30**, 366–372.

146 Stringel, G., Mercer, S., Bass, J. (1984) Surgical management of persistent chylothorax in children. *Canadian Journal of Surgery* **27**, 543–546.

147 Stringer, M.D., Goldstein, R.B., Filly, R.A. *et al.* (1995) Fetal diaphragmatic hernia without visceral herniation. *Journal of Pediatric Surgery* **30**, 1264–1266.

148 Suen, H.C., Bloch, K.D., Donahoe, P.K. (1994) Antenatal glucocorticoid corrects pulmonary immaturity in experimentally induced congenital diaphragmatic hernia in rats. *Pediatric Research* **35**, 523–529.

149 Sumner, E., Frank, J.D. (1981) Tolazoline in the treatment of congenital diaphragmatic hernias. *Archives of Disease in Childhood* **56**, 350–353.

150 Sweed, Y., Puri, P. (1993) Congenital diaphragmatic hernia: influence of associated malformations on survival. *Archives of Disease in Childhood* **69**, 68–70.

151 Tannuri, U., Maksoud-Filho, J.G., Santos, M.M. *et al.* (1998) The effects of prenatal intraamniotic surfactant or dexamethasone administration on lung development are comparable to changes induced by tracheal ligation in an animal model of congenital diaphragmatic hernia. *Journal of Pediatric Surgery* **33**, 1198–1205.

152 The Neonatal Inhaled Nitric Oxide Study Group (NINOS). (1997) Inhaled nitric oxide and hypoxic respiratory failure in infants with congenital diaphragmatic hernia. *Pediatrics* **99**, 838–845.

153 Thebaud, B., Mercier, J.-C., Dinh-Xuan, A.T. (1998) Congenital diaphragmatic hernia. A cause of persistent pulmonary hypertension of the newborn which lacks an effective therapy. *Biology of the Neonate* **74**, 323–336.

154 Thibeault, W.D., Haney, B. (1998) Lung volume, pulmonary vasculature and factors affecting survival in congenital diaphragmatic hernia. *Pediatrics* **101**, 289–295.

155 Thorpe-Beeston, J.G., Gosden, C.M., Nicolaides, K.H. (1989) Prenatal diagnosis of congenital diaphragmatic hernia: associated malformations and chromosomal defects. *Fetal Therapy* **4**, 21–28.

156 Thorup, J., Pedersen, P.V., Nielsen, O.H. (1986) Late return of function after intrathoracic torsion of the spleen in congenital diaphragmatic hernia. *Journal of Pediatric Surgery* **21**, 722–724.

157 Thurlbeck, W.M., Kida, K., Langston, C. *et al.* (1979) Postnatal lung growth after repair of diaphragmatic hernia. *Thorax* **34**, 338–343.

158 Tibboel, D., Gaag, A.V.D. (1996) Etiologic and genetic factors in congenital diaphragmatic hernia. *Clinics in Perinatology* **23**, 689–699.

159 Tracy, T.F., Bailey, P.V., Sadiq, F. *et al.* (1994) Predictive capabilities of preoperative and postoperative pulmonary function tests in delayed repair of congenital diaphragmatic hernia. *Journal of Pediatric Surgery* **29**, 265–270.

160 UK Collaborative ECMO Trial Group. (1996) UK collaborative randomized trial of neonatal extracorporeal membrane oxygenation. *Lancet* **348**, 75–82.

161 van Meurs, K.P., Robbins, S.T., Reed, V.L. *et al.* (1993) Congenital diaphragmatic hernia: long term outcome in neonates treated with extracorporeal membrane oxygenation. *Journal of Pediatrics* **122**, 893–899.

162 Wayne, E.R., Campbell, J.B., Burlington, J.D., Davis, W.S. (1974) Eventration of the diaphragm. *Journal of Pediatric Surgery* **9**, 643–651.

163 Whittle, M.J., Gilmore, D.H., McNay, M.B. *et al.* (1989) Diaphragmatic hernia presenting in utero as a unilateral hydrothorax. *Prenatal Diagnosis* **9**, 115–118.

164 Wiener, E., Owens, L., Salzberg, A. (1973) Chylothorax after Bochdalek herniorrhaphy in a neonate. *Journal of Thoracic and Cardiovascular Surgery* **65**, 200–205.

165 Wilcox, D.T., Glick, P.L., Karamanoukian, H.L. *et al.* (1995) Perfluorocarbon associated gas exchange improves pulmonary mechanics, oxygenation, ventilation and allows nitric oxide delivery in the hypoplastic lung congenital diaphragmatic hernia lung model. *Critical Care Medicine* **23**, 1858–1863.

166 Wilcox, D.T., Glick, P.L., Karamanoukian, H.L. *et al.* (1997) Partial liquid ventilation and nitric oxide in congenital diaphragmatic hernia. *Journal of Pediatric Surgery* **32**, 1211–1215.

167 Williams, O., Greenough, A., Rafferty, G.F. (2003) Extubation failure due to phrenic nerve injury. *Archives of Disease in Childhood* **88**, F72–73.

168 Wilson, J.M., Lund, D.P., Lillehei, C.W. *et al.* (1992) Delayed repair and preoperative ECMO does not improve survival in high-risk congenital diaphragmatic hernia. *Journal of Pediatric Surgery* **27**, 368–375.

169 Wilson, J.M., Thompson, J.R., Schnitzer, J.J. *et al.* (1993) Intratracheal pulmonary ventilation and congenital diaphragmatic hernia: a report of two cases. *Journal of Pediatric Surgery* **28**, 484–487.

170 Wohl, M.E.B., Griscom, N.T., Streidel, D.J. *et al.* (1977) The lung following repair of congenital diaphragmatic hernia. *Journal of Pediatric Surgery* **90**, 405–414.

171 Wung, J.T., Sahni, R., Moffitt, S.T. *et al.* (1995) Congenital diaphragmatic hernia: survival treated with very delayed surgery, spontaneous respiration and no chest tube. *Journal of Pediatric Surgery* **30**, 406–409.

172 Zaccara, A., Turchetta, A., Calzolari, A. *et al.* (1996) Maximal oxygen consumption and stress performance in children operated on for congenital diaphragmatic hernia. *Journal of Pediatric Surgery* **31**, 1092–1095.

173 Zhang, S., Garbutt, V., McBride, J.D.T. (1996) Strain-induced growth of the immature lung. *Journal of Applied Physiology* **86**, 1471–1476.

Abnormalities of the skeleton

ANNE GREENOUGH

Skeletal disorders may present with neonatal respiratory distress, which is usually lethal. Respiratory distress results from abnormal lung growth due to restriction by limited rib growth (osteochondrodysplasias), upper airway obstruction (diastrophic dysplasia) and/or abnormal bone, cartilage or collagen development leading to a small or abnormal thoracic cage (hypophosphatasia, achondrogenesis and osteogenesis imperfecta) (Tables 35.1 and 35.2). Rarely, 'localized' severe sternal or vertebral anomalies can so alter the structure of the thoracic cage as to impair lung function.

ANTENATAL ASSESSMENT OF THE THORAX IN SKELETAL DYSPLASIA

Measurement of the size of the thoracic cage using ultrasound is particularly important in the evaluation of any fetus with a skeletal dysplasia, as the outcome of affected infants with a small thorax is extremely poor. Thoracic dimensions can be quantified by measuring the circumference of the thorax at the level of the four chamber view of the heart. Nomograms have been developed relating thoracic circumference to gestational age (p. 451). The dysplasias in which marked limb shortening is associated with a small thorax include achondroplasia, achondrogenesis, congenital hypophosphatasia, asphyxiating thoracic dystrophy, short rib-polydactyly syndromes and 'congenital' forms of osteogenesis imperfecta.[29] All except asphyxiating thoracic dystrophy (ATD) are lethal in the neonatal period.

Sharony et al.[49] examined the accuracy of prenatal diagnosis of skeletal dysplasias in a total of 226 fetuses and

Table 35.1 *Skeletal abnormalities associated with polydactyly or syndactyly*

	Other features	Inheritance
Asphyxiating thoracic dystrophy	Bell-shaped chest Short ribs	Autosomal recessive
Ellis and van Creveld	Small thorax Cardiac defects Nail hypoplasia	Autosomal recessive
Short rib syndrome:		
Saldino and Noonan (type 1)	Narrow thorax Cardiac defects Polycystic kidneys	Autosomal recessive
Majewski (type 2)	Narrow thorax Short limbs Cleft lip and palate	Autosomal recessive

stillbirths referred because of suspected skeletal dysplasia. Only 15 of the 226 cases (7 percent) did not have a skeletal dysplasia or an obvious dysmorphic syndrome. The majority of cases were sporadic. Forty-six percent of the cases were detected by routine ultrasonography between 16 and 24 weeks of gestation, 30 percent because of pregnancy complications and 18 percent because of a family history. Intrauterine radiographs were helpful in making a specific diagnosis and differentiating between lethal and non-lethal disorders. The most common final diagnosis was osteogenesis imperfecta and the most accurately diagnosed abnormality was thanatophoric dwarfism. Heterozygous achondroplasia, however, is the most common type of neonatal skeletal dysplasia. It is not diagnosable before

Table 35.2 *Skeletal abnormalities associated with short limbs*

	Other features	Inheritance
Very short limbs		
Thanatophoric dwarfism	Narrow thorax	?recessive
	Large head	?spontaneous
	Cardiac defects	
Short rib syndrome	Small chest	Autosomal recessive
Type I	Narrow thorax	Autosomal recessive
Type II	Cleft lip and palate	Autosomal recessive
	Polydactyly	
Diastrophic dysplasia problems	Upper airway including cleft palate, kyphoscoliosis, talipes	Autosomal recessive
Hypophosphatasia	Small stature	Autosomal recessive
	Short ribs	
	↓alkaline phosphatase	
Achondrogenesis	Small stature	Autosomal recessive
	Large cranium	
	Under-ossification of skeletal structure	
Osteogenesis imperfecta	Blue sclerae	Autosomal recessive
	Multiple fractures	
Moderately short limbs		
Ellis and van Creveld	Small thorax	Autosomal recessive
	Cardiac defects	
	Polydactyly	
Achondroplasia	Small chest	Autosomal dominant
	Large head	
	Short trident hand	
Camptomelic dysplasia	Small chest	Autosomal recessive
	Large head	
	Bowed long bones	

24 weeks of pregnancy, the mothers usually have a normal pregnancy[11,28] and it is not associated with perinatal death.

OSTEOCHONDRODYSPLASIAS

In these conditions, neonatal respiratory distress is primarily due to limited rib growth which drastically reduces intrathoracic volume. The prevalence at birth has been estimated to be between 2.29 and 4.7 per 10 000.[4,18,41,57]

Asphyxiating thoracic dystrophy (ATD)

ATD, first described by Jeune,[26] is the most common of the small chest syndromes. This generalized chondrodystrophy mainly affects the thoracic cage, producing a small bell-shaped thorax. Associated anomalies include polydactyly, abnormal dentition, hypoplasia of the abdominal wall muscles and renal abnormalities such as cystic tubular dysplasia and/or glomerular sclerosis.[22] It is inherited as an autosomal recessive.

CLINICAL SIGNS

The majority of affected children have symptoms from birth. Many patients will require respiratory support from birth, frequently at very high peak inflating pressures and inspired oxygen concentrations. Sadly, those babies frequently die in the early neonatal period or require long-term respiratory support, often including tracheostomy and ventilation. Those less severely affected may die in the first year of life of respiratory failure often brought about by a relatively trivial infection. Chronic nephritis leading to renal failure can occur. Although renal insufficiency may be evident by 2 years of age, survival to the fourth decade has occurred.

DIFFERENTIAL DIAGNOSIS

The short long bones, the square iliac bones and underdeveloped bones may be confused with achondroplasia, thanatophoric dwarfism or achondrogenesis, but in the latter conditions the long bones are shorter and more abnormal in appearance. In addition, in ATD the upper ends of the femur do not have the same bulbous appearance as is found in achondroplasia. Further distinguishing features are the premature appearance of the proximal femoral epiphysis in ATD and that the development of the vertebral bodies and spinal canal are normal. In other conditions mentioned above, there can be foramen magnum constriction, underdevelopment of the vertebral bodies and narrowing of the spinal canal.

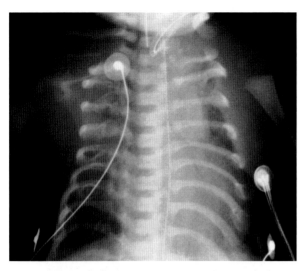

Figure 35.1 *Asphyxiating thoracic dystrophy. Classical short ribs with resultant narrowing of both transverse horizontal and posterior axes of the chest; underlying pulmonary hypoplasia is present.*

Thoracic dysplasia in an isolated form, similar to that seen in ATD, has been documented;[43] this may represent a simple variant or a different entity.

DIAGNOSIS

Prenatal diagnosis using ultrasonography has been successfully accomplished at 18 weeks of gestation.[8]

Radiology

The ribs are short with flared and irregular costochondral junctions (Figure 35.1). The limbs may be shortened. There are wide irregular metaphyses of the long bones and often a pyriform deformity of the epiphyses of the short tubular bones. There are hypoplastic iliac wings and horizontal acetabular roofs with spur-like projections at the lower margins of the sciatic notches. There is early ossification of the capital femoral epiphysis.

MANAGEMENT

A variety of maneuvers have been attempted to increase the chest wall dimensions and allow for lung expansion. Bone grafts were used to increase the size of the thoracic cage in one child.[2] Acrylic prostheses have also been used for the same purpose.[60] Others have favored long-term continuous positive airway pressure via a tracheostomy.[64] Portable systems of supplying positive end expiratory pressure have been designed to facilitate long-term management.[7]

PROGNOSIS

The prognosis is better if the child survives the first year of life, providing there is no associated severe renal disease.[39] Only a proportion of affected children have abnormal lung growth. Several children dying in early childhood of renal failure have been demonstrated to have normal lungs.[39,65]

Ellis and van Creveld syndrome

Ellis and van Creveld described infants with small stature of prenatal onset.[10] Characteristic features are short distal extremities, ectodermal dysplasia, polydactyly and nail hypoplasia. The patients have a small thorax and half have a cardiac defect, commonly an atrial septal defect. The syndrome is inherited as an autosomal recessive.

DIFFERENTIAL DIAGNOSIS

The form of Ellis and van Creveld syndrome which presents in the neonatal period has skeletal abnormalities similar to those seen in asphyxiating dystrophy. The conditions can, however, be differentiated as the polydactyly is on the medial (ulnar) side of the hand in Ellis and van Creveld syndrome, but on the lateral (radial) in asphyxiating dystrophy. Congenital heart disease is a more consistent finding in Ellis and van Creveld syndrome than in ATD, but the thoracic cage deformity is more pronounced in the latter disorder.

DIAGNOSIS

The small thorax, short limbs, polydactyly and congenital heart disease detected by ultrasonography are strongly suggestive of the diagnosis.

PROGNOSIS

Approximately half of affected patients die in early infancy as a consequence of cardiorespiratory problems. The majority of survivors are of normal intelligence; eventual stature is in the region of 43–60 inches. There is usually some limitation of hand function and dental problems are frequent.

Blomstrand chondrodysplasia

The main findings in this lethal osteochondrodysplasia are osteosclerosis and advanced skeletal maturation.[13] The chest is very short and narrow and there is pulmonary hypoplasia. Aortic coarctation is also frequently found. Autosomal recessive inheritance has been proposed because of parental consanguinity of affected children in all reported cases.

DIAGNOSIS

There is craniofacial disproportion, a short base of the skull and severe mandibular hypoplasia. The ribs are shortened with diffuse widening and exaggerated thickening at their anterior ends. The vertebral bodies are small and dense, with notches on the superior and inferior faces. The long bones are severely shortened (micromelia). The histopathological finding of advanced skeletal maturation corroborates the radiological findings.

Achondroplasia

Achondroplasia is the most common chondrodysplasia with a frequency of 1 in 26 000. It is inherited as an autosomal dominant; approximately 90 percent of cases are fresh mutations. Older paternal age has been a contribution in fresh mutations.

PATHOLOGY

Histological evaluation at the epiphyseal line discloses shorter cartilage columns which lack the usual linear arrangement and some cartilage cells appear to be undergoing a mucinoid degeneration.

CLINICAL SIGNS

It can cause respiratory distress in the neonatal period.[1,24] Respiratory problems are secondary to a small chest and upper airway obstruction which may cause sleep-disordered breathing. Apnea secondary to cervical spinal cord and lower brainstem compression can occur.[56] Affected patients have short trident hands (their fingers being similar in length), mild hypotonia and hydrocephalus secondary to a narrow foramen magnum.[19]

DIAGNOSIS

Antenatal
Although the femoral length may be within the normal range during the second trimester, the ratio between femur and biparietal diameter is predictive.[28]

Radiology
There are small, cuboid-shaped vertebral bodies with short pedicles. There may be lumbar lordosis, narrowed spinal canal, mild thoracolumbar kyphosis with anterior breaking of the first and/or second lumbar vertebra, small iliac wings and short tubular bones (Figure 35.2). The extremities are characteristically short and there is marked flaring of the metaphyses. The skull is enlarged with underdevelopment of the bone, frontal and biparietal bossing.

MANAGEMENT

Early sitting and walking should be avoided as the large head presents an excessive load onto the hypotonic spine.[51] Exercises may help to flatten the lumbosacral curve. Mandibular teeth may need to be removed because of overcrowding.

PROGNOSIS

Neurological complications occur due to spinal cord and/or root compression associated with disk compression, kyphosis or stenosis of the spinal canal. Approximately 46 percent of patients have spinal complications. The mean adult height is 131 cm in males and 124 cm in

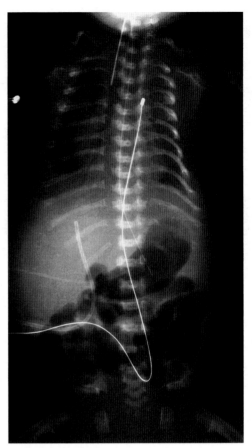

Figure 35.2 *First child of two unrelated adults, both with achondroplasia. Note the narrow chest and short ribs. Umbilical artery catheter and umbilical venous catheter are present, both in non-optimum positions.*

females. Osteoarthritis occurs in adults. Short Eustachian tubes lead to middle ear infection.

Thanatophoric dwarfism

Thanatophoric dwarfism, a chondrodystrophy, is a severe form of achondroplasia. The inheritance of the condition is uncertain; it may be recessive or a spontaneous mutation. The incidence appears to be about one in 64 000.

CLINICAL SIGNS

Affected children have very short limbs and a narrow thorax (Figure 35.3). Feeble fetal activity and/or polyhydramnios are frequently described. There is severe growth deficiency with a large cranium. The infants are hypotonic and may have hydrocephalus, patent ductus arteriosus, atrial septal defect, hydronephrosis, imperforate anus and radioulnar synostosis.

DIAGNOSIS

Antenatal
Polyhydramnios, beginning in the second trimester, is a frequent finding.[42] The most prominent findings are

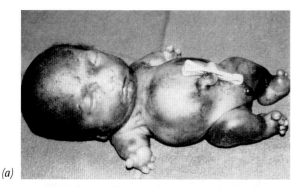

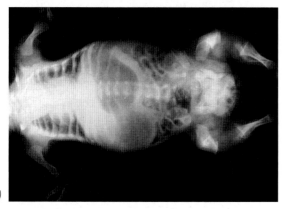

(a)

(b)

Figure 35.3 *Thanatophoric dwarfism. (a) Note the large head, small thorax and very short limbs. (b) Abnormal bell-shaped chest, vertebral bodies and abnormal long bones.*

shortening of long bones, bowed femurs and severe thoracic hypoplasia with redundant soft tissues. A cloverleaf skull is found in 11 percent of cases.[25]

Radiology
The infants have short fingers, bowed long bones, narrow short ribs and underdeveloped, very flat vertebrae.

PROGNOSIS

Death from respiratory failure occurs at delivery or usually within a few hours, although one infant survived for 26 days[40] and a second for 10 weeks.[36]

Camptomelic dysplasia

Infants have bowed tibiae, hypoplastic scapulae and flattened facies.[53] They have a small chest with slender and/or decreased number of ribs and kyphoscoliosis. They are short, with a large head, hydrocephalus and the olfactory tract is absent. Tracheobronchial cartilage underdevelopment can lead to respiratory distress.[33] Inheritance is autosomal recessive.

DIAGNOSIS

Antenatal
Bowing of the long bones can be detected ultrasonographically.[66]

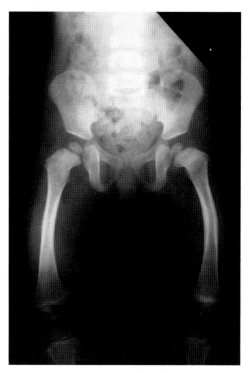

Figure 35.4 *Camptomelic dwarfism. Note the bowed femurs.*

Radiology
The characteristic feature is the multiple bowing abnormalities of the long bones (Figure 35.4).[58] The bones may be of normal length or shortened and fatter than usual. Widening of the interpedicular space in the upper lumbar region and hypoplasia of the lower cervical spine have also been noted.

PROGNOSIS

The majority die in the neonatal period because of respiratory insufficiency. If they survive the neonatal period, they have feeding problems, failure to thrive and evidence of serious central nervous system deficiency including apneic spells. A 17-year-old with the condition has been reported.

Jarcho–Levin syndrome

Spondylothoracic or spondylocostal dysostosis is a rare entity with variable clinical severity. It has been variously termed costovertebral dysplasia, spondylothoracic dysostosis and occipito-facial-cervico-thoracic-abdomino-digital syndrome. Inheritance is autosomal recessive with an increased incidence in Puerto Ricans.[67] It is a rare form of short-limbed dwarfism characterized by extensive vertebral and chest wall abnormalities. Patients are of short stature, with neck and thoracic cage deformities and multiple vertebral anomalies at all levels including butterfly vertebrae, hemivertebrae and fused hypoplastic vertebrae (Figures 35.2 and 35.5). The small size of the thorax in

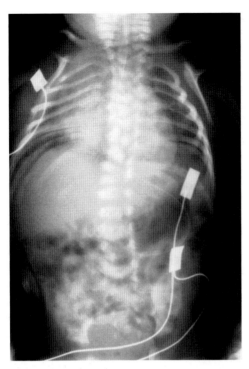

Figure 35.5 *Jarcho–Levin syndrome. Note the abnormal vertebrae and the crowded ribs on the right side of the thorax.*

newborns often leads to fatal respiratory compromise. Associated anomalies include severe cardiomyopathy[61] and cardiac abnormalities,[50] including aortic root dilatation.[14]

DIFFERENTIAL DIAGNOSIS

Spondylocostal dysostosis (COVESDEM; costo-vertebral segmentation defect with mesomelia) syndrome.

DIAGNOSIS

Prenatal diagnosis

This condition has been detected as early as 12 weeks of gestation in a family known to carry the disease.[9] Prenatal sonography demonstrates fanned-out ribs from fused vertebral bodies. Other abnormalities include neural tube defects, Arnold–Chiari malformations and urinary tract malformations.

Radiology

Radiology shows severe vertebral anomalies, hemivertebrae (Figure 35.5) neural arches, missing vertebral bodies, fan-shaped appearance of the ribs in the posteroanterior direction with posterior convergence of the ribs.

PROGNOSIS

Restrictive lung disease is usually the cause of early death, although survivors into adulthood have been described.[21,50] Aggressive neonatal care facilitated by antenatal diagnosis

has been claimed to lead to an excellent outcome.[32] It has been suggested, however, that the spinal abnormalities may not be as benign as previously reported. Sagittal, as well as frontal, plane deformities may exist secondary to multiple hemivertebrae and spinal fusion may be required to effect spinal stabilization.[37] A 61-year-old woman with Jarcho–Levin syndrome who underwent corrective surgery for an atrial septal defect and anomalous pulmonary venous return has been reported.[50]

SHORT RIBS (TABLE 35.3)

Saldino and Noonan syndrome[48]

This is short rib syndrome type I with or without polydactyly. There may be cardiac defects including transposition of the great vessels, double outlet left ventricle, endocardial cushion defect and hypoplastic right heart. Polycystic kidneys and imperforate anus may also occur. It is inherited as an autosomal recessive.

RADIOLOGY

Infants have short horizontal ribs, notch-like ossification defects around the periphery of the vertebral bodies. There are short limbs, short stature, polydactyly and syndactyly.

PROGNOSIS

Death from respiratory insufficiency secondary to pulmonary hypoplasia occurs in all infants within the first few hours after birth.

Majewski syndrome

Majewski *et al.*[35] described four infants with short-limbed dwarfism who died soon after birth because of respiratory insufficiency due to pulmonary hypoplasia. This is also called short rib syndrome type II and may be associated with polydactyly (Figure 35.6). Infants have a narrow thorax, short horizontal ribs and high clavicles. They suffer from short stature with disproportionately short limbs. Associated abnormalities include ambiguous genitalia, hypoplasia of the epiglottis and larynx, multiple glomerular cysts and focal dilation of the distal tubules of the kidney, midline cleft lip, cleft palate, low-set, small malformed ears, polydactyly, disproportionately short oval-shaped tibiae. Inheritance is autosomal recessive.

Other short rib skeletal dysplasias

There are at least 24 syndromes characterized by a combination of short ribs and micromelia, approximately half of which are lethal.[52]

Table 35.3 *Skeletal 'conditions' associated with rib abnormalities*

Skeletal condition	Features	Inheritance
Asphyxiating thoracic dystrophy	Bell-shaped chest, short ribs, nephritis or nephropathy	Autosomal recessive
Ellis and van Creveld syndrome	Small thorax, polydactyly or syndactyly, cardiac defects	Autosomal recessive
Jarcho–Levin syndrome	Small thorax, multiple vertebral anomalies, cardiomyopathy, neural tube defects, renal malformations	Autosomal recessive
Short rib syndrome		
Type I (Saldino and Noonan)	Narrow thorax, cardiac defects, polycystic kidneys	Autosomal recessive
Type II (Majewski)	Narrow thorax, short limbs, cleft lip and palate	Autosomal recessive
Thanatrophic dwarfism	Narrow thorax, large head, cardiac defects	Spontaneous
Hypophosphatasia	Small stature, short ribs	Autosomal recessive
Achondroplasia	Small chest, large head	Autosomal recessive
Osteogenesis imperfecta	Blue sclera, multiple rib fractures	Autosomal recessive

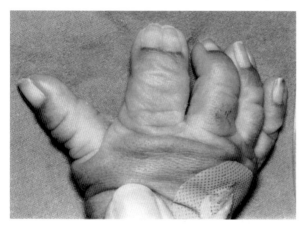

Figure 35.6 *Syndactyly of Majewski syndrome.*

DIASTROPHIC DYSPLASIA

Diastrophic dysplasia may be complicated by respiratory problems[30] due to upper respiratory obstruction, because of cleft palate and micrognathia or laryngeal stenosis. Infants are of short stature, there is scoliosis with or without kyphosis, talipes, limitation of flexion of the interphalangeal joints and dislocation of the hips. The first metacarpal is unduly small with a proximal thumb and there is variable webbing at joints. Ossification is generally delayed and disturbed in patients with diastrophic dysplasia; when ossifying nuclei do appear they show abnormal configuration with flattening and stippling.[46] Soft cystic masses in the auricle develop into hypertrophic cartilage in early infancy in 84 percent of patients. It is inherited as an autosomal recessive.

Radiology

Characteristic abnormalities include short bones, particularly the thumb and an almost oval first metacarpal. The long bones are flared and dislocation of the radial heads and hips can occur in infancy.[6] In older patients the manubrium appears as an asymmetrical club.[46] There is delayed appearance of epiphysis in long bones and deformed hip joints.[62]

Prognosis

The mortality in early infancy is as high as 25 percent.

HYPOPHOSPHATASIA

Hypophosphatasia is characterized by small stature, a poorly mineralized cranium (Figure 35.7a) and hypoplastic fragile bones (Figure 35.7b). Patients have short ribs with a rachitic rosary and small thoracic cage. The disease is a consequence of severe deficiency of tissue and serum alkaline phosphatase and as a consequence normal bone mineralization does not take place. It has an autosomal recessive inheritance.

Diagnosis

ANTENATAL

This can be made by an alkaline phosphatase assay on a chorion villus sampling specimen taken during the first trimester.

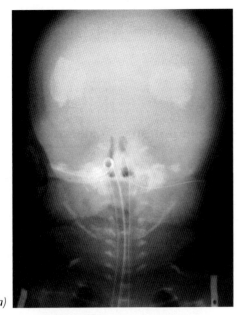

(a)

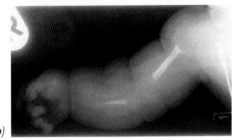

(b)

Figure 35.7 *Hypophosphatasia. Classical radiological appearance of osteopenia with irregular metaphyseal defects: (a) defective mineralization of the skull vault; (b) affecting the radius, ulnar and humerus.*

POSTNATAL

Affected infants have a low alkaline phosphatase in the blood and a raised phosphoethanolamine in the urine.

Radiology

The bones are extremely poorly ossified and pathological fractures are common. There is excessive wormian bone formation. There is defective mineralization of the skull vault, sutural widening occurs consequent to the poor mineralization, craniosynositosis may develop.

Prognosis

Death secondary to respiratory insufficiency during early infancy is usual.

ACHONDROGENESIS

Achondrogenesis (types 1a and 1b) are due to a severe defect in the development of cartilage and bone. Infants have small stature, large cranium for gestational age and severe micromelia. The skull vertebral bodies are poorly ossified and the ribs are extremely short. Multiple fractures occur in type 1a, but not 1b. It is inherited as an autosomal recessive.

Diagnosis

ANTENATAL

The most typical ultrasonographic findings are micromelia and extreme thoracic hypoplasia in association with absence of vertebral body ossification.[42] There may also be polyhydramnios and hydrops.

POSTNATAL
Radiology
There is absence of vertebral body ossification. This may affect just the lower regions of the spine but often is extensive.

Prognosis

It is a lethal disorder. Infants are stillborn or die shortly after birth due to pulmonary hypoplasia resulting from the restricted thoracic cavity.

OSTEOCHONDRODYSPLASIA WITH OSTEOPETROSIS

Cleidocranial dysostosis

This condition encompasses defects of the clavicle, late ossification of the cranial sutures and delayed eruption of the teeth. Partial to complete aplasia of the clavicle with associated muscle defects and a small thorax with short oblique ribs may lead to respiratory distress in early infancy. It usually has an autosomal dominant inheritance.

CONNECTIVE TISSUE DISORDERS

Osteogenesis imperfecta type II

This disease is characterized by short limbs, short, broad long bones, radiological evidence of severe osseous fragility and defective ossification. There is prenatal short-limbed growth deficiency, poorly mineralized soft calvarium with large fontanelles and multiple wormian bones. The infants have deep blue sclerae, short thick long bones with multiple fractures, flattened vertebrae, hypotonia and hydrops. In 90 percent of cases an abnormal type I collagen molecule is found. This condition is likely to represent the sporadic mutation of a dominant gene with a recurrence risk of 6 percent. Occasional cases are inherited as autosomal recessive.

DIAGNOSIS

Antenatal
Ultrasonography demonstrates long bone deformities.[23]

Radiology
The entire skeleton is affected, the diaphyses of the long bones are thin and fragile. There may be multiple intra-uterine fractures with prenatal bowing.

PROGNOSIS

Infants are stillborn or die in early infancy of respiratory failure.

STERNAL DEFECTS

Pectus excavatum

This is the most common sternal defect, perhaps occurring in one in 300 births.[44] It is sometimes associated with the Pierre Robin, Marfan or Turner syndromes. It is extremely rare for severe deformity to occur until at least several months of age. In one series,[63] 37 percent of patients had a positive family history of some type of anterior thoracic deformity, with or without scoliosis. The deformity involves the anterior wall below the angle of Louis, the first and second ribs; corresponding costal cartilages and manubrium are essentially normal. In response to some unknown stimulus, the lower cartilages grow too rapidly, a concave deformity ensues and the lower sternal segments are forced inward.[63]

MANAGEMENT

Operative correction is only necessary if the deformity is progressing as documented by serial photography, electrocardiogram, echocardiography and pulmonary function tests. Although the results of operative correction are excellent, in more than 80 percent of patients, recurrences are possible during later active growth.

Sternal clefts

Clefts of the sternum vary from minor separation to complete diastasis of the paired right and left sternebral growth. The most dramatic cases involve incomplete ingrowth of all precordial soft tissues. Lower sternal clefts are associated with defects of the abdominal wall (exomphalos), ventral diaphragm, pericardium and heart (usually Fallot's tetralogy) (pentalogy of Cantrell).

'DOUBLE-LAYERED' MANUBRIUM

The manubrium sterni is abnormal in almost all patients with diastrophic dysplasia (p. 511). The majority have accessory ossification centers, usually located ventral to the central part of the manubrium (a double-layered manubrium).[46] In older patients, the manubrium bulges forward, resembling an asymmetric club.

RIB DEFECTS (TABLE 35.3)

Abnormal rib configuration

Abnormal rib configuration may be associated with pulmonary hypoplasia. This particularly occurs in ATD (p. 506), but some infants with isolated rib abnormalities (Figures 35.8 and 35.9) can also be affected.

Poland's syndrome

Poland's syndrome (Figure 35.10) consists of unilateral deficiency of the second to fourth ribs, absence of pectoralis minor, the costal portion of pectoralis major and the breast. The condition is evident from birth, but is only associated with mild paradoxical breathing and visible cardiac pulsation.

Trauma

The ribs can be damaged prior to birth if an invasive procedure is performed. Thoracoamniotic shunt insertion is perhaps the most common of such procedures and is performed to drain fetal pleural effusions,[38] relieving pressure on the ipsilateral lung and permitting lung growth.[3]

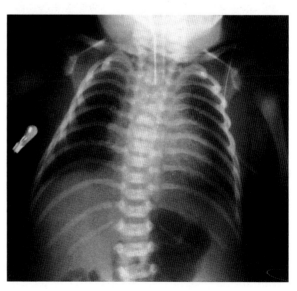

Figure 35.8 *Pulmonary hypoplasia associated with short ribs.*

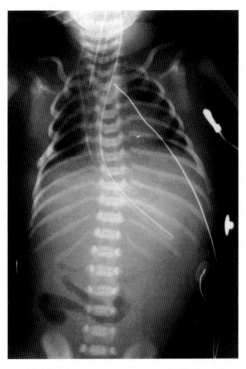

Figure 35.9 *Small volume lungs associated with abnormal ribs on the right.*

procedure can inflict permanent damage to the developing fetal rib bone and cartilage (Figure 35.11). Cardiac surgery performed early in infancy may cause similar problems (Figure 35.12). Rib fractures are occasionally seen as the result of birth trauma, but frequently go unnoticed until observation of a callus at a later date. If a number of ribs are fractured, however, the infant will exhibit respiratory difficulties at birth. Rib fractures are the commonest pathological fractures in patients with metabolic bone disease of prematurity[15] and then usually occur 4–8 weeks after birth; fractures of the distal ends of long bones may also occur.[27] Copper deficiency should be excluded.[59] Physiotherapy using a vibrating toothbrush can cause rib fractures in osteopenic infants.[68] The combination of respiratory distress, chronic chest abnormalities and rib fractures has been termed 'rachitic respiratory distress'.[16]

Metabolic bone disease

Metabolic bone disease in preterm infants is initially characterized by biochemical abnormalities and then reduced bone mineralization (Figure 35.13), which results in abnormal bone remodeling. In extreme forms, there is craniotabes and fractures of both ribs and the distal ends

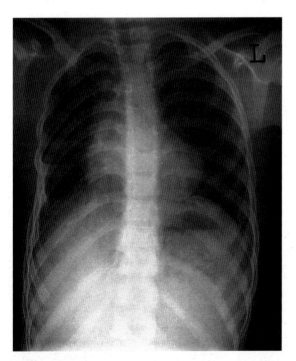

Figure 35.10 *Chest radiograph demonstrating an abnormal rib configuration affecting the right hemothorax. This skeletal abnormality is a recognized feature of Poland's syndrome. The infant also had an equilobar centrally placed liver.*

Rib formation and primary ossification commence at around 6 weeks of gestation, primary ossification ending at the fourth fetal month. Thus, as secondary ossification does not begin until adolescence,[31] an invasive antenatal

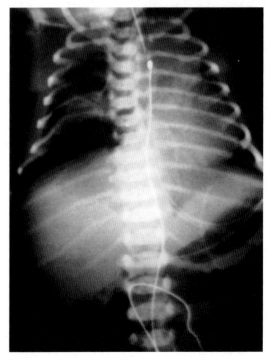

Figure 35.11 *Deformity of the fifth and sixth ribs resulting from insertion of a thoracoamniotic shunt to drain a pleural effusion associated with a congenital cystic adenomatoid malformation of the lung. (Reproduced with permission from Hannam, S., Greenough, A., Karani, J. (2000) Rib abnormalities arising before and after birth. European Journal of Pediatrics* **159**, *264–267. Copyright Springer-Verlag).*

of bones.[27] Preterm infants, regardless of their respiratory status, are severely undermineralized when compared to infants born at full term.[47,55] Anterior cupping of the ribs in preterm infants is often marked, but without other abnormalities should not be interpreted as due to rickets or bony dysplasias. Osteopenia has been reported as a complication of neonatal chronic lung disease,[54] although others have suggested that factors other than the presence or absence of chronic lung disease are responsible for the marked delays in bone mineralization in very low birthweight (VLBW) infants.[17] Pathological fractures can occur as a complication of chronic lung disease.

Intrauterine hypotonia

'Ribbon-like' or gracile ribs occur in conditions associated with generalized hypotonia due to a lack of intrauterine intercostal muscle contraction.[5] In both trisomies 13 and 18 gracile ribs can be found without evidence of underlying pulmonary hypoplasia.[45] In addition, in trisomy 18, frequently only 11 ribs are present. In congenital myotonic

dystrophy, the ribs are often initially thin and poorly mineralized (Figure 35.14), but this improves with increasing postnatal age.[12] Gracile ribs are also seen in myotubular myopathy (Figure 35.15). A similar appearance is sometimes noted in congenital hypothyroidism[5] and reflects a general immaturity of the skeleton. The ribs of very premature infants are often fragile with pronounced posterior thinning.

Multiple congenital abnormalities

Rib abnormalities can be associated with many other congenital abnormalities. Abnormal ribs in association with abnormal vertebrae (hemivertebra or butterfly vertebra) suggest the VATER syndrome (vertebral, anal, tracheal, esophageal and renal anomalies).

Miscellaneous syndromes with rib abnormalities

Rib hypoplasia can occur with partial or complete absence of the pectoralis major muscle and abnormalities of the upper extremity with or without dextrocardia (Poland's syndrome) (p. 513). Metaphyseal dysostosis – thymolymphopenia syndrome – and the related Schwachmann– Diamond syndrome, are also both associated with rib abnormalites. Radiological examination

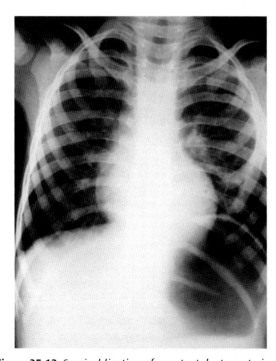

Figure 35.12 *Surgical ligation of a patent ductus arteriosus was performed at 3 weeks of age in an infant born at 25 weeks of gestation. At 3 years a swelling on his left anterior chest wall became more pronounced; the chest radiograph demonstrates the swelling was due to abnormal clustering of the third, fourth and fifth ribs on the left with abnormal development of the fifth rib. (Reproduced with permission from Hannam, S., Greenough, A., Karani, J. (2000) Rib abnormalities arising before and after birth.* European Journal of Pediatrics **159**, 264–267. Copyright Springer-Verlag.)

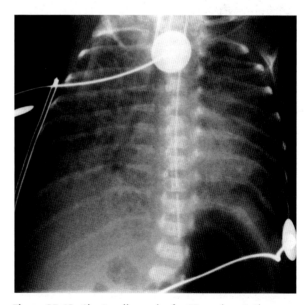

Figure 35.13 *Chest radiograph of a 32-week gestation infant demonstrating rib narrowing and severe osteopenia of prematurity. The infant had liver failure and associated malabsorption. (Reproduced with permission from Hannam, S., Greenough, A., Karani, J. (2000) Rib abnormalities arising before and after birth.* European Journal of Pediatrics **159**, 264–267. Copyright Springer-Verlag.)

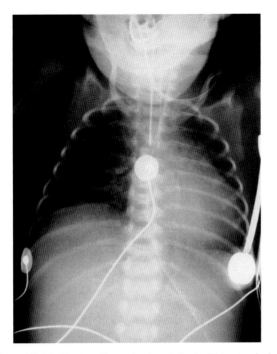

Figure 35.14 *Chest radiograph of an infant with congenital myotonic dystrophy. Note raised right hemidiaphragm. The infant required intubation at birth because of hypotonia and poor respiratory effort. Examination of the grandmother, aunt and mother revealed previously undetected features of myotonic dystrophy. (Reproduced with permission from Hannam, S., Greenough, A., Karani, J. (2000) Rib abnormalities arising before and after birth.* European Journal of Pediatrics *159, 264–267. Copyright Springer-Verlag.)*

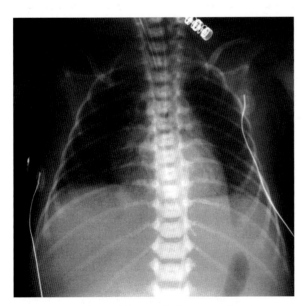

Figure 35.15 *Infant with myotubular myopathy who presented at birth with absent respiratory effort and lack of spontaneous respiratory effort. Note again the gracile ribs.*

in the former condition reveals rachitic-like bony changes resulting from metaphyseal dysplasia, with cupping and widening of the anterior ends of the ribs. In Schwachmann–Diamond syndrome the ribs are also short with pronounced cupping. A new type of lethal micromelic short rib skeletal dysplasia characterized by short limbs and distinctive triangular-shaped humeri has been reported in two brothers.[52]

Infection

Bacterial and viral bony infection rarely affects the ribs. In congenital syphilis; however, widespread involvement of the skeleton and ribs can occur.[34]

REFERENCES

1 Barnes, N.D., Glover, W.J., Hull, D., Milner, A.D. (1969) Effects of prolonged positive pressure ventilation in infancy. *Lancet* **2**, 1096–1099.

2 Barnes, N.D., Hull, D., Milner, A.D., Waterson, D.J. (1971) Chest reconstruction in thoracic dystrophy. *Archives of Disease in Childhood* **46**, 833–837.

3 Blott, M., Nicolaides, K.H., Greenough, A. (1988) Pleuroamniotic shunting for decompression of fetal pleural effusions. *Obstetrics and Gynecology* **71**, 798–800.

4 Camera, G., Mastroiacovo, P. (1982) Birth prevalence of skeletal dysplasias in the Italian Multicentric Monitoring System for Birth Defects. In Papadatos, C.J., Bartsocas, C.S. (eds), *Skeletal Dysplasias*. New York: Alan R Liss, 441–449.

5 Chassevent, J., Sauvegrain, J., Besson-Leaud, M., Kalifa, G. (1978) Myotonic dystrophy (Steinert's disease) in the neonate. *Radiology* **127**, 747–749.

6 Cremin, B.J., Jarrett, J. (1970) Diastrophic dwarfism. *Australasian Radiology* **14**, 84–87.

7 Eddes S., Moulden, A., Winter, R.J. (1992) Positive end expiratory pressure via a portable system in thoracic dystrophy. *Archives of Disease in Childhood* **67**, 136–137.

8 Elejalde, B.R., de Elejalde, M.M., Pausch, D. (1985) Prenatal diagnosis of Jeune syndrome. *American Journal of Medical Genetics* **21**, 433–438.

9 Eliyahu, S., Weiner, E., Lahau, D., Shalev, E. (1997) Early sonographic diagnosis of Jarcho-Levin syndrome: a prospective screening program in one family. *Ultrasound in Obstetrics and Gynecology* **9**, 314–318.

10 Ellis, R.W.B., van Creveld, S. (1940) A syndrome characterized by ectodermal dysplasia, polydactyly, chondro-dysplasia and congenital morbus cordis. Report of 3 cases. *Archives of Disease in Childhood* **15**, 65–84.

11 Filly, R.A., Golbus, M.S., Carey, J.C., Hall, J.G. (1981) Short-limbed dwarfism: ultrasonographic diagnosis by mensuration of fetal femoral length. *Radiology* **138**, 653–656.

12 Fried, K., Pajewski, M., Mundel, G. *et al.* (1975) Thin ribs in neonatal myotonic dystrophy. *Clinical Genetics* **7**, 417–420.

13 Galera, M.F., Patricio, F.R.S., Lederman, H.M. *et al.* (1999) Blomstrand chondrodysplasia: a lethal sclerosing skeletal dysplasia. *Pediatric Radiology* **29**, 842–845.

14 Galguera, M.A., Garcia, F.L., Bauza Rossi, J., Vazquez de Corral, L. (1997) Jarcho-Levin syndrome: a new case report

with unusual unexplained aortic root dilatation. *Boletin Asociacion Medica de Puerto Rico* **89**, 134–136.

15 Geggel, R.L., Pereira, G.R., Spackman, T.J. (1978) Fractured ribs: unusual presentation of rickets in premature infants. *Journal of Pediatrics* **93**, 680–682.

16 Glasgow, J.F., Thomas, P.S. (1977) Rachitic respiratory distress in small preterm infants. *Archives of Disease in Childhood* **52**, 268–273.

17 Green, F.R., McCormick, A. (1987) Bone mineral content and growth in very low birthweight premature infants. Does bronchopulmonary dysplasia make a difference? *American Journal of Diseases in Children* **141**, 179–183.

18 Gustavason, K.H., Jorulf, H. (1975) Different types of osteochondrodysplasia in a consecutive series of newborns. *Helvetica Paediatrica Acta* **30**, 307–314.

19 Hall, J.G., Horton, W., Kelly, T., Scott, C.I. (1982) Head growth in achondroplasia. Use of ultrasound studies. *American Journal of Medical Genetics* **13**, 105.

20 Hannam, S., Greenough, A., Karani, J. (2000) Rib abnormalities arising before and after birth. *European Journal of Pediatrics* **159**, 264–267.

21 Hayek, S., Burke, S.W., Boachie-Adjei, O., Bisson, L.J. (1999) Jarcho-Levin syndrome: report on a long-term follow-up of an untreated patient. *Journal of Pediatric Orthopaedics* **8**, 150–153.

22 Herdeman, R.C., Langer, L.O. (1968) The thoracic asphyxiant dystrophy and renal disease. *American Journal of Diseases in Children* **116**, 192–201.

23 Hobbins, J.C., Bracken, M.B., Mahoney, M.J. (1982) Diagnosis of fetal skeletal dysplasias with ultrasound. *American Journal of Obstetrics and Gynecology* **142**, 302–312.

24 Hull, D., Barnes, N.D. (1972) Children with small chests. *Archives of Disease in Childhood* **47**, 12–19.

25 Isaacson, G., Blakemore, K.J., Chervenak, F.A. (1983) Thanatophoric dysplasia with clover leaf skull. *American Journal of Diseases in Children* **137**, 896–898.

26 Jeune, M., Carron, R., Bernard, C., Loaec, Y. (1954) Polychondrodystrophie avec blocage thoracique d'evolution fatale. *Pediatrie* **9**, 390–397.

27 Koo, W.W., Sherman, R., Succop, P. *et al.* (1988) Sequential bone mineral content in small preterm infants with and without fractures and rickets. *Journal of Bone and Mineral Research* **3**, 193–197.

28 Kurtz, A.B., Filly, R.A., Wapner, R.J. *et al.* (1986) In utero analysis of heterozygous achondroplasia: variable time of onset as detected by femur length measurements. *Journal of Ultrasound in Medicine* **5**, 137–140.

29 Lachman, R.S., Rappaport, V. (1990) Fetal imaging in the skeletal dysplasias. *Clinics in Perinatology* **17**, 703–722.

30 Lamy, M., Maroteaux, P. (1960) Le nanisme diastrophique. *Presse Medicale* **68**, 1977–1980.

31 Larsen, W.J. (1993) *Human Embryology*. New York: Churchill Livingstone.

32 Lawson, M.E., Share, J., Benacerraf, B., Krauss, C.M. (1997) Jarcho-Levin syndrome: prenatal diagnosis, perinatal care and follow-up of siblings. *Journal of Perinatology* **17**, 407–409.

33 Lee, F.A., Isaacs, H., Straus, J. (1972) The camptomelic syndrome. *American Journal of Diseases in Children* **124**, 485–496.

34 Lilien, L.D., Harris, V.J., Pildes, R.S. (1977) Congenital syphilitic osteitis of scapulae and ribs. *Pediatric Radiology* **6**, 183–185.

35 Majewski, F., Pfeiffer, R.A., Lenz, W. *et al.* (1971) Polysyndaktylie, verkurzte Gliedmassen und Genitalfehlbildungen: Kennzeichen eines selbstandigen Syndroms [Polysyndactyly, short limbs, and genital

malformations – a new syndrome?]. [German]. *Zeitschrift fur Kinderheilkunde* **111**, 118–138.

36 Moir, D.H., Kozlowski, K. (1976) Survival in thanarophoric dwarfism. *Pediatric Radiology* **5**, 123–125.

37 Mooney, J.F.R., Emans, J.B. (1995) Progressive kyphosis and neurologic compromise complicating spondylothoracic dysplasia in infancy (Jarcho-Levin syndrome). *Spine* **20**, 1938–1942.

38 Nicolaides, K.H., Azar, G.B. (1990) Thoraco-amniotic shunting. *Fetal Diagnosis and Therapy* **5**, 153–164.

39 Oberklaid, F., Danks, D.M., Mayne, V., Campbell, P. (1970) Asphyxiating thoracic dysplasia. *Archives of Disease in Childhood* **52**, 758–765.

40 O'Mally, B.P., Parker, R., Saphyakhajon, P., Oizilbash, A.H. (1972) Thanatophoric dwarfs. *Journal of the Canadian Association of Radiologists* **23**, 62–69.

41 Orioli, I.M., Castilla, E.E., Barbosa-Neto, J.G. (1986) The birth prevalence rates for the skeletal dysplasias. *Journal of Medical Genetics* **23**, 328–332.

42 Pilu, G., Rizzio, N., Perolo, A. (1983) Anomalies of the skeletal system. In Chervenak, F.A., Isaacson, G.C., Campbell, S. (eds), *Ultrasound in Obstetrics and Gynecology*. Boston, MA: Little Brown and Company, 981–997.

43 Rabustika, S.E., Lowe, L., Kadison, H.I. (1973) Isolated thoracic dysotosis. *Radiology* **106**, 161–165.

44 Ravitch, M.M. (1977) *Congenital Deformities of the Chest Wall and their Operative Correction*. Philadelphia, PA: W.B. Saunders.

45 Reeder, M.M., Felson, B. (1975) Comprehensive lists of roentgen differential diagnosis. In Reeder, M.M., Felson, B. (eds), *Gamuts in Radiology*. Cincinnati: Audiovisual Radiology of Cincinnati Inc., Gamut D-114.

46 Remes, V.M., Helenius, I.J., Marttinen, E.J. (2001) Manubrium sterni in patients with diastrophic dysplasia – radiological analysis of 50 patients. *Pediatric Radiology* **31**, 555–558.

47 Ryan, S., Congdon, P.J., Horsman, A. *et al.* (1987) Bone mineral content in bronchopulmonary dysplasia. *Archives of Disease in Childhood* **62**, 889–894.

48 Saldino, R.M., Noonan, C.D. (1972) Severe thoracic dystrophy with striking micromelia, abnormal osseous development including the spine and multiple visceral anomalies. *American Journal of Roentgenology, Radium Therapy and Nuclear Medicine* **114**, 257–263.

49 Sharony, R., Browne, C., Lachman, R.S., Rimoin, D.L. (1993) Prenatal diagnosis of the skeletal dysplasias. *American Journal of Obstetrics and Gynecology* **169**, 668–675.

50 Shimizu, K., Arai, H., Sakamoto, T. *et al.* (1997) Jarcho-Levin syndrome associated with atrial septal defect and partial anomalous pulmonary venous return: a case report. *Journal of Cardiac Surgery* **12**, 198–200.

51 Siebens, A.A., Hungerford, D.S., Kirby, N.A. (1978) Curves of the achondroplastic spine: a new hypothesis. *Johns Hopkins Medical Journal* **142**, 205–210.

52 Slaney, S.F., Sprigg, A., Davies, N.P., Hall, C.M. (1999) Lethal micromelic short-rib skeletal dysplasia with triangular-shaped humerus. *Pediatric Radiology* **29**, 835–837.

53 Spranger, J., Langen, L.O., Maroteaux, P. (1970) Increasing frequency of a syndrome of multiple osseous defects? *Lancet* **2**, 716.

54 Steichen, J.J., Gratton, T.L., Tsang, R.C. (1980) Osteopenia of prematurity: the cause and possible treatment. *Journal of Pediatrics* **96**, 528–534.

55 Steichen, J.J., Asch, P.A., Tsang, R.C. (1988) Bone mineral content measurement in small infants by single photon absorptiometry: current methodological issues. *Journal of Pediatrics* **113**, 181–187.

56 Stokes, D.C., Phillips, J.A., Leonard, C.O. *et al.* (1983) Respiratory complications of achondroplasia. *Journal of Pediatrics* **102**, 534–541.

57 Stoll, C.B., Dott, B., Roth, M.-P., Alembik, Y. (1989) Birth prevalence rates of skeletal dysplasias. *Clinical Genetics* **42**, 199–217.

58 Storer, J., Grossman, H. (1974) The camptomelic syndrome. Congenital bowing of the limbs and other skeletal and extraskeletal anomalies. *Radiology* **111**, 673–681.

59 Thomas, P.S. (1977) Rib fractures in infancy. *Annals of Radiology* **20**, 115–122.

60 Todd, D.W., Tinguely, S.J., Norberg, W.J. (1986) A thoracic expansion technique for Jeune's asphyxiating thoracic dystrophy. *Journal of Pediatric Surgery* **21**, 161–163.

61 Ughi, M., Visco, G., Rubin, R. *et al.* (1998) Description of a case of spondylo-thoracic dysplasia or Jarcho-Levin syndrome. *Pediatria Medica e Chirurgica* **20**, 353–355.

62 Vaara, P., Peltonen, J., Poussa, M. *et al.* (1998) Development of the hip in diastrophic dysplasia. *Journal of Bone and Joint Surgery British Volume* **80**, 315–320.

63 Welch, K.J. (1980) Chest wall deformities. In Holder, T.M., Ashcraft, K.W. (eds), *Pediatric Surgery*. Philadelphia, PA: W.B. Saunders, 162–182.

64 Wiebicke, W., Pasterkamp, H. (1988) Long term continuous positive airway pressure in a child with asphyxiating thoracic dystrophy. *Pediatric Pulmonology* **4**, 54–58.

65 Williams, A.J., Vawter, G., Reid, L.M. (1984) Lung structure in asphyxiating thoracic dystrophy. *Archives of Pathology and Laboratory Medicine* **108**, 658–661.

66 Winter, R., Rosenkranz, W., Hoffmann, H. *et al.* (1985) Prenatal diagnosis of camptomelic dysplasia by ultrasonography. *Prenatal Diagnosis* **5**, 1–3.

67 Wong, G., Levine, D. (1998) Jarcho-Levin syndrome: two consecutive pregnancies in a Puerto Rican couple. *Ultrasound in Obstetrics and Gynecology* **12**, 70–73.

68 Wood, B.P. (1987) Infants ribs: generalized periosteal reaction resulting from vibrator chest physiotherapy. *Radiology* **162**, 811–812.

36

Respiratory problems of infants with neurological disease

JANET M RENNIE

Although the vast majority of ventilator days are occupied by infants suffering from RDS and its complications, perhaps 5–10 percent of the workload of a neonatal intensive care unit involves ventilating babies with normal lungs who have neurological disease. These infants are important not only because accurate diagnosis is vital in order to avoid iatrogenic lung injury from barotrauma, but also because, quite often, their neurological disease is incurable and their continued survival depends on long-term artificial ventilation. This creates ethical problems, which can be almost insurmountable. As well as this difficult group there are a small number of infants whose stridor or apnea is a manifestation of a CNS disorder. The respiratory manifestations of CNS disorders include apnea, stridor, respiratory failure and failure to wean from artificial ventilation. Neurological disease at any level within the CNS can cause respiratory problems, and it can be helpful to consider the cortex, brainstem, spinal cord, peripheral nervous system and muscle in a hierarchical system (Table 36.1).

CORTICAL DISORDERS CAUSING RESPIRATORY PROBLEMS

In the neonate, the two most common problems in this category are hypoxic ischemic CNS damage, and intracranial hemorrhage. There is often damage to both the cortex and brainstem in these cases.

Hypoxic ischemic cerebral injury and temporal lobe seizures affecting respiration

In a term baby, the seizures of hypoxic ischemic encephalopathy can manifest purely as apnea. The diagnosis of apneic seizure should be strongly suspected in a full-term infant delivered after a period of intrapartum hypoxia, with depressed Apgar scores and an early metabolic acidosis who develops apneic attacks during the first 24 hours after birth. If the infant occasionally shows abnormal eye movements, lip smacking or limb automatisms, then the diagnosis is probable, and can be confirmed with EEG monitoring. Cerebral function monitoring may not reveal localized or short seizures. Watanabe et al.[38] described apneic seizure in 21 neonates, 19 of whom were full term. The most common associated neurological diagnoses were hypoxic ischemic encephalopathy and meningitis, although one or two infants had intracranial hemorrhage. Eight of the infants had no other seizure manifestation apart from apnea, and it was interesting that the apneic seizures were never seen in quiet sleep, being most common during active sleep. This is in marked contrast to non-convulsive apnea, which is more common in quiet sleep. The most typical electrical discharge was rhythmic alpha waves in the temporal region (14 of 21), although some infants had occipital discharges. Our experience has confirmed the association between temporal lobe seizures and apnea (Figure 36.1). When trying to distinguish between convulsive and non-convulsive

Table 36.1 *Classification of CNS disorders which can give rise to respiratory problems in babies*

Level of CNS	Specific disorder
Cortex	Hypoxic-ischemic damage
	Temporal lobe seizures causing apnea
	Intracranial hemorrhage
Brainstem respiratory center	Olivopontocerebellar hypoplasia
	Drugs depressing the respiratory center
	Arnold–Chiari malformation
	Dandy–Walker malformation
	Joubert's syndrome
	Central alveolar hypoventilation (Ondine's curse)
	Immature respiratory center
	Brainstem 'stroke' or hemorrhage
Brainstem output to glossopharyngeal, vagus and hypoglossal nerves	Bulbar palsy with stridor – congenital or due to hypoxia-ischemia
Peripheral nervous system	Spinal cord injury from hemorrhage, infarction or compression (osteogenesis imperfecta)
	Spinal muscular atrophy (usually type I, Werdnig–Hoffman disease)
	Syringomyelia
	Phrenic nerve palsy (with and without Erb's palsy)
	Laryngeal nerve palsy
Polyneuritis	Infantile Guillain–Barré syndrome ? botulism
Neuromuscular junction	Myasthenia gravis
	Infantile botulism
Muscle disease (intercostals, diaphragm)	Dystrophia myotonica
	X-linked myotubular myopathy
	Nemaline myopathy
	MELAS
	Metabolic muscle disorders, e.g. Carnitine deficiency, Cytochrome C oxidase deficiency

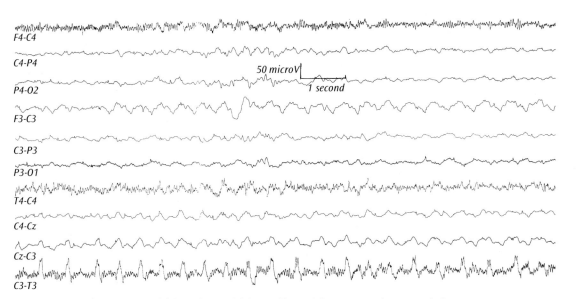

Figure 36.1 *EEG showing a temporal lobe seizure which manifest solely as apnea in a term baby.*

apnea with EEG it is important to remember that in a genuine apneic seizure breathing ceases within seconds of the electrical discharge, whereas prolonged apnea is sometimes associated with secondary depression of the amplitude of the EEG.

The diagnostic yield of monitoring apneic preterm babies with EEG is low, because in this group the diagnosis is far more likely to be apnea of prematurity (Chapter 23). Fenichel has suggested that apnea which began without bradycardia was more likely to be convulsive.[9] Treatment of apneic seizures should be along conventional lines with phenobarbital (phenobarbitone) as the first choice anticonvulsant. Affected infants are likely to require ventilation.

It is rare for the brainstem to be so damaged by hypoxia-ischemia that babies are rendered apneic. 'Brainstem death' is not a diagnosis which is usually made in the newborn.[1,36] Babies with hypoxic-ischemic encephalopathy who do not breathe at all without a ventilator are usually either very sedated by anticonvulsant drugs or very hypocapnic. As a consequence, the diagnosis of hypoxic brainstem damage should be made with caution and only when anticonvulsant drug levels are known and the arterial carbon dioxide tension has been allowed to rise to 8 kPa (60 mmHg) or more. Testing for apnea in this situation must continue for 10 minutes or more, in an infant who was well oxygenated at the start of the test. By contrast, involvement of bulbar musculature is common in hypoxic-ischemic encephalopathy. Infants with severe bilateral basal ganglia injury often have an associated bulbar palsy, probably due to associated brainstem involvement, with difficulty swallowing and clearing upper airway secretions and maintaining upper airway patency as a result.[5] Bulbar palsy can be very disabling, necessitating tube feeding and frequent suction with the ever-present risk of aspiration.

Intracranial hemorrhage affecting respiration

A massive, catastrophic intracranial hemorrhage can cause acutely raised intracranial pressure and 'coning', although this is very rare in infants who have open sutures and fontanelles. The infant with this condition, usually born prematurely, deteriorates suddenly, with apnea, seizures, fixed dilated pupils or skew deviation of the eyes, and a bulging fontanelle. The diagnosis is easily confirmed with cranial ultrasound, and the prognosis is grim. MRI-confirmed coning can occur in an infant with a subdural hematoma resulting from a tentorial tear after Ventouse delivery (personal observation).

BRAINSTEM DISORDERS CAUSING RESPIRATORY PROBLEMS

The brainstem respiratory control system contains the neurons of the dorsal and ventral respiratory group, and there is also a pontine respiratory group (page 38). These neurons receive inputs from the peripheral and central chemoreceptors, and the peripheral stretch receptors, together with input from the cortex. These neurons have the property of spontaneous oscillation, and hence respiration is an automatic and involuntary process which continues during sleep. Damage to the brainstem respiratory

center produces serious respiratory problems, and can occur in association with cortical hemorrhage and raised intracranial pressure as a part of coning (see above) or in association with other neurological problems, which are discussed below.

Central alveolar hypoventilation (Ondine's curse)

Alveolar hypoventilation in the absence of lung or neuro-muscular disease is very uncommon. There are perhaps 200 children alive worldwide with this condition. Ondine was a water nymph, who cursed her mortal husband when she found him to be unfaithful, allowing him to breathe only when awake. An infant afflicted with central alveolar hypoventilation has shallow breathing and cyanosis when asleep, but a normal respiratory pattern when awake. When asleep, their tidal volume is so low that it is often less than the physiological dead space, hence the cyanosis. These infants have carbon dioxide levels in sleep which are consistently higher than 8 kPa (60 mmHg), and they are hypoxic at the same time. This unusual pattern of ventilation can take some time to recognize, particularly as autoresuscitation (gasping) is absent. Infants with this condition also have absent ventilation sensitivity to hypoxia and hypercapnia even when they are awake. There is an association with Hirschsprung's disease, ganglioneuroblastoma and neuroblastoma.[6] This link suggests a common abnormality of neural crest cells; a neurocristopathy.

Children with central hypoventilation syndrome can survive many years if they are offered appropriate support, usually home ventilation. Negative pressure ventilation and diaphragmatic pacing have been tried. Marcus et al.[19] described 12 long-term survivors (aged 7.5 years), all of whom had tracheostomies and were receiving some form of ventilatory support. Most had adequate growth and nutrition, although five had gastrostomy tubes. Eight of the nine had developmental scores more than one standard deviation below the mean for their age, and two had scores less than 70. Five of the children had suffered at least one seizure associated with hypoxia, and one had a hemiplegia after a stroke. Weese-Mayer et al.[39] described 22 children (of a cohort of 32) who survived up to 14 years; hypotonia or major motor delay was apparent in all, and their performance was below average.

Olivopontocerebellar hypoplasia

The terms olivopontocerebellar hypoplasia and ponto-cerebellar hypoplasia are used interchangeably. These usually recessively inherited disorders present with marked neurological abnormalities including apnea in the neonatal period. There are other forms of cerebellar hypoplasia

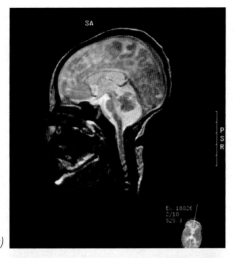

(a)

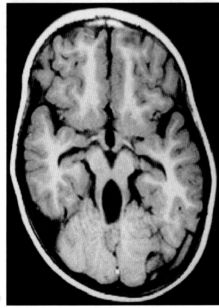

(b)

Figure 36.2 *(a) MRI showing hypoplastic pons and cerebellum in a baby who was ventilator dependent. (b) MRI showing the 'molar tooth' sign in Joubert's syndrome. (Reproduced with permission from Pediatric Neurology, 20, Sztriha, L., Al-Gazali, L., Aithala, G.R., Nork, M., Joubert's syndrome: new cases and review of clinicopathological correlation, 274–281, 1999, with permission of Elsevier Science.)*

which present in later childhood with ataxic cerebral palsy, and which are inherited in different ways. Babies with pontocerebellar hypoplasia have high tone and may be so jittery that initially a diagnosis of hyperreflexia might be considered. They have an inability to feed, and deteriorate rapidly with seizures and extrapyramidal signs. MRI reveals the very hypoplastic pons and cerebellum (Figure 36.2a). There is no treatment for this condition, which eventually proves fatal. Autopsy reveals the lack of neurons in the inferior olive.

Joubert's syndrome

In contrast to olivopontocerebellar hypoplasia, the complete absence of the cerebellar vermis in Joubert's syndrome is associated with an effortless panting tachypnea complicated by apneic attacks. The first cases were four siblings.[14] Babies with Joubert's syndrome can breathe up to 200 times a minute; the clinical clue to the diagnosis can be the presence of associated jerky eye movements or rapid movements of the protruded tongue. Joubert's original cases had periods of hyperpnea interspersed with episodic apnea ('cluster breathing'). A characteristic facies has been described with high forehead, epicanthic folds, upturned nostrils, and an open 'rhomboid' mouth. MR or CT reveals the absent cerebellar vermis. Some families have an associated retinal dysplasia, which breeds true.[15] Antenatal diagnosis is now possible, and postnatal diagnosis is best confirmed with MRI. The lack of a vermis means that the cerebellar hemispheres are separated by a cleft apparent in the coronal plane (the 'buttocks' sign); and the elongated superior cerebellar peduncles and enlarged fossa between them gives the appearance of a molar tooth in the axial plane (Figure 36.2b).[32] If the diagnosis is not made in infancy, the increased respiratory rate tends to resolve over the first year or so. The prognosis for neurodevelopment is poor, with virtually all children in the severely impaired range. The disorder is inherited as an autosomal recessive trait.

Dandy–Walker malformation

Babies with the Dandy–Walker malformation (hydrocephalus, cerebellar hypoplasia with absent vermis, and large posterior fossa cyst) have a tendency to apnea, and can also have abnormal respiratory patterns similar to those with Joubert's syndrome. This is not surprising because this group of disorders is characterized by a complete or partial hypoplasia of the cerebellar vermis, and there is usually a posterior fossa cyst formed from the fourth ventricle and the cisterna magna.

Arnold–Chiari malformation

The Arnold–Chiari malformation is associated with abnormal function of the ninth, tenth and twelfth cranial nerves due to defective myelination or hypoplasia of the brainstem nuclei, resulting in a blunting of respiratory drive and apnea. There may be reflux and stridor because of vocal cord paralysis. Babies with spina bifida often have difficulty swallowing (with an increased risk of reflux), and can be troubled by apneic attacks particularly during sleep.[37] Disordered breathing during sleep contributes to an excess of deaths in affected spina bifida babies.[16] In total, bulbar involvement, vocal cord paralysis or dysphagia affects between 5 and 20 percent of babies with the Arnold–Chiari type II malformation. In a prospective study using a pneumogram and a carbon dioxide challenge, it proved impossible to predict which babies would be affected.[26]

Drug depression of the respiratory center

Morphine and fentanyl are both now widely used as analgesics in neonatal intensive care units, and pethidine remains the most commonly used narcotic analgesic given during labor. Both these drugs can cause respiratory depression. Pethidine crosses the placenta, with a plateau level in the fetus between 1 and 5 hours after maternal intramuscular administration.[34] The maternal concentration peaks at 30–60 minutes. This is the explanation for the clinical observation that neonatal respiratory depression is seen in babies born more than an hour and less than 6 hours after maternal administration. The maximal effect is seen after 2–3 hours.[3] Affected infants have a lower respiratory rate, lower alveolar ventilation, and a higher $PaCO_2$ than unaffected infants. Naloxone (Narcan) is a specific opiate antagonist and can be used to reverse the effect of maternal opiate administration on the neonatal respiratory center. Naloxone is not a substitute for effective resuscitation, and should only be given after the circulation is restored and respiratory support is in place. Neonatal naloxone is now known to be ineffective, because the concentration of 20 μg/ml is too low to achieve therapeutic levels in a reasonable volume of administration. Adult strength naloxone should always be given. The drug acts more quickly when given intravenously, but the effect is more transient (about 90 minutes) when this route is used. The recommended dose of naloxone is 100 μg/kg (0.25 ml/kg of 'adult' strength naloxone which contains 400 μg/ml), although some have suggested that this could safely be doubled.[4] When given intramuscularly, the drug forms a depot which can lessen the effects of maternal pethidine on neonatal behavior for about 24 hours.[40] Naloxone should not be given to infants of opiate-addicted mothers because it can precipitate acute withdrawal. There is not usually any need to reverse morphine when it is used as an analgesic for infants who are in pain, because they tend to be ventilated postoperatively or because they are very ill at the time (for example, with necrotizing enterocolitis). If morphine-induced respiratory depression is thought to be inhibiting withdrawal from artificial ventilation, then the dose can be weaned.

Immature respiratory center

This is the most common cause of apnea in preterm babies.

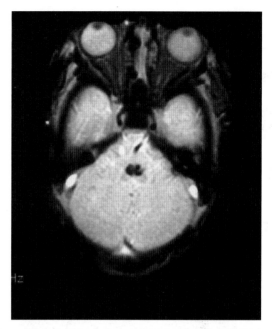

Figure 36.3 *Brainstem hemorrhage seen on axial MRI in a baby who required prolonged ventilation. The infant had widespread petechiae and a low platelet count.*

Brainstem stroke or hemorrhage

Bleeding into the cerebellum and the brainstem usually occurs during difficult breech delivery or forceps extraction, and the infants present in a similar manner to that described above in the section on intracranial hemorrhage. There are signs of brainstem compression, with apnea and bradycardia, a full fontanelle, and eye signs. The diagnosis can be made with ultrasound but this technique is not reliable and if there is a high index of suspicion, CT or MRI (Figure 36.3) should be arranged. The prognosis for preterm infants is very poor, but some term babies have survived, usually with neurological deficits.

DISORDERS AFFECTING THE CRANIAL NERVES SUPPLYING THE BULBAR MUSCLES

Bulbar palsy

A bulbar palsy (often caused by hypoxic-ischemic damage to the basal ganglia, thalami and brainstem) can result in respiratory symptoms due to a failure to swallow secretions. Aspiration is common in this situation, and infants can have stridor because of laryngeal nerve involvement. Congenital absence of the cranial nerve nuclei can cause stridor for the same reason, and babies with congenital absence of the cranial nerve nuclei (Möbius syndrome) can present with significant respiratory difficulties and die.[10,12]

DISORDERS AFFECTING THE PERIPHERAL NERVOUS SYSTEM

Spinal cord injury

Fortunately, neonatal high spinal cord injury is extremely rare, and, now that most fetuses known to be presenting by the breech are delivered by elective cesarean section, the incidence is likely to fall further. There are two patterns of injury. The first involves traction during breech delivery and this results in injury to the lower cervical and upper thoracic spinal cord. The second pattern follows rotational injury during instrumental cephalic delivery, and this results in a high cervical cord injury.[21] Cesarean section does not completely protect against cervical cord damage in fetuses with breech presentation, particularly those whose neck is hyperextended. A case of C4–5 damage was described in a baby with cephalic presentation who was delivered by cesarean section.[23] The typical clinical presentation, however, is of an infant born vaginally by the breech who has a flaccid weakness and areflexia. The respiratory movements are paradoxical due to a dependence on diaphragmatic breathing. A survey of five Canadian centers between 1972 and 1991 revealed 22 such cases.[18] The long-term outcome was poor in the group who had no respiratory movement within 24 hours. MRI is the investigation of choice, and provides *in vivo* evidence of the underlying pathology, previously described.[22,35] Operative intervention is rarely indicated; some children have been fitted with phrenic pacemakers. Compression of the spinal cord from osteogenesis imperfecta has been described.

Phrenic nerve palsy

Phrenic nerve injury can occur in association with Erb's palsy as a stretch injury to the brachial plexus at birth (80–90 percent of cases), or the nerve can be damaged during the insertion of chest drains or during intrathoracic surgery.[24] Damage to the nerve in the neck from dissection for the insertion of ECMO cannulas or to insert an internal jugular venous cannula has been described.[27,30] The resulting diaphragmatic palsy can cause significant respiratory problems, particularly in preterm babies who are ventilator-dependent. Full-term infants with Erb's palsy and associated phrenic nerve damage usually do well without treatment unless the lesion is bilateral. The typical clinical presentation is of a large infant delivered with shoulder dystocia who has a clinical Erb's palsy (or a flaccid arm) and whose chest radiograph shows an elevated left hemidiaphragm (page 498). The phrenic nerve is involved in about 5 percent of brachial plexus palsy cases, and should be looked for specifically. Involvement of the phrenic nerve has no bearing on the prognosis of the nerve palsy in general. Treatment options include CPAP (or negative pressure ventilation), diaphragmatic plication (page 499), nerve grafting, and electrical pacing.

Laryngeal nerve palsy

Damage to the laryngeal nerve during intrathoracic surgery can result in stridor, and the same is true if there is congenital absence of the cranial nerve nuclei or a brainstem hemorrhage.

Syringomyelia

Syringomyelia does not usually present in the neonatal period, but infants with the Arnold–Chiari malformation or trauma to the spinal cord can develop a syrinx which presents with neurological and respiratory symptoms later on.

Spinal muscular atrophy

Spinal muscular atrophy (SMA) type I (Werdnig–Hoffman disease) can present in the neonatal period. This severe anterior horn cell degeneration has autosomal recessive inheritance. SMA type I is clinically apparent at birth in about a third of cases, and the mothers often give a history of reduced fetal movement. There can be respiratory depression at birth, asphyxia, or respiratory distress. Rarely, infants have presented acutely after respiratory tract infections, leading to confusion with Guillain–Barré syndrome.[28] The characteristic clinical picture is of a weak, areflexic infant who adopts a frog-like posture, but whose facial expression remains alert. The internal rotators of the shoulders are usually involved, and the resulting 'jug-handle' posture of the arms is a consistent feature.[7] The chest radiograph (Figure 36.4) can show the thin ribs

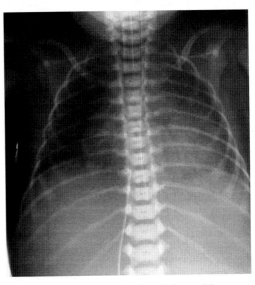

Figure 36.4 *Chest radiograph of an infant with neuromuscular disease showing thin (gracile) ribs.*

which suggest neuromuscular disease.[25] The diagnosis is confirmed by genetic studies which reveal a homozygous deletion of exon seven and eight of the SMA genes, which are in the q11–q13 region of chromosome 5. The creatinine kinase level is normal. EMG can help in diagnosis. The prognosis for infants who present in the first few weeks is dismal, with most dying by 3 months and hardly any surviving beyond 2 years.

POLYNEURITIS

Neonatal Guillain–Barré syndrome

This is fortunately extremely rare. A case born to an affected mother has been reported.[17] A woman who required ventilation for the disease in the twenty-ninth week of pregnancy gave birth at 38 weeks. The boy was initially unaffected, but presented on the twelfth day with hypotonia and respiratory distress for which he required ventilation but recovered after 2 weeks. Lumbar puncture showed an increased CSF protein without excess cells and the creatine kinase (CK) level was high.

DISORDERS OF THE NEUROMUSCULAR JUNCTION

Myasthenia gravis

About 10–20 per cent of babies born to myasthenic mothers develop transient neonatal myasthenia due to passive transfer of acetylcholine receptor antibodies. The mother can be in remission, and the occasional baby has been born to a previously undiagnosed mother. Affected babies develop weakness with difficulty in feeding and swallowing, usually within a few hours of birth and never after more than 3 days.[8] One-third require artificial ventilation. The diagnosis can be confirmed with a Tensilon test: 0.03 mg/kg of edrophonium (Tensilon) is given as a test dose, which should be followed by 0.15 mg/kg given intravenously. Atropine should be available in case of increased saliva threatening the airway, and the test should be done in intensive care with full monitoring, because arrhythmias have been described. Acetylcholine receptor (AchR) antibodies can be detected in the blood of both mother and baby. The EMG is characteristic but difficult to perform. Mutations in the AchR subunit genes are now recognized.[8] Management is support, including tube feeding, suction and ventilation, together with anticholinesterase drugs, which have proved life saving in the neonate. The usual therapy is neostigmine 0.4 mg/kg orally 30 minutes before feeds; the intramuscular dose is 10 times smaller. Pyridostigmine 4–10 mg by mouth every 4 hours prior to feeds is an alternative. Intravenous

immunoglobulin has been tried, but was ineffective in one case,[33] and exchange transfusion also fails to help, in contrast to older children and adults. Most cases resolve after 2–3 weeks, with no recurrence, and the long-term prognosis is excellent.

There are other congenital myasthenic syndromes which affect babies born to non-myasthenic mothers. These syndromes are probably all inherited as autosomal recessive traits. Some are caused by deficiency of the end plate receptors, but there are many others. These disorders have been classified by Shillito and colleagues.[31] The disorders are managed along the same lines as transient neonatal myasthenia, but clearly treatment in this group needs to be lifelong. Although these disorders are rare, some cases are probably missed and it is important to consider congenital myasthenia in a baby who required resuscitation and who then remains weak with difficulty in feeding and swallowing secretions.

Infantile botulism

Most cases of this disorder have been described in the USA, where a link with botulinum spores in honey was identified. Affected babies usually present at 2–4 weeks of age, after they have ingested botulinum toxin contained in dirt, dust or honey. Babies become floppy, constipated and cannot feed. The paralysis is descending, the opposite to Guillain–Barré syndrome, and there is ptosis and an absent pupil response. There is no specific treatment, and general intensive care support is required. Aminoglycoside antibiotics should be avoided.

MUSCLE DISEASE

Muscle disorders can present in the neonatal period with fulminant respiratory failure, floppiness, or difficulty in feeding. Myotubular myopathy and nemaline myopathy typically present with respiratory difficulty, but other disorders can mimic these. Mothers who are severely affected with myotonic dystrophy often give birth to affected babies who can require prolonged ventilation.

Dystrophia myotonica

Affected babies are hypotonic and have difficulty in feeding and breathing, there is often talipes. The main clue to the diagnosis is an affected mother, and once the suspicion is raised then confirmation can be sought by demonstrating the presence of CTG triplet repeat expansions on chromosome 19. Babies who are severely affected require ventilation, and in them the prognosis is worse. All cases admitted to the Hammersmith Hospital between 1982 and 1989 who required ventilation for longer than 4 weeks died before the age of 15 months.[29] In babies who survive, there is a significant risk of developmental delay with intellectual and motor impairment. Ventricular dilatation has been seen on MRI.[20]

X-linked myotubular myopathy

This congenital myopathy typically presents in male infants at birth, with severe hypotonia and respiratory distress. The disorder is usually fatal, although some long-term ventilator-dependent survivors have been described.[11] The diagnosis is confirmed by muscle biopsy which reveals central nuclei resembling fetal myotubules (hence the name). The genetic locus has been recognized and the gene encodes for a protein, myotubularin.

Nemaline myopathy

Neonatal presentation of this disease usually implies a poor prognosis although exceptions are described.[2] Mutations in the muscle alpha-skeletal-actin gene are now recognized.[13]

Mitochondrial encephalopathy, lactic acidosis and stroke-like episodes (MELAS)

This rare disorder usually presents in childhood or adult life, but neonatal cases have been recognized. The diagnosis is usually revealed by MRI, which shows abnormal T_2 signal in the periventricular white matter with the deep grey matter nuclei being involved early on. Multiple migrating infarct-like lesions, which are not limited to a specific vascular territory, are highly suggestive of the diagnosis.

Metabolic muscle disease: cytochrome C oxidase deficiency, carnitine deficiency

These rare disorders can present in the neonatal period with respiratory difficulty.

REFERENCES

1 Ashwal, S. (1997) Brain death in the newborn. *Clinics in Perinatology* **24**, 859–882.
2 Banwell, B.L., Singh, N.C., Ramsay, D.A. (1994) Prolonged survival in neonatal nemaline rod myopathy. *Pediatric Neurology* **10**, 335–337.
3 Belfrage, P., Boreus, I.O., Hartvig, P., Iresteddt, L., Raabe, N. (1981) Neonatal depression after obstetrical analgesia with pethidine. The role of the injection–delivery time interval and of the plasma concentrations of pethidine and norpethidine. *Acta Obstetrica et Gynaecologia Scandinavica* **60**, 43–49.

4 Brice, J.E.H., Moreland, T.A., Walker, C.H.M. (1979) Effects of pethidine and its antagonists on the newborn. *Archives of Disease in Childhood* **54**, 356–361.
5 Cowan, F. (2000) Outcome after intrapartum asphyxia in term infants. *Seminars in Neonatology* **5**, 127–140.
6 Croaker, D.T., Shi, E., Simpson, E., Cartmill, T., Cass, D.T. (1998) Congenital central hypoventilation syndrome and Hirschsprung's disease. *Archives of Disease in Childhood* **78**, 316–322.
7 Dubowitz, V. (1995) Disorders of the lower motor neurone: the spinal muscular atrophies. In Dubowitz, V. (ed.), *Muscle Disorders in Childhood*, 2nd edition. London: W.B. Saunders, 325–369.
8 Engel, A.G., Ohno, K., Sine, S.M. (1999) Congenital myasthenic syndromes. *Archives of Neurology* **56**, 163–167.
9 Fenichel, G.M., Olson, B.J., Fitzpatrick, J.E. (1980) Heart rate changes in convulsive and non-convulsive apnea. *Annals of Neurology* **7**, 577–582.
10 Fujita, I., Koyanagi, T., Kukita, J. *et al.* (1991) Moebius syndrome with central hypoventilation and brainstem calcification: a case report. *European Journal of Pediatrics* **150**, 582–583.
11. Herman, G.E., Finegold, M., Zhao, W., de Gouyon, B., Metzenberg, A. (1999) Medical complications in long-term survivors with X-linked myotubular myopathy. *Journal of Pediatrics* **134**, 206–214.
12 Igarashi, M., Rose, D.F., Storgion, S.A. (1997) Moebius syndrome and central respiratory depression. *Pediatric Neurology* **16**, 237–240.
13 Ilkovski, B., Cooper, S.T., Nowak, K., Ryan, M.M., Yang, N., Schnell, C. (2001) Nemaline myopathy caused by mutations in the muscle alpha-skeletal actin gene. *American Journal of Human Genetics* **68**, 1333–1343.
14 Joubert, M., Eisenring, J.-J., Robb, J.P., Andermann, F. (1969) Familial agenesis of the cerebellar vermis. *Neurology* **15**, 813–825.
15 King, M.D., Dudgeon, J., Stephenson, J.B.P. (1984) Joubert's syndrome with retinal dysplasia: neonatal tachypnoea as the clue to a genetic brain–eye malformation. *Archives of Disease in Childhood* **59**, 709–718.
16 Kirk, V.G., Morielli, A., Brouillette, R.T. (1999) Sleep disordered breathing in patients with myelomeningocele: the missed diagnosis. *Developmental Medicine and Child Neurology* **41**, 40–43.
17 Luijckx, G.J., Vles, J., de Baerts, M., Buchwald, B., Troost, J. (1997) Guillain–Barré syndrome in mother and newborn child. *Lancet* **349**, 27.
18 MacKinnon, J.A., Perlman, M., Kirplani, H. (1993) Spinal cord injury at birth: diagnostic and prognostic data in twenty-two patients. *Journal of Pediatrics* **122**, 431–434.
19 Marcus, C.L., Jansen, M.T., Poulsen, M.K. *et al.* (1991) Medical and psychosocial outcome of children with congenital central hypoventilation syndrome. *Journal of Pediatrics* **119**, 888–895.
20 Martinello, F., Piazza, A., Pastorello, E., Angelini, C., Trevisan, C.P. (1999) Clinical and neuroimaging study of central nervous system in congenital myotonic dystrophy. *Journal of Neurology* **246**, 186–192.
21 Menticoglou, S.M., Perlman, M., Manning, F.A. (1995) High cervical spinal cord injury in neonates delivered with forceps: report of 15 cases. *Obstetrics and Gynecology* **86**, 589–594.
22 Mills, J.F., Dargaville, P.A., Coleman, L.T., Rosenfeld, J.V., Ekert, P.G. (2001) Upper cervical spinal cord injury in neonates: the use of magnetic resonance imaging. *Journal of Pediatrics* **138**, 105–108.

23 Morgan, C., Newell, S.J. (2001) Cervical spinal cord injury following cephalic presentation and delivery by caesarean section. *Developmental Medicine and Child Neurology* **43**, 274–276.

24 Odita, J.C., Khan, A.S., Dinscoy, M., Kayyali, M., Masoud, A., Ammari, A. (1992) Neonatal phrenic nerve paralysis resulting from intercostal drainage of pneumothorax. *Pediatric Radiology* **22**, 379–381.

25 Osborne, J.P., Murphy, E.G., Hill, A. (1983) Thin ribs in chest X ray: a useful sign in the differential diagnosis of the floppy newborn. *Developmental Medicine and Child Neurology* **25**, 343–345.

26 Petersen, M.C., Wolraich, M., Sherbondy, A., Wagener, J. (1995) Abnormalities in control of ventilation in newborn infants with myelomeningocele. *Journal of Pediatrics* **126**, 1011–1015.

27 Pleasure, J.R., Shashikumar, V.L. (1990) Phrenic nerve damage in the tiny infant during vein cannulation for parenteral nutrition. *American Journal of Perinatology* **7**, 136–138.

28 Ravid, S., Topper, L., Eviatar, L. (2001) Acute onset of infantile spinal muscular atrophy. *Pediatric Neurology* **24**, 371–372.

29 Rutherford, M.A., Heckmatt, J.Z., Dubowitz, V. (1989) Congenital myotonic dystrophy: respiratory function at birth determines survival. *Archives of Disease in Childhood* **64**, 191–195.

30 Schumacher, R.E., Weinfeld, I.J., Bartlett, R.H. (1989) Neonatal vocal cord paralysis following extracorporeal membrane oxygenation. *Pediatrics* **84**, 793–796.

31 Shillito, P., Vincent, A., Newson-David, J. (1993) Congenital myasthenic syndromes. *Neuromuscular Disorders* **3**, 183–190.

32 Sztriha, L., Al-Gazali, L., Aithala, G.R., Nork, M. (1999) Joubert's syndrome: new cases and review of clinicopathological correlation. *Pediatric Neurology* **20**, 274–281.

33 Tagher, R.J., Baumann, R., Desai, N. (1999) Failure of intravenously administered immunoglobulin in the treatment of neonatal myasthenia gravis. *Journal of Pediatrics* **134**, 233–235.

34 Tomson, G., Garle, R.I., Thalme, B., Nisell, H., Nylund, L., Rane, A. (1982) Maternal kinetics and transplacental passage of pethidine during labour. *British Journal of Clinical Pharmacology* **13**, 653–659.

35 Towbin, A. (1970) Central nervous system damage in the human fetus and newborn infant. *American Journal of Diseases of Childhood* **119**, 529–542.

36 Volpe, J.J. (1987) Brain death determination in the newborn. *Pediatrics* **80**, 293–295.

37 Ward, S.L., Jacobs, R.A., Gates, E.P., Hart, L.D., Keens, T.G. (1986) Abnormal ventilatory patterns during sleep in infants with myelomeningocele. *Journal of Pediatrics* **109**, 613–614.

38 Watanabe, K., Hara, K., Miyazaki, S., Hakamada, S., Kuroyanagi, M. (1982) Apneic seizures in the newborn. *American Journal of Diseases of Children* **136**, 980–984.

39 Weese-Mayer, D.E., Silvestri, J.M., Menzies, L.J., Morrow-Kenny, A.S., Hunt, C.E., Hauptman, S.A. (1992) Congenital central hypoventilation syndrome: diagnosis, management and outcome in 32 children. *Journal of Pediatrics* **120**, 381–387.

40 Wiener, P.C., Hogg, M.I.J., Rosen, M. (1977) Effects of naloxone on pethidine-induced neonatal depression. *British Medical Journal* **2**, 228–231.

Appendices

Appendix 1: Normal data for lung function in term infants during the neonatal period

SIMON HANNAM

Measurement	No. of infants studied	Mean	Standard deviation	Range
Tidal volume (ml/kg)	266	4.8	1.0	2.9–7.9
Respiratory rate (bpm)	266	50.9	13.1	25–104
Minute volume (ml/kg/min)	266	232	61.4	——
Dynamic compliance (ml/cmH$_2$O/kg)	266	1.72	0.5	0.9–3.7
Total pulmonary resistance (cmH$_2$O/l/s)	266	42.5	1.6	3.1–171
Work of breathing (G.cm)	266	11.9	7.4	1.1–52.6
Expiratory time (s)	291	0.57	0.17	0.27–1.28
Inspiratory time (s)	291	0.51	0.10	0.28–0.87
Time to maximum expiratory flow/total expiratory time (s)	291	0.51	0.12	0.18–0.83
Static compliance (ml/cmH$_2$O/kg)	289	1.25	0.41	0.43–2.07
Respiratory system resistance (cmH$_2$O/l/s)	299	63.4	16.6	34.9–153.3
Time constant of respiratory system (s)	299	0.24	0.10	0.08–1.1
FRC$_{pleth}$ (ml/kg)	271	29.8	6.2	14.5–15.6

All data are from Milner *et al.* (1999) Effects of smoking in pregnancy on neonatal lung function. *Archives of Disease in Childhood* **80**, F8–F14. The tidal volume and volume were measured by a type 00 Fleisch Pneumotachograph and intrathoracic pressure with a 4 cm esophageal balloon. Babies were supine in quiet sleep. Dead space was eliminated by a bias flow of air.

Appendix 2: Normal blood gas values

SIMON HANNAM

	PaO_2 Term		Preterm		$PaCO_2$ Term		Preterm		H^+ Term		Preterm	
	kPa	mmHg	kPa	mmHg	kPa	mmHg	kPa	mmHg	nmol/l	pH	nmol/l	pH
15 minutes	11.6	87			3.7	28			48	7.32		
30 minutes	11.4	86			4.3	32			43	7.37		
60 minutes	10.8	81			4.1	31			40	7.40		
1–6 hours	8–10.6	60–80	8.0–9.3	60–70	4.7–6	35–45	4.7–6	35–45	46–49	7.31–7.34	42–48	7.32–7.38
6–24 hours	9.3–10	70–75	8.0–9.3	60–70	4.4–4.8	33–36	3.6–5.3	27–40	37–43	7.37–7.43	35–45	7.36–7.45
48 hours–1 week	9.3–11.3	10.0–10.6	10–10.6	75–80	4.4–4.8	33–36	4.3–4.5	32–36	42–44	7.36–7.38	40–48	7.32–7.40
2 weeks					4.8–5.2	36–39	5.1	38	43	7.37	48	7.32
3 weeks					5.3	40	5.1	38	42	7.38	49	7.31
1 month					5.2	39	4.9	37	41	7.39	49	7.31

The values at 15, 30 and 60 minutes of age are from unpublished observations on term infants (Roberton). Data from 1 hour to 1 week are drawn from the literature on arterial samples. Data beyond 1 week are on capillary samples.
Reproduced with permission from Roberton, N.R.C. (1993) *Manual of Neonatal Intensive Care*. London: Arnold.

Appendix 3: Pharmacopeia

SIMON HANNAM

Drug	Route	Dose	Notes	Dose interval
Aciclovir	i.v.	10 mg/kg per dose	Infuse over 1 hour. Reduce if creatinine raised	12 hourly (<7 days old); 8 hourly (>7 days old)
	Oral	10–20 mg/kg		6 hourly for 2 weeks
Adenosine	i.v. by rapid bolus	100 µg/kg per dose. Max 300 µg/kg per dose	Try iced water first. Half-life is less than 10 s. May cause bronchoconstriction	Repeatable
Adrenaline (Epinephrine)	i.v.	0.1–0.3 ml/kg of 1:10 000	For resuscitation	Repeatable
	ETT	0.1–1.0 ml/kg of 1:10 000		
	Infusion	0.05–0.5 µg/kg/min (max 1.5 µg/kg/min)	For hypotension	
	Nebulized	0.5 ml/kg (1:1000) made up to 2.5 ml with normal saline	For upper airway obstruction due to edema	
Amoxycillin	i.v., i.m., oral	50 mg/kg per dose	Double dose in severe infections	12 hourly; 8 hourly if term and >7 days old
Ampicillin	i.v., i.m., oral	50 mg/kg per dose	Double dose in severe infections	12 hourly; 8 hourly if term and >7 days old
Atracurium	Infusion i.v. bolus	5–10 µg/kg/min; 500 µg/kg	Can be reversed with neostigmine	
Atropine	i.v., s.c., i.m.	10–15 µg/kg		Single dose
Beractant (Survanta)	ETT	100 mg/kg (equivalent to 4 ml/kg)		Maximum of four doses may be given within 48 hours at intervals of at least 6 hours
Budesonide	Via spacer	200 µg		12 hourly
	Nebulized	0.5–1.0 mg		12 hourly
Caffeine citrate	i.v., oral	20 mg/kg, then	Loading	Once only
		5 mg/kg per dose	Maintenance. 1 mg caffeine citrate is equivalent to 0.5 mg caffeine base. Levels need monitoring. Aim for 6–14 mg/l	24 hourly

(Continued)

Drug	Route	Dose	Notes	Dose interval
Calcium gluconate	i.v.	2 ml of 10% solution/kg (i.e. 200 mg/kg per dose)	Give slowly over 5–10 minutes For arrhythmias Beware of extravasation	
Captopril	Oral	10 µg/kg	Increase slowly to a maximum of 2 mg/kg/day	8 hourly
Cefotaxime	i.v., i.m.	50 mg/kg per dose	Double in severe infections	12 hourly; 8 hourly if term and >7 days old
Ceftazidime	i.v.	25 mg/kg per dose		12 hourly; 8 hourly if term and >7 days old
Chloral hydrate	Oral	30–50 mg/kg		Max 4 doses/day
Chlorothiazide	Oral	10–20 mg/kg per dose	Usually given with spironolactone	12 hourly
Cimetidine	Oral	5 mg/kg (prophylaxis) 5 mg/kg (treatment)		12 hourly 6 hourly
Dexamethasone	i.v., oral	0.25 mg/kg for 3 days then 0.15 mg/kg for 3 days then 0.05 mg/kg for 3 days	For BPD. If no response after 3 days, stop	12 hourly
	iv	0.25 mg/kg	For laryngeal edema. Start 4 hours prior to extubation	12 hourly, give for a maximum of 48 hours
Diamorphine	i.v. i.v. infusion	50 µg/kg (load) 15 µg/kg/h	Over 30 minutes. Maintenance In severe renal impairment, reduce dose by 50–75%	Once only
Dobutamine	i.v. infusion	5–15 µg/kg/min		
Dopamine	i.v. infusion	Low dose 2–5 µg/kg/min High dose 6–10 µg/kg/min	Improves renal and gut perfusion For hypotension	
Doxapram	i.v.	2.5 mg/kg	Loading dose over 10 minutes	Once only
	i.v. infusion Oral	0.25 mg/kg/h (max 1.5 mg/kg/h) 6 mg/kg per dose	Maintenance Best after i.v. loading dose	6 hourly
Erythromycin	i.v., oral	15 mg/kg per dose	Give over 1 hour if i.v.	8 or 12 hourly
Fentanyl	i.v. infusion	5 µg/kg, stat 5 µg/kg/h	Only use in ventilated infants	
Flucloxacillin	i.v., oral, i.m.	50 mg/kg per dose	Double in severe infections	12 hourly; 8 hourly if term and >7 days old

Drug	Route	Dose	Notes	Frequency
Frusemide	i.v., oral	1–2 mg/kg per dose	Can cause hypokalemia, hyponatremia and nephrocalcinosis	12 or 24 hourly
Gaviscon	Oral	0.25 to 0.5 sachet per feed		
Gentamicin	i.v., i.m.	2.5 mg/kg	Levels need to be monitored Trough level: 0.5–1 mg/l Peak level: 5–10 mg/l	GA <28 weeks: 24 hourly GA 29–35 weeks: 18 hourly GA >35 weeks: 12 hourly Term and >7 days old: 8 hourly
Hydrocortisone	i.v. Oral i.v.	25 mg/kg 2.5 mg/kg 2.5 mg/kg	Addisonian crisis Maintenance Refractory hypotension	Once 6 hourly 4 hourly for two doses then 6 hourly
Indomethacin	i.v., oral i.v., oral	0.1 mg/kg or 0.2 mg/kg	For 7 days For 3 doses only	24 hourly (<7 days old) 12 hourly (>7 days old)
Ipratropium bromide	Nebulized Inhaler	10 μg/kg 40 μg	Dilute to 2 ml with sterile, 0.9% saline	4 to 6 hourly 12 hourly
Isoprenaline	i.v. infusion	0.1–0.5 μg/kg/min	For heart block or shock	
Magnesium sulfate	i.v.	200 mg/kg over 20 minutes, then, 20–50 mg/kg/h infusion	For pulmonary hypertension	
Midazolam	i.v.	150 μg/kg as bolus, then, 30–60 μg/kg/h as infusion		
Morphine	i.v. bolus i.v. infusion	100 μg/kg 10–40 μg/kg/h (ventilated infant)		
Naloxone	i.v. (i.m.)	100 μg/kg	Short half-life so dose may need repeating	
Neostigmine	i.v. i.m. i.v.	50 μg/kg 0.15–0.3 mg/kg 80 μg/kg (after 20 μg/kg of atropine)	For diagnosis of myasthenia gravis For treatment of myasthenia gravis For reversal of pancuronium	Once only 6 hourly (starting dose) Once only
Nitric oxide	Inhaled	1–40 ppm	For use in pulmonary hypertension. Monitor clotting and methemoglobin levels	
Noradrenaline (Norepinephrine)	Via central vein	0.1 μg/kg/min of noradrenaline *base* (max 1.5 μg/kg base per min)	For maintenance of blood pressure in septic shock	
Pancuronium	i.v. (i.m.)	Initial dose 100 μg/kg	Dose may be increased. Synergism with aminoglycosides. Renally excreted. Effects can be reversed with neostigmine and atropine	Usually 4 to 6 hourly

(Continued)

Drug	Route	Dose	Notes	Dose interval
Paracetamol	Oral, p.r.	24 mg/kg per dose (max 60 mg/kg/day)		8 hourly
Penicillin G (benzylpenicillin)	i.v., i.m.	50 mg/kg per dose		12 hourly (<7 days old); 8 hourly (1–3 weeks); 6 hourly (>4 weeks)
Pethidine	i.v., i.m.	1 mg/kg		12 hourly
Phenobarbitone (phenobarbital)	i.v., i.m.	20 mg/kg, can use 30–40 mg/kg in ventilated infants	Loading dose	Once only
	i.v., oral	5 mg/kg	Maintenance Need to monitor levels Aim for 15–40 mg/l	24 hourly
Phenytoin	i.v. *only*	20 mg/kg (give over 20 minutes with ECG)	Loading dose	Once only
		2.5 mg/kg	Maintenance Need to monitor levels Aim for 10–20 mg/l	12 hourly
Poractant alfa (Curosurf)	ETT	100–200 mg/kg, then, 100 mg/kg	Initial Depends on respiratory status of infant	Once only 12 hourly (up to 4 doses)
Prostacyclin (epoprostenol, PGI₂)	i.v. infusion	2–22 ng/kg/min	Can cause severe hypotension	
Prostaglandin E₂	i.v. infusion	0.6 µg/kg/h	Preferred prostaglandin for duct-dependent cardiac malformations Apnea can occur	
Ranitidine	i.v.	0.5 mg/kg per dose given slowly to avoid arrhythmias		6 hourly
	i.v. infusion	0.25 mg/kg, then 0.05 mg/kg/h	Loading dose Maintenance	Once only
Salbutamol	Nebulized i.v.	2.5 mg diluted to 2 ml with 0.9% saline 4 µg/kg over 20 minutes	For wheeze For hyperkalemia	3 to 4 hourly

Drug	Route	Dose	Notes	Frequency
Sodium bicarbonate	i.v.	If 8.4% solution, dilute with equal parts of dextrose to give 4.2% and then give 2 ml/kg	For correction of metabolic acidosis 1 ml of 8.4% solution contains 1 mmol of bicarbonate Infuse over 30 minutes	
Spironolactone	Oral	1–2 mg/kg		12 hourly
Streptokinase	i.v.	3000 units/kg, then,	Loading dose, infuse slowly	Once only
	i.v. infusion	500–1000 units/kg/h maintenance	Maintenance Monitor fibrinogen levels, if <1 g/l, stop	
Surfactant	See beractant and poractant alfa			
Suxamethonium	i.v.	1–2 mg/kg	Atropine should be given prior to suxamethonium to reduce associated bradycardia	Single dose
Theophylline	Oral	4 mg/kg, then,	Loading dose	Once only
		2 mg/kg	Maintenance Levels need monitoring, aim for 8–12 mg/l	12 hourly
Tissue plasminogen activator	i.v.	0.5 mg/kg over 10 minutes, then,	For dissolving clots	
	i.v. infusion	0.2 mg/kg/h	For not more than 3 hours	
Tolazoline	i.v.	1–2 mg/kg bolus	Can cause severe hypotension which may be countered by using in conjunction with dopamine	Once only
	i.v. infusion	0.2–0.3 mg/kg/h (max 1.0 mg/kg/h		
Urokinase	i.v. infusion	200 U/kg	Infuse for total of 24 hours	
Vancomycin	i.v.	15 mg/kg	Infuse over 1 hour Levels need monitoring	24 hourly (<28 weeks GA) 18 hourly (29–32 weeks GA) 12 hourly (>33 weeks GA) 12 hourly (term, >7 days old)

Abbreviations: GA, gestational age; kg, kilograms; l, liter; mg, milligrams; μg, micrograms. ng, nanograms
Solutions: A 1:100 (1%) weight for volume (w/v) solution contains 1 g of substance in 100 ml of solution. A 1:1000 solution contains 1 mg in 1 ml. A 1:10 000 solution contains 100 μg in 1 ml.
References: *Children Nationwide Regional Neonatal Unit Formulary*, London; *Northern Neonatal Network 1998*; *Neonatal Formulary*, BMJ Books, London.

Index

Note: page numbers in **bold** indicate tables